PLATE I

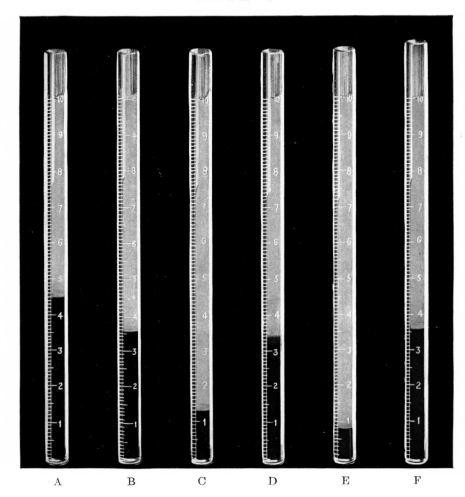

A   B   C   D   E   F

THE APPEARANCE OF CENTRIFUGED BLOOD IN VARIOUS CONDITIONS

(Oxalated venous blood was placed in hematocrit tubes and centrifuged at 3000 revolutions per minute for one-half hour.)

A. Normal blood.

B. Simple anemia due to chronic infection.

C. Chronic posthemorrhagic anemia. The blood plasma is very pale.

D. Chronic myelocytic leukemia. There is a thick layer of white corpuscles and platelets above the red corpuscles.

E. Pernicious anemia. Note the small amount of packed red corpuscles, the very narrow layer of leukocytes and platelets, and the coloring of the blood plasma due to increased bilirubinemia.

F. Infectious hepatitis and slight anemia. In this case the coloring of the blood plasma is due to biliary obstruction rather than to increased blood destruction. *(Wintrobe, Tice Practice of Medicine, courtesy of W. F. Prior Company.)*

CLINICAL HEMATOLOGY

By

Maxwell M. Wintrobe, M.D., Ph.D., D.Sc. (Hon.)

Professor and Head, Department of Medicine and Director Laboratory for the Study of Hereditary and Metabolic Disorders, University of Utah, College of Medicine, Salt Lake City, Utah; Formerly Associate in Medicine, Johns Hopkins University, Associate Physician, Johns Hopkins Hospital, and Physician-in-Charge, Clinic for Nutritional, Gastro-Intestinal and Hemopoietic Disorders, Baltimore, Maryland

Fifth Edition, Thoroughly Revised
265 Illustrations in Black and White
50 Illustrations in Color on 19 Plates

Lea & Febiger

Philadelphia

TO MY WIFE
AND IN MEMORY OF OUR SON, PAUL

Preface to the Fifth Edition

THE fundamental contributions which have been and continue to be made in the field of hematology attest to the ingenuity and industry of the investigators and demonstrate the comprehensive character of the field. Once a discipline limited to morphology, hematology now has grown in depth and in breadth; in depth to the molecular level and in breadth to the fields of human genetics and anthropology. Many other disciplines are embraced within this range.

No wonder, then, that in spite of the overwhelming quantity of literature which has been published in the five years intervening since the publication of the fourth edition, the effort of reviewing and digesting the important contributions to the field of hematology has been well repaid. It may be added that, seen individually as they have been published, these sometimes have failed to impress one as much as they should; fitted together, some as bricks and stones and a few as keystones which serve to complete the bridge of knowledge which joins facts until then of uncertain significance, each observation stands out in a truer light. Vague details take shape and understanding advances. A comparison with the first edition of this work, published twenty years ago, gives some indication of the growth of the field and, incidentally, provides a glimpse of the advances in medicine as a whole in that interval. It is noteworthy how much has depended on the successive discovery of various techniques whereby some of the secrets of nature have been pried loose.

As before, the whole text has required careful review and much has needed modification, some of it very extensively. In many respects, only the skeleton is the same as before. Many sections have been completely rewritten and a number of new topics have been added, in keeping with the progress of hematology. Numerous new illustrations have been included and a number of older ones have been discarded. This applies also to the color plates; here advantage has been taken of the development of color photomicrography. New tables have been designed and the bibliography has been completely revised.

Certain explanations may prove helpful. In preparing this book the writer has had in mind the beginning student, the discerning technician, the advanced postgraduate, the clinician, the teacher, and even the biochemist and the sophisticated hematologist. For this reason certain details will be found and some illustrations have been retained because it is thought that they have value for certain potential readers although they may not be useful to others. Here it may also be explained that this book is not designed primarily as a laboratory manual and that, for this reason, laboratory techniques are not all discussed in one section, in an appendix. The intent, rather, is to indicate the principles and objectives of a procedure, its value and its pitfalls. Details are given concerning the simpler procedures, many of which every physician should be able to carry out himself. In addition, enough detail has been provided concerning other techniques to allow the reader to gain a thorough understanding of the method. When possible, these techniques have been described in connection with the kind of information which they are designed to provide; in context rather than in appendix.

It probably needs only to be mentioned

that the bibliography, voluminous as it is, must necessarily represent only a small proportion of the papers which have been published. Omissions should not be construed as implying lack of appreciation of the worth of the papers not cited. In general, the attempt has been made to limit the bilbiographic references to the most recent ones dealing with the topic concerned, or to especially pertinent or historical ones. Additional references will be found in the papers quoted, some of which have been selected because of their value in this regard.

As in the past the author is greatly indebted to his associate, Dr. George E. Cartwright, for his criticism and advice. Dr. Paul Didisheim has been most helpful in the area of coagulation and the hemorrhagic disorders. The technical procedures which are described are those employed in our coagulation laboratory under his direction. Dr. Robert L. Hill also has been most generous of his time and help, especially in connection with the fascinating problems of the normal and abnormal hemoglobins. To Dr. Arthur Haut and his assistant, Miss Doris Kurth, the author is deeply indebted for their skill and many hours of labor in providing essentially all of the new illustrative material including, especially, the color photomicrographs.

A number of workers in the field of the hemoglobinopathies have graciously supplied information, some as yet unpublished, and have been helpful in many ways. The author is especially indebted to Dr. Hermann Lehmann, Dr. Richard T. Jones, Dr. E. M. Shooter and Dr. S. Park Gerald, as well as to Dr. Corrado Baglioni, Dr. A. O. W. Stretton and Dr. Phillip Sturgeon.

For proofreading the author thanks his wife, as well as Drs. Robert C. Edmondson, Otto P. Haab, G. Richard Lee and Dane R. Boggs. To them he is also indebted for many helpful suggestions.

Inexhaustible energy, infinite patience and sincere dedication are a few of the attributes of his secretary, Miss Alida Woolley, for which the author expresses appreciation. Last but not least, thanks are due to his associates in the Department of Medicine, as well as to his wife, for their understanding and indulgence.

It is a special pleasure to express the author's appreciation of the skill and the wholehearted and unstinting cooperation of the publishers, Lea and Febiger, and their staff, especially Mr. Victor J. Boland.

MAXWELL M. WINTROBE

Salt Lake City, Utah

Preface to the First Edition

As knowledge is gained and a subject is better understood, it should become more simple rather than more difficult. Yet hematology has appeared to the average physician to grow constantly more complex, in spite of the fact that great progress has been made in this field and a clearer concept of the factors governing hematopoiesis as well as of the disorders of blood formation has been evolved.

The introduction of new methods, the description of new disease syndromes and the application of new terms have contributed to the apparent complexity of the subject. The literature, moreover, has grown voluminous and the task of the physician who must keep abreast of many fields is overwhelming.

To bring together the accumulated information in the field of hematology in a systematic and orderly form, to sift the important from the less significant, to describe the newer methods which are of practical value and to make note of those which are less essential, to outline details of differential diagnosis, to describe the indications for and methods of treatment, and to make clear as far as present knowledge permits the nature of the underlying physiological disturbances, are the objects of this book.

To fulfill these objects a book must be comprehensive, complete and authoritative. To this end thousands of publications have been consulted. This information has been so organized that it should be readily accessible. In addition, a bibliography of some 2400 references is provided in order that the interested reader may obtain still more information if he so wishes. The bibliographies are found at the end of each chapter and the text of the chapter serves as an index to the contents of each bibliography. Monographs and articles furnishing more complete bibliographies are so designated.

Emphasis is placed on the importance of accurate diagnosis as a prerequisite to efficacious treatment. The use of therapeutic measures without discrimination and the administration of "shotgun" antianemic remedies indicate the need for a clear understanding of the indications for liver, iron, vitamins and other substances. The effective employment of these and other therapeutic agents is discussed in detail.

Laboratory procedures of value in diagnosis are in the main quite simple and can be carried out in the office of the average physician. They are considered in detail. A departure from the usual custom has been made, however, in that the technical methods are not all grouped in a single section but are described in the various chapters of which they logically form a part. This is done because the objects and principles of a laboratory test must be thoroughly understood if it is to be well performed and correctly interpreted. Only those procedures which do not come within the scope of the various specific chapters are described in the chapter on methods. The vital importance of technical precision is stressed and the limits of accuracy of various procedures are indicated.

There is in this book no departure from accepted terminology. Instead, an attempt is made to give a clear interpretation of the terms now employed. Furthermore, no glossary of hematological terms has been prepared. It is believed that the meaning of a name or descriptive phrase is best expressed in the text where it is used. The index serves as the key to the definitions of the various terms.

In a book on hematology adequate illustration is essential. Nevertheless the cost must not be prohibitive to the student and physician. The excellent illustrations which have been published by a number of writers prove that much of the essential detail of cells, including even the leukocytes, can be demonstrated in engravings without the aid of color. For these reasons colored plates have been used sparingly in this book and serve to amplify rather than to displace illustrations in black and white. This saving in expense has permitted the inclusion of many illustrations of clinical features which have been neglected in most books on hematology.

Although it forms no part of clinical hematology, an Appendix giving the blood findings in 46 species of animals, including non-mammals, as well as a bibliography of literature on comparative hematology, is included in this book because I have been called upon to supply such information frequently and know that it is not readily accessible elsewhere. Many of the blood determinations have been made in our own laboratories.

Photographs, drawings and roentgenograms of patients have been used freely for illustration, through the courtesy of Dr. Warfield T. Longcope, my chief, to whom I am also indebted for the opportunity to study all of the cases with hemopoietic disorders on the medical service and to use the records which have been accumulated with great care over a period of many years. Dr. Edwards A. Park has very kindly allowed me the privilege of seeing many patients in the Department of Pediatrics.

It is with pleasure that I express my gratitude to those students of the Department of Art as Applied to Medicine of the Johns Hopkins University who have prepared many of the drawings which are reproduced here. Thanks are due particularly to Miss Laura Ornstedt, Miss Dagmar Haugen, Miss Marjorie Hoag and Miss C. M. Shackleford. I am also indebted to W. F. Prior Company, Inc., for permission to reproduce a number of the plates prepared under my direction which appear in Tice's Practice of Medicine.

I am particularly grateful to Dr. Oliver P. Jones for his helpful advice and criticism and to my many associates at the Johns Hopkins Hospital for the same reasons, including especially Dr. J. William Pierson and his staff in the Department of Roentgenology, Dr. Alan M. Chesney, Dr. Arnold Rich, and Dr. Harry Eagle. Thanks are due also to Dr. Edward A. Gall, Dr. Jacob Furth and Dr. Samuel Richman, and to the authors and publishers of articles from which illustrations have been reproduced. These are acknowledged in the text. The hundreds of investigators who have generously furnished reprints of their papers have made my task very much easier and I have thought of their kindness many times as this book was being written.

My wife has been my chief assistant in the preparation of the manuscript and in the reading of proofs, and my debt to her for this and for her patience and encouragement is great. Mrs. Norma Strobel, my secretary, Dr. Conrad Acton and the members of my laboratory staff gave valuable assistance in the preparation of the manuscript and charts. The staff of Messrs. Lea & Febiger have been both patient and skilful in their work of publication.

M. M. Wintrobe

Baltimore, Maryland

Contents

CHAPTER 3

THE ERYTHROCYTE—(Continued)

Biochemical Considerations and Kinetics.
Porphyrias and Disorders Usually Accompanied by Cyanosis

CHAPTER 4

THE LEUKOCYTES

CHAPTER 5

BLOOD PLATELETS AND COAGULATION

CHAPTER 6

THE BLOOD AS A WHOLE

CHAPTER 7

BLOOD GROUPS AND BLOOD TRANSFUSION

CHAPTER 8

THE PRINCIPLES AND TECHNIC OF BLOOD EXAMINATION

CHAPTER 9

ANEMIA: GENERAL CONSIDERATIONS AND TREATMENT

CHAPTER 10

PERNICIOUS ANEMIA AND RELATED MACROCYTIC ANEMIAS

CHAPTER 11
THE NORMOCYTIC ANEMIAS

Acute Post-hemorrhagic, Primary Refractory, Simple Chronic Anemia, Myelofibrosis and Myelophthisic Anemia

CHAPTER 12

Normocytic Anemias—(*Continued*): Hemolytic Anemias

CHAPTER 13

SICKLE CELL DISEASE, THALASSEMIA AND THE ABNORMAL HEMOGLOBIN SYNDROMES

CHAPTER 14

Hypochromic Microcytic (Iron Deficiency) Anemia

CHAPTER 15

Anemia and Other Disorders in Infancy and Childhood

CHAPTER 16

POLYCYTHEMIA

CHAPTER 17

THE PURPURAS

CHAPTER 18

Hemophilia and Other Hemorrhagic Disorders

CHAPTER 19

LEUKEMIA

CHAPTER 20

Tumors and Tumor-like Conditions Involving the Blood-forming Organs

CHAPTER 21

AGRANULOCYTOSIS AND INFECTIOUS MONONUCLEOSIS

APPENDIX A

APPENDIX B

Plates

CLINICAL HEMATOLOGY

Chapter 1

The Origin and Development of the Cells of the Blood in the Embryo, Infant and Adult

BLOOD FORMATION IN THE EMBRYO

THE matrix from which the blood cells are derived is the embryonic connective tissue, the mesenchyme. In the human embryo blood cells are first formed in the numerous blood islands of the yolk sac.[3] Later hematopoiesis appears in areas of mesoblastic tissue within the embryo but in these sites blood island development never reaches any considerable proportions.[10,16]

The cells of these blood islands, according to Maximow,[16] differentiate in two directions, the peripheral cells to form the walls of the first blood vessels (primitive endothelium) and those centrally situated to become the **primitive blood cells.** The latter have been described as possessing a more or less basophilic cytoplasm, a relatively large nucleus with an open, spongy chromatin network and several nucleoli.[15,16] In supravital preparations mitochondria are absent or very fine.[7] This distinguishes the cells from the lymphocytes of the blood in which the mitochondria are characteristically large and rod-shaped. The primitive cell just described has been called the primary wandering cell (Saxer), a large lymphocyte (Maximow), hämatogone (Mollier), hemocytoblast (Bloom, Maximow, Jordan), lymphoidocyte (Pappenheim), hemohistioblast (Ferrata, di Guglielmo) and mesameboid cell (Minot). It has been shown to have the potentiality of forming erythroblasts, granulocytes and megakaryocytes. Normally, primitive blood cells are present in small numbers and are difficult to identify in marrow smears. They are fragile and easily broken up. In pathological states when there is marrow hyperplasia, they may be more numerous and may be observed in groups or even as syncytia.

Hemoglobin-containing cells are the most predominant of the first blood cells

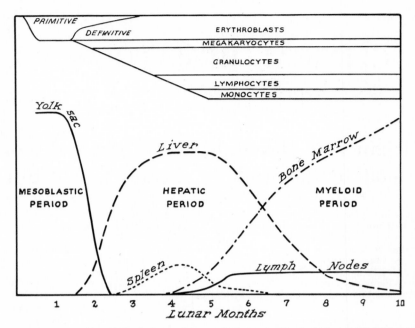

F‍IG. 1–1.—Stages of hemopoiesis in the embryo and fetus, indicating the comparative participation of the chief centers of hemopoiesis and the approximate times at which the different types of cells make their appearance.

formed (Kolliker, Naegeli). These **primitive erythroblasts** possess abundant cytoplasm, which may be polychromatophilic, and the chromatin in the nucleus is cloudy and coarse.[13] There may be several prominent nucleoli in the youngest cells. The primitive erythroblasts are similar to and were regarded by Ehrlich, probably erroneously, as identical with pernicious anemia megaloblasts (see Fig. 2–1, p. 87 and p. 513). At first spherical in shape (Maximow), they later become bell-shaped—Minot's ichthyoid type of erythrocyte.[15] Knoll estimated the volume of the primitive erythroblasts to be 1800 to 2400 c.μ. As development continues, these large cells gradually disappear and are replaced by smaller cells of the **definitive or normoblastic generation.**[3,15]

During the earliest stage of blood formation, cells resembling the leukocytes of adults are rarely found.[3,15,16]

The very first leukocytes, according to Maximow, are the undifferentiated primitive cells. The primary blood plasma in his opinion is secreted by the island cells when the free blood cells are formed.

The exact duration of this first or **mesoblastic period of hematopoiesis** is not known. The blood islands are demonstrable in the 2.25 mm. embryo and are absent at the 5 mm. stage.[15] Throughout this period no bloodforming organ is present and most of the cells are formed outside the embryo. Intravascular blood formation in the yolk sac can be observed as long as the 20 mm. stage. It is markedly diminished in a human embryo of nine weeks (Fig. 1–1).[3]

The **hepatic period of hematopoiesis** commences in the embryo of 5 to 7 mm.[15] The blood cells here are thought by most investigators to be derived from undifferentiated, polyvalent mesenchyme which has spread out between the liver cells. Nests of definitive erythroblasts, smaller than those found in blood islands and possessing relatively little cytoplasm, appear extravascularly. The nuclear chromatin pattern is relatively coarse, the chromatin masses may be radially arranged, and the parachromatin is very acidophilic (Fig. 2–1). At the same time (second month) granular leukocytes, identifiable by their positive oxydase reaction, can be demonstrated. Megakaryocytes can also be made out in the liver, as well as in the yolk sac. Small lymphocytes and the monocytes of adult blood, according to most observers,[7,15,19] are not found. The granulocytes increase in number so that by the fourth month of fetal life they are quite numerous.

Erythropoiesis in the *spleen* is at first more pronounced than leukopoiesis but it is short-lived, commencing two months after blood formation appears in the liver and terminating at about the fifth month of fetal life. It may persist to a slight degree until birth. The spleen, however, is chiefly concerned with lymphopoiesis. Hematopoiesis in the *thymus* is of brief duration. It is not limited to the production of lymphocytes, for a few myelocytes and definitive erythroblasts are present.[10]

The final or **myeloid period of hematopoiesis** begins approximately at the fifth month, being initiated with the establishment of placental circulation.[17] The mesenchyme causes resorption of the cartilage of the bone primordia, producing centers of blood formation. At first the liver is chiefly occupied in erythropoiesis and the bone marrow in leukocyte formation, but soon the bone marrow takes over all hematopoietic activity and this function of the liver disappears. By the growth of the myeloid cells, the fixed mesenchymal cells are reduced to a very scant reticular stroma.[16] This remains, nevertheless, throughout life with all of its potentialities intact.

3

These multipotential cells of the mesenchyme persist not only in the bone marrow, but also line the intralobular capillaries of the liver (Kupffer cells), the venous sinuses of the spleen and the sinuses of the lymph nodes, and are found in the walls of the intestine, in the serous membranes and possibly in endocrine glands such as the adrenals, as well as in the form of free macrophages. Individually they have been given a variety of names—resting wandering cells (Maximow), macrophages (Evans), clasmatocytes (Ranvier), hemohistioblasts (Ferrata). Together they form an important group of cells which is commonly known by the name suggested by Aschoff and Kiyono, *the reticulo-endothelial system*

THE BLOOD OF THE FETUS

As already stated, the first cells to appear in the blood of the fetus are chiefly primitive **erythroblasts.** In the embryo of 6.5 to 8 mm. the **erythrocyte count** is given as 366,900 per c.mm.[15] Of these cells, 92 per cent are very large, primitive erythroblasts ("first generation"). The smaller erythroblasts of the second or definitive generation become numerous during the hepatic period of hematopoiesis and gradually replace the more primitive cells.[3] The latter disappear from the circulation either by degeneration or by being phagocytized. Thus in the embryo of 19 to 28 mm. (end of second month), they form only 53 per cent of all erythroblasts. By the fourth month the first generation of cells has been completely replaced by the second or normoblastic generation.

The erythrocyte count of fetal blood increases rapidly at first and then more slowly[20,22] (Fig. 1–2) but it is only after birth that the counts found in adults are attained (see p. 109). At the same time the size and hemoglobin content of the corpuscles decrease. The volume of packed red cells and the hemoglobin per

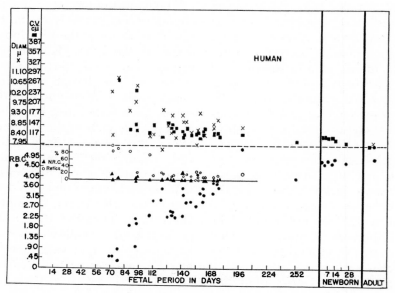

FIG. 1–2.—The red corpuscles of human fetuses of different ages compared with those of the newborn and adult. Erythrocyte counts are represented by solid circles; mean corpuscular volumes by squares; mean erythrocyte diameters (measured in wet preparations) by crosses; proportion of nucleated red corpuscles by black triangles and proportion of reticulocytes by open circles. (Wintrobe and Shumacker, Jour. Clin. Investigation.)

100 ml. of blood change less since they are the resultants of the erythrocyte count and the volume and hemoglobin content of the cells (Table 1–1).

At first all the erythrocytes are nucleated but they are rapidly replaced by non-nucleated forms and by the middle of the third month the erythroblasts make up no more than 8 per cent of all the erythrocytes. At this period, however, reticulocytes are still very numerous. Their number decreases more slowly than the number of nucleated red cells (Fig. 1–2, Table 1–1). The possible significance of the changes in the number and size of the erythrocytes in the fetus in relation to the so-called pernicious anemia of pregnancy is discussed elsewhere (p. 513).

The **hemoglobin** in fetal and cord blood differs from that of adult blood in a number of ways. It has been suggested that in early fetal life (10 to 20 weeks) a *primitive or embryonal* type of hemoglobin

is formed which is slower in electrophoretic mobility than adult hemoglobin and is under separate genetic control.[11] The existence of such a distinct hemoglobin is in doubt,[15a] but has not been excluded.[3b,26] The existence of a true *fetal hemoglobin* (Hb–F) is unquestioned.[22] This differs from adult hemoglobin (Hb–A) in varying degrees of subtlety in most properties; for example, in crystal form and x-ray diffraction, greater solubility, immunological specificity and readier oxidation. The basis for the differences lies in the globin, rather than the heme, Hb–F containing isoleucine, which is not present in Hb–A, and differing in other respects in amino acid composition (Table 3–4, p. 158). The pair of α-peptide chains in Hb–A and Hb–F are identical[12] but the pair of β-peptide chains in Hb–A differ so much from the corresponding pair in Hb–F that the latter have been designated γ-peptide chains.

In addition to Hb–F, cord blood has

Table 1–1.—Blood Values in 30 Human Fetuses

Age (days)	Full (mm.)	Cr.-R. (mm.)	Wt. (gm.)	R.B.C. ×10⁶	Hgb. (gm.)	Ht. (ml.)	C.V. (c.μ)	C.H. (γγ)	C.C. (%)	Icterus index	Fresh (μ)	Stained (μ)	N.R.C. (%)	Retics. (%)	W.B.C. ×1000 (p.c.mm.)
71	53	37	5.1	0.49	..	..	..	..	..	..	10.35	9.40	17.0	100	
72	57	43	5.7	0.49	..	..	..	..	..	..	8.41	7.34	3.0	87	7.8
78	..	..	8.7	0.31											
78	71	53	9.2	0.88	..	25.0	285	..	..	..	10.96	9.18	7.6	94	
88	..	..	..	1.82	..	..	136	..	..	15?	9.51	8.98	..	82	
95	..	88	..	0.95	8.0	22.8	249	93	36	7	..	7.86	0.3		
95	115	78	..	2.20	10.9	33.5	152	49	32	25?	9.90	8.45	1.4		
96	128	90	44	1.96	9.1	26.2	134	47	34	7	10.64	9.37	4.0	18	2.0
109	154	109	73	2.29	6.0	29.0	126	35	31	20	8.39	8.29	0.5	75	3.1
112	172	120	87	2.94	13.1	44.0	150	45	30	35	8.49	7.72		12	15.5
120	215	95	185	3.00	10.5	34.0	113	35	31	..	7.80	8.40	1.2	18	6.6
121	205	138	148	3.53	13.1	40.3	113	37	32	17?	9.56	7.62	..	19	12.2
126	222	155	..	2.29	10.9	36.2	154	48	31	20	8.85	7.70	0.9		
128	135	115	..	2.59	10.8	36.0	138	42	30	7	8.55	7.96	0.4	9	
131	220	150	245	2.46	10.2	32.5	132	42	32	30	..	7.54	0.6	18	11.4
133	218	160	255	2.24	11.3	32.0	139	51	36	..	8.30	7.90			
140	250	175	290	2.30	8.7	30.0	130	38	29	10	9.30	8.50	0.7	22	17.0
141	245	165	323	3.52	14.6	40.7	116	42	36	11	9.04	8.70	..	9	10.7
142	250	170	330	3.23	11.9	40.0	124	38	30	17	..	7.58	..	..	12.9
144	255	176	325	2.89	12.0	39.0	140	42	30	13	9.02	8.53	..	15	5.9
149	270	180	362	2.91	12.8	36.1	125	44	35	20	8.70	7.50	0.3	10	12.2
154	292	180	411	2.76	11.0	34.6	125	40	32	8	8.00	7.68	0.6	18	14.0
155	295	202	515	4.13	17.6	52.0	126	33	34	12	8.69	8.10	0.2	14	4.4
160	280	..	700	2.94	11.0	36.0	122	38	31	4	..	7.17	..	..	3.4
160	297	202	551	3.54	13.9	46.1	130	39	30	25	..	8.30	0.9	6	1.6
161	300	190	540	3.25	14.6	44.5	136	45	33	5	8.40	8.10	0.2	6	8.6
170	320	215	626	3.86	14.7	48.1	124	42	30	16	8.81	8.05	1.0	7	17.4
170	315	215	624	3.30	12.4	40.1	121	37	31	15	8.86	7.11	0.2	6	3.2
175	340	230	640	3.75	14.6	47.0	125	39	32	..	9.14	7.60	0.3	12	6.0
177	320	200	960	3.51	14.1	41.2	116	40	34	..	..	7.88	0.3	..	8.8

Ht. = volume of packed cells per 100 ml. blood; C.V. = mean corpuscular volume. CH. = mean corpuscular hemoglobin; C.C. = mean corpuscular hemoglobin concentration.

been found to contain two minor components (10 per cent), designated F_1^{1a} and F_{II}.

The oxygen dissociation curve for fetal hemoglobin lies to the left of that for maternal blood; *i.e.*, there is a greater affinity for oxygen. It is uncertain, however, whether this is attributable to the differences in the molecule itself or to other factors, such as the ionic environment, red cell permeability and blood pH.[1]

Hb–F is more stable to alkali than Hb–A. Thus, when alkali is added to a sample of blood, adult hemoglobin is rapidly converted to brown alkaline hematin, while that of fetal blood remains bright red for a considerable period. The rate of alkali-denaturation has consequently been used as a means for the quantitative estimation of Hb–F (method of Brinkman and Jonxis), the measurement depending on the conversion of HbO_2 into alkaline hematin. Since this conversion is associated with a change of color from red to brown, it can be followed spectrophotometrically or colorimetrically at wave lengths appropriate to either oxyhemoglobin or the product. However, the method is reliable only to about 10 per cent Hb–F. In the modification of Singer, Chernoff and Singer,[20] the alkaline hematin formed after one minute is separated and the oxyhemoglobin remaining in solution is read as Hb–F. This method (p. 719) provides a measure of levels below 10 per cent but not below 2 per cent Hb–F. More sensitive (down to the 1 per cent level or less) is a combined residue and spectrographic method[1c] and even more exact would be the assay for isoleucine. In the identification of Hb–F paper electrophoresis has limited usefulness but starch-gel electrophoresis permits good separation. Column chromatography, using Amberlite IRC–50 cationic exchange resin, is valuable.[22]

Attempts have been made to identify the different kinds of hemoglobin described above with the different sites of hemopoiesis during the development of the embryo and fetus. This has not met with success for Hb–A has been observed even as early as the 13-week fetus.[21] However, in the 20-week fetus 94 per cent of the hemoglobin is Hb–F and at birth 55 to 85 per cent. The amount present at birth has been found to be related to gestational age.[5] During the first year of life, the proportion of Hb–F decreases rapidly, no more than 10 per cent persisting four months after birth. In two-thirds of children within the age range six months to ten years the Hb–F level was found to be less than 1 per cent, frequently nil.[1c] In the remainder, however, some Hb–F, in trace amounts (0.4 to 1 per cent), persisted up to ten years of age. No Hb–F was detected, even by the more sensitive combined method, in normal adults.

The physiological significance of fetal hemoglobin is uncertain. It is possible that its production represents an adaptation to the fetal encironment in which oxygen and glucose are at a premium. When reticulocyte-rich suspensions of red cells from umbilical cord blood were incubated *in vitro* it was observed that conditions of hypoxia, or glucose deficiency, favored the formation of fetal hemoglobin as compared to adult hemoglobin.[1b]

Some have postulated that the production of fetal hemoglobin is determined by genes non-allelic with those regulating adult hemoglobin formation. Postnatally fetal hemoglobin is formed when the production of adult hemoglobin seems to be suppressed. Fetal hemoglobin is found in association with a number of hereditary hemoglobinopathies, as will be discussed in a later chapter (p. 668). Furthermore, in some of the latter, "abnormal" forms of fetal hemoglobin ("fast fetal," Bart's, "Alexandra") have been described. In addition, in certain other disorders of the blood, the presence of Hb–F has been demonstrated.[1c] This is true particularly in pernicious anemia and, in this disease, continued synthesis of Hb–F was observed during the initial stages of response to specific therapy with vitamin B_{12}. In view of the resemblance of megaloblasts to the primitive embryonic erythroblasts, already alluded to, this is of special interest. In addition, in refractory normoblastic anemias of non-hereditary character Hb–F was found in about one-third of cases. In congenital hemolytic anemias, only rarely were more than traces of Hb–F demonstrated and in conditions in which fetal sites of extramedullary hemopoiesis were reactivated, Hb–F formation was not a feature. In some children with variants of myeloid leukemia, appreciable proportions of Hb–F were encountered, and low levels were found in some cases of adult erythroleukemia.

Leukocytes, which are either absent from the blood of the earliest embryos, or extremely rare, number about 1000 per c.mm. in embryos 12 to 18 mm. in length (second month).[15] Of these cells 75 per cent are "myeloblasts" and the remainder are granulocytes. The total

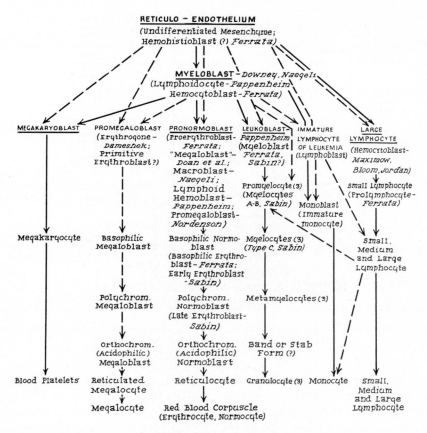

FIG. 1–3.—Origin and relation of blood cells under normal, pathological and experimental conditions, according to the modified neo-unitarian theory of Downey (arranged by Dr. Oliver P. Jones). The solid lines indicate the relation of blood cells in the normal human adult. The broken lines represent the various possibilities under pathological and experimental conditions.

count is said to rise gradually and to be due more to an increase of granulocytes than of younger cells.[15] In our own observations no clear-cut pattern was evident (Table 1–1). Lymphocytes morphologically similar to those found in the blood of adults do not appear until the fourth month of fetal life[25] and monocytes appear for the first time during the fifth month.[15]

THE INTERRELATIONSHIP OF THE BLOOD CELLS

Perhaps the most disputed issue in hematology concerns the interrelationship of the blood cells. Several schools of thought regarding this subject have arisen. According to the **monophyletic school** (Maximow,[16] Dantschakoff, Weidenreich, Jordan,[14] Bloom[3]) the lymphocyte of lymphatic tissue is identical with the primitive blood cell and is thus totipotential, giving rise under proper stimulation to any other type of blood cell, whether erythrocyte or leukocyte, granulocyte or monocyte. This change can be a direct one or the small lymphocyte of the blood may be first modified to a larger lymphoid cell (hemocytoblast of Maximow). *Neo-unitarians* such as Downey maintain that the lymphocyte of normal

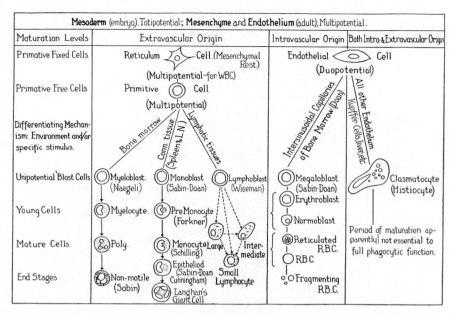

Fig. 1–4.—Origin of the cells of the blood, according to the complete polyphyletic school. (Wiseman, courtesy of Jour. Am. Med. Assn.)

blood does not usually change to some other type of cell but the developmental potentialities of the lymphocytes are such that this may occur in an abnormal environment (tissue cultures, experimental and pathological conditions) (see Fig. 1–3). Under normal conditions only the myeloblast functions as a myelopotent cell and cells morphologically identical with it are not present in adult lymph nodes.

Proponents of the **polyphyletic theory** have described a number of "blast cells" which are said to be the precursors of the completely differentiated cells of the blood. According to the number of "blast" cells which are recognized, the polyphyletists have been distinguished as dualists, trialists, and "complete" polyphyletists. The classical *"dualists"* (Ehrlich, Schridde, Naegeli) made a sharp morphological distinction between the basophilic stem cells in the myeloid and lymphatic tissues (myeloblasts and lymphoblasts). According to Naegeli the

precursors of the blood cells are (1) the lymphoblast, the ancestor of the lymphocytes; (2) the myeloblast, from which the myelocytes and granulocytic series of cells, as well as the monocytes and the megakaryocytes are derived; and (3) the pro-normoblast whence the red cells arise. This theory was modified by Schilling who asserted that the monocytes are quite separate from the myeloid elements and develop from reticuloendothelial cells, especially those lining the venous sinuses of the liver and spleen (*"trialistic"* theory).

Sabin and her co-workers[7,19,24] offered evidence for a theory of *complete polyphyletism*, according to which a stem cell for each of the cells of the blood is described. A new blast cell was introduced, the monoblast, which gives rise to the monocyte. These investigators assigned different functions to the primitive reticulum cells and the endothelial cells. The former give rise to multipotential, freely moving cells which, according to environment and specific stimulation, produce myeloblasts, lymphoblasts or monoblasts and these in turn differentiate to the stage of complete maturity. The erythrocytic series of cells is derived from endothelial cells lining the intersinusoidal capillaries of the bone marrow. Of endothelial origin also are the giant macrophages, clasmatocytes or histiocytes (see (Fig. 1–4).

The various theories of blood cell origin were discussed fully by a number of writers in Downey's Handbook of Hematology.[8] One of the main points of disagreement has been in regard to what constitutes a lymphocyte and whether this cell is capable of development along a variety of lines. Differences in technics, such as the use of sections and wet preparations as compared with dry, stained smears and imprints, have resulted in different interpretations. Some observers (Schridde, Naegeli, Ferrata, Knoll[15]), for example, have asserted that lymphocytes are not found in the early embryo and that they appear only with the formation of lymph nodes, about two months after the first granulocytes. This favors the polyphyletic concept. Other workers, however, while agreeing that in the early stages of development there is only one hemopoietic tissue, contend that this tissue produces both myeloid and lymphocytic elements.[2] If this is true the essential unity of myeloid and lymphocytic cells is indicated. Again, the description[24] of a definitive life cycle for the lymphocyte, corresponding to that of granulocytes, was not accepted by Downey and Stasney[9] who held that cytoplasmic basophilia, one of the criteria for the recognition of "young" lymphocytes, is not necessarily an index of cellular immaturity.

Furthermore, observations based on the study of living cells have not all been in agreement with conclusions drawn with the aid of other methods of study. Thus Maximow believed that the so-called endothelial cell of hematopoietic potency is simply a flattened reticulum cell.[16] On the other hand, Aschoff, Cunningham and Doan stressed differences in the behavior of reticulum and endothelial cells with respect to particulate matter.[7] There is even disagreement regarding the changes occurring in tissue cultures, Bloom contending that he observed the transformation of lymphocytes to monocytes, whereas the Lewises found no relationship whatever between these cells in tissue culture. We found that cells obtained from cases of acute myeloblastic and lymphoblastic leukemia showed striking differences in appearance and motion in tissue culture and differed in turn from monocytes (see Chapter 4, p. 215).

In clinical experience it is common for a single cell type to multiply to the exclusion of other forms, as is seen in reactions to infections and in other conditions causing changes in leukocytes, and occurs in chronic myelocytic and lymphocytic leukemias and, less frequently, in monocytic leukemia. This might be interpreted as strong evidence favoring the polyphyletic point of view. Yet it must be admitted that one frequently finds a few cells, sometimes even in normal blood, which possess characteristics suggesting intermediate forms. In some cases of acute leukemia it is certainly difficult to classify every cell with assurance and one simply assumes that all the abnormal cells belong to a single cell type. That this assumption is not necessarily correct is suggested by the findings in a form of "monocytic" leukemia in which myelocytes as well as monocytes are found (see p. 936). One is forced, therefore, to hesitate in accepting wholeheartedly the polyphyletic theory and to give serious consideration at least to the modified monophyletic theory of Downey as outlined in Figure 1–3. In the writer's opinion a dogmatic viewpoint on the interrelationship of the blood cells is not justified at this time.

POST-NATAL HEMATOPOIESIS

As already indicated, blood formation after birth is confined, under normal conditions, to the bone marrow. The three main cellular functions, erythropoiesis, leukopoiesis and thrombocytopoiesis, are in part independent of one another, in part reflect one another. Thus infection usually stimulates leukopoiesis but impairs erythropoiesis. On the other hand, the sudden loss or destruction of blood stimulates the production of all three components. The regeneration of the blood elements involves not only the multiplication of precursor cells but also the evolution of the definitive characteristics of each type and the release of the mature elements. It is obvious, therefore, that a thorough knowledge of the anatomy, cytology, cytochemistry and physiology of the bone marrow is essential for an understanding of hematology. Unfortunately, there still are many gaps in what is known today.

Structure of the Bone Marrow.— Encased within all the bones of the body and enclosed by the endosteum, the bone marrow consists of a variety of blood cells and their precursors, as well as fat cells, blood vessels and a framework of reticulum. The last is connected with the endosteum and closely bound with the blood vessels. It consists of a loose fibrous syncytium as well as reticulum cells with pale nuclei poor in chromatin. Most of these cells are fixed, but they are capable of rounding off to become large free macrophages. No lymph vessels have been demonstrated in bone marrow, and nerves have been demonstrated only in connection with the larger divisions of the blood vessels. Lymph follicles like those in the spleen have been observed in bone marrow and are considered by

most investigators to be normal constituents.[30,69,92]

The *vascular supply* of the bone marrow is derived from the nutrient artery. As visualized by vital microscopy of intact bone marrow in the rabbit[34] the arterioles derived from the nutrient artery divide dichotomously into capillaries. The latter run into sinusoids, which are sometimes hexagonal, sometimes spindle-shaped. Sinusoids sometimes unite to form sinusoidal systems. The sinusoids are ultimately drained by venules into collecting venules, which empty into the vein accompanying the nutrient artery. Capillaries stemming from marrow arterioles enter the Haversian canals to supply endosteal parts of the diaphyseal bone.

The sinusoids vary rhythmically in degree of dilatation. The vascular system of the bone marrow is unique in that the entire capillary bed can never be dilated at one time. Sabin and her co-workers,[92] studying the marrow of pigeons, concluded that regeneration of marrow begins in the collapsed vessels. They found that the endothelial cells swell, divide and differentiate to form erythroblasts. They claimed that the erythrocytic series is produced intravascularly whereas the leukocytes are formed extravascularly. However, later embryological studies showed that endothelium is not essential for the production of erythroblasts[3] and many workers regard the origin of all the cells of the blood to be extravascular.[6]

The number of fat cells found in the bone marrow varies with the age of the individual and the requirements of the occasion. The fat acts as a sort of buffer which occupies unneeded space but, being in a much more labile state than the general adipose tissues of the body, it can be readily displaced by hematopoietic tissue. The fat cells are probably reticulum cells which have stored fat. In pigeons under experimental conditions,

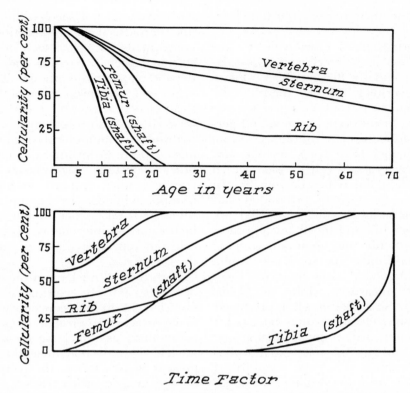

Fig. 1–5.—The amount of cellular red marrow in different bones at various ages (above) and the relative response to stimuli in these bones (based on the data of Custer and Ahlfeldt, J. Lab. and Clin. Med.)

fatty marrow has been observed to become completely cellular in 48 hours.[45,92]

It has been calculated that there are 0.56 gm. of marrow per gram of blood and that the bone marrow amounts to from 3.4 to 5.9 per cent of the body weight[80] or 1600 to 3700 gm. That is, it roughly equals the weight of the liver. In the adult only half the bone marrow, approximately, is red and the other half is fatty.

During the first few years of life the marrow of practically all the bones is red and cellular. Between the ages of five and seven years, fat cells begin to appear between the blood cells in the marrow and with progressing age the active marrow gradually recedes from the distal portions of the skeleton towards the trunk. At about the age of eighteen actively hematopoietic marrow is found only in the vertebrae, ribs, sternum, bones of the skull, the innominate bone and to some extent in the proximal epiphyses of the femur and humerus. This change is shown in Figure 1–5 which is based on a study of 100 cases.[45]

PROLIFERATION OF CELLS IN THE BONE MARROW

The numbers of red corpuscles, leukocytes and platelets in the circulation are remarkably constant under normal conditions and the changes which take place in various physiological and pathological states are quite predictable. This indicates that the production of cells in the marrow is finely balanced and that powerful mechanisms exist which govern the proliferation of cells in the bone marrow and their release into the circulation.

The formation of blood cells by the marrow was first described in 1868 by Neumann and by Bizzozero.[8,34] Flemming[8] described mitosis there. The multiplication of cells destined for the circulating blood occurs chiefly, and perhaps exclusively, by mitotic division. Many schemes have been devised concerning the types of cell division which take place in the bone marrow.[106] In any scheme, it must be postulated that in a given series of cells some that are morphologically and biochemically most primitive divide and maintain somatic genetic continuity, the so-called "alpha cells" of Osgood.[84] The majority, however, have measured, finite life spans ("n cells"). Since the "n cell" is produced by the alpha cell, there must be a point of bifurcation, a division producing one alpha cell and one "n" cell. No morphologic distinction has been established between the "primitive proliferating pool" of alpha cells and the finite "n" cells.

Metabolism of the Bone Marrow. [74]—Growth, whether it takes place by division or by enlargement of the cell, depends on the new formation of the fundamental substances of the cell and requires systems for energy production. Study of the metabolism of the bone marrow presents a comparatively unique problem because of the heterogeneous populations of cells contained therein and the considerable differences in their metabolic activity. Fortunately technics have been developed which permit study of metabolism at the cellular level. These include cytochemical procedures, ultraviolet absorptiometry, micro-interferometry, and autoradiography. In addition, the successful maintenance of bone marrow cells *in vitro* in suspension cultures has facilitated the study of their metabolism.

Substances manufactured by the cells of the bone marrow include proteins, carbohydrates, polysaccharides, lipids and and steroids. Cell proliferation and the constituents of cells, such as the cell stroma, special enzymes and secretions depend on protein synthesis. The energy required for the production of the various substances and energy needed for mitosis is derived from breakdown of carbohydrates, through glycolysis in some cells and respiration in others. Oxidation of other foodstuffs also occurs and the energy is then trapped in high-energy phosphate bonds. In relation to mitosis, these steps take place in the antephase, before any visible changes occur in the cell and represent a sort of charging of the "batteries."

Both the cell nuclei and the cytoplasm of young, actively growing cells contain nucleic acids in high concentration, these being attached to proteins or protein-like compounds as "nucleo-proteins." The nucleic acids are polynucleotides and are present in two forms, the pentose series or ribonucleic acids (RNA) and the deoxypentose series or deoxyribonucleic acids (DNA). Both types yield the purine bases guanine and adenine, the pyrimidine base cytosine, and phosphoric acid, but DNA contains the pyrimidine base thymine in addition to 2-desoxyribose whereas RNA yields uracil and *d*-ribose. The purines are probably derived from the liver, rather than being synthesized *de novo* in the bone marrow.[75]

Chromosomes and the chromatin of resting cells contain an abundance of DNA. In bone marrow tissue cultures it has been found that DNA synthesis takes place in the second half of the interphase between mitoses and is complete three to four hours before mitosis.[74] The Feulgen reaction, widely used in chemical studies, is regarded as a specific test for DNA.

The nucleoli, on the other hand, contain RNA. They are Feulgen negative. RNA is also found in cytoplasm, especially in the mitochondria and microsomes. Light areas in basophilic cytoplasm, previously described as hyaloplasm or paraplasm, represent, for the most part, the negative images of underlying mitochondria.[68] These structures are the sites of important enzymatic activities and probably function as centers for protein synthesis. There is evidence that the cellular RNA is formed in nuclei and migrates into the cytoplasm later.[110] This suggests that RNA is a direct product of gene action.

The presence of nucleoli, the "organizing centers" of the cells,[74] is correlated with the capacity for cell proliferation, their absence signifying the termination of development.[73] The decreasing growth activity of the individual cell during maturation is regulated by a specific part of the chromatin, the nucleolus-associated chromatin or heterochromatin, the nucleolus being ultimately replaced by this. It has been observed that the resting nuclei of all the cell types of the red and white series in the bone marrow show a striking similarity in that in the earliest phases they have Feulgen-negative nucleoli, while later these diminish and disappear on the formation of Feulgen-positive heterochromatic bodies.[73] The ribonucleic acids (RNA) of nucleolus and cytoplasm, together with the nucleolus-associated chromatin, appear to be closely related not only to the proliferation of the young marrow cells but also to the synthesis of their characteristic cytoplasmic contents,[108] namely hemoglobin in the red series and the complex enzyme systems of the specific granules in the granulocytes.

By applying Caspersson's microspectrographic method for the detection of nucleic acids to bone marrow cells, Thorell[99] found that the main cellular protein synthesis connected with growth in normoblasts takes place during the earliest developmental stage and at this time the ribonucleic acids (RNA) are actively involved. When cellular growth activity ceases, the concentration of these substances decreases rapidly and the main synthesis of hemoglobin begins, the cellular content of hemoglobin rising rapidly from an amount less than 2 $\gamma\gamma$ up to 28$\gamma\gamma$ ultimately. By the time the cytoplasm is polychromatophilic the concentration of ribonucleic acids has decreased to one-tenth of its maximum value (Fig. 1–6). Studies of cells in bone marrow cultures, however, indicate that small amounts of RNA can still be demonstrated by staining methods in polychromatophilic cells which are largely hemoglobinized.[87] Only a trace of RNA remains in the orthochromatic normoblast and the last vestiges are found in the reticulum of reticulocytes.

In the bone marrow cells in pernicious anemia, on the other hand, Thorell found that the RNA of the cytoplasm and nucleolar apparatus failed to disappear although hemoglobin formation took place. In contrast, in hemorrhagic anemia the decrease in RNA proceeds normally even though hemoglobin synthesis is impaired due to lack of iron. In leukemia, as in pernicious anemia, the cells accumulate very high concentrations of RNA in the cytoplasm and nucleolar apparatus and fail to show the rapid decline in RNA which occurs in normal bone marrow cells.

In studying cells during the cycle of mitosis, Koller[72] observed that DNA is attached at specific loci to the polypeptide chain which represents the permanent chromosome fiber. Maximum spiralization of the chromosomes at metaphase is associated with maximum attachment or "charge." Beginning in late anaphase and proceeding through telophase, detachment of nucleic acid charge occurs and this is associated with despiralization of the chromosome thread. The rate of nucleic acid detachment along the chromosome fiber differs, however, the regions which have a different cycle being called heterochromatic.

Differences have been found between

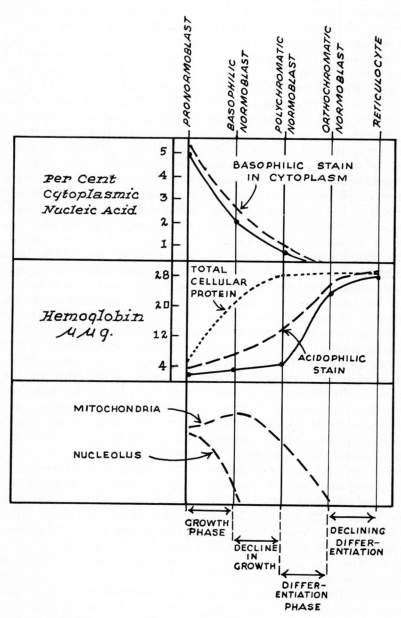

Fig. 1–6.—The development, differentiation and maturation of the erythroblast (modified from Thorell). Only the full lines represent quantitative data. It will be noted that considerable protein synthesis takes place during the growth phase. The nucleolus then disappears and, as the concentration of RNA decreases, hemoglobin begins to appear and increases rapidly in amount.

normal and abnormal cells and changes have been described as the consequence of irradiation and the action of certain chemical agents. Thus, an intensive hyperfunction of the heterochromatin appears to be characteristic of cancer cells and is responsible for stimulating protein synthesis and nucleic acid metabolism. There is evidence that RNA can be transformed into DNA. Such a transformation may be prevented by radiation of dividing cells, resulting in an accumulation of RNA in the cytoplasm.[81] Although the enzymes of the cytoplasm seem to be well protected from the effect of radiation, the nucleus can be damaged and thereby cytoplasmic activity can be disturbed to such a degree that mitosis is greatly delayed and the cell may die without going through mitosis. A marked reduction of the mitotic index has been observed; its degree was related to the dose.[54] After irradiation, chromosomes clump and stick together at metaphase and form bridges at anaphase and telophase.[72] According to Koller,[72] the nitrogen mustards act chiefly during the resting phase and probably break the chromosomes, causing sticking during mitotic division. Chemical carcinogens are considered to act directly or indirectly on those particular processes which underlie or regulate cell division and also chromosome organization.

Thus the balanced production of the cells in the bone marrow appears to depend on a highly adapted chemical system. It has been suggested that, since the nucleic acids govern cell division, the difference in their concentration between red and white cell precursors may be responsible for the proportion of red and white cells in the blood.[73] Furthermore, it is possible that under stress of pathological conditions, competition may take place within the cell, or between cells, for substances essential to the maintenance of this equilibrium.

In subsequent chapters further details

of cytology and cytochemistry will be considered in relation to hemoglobin formation (p. 122), the different types of leukocytes (p. 234), the pathogenesis of various types of anemia (p. 524), the nature of leukemia (p. 908) and the effects of radiation (p. 556) and of chemotherapeutic agents (p. 963).

Multipliction and Maturation of Cells in the Bone Marrow.—The production of cells destined for the blood depends first on mitosis and subsequently on the maturation of the respective lineages of cells. As a result, growth is at first logarithmic (exponential) and then becomes arithmetic. As stated earlier, many schemes have been devised in postulating the types of cell division in bone marrow, but facts are limited. It is assumed that certain cells maintain somatic genetic continuity and remain as primitive or stem cells ("alpha cells") but it is not known how many are involved in this "primitive proliferative pool" or how many mitoses the remaining cells undergo before maturation occurs and no further division takes place. Here the labeling of cells with tritiated thymidine is extremely helpful in that this identifies the cells which are synthesizing DNA and are capable of division but this obviously answers only one of the problems inherent in any study of the dynamics of blood formation. Thus, it must be recognized that the stages in the development of a cell which have been designated arbitrarily for the convenience of discussion are purely artificial and that, within these arbitrary bounds it would be impossible to state how many divisions occur. Furthermore, it does not necessarily follow that the number of divisions is always the same, nor is there any information concerning the number of cells which have undergone one or more divisions and then have failed to proceed further and have died.

The study of cell proliferation necessitates determination of the types of cells undergoing mitosis, as well as the rate of mitosis and the time intervals involved in the various stages of cell growth. Following mitosis, a "resting" phase takes place before mitosis is initiated again. This is known as the intermitotic time. The various steps have been designated (1) the period of mitosis, (2) the postmitotic rest period, (3) the period during which the synthesis of DNA is taking place (p. 42) and (4) a premitotic rest period.

The frequency of mitotic division is indicated by the *mitotic index*; that is, the number of cells in mitosis divided by the total number of cells in the population. The mitotic time together with the intermitotic time represents the *generation time*. A valuable method for estimation of *mitotic time* is based on the arrest of mitosis by subjecting cells to the action of spindle poisons, such as colchicine.[49,72a] These agents totally or partially destroy the fibrillar structure of the spindle; as a consequence the chromosomes remain in a state of pseudometaphase or "*stathmokinesis*."[31] A comparison of the number of dividing cells at a given time in a nontreated animal with that in a colchicine-treated animal makes it possible to calculate mitotic time.

If the duration of mitosis (mitotic time) is known, the *turnover time* can be calculated. The last may be defined as the average time needed to renew the cells of a particular type[72a] and thus, in essence, represents the average time spent in that state ("compartment"). This is calculated by dividing the mitotic time by the mitotic index.

The determination of mitotic index and of the other rates mentioned above presents a number of problems, such as difficulties in the identification of cell types when in mitosis, the possibility that diurnal variations occur and, in man, limitations in the number of samples obtainable and the types of studies which can be conducted. It is natural that published data should differ somewhat.

In the most recent study, carried out in nine healthy males, 8.86 mitoses per 1000 cells were found, that is, a mitotic index of 0.9 per cent.[54,70a] The mitotic figures in the preparations examined were divided as follows: prophase 39 per cent, metaphase 38 per cent, anaphase 17 per cent, telophase 5.5 per cent.[54] This is in good agreement with earlier studies.[67]

The relative contributions of erythroid and myeloid cells to the overall mitotic index indicated that 69.4 per cent or 6.15 mitoses per 1000 cells were erythroid and the remainder, 2.54, were neutrophil precursor mitoses.[70a] This differs from earlier widely cited data.[67] Polychromatic normoblasts were observed to give rise to about two-thirds of all erythroid mitoses. Typical small orthochromatic normoblasts were not found to label with tritiated thymidine and hence presumably do not undergo mitosis. In the myeloid series, myelocyte mitoses appeared to contribute somewhat more than two-thirds of all the myeloid mitoses.

An attempt was also made to determine the percentage of mitotic cells among each of the various cell types ("specific mitotic index"). The following data were obtained, per 1000 cells: myeloblast 2.52, promyelocyte 1.49, myelocyte 1.10, proerythroblast 2.53, basophilic normoblast 4.94 and polychromatic normoblast 5.65.[70a]

Estimates of the time required for normal mitosis in erythroblasts are in the range of 0.5 to 1.5 hours[86] but figures as high as three hours have been cited.[106] In the latter study the times for the various steps in mitosis in the early erythroblast were calculated to be as follows: prophase 43 to 54 minutes; metaphase 25 to 31 minutes; anaphase 32 to 40 minutes; telophase 20 to 25 minutes.[106] Mitoses in later forms were estimated to be twice as fast. The time required for mitosis of granulocyte precursors has been estimated to be between 0.5 and 1.5 hours.[3a,42]

Turnover time was calculated by Killman et al.[70a] to be 19.8 to 39.7 hours for myeloblasts, 33.5 to 44.6 hours for promyelocytes, 58.3 to 64.1 hours for myelocytes and 129.1 to 142 hours for the later, non-proliferating neutrophilic leukocytes. These figures are intermediate between those obtained in earlier calculations by others.[78,86] For the erythroid series the following figures were obtained: proerythroblast 19.8 to 39.6 hours, basophilic normoblast 13.6 to 16.3 hours, polychromatic normoblast 10.8 to 11.5 hours and, for the non-proliferating orthochromatic normoblasts, 15.5 to 16.6 hours. This is in reasonably good agreement with earlier estimates.[48a,86] These calculations were based on a mitotic time of one hour and are subject to the limitations already mentioned. They can only be considered to be approximations.

Estimates have also been made of the total number of cells in the bone marrow on the basis of the above data. For a normal man the figures would be: total number of erythroid precursors 4.5 × 10^9/Kg.; total number of marrow neutrophils and neutrophil precursors, 10.7 × 10^9/Kg.[70a] These are in good agreement with the data of others (5.0 and 11.4 × 10^9 cells/Kg., respectively).[48a]

Calculations such as these are important in the study of the kinetics of cellular proliferation. The details of erythrokinetics and of leukokinetics will be dealt with in the chapters concerned with the erythrocyte (p. 180) and the leukocytes (p. 240), respectively.

Little quantitative information is available regarding *megakaryocytes*. Divisions of megakaryocytes are infrequent. The mitotic index may be 0.5 to 1 per cent.[106] On morphological grounds it is apparent that these cells can undergo endomitotic divisions and the nucleus can divide into two, four or more nuclei. Polyploidy is also not unusual.[106]

The Release of Mature Elements. The *method of entrace of cells* into the circulation is not clear. The view[92] that red blood cells arise within the endothelial lining while leukocytes are formed extravascularly, has been mentioned already. According to this theory, the intersinusoidal capillaries open intermittently to release mature cells and then close again to form more cells. One of the reasons presented to support this theory is the fact that the red cells possess no means of locomotion and could not reach the blood stream if they were produced outside the vessels. Others[64] hold that all blood formation is extravascular, the new cells being released into the circulation by diapedesis or by temporary dissolution of the capillary wall. The immature cells are described as being embedded in a thick jelly-like substance which is liquefied as the cells become mature, thus permitting them to enter the blood stream. In the case of leukocytes it is assumed that they reach the blood vessels by their own action. The fact that the marrow is confined within a limited space may contribute to the expulsion of cells into the circulation.

Sabin and her associates[92] found that granulocytes enter the blood stream rhythmically with small hourly accessions and a larger daily rise in the afternoon and again at midnight. These observations have been challenged, however, and the subject requires further study.

Factors Which Govern the Formation, Maturation and Release of Blood Cells into the Blood Stream.—It is evident that a well balanced mechanism exists which maintains the blood at "normal," controls the normal sex differences in erythrocyte levels and mediates the response to a variety of normal and abnormal situations. Little is known about this mechanism, however. Chemotactic factors (p. 236) probably play a role in calling forth leukocytes. Erythropoietic activity has been regarded as being regulated by the oxygen content of arterial blood. It is true that anoxemia produced by a variety of causes leads to erythrocytosis (p. 788), and high tensions of inspired oxygen have been observed to depress erythropoiesis in hemolytic anemia, in pernicious anemia and even in normal subjects (see p. 688). However, it appears that the effect of anoxia is not mediated directly through alterations in oxygen saturation or tension in the bone marrow blood.[60] For this and other reasons it has been postulated that the effect of anoxia is transmitted to the bone marrow by some intermediate mechanism. The nervous system, the endocrine glands,[58] the spleen and plasma factors have been proposed by various investigators as playing this role in the regulation of hemopoiesis.

Irritation of the **diencephalon** in the region of the corpus striatum, the thalamus and the hypothalamus has been shown to produce in rabbits a pronounced leukocytosis with the appearance of many immature forms.[91] It has been claimed that the bone marrow can be stimulated directly through the parasympathetic system and inhibited *via* sympathetic fibers and that there is an interplay between the nervous system and hormonal factors.[82] These and other studies implicating the nervous system have not been very convincing.[60] On firmer ground is the evidence that certain hormones are involved in the control of hemopoiesis, particularly those of the gonads, the thyroid, adrenal cortex and anterior pituitary.

Role of Hormones in Control of Hemopoiesis.—*Anemia* usually accompanies hypothyroidism in man (p. 519), adrenal cortical insufficiency (Addison's disease, p. 581) and anterior pituitary insufficiency (Simmonds' disease) and polycythemia is associated with adrenal cortical hyperfunction[62] (Cushing's syndrome, p. 793). From this it may be inferred that the endocrine glands may influence hemopoiesis.

Many experimental studies in animals indicate that such a relationship exists.[58] Thus, castration in male rats is associated with a decrease in the red cell count whereas this causes an increase in female rats.[58] In castrated females the administration of estradiol benzoate caused a drop in the elevated counts while testosterone produced a rise to normal in castrated males. It has been observed, furthermore, that the normal sex differences of male and female rats can be accentuated by the administration of a gonadotropic extract, in male rats even when the hypophysis was removed. In these different experiments bone marrow hypo- and hyperplasia were observed which reflected the behavior of the red cell counts. Similar though less complete observations have been made in the rabbit, in the bird and in certain other species, including man.[46,70]

In rats thyroidectomy or the prolonged administration of thiouracil is associated with decreased iron utilization for hemoglobin formation.[33] In the same species hypophysectomy induces moderately severe anemia. This can be duplicated by removal of both the thyroid and the adrenals and can be decreased by administration of thyroxine and cortisone. The anemia is entirely prevented by a combination of thyroxine, testosterone proprionate and a high protein diet.[38] This anemia is not associated with shortened red cell survival but is associated with decreased marrow uptake of radioactive iron.[32] It has been attributed to a decrease in erythrocyte production rate. Administration of growth hormone has failed to prevent the development of this anemia.[38] The claim that an extract of sheep pituitary is capable of producing reticulocytosis and the appearance of normoblasts in the blood, correcting the anemia, preventing neonatal anemia and even, in the normal, producing polycythemia,[37] has not been confirmed by others.[38] It has been suggested that the loss of thyrotropic and adreno-corticotropic hormones, and possibly of growth hormone, which results from hypophysectomy causes decreased need for oxygen by the tissues which, in turn, leads to a decrease in the rate of erythro-poiesis.[38]

It is now well established that the pituitary adrenocorticotropic hormone (ACTH) through its effect on adrenal secretion evokes a *leukocytic response* in man, as well as in various species of animals. Single injections of ACTH in mice, rats and rabbits produce within a few hours, an absolute lymphopenia, a reaction which fails to occur in adrenal-ectomized animals.[48b] Adrenocortico-steroids produce the same response in intact and in adrenalectomized animals. Similar changes have been observed in man.[46] A single, intramuscular dose of 25 mg. of ACTH administered to human subjects with unimpaired adrenal func-tion, is followed by an increase of circulat-ing neutrophils and a decrease of circu-lating lymphocytes and eosinophils. The latter changes do not take place in the absence of a functionally competent adrenal cortex but the neutrophilic re-sponse still occurs. Consistent with these observations is the fact that, in patients with Cushing's syndrome, leukocytosis due to an absolute and relative increase in neutrophils and a relative and usually absolute lymphocytopenia are found. In contrast, in Addison's disease and pan-hypopituitarism, neutropenia and rela-tive lymphocytosis are present (p. 581).

Striking degenerative changes can be demonstrated in lymphoid tissue follow-ing the administration of adrenocortico-steroids and there are observations which indicate that cortisol has a direct effect on the lymphocytes.[48b] Shedding of the lymphocyte cytoplasm, pyknosis and karyorrhexis of the cells and inhibition of mitosis and heteroplasia have been de-scribed. The effect on the eosinophilic leukocytes has been attributed to pro-longation of mitosis and lengthening of the intermitotic time.[49]

Other hormones have less influence on leukocytes. A relative and absolute increase in lymphocytes and an increase in eosinophils may be encountered in hyperthyroidism (p. 261) and such changes in the blood of rats have been reported to follow the injection of thyroxine.[29] Thyroidectomy in rats is associated with leukopenia which is characterized chiefly by eosinopenia and lymphocytopenia.[29] The latter changes can be prevented by the simultaneous removal of the adrenals.

There is less evidence of an influence of hormones on *platelets*. A decrease in platelets is alleged to occur during the two-week period prior to menstruation (p. 284) but this is not well established.

For many years investigators were reluctant to accept the claim that the endocrine organs influence hematopoiesis. This was in large measure due to the fact that the changes observed were of small degree, especially in comparison with the changes in the blood which are associated with deficiencies of substances essential for blood formation, such as iron, folic acid, pyridoxine and vitamin B_{12}. More recently, better controlled studies and the availability of more purified hormone preparations have yielded more convinc-ing results. It has also come to be appreciated that only small variations can be expected to occur under the influence of *controlling* factors as distin-guished from the influence of substances which are used in the production of the blood cells. The failure of "specific" substances such as iron or vitamin B_{12} to cause an increase in blood values in normal persons or animals indicates that they are not governing factors in erythro-cyte formation but are, rather, building blocks which form part of the substance of the red corpuscle or agents which are concerned with its construction.

Plasma Factor(s).[51,57,60,65]—In 1906 Carnot and Déflandre proposed that the circulating blood carries an erythropoietic stimulating substance, "hémopoiétine."[60] Their work was ignored, in part because they provided scanty experimental data to support their view, and also because the concept of Miescher (1893) was generally accepted; namely, that erythropoiesis in the bone marrow is controlled by the level of oxygen in the marrow substance.

The report in 1950 that normoblastic hyperplasia of the bone marrow developed in both partners of parabiotic pairs of rats only one of which was subjected to hypoxia,[90] renewed interest in the possibility that the hypoxic stimulus is mediated through a hormone-like factor in the blood. The work of a number of investigators since that time has furnished convincing evidence of the presence of one or more such *erythropoietic-stimulating factors (ESF)*, (*"erythropoietin"*).[57,65]

Thus, to cite a few examples, it was shown that nursing mice kept at low oxygen tension except when suckling their young secrete in the milk a substance that causes polycythemia in the nurslings;[60] the intravenous injection into normal recipients of larger amounts of plasma from anemic animals than were used in Carnot's studies was found to produce more impressive reticulocytosis than had been observed before, and the quantity of circulating hemoglobin increased as well;[51,57] it was shown that erythropoiesis can be suppressed by transfusing normal animals, and a profound decrease in red cell iron turnover can be induced thereby.[50] Multiple transfusions in human subjects were shown to suppress erythropoiesis.[48,95,100] "Dilution anemia," produced in rabbits by injecting dextran and thereby causing hypervolemia without a reduction in red cell mass, did not interfere with red cell production, thus suggesting that it is the tissue tension of oxygen and not the oxygen content per unit of blood which regulates red cell production.[51]

Furthermore, that this is not due to the oxygen tension in the bone marrow but is related to the oxygen tension of an extramedullary organ or cellular system was suggested by the observation that the erythropoietic activity of bone marrow, *in vitro*, was depressed rather than stimulated by a reduction in the oxygen tension. In a patient with regional hypoxia secondary to patent ductus arteriosus and reversal of flow through the shunt, erythroblastic hyperplasia was found in bone marrow supplied by blood with a normal saturation of oxygen and was not confined to the area of regional hypoxia.[97]

A large variety of techniques have been developed for the assay of erythropoietin.[57] Although none is as yet completely satisfactory,[65] a number are based on the observation that hypophysectomy, transfusion-induced polycythemia or acute starvation are effective means of bringing about suppression of erythropoiesis. The reticulocyte response of the polycythemic mouse or the stimulation of the incorporation of Fe^{59} into the red cells of the acutely starved rat are among the simpler methods for the measurement of the quantity of erythropoietin in a sample of plasma. By such assay procedures it has been possible, to some extent, to characterize the plasma factor and to show that it is protein in nature, appreciably heat resistant, nondialyzable, nonultrafiltrable, nonprecipitable by perchloric acid or boiling, but precipitable with 70 to 80 per cent saturated ammonium sulfate or 60 to 80 per cent ethanol. It contains sialic acid and has an electrophoretic mobility characteristic of alphaglobulins. Activity is destroyed by proteolytic enzymes. Thus erythropoietin appears to be a small molecular weight glycoprotein, possibly with an associated active polypeptide grouping.[57] The claim that there are two humoral erythropoietic factors, one thermostable and ether-soluble which governs the mitotic or proliferative activity of erythrocytic precursors and the other thermolabile and ether-insoluble which augments hemoglobin synthesis,[77] is as yet unconfirmed.

Interesting observations have been made concerning the site of erythropoietin production. It was observed that the reduction of marrow and lymphatic tissue to a reticulum stroma by roentgen irradiation or by the administration of nitrogen mustards does not impair the capacity of animals to respond to anemic stimuli by increasing the circulating level of erythropoietin.[65] This led to the testing of heated extracts of liver, spleen, thymus, lung, brain and skeletal muscle, and these, like marrow or red cells from anemic animals were found to be devoid of erythropoietic activity.[57] Finally the extirpation of various organs before measuring the liberation of erythropoietin in response to stimuli such as phlebotomy or cobalt revealed no inhibition of response, except when the kidneys were removed.[65] Furthermore, it was found that nephrectomized dogs, kept alive by peritoneal dialysis, had a severely suppressed rate of erythropoiesis whereas ureter-ligated dogs underwent only a minimal depression in this regard.[83] These experiments have been confirmed in dogs[98] and in rats.[90] Thus the kidney appears to be directly or indirectly concerned with the production of erythropoietin. It has been postulated that the presence of functioning renal (tubular) tissue is necessary for a normal erythropoietic response.[90] Renal extracts have been reported to possess erythropoietic stimulating action;[98] other investigators were not so successful.[65] Some evidence has been presented which suggests that the adrenocorticotropic hormone, by an extra-adrenal mechanism, stimulates the secretion of the kidney factor.[84]

It is postulated that the dynamic equilibrium of the erythron is controlled by erythropoietin through a very sensitive system which monitors and responds to the natural disappearance of red cells

and reacts to the internal stresses of the body in health and disease and to changes in external environment, such as ascent to high altitude.[65] As stated earlier the relationship of oxygen demand to supply may govern the rate of red cell production. It has been suggested that erythropoietic depression occurs in hypophysectomized or in starved animals because of a reduced tissue requirement for oxygen. Transfusion-induced polycythemia has a similar effect. The erythropoietic response to hypoxia may be mediated in the bone marrow by changing undifferentiated stem cells to differentiated pronormoblasts.[51] This may be the effect of erythropoietin.[28] It is possible that erythropoietin, formed in the kidneys, is utilized and/or destroyed in the hemopoietic organs;[96] or, perhaps, an inhibitor is normally inactivated by the kidneys.[90] The significance of the demonstration of erythropoietin in the urine[101] is obscure.

Assays of erythropoietin levels in plasma have revealed high titers in some patients with hypoplastic anemias, in Cooley's anemia, in some cases of leukemia associated with anemia, in subjects with secondary polycythemia and in some cases of polycythemia vera, as well as in the cord blood plasma of the newborn.[57] Low levels have been observed in anemic patients with chronic renal disease.[65] On the whole, however, results have been conflicting and contradictory. From the studies made so far no correlation can be drawn between the intensity of anemia or the duration of the condition in the patient and the amount of erythropoietin detectable in plasma. The quantity circulating in the blood is variable. It is clear that much more needs to be learned about the factors which govern the production, destruction and excretion of erythropoietin than is known at present.

The hope that erythropoietin might be obtainable in large amounts and might prove useful in the treatment of certain forms of anemia has not materialized so far. Such therapeutic trials as have been carried out have been disappointing. Thus, its administration to several patients with congenital hypoplastic anemia has produced no benefit.[57] However, the clinical applications of the intriguing observations on erythropoietin have as yet been barely touched upon.

The results of the studies of factors which stimulate erythropoiesis have led to a search for humoral factors regulating the production and release of *leukocytes*[59, 93a] and of *platelets*.[69a]

Role of the Spleen.—For many years a controlling role in hematopoiesis has been attributed to the spleen. The functions of that organ will be discussed elsewhere (p. 1046) but it may be stated here that no conclusive evidence has yet been furnished to support the claim that the spleen governs erythropoiesis. There are, however, data that suggest that the spleen may influence the liberation of leukocytes from the bone marrow and may affect the rate of thrombopoiesis (see p. 1050).

Functional Capacity of the Bone Marrow.[71]—Various experimental approaches have been employed to estimate the number of marrow precursors of the circulating blood elements. In man the amount of total hematopoietic tissue has been reported to range from 12 to 34 $\times$ 10^9 marrow cells per Kg.[48a] Of this the erythroid marrow has been estimated to make up approximately 4 to 8 $\times$ 10^9 cells and the granulocytes 8 to 25 $\times$ 10^9 cells per Kg. It has been calculated that 900 billion erythrocytes are produced daily by the bone marrow[30] and that, in response to the stimulus of increased blood destruction, the well nourished, hyperplastic bone marrow of otherwise healthy men is capable of producing about seven times the normal output of hemoglobin.[43] Quantitative aspects of hemoglobin production and destruction will be considered further in a later chapter (p. 180).

The magnitude and duration of the neutrophilic leukocytosis which is observed in some types of infection gives some concept of the granulopoietic functional capacity of the bone marrow. It has been estimated that the myeloid reserve in the marrow of guinea pigs is 100 times the number of granulocytes in the blood.[109]

The transformation of fatty to red marrow usually begins at the margin of the myeloid cavity and extends toward the center. Generally this occurs in the bones in inverse order to that followed in the development of fatty marrow with progressing age, except in the case of the marrow of the femur, which seems to be more labile than that of the rib (Fig. 1–5). The rapidity with which this change occurs in the human is not known. It is noteworthy that the extent and even the site of hyperplasia of the bone marrow varies considerably even in the presence of apparently similar degrees of stimulation.[45]

An interesting explanation to account for the distribution of red and yellow bone marrow was offered by Huggins *et al.*[63] Observing that bone marrow is largely confined to the proximal skeleton, they demonstrated that the temperature of the marrow in the extremities is lower than that of marrow in the bones of the body trunk. They suggested that the lowered temperature is the cause of the disappearance of cellular marrow from the bones of the extremities. By several experimental procedures in animals, they produced elevation of the temperature of distal parts and were able to show that red marrow developed in such bones.

Extramedullary Hematopoiesis. — The normal formation of the cells of the blood in the bone marrow exclusively may occasionally be supplemented by the development of foci of hematopoiesis in other tissues. These occur particularly in the spleen and lymph nodes and less frequently in the liver but they have also been discovered in the suprarenal gland, in cartilage, in the broad ligament, in organizing thrombi and in adipose tissue in various locations.[124] Nodules and even large tumors of heterotopic bone marrow have been described. Whether the diffuse reaction of granulocytic cells in the connective tissues in response to infection and to mechanical irritation, (acute splenic tumor) should also be classed under the head of extramedullary hematopoiesis, is debatable.[121]

Extramedullary hematopoiesis is found in association with severe anemia, particularly in the anemia of infants and young children.[121] Tumors of such tissue have been observed in the hiluses of the kidney in erythroblastic anemia. In pernicious anemia during relapse, nodules of erythrogenic tissue are regularly found in the spleen and liver.[128,129] In association with macrocytic anemia of other types, and particularly in the macrocytic anemia of liver disease,[140] these foci are found in the spleen. Similar findings have been noted in osteosclerosis[123] and myelofibrosis[122] and in cases with invasion of the bone marrow (carcinoma,[121,127] Hodgkin's disease[140]) even when the anemia was normocytic and not very severe, as well as in erythremia and in cases in which bone marrow hypofunction followed injury by some toxin (see p. 571).[140] In the last-mentioned type of case, splenomegaly has often been so pronounced as to suggest a diagnosis of leukemia. Heterotopic bone marrow has been described in hemolytic jaundice [126] and such tumors have been observed in adipose tissue in cases of severe sepsis with anemia.[120,121] Extramedullary blood formation in the spleen, lymph nodes and liver is a regular occurrence in leukemia. [127,131] Experimentally it has been produced by repeated bleeding and by chronic poisoning with blood-destroying substances[121] as well as by the intravenous injection of the cellular constituents of the bone marrow.[130]

The nodules of blood-forming tissue may be composed of normoblasts or their precursors, or myelocytes, megakaryocytes, or all three strains of cells. It is a moot point whether these cells arise from lymphocytes in the blood, as the unitarians hold,[127] or from undifferentiated hemocytoblasts, or by an alteration of clasmatocytes or other partially or completely differentiated cells. Most hematologists hold that extramedullary hematopoiesis is a compensatory phenomenon and the readiness with which this change occurs in infants and young children, in whom the bone marrow has little or no room for expansion, is cited as evidence. It has been suggested that the immature cells found outside the bone marrow, not being held within a framework encased in bone, are dislodged more readily during the movements of organs such as the spleen and consequently appear in the circulating blood.[64]

THE STUDY OF THE BONE MARROW

Normal cellular marrow is soft and semi-fluid during life and consequently can be removed for examination. Marrow biopsy was performed in 1903 by Pianese who punctured the epiphysis of the femur by means of a trocar, and in 1908 by Ghedini who trephined the tibia in its upper third.[188] The latter's method was employed for a number of years but it soon became evident that active marrow is not always found in this bone.

The first real impetus to bone marrow biopsy came from Seyfarth's studies in 1923.[188] He trephined the sternum, choosing this site because of the accessibility and thinness of the bone and the likelihood of finding active marrow within it. Aspiration of the bone marrow was first proposed by Arinkin[151] in 1929 and, since then, with improvements in technic, this procedure has gained preference over trephining. Bone marrow

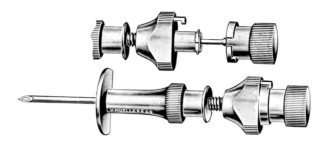

FIG. 1–7.—University of Illinois Sternal Needle with adjustable guard, special locking device for the stylet and Luer-Lok hub set into the needle. (Courtesy of V. Mueller and Co., Chicago.)

aspiration can be repeated and does not entail the trouble and expense of an operating room procedure. Trephine biopsies are now performed, as a rule, only when repeated aspirations at various sites have failed to yield adequate samples of marrow. The study of the bone marrow has attracted wide attention and is the subject of a number of monographs.[45,158,169,180a,187,188]

Technic. — For marrow aspiration many types of *needles* have been used. Although a short-beveled, 18-gauge spinal puncture needle 3 to 4 cm. in length with a lumen of 1 to 2 mm. in diameter can be used, it is much better to obtain one of the special needles devised for the purpose. It is advisable to have an adjustable guard attached to the needle so that the operator may know the depth penetrated. A very satisfactory needle[170] is shown in Figure 1–7.

Various *sites* may be used for the puncture. The *sternum* is very satisfactory. The upper portion of the bone, between the second and third ribs is most suitable because the bone is less likely to bend or give at this point. The lower third of the sternum is unsatisfactory because congenital abnormalities in this region are common. Arinkin[151] inserted the needle into the manubrium, but this is more likely to contain fat than the body of the sternum.

The operator should scrub, as for any surgical procedure. Some also wear sterile gloves. If the patient is apprehensive it is well to administer a sedative a half hour before the procedure. The skin over the mid-sternum is washed, and shaved if necessary. Iodine and alcohol or other suitable antiseptics are applied and sterile towels are laid closely around the selected site of aspiration. The skin is infiltrated in the region of the second to fifth intercostal spaces with procaine. The hypodermic needle is next passed more deeply until the bone is touched. Procaine is then injected under the periosteum. For penetration of the body of the sternum, the guard is set at 1 cm. if the patient is an adult or at 0.2 to 0.6 cm. if a child. The outer lamina of the body of the sternum varies considerably in thickness, ranging from 0.2 to about 5 mm. Alternatively, the thickness of the skin and subcutaneous tissue over the site selected for puncture may be gauged by marking the needle used for injecting the local anesthetic when the needle is held at right angles to the surface of the sternum. The aspiration needle illustrated in Figure 1–7 has a guard with a threaded shank which moves upward 1 mm. for each complete turn. In setting the guard, 2 to 3 mm. should be allowed for thickness of the cortex of the sternum in adults.

The needle is pushed vertically with a light rotating or boring motion into the

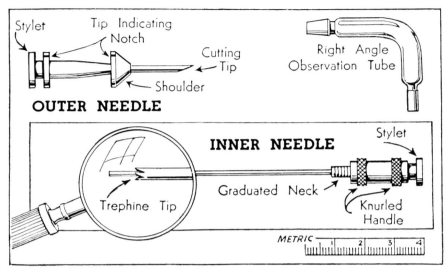

FIG. 1–8.—Puncture biopsy needle of Turkel and Bethell. Two needles with stylets: an outer guiding or splitting needle of 14-gauge, 20 mm. long, and an inner trephine needle and stylet, 17-gauge.

sternum between the levels of the second and third ribs in the midline or slightly to the side of the midline. If necessary, it may be tapped gently with a mallet. Rotation of the needle may aid penetration. A "give" is felt when the marrow cavity is entered. The needle may be passed about 1 or 2 mm. into the cavity for it is normally about 5 to 15 mm. in depth.

Turkel and Bethell[193] described an instrument which permits one to obtain small specimens of marrow without making an incision in the skin (Fig. 1–8). The same equipment can be used for administration of fluids through bone marrow (p. 358).

The site for puncture is the same as that chosen for sternal puncture (see above) and the skin is prepared in the same manner. The outer needle, with stylet in place, is inserted through the skin with the tip of the needle in the direction of the face of the patient and at an angle of 45 degrees (Fig. 1–9), until the point of the needle just engages the anterior lamella of the sternum. The stylet is then replaced by the inner trephine

needle and its stylet (Fig. 1–8). The stylet is then removed, leaving the inner needle in place. While holding the head of the outer needle with the fingers of one hand, the head of the inner needle is turned with the fingers of the other with a to-and-fro motion, at the same time exerting gentle inward pressure. Entrance of the cutting tip into the sternal cavity is signified by a sudden release of resistance. The cutting action is continued by exerting slight pressure, until the neck of the inner needle is completely within the head of the outer needle (6 cm.). When a specimen of marrow is desired the inner needle is revolved several times without further insertion, in order to insure detachment of the plug from the surrounding marrow. The inner needle and then the outer needle is removed. The point of insertion is covered with a collodion dressing. The biopsy core is removed from the needle by inserting the stylet into the inner needle, and is placed in fixative solution.

When it is desired to infuse solutions into the marrow, the outer needle is pushed in so that its tip enters the mar-

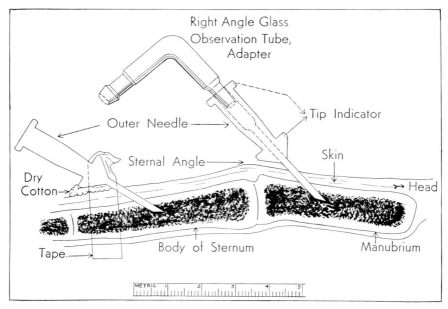

FIG. 1–9.—Two suitable positions for Turkel needle in sternum. A convenient adapter for use when the needle is employed for infusion is also shown.

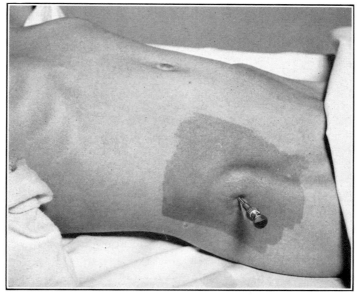

FIG. 1–10.—Iliac-crest puncture, showing the position of the needle.
(Courtesy of Rheingold *et al.*, New Eng. J. Med.)

row cavity and becomes firmly fixed in the sternum. The inner cutting needle is then removed. With the aid of a syringe, about 1 ml. of marrow is withdrawn. A complaint of pain at this point indicates that suction has been made in the marrow cavity. The infusion apparatus may now be attached. A suitable glass adapter is supplied.

Other satisfactory sites for aspiration biopsy of the marrow include the iliac crests, spinous processes, ribs[180] and, in children, the heads of the tibiae. For *iliac crest* puncture (Fig. 1–10), the skin about the anterior, superior spine is cleansed as for sternal puncture and the skin, subcutaneous tissues and periosteum are infiltrated with procaine in a small area just below the iliac crest. The bone marrow needle is then pushed into the ilium distal to the crest. As in the case of the sternum, entry of the marrow cavity is usually signalled by a sense of "give." Alternatively, bone marrow may be aspirated from the *anterior, superior iliac spine* by passing the needle into the center of the oval protuberance, pointing slightly cephalad.[168] Others prefer the *posterior ilium*,[160] where multiple aspirations are easily made.[156]

Spinous process puncture may be performed with the patient in the sitting position,[171] leaning forward slightly. The third or fourth lumbar vertebrae are preferred as these are likely to present the broadest spinous process but the lower thoracic and first and second lumbar may also be used. After appropriate skin sterilization and anesthetization of the skin, subcutaneous tissues and periosteum, the needle, with the guard set at about 1.5 cm., is pushed through the skin and inserted with a rotary motion into the spinous process, midway between the upper and lower border. When the needle is firmly fixed in the bone, the stylet is removed and suction is applied with a syringe. Occasionally the needle must be advanced a few millimeters at a

time to secure marrow. In children particularly, it may be better to have the patient lying face downward[180] rather than in the sitting position, since the patient then lies in a relatively fixed and comfortable position and cannot move as readily when pressure is applied. Instead of puncturing the tip of the spinous process directly, the needle can be introduced at one side of it.[155] It is then passed medially, entering the bone anteriorly to the tip, at a point where the cortex is less thick.

In children from birth to two years of age, the most suitable site for aspiration of bone marrow is the flat triangular area at the proximal end of the medial surface of the *tibia*, just below the tubercle and medial to the tibial tuberosity.[160] The iliac crest is technically superior to the sternum in children two to eleven years of age.[189]

Whatever site is used, when the marrow cavity has been entered, the stylet is removed from the needle and a sterile, 5 ml. tight-fitting syringe is attached. The plunger is slowly withdrawn, firmly but gently, until the first drop of marrow appears. Momentary pain is usually experienced by the patient when suction is applied, provided the needle is in the marrow cavity. As soon as one drop of marrow appears in the syringe, the syringe is removed from the needle and passed to an assistant who prepares several smears. A second dry, sterile syringe may be attached and 1.0 ml. of marrow, or more, is withdrawn. This provides material for concentration of cells if they are scarce (see below) and for selection of marrow particles. The material obtained is placed in a paraffin-lined vial containing a minute amount of heparin or versenate and gently rotated to achieve mixing.

If no marrow is obtained, the stylet may be replaced and the marrow penetrated more deeply. If this is unsuccessful it is probably better to try another site

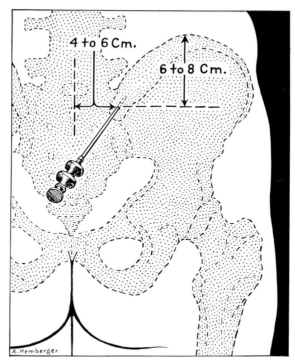

4 to 6 Cm.

6 to 8 Cm.

A. Hemberger

Fig. 1–11.—Schematic diagram of Vim-Silverman needle in place. In most adults the position of the posterior superior iliac spine may be verified by using as a landmark the point of intersection of a vertical line drawn 4 to 6 cm. from the midline with a horizontal line drawn 6 to 8 cm. from the highest portion of the iliac crest. The needle is directed slightly superiorly and laterally as indicated. (Brody and Finch, Am. J. Med. Sc.)

than to attempt dislodgment of cells by introducing a small quantity of the patient's plasma. When the puncture needle is removed, the wound may be sealed with collodion. A tight, sterile dressing should be applied.

The Vim-Silverman needle ($2\frac{3}{8}$ in.), inserted into the posterior iliac crest just cephalad to the posterior superior spine, has been found to produce specimens in cases of "dry tap"[158a,174] (Fig. 1–11). Others prefer a Sacker-Nordin needle.[182a]

Comparisons of marrow obtained from the sternum, vertebra, rib and pelvic bone have shown good agreement.[152,176]

Similar procedures, slightly modified, may be used in *laboratory animals*. Sundberg[190] described the aspiration of tibial bone marrow in small animals.

A simple technic was outlined,[173] also, for the study of the whole femoral marrow where it is desired to determine the quantitative relationship of the various types of cells to one another and the relative proportions of cells, fat and sinuses.

Preparation of Aspirated Material. —*Smears* made promptly from the freshly drawn marrow in the same manner as blood smears are the most satisfactory preparations for the study of cell morphology. If *Wright's stain* is used, it may be found advisable to dilute the stain with an equal quantity of absolute methyl alcohol. This is allowed to remain on the smear for two minutes and then water is added, the mixture being allowed to remain from four to eight minutes (p. 414). Schleicher[183] described a good method in detail. The *May-Grünwald-Giemsa stain* also gives satisfactory results. The slide is flooded for two minutes with the May-Grünwald stain. An equal number of drops of buffered distilled water is then added while the slide is agitated. The diluted stain is allowed to remain on the slide for two minutes. It is then drained off and the slide is covered with Giemsa stain, double strength (2 drops of stock solution to 1 ml. of buffered distilled water) for ten to twelve minutes. Finally the preparation is rinsed in neutral distilled water until the water runs clear. It is then placed in a vertical position to dry. Wright's stain may be used instead of the May-Grünwald. Bone marrow smears may also be stained by the peroxidase method (see p. 417), alkaline phosphatase method (p. 418) or Prussian blue method (p. 60).

Imprints.—In order to gain some idea of the relation of the various cells to one another, it is useful to select one or two particles of marrow from the aspirated material and to make several rows of imprints on clean slides. This is done by picking up one or more gross marrow units with the cut end of a wooden applicator and, holding this vertically to the slide surface, the tissue is touched to the glass with the slightest smearing motion.[184] The slide is then waved vigorously through the air to ensure rapid drying. This is stained in the same manner as blood smears. Imprints have special value because cells of primitive type tend to be present in syncytial masses or compact clusters and thus may be missed if only the more fluid portions of the marrow are examined.

Teased and Supravital Preparations.—Teased preparations are useful for observing motility of marrow cells. A drop of marrow is gently mixed with a small quantity of serum on a cover glass, this is inverted into the chamber of a hanging drop slide, and the preparation is examined in a warm-stage microscope. Supravital staining offers an opportunity to study partially stained and yet living cells. On slides prepared with a dry film of stain (double quantity, see p. 410), small portions of bone marrow are flattened out under a cover glass by gentle pressure. Areas bounded by fat cells in which each marrow cell can be seen, are examined.

Preparation of Sections from Aspirated Material.—Aspiration of bone marrow is so much more practical a procedure than trephine biopsy, that various technics, chiefly modifications of the technic of Amprino and Penati,[150] have been devised for securing material for making sections. A simple technic[154] is as follows: A small amount of powdered topical thrombin is placed on a clean glass slide, mixed into solution with a drop of water and allowed to dry. Gross marrow particles are carefully picked out from the paraffin-lined vial into which the aspirated material was placed. By holding the vial against a light source and by slowly rotating it, the units are encouraged to stick to the paraffin. Thus they are easily seen. They are transferred to the thrombin-coated area on the slide and are gently manipulated until they are in contact with one another. To this are added three or four drops of the heparinized plasma obtained from the centrifuged specimen (see below). The presence of the thrombin causes clotting of the plasma. The marrow particles are included in the plasma clot that is formed and this firm mass is next lifted from the slide and dropped into a vial containing the fixing solution[185] (10 ml. neutral formaldehyde [40 per cent] in 90 ml. physiological sodium chloride solution). This is replaced after ten minutes with fresh fixing fluid, which should be renewed again if necessary until the fluid is clear. Complete fixation occurs within one hour. The units are then transferred into graded alcohols, 50, 75, 85, 95 per cent, for one-half hour each, and then into absolute alcohol, dioxan or acetone, for fifteen minutes. The specimens are kept in paraffin for one or two hours. The units are then blocked, sectioned about five micra in thickness and stained with hematoxylin and eosin.[157,186]

Concentrated Preparations.—The material collected in the paraffin-lined vial can be used for making cell counts, but little is to be gained by the effort. It is of some interest to centrifuge the material in a hematocrit (5 minutes, 1000 R.P.M.), as is done with blood (p. 379), since thereby four layers may be distinguished: fat, plasma, nucleated cells, red corpuscles. Measurement of the size of these layers is of very limited value (see below) but, when few cells are found in the smears made from the uncentrifuged, fresh specimens, it is useful to prepare smears from the concentrated material of the nucleated cell layer. This is done by aspirating an equal amount of plasma and nucleated cells from the appropriate layers in the hematocrit, mixing these in a paraffin-coated watch glass and making smears which are then stained in the usual manner. Since the cells found in such preparations were not fixed immediately on removal from the body, interpretation of unusual findings must be made cautiously because artifacts are easily produced *in vitro*.

Hemosiderin in Bone Marrow.— To demonstrate hemosiderin granules, particles of marrow must be examined. These may be obtained as described above. More specifically,[178] one may prepare a sterile syringe containing 3 ml. of a solution of 4 per cent sodium citrate. This is attached to the marrow aspiration needle and 3 ml. of material is withdrawn from the marrow. The mixture is then placed on a large watch glass, particles of marrow are identified, picked out with a capillary pipet and smeared on cover glasses.

The unstained preparation is examined first under low power magnification with reduced illumination in order to locate an area of marrow tissue. This is then examined under oil immersion magnification. The hemosiderin appears as golden yellow refractile granules, varying from a fraction to several micra in diameter.

The marrow hemosiderin may be more easily identified after staining with Prussian blue. The stain for this purpose is prepared by adding concentrated hydrochloric acid to 20 ml. of a 20 per cent solution of potassium ferrocyanide in distilled water until a white precipitate is formed. The solution is then filtered and the smears covered with the filtrate for 30 minutes, after which they are examined as described above.

In the stained preparation the granules are blue in color. Normal marrow usually contains a few small granules distributed throughout the preparation. In patients with reduced iron stores (iron deficiency) the number of granules is reduced. In patients with large iron stores (infection, cirrhosis, hemochromatosis, pernicious anemia, malignancy, uremia, hemolytic anemia) the number of granules is increased. Not infrequently artifacts will also stain, usually in proportion to the amount of iron present. Thus, in iron deficiency pale yellow granules which do not take the iron stain are sometimes seen. These are probably protein granules of hemosiderin which contain absorbed bilirubin but not iron.

More sensitive but more exacting procedures are also available.[167]

Trephining.—The technic is simple. The patient is prepared as for an operation and the operator wears sterile gown and gloves. The skin over the midsternum, after iodine and alcohol have been applied, is infiltrated in the region of the third to fifth intercostal spaces with 1 per cent procaine. After five to ten minutes, an incision about 4 cm. in

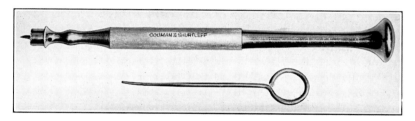

FIG. 1–12.—Bone marrow trephine (slightly less than actual size), and stylet for extraction of the plug of bone from the "crown" (made by Codman and Shurtleff, Boston). (Dameshek, Am. Jour. Med. Sci.)

length is made in the midline and the edges of the wound are retracted. The subperiosteal space is then infiltrated with procaine and a cruciate incision in the periosteum is made. Each flap of periosteum is next retracted by means of a small periosteum elevator. A bone marrow trephine is now placed over the bare surface of the bone and slight pressure and a rotating motion are made. The trephine may also be tilted slightly back and forth in sagittal and transverse planes in order to break the fine trabeculae of the underlying cancellous bone. A "give" is felt when the bone marrow cavity is entered. The trephine is then removed, together with its enclosed plug of bone. This is placed in fixative solution. The open marrow cavity is next scooped out by means of a fine curet and soft marrow is thus obtained. This is used for supravital staining, touch preparations and smears. The cavity is packed with gauze until bleeding has ceased and the four flaps of periosteum are then brought in apposition and held together by a simple suture. It is rarely necessary to pack bone wax into the marrow cavity to stop bleeding. The skin wound and subcutaneous tissue are approximated with interrupted No.00 catgut, or horsehair sutures. Sterile dressings are applied.

Seyfarth's trephine, as modified by Dameshek (Fig. 1–12), possesses a saw-toothed crown, 5 mm. in diameter and 5 mm. long to the beveled edge. A central protruding edge is present, and small holes at the base of the crown allow entrance of a stylet for the purpose of extracting the bone marrow after biopsy.

Preparation of Trephined Material.— *Fixation.* — Custer[45] recommends Zenker-formol solution composed of 9 parts of freshly prepared Zenker solution (without acetic acid) to which one part of neutral formol (40 per cent formaldehyde over magnesium carbonate) is added within one-half hour after the tissue has been placed in the Zenker solution. The tissue is kept in the fixing solution for four to six hours and is then washed for twelve to twenty-four hours in running water.

Decalcification.—The cortex of bone should be trimmed away. Custer[45] recommends a solution of equal parts of 85 per cent formic acid and 20 per cent sodium citrate. Six hours is usually sufficient for decalcification. The tissue is then washed for four hours in running water.

Dehydration, Embedding, and Staining.— After decalcification and washing, Custer[45] transfers through 95 per cent alcohol (twelve hours), absolute alcohol (six hours), chloroform (forty-five minutes), chloroform and paraffin (thirty minutes in oven), paraffin (40 to 42° C.) (fifteen to twenty minutes), paraffin (53 to 56° C.) (two changes totaling thirty minutes) and finally embeds in paraffin with the marrow surface downwards. The tissue is blocked and cut in the usual fashion, preferably not over 5 micra in thickness, mounted on albuminized slides and placed in the oven for at least two hours and preferably overnight. Paraffin is removed by two changes of xylol, following which the slides are transferred through the following solutions: 95 per cent alcohol, 95 per cent alcohol and iodine (cherry-red solution) until the mercury of the fixative is removed, 95, 70, 50, and 30 per cent alcohol and finally through three changes of distilled water to insure removal of all alcohol. Slides are then placed in Azure II-Eosin stain mixtures which are prepared as follows:

Solution I

Eosin für Blut (Grübler) . . . . . 1 gm.
Distilled water . . . . 1 liter

Solution II

Azure II (National Anilin Chemical Co.) 1 gm.
Distilled water . . . . 1 liter
  Mix solutions as follows in the indicated order:
1. Distilled water . . . . 80 ml.
2. Solution I . . . . 20 ml.
3. Solution II . . . . 10 ml.

Stain from late afternoon until the following morning. Differentiate, controlling differentiation under the microscope:

1. Alcohol, 95 per cent, until blue stain ceases to come off in a cloud.

2. Alcohol, 95 per cent, until differentiation is complete (bone trabeculae, red blood cells, eosinophil granules, are the landmarks and should be red; nuclei should be sharp and brilliant blue).

3. Transfer rapidly through two changes of absolute alcohol for dehydration.

4. Xylol (three changes) until clear. At this time check stain under high dry power; if underdifferentiated, slide can be carried back into alcohol; if overdifferentiated, it is practically useless. Decolorizing in acid-alcohol and restaining are possible but results do not justify the effort; it is better to cut new sections.

The *Maximow technic*, employing hematoxylin eosin-azure II, is time consuming but furnishes material which permits as accurate recognition of cell types in sections as is possible in dry smears.[157]

Dangers and Limitations of Marrow Biopsy. — Although potentially marrow biopsy may permit infection or hemorrhage, the former has not been reported and bleeding is very uncommon. A number of cases of death from cardiac tamponade have been reported.[162] Marrow puncture is contraindicated in hemophilia. The procedure should cause little discomfort and may be classed with such routine examinations as spinal puncture and pleural tap. The most important criticism of bone marrow biopsy is that only a small and not necessarily representative sample of marrow is obtained. Lesions which are patchy in character, such as those of Gaucher's disease or multiple myeloma, may be completely missed. This criticism applies to the trephining as well as to the puncture technic, but refers of course more to the latter than to the former. The youngest cells are likely to be more adherent to one another and to the bone spicules than mature forms. The preparation and study of imprints and of sections of marrow particles, as already described, help to meet these objections. Aspiration of marrow, especially in inexperienced hands, may yield no marrow whatever or lead to an erroneous diagnosis. Nevertheless, the procedure is commendable for its simplicity and because it offers the possibility of frequently repeated examinations. Especially when one considers the theoretical limitations of marrow puncture, it is remarkable how valuable a procedure it is when it is applied with discrimination and understanding.

Bone Marrow Examination at Autopsy.—Bone marrow examinations as generally carried out postmortem are unsatisfactory. To secure good preparations, bone marrow should be removed, if possible, within two hours postmortem.[181] However, if marrow is scooped out and is suspended in a viscous medium, such as bovine albumin, changes in the cells usually attributed to autolysis are prevented and satisfactory material can be obtained a day or longer after death.[153] Because the cellular state of the marrow varies widely in different bones, it is best to obtain specimens from several bones. If but one specimen of marrow is to be taken, the *mid-femur* rather than the tibia is recommended because the marrow of the femur is more labile than that of the tibia or even that of the rib.[45] A mid-portion of the shaft is exposed through a horseshoe incision through skin, fascia and muscle. Parallel saw-cuts are made halfway through the bone about 3 inches apart, and the cortex between the two cuts is chiseled off. When the marrow cavity is exposed, a pencil of marrow may be lifted out intact with a gouge or similarly curved instrument.

If a second specimen of marrow may be taken, the *vertebra* is recommended. A thin wedge of lumbar vertebra is removed. This will afford a specimen for study of the cell content of red marrow at a site where it is normally present, whereas the femur marrow indicates the degree of response of the blood-forming organs to stimulation. Whenever possible, however, specimens of the tibia, rib and sternum should also be obtained. The marrow from the tibia is removed in the same way as that of the femur. The sternum specimen is best obtained from the gladiolus by transverse cuts not over 5 mm. apart. Because rib marrow is easily squeezed out of the myeloid cavity, it is best to cut a piece of the rib 5 to 7 mm. in length with a fine hacksaw and section the bone intact.[45]

The Normal Bone Marrow.—Erythrocyte counts and hemoglobin determinations, as made on the material obtained by sternal puncture, are stated to be about the same as those of blood or slightly lower, while the leukocyte counts have been reported as ranging from 10,000 to 190,000 per c.mm.[188] The leukocyte counts tend to be higher the less the amount of marrow withdrawn because the removal of large quantities of marrow probably leads to the flow of blood into the marrow cavity. Since absolute counts of marrow cells are subject to wide fluctuations they are of little value.[179]

The morphology of the various cell types will be described in the succeeding chapters (2, 4, 5). It is illustrated on Plate XIV*E*, page 924. Mention has been made already (p. 38) of the primitive blood cells or *reticulum cells*. In film preparations of marrow, these vary between 20 and 30 μ in diameter (Plate II, *C*). Their cytoplasm is palely basophilic and abundant, and may contain a few azurophil granules. The nucleus is large, round or oval and presents a pale-staining, fine chromatin pattern and one or more round or oval nucleoli. In a somewhat later stage, this cell of somewhat variable outline develops a more deeply basophilic cytoplasm. The nuclear chromatin pattern is finely stranded and stippled. One or more nucleoli are present.

Osteoblasts and osteoclasts must be differentiated from the cells of the bone marrow since they may be mistaken for cells of the plasmocyte series and megakaryocytes, respectively. *Osteoblasts* are oval cells, sometimes elongated, 25 to 50 μ in diameter, with rather blurred outlines. The cytoplasm most frequently takes a light blue stain, may contain a few azurophilic granules and is occasionally fenestrated. The nucleus as a rule lies eccentrically and is composed of clumped or trabeculated chromatin and distinct parachromatin. It contains 1 to 3 nucleoli. Sometimes the nucleus appears to lie wholly or partially outside the cytoplasm.

Osteoclasts or *polykarocytes* are giant cells, their diameters often exceeding 100 μ. Their outlines are distended and not very clear, and fragmentation is observed frequently. The cytoplasm is cloudy and finely granular in the marginal portions and may stain from weakly basophilic to strongly acidophilic. It may contain numerous azurophilic granulations of various sizes. These cells contain several nuclei scattered loosely over the whole cell and not touching one another. The nuclear chromatin is dense. One nucleolus is present in each nucleus.

Osteoblasts and osteoclasts are seen most frequently and in largest numbers in fetal marrow. In disease they have been observed especially frequently in association with metastatic malignancies, acute leukemia, myelofibrosis and secondary osteoporosis.[164a] These cells are illustrated in Plate II (*A* and *B*).

For the *marrow differential count*, 300 to 500 cells should be examined. Even when large numbers of cells are counted, considerable variations will be found not only between specimens removed at different times but between several preparations of the same material. The values given as normal by a number of investigators vary widely.[169,176,187] The figures shown in Table 1–2 represent the range which may generally be expected in bone marrow removed from normal adults but they cannot be considered as being very exact.

The figures given by Osgood and Seaman[176] differ in that their values for myeloblasts (0 to 2.4), promyelocytes (0 to 3) and erythroblasts (3 to 21) are lower, and those for lymphocytes (7 to 30) are higher than those given in Table 1–2. Custer[45] accepts as normal a higher proportion of myelocytes (up to 34 per cent) and expects fewer polymorphonuclear neutrophils (up to 20 per cent) and lymphocytes (up to 7 per cent) than are shown in Table 1–2.

The composition of the bone marrow in the fetus has been described already. Glaser, Limarzi and Poncher[164] examined the bone marrow of 151 normal infants, children and young adults from birth to 20 years of age and reviewed the literature. Marked variations occur during the first year of life and particularly during the first month. The cells of the erythroid series show a sharp decrease in number during the first days of life and reach essentially stable values (23 per cent) by the end of the first month. The myeloid series, on the other hand, has been found to increase during the first two weeks of life, following which a sharp drop occurs about the third week. At the end of the first month, values are established which are close to the average percentage as calculated for the period from 1 to 20 years (61 per cent). Lymphocytes increase in number during the first weeks of life, even to 40 per cent, and then gradually decrease during the first and second year, thereafter fluctuating little about the average (16 per cent). The myeloid-erythroid ratio is low at birth (1.85:1), increases rapidly during the first two weeks to values as high as 11:1 and then gradually decreases to the 1 to 20 years average (2.95:1) during the first year. In the adult the normal M:E ratio is about 3 or 4:1.

During normal pregnancy quantitative changes in the cellular components of the bone marrow occur which are maximal in the third trimester.[172] There is an increase of normoblastic erythropoiesis and, to a lesser extent, of granulopoiesis, with some increase of immature cells as compared with the marrow of non-pregnant persons. A return towards normal

PLATE II

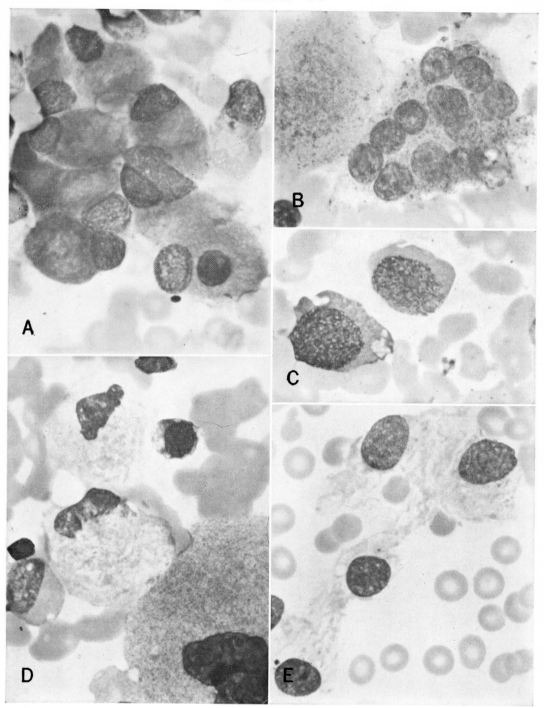

Giant cells found in bone marrow: A, Osteoblasts; B, a multinucleated osteoclast. A small amount of megakaryocyte cytoplasm can be seen in the upper left corner; C, two reticulum cells; D, two Gaucher cells. Their pale cytoplasm contrasts with the deep blue cytoplasm of the megakaryocyte in the lower right hand corner. E, shows endothelial cells in a blood smear from the lining of a vein. Venous blood was used for the smear. (Wright's stain, × 1220).

Table 1–2—*Relative Number of Nucleated Cells in Normal Bone Marrow*

	Range	Average
Myeloblasts	0.3– 5.0	2.0
Promyelocytes ("undifferentiated myelocytes," "progranulocytes")	1.0– 8.0	5.0
Myelocytes: Neutrophilic	5.0–19.0	12.0
Eosinophilic	0.5– 3.0	1.5
Basophilic	0.0– 0.5	0.3
Metamyelocytes ("juvenile" forms)	13.0–32.0	22.0
Polymorphonuclear neutrophils	7.0–30.0	20.0
Polymorphonuclear eosinophils	0.5– 4.0	2.0
Polymorphonuclear basophils	0.0– 0.7	0.2
Lymphocytes	3.0–17.0	10.0
Plasma cells	0.0– 2.0	0.4
Monocytes	0.5– 5.0	2.0
Reticulum cells	0.1– 2.0	0.2
Megakaryocytes	0.03–3.0	0.4
Pronormoblasts (macroblasts)	1.0– 8.0	4.0
Normoblasts (basophilic, polychromatophilic and acidophilic)	7.0–32.0	18.0

begins early in the puerperium but is not completed even at six weeks postpartum.

Centrifuged specimens of normal marrow will usually reveal about 3 volumes per cent to be made up of fat and about 5 to 6 per cent is occupied by nucleated cells. In marrow aplasia the nucleated layer is reduced in size and in erythroid hyperplasia it may be greatly increased (up to 20 and even 40 per cent), while in leukemia even greater amounts of nucleated cells may be found. This method, however, is a crude and unreliable index of fat content or of cellular composition.[154]

The Bone Marrow in Disease.[161, 169,177]—In many disorders gross as well as microscopic changes may occur in the bone marrow. The bone marrow has been the subject of study since 1868, when Neumann and Bizzozero independently discovered the hematopoietic function of this tissue. The "raspberry jelly-like" character of the bone marrow in pernicious anemia was described by Cohnheim (1876). In anemia the extension of red marrow may be so great that not only is fat displaced, but the bony trabeculae in the marrow and even the bone itself may be encroached upon, producing thereby changes which can be demonstrated in roentgenograms of the bones (see Chapter 12). Some writers distinguish between hyperplasia of the bone marrow and dysplasia, the latter term referring to the formation of abnormal cells (*e.g.*, pernicious anemia). On the other hand, bone marrow function may be reduced in degree (hypoplasia) or even be totally absent (aplasia). Again, gelatinous marrow composed of an albuminoid substance may displace the fat. This has been observed in starvation and in wasting diseases. In dystrophic diseases and in osteomalacia and chronic inflammation, the bone marrow changes into fibrillar connective tissue.[166]

In the cytological examination of the bone marrow, consideration should be given to the following:

1. The Myeloid: Erythroid (M:E) Ratio.—If *the proportion of leukocytes* of the myeloid series to nucleated red cells *is increased*, an infection stimulating leukopoiesis, leukemia or a leukemoid reaction may be suspected; or the altered ratio may be due to a decrease of the nucleated red cells.

If the proportion of nucleated red cells is increased, the change may be due to a reduction in the quantity of the myeloid leukocytes, as in agranulocytosis or, as is more often the case, there is hyperplasia of the erythropoietic tissue. The latter may be *normoblastic* in type and may be due to blood loss, increased blood destruction or iron deficiency, or may be associated with polycythemia vera, thalassemia, plumbism or cirrhosis of the liver; or it may be *megaloblastic*, as occurs in pernicious anemia, sprue and other related disorders (p. 481).

A normal M:E ratio is found not only in normal marrow but also in certain pathological conditions, such as myelosclerosis. It is important to recognize that an aspirated sample of marrow cannot be relied upon to indicate the degree of cellularity of the marrow and may be quite misleading in this respect. The M:E ratio is likely to be normal also, in many instances, in those disorders in which the discovery of certain cells of diagnostic significance is the important feature; *e.g.*, multiple myeloma. A normal M:E ratio may be encountered also in aplastic anemia but there a relative increase in lymphocytes is usually observed.

Some European hematologists prefer a ratio in which mature leukocytes are excluded from the count.[6] The ratio in normal marrow ranges, then, from 0.56:1 to 2.67:1. In most anemias the ratio is below unity.

2. The **presence of cells** which are *normally not found* in the bone marrow or are not normally present in the numbers actually observed, such as lymphocytes, plasma[159] or "myeloma" cells, reticulum cells, tumor cells, and Gaucher's cells. (See Plates II and III.)

In disorders associated with pronounced hyperglobulinemia, not only is an increase of plasma cells found, but some of the plasma cells and plasmacytoid reticulum cells may contain within their cytoplasm (1) many hyaline, bluish, transparent vesicles of different sizes which may be so numerous that they completely obscure the cytoplasm and may cover parts of the nucleus, the so-called "*morular* (berry) cells" of Mott; or (2) globular bodies of different sizes, which may be few in number or very numerous ("*grape cell*" of Stich).[199] The latter must be distinguished from Russell bodies which are fuchsinophilic in Romanowsky stains, rather than gray-blue. The inclusions appear to be protein in nature.

3. The quantity and morphology of the **megakaryocytes.**

4. The presence of **parasites:** Leishmania, histoplasma capsulatum, malaria.

5. The presence of **focal lesions:** brucellosis, sarcoidosis, *etc.*

6. If little material has been obtained by aspiration, and if repeated punctures at different sites give similar results, **trephine biopsy** is indicated for the bone marrow may be aplastic or fibrotic (Fig. 11–13, p. 585) or may be so involved in metastases that little material can be aspirated.[196]

It is natural that a procedure such as marrow aspiration, once established as a

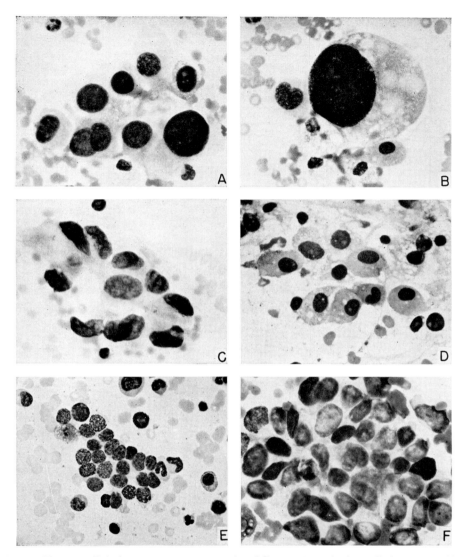

FIG. 1–13.—Tumor cells in bone marrow smears: *A* and *B*, mucus producing cells from case of broncho-genic carcinoma; *C*, mucoid carcinoma of the colon; *D*, hypernephroma; *E* and *F*, small and large cell metastases from neuroblastomas. All × 380. (Jonsson and Rundles, courtesy of Blood.)

useful diagnostic aid, should come to be expected to solve all hematologic problems. It must be emphasized, therefore, that, while this method of study is at all times interesting and affords a more complete picture of the reaction of the hemopoietic tissues than can be gained from examination of the blood alone, it can be expected to *yield information of crucial importance only in* a limited number of conditions. These may be listed as follows:

1. Those disorders of the hemopoietic system in which no changes of crucial diagnostic value are to be found in the blood and those in which these changes

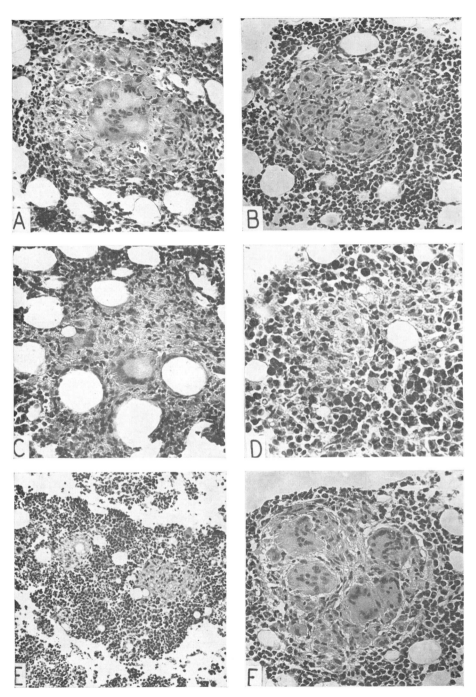

Fig. 1–14.—Granulomatous lesions in sternal bone marrow. (A) Miliary tuberculosis (× 205); (B) sarcoidosis (× 225); (C) Hodgkin's disease (× 285); (D) infectious mononucleosis (× 350; (E) granulomatous hepatitis (× 235); (F) acquired hemolytic anemia, history of undulant fever seven years before (× 145); hematoxylin and eosin stain. (Courtesy of Dr. Gertrude L. Pease[34d] and Grune and Stratton).

Table 1–3.—*Conditions in Which Various Types of Reaction May be Observed, as Demonstrated by Bone Marrow Aspiration*

M:E Ratio Increased

Myeloid Forms of Leukemia
The Majority of Infections
Leukemoid Reaction
Decrease in Nucleated Red Cells

M:E Ratio Normal

Normal Marrow
Myelosclerosis
Multiple Myeloma, *etc.*
Aplastic Anemia

Non-Myeloid Cells Increased

Other Forms of Leukemia
Multiple Myeloma
Metastases from Carcinoma, *etc.*
Gaucher's Disease, Niemann-Pick Disease
Aplastic Anemia (usually relative increase only)
Infectious Mononucleosis

M:E Ratio Decreased

Decrease in Myeloid Cells (Agranulocytosis)
Increase in Erythroid Cells due to either

Normoblastic Hyperplasia

Hemorrhagic Anemias
Iron Deficiency Anemia
Hemolytic Anemias
Thalassemia
Cirrhosis of the Liver
Polycythemia Vera
Plumbism
Anemia of Chronic
    Renal Disease

OR *Megaloblastic Hyperplasia*

Pernicious Anemia
Sprue, Idiopathic Steatorrhea, Resection of
    Small Intestine (certain cases)
Tropical Macrocytic Anemia
Non-tropical Nutritional Macrocytic Anemia
Macrocytic Anemia with *Diphyllobothrium* Infes-
    tation
Megaloblastic Anemia of Infancy
Megaloblastic Anemia of Pregnancy
"Refractory Megaloblastic" Anemia
"Achrestic" Anemia

are not of sufficient degree to permit more than very tentative conclusions to be drawn. Thus pancytopenia (anemia with leukopenia and thrombocytopenia) may be due to a number of different causes (p. 549). If it is the result of leukemia in the "aleukemic" form, aspiration of marrow will permit an unequivocal diagnosis to be made.

2. Certain conditions in which characteristic evidence is frequently found in the bone marrow but is rarely or never discovered in the blood. Multiple myeloma (Fig. 20–24, and Plate XVIII, p. 1070), Gaucher's disease (Fig. 15–3, p. 773) and Niemann-Pick disease (Fig. 15–4, p. 775) are examples of disorders in which cells of critical diagnostic importance are likely to be found in the bone marrow and kala-azar (Fig. 20–21, p. 1057) and histoplasmosis are examples

of infections in which the causative agent is demonstrable by this means. Sometimes malarial parasites may be found by marrow aspiration when they cannot be demonstrated in the blood.[165]

3. Tumor cells, metastatic from carcinoma of the prostate,[182] breast, lung, kidney and other tissues, as well as in neuroblastoma,[163] have been demonstrated by marrow aspiration,[175,192] especially if fixed tissue sections of aspirated material have been made,[196] when the diagnosis would otherwise have been obscure or uncertain. The tumor cells often form a syncytium, which is easily differentiated from the loosely arranged cells of the normal bone marrow. In smears of marrow they are often found in groups or clumps (Fig. 1–13 and Plate III. Also Fig. 11–14, p. 589). In sections they may be found as isolated nodules

Table 1–4.—Representative Differential Counts of Bone Marrow Obtained by Puncture

Types of cells	Leukemia acute[1,2]	Leukemia[2] chronic myelocytic	Leukemia[2] chronic lymphocytic	Multiple myeloma[3]	Pernicious anemia	Hemolytic anemia	Iron deficiency anemia	Purpura hemorrhagica[4]
Myeloblasts	50.0 95.0	4.0		0.5	0.8	0.8	0.5	
Promyelocytes		10.0	0.8	1.8	2.7	3.0	2.0	1.5
Myelocytes								
Neutrophilic		26.0	1.5	1.8	7.7	8.0	9.0	8.0
Eosinophilic		2.0	0.7		0.8	2.0	0.8	
Basophilic		0.4	0.2		0.3			
Metamyelocytes		22.0	8.0	3.3	14.5	18.0	15.0	15.3
Polymorph. Neut.		29.0	8.5	62.0	14.5	9.0	28.0	31.0
" Eosin.		0.8	1.0	3.5	0.5	0.6	0.2	0.5
" Baso.		0.4	3.0	1.2	0.2			0.2
Lymphocytes		1.4	60.0	13.0	9.5	10.0	1.0	2.5
Plasma cells				4.5[3]	0.2	0.4	0.7	0.8
Monocytes		0.2		0.2	0.3			
Reticulum cells		1.2	1.5	1.0	2.0	2.6	0.8	
Mitotic figures		0.2	0.3		2.7	1.0		
Abnormal cells								
Megakaryocytes								0.2[4]
Megaloblasts					40.0			
Pronormoblasts			0.2			5.0		4.0
Normoblasts		2.4	14.3	9.0	3.0	43.0	40.0	36.0
Myel.:Eryth. Ratio		40:1	1.5:1	8:1	1:1.5	1:1	1.4:1	1.5:1

[1] The immature forms are listed in the table as myeloblasts merely as a matter of convenience. In acute lymphoblastic leukemia the cells are lymphoblasts, not myeloblasts. Often it is difficult to distinguish the various immature leukocytic cells seen in acute leukemia. The essential point is the great preponderance of very young forms.

[2] The bone marrow picture in "aleukemic leukemia" is similar to that of leukemia of the various types, whether or not changes can be demonstrated in the blood.

[3] The characteristic cells in multiple myeloma differ somewhat from typical plasma cells in that the nuclear chromatin is relatively fine, and the wheel-spoke arrangement of the chromatin is not present; the cytoplasm is basophilic and bright blue, not blue-green as in the plasma cell. A perinuclear clear zone is unusual.

[4] Although the number of megakaryocytes may not appear to be increased, in typical purpura hemorrhagica the majority (64 per cent in the case cited) have no platelets about them and most of the remainder (32 per cent) have very few.

or may replace the bone marrow. The cells are usually large, with vesiculated nuclei and scanty cytoplasm. Their cytoplasm may be basophilic and mitotic figures may be found. One or more prominent nucleoli are frequently visible.

4. The study of sections made from aspirated material has, in certain cases, made possible the demonstration of lesions of brucellosis,[191] miliary tuberculosis,[185] histoplasmosis[177] and sarcoidosis in the bone marrow,[154] as well as Hodgkin's disease (Fig. 1–14). In these various disorders, therefore, bone marrow aspiration is indicated.

It is rare that clinical blood and other laboratory procedures fail to make possible an unequivocal diagnosis of one of the megaloblastic anemias. Only in those cases in which doubt still remains, need marrow aspiration be regarded as necessary. The introduction of marrow aspiration in pediatric practice can be credited, however, with hav-

PLATE   III

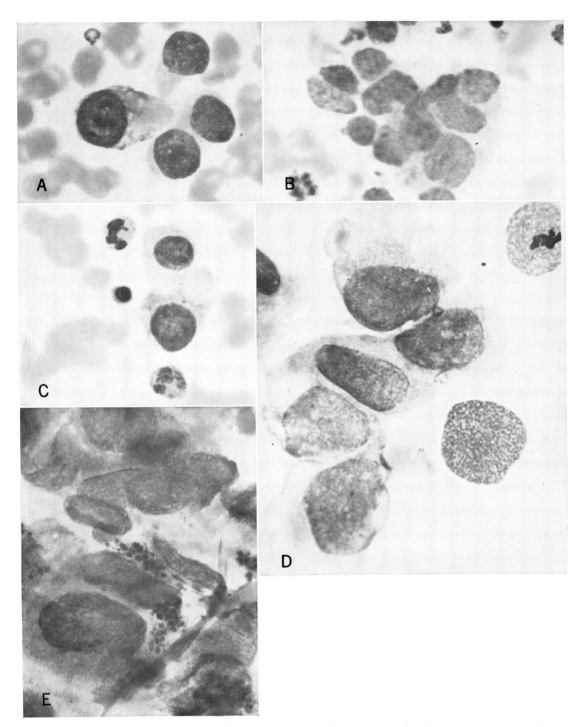

Tumor cells from bone marrow: A, carcinoma of the colon; B, carcinoma of the lung; C, carcinoma of the breast. (Wright's stain, × 1220). Cellular detail, especially in B, is obscured but the grouping of the cells is characteristic. D, photographed by Drs. Avery A. Sandberg and Edwin Gordy, gives good detail of cells from a case of carcinoma of the breast (Wright-Giemsa stain, × 1400). E, adenocarcinoma probably of renal origin (Wright's stain, × 1220).

ing contributed in large measure to the recognition of megaloblastic anemia of infancy.

Hemolytic anemias, hypochromic anemias and other types of anemia should rarely require marrow aspiration for their recognition or differentiation. In the differential diagnosis of the purpuras, marrow aspiration is helpful in confirming a diagnosis which, however, should be possible to make usually by more routine clinical and blood examinations.

In Table 1–4 representative findings in a number of conditions are listed. These must be regarded only as examples of what may be expected in typical cases and do not give the range of variation in disease. The details of the pathological changes which may be encountered in the various disorders of the blood will be discussed in subsequent chapters.

SPLEEN AND LYMPH NODE EXAMINATION

American hematologists have been slow in adopting biopsy procedures. This was true of bone marrow examination and is still the case with splenic and lymph node punctures. Splenic puncture was employed as a means of obtaining material for bacterial culture by Widal and his school at the turn of the century and has been used as an aid in the study of splenomegalies in Europe and in Asia since that time.[208] Lymph node examinations have also been practiced by Europeans for a number of years.[200,203]

Moeschlin[208] recommends that splenic puncture be carried out only when there is distinct splenic enlargement and that it be performed with strictest aseptic technic. The procedure is contraindicated in patients with hemorrhagic manifestations, in those with painful splenomegaly (infarct, *etc.*) or enlargement due to acute sepsis, and in patients who are lethargic or cannot cooperate.

Technic.[208]—The spleen should be carefully outlined. If it is not palpably enlarged, it must be outlined by percussion and the patient should also be examined fluoroscopically. By giving 10 grams of bicarbonate in a little water followed by a small amount of lemon juice, a bubble of air is produced in the stomach and then the spleen can be seen lying between the gastric gas bubble and the diaphragm.

Moeschlin performs splenic puncture in the ninth or tenth rib interspace in the midaxillary line during complete inspiration (Fig. 1–15). The latter is strongly recommended because a reflex inspiratory descent of the diaphragm is sometimes produced as the needle enters the abdominal cavity and, if the puncture is being done during expiration, there is a risk of rupturing the spleen. Puncture of adjacent organs is avoided by using the site recommended. Puncture through the abdominal wall is not desirable as this, even under the best of circumstances, runs the risk of puncture of viscera or displacement of the needle by contraction of the abdominal muscles.

The patient lies flat on his back without pillows under the head. The splenic area is outlined and the lowest limit of pulmonary resonance during full inspiration is determined by light percussion. A site 5 centimeters below this level is marked. This is where the needle will be inserted. The skin is then painted with an appropriate antiseptic and draped with a sterile eyecloth.

Anesthesia is carried out by means of a fine needle, 10 centimeters long and attached to a 5 ml. record syringe containing 4 ml. of 2 per cent procaine solution. A cutaneous wheal is produced and then the underlying tissues are infiltrated perpendicularly to the skin surface to a depth of 1 to 2 cm. The patient is asked to breathe rapidly but superficially while the needle is slowly pushed more and more deeply, 1 ml. at

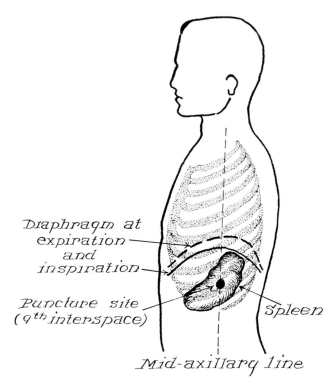

Diaphragm at
expiration
and
inspiration

Puncture site
(9ᵗʰ interspace)

Spleen

Mid-axillary line

Fig. 1–15.—Splenic puncture. The preferred site of puncture is indicated
(after Ferris and Hargraves, courtesy of Arch. Surg.)

a time, until slight pain is produced. The development of pain indicates that the peritoneum has been penetrated. The needle is finally pushed 1 to 2 mm. further until a scratching sensation is felt as it rubs against the spleen. The depth from the skin to this point is marked on the needle.

On the splenic puncture needle a distance is marked by setting the guard in a position which is equal to the depth marked on the anesthesia needle plus 2 cm. The latter makes it possible to penetrate the spleen to a depth of 2 cm. and no more. This prevents too deep penetration of the spleen and avoids damage to the larger vessels of that organ. These enter at the hilum and end in a fine mesh-work at the subcapsular region.

For splenic puncture a needle 12 to 15 centimeters long and 1.2 to 2.0 milli-meters in diameter is recommended. There should be a ground-in stylet and the bevel must not be steep but it should be extremely sharp. A movable guard should be attached to the needle. A 20 ml. record syringe is preferred to a smaller one since this permits stronger suction. The needle and syringe must be dry.

In performing the puncture, the needle is pushed through the marked spot on the skin, the stylet is then removed and the syringe is attached. The patient is told to take a deep breath, close his mouth, and pinch his nose. The needle is then pushed in rapidly to the hilt of the guard. Aspiration is carried out quickly but strongly one or two times. The needle is then withdrawn but, before doing this, negative pressure is gradually released by permitting the plunger to come back slowly. If this is not done, the negative pressure will bring blood or the anesthetic agent into the syringe and ruin the preparations.

It is important that the patient hold his breath throughout the whole procedure. It is necessary to practice the steps which are required of a patient before performing the puncture. Following the procedure, the patient must remain in bed, lying flat on his back for one hour. At the end of this time he may be given a meal but is asked to remain in bed for another six hours.

Moeschlin has performed successfully many hundred splenic punctures by this technic, without accident. Others[215] have used without trouble a 20 gauge needle to aspirate even intercostally in the area of maximal dullness when the spleen has not been palpably enlarged. With such a needle it was not found necessary to use a preliminary local anesthetic.

Biopsy with the Vim-Silverman needle is more dangerous and several deaths have occurred.[202] Sections obtained with such a needle are especially useful in disorders such as amyloidosis or sarcoidosis in which architecture is more important than individual cell morphology.

Indications and Interpretation.—The material obtained by splenic puncture usually consists of 1 to 3 drops of rather bloody fluid in the needle and a few fragments of tissue. Microscopically 60 to 90 per cent of the cells are found to be lymphocytes. The remainder include granulocytes and reticulo-endothelial cells. The latter are mainly derived from the sinuses. Moeschlin's "pulp cells" (Fig. 1–16) have not been observed in gland or marrow punctures. Other important elements include typical plasmacytoid reticulum cells identical with those of the marrow and large lymphatic plasma cells of the same type as is seen in gland punctures.

Although differential counts (splenograms) can be carried out, an exact splenogram is not usually necessary. Careful examination of films will give a sufficiently accurate idea of the distribution of the cells and will reveal the presence of abnormal ones.

Splenic puncture is useful in the diagnosis of disorders due to parasites, such as leishmaniasis and malaria; it may serve to differentiate one of the fat storage disorders from atypical leukemia or splenic neutropenia, and it may be useful in distinguishing leukemoid reactions from true leukemia.[215] It has also been possible by this means to demonstrate Dorothy Reed cells in the spleen in cases of abdominal Hodgkin's disease and epithelioid cells in cases of tuberculosis and of brucellosis.[208] In other conditions, the procedure has less importance. In cirrhosis of the liver and in spleno-portal thrombosis, the splenogram is practically normal, even though the spleen may be greatly enlarged. It is likely to be unusually bloody. In hemolytic anemias a fairly normal picture has been observed although, as the result of increased blood destruction, hemosiderin-containing macrophages may be quite numerous and some erythroblasts may be observed during periods of exacerbation. Moeschlin did not find signs of phagocytosis of red corpuscles. In pernicious anemia, megaloblasts are plentiful in the spleen.

In inflammatory splenomegalies, hemopoietic foci in the spleen have been described.[208] In acute inflammatory reactions, lymphocytes are reduced in number while neutrophils, including stab cells and myelocytes, are increased as are also the pulp cells and macrophages. Only an occasional erythroblast is seen. In chronic inflammatory splenomegalies, in addition to these changes, the monocytes, plasmacytoid reticulum cells and sometimes erythroblasts are increased in number. Cells from these foci may enter the blood in sufficient numbers to arouse, together with the splenomegaly and leukocytosis, a suspicion of early chronic

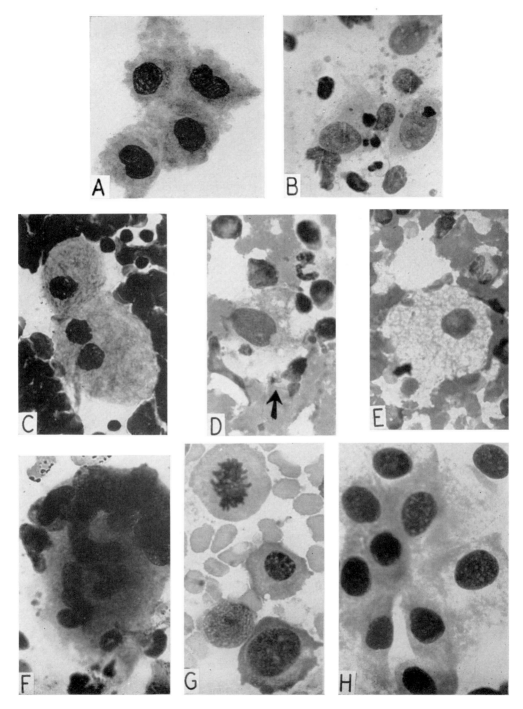

Fig. 1–16.—Cells obtained by splenic puncture (Courtesy of Dr. S. Moeschlin). *A*, splenic pulp cells; *B*, Dorothy-Reed cells in Hodgkin's disease; *C*, Gaucher cells; *D*, spleen macrophage with vacuolated cytoplasm; *E*, Niemann-Pick cell; *F*, multinucleated epithelioid cell in tuberculosis; *G*, megaloblasts, pernicious anemia; *H*, hypernephroma cells, from tumor mistaken for spleen.

myelocytic leukemia. In leukemia, however, myelocytes form 20 to 60 per cent of the cells whereas in chronic inflammatory splenomegaly they do not rise above 1 to 5 per cent. Even in cases of myelofibrosis with myeloid metaplasia, the persistence of large numbers of lymphocytes (50 to 60 per cent) distinguishes the condition from myelocytic leukemia.

Lymphocytic leukemias are characterized by an almost purely lymphocytic picture (92 to 99 per cent). The cells often vary greatly in size and lymphoblasts in mitosis may be prominent. Normally mitoses in lymphocytes are rare, their mitotic index having been found to be 50 times less than that of granulocytes. In cases of lymphoid leukemia, the mitoses may be increased 15 or 30 times the normal, although this does not occur in all cases.

In infectious mononucleosis at the height of the disease, a considerable excess of reticulo-endothelial cells, some in mitosis, with transitions between them and the typical infectious mononucleosis cells have been described. In infectious hepatitis, many of the immature precursors of the lymphatic plasma cells that are found in the blood have been observed.

Lymph node puncture[200,203] is especially helpful in the differential diagnosis of the various lymph node disorders and metastases of malignant tumors. In Hodgkin's disease, Reed-Sternberg cells, monocytoid cells, eosinophils, polymorphonuclear neutrophils and large lymphoid cells will be found.[210] In lymphosarcoma similar large lymphoid cells with large nuclei, rare nucleoli, scant cytoplasm and prominent mitotic figures are observed but the other cells found in Hodgkin's nodes are lacking. In lymphoid leukemia, in contrast, small lymphocytes are found in the chronic form and lymphoblasts are seen in acute leukemia. In lymphadenitis, polymorphonuclear neutrophils are pres-

ent in numbers roughly corresponding to the acuteness of the inflammatory process. In nodes harboring metastatic malignancy, the carcinoma cells are usually found in clusters and mitotic figures are prominent.

The procedure is simple. The overlying skin is cleansed and sterilized. No anesthetic is necessary. Using a 20-gauge sterile needle and dry syringe, the operator grasps the node securely between the thumb and index finger of the left hand and pierces the node. The tissue is aspirated rapidly and the needle is then withdrawn. Smears of the aspirate are made on a clean slide and stained with Wright's stain.

THE INHERITANCE OF ABNORMALITIES OF THE BLOOD[226,229]

Of the disorders of man which are recognized as being hereditary in origin, a remarkably large number involve the hemopoietic system. It is necessary, therefore, that the hematologist understand the principles of genetics and that he appreciate their application to human disorders. While details concerning the various hemopoietic disorders may be left for consideration in relation to each condition, certain principles may be discussed here.

In man the nucleus of the spermatozoon and that of the ovum contain 23 chromosomes each. The inherited traits of man have as their ultimate basis the nucleoproteins of the total of 46 chromosomes derived from the union of the spermatozoon and the ovum. The chromosomes may be visualized as a continuum of tremendously elongate nucleic acid strands. These are differentiated into thousands of specific subdivisions, known as *genes*. The character of a particular gene depends on the precise sequence of the constituents of the nucleic acid strands at that particular area in the chromosome. The site on a chromosome at which a gene occurs is known as a *locus*.

The various genes afford the *potentialities* for the development of certain characters, provided external conditions as well as the assemblage of other genes present within the genetic material are suitable. It is a common misconception that a given gene is *the* gene for this or that character. Those concerned with human genetics must be cognizant of the fact that not only is the transmission of a particular gene necessary for the inheritance of a certain characteristic, but that other factors, both of external and internal environment, help to determine whether or not the characteristic will be *expressed*.

In the union of chromosomes which occurs following fertilization of the ovum, for every maternal one there is ordinarily a corresponding ("homologous") paternal one. With the exception of the sex chromosomes, the likeness between each two homologous chromosomes extends to their string of contained genes so that, ordinarily, for each gene in a maternal chromosome there is a corresponding gene present, in the same place in the line, in the homologous paternal chromosome. Here and there, however, there is apt to be found in the line of genes a *mutant* gene. The various alternative forms of a gene which may occur at a given locus on a chromosome are known as *alleles*. Where there is a conjunction of two different alleles, the condition is called *heterozygous*. When there are two like alleles, whether they are both normal or, as occurs very rarely, both mutant, the condition is called *homozygous*.

The expression of the characteristic determined by the genes in question depends on whether the influence of a particular gene in heterozygous alleles is greater than that of its partner, that is whether it is "*dominant*," or has little influence and is, thus, "*recessive*." The influence of a mutant gene may be recessive or dominant as compared with that of its normal allele. Some genes have constant expressivity, regularly producing the same degree of manifestation of the character, while others with variable expressivity result in different manifestations of the trait from person to person.

In relation to the blood disorders, the phenomenon of "*crossing over*," a condition in which a pair of chromosomes closely twisted about each other during meiosis (to be distinguished from mitosis) undergo a break and exchange of segments at certain points, has not been proved so far to be involved in the transmission of inherited abnormalities. However, the process of *linkage* must be considered, especially as it applies to the sex chromosomes. When genes for two characteristics are in the same chromosome they are regarded as being *linked*. If their loci in the chromosome are close together, the linkage will be easily detected. If they are far apart, linkage will be most difficult to detect. Linkage in the sex chromosome is more easily demonstrable, however. In mammals the female is homozygous for the chromosomes (the X's) that determine sex (Fig. 1–17). The male, on the other hand, is heterozygous, having one X like that in the female and another different chromosome called the Y. By the process of segregation, 50 per cent of the spermatozoa get the male's X and these, fertilizing an egg, which always has an X itself, form an individual with two X's, which becomes a female. The other 50 per cent of the spermatozoa get the male's Y, which with the X chromosome of the egg forms an XY individual, a male.

Of special significance here is the fact that characters dependent on genes in the X chromosome must be *linked* with sex in their heredity. If the genes in question are in that section of the X which is missing in the Y chromosome, that is, the non-homologous portion, there can be no crossing over from the X to the Y chromosome. Such genes are regarded,

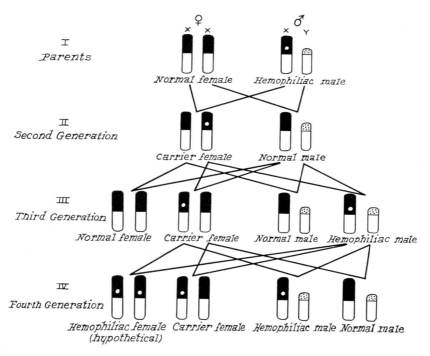

Fig. 1–17.—The mode of inheritance of completely sex-linked, recessive characters through the X-chromosome. The X-chromosome is represented as a full length rod, the portion differing from the Y-chromosome being represented as solid black. The sex-linked abnormality appears as a white spot in the black portion of the X-chromosome.

therefore, as being completely sex-linked. If the genes in question are present in other parts of the X so that crossing over with the corresponding part of the Y can take place, they are said to be only partially sex-linked. Completely sex-linked characters will always be evident in a male possessing the genes for them in his X, even if those genes are recessive ones, since there is no corresponding section of an X which contains normal genes to dominate over them. On the other hand, in the female such a characteristic, if recessive, can show itself only if the gene for it is present in both her X's, an occurrence which is very rare since intermarriage between brothers and sisters, as outlined in figure 1–17, is not human practice and a similar union between two affected families would be very rare. Even in the absence

of such a mating, however, the female may transmit the gene to her offspring since it is present in one of her X's. Where this is transmitted to a male, it manifests itself since there is no normal X to dominate it; if transmitted to a female it is not manifest but can still be transmitted again by her. Hemophilia is a well known example of an inherited sex-linked recessive trait.

The ready availability of the blood cells for examination has been of great importance from the standpoint of advancing our knowledge of the role of inheritance in the transmission of certain normal characteristics as well as of many disorders. Furthermore, the impact of the investigations in hematology has been felt in the fields of biochemistry and genetics, as well as in many other areas. Thus, advantage could be taken of the fact that the hereditary hemoglobin-opathies, transmitted as autosomal dominants, can be recognized in the heterozygote. Their investigation led to clarification of the structure of globin, which is now recognized as being composed of two pairs of polypeptide chains, each probably under the control of a different gene. Study of the abnormal hemoglobins provided the first clues concerning the effects of gene mutations on protein structure and led to the important observations on the significance of amino acid sequences which are discussed in Chapter 3 (p. 157). The study of hemolytic anemias, on the other hand, led to investigation of the metabolism of the red cell and the recognition of heritable enzymic defects in the red corpuscle (p. 632).

As these advances apply to the different topics dealt with in this book they will be discussed in the following pages. They encompass a very wide range; yet many details remain to be filled in. Thus, although the inheritance of the ABO serological blood types is clear, that of the Rh system is still a matter of dispute (p. 340). The mode of inheritance of hemophilia (Fig. 1–17) is so well established that it serves as a standard example in courses in human genetics. However, whether this disease is due to the lack of an essential protein or to other causes, remains to be seen (p. 863). Again, it is commonly said that hereditary spherocytosis is inherited as if due to a dominant gene and that the carrier, like the individual with the manifest disease, is a heterozygote. However, the effects of this gene when homozygous are unknown and other uncertainties remain. The same can be said about ovalocytosis and hereditary hemorrhagic telangiectasia, both of which are inherited as dominant traits.

In addition to the disorders which can be readily studied because the carriers actually manifest the abnormality, there are conditions in which the carrier appears normal and yet his or her genetic constitution includes determiners for the disease in question which fail to find expression for various reasons, such as as environmental factors, dominance relations, reduced "penetrance" of the gene, and so on. Thus, in pernicious anemia a single dominant autosomal gene may be responsible for the inheritance of a reduced capacity to absorb vitamin B_{12} but many factors undoubtedly influence the expression of the gene (p. 470). A number of disorders of the blood probably fall in this category.

It can be expected that the future will yield additional details as investigations are pursued. Much less is known about inherited abnormalities of leukocytes (p. 224) or of platelets than of red cells but a beginning has been made in the study of qualitative platelet disorders, such as thrombasthenia (p. 847). Much has been learned concerning the factors involved in the process of coagulation (p. 289) and more is being uncovered regarding the inheritance of important serum factors, such as the haptoglobins (p. 168).

BIBLIOGRAPHY

Blood of the Embryo and Fetus

1. ALLEN, D. W., WYMAN, J., JR. and SMITH, C. A.: The Oxygen Equilibrium of Fetal and Adult Human Hemoglobin, J. Biol. Chem., 203, 81, 1953.
1a. ALLEN, D. W., SCHROEDER, W. A. and BALOG, JOAN: Observations on the Chromatographic Heterogeneity of Normal Adult and Fetal Human Hemoglobin, J. Am. Chem. Soc., 80, 1628, 1958.
1b. ALLEN, D. W. and JANDL, J. H.: Factors Influencing Relative Rates of Synthesis of Adult and Fetal Hemoglobin in Vitro, J. Clin. Invest., 39, 1107, 1960.
1c. BEAVEN, G. H., ELLIS, M. J. and WHITE, J. C.: Studies on Human Foetal Haemoglobin, Brit. J. Haemat., 6, 1 and 201, 1960.
2. BLOOM, W.: The Hemopoietic Potency of the Small Lymphocyte, Folia haemat., 33, 122, 1926.

3. BLOOM, W. and BARTELMEZ, G. W.: Hematopoiesis in Young Human Embryos, Am. J. Anat., 67, 21, 1940.

3a. BOLL, I.: Morphologische Studien zum Verhalten von Knochenmarkzellen in vitro, Folia haemat., 3, 58, 1958.

3b. BUTLER, ELIZABETH A., FLYNN, F. V. and HUEHNS, E. R.: The Haemoglobin of Foetal Blood, Clin. Chim. Acta, 5, 571, 1960; Nature, 189, 496, 1961.

4. CHERNOFF, A. I. and SINGER, K.: Studies on Abnormal Hemoglobins. IV. Persistence of Fetal Hemoglobin in the Erythrocytes of Normal Children, Pediatrics, 9, 469, 1952.

5. COOK, C. D., BRODIE, H. R. and ALLEN, D. W.: Measurement of Fetal Hemoglobin in Newborn Infants. Correlation with Gestational Age and Intrauterine Hypoxia, Pediatrics, 20, 272, 1957.

6. DACIE, J. V. and WHITE, J. C.: Erythropoiesis with Particular Reference to Its Study by Biopsy of Human Marrow, J. Clin. Path., 2, 1, 1949.

7. DOAN, C. A.: Current Views on the Origin and Maturation of the Cells of the Blood, J. Lab. & Clin. Med., 17, 887, 1932.

8. DOWNEY, H.: Handbook of Hematology, New York, Paul B. Hoeber, Inc., 1938.

9. DOWNEY, H. and STASNEY, J.: Infectious Mononucleosis, J. A. M. A., 105, 761, 1935.

10. GILMOUR, J. R.: Normal Haemopoiesis in Intra-uterine and Neonatal Life, J. Path. & Bact., 52, 25, 1941.

11. HALBRECHT, I. and KLIBANSKI, C.: Identification of a New Normal Embryonic Haemoglobin, Nature, 178, 794, 1956; ibid., 179, 477, 1957; Am. J. Clin. Path., 29, 340, 1958; Nature, 183, 327, 1959.

12. HUNT, J. A.: Identity of the α-chains of Adult and Foetal Human Haemoglobins, Nature, 183, 1373, 1959.

13. JONES, O. P.: Cytology of Pathologic Marrow Cells with Special Reference to Bone-marrow Biopsies, in Downey, H., Handbook of Hematology, New York, Paul B. Hoeber, Inc., 3, 2043, 1938.

14. JORDAN, H. E.: The Significance of the Lymphoid Nodule, Am. J. Anat., 57, 1, 1935.

15. KNOLL, W.: Die Blutbildung beim Embryo, in Handbuch der allgemeinen Hämatologie, Hirschfeld, H., und Hittmair, A., Berlin, Urban & Schwarzenberg, 1 (1st half), 553, 1932; Acta haemat., 2, 369, 1949.

15a. MATSUDA, G., SCHROEDER, W. A., JONES, R. T. and WELIKY, N.: Is There an "Embryonic" or "Primitive" Human Hemoglobin? Blood, 16, 984, 1960.

16. MAXIMOW, A. A.: Relation of Blood Cells to Connective Tissues and Endothelium, Physiol. Rev., 4, 533, 1924.

17. MICHELS, N. A.: Erythropoiesis, Haematologica, 45, 75, 1931 (Bibliography).

18. OSGOOD, E. E.: Number and Distribution of Human Hemic Cells, Blood, 9, 1141, 1954.

19. SABIN, F. R., MILLER, F. R., SMITHBURN, K. C., THOMAS, R. M. and HUMMEL, L. E.: Changes in the Bone Marrow and Blood Cells of Developing Rabbits, J. Exper. Med., 64, 97, 1936.

20. SINGER, K., CHERNOFF, A. I. and SINGER, L.: Studies on Abnormal Hemoglobins. I. Their Demonstration in Sickle Cell Anemia and Other Hematologic Disorders by Means of Alkali Denaturation, Blood, 6, 413, 1951.

21. WALKER, J. and TURNBULL, E. P. N.: Haemoglobin and Red Cells in the Human Foetus, Lancet, 2, 312, 1953; Arch. Dis. Childhood, 30, 111, 1955.

22. WHITE, J. C. and BEAVEN, G. H.: Foetal Haemoglobin, Brit. M. Bull., 15, 33, 1959.

23. WINTROBE, M. M. and SHUMACKER, H. B., JR.: Comparison of Hematopoiesis in the Fetus and During Recovery from Pernicious Anemia, J. Clin. Invest., 14, 837, 1935; Am. J. Anat., 58, 313, 1936.

24. WISEMAN, B. K.: The Origin of the White Blood Cells, J. A. M. A., 103, 1523, 1934.

25. ZANATY, A. F.: Erythrokonten und Erythropoese bei der Biermerschen Anämie und bei den Embryonen, Arch. path. Anat., 293, 794, 1934.

26. ZILLIACUS, H.: Human Embryo Haemoglobin, Nature, 188, 1102, 1960.

Post-Natal Hematopoiesis

28. ALPEN, E. L., LAJTHA, L. G. and VAN DYKE, D. C.: Lack of Direct Effect of Erythropoietin on Human Erythroid Cells in vitro, Nature, 184, 1228, 1959.

29. ASCHKENASY, A.: Effets de la thyroidectomie, seule ou combinée à la surrénalectomie, sur les leucocytes sanguins chez le rat, J. physiol., Paris, 48, 376, 1956; Sang, 27, 97, 1956; ibid., 27, 759, 1956; ibid., 28, 400, 485, 1957; Semaine d. hôp., Paris, 34, 683, 1958.

30. ASKANAZY, M.: Knochenmark, in Henke, F. and Lubarsch, O., Handbuch der speziellen pathologischen Anatomie, Berlin, Julius Springer, vol. 1, part 2, 1927.

31. ASTALDI, G. and MAURI, C.: New Criteria for the Evaluation of the Bone-marrow Cells Mitotic Activity, Sang, 21, 378, 1950;

Minerva med., *49*, 3677, 1958; Haemat. latina, *2*, 17, 1959.

32. AUSTONI, M. E., ZILIOTTO, A. und CARENZA, P.: Hypophyse und Eisenstoffwechsel. Die Aufnahme des Fe[59] in Knochenmark, Blut und in verschiedenen Organen hypophysektomierter Ratten, Wien. Ztschr. inn. Med., *37*, 10, 1956; Folia endocrinol., *9*, 577, 1956.

33. AUSTONI, M., ZILIOTTO, D., CARENZA, P. and ODEBLAD, E.: Thyroid and Iron Metabolism. III. The Fe[59]-uptake by Bone Marrow, Blood and Various Organs of Rats Treated with Propylthiouracil (Scintillation Counting and Autoradiography), Acta med. scandinav., *162*, 1, 1958.

34. BRÅNEMARK, P.-I.: Vital Microscopy of Bone Marrow in Rabbit, Scandinav. J. Clin. & Lab. Invest. (supp. 38), *11*, 5, 1959.

37. CONTOPOULOS, A. N., VAN DYKE, D. C., SIMPSON, M. E., GARCIA, J. F., HUFF, R. L., WILLIAMS, B. S. and EVANS, H. M.: Increase in Circulating Red Cell Volume after Oral Administration of Pituitary Anterior Lobe, Blood, *8*, 131, 1953; Proc. Soc. Exper. Biol. & Med., *86*, 729, 1954; Acta haemat., *11*, 203, 1954; Endocrinology, *55*, 808, 1954; Blood, *10*, 115, 1955.

38. CRAFTS, R. C. and MEINEKE, H. A.: Influence of the Pituitary on Hemopoiesis, Am. J. Clin. Nutrition, *5*, 453, 1957.

42. CRONKITE, E. P., FLIEDNER, T. M., BOND, V. P. and ROBERTSON, J. S.: Anatomic and Physiologic Facts and Hypotheses about Hemopoietic Proliferating Systems, *in The Kinetics of Cellular Proliferation*, edited by F. Stohlman, Jr., New York, Grune & Stratton, 1959, p. 1.

43. CROSBY, W. H. and AKEROYD, J. H.: The Limit of Hemoglobin Synthesis in Hereditary Hemolytic Anemia, Am. J. Med., *13*, 273, 1952.

45. CUSTER, R. P.: Studies on the Structure and Function of Bone Marrow, J. Lab. & Clin. Med., *17*, 951, 960, 1932; Am. J. M. Sc., *185*, 617, 1933; *Atlas of the Blood and Bone Marrow*, 1949, W. B. Saunders Co., Philadelphia.

46. DAUGHADAY, W. H., WILLIAMS, R. H. and DALAND, GENEVA A.: The Effect of Endocrinopathies on the Blood, Blood, *3*, 1342, 1948.

47. DAVIDSON, J. N., LESLIE, I. and WHITE, J. C.: The Cytoplasmic Basophilia of Marrow Cells: The Distribution of Nucleic Acids, J. Path. & Bact., *60*, 1, 1948.

48. DONEGAN, C. C., JR., MACILWAINE, W. A. and LEAVELL, B. S.: Hematologic Studies on Patients with Sickle Cell Anemia following Multiple Transfusions, Am. J. Med., *17*, 29, 1954.

48a.DONOHUE, D. M., GABRIO, BEVERLY W. and FINCH, C. A.: Hematopoietic Cells of the Marrow, J. Clin. Invest., *37*, 1564 and 1571, 1958.

48b.DOUGHERTY, T. F.: Adrenal Cortical Control of Lymphatic Tissue Mass, *in The Kinetics of Cellular Proliferation*, edited by F. Stohlman, Jr., New York, Grune & Stratton, 1959, p. 264.

49. DUSTIN, P., JR.: Cortisone et stathmocinéses; à propos de recherches sur l'éosinopénie hormonale, Sang, *28*, 581, 1957.

49a.DUSTIN, P., JR.: The Quantitative Estimation of Mitotic Growth in the Bone Marrow of the Rat by the Stathmokinetic (Colchicinic) Method, *in The Kinetics of Cellular Proliferation*, edited by F. Stohlman, Jr., New York, Grune & Stratton, 1959, p. 50.

50. ELMLINGER, P. J., HUFF, R. L. and ODA. J. M.: Depression of Red Cell Iron Turnover by Transfusion, Proc. Soc. Exper. Biol. & Med., *79*, 16, 1952.

51. ERSLEV, A.: Humoral Regulation of Red Cell Production, Blood, *8*, 349, 1953; *ibid.*, *9*, 1055, 1954; *ibid.*, *10*, 616 and 954, 1955; *ibid.*, *14*, 386, 1959.

54. FLIEDNER, T. M., CRONKITE, E. P., BOND, V. P., RUBINI, J. R. and ANDREWS, G.: The Mitotic Index of Human Bone Marrow in Healthy Individuals and Irradiated Human Beings, Acta haemat., *22*, 65, 1959.

57. GORDON, A. S.: Hemopoietine, Physiol. Rev., *39*, 1, 1959; *in* Ciba Foundation Symposium on Haemopoiesis, edited by G. E. W. Wolstenholme and Maeve O'Connor, J. & A. Churchill Ltd., London, 1960, p. 325.

58. GORDON, A. S. and CHARIPPER, H. A.: The Endocrine System and Hemopoiesis, Ann. New York Acad. Sc., *48*, 615, 1947 (Bibliography); Acta haemat., *15*, 249, 1956.

59. GORDON, A. S. *et al.*: Humoral Regulation of Leukocyte Numbers, Tr. New York Acad. Sc., *23*, 39, 1960.

60. GRANT, W. C. and ROOT, W. S.: Fundamental Stimulus for Erythropoiesis, Physiol. Rev., *32*, 449, 1952; Blood, *10*, 334, 1955.

62. GÜNTHER, H.: Über die Beziehung endokriner Organe zur Entstehung der Polyglobulie und über klinische Typen hormonal bedingter Polyglobulia, Endokrinologie, *4*, 96, 1929.

63. HUGGINS, C. and BLOCKSOM, B. H.: Changes in Outlying Bone Marrow Accompanying a Local Increase of Temperature within

Physiological Limits, J. Exper. Med., *64*, 253, 1936.

64. ISAACS, R.: The Physiological Histology of Bone Marrow, Folia haemat, *40*, 395, 1930.

65. JACOBSON, L. O., GURNEY, C. W. and GOLD-WASSER, E.: The Control of Erythropoiesis, Advances in Internal Medicine, *10*, 297, 1960.

66. JACOBSON, L. O., MARKS, E. K., GASTON, E. O. and GOLDWASSER, E.: Studies on Erythropoiesis. XI. Reticulocyte Response of Transfusion-Induced Polycythemic Mice to Anemic Plasma from Nephrectomized Mice and to Plasma from Nephrectomized Rats Exposed to Low Oxygen, Blood, *14*, 635, 1959; J. Lab. & Clin. Med., *53*, 446, 1959; Blood, *14*, 644, 1959.

66a. JANDL, J. H.: The Agglutination and Sequestration of Immature Red Cells, J. Lab. & Clin. Med., *55*, 663, 1960.

67. JAPA, J.: A Study of the Mitotic Activity of Normal Human Bone Marrow, Brit. J. Exper. Path., *23*, 272, 1942.

68. JONES, O. P.: Mitochondria and Their Relation to the So-called Hyaloplasm, J. Lab. & Clin. Med., *32*, 700, 1947.

69. JORDAN, H. E. and ROBESON, J. M.: The Production of Lymphoid Nodules in the Bone Marrow of the Domestic Pigeon following Splenectomy, Am. J. Anat., *71*, 181, 1942.

69a. KELEMEN, E., CSERHÁTI, I. and TANOS, B.: Demonstration and Some Properties of Human Thrombopoietin in Thrombocythaemic Sera, Acta haemat., *20*, 350, 1958.

70. KENNEDY, B. J. and GILBERTSEN, A. S.: Increased Erythropoiesis Induced by Androgenic-Hormone Therapy, New England J. Med., *256*, 719, 1957.

70a. KILLMANN, S. A., CRONKITE, E. P., FLIEDNER, T. M. and BOND, V. P.: Erythro- and Granulocytopoietic Turnover in Human Bone Marrow Estimated from Mitotic Indices, Blood, *17*, 1961.

71. KINDRED, J. E.: A Quantitative Study of the Hemopoietic Organs of Young Adult Albino Rats, Am. J. Anat., *71*, 207, 1942.

72. KOLLER, P. C.: The Experimental Modification of Nucleic Acid Systems in the Cell, Symposia of the Society for Experimental Biology, No. I, 1947, p. 270.

72a. LEBLOND, C. P.: Classical Technics for the Study of the Kinetics of Cellular Proliferation, *in The Kinetics of Cellular Proliferation*, edited by F. Stohlman, Jr., New York, Grune and Stratton, 1959, p. 31.

73. LA COUR, L. F.: Mitosis and Cell Differentiation in the Blood, Proc. Royal Soc. Edinburgh, *62*, 73, 1944.

74. LAJTHA, L. G.: Bone Marrow Cell Metabolism, Physiol. Rev., *37*, 50, 1957.

75. LAJTHA, L. G. and VANE, J. R.: Dependence of Bone Marrow Cells on the Liver for Purine Supply, Nature, *182*, 191, 1958.

77. LINMAN, J. W., BETHELL, F. H. and LONG, M. J.: Factors Controlling Hemopoiesis: Experimental Observations on Their Role in Polycythemia Vera, Ann. Int. Med., *51*, 1003, 1959.

78. MAUER, A. M., ATHENS, J. W., WARNER, H. R., ASHENBRUCKER, HELEN, CARTWRIGHT, G. E. and WINTROBE, M. M.: An Analysis of Leukocyte Radioactivity Curves Obtained with Radioactive Diisopropylfluorophosphate (DFP^{32}), *in The Kinetics of Cellular Proliferation*, edited by F. Stohlman, Jr., New York, Grune & Stratton, 1959, p. 231.

79. MAZIA, D. and PRESCOTT, D. M.: Nuclear Function and Mitosis, Science, *120*, 120, 1954.

80. MECHANIK, N.: Untersuchungen über das Gewicht des Knochenmarkes des Menschen, Ztschr. f. d. ges. Anat., *79*, 58, 1926.

81. MITCHELL, J. S.: Disturbance of Nucleic Acid Metabolism Produced by Therapeutic Doses of X- and Gamma-Radiations, Brit. J. Exper. Path., *23*, 309, 1942.

82. MOESCHLIN, S.: Nervous Regulation of Hematopoiesis, Proceedings of the Fourth International Congress of the International Society of Hematology, New York, Grune & Stratton, 1952, p. 41.

83. NAETS, J. P.: Erythropoiesis in Nephrectomized Dogs, Nature, *181*, 1134, 1958; *ibid., 182*, 1516, 1958; *ibid., 184*, 371, 1959; Proc. Soc. Exper. Biol. & Med., *102*, 387, 1959; J. Clin. Invest., *39*, 102, 1960; Blood, *16*, 1770, 1960.

84. OSNES, S.: Influence of the Pituitary on the Erythropoietic Principle Produced in the Kidney, Brit. M. J., *1*, 1153, 1960.

85. OSGOOD, E. E.: A Unifying Concept of the Etiology of the Leukemias, Lymphomas, and Cancers, J. Nat. Cancer Inst., *18*, 155, 1957; and *in The Kinetics of Cellular Proliferation*, edited by F. Stohlman, Jr., New York, Grune & Stratton, 1959, p. 282.

86. PATT, H. M.: A Consideration of Myeloid-Erythroid Balance in Man, Blood, *12*, 777, 1957.

87. POWSNER, E. R. and BERMAN, L.: Correlation of Radioactive Hemin Formation with Morphologic Alterations in Cultures of Human Bone Marrow, Blood, *14*, 1213 1959.

6

90. REISSMANN, K. R.: Studies on the Mechanism of Erythropoietic Stimulation in Parabiotic Rats during Hypoxia, Blood, *5*, 372, 1950; *ibid.*, *16*, 1411, 1960.

91. ROSENOW, G.: The Nervous-Humoral Regulation of the Leukocytes, Acta haemat., *5*, 1, 1951.

92. SABIN, F. R.: Bone Marrow, Physiol. Rev., *8*, 191, 1928 (Bibliography).

93. SHEMIN, D. and RITTENBERG, D.: The Life Span of the Human Red Blood Cell, J. Biol. Chem., *166*, 627, 1946.

93a.SHEN, S. S. and HOSHINO, T.: Study of Humoral Factors Regulating the Production of Leukocytes, Blood, *17*, 434, 1961.

94. STEDMAN, E. and STEDMAN, ELLEN: The Cytological Interpretation of the Feulgen Reaction, Biochem. J., *47*, 508, 1950.

95. SMITH, C. H., SCHULMAN, I., ANDO, R. E. and STERN, G.: The Suppression of Hematopoiesis by Transfusions, Blood, *10*, 707, 1955.

96. STOHLMAN, F., JR.: Observations on the Physiology of Erythropoietin and Its Role in the Regulation of Red Cell Production, Ann. New York Acad. Sc., *77*, 710, 1959; Proc. Soc. Exper. Biol. & Med., *100*, 40, 1959.

97. STOHLMAN, F., JR., RATH, C. E. and ROSE, J. C.: Evidence for a Humoral Regulation of Erythropoiesis, Blood, *9*, 721, 1954.

98. SUKI, W. and GROLLMAN, A.: Role of the Kidney in Erythropoiesis, Am. J. Physiol., *199*, 629, 1960.

99. THORELL, B.: *Studies on the Formation of Cellular Substances during Blood Cell Production*, Diss. med. Stockholm. Karolinska Institutet, Henry Kimpton, London, 1947.

100. TINSLEY, J. C., MOORE, C. V., DUBACH, RUBENIA, MINNICH, VIRGINIA and GRINSTEIN, M.: The Role of Oxygen in the Regulation of Erythropoiesis, J. Clin. Invest., *28*, 1544, 1949.

101. VAN DYKE, D. C., GARCIA, J. F., SIMPSON, M. E., HUFF, R. L., CONTOPOULOS, A. N., and EVANS, H. M.: Maintenance of Circulating Red Cell Volume in Rats after Removal of the Posterior and Intermediate Lobes of the Pituitary, Blood, *7*, 1017, 1952; Proc. Soc. Exper. Biol. & Med., *81*, 574, 1952; *ibid.*, *82*, 287, 1953; *ibid.*, *96*, 541, 1957.

105. WEICKER, H.: Die Erythroblastenmitosen, Ztschr. klin. Med., *151*, 407, 1954.

106. WEICKER, H.: Zellteilung und Zellteilungsstörungen, *in Handbuch der gesamten Hämatologie*, edited by Heilmeyer, L. and Hittmair, A., Munchen, Urban & Schwarzenberg, 1957, p. 148.

108. WHITE, J. C.: The Cytoplasmic Basophilia of Bone-Marrow Cells, J. Path. & Bact., *59*, 223, 1947.

109. YOFFEY, J. M.: Bone Marrow, Brit. M. J., *2*, 193, 1954.

110. ZALOKAR, M.: Nuclear Origin of Ribonucleic Acid, Nature, *183*, 1330, 1959.

Extramedullary Hematopoiesis

120. BLAISDELL, J. L.: Extramedullary Hematopoiesis in a Retroperitoneal Tumor, Arch. path. Anat., *16*, 643, 1933.

121. BRANNAN, D.: Extramedullary Hematopoiesis in Anemia, Bull. Johns Hopkins Hosp., *41*, 104, 1927.

122. CLOSE, A. S., TAIRA, Y. and CLEVELAND, D. A.: Spinal Cord Compression Due to Extramedullary Hematopoiesis, Ann. Int. Med., *48*, 421, 1958.

123. DONHAUSER, J. L.: The Human Spleen as an Haemoplastic Organ, as Exemplified in a Case of Splenomegaly with Sclerosis of the Bone Marrow, J. Exper. Med., *10*, 559, 1908.

124. FRESEN, O.: Zur Nosologie und Struktur dystoper markartiger Blutbildungsherde, Acta haemat., *22*, 20, 1959.

126. HARTFALL, S. J. and STEWART, M. J.: Massive Paravertebral Heterotopia of Bone Marrow in a Case of Acholuric Jaundice, J. Path. & Bact., *377*, 455, 1933.

127. JORDAN, H. E.: Extramedullary Erythrocytopoiesis in Man, Arch. Path., *78*, 1, 1934; Physiol. Rev., *22*, 375, 1942.

128. LYALL, A.: Massive Extramedullary Bone Marrow Formation in a Case of Pernicious Anemia, J. Path. & Bact., *41*, 469, 1935.

129. MEYER, E. and HEINEKE, A.: Uber Blutbildung in Milz und Leber bei schweren Anämien, Verhandl. d. deutsch. path. Gesellsch., *9*, 224, 1905.

130. OSOGOE, B. and OMURA, K.: Transplantation of Hematopoietic Tissues into the Circulating Blood, Anat. Rec., *108*, 663, 1950.

131. SCHILLER, W.: Local Myelopoiesis in Myeloid Leukemia, Am. J. Path., *19*, 809, 1943.

140. WINTROBE, M. M.: Relation of Disease of the Liver to Anemia, Arch. Int. Med., *57*, 289, 1936.

Examination of Bone Marrow

150. AMPRINO, R. and PENATI, F.: L'allestimento di preparati istologici di midollo osseo dal materiale estratto con la puntura dello sterno secondo Arinkin, Minerva med., *25*, 463, 1934.

151. ARINKIN, M. J.: Intravitale Untersuchungsmethodik des Knochenmarks, Folia haemat., *38*, 233, 1929.

152. Bennike, T., Gormsen, H. Møller, B.: Comparative Studies of Bone Marrow Punctures of the Sternum, the Iliac Crest and the Spinous Process, Acta med. scandinav., *155*, 377, 1956.

153. Berenbaum, M. C.: The Use of Bovine Albumin in the Preparation of Marrow and Blood Films, J. Clin. Path., *9*, 381, 1956.

154. Berman, L. and Axelrod, A. R.: Aspiration of Sternal Bone Marrow, Am. J. Clin. Path., *17*, 61, 551, 557 and 631, 1947; *ibid.*, *18*, 898, 1948; *ibid.*, *23*, 385, 1953.

155. Bickel, G. and Della Santa, R.: La ponction spinovertébrale, Acta haemat., *2*, 133, 1949.

156. Bierman, H. R. and Kelly, K. H.: Multiple Marrow Aspiration in Man from the Posterior Ilium, Blood, *11*, 370, 1956.

157. Block, M., Smaller, V. and Brown, J.: An Adaptation of the Maximow Technique for Preparation of Sections of Hematopoietic Tissues, J. Lab. & Clin. Med., *42*, 145, 1953.

158. Bover, G. F.: *El Diagnostico por la Puncion Esternal*, Madrid, Ed. Morata, 1946.

159. Clark, H. and Muirhead, E. E.: Plasmacytosis of Bone Marrow, Arch. Int. Med., *94*, 425, 1954.

160. Emery, J. L.: The Technique of Bone Marrow Aspiration in Children, J. Clin. Path., *10*, 339, 1957.

161. Fieschi, A.: Semiologie des Knochenmarks, Ergebn. d. inn. Med. u. Kinderheilk, *59*, 382, 1940 (Bibliography).

162. Fortner, J. G. and Moss, E. S.: Death following Sternal Puncture, Ann. Int. Med., *34*, 809, 1951.

163. Gaffney, P. C., Hansman, Charlotte F. and Fetterman, G. H.: Experience with Smears of Aspirates from Bone Marrow in the Diagnosis of Neuroblastoma, Am. J. Clin. Path., *31*, 213, 1959.

164. Glaser, K., Limarzi, L. R. and Poncher, H. G.: Cellular Composition of the Bone Marrow in Normal Infants and Children, Pediatrics, *6*, 789, 1950 (Bibliography).

164a. Hanicki, Z. and Libánský, I.: The Cytomorphology of Osteoblasts and Osteoclasts, Acta haemat., *21*, 366, 1959.

165. Jacobson, B. M. and Russell, H. K.: Sternal Puncture in Diagnosis of Malaria, U. S. Naval Med. Bull., *45*, 429, 1945.

166. Jaffé, R.: The Bone Marrow, J. A. M. A., *107*, 124, 1936.

167. Kerr, L. M. H.: A Method for the Determination of Non-Haem Iron in Bone Marrow, Biochem. J., *67*, 627, 1957.

168. Leffler, R. J.: Aspiration of Bone Marrow from the Anterior Superior Iliac Spine, J. Lab. & Clin. Med., *50*, 482, 1957.

169. Leitner, S. J.: *Bone Marrow Biopsy*, New York, Grune & Stratton, 1949 (Bibliography).

170. Limarzi, L. R. and Bedinger, P. L.: A Modified and Improved Sternal Puncture Needle, Am. J. Clin. Path., *18*, 913, 1948.

171. Loge, J. P.: Spinous Process Puncture, Blood, *3*, 198, 1948.

172. Lowenstein, L. and Bramlage, Catherina A.: The Bone Marrow in Pregnancy and the Puerperium, Blood, *12*, 261, 1957.

173. Mayer, E. and Ruzicka, A. Q.: A Method for Studying Numerical and Topographic Problems in the Whole Femoral Marrow of Rats and Guinea Pigs with the Use of Undecalcified Sections, Anat. Rec., *93*, 213, 1945.

174. McFarland, W. and Dameshek, W.: Biopsy of Bone Marrow with the Vim-Silverman Needle, J. A. M. A., *166*, 1464, 1958.

175. Motulsky, A. G. and Rohn, R. J.: The Bone Marrow in Metastatic Malignant Melanoma, J. Lab. & Clin. Med., *41*, 526, 1953.

176. Osgood, E. E. and Seaman, A. J.: The Cellular Composition of Normal Bone Marrow as Obtained by Sternal Puncture, Physiol. Rev., *24*, 46, 1944 (Bibliography).

177. Pease, G. L.: The Significance of Granulomatous Lesions in Bone Marrow Aspirations, Am. J. Clin. Path., *22*, 107, 1952; *ibid.*, *25*, 654, 1955; Blood, *11*, 720, 1956.

178. Rath, C. E. and Finch, C. A.: Sternal Marrow Hemosiderin, J. Lab. & Clin. Med., *33*, 81, 1948.

179. Reich, C. and Kolb, E. M.: A Quantitative Study of the Variations in Multiple Sternal Marrow Samples Taken Simultaneously, Am. J. M. Sc., *204*, 496, 1942.

180. Rheingold, J. J., Weisfuse, L. and Dameshek, W.: Multiple Sites for Bone-Marrow Puncture, New England J. Med., *240*, 54, 1949; Med. Ann. District of Columbia, *19*, 61, 1950.

180a. Rohr, K.: *Das Menschliche Knochenmark*, Ed. 3, Georg Thieme, Stuttgart, 1960.

181. Rohr, K. and Hafter, E.: Untersuchungen über postmortale Veränderungen des menschlichen Knochenmarks, Folia haemat., *58*, 38, 1937.

182. Rundles, R. W. and Jonsson, U.: Metastases in Bone Marrow and Myelophthisic Anemia from Carcinoma of the Prostate, Am. J. M. Sc., *218*, 241, 1949; Blood, *6*, 16, 1951.

182a. Sacker, L. S. and Nordin, B. E. C.: A Simple Bone Biopsy Needle, Lancet, *1*, 347, 1954.

183. SCHLEICHER, E. M.: Staining Aspirated Human Bone Marrow with Domestic Wright Stain, Stain Technol., *17*, 161, 1942.

184. ——— Method for Making Imprints and Direct Smears from Gross Marrow Units, Am. J. Clin. Path., *15* (Tech. Supp. *9*), 8, 1945; *ibid.*, *20*, 476, 1950.

185. ——— Miliary Tuberculosis of the Bone Marrow, Am. Rev. Tuberc., *53*, 115, 1946.

186. ——— An Improved Hematoxylin-Eosin Stain for Sections of Marrow Units, Stain Technol., *28*, 119, 1953.

187. SCHULTEN, H.: *Die Sternalpunktion als diagnostische Methode*, Leipzig, Georg Thieme, 1937.

188. SEGERDAHL, E.: *Uber Sternalpunktionen*, Uppsala, Appelbergs Boktryckeriaktiebolag, 1935 (Bibliography).

189. STURGEON, P.: Volumetric and Microscopic Pattern of Bone Marrow in Normal Infants and Children, Pediatrics, *7*, 577, 652 and 775, 1951.

190. SUNDBERG, R. D. and HODGSON, R. E.: Aspiration of Bone Marrow in Laboratory Animals, Blood, *4*, 557, 1949.

191. ——— and SPINK, W. W.: The Histopathology of Lesions in the Bone Marrow of Patients Having Active Brucellosis, Blood, Supp. I, 7, 1947.

192. TISCHENDORF, W. and FRANK, A.: Tumorzellen im Knockenmark-, Lymphknoten- und Organpunktat, Deutsches Arch. klin. Med., *186*, 534, 1940.

193. TURKEL, H. and BETHELL, F. H.: A New and Simple Instrument for Administration of Fluids through Bone Marrow, War Med., *5*, 222, 1944.

196. WEISBERGER, A. S. and HEINLE, R. W.: Metastatic Carcinoma in Sternal Bone Marrow, Am. J. M. Sc., *217*, 263, 1949; Arch. Int. Med., *91*, 212, 1953.

199. ZLOTNICK, A.: The "Morular Cell" and the "Grape Cell" in Bone Marrow and Peripheral Blood, Blood, *11*, 1140, 1956.

Splenic and Lymph Node Examination

200. ANDRE, R. and DREYFUS, B.: *La Ponction Ganglionaire*, Langres, Expansion Scientifique Francaise, 1954.

202. BLOCK, M. and JACOBSON, L. O.: Splenic Puncture, J. A. M. A., *142*, 641, 1950.

203. BOVER, G. F.: *El Diagnostico por la Puncion Ganglionar*, Valencia, Libreria de F. Garcia Muñoz, 1947.

208. MOESCHLIN, S.: *Spleen Puncture*, London, Wm. Heinemann, Ltd., 1951.

210. MORRISON, M., SAMWICK, A. A., RUBINSTEIN, J., STICH, M. and LOEWE, L.: Lymph Node Aspiration. Clinical and Hematologic Observations in 101 Patients, Am. J. Clin. Path., *22*, 255, 1952.

212. SHIELDS, J. W. and HARGRAVES, M. M.: An Evaluation of Splenic Puncture, Proc. Staff Meet., Mayo Clin., *31*, 440, 1956.

213. TISCHENDORF, W.: Uber die Verwertbarkeit der Lymphdrusenpunktate zur Differentialdiagn. d. Lkt. Erkrankungen, Dstch. Archiv. f. Klin. Med., *183*, 448, 1939.

215. WATSON, R. J., SHAPIOR, H. D., ELLISON, R. R. and LICHTMAN, H. C.: Splenic Aspiration in Clinical and Experimental Hematology, Blood, *10*, 259, 1955.

The Inheritance of Abnormalities of the Blood

220. ALLISON, A. C. and BLUMBERG, B. S.: Dominance and Recessivity in Medical Genetics, Am. J. Med., *25*, 933, 1958.

225. NEEL, J. V.: The Clinical Detection of the Genetic Carriers of Inherited Disease, Medicine, *26*, 115, 1947; Am. Jour. of Hum. Genetics, *6*, 208, 1954; Pediat. Clin. North America, *4*, 325, 1957.

226. NEEL, J. V. and SCHULL, W. J.: *Human Heredity*, 1954, Univ. of Chicago Press, Chicago, Ill.

229. STERN, C.: *Human Genetics*, 1949, W. H. Freeman and Co., San Francisco, Calif

Chapter 2

The Erythrocyte

DISCOVERY OF THE ERYTHRO-CYTE AND EARLY STUDIES

"Small round globules" were described in human blood by the Dutch microscopist, Leeuwenhoek in 1673, but the "ruddy globules" were probably first observed by Swammerdam fifteen years earlier. Malpighi (1665) mistook them for fat globules "looking like a rosary of red coral." Leeuwenhoek made a thorough study of these red bodies, and attributed the color of blood to them.

One hundred years later, William Hewson recognized that these red particles are really flat discs rather than globules and suggested that they "must be of great use" in the body economy. The presence of iron in blood was demonstrated by Menghini in 1747, and Funke isolated hemoglobin in crystalline form in 1851. It was not, however, until 1867 that Hoppe-Seyler demonstrated that hemoglobin has the property of readily taking up and discharging oxygen. It was then that the functional significance of hemoglobin and of the particles in which it is carried, became clear.

During the latter half of the nineteenth century, many studies of the erythrocyte were made. Vierordt (1852) and Welcker (1854) made the first blood counts. Their laborious technic was considerably improved by the invention of the counting chamber and diluting pipet. At the same time, attention was given to methods for measuring the coloring matter of the blood. Vierordt devised a spectroscopic method and Welcker described a colorimetric method. In the first monograph on hemoglobin, Preyer in 1871 referred to several spectroscopic, chemical and colorimetric methods.[14]

Neumann, in 1868, demonstrated that the red corpuscles are formed in bone marrow, arising there from colorless, nucleated elements.[33] With the introduction of the anilin dyes which followed Ehrlich's studies of 1877 and later, the morphological study of the blood and tissues received attention. At the same time interest was aroused in the variations in the size and hemoglobin content of erythrocytes in anemia and in methods for their measurement. These will be described later.

NORMAL DEVELOPMENT OF THE ERYTHROCYTE

The formation of erythrocytes in the embryo and after birth has been described already and their relationship to other cells of the blood has been discussed (Chapter 1). From the multipotential cell of the bone marrow (hemocytoblast,

(85)

p. 37) development follows as a result of a series of mitotic divisions. By measuring nuclei and cells, counting mitoses and chromosome numbers and by a series of calculations, Weicker[47d] concluded that diploid proerythroblasts reproduce themselves by generative division and, simultaneously, they produce erythroblasts which are incapable of reproducing themselves. There follow four erythroblastic generations, each of which is derived from the previous one by halving the nuclear volume and becoming more and more hypoploid. Time relationships and other quantitative aspects of erythropoiesis will be dealt with in a later section (p. 93).

On morphological grounds a number of stages in the development of the erythrocyte have been described. To designate these a variety of terms has been employed. The original terminology will be used here but synonymous terms as applied by various authors will also be given.

Erythroblast was a term used by Ehrlich to refer to all forms of nucleated red corpuscles, pathological as well as normal and is so used here. He considered erythroblasts as being of two main types, a normal or normoblastic series and a pathological or megaloblastic series. The latter he had observed in pernicious anemia during relapse as well as in early embryonic blood. Certin aworkers, however, notably Sabin and her school, have used the term megaloblast in a less restricted sense. The term megaloblast will be used in this book in the sense given it by Ehrlich and followed by Naegeli, Ferrata, Downey, Jones and others[33] (see p. 93).

Four stages in the development of the normoblast can be recognized.

1. **Pronormoblast.**—The pronormoblast (macroblast of Naegeli, proerythroblast of Ferrata, megaloblast of Sabin, lymphoid hemoblast of Pappenheim, "rubriblast,"[4] "prorubricyte"[4]) is a round or oval cell of moderate size (12 to 15μ) or larger (14 to 19μ) which possesses a relatively large nucleus and a thin rim of basophilic cytoplasm. The nucleus is composed of relatively thick strands of chromatin, which has a tendency to clump. The nucleus of the youngest cells in this group, however, may differ but little from that of the myeloblast. Nucleoli are present and may be prominent. There is a very thin or delicate nuclear membrane. At this stage no true hemoglobin can be made out in the cell because of the basophilia and consequently its classification as a member of the red cell series is difficult. As compared with that of myeloblasts and lymphoblasts, the cytoplasm has a tendency to be more homogeneous and condensed; it may appear "thick." The chromatin is somewhat more coarse. In supravitally stained preparations a number of rod-shaped mitochondria are seen in the cytoplasm as well as a slight tint of hemoglobin. In normal marrow these cells are scarce (Plate IV, *11*).

2. **Basophilic Normoblast.** — The basophilic normoblast (basophilic erythroblast of Ferrata, early erythroblast of Sabin, "rubricyte"[4]) (Fig. 2–1, *3 a*) is similar to the pronormoblast except that the nucleoli have disappeared and the cytoplasm may be even more basophilic. The chromatin has the appearance of coarse, granular material, and there is thus little resemblance to the myeloblast. The nuclear structure may assume a wheel-spoke arrangement ("Radkern"). Unlike what is found in plasma cells there is a sharp contrast between chromatin and parachromatin (Plate IV, *12*).

3. **Polychromatic Normoblast.** — The first faint blush of hemoglobin, as indicated by a few pink spots near the nucleus in dry fixed preparations, introduces the next stage which is called the polychromatic normoblast (late erythroblast of Sabin) (Fig. 2–1, *3 b*). The role of ribonucleic acid in the synthesis of the

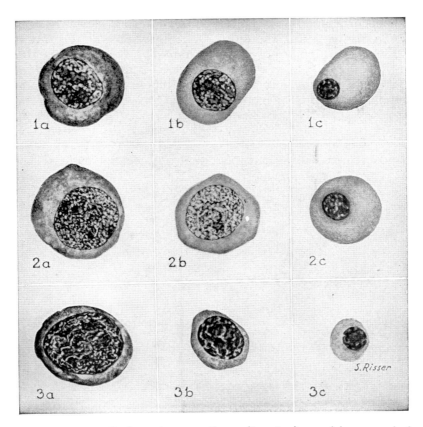

Fig. 2–1.—Nucleated red cells from the rat yolk sac (1 *a*, *b*, *c*), pernicious anemia bone marrow (2 *a*, *b*, *c*) and embryonic rabbit liver (3 *a*, *b*, *c*). Series 3 represents basophilic (*a*), polychromatic (*b*) and orthochromatic (*c*) normoblasts; Series 2 shows megaloblasts in the same order and Series 1 illustrates the appearance of the primitive erythroblasts found in the yolk sac. Dry imprints. May-Grünwald-Giemsa stain, prepared by Dr. A. Kirschbaum. × 1400. (O. P. Jones *in* Downey's *Handbook of Hematology*, courtesy of Paul B. Hoeber, Inc.)

hemoglobin was discussed elsewhere (p. 42). Further differentiation of the cell takes the form of gradual elaboration of hemoglobin at the expense of decreasing basophilia, as well as increasing condensation of nuclear chromatin. Irregular lumps of chromatin are formed, which may stain very deeply. Nucleoli are no longer visible. The nucleus becomes smaller (7 to 9 μ) as may the cell as a whole (12 to 15 μ) (Plate IV, *13*). When supravitally stained, the maximum number of mitochondria will be found in the early phases of this stage, but as hemo-

globin becomes more plentiful, mitochrondria decrease in number.

Sabin found that, in normal marrow, "early erythroblasts" make up about 1 to 4 per cent of all the nucleated red cells while the late forms account for about 26 to 29 per cent.

4. Orthochromatic (Acidophilic) Normoblast. — When the basophilic spongioplasm is not readily demonstrable and the cytoplasm possesses almost its full complement of hemoglobin, the cell is termed an orthochromatic (acidophilic) normoblast (Fig. 2–1, *3 c*) (Plate IV, *14*,

15). Strictly speaking, normoblasts are rarely fully orthochromatic but this term is convenient in distinguishing the more acidophilic from the distinctly polychromatic stage.

In its final stage the nucleus of the normoblast undergoes pyknotic degeneration ("metarubricyte").[4] The chromatin becomes greatly condensed and the nucleus shrinks. It may appear to be an almost homogeneous mass. The nucleus may assume various bizarre forms such as buds, rosettes, clover leaves, or double spheres, or only a faint ring may remain (Plate IV, *16, 17*). That the changing pattern of the nuclear chromatin is not an artifact produced by fixation has been shown by studies with the electron microscope.[43a] Distortions of this process have been described.[15a] Finally the nucleus is lost.[5a] It is generally thought that this occurs by extrusion,[18,43c] but

---

LEGEND FOR PLATE IV

NORMAL AND ABNORMAL ERYTHROCYTES AND PLATELETS

(WRIGHT'S STAIN 1 MM-1μ)

1. Normal red corpuscles (normocytes).
2. Small red corpuscles (microcytes).
3. Large red corpuscles (macrocytes).
4. Exceptionally large red corpuscle (megalocyte) from a case of pernicious anemia.
5. Abnormally shaped red corpuscles (poikilocytes) from cases of pernicious anemia, chronic post-hemorrhagic anemia and sickle cell anemia.
6. Reticulocytes, stained with cresyl blue, as well as Wright's solution, to show the granulo-reticulo-filamentous network.
7. Red corpuscles showing polychromatophilia (diffuse basophilia).
8. Red corpuscles showing basophilic stippling (punctate basophilia); *a*, *b* and *c* are from a case of pernicious anemia, *d* from a case of lead poisoning. The stippling in *d* in much finer than in the other cells; *c* contains a large nuclear fragment; *b* and *d* are diffusely basophilic.
9. Red corpuscles containing Cabot ring bodies. The cytoplasm of *a* and *c* is diffusely basophilic and contains fine "chromatin dust."
10. Basophilic red corpuscles containing 3 Howell-Jolly bodies, a Cabot ring body and fine "chromatin dust."
11 to 18 inclusive. *Normoblasts*, 11 to 17 from the bone marrow of cases of hemolytic anemia, 18 from a case of hypochromic microcytic anemia.
11. Pronormoblast. There are a few tiny nucleoli in the nucleus. The cytoplasm is deeply basophilic but hemoglobin formation is just commencing at the four o'clock position.
12. Basophilic normoblast. There are no nucleoli, the cytoplasm is less deeply basophilic than that of cell 11. There is beginning hemoglobin formation in the upper portion of the cell.
13. Polychromatic normoblast.
14, 15, 16 and 17. Orthochromatic normoblasts. In 16 and 17 there is karyorrhexis. In 17 there is also punctate basophilia.
18. Basophilic "microblast," to be distinguished from a lymphocyte by the opaque grayish-blue color of the cytoplasm and the small size of the cell.
19 to 23, inclusive. *Megaloblasts* from the bone marrow of cases of pernicious anemia.
19. Promegaloblast. Note that the chromatin appears finely granular and is much more homogeneous than that of the pronormoblast (No. 11). The nucleoli are barely perceptible.
20. Basophilic megaloblast. Note the finely divided, mesh-like chromatin, so characteristic of the megaloblast. Compare with cell 12.
21 and 22. Polychromatic megaloblasts. Not only is the color of the cytoplasm changing as compared with that of cells 19 and 20 but the chromatin is becoming aggregated into larger masses. It continues to be rather homogenous.
23. Orthochromatic megaloblast containing two Howell-Jolly bodies.
24. Giant platelet.
25. A few platelets of normal size and one exceptionally large one.

PLATE IV

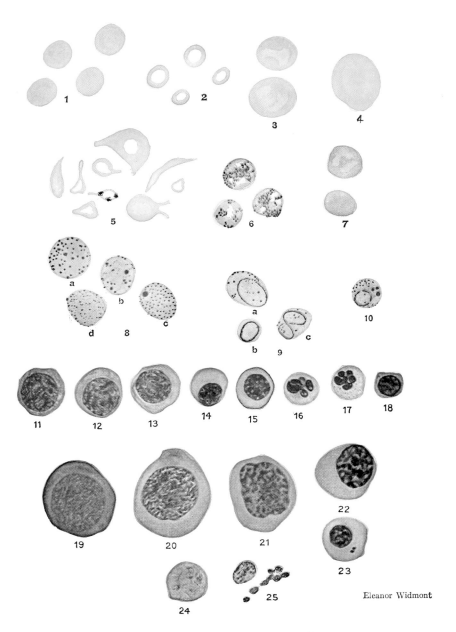

NORMAL AND ABNORMAL RED CELLS AND PLATELETS

(WRIGHT'S STAIN. 1 MM. $= 1\ \mu$)

(Wintrobe, Tice Practice of Medicine, courtesy of W. F. Prior Company)

some have maintained that the nucleus is destroyed by intracellular karyolysis.[8] By electron microscopy hemoglobin has been observed to be deposited in the nucleus while the nucleo-cytoplasmic boundary gradually disappears.[37b] Mitochondria are no longer found.

Orthochromatic normoblasts, together with the moderately polychromatic forms, make up 65 to 80 per cent of the nucleated red cells in the bone marrow.

5. **Basophilia, Diffuse and Punctate, and Reticulocytes.**—Even after the nucleus has been lost, the remnants of the cytoplasmic basophilic substance (RNA) persist for a short time. Methyl alcohol, or similar fixative agents used in staining, cause a uniform precipitation of the basic staining substance and the intensity of the stain is roughly proportional to the amount present. After staining, the cells may appear uniformly blue or gray **(diffuse basophilia)** but more often various shades of basophilia are intermingled with pink staining portions (*polychromatophilia* or *polychromasia*) (Plate IV, 7). The effects of overstaining, which affects all the red corpuscles in the smear, must be distinguished from true basophilia which is found only in a small proportion of the cells.

Punctate basophilia or **basophilic stippling** is the term applied when there are bluish or bluish-black granules in red corpuscles stained by one of the Romanowsky methods (Plate IV, 8). The granules may be fine or coarse, are usually uniform and round but may be angular, and have been seen in the unstained condition as well as by dark-field illumination.[34]

Staining by special methods demonstrates a third type of basophilia, the "substantia granulo-filamentosa" (Cesaris-Demel). These "skein cells" (Plate IV, 6) were first observed by Ehrlich and their significance was appreciated by Theobald Smith, but only much later did **"reticulocytes"** as they came to be

called, assume a position of importance in hematological technology.

"Stippling" is closely associated with polychromasia and may appear in the same cell. Rapid fixation is said to produce a high proportion of polychromatic corpuscles and few stippled cells, whereas prolonged staining has the opposite effect.[8] There is a close parallelism between the numbers of polychromasic and reticulated cells in various samples of blood, although the proportions are not always similar. It has been reported that, with methylene blue and thionin, the structures appearing in other stains as basophilic stippling stain blue, while the basophilic substantia granulo-filamentosa stains red.[34]

The occurrence of stippling in cases of poisoning by heavy metals (lead, bismuth, zinc, silver, mercury) in the absence of a degree of anemia which might be expected to stimulate the liberation of many young cells suggests that these metals damage the erythrocytes. In view of the fact that there is a close numerical relation between the numbers of reticulocytes and of stippled cells in cases of plumbism,[8,40] it is plausible to assume that the membrane of the cells has been injured by the metal and the basophilic substance of young red corpuscles is, in consequence, precipitated even by stains applied after fixation. It is noteworthy that punctate basophilia is found not only in cases of heavy metal poisoning but it is to be seen under a great variety of circumstances, including anemias of various types and, in occasional cells (0.01 per cent), even in the blood of normal persons.[10] It is claimed that stippling can be produced *in vitro*.[9d]

Unlike the granules in "stippled" red corpuscles, those of *reticulocytes* cannot be seen, even by darkground illumination or by phase microscope unless stained. They are brought out by "supravital staining;" *i.e.* mixture of appropriate dyes with blood while wet or before it has dried.

Brilliant cresyl blue, Janus green, Nile blue sulfate, neutral red[39] and, best of all, new methylene blue (Color Index 927)[3] cause a flaky precipitation of the basophilic substance.[38] About 30 seconds is required for the dye to penetrate the wet red corpuscles.[32] If the blood is then allowed to dry, the reticulum will persist for a time but a more permanent preparation can be made by counterstaining with Wright's stain, or any other Romanowsky stain. In counterstaining, the "vital dye" is replaced by the methylene blue of the counterstain.[38]

The reticulum may appear as a narrow band traversing the cell, it may be evenly distributed throughout the cell or it may be so densely packed as to give the appearance of a nucleus. Generally speaking, there is a large amount of reticulum in reticulocytes close to the nucleated stage of the red corpuscle and very little in those which are nearly mature. In "old" reticulocytes only a few granules or scattered threads may be found.[16] The shape and density of the network also depend, however, on a number of physical factors. Thus the stronger the concentration of the dye, the larger and less broken up is the reticulum.[8] Drying of the film tends to produce a fine reticulum. Heating tends to destroy the reticulum, only rods and granules being demonstrable. A change in the pH of the staining mixture towards the acid side results in a finely granular reticulum whereas treatment with dilute alkali produces a stippled form.[39] Strong fixing agents tend to produce diffuse basophilia rather than reticulation. Certain substances such as glucose and sodium salts, inhibit the staining of reticulocytes.[17] Crenation of red corpuscles is said to obstruct the passage of dye into the cells.[8]

The substantia granulo-filamentosa of reticulocytes has been shown by electron microscopy to be the product of the action of lipophilic dyes, which cause coagulation of endoplasmic reticulum granules.[45d] Rod-like or filamentous mitochondria with typical cristae can be seen in reticulocytes as well, but these in themselves probably do not form the filamentous structure of reticulocytes.

Reticulocytes are larger than fully matured red corpuscles. The difference in size is sufficiently great to be appreciated without measurement. In other respects, however, they conform to the general pattern of the red corpuscles; thus the reticulocytes in hereditary spherocytosis are large in comparison to their fellows but they are considerably smaller than those found in the blood of cases of pernicious anemia. When reticulocyte increases occur in cases of anemia a corresponding increase in mean corpuscular volume can be demonstrated, whether the anemia be macrocytic or microcytic.[49a] (Fig. 2–2).

Reticulocytes are more adhesive than adult corpuscles and move about in currents at a much slower rate than mature cells.[8] This adhesive property, like that described for more primitive cells,[21] may account for their tendency to remain within the bone marrow under normal conditions (p. 1049). Their specific gravity is lower than that of adult corpuscles[27] and they tend to collect in the upper portions of suspensions of corpuscles. They vary in their resistance to hypotonic solutions.[6]

Enumeration of Reticulocytes.—The stain is prepared by dissolving 1 Gm. brilliant cresyl blue in 100 ml. normal (0.85 per cent) saline, to which 0.4 Gm. sodium citrate has been added. New methylene blue (Color Index 927) was found to be superior to the classical brilliant cresyl blue because of its uniform performance and the sharp, blue staining of the reticulum.[3] This is prepared by dissolving 0.5 Gm. of the dye in 100 ml. distilled water, to which 1.6 Gm. potassium oxalate has been added.

Equal quantities of dye solution and

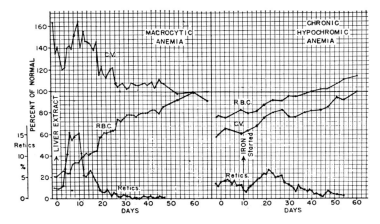

FIG. 2-2.--Influence of increase in reticulocytes on mean corpuscular volume. The chart on the left represents the blood of a case of pernicious anemia treated with liver; that on the right, a case of chronic hypochromic anemia treated with iron. In each case the mean corpuscular volume (C.V.) and the red cell count (R.B.C.) are represented in proportion to their respective average normal values, and reticulocytes are recorded directly. In each case there was a rise in mean corpuscular volume corresponding to the increase in the number of reticulocytes.

blood may be mixed in a capillary pipet, in a small test tube or on a porcelain plate but, *simplest of all*, a drop of blood is placed on a clean glass slide, about twice as much dye solution is added and mixed with the blood and a cover slip is placed on the mixture. Gentle pressure is exerted to produce a thin film of blood, any excess stain and blood is drawn off with a piece of filter paper and the preparation is sealed with petroleum jelly. After the preparation has stood for 5 to 10 minutes, the proportion of reticulated red corpuscles to total red corpuscles is determined. All red corpuscles that contain blue staining threads or granules are counted. In "old" reticulocytes, only a few blue granules or scattered threads will be found, but these should be classed as reticulocytes. The percentage in 500 or, better still, 1000 red corpuscles is counted. An accurate estimate can be made only if the red corpuscles are distributed evenly, without overlapping clumps or rouleaux. There should be no visible conglomeration at the free edges.[32] To attain these objectives the cover glass

must be perfectly flat and the blood must be spread quickly. Counting is facilitated by placing into the eyepiece of the microscope a piece of paper in which a perforation about $\frac{1}{4}$ inch square has been made. Miller's ocular micrometer is a useful adjunct.[3a] Crenated red corpuscles should not be confused with reticulocytes. Their spine-like projections, although refractile, do not stain with brilliant cresyl blue.

In Dameshek's platelet counting preparation (p. 282) reticulocytes may be enumerated as well.

Permanent reticulocyte preparations can be made only by using the "dry," as distinguished from the "wet" method described above, but the method is less reliable. A 0.5 per cent solution of dye in absolute alcohol is prepared. This is spread on cover glasses. Previous warming of the glassware facilitates even spreading. The thin film of dye is polished by gently rubbing the cover glass, face downwards, on smooth paper. Reticulocyte preparations are made by placing a drop of blood on a plain cover glass, inverting this over a prepared cover glass and, when the blood has turned a deep blue-brown color, making blood smears in the usual manner. They are allowed to dry and then are counter-stained with Wright's or any other Romanowsky stain in the usual manner for staining blood smears.

The *margin of error* in reticulocyte counting is great. This is greatest when counts are made on different preparations by different observers and are even large when they are done on the same prepara-tion by different observers. The range of values may be as great as 100 per cent above or below the mean value. Repeated reticulocyte counts by the same observer on the same specimen of blood vary less. It is desirable, therefore, that the same observer make all of the counts on any one patient.

Methods for enumerating reticulocytes in a counting chamber[13] have not been very satisfactory because, with the mag-nification which can be used with the ordinary objective, reticulocytes cannot be made out readily. Björkman,[26] how-ever, has introduced a technic whereby reticulocytes are first stained in a capil-lary pipet, as described above, and after-wards are fixed in a diluent consisting of 0.30 per cent potassium thiocyanate (KSCN) in 0.05 normal sulfuric acid. The fixation process is attended by an escape of hemoglobin from the red cells which allows them to show up more clearly than otherwise.

Numbers and Significance of Reticulocytes.— There is a significant pool of reticulo-cytes in the bone marrow. They have been found to be approximately equal numerically to the number of nucleated red cells.[43b] In contrast to diffusely basophilic or stippled red corpuscles, which are very infrequent in the blood of *normal* persons, appreciable numbers (0.5 to 1.5 per cent) of reticulocytes are normally found. In the embryo, very high values are present (6 to 50 per cent

or higher, p. 35). High values (2 to 6 per cent) are also found in the newborn infant[13,39] but these immature forms dis-appear rapidly and values similar to those in adults are found at the end of 2 to 5 days.[25] Reticulocytes have been reported to be increased during the spring months[13] but a diurnal variation has not been established. Reticulocytosis noted in pregnancy and in the pre-mature infant is usually associated with anemia and thus represents a response of the hemopoietic system. The significance of reticulocytosis in association with de-mands upon the hemopoietic system will be discussed below (p. 114).

In man most red corpuscles are fully matured when they leave the bone mar-row but in other species larger propor-tions pass out as reticulocytes. Reticulo-cytes can probably mature in the circu-lating blood. It is well known that reticulocytes can be demonstrated in oxalated blood as long as 24 hours after it has been collected; if the blood is kept at a low temperature, the reticulum can be demonstrated for as long as six months.[17] On the other hand, if incubated at body temperature, or *in vivo*, as was done in the pleural cavity of a rabbit, there is a progressive decrease in the proportion of reticulocytes.[16] This has been attrib-uted to maturation.

Hemoglobin synthesis proceeds in re-ticulocytes;[2,29] in fact, it has been found that this occurs most actively at the very moment of denucleation and that heme synthesis is conducted by the mito-chondria and globin synthesis by the endoplasmic reticulum.[45d] By means of the electron microscope it has been shown that granules of iron are ab-sorbed by pinocytosis, accumulate in the mitochondria of the erythroblast and are utilized in hemoglobin synthesis. In reticulocytes, iron from the iron-binding protein of plasma is taken up by iron receptors of the reticulocyte membrane by an energy-dependent process.[23] The metal first accumulates in the particulate matter of the cell: stroma, mitochrondria and microsomes. When released from this it is first associated with non-hemoglobin protein, presumably as a step prior to incorporation in hemoglobin.

The "life-span" of reticulocytes will be discussed below.

6. **Mature Red Corpuscle.**—The mature red corpuscle in the unstained state appears greenish-yellow and is circular or slightly oval, with a thinner central area. On the edge it appears biconcave but occasionally it is found to be concavo-convex, bell-shaped or even spherical. Erythrocytes characteristically collect in rouleaux, like a column of coins. This is probably the effect of surface tension phenomena.[30] For further discussion of the mature corpuscle see page 95.

Maturation Time of Erythroblasts and Reticulocytes.—As well as can be judged from available data derived from radio-iron studies and from estimates of the number of cells in each phase normally present in bone marrow, and on the basis of an erythrocyte life span of 120 days (p. 163), the entire process of maturation of the erythroblast to the mature erythrocyte in man probably occupies about four or five days. The doubling time of the nucleated red cells in the marrow is probably of the order of 36 to 44 hours.[11a] Perhaps a third or half of this time represents the generation time (p. 46) of the pronormoblast.[1a] Studies with tritiated thymidine indicate a generation time for the polychromatic normoblast of 15 to 18 hours and possibly a shorter time for the orthochromatic normoblast.[2g] The marrow reticulocyte time may be about 36 to 44 hours, or less, while the time for maturation of reticulocytes in the circulation is about 24 to 29 hours.[11a] These data are in agreement with clinical experience. Thus, in pernicious anemia the maximal reticulocyte response to a

highly effective therapeutic agent occurs in four to six days (p. 452). After hemorrhage, the reticulocyte response begins by the third or fourth day. It seems likely that the increased rate of erythropoiesis in response to various stimuli is not mediated by shortening the generation time of the pronormoblast but more probably is the result of a rapid increase in the rate of differentiation of the multipotential stem cell.[1a]

THE MEGALOBLAST SERIES

As already stated, the term megaloblast was used by Ehrlich to refer to a type of erythroblast seen in pernicious anemia during relapse. This cell differs from the normoblast series not only in size, which is a relatively unimportant difference, but in the structure of the nucleus. The latter has so fine and delicate a structure that the chromatin presents the appearance of fine meshwork or a scroll design (Fig. 2–1 and Plate V). Stages in the development of this cell may be observed which are similar to those found in the normoblast series; namely, (1) **promegaloblast** (erythrogone of Dameshek, "pernicious anemia type rubriblast or prorubricyte"[4]) (Plate V, *A*), a cell 19 to 27 μ in diameter, in which the nuclear chromatin is distributed uniformly without any tendency to clumping, 3 to 5 nucleoli are present and the cytoplosm is usually basophilic (Plate IV, 19). As compared with the pronormoblast there is more cytoplasm in proportion to the amount of nuclear material and there may be perinuclear light areas of hyaloplasm. This cell is similar to the primitive erythroblast of the early embryo; (2) the **basophilic megaloblast** (Plate III, 20) similar to the above cell and possessing an intensely basophilic cytoplasm and no nucleoli ("pernicious anemia type rubricyte"[4]) (Fig. 2–1, *2 a*, and Plate V); (3) the **polychromatic megaloblast** (Plate IV,

21, 22) in which beginning hemoglobin formation can be perceived and the cytoplasm becomes multicolored (Fig. 2–1, 2 *b*, Plate V); and (4) the **orthrochromatic megaloblast** in which the cytoplasm approaches the uniform color of fully developed hemoglobin (Fig. 2–1, 2*c*, Plate V). The nucleus in this stage may show clumping of chromatin, but rarely to the extent seen in orthochromatic normoblasts. In the most mature form the nucleus is shrunk and eccentric, occupying only about a fifth of the area of the cell. This form is difficult to distinguish, except by its size, from the orthochromatic normoblast. In general the cytoplasm is more intensely acidophilic and more abundant in proportion to the nucleus than in normoblasts (Plate IV, *23*).

The chief characteristic of these cells which distinguishes them from the normoblast series is that the fine nature of the nuclear chromatin persists without any tendency to clumping as the cell matures (Plate V). In the later stages the nucleus may have a sieve-like appearance with round areas of parachromatin between the chromatin strands, but there is no "Radkern" and no formation of clumps.[24]

The megaloblast, like the normoblast, is derived, according to various views, from indifferent mesenchyme (reticulum) (Fieschi,[11] Downey) or from the myeloblast (hemocytoblast) (Ferrata, Storti, Jones). Other hematologists, such as Sabin and Doan, have denied the special character of the megaloblast and regard the cell as representing an early stage in the development of the normal erythroblast (see Fig. 1–4). Downey[9b] admitted the difficulty in classifying the earliest erythroblasts as normoblastic or megaloblastic but, with the Italian school of hematologists, and with Naegeli, Jones[24] and others[22] he concluded on the basis of an exhaustive study of slides from sternal aspirations in treated and untreated cases of pernicious anemia and other disorders that megaloblasts and normoblasts constitute two separate series of erythrocytes which can usually be distinguished without difficulty after they have reached the "pro" or later stages of development. With this view the writer agrees. There is less reason to regard the primitive erythroblast of the early embryo (Fig. 2–1, *1 a, b, c*) as the same as the megaloblast,[2b] as Ehrlich assumed.

The rapidity with which the megaloblastic marrow of pernicious anemia can be transformed to a normoblastic one on administration of liver extract or vitamin B_{12} (p. 455) has led to the view that the megaloblast is a reversible morbid modification of the erythroblast.[47c] Although the changes associated with therapy could be accounted for by postulating that megaloblasts are speeded up in maturation and disappear, being replaced by normoblasts,[9b] *in vitro* cultures of bone marrow support the former explanation. It has been observed by a number of investigators that megaloblasts can be transformed in cultures to normoblasts by the addition of normal serum, or vitamin B_{12} together with its binding protein[40b] or folinic acid[47a] whereas the reverse of this can be produced by culturing cells in concentrated pernicious anemia serum.[30a]

A characteristic feature of the megaloblast is asynchronism between nuclear and cytoplasmic maturation. As the cell matures the delicate, unclumped nature of the nuclear chromatin persists whereas the cytoplasm becomes more and more eosinophilic. The degree of megaloblastic change differs more or less in proportion to the degree of deficiency of the hemopoietic principle and hence is proportional to the severity of the anemia. Thus, when the anemia is not severe, in patients who have received inadequate amounts of vitamin B_{12} or folic acid, or when there is an associated

PLATE V

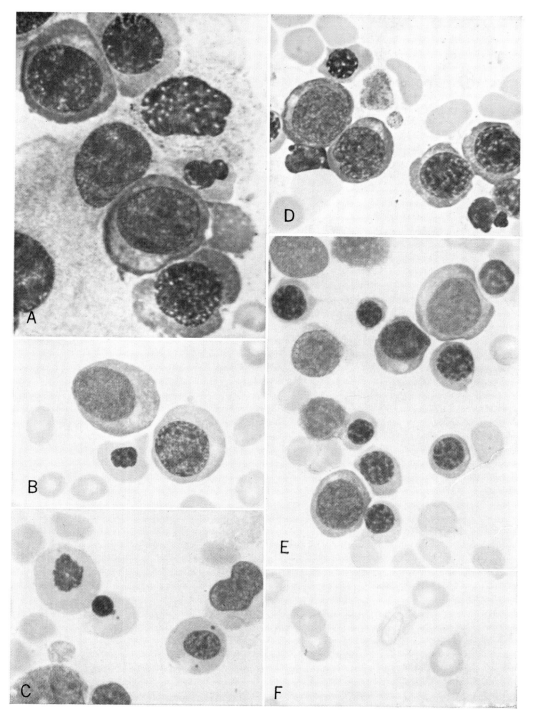

Nucleated red cells from human bone marrow (Wright's stain, × 1220). *A, B* and *C* are *megaloblasts* from cases of pernicious anemia showing various degrees of maturity, the most immature forms being found in *A. D* and *E* are *normoblasts*. The more immature forms are found in *D. F* shows a Cabot ring in a red corpuscle in a blood smear.

iron[13a] or ascorbic acid[40a] deficiency *"intermediate" megaloblasts*[5a] may be observed in bone marrow which do not possess all the typical features of megaloblasts. Such cells present difficulties in differential diagnosis. They must be distinguished from "macronormoblasts," cells in which the nuclear chromatin is coarse. They may show less asynchronism between the maturation of the nucleus and that of the cytoplasm than is seen in typical megaloblasts. Their morphology, nevertheless, differs from that of typical normoblasts and it is assumed that the morphological changes imply a lack of essential building materials.

In the bone marrow of cases of anemia, *giant orthochromatic erythroblasts*[45b] 16 to 40 μ in diameter and containing lobulated, multilobed or fragmented nuclei are sometimes found. These do not appear to be diagnostic of any specific disease and are not necessarily related to megaloblasts.[2a]

THE MATURE RED CORPUSCLE

Structure.—The manner in which hemoglobin is held within the corpuscles and the forces which cause the erythrocyte to maintain its biconcave shape, are poorly understood.[1b] That red corpuscles are flexible, elastic structures can be readily observed if they are watched flowing in the smaller blood vessels. Some investigators maintain that the erythrocyte is composed of a homogeneous, jelly-like substance in the meshes of which hemoglobin is held.[34] Favoring this conception is the observation that red corpuscles can be divided without loss of their contents. Opponents of this theory argue that tampering with the cell causes coagulation of its contents. Others have attempted to show that the erythrocyte possesses a definite, histological membrane within which hemoglobin is held in the form of a hydrophil gel.[27] So far the electron microscope[17b] has given somewhat ambiguous evidence regarding the thickness of the surface layers of the red corpuscle and uncertain information regarding fine structure.[42a] It seems that there is a highly oriented lipid and protein surface ultrastructure surrounding a quantity of hemoglobin which has an orientation more definite than the randomness of a solution. The orientation and thickness of the protein layer are uncertain. The surface ultrastructure may, by acting as a preferential barrier to diffusion, play a large part in determining the difference between the composition of the red cell interior and that of the surrounding medium.[42] The components of either the surface or of the interior may be so arranged as to give the corpuscle its characteristic shape. Ponder[42a] is less certain than formerly of the existence of a palisade arrangement of lipids.

In the interior the hemoglobin molecules must be packed very intimately. Although there are many other constituents (see p. 123), these make up no more than 5 per cent of the dry substance of the red corpuscle. The concentration of hemoglobin is about 34 per cent. It has been calculated that any further increase in concentration would lead to mutual hindrance in the rotation of the molecules and would be likely to affect the reaction rates.[41a]

Because of its biconcave shape the surface area of the red corpuscle is difficult to determine with exactness but it is probably of the order of 140 square microns. It is of interest that the total surface area of the red cells of an average man is about 3820 square meters, 2000 times greater than his total body surface. In spite of this amazingly large surface area, only about 2 per cent of the total hemoglobin in red corpuscles can be anchored at the surface of the red cell, there being approximately 300,000,000 molecules of hemoglobin in each red

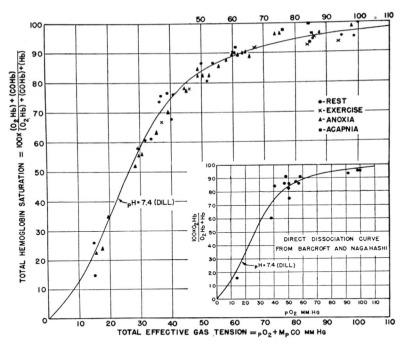

Fig. 2–3.—Human oxyhemoglobin dissociation *in vivo* (Riley *et al.*, J. Clin. Invest.).

corpuscle. On the basis of these calculations, Drabkin discards the theory of membrane-bound hemoglobin. He regards hemoglobin as being present in solution in the red cell.

Function of the Erythrocyte.— Oxygen is transported in erythrocytes by combination with the hemoglobin molecule. The amount of oxygen which combines with hemoglobin varies with the tension of this gas, more entering into combination at high than at low pressures (Fig. 2–3). In the lung capillaries oxygen diffuses into the erythrocyte to form oxyhemoglobin. The carbon dioxide, which exists within the cells chiefly as sodium bicarbonate, loses its sodium to the hemoglobin molecule and diffuses out of the cell. In the tissues, loss of oxygen is promoted by the surrounding low oxygen tension as well as through the action of carbon dioxide. This gas passes into the plasma and cells at relatively high tension, which drives off the oxygen. At the same time,

base is liberated to join with the carbon dioxide.

One of the most striking examples of the importance of the evolutionary process, as well as of the efficiency of the body economy, is found in the mammalian erythrocyte. The essential chemical nature of life is a process of combustion for which a constant supply of oxygen and a simultaneous removal of carbon dioxide are required. In man at rest about 250 ml. of oxygen are absorbed and 200 ml. of carbon dioxide are produced per minute. During exercise these quantities increase tenfold. If the respiratory gases were carried in physical solution in the plasma, our activity could only be one-fiftieth of that actually possible. The development of hemoglobin makes possible the transportation of a hundred times as much oxygen as could be carried by the plasma alone.

In the majority of invertebrates, oxygen-carrying pigment is transported freely in the plasma without the aid of cor-

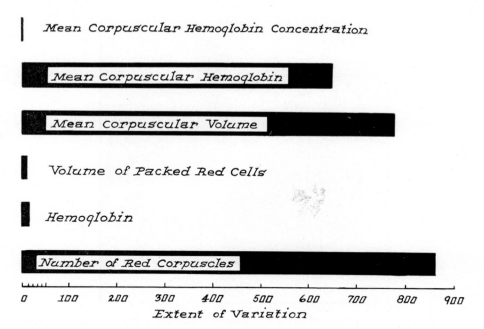

FIG. 2–4.—The red corpuscles of various vertebrates vary greatly in number per c.mm. as well as in mean corpuscular volume and mean corpuscular hemoglobin. However, there is comparatively little variation in volume of packed red cells or in hemoglobin per 100 ml. blood and almost none in mean corpuscular hemoglobin concentration.

puscles. This is a relatively inefficient method. Hemoglobin, as a protein free in the plasma, exerts an osmotic pressure about five times as much as that produced by the plasma proteins. By the inclusion of this pigment in corpuscles the viscosity of the blood is maintained at a low level, water is not drawn from the tissues by it, and the flow of blood containing such a large amount of protein is made possible.[1c] It is thought, furthermore, that hemoglobin functions more efficiently in a phosphate medium and at the hydrogen-ion concentration which is found in the red corpuscle.

Red Corpuscles of Various Mammals and Lower Vertebrates.—Differences in number, size and morphology of the red blood corpuscles of the lower vertebrates and those of the mammalia, furnish further evidence of the efficiency attained through the evolutionary process. Differences in the mass of red cor-

puscles, as represented by the volume of packed red cells, are relatively small throughout the vertebrate phylum[49] (Fig. 2–4). Correspondingly, the range in amount of hemoglobin per unit volume of blood is small, being actually no greater than the physician encounters in anemia. There is, in other words, a relatively constant amount of hemoglobin available for the transportation of oxygen in all vertebrates. However, the differences in the number and kind of vehicles which transport this hemoglobin are extraordinarily great. In the vertebrate phylum, erythrocyte counts as low as 21,250 per c.mm. (in a tailed amphibian, Amphiuma) and as high as 17,920,000 per c.mm. (in the goat) have been found.[49] The size of the red corpuscles is inversely proportional to the red cell count, the corpuscles of one of the tailed amphibia measuring almost 15,000 c.μ, while those of the goat measure

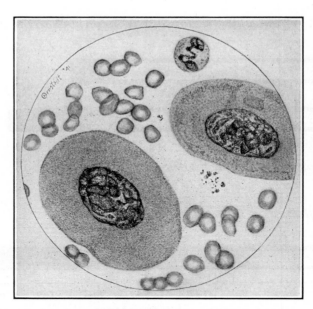

Fig. 2–5.—The giant nucleated erythrocytes of a tailed amphibian (*Amphiuma means*) compared with human red corpuscles. A polymorphonuclear leukocyte is also shown. Drawing of a slide stained with Wright's and magnified × 960.

19 c. μ. In Figure 2–5, the red corpuscles of human blood and those of the "Congo Snake," a tailed amphibian, are compared. (See also Table A–2, p. 1130).

The excessively large corpuscles of the lower vertebrates probably are transported less readily through the blood vessels than the smaller corpuscles of mammalia. What is still more important, the small size of the corpuscles of mammals is adapted for the maximal development of surface. For the gaseous exchanges which occur through the mediation of the erythrocyte, this is extremely important.

The biconcave shape of the erythrocyte has been shown to be the best shape whereby in- and out-going gases may reach and leave all parts of the corpuscle with the least variation in time.[15] Another source of efficiency is the absence of a nucleus. Although the red corpuscle is by no means metabolically inert, as was once assumed (see p. 122), its oxygen consumption is only 0.5 per cent of that of nucleated red cells[26] and less even than that of reticulocytes.[43]

ABNORMAL FORMS OF THE ERYTHROCYTE

Close inspection of normal blood reveals the fact that not all the cells are exactly alike, even in wet films in which they have been subjected to a minimum of trauma. In the presence of disease, the most common alteration from the normal is an exaggeration of the usual variation in size. This is referred to as **anisocytosis.** Cells smaller than 6 μ in diameter are spoken of as **microcytes,** while those larger than 9 μ are called **macrocytes.**

Variation in shape, or **poikilocytosis,** may also occur. The abnormal cells may assume a great variety of bizarre forms (Plate IV, *5*). In most cases of anemia elliptical red corpuscles are found[12] and sometimes more than 25 per cent of the cells may be elliptical (p. 102). **Spherocytes** are relatively small corpuscles which stain bright red and show no central pallor. These are characteristically seen in hereditary spherocytosis and are also found in other forms of hemolytic anemia (see p 604). **Schistocytes** are red cell fragments and are also seen in hemolytic anemias.

Alterations in the shape of red corpuscles which occur in anemia must be distinguished from those produced artificially by trauma during the preparation of the blood film. Under the latter head comes *"crenation,"* which refers to the shrinkage of cells in a hypertonic medium with the formation of irregular margins and a varying number of prickly points. In wet films, when these points are examined from above, they may give the impression of cellular inclusions. Somewhat resembling this is a peculiar poikilocyte, often triangular or crescentic, with one or more spiny projections along its periphery (**"burr cell"**) which has been found in a small proportion of the total red cell population in azotemia especially,[1] but also in cases of carcinoma of the stomach and bleeding peptic ulcer.[45c] Another abnormal form has been observed to make up 70 to 80 per cent of the red corpuscles in the offspring of consanguineous marriages in several different families[9c,35,45e] and was associated with a neurologic disorder, retinitis pigmentosa, a celiac syndrome with hypocholesterolemia and other biochemical abnormalities.[35] These red corpuscles had several, irregularly spaced, large and coarse projections on their their surface which varied in width and length. Many resembled spherocytes with pseudopods, hence the name **acanthrocyte** (thorny red cell). There was no evidence of an exaggerated hemolytic process *in vivo* in these individuals even though the acanthrocytes exhibited a markedly increased lipolecithin and

mechanical fragility. Heat and acid fragility were normal and osmotic fragility was slightly decreased. The condition has been attributed to a mutant recessive allele for a gene which controls the normal architecture of the red corpuscle.

Degeneration of red corpuscles may be only partial and such a change may, in wet films particularly, suggest inclusions or even a nucleus. The most common form is a round or elliptical body (**Maragliano body**) which looks like a vacuole and occupies the center or the periphery of the corpuscle. Changes in the size or position of the body often lead to confusion with early forms of malarial parasites. Rod-like hyaline areas (**bacillary degenerations**) with a vibratory motion, and dark bodies in the center of the red corpuscles (**Ehrlich's hemoglobinemic degeneration**) are further sources of confusion.

Degeneration bodies in red corpuscles may be distinguished from actual inclusions by changing the focus of the microscope. When the structure in question is a degeneration body, it will appear to vary in size as the focus is changed and may even be made to look bigger than the corpuscle. A nucleus or parasite, on the other hand, will simply become more or less distinct.

Still another degeneration form is the "crescent" or "selenoid" body[4a] ("corps en demi-lune") or **"achromocyte,"**[47e] an artifact in the shape of a quarter moon which stains more faintly than intact red corpuscles. It is probably derived from the rupture of red corpuscles and should not be confused with sickle cells.

Because of their biconcave shape, red corpuscles normally appear more pale in the center than at the periphery. **Hypochromia,** hypochromasia or "achromia" are terms used to describe cells in which this normal pallor is increased. The central colorless area may even encroach upon the peripheral colored zone to such an extent that only a narrow rim of coloring matter remains (*pessary forms*).

In macrocytes the central pallor is less marked than in normocytes and may disappear completely. The cells may appear unusually dark. This is not the reverse of hypochromia, however, for the mean corpuscular hemoglobin concentration indicates that the increase in the hemoglobin content of macrocytes is parallel with and not in excess of the increase in size. Consequently, the term hyperchromia should not be used. The central pallor is absent because macrocytes are thicker than normocytes.

A peculiar combination of poikilocytosis and hypochromia may be seen in hypochromic anemia, sickle cell anemia, thalassemia and, especially, in the hemoglobin C abnormality (p. 690). In these conditions one may find corpuscles with a central rounded area of pigmented material, surrounded by a clear ring without pigment, outside of which is the pigmented border of the corpuscle. The terms **"target"** or **"Mexican hat"** cell and **leptocyte** have been used in referring to such corpuscles (Fig. 2–6 and Fig. 13–14, p. 692). They are also frequently found in the presence of jaundice, even in the absence of anemia and may be seen in association with liver disease in the absence of jaundice. Following splenectomy many are found in the blood. Target cells have been produced *in vitro* by suspending normal erythrocytes in plasma or serum rendered hypertonic. Those found in cases of sickle cell anemia may be converted to cells of relatively normal appearance by suspending them in the patient's own plasma rendered hypotonic by dilution with distilled water. Thus it appears that the target cell is one whose envelope is large in relation to its contents.[47b] In this respect the spherocyte is exactly the opposite. Target cells probably sometimes represent cells formed poorly as the

result of faulty materials (abnormal hemoglobin, lack of iron); altered conditions in the cell environment such as those associated with jaundice and dehydration can produce cells of similar appearance.

Very occasionally one may encounter **nuclear remnants** in red corpuscles (Plate IV, *9* and *10*). These are seen more readily in stained preparations than in the wet unstained film. They may take the form of fine bluish dots ("*chromatin particles*"), spherical, eccentrically placed granules about 1 μ in diameter (*Howell-Jolly bodies*) or bluish thread-like rings and convolutions (*Cabot's rings*) (Plate V,*F*). The nuclear derivation of these structures is suggested by the fact that they can be stained with stains specific for chromatin such as methyl green.[34] Howell-Jolly bodies have been observed after splenectomy, in cases of splenic atrophy or of congenital absence of the spleen, in hemolytic anemia, in pernicious anemia and sprue, in thalassemia and in leukemia. It is also not unusual to find them in the later stages of maturing erythroblasts, especially megaloblasts.[19a] It is likely that they are produced by abnormal mitosis when single chromosomes become detached and fail to take part in the formation of the interphase nucleus. Cabot rings are found in the same disorders but their source is less clear. It has been claimed that they are artifacts resulting from damage to the lipoprotein constituents of the surface layer of the red corpuscle.[45a]

Granules which stain with neutral red in supravital preparations, and black in stained blood films,[34] have been found in 0.3 to 0.7 per cent of red corpuscles in normal blood.[20] They appear as single brilliant refractive bodies about 0.5 μ in diameter and, unlike Howell-Jolly bodies, do not take nuclear stains or cresyl blue.

Under the title of **siderocytes,**[9] Grüneberg described red cells in which blue granules, 1 to 20 or more in number, could be demonstrated by the Prussian blue reaction. He found them in small numbers in the blood of normal rat, mouse and human embryos, and in large numbers in mice with a congenital anemia. Siderocytes have since been found in human blood, but they are not seen in significant numbers in the peripheral blood in health. They may be seen in marrow blood[2d] and are present in health in many normal normoblasts, sometimes as a ring about the nucleus.[24a] A higher proportion of siderocytes is found among reticulocytes than in adult red corpuscles. They are usually present in considerable numbers in the peripheral blood after splenectomy. The greatest numbers have been seen in cases of hemolytic anemia with high reticulocyte counts persisting after splenectomy but they are also found in other anemias, except when there is iron deficiency (Fig. 2–6).

These iron-containing granules may appear as basophilic granules ("*Pappenheimer bodies*," p. 626) when blood films are stained by Romanowsky dyes, possibly because the iron in such cells is associated with basophilic staining material. However, the granules of diffuse punctate basophilia differ from siderotic granules, for few of the granules seen in red cells with basophilic stippling are iron-containing.[5] The siderotic granules vary in number and tend to be large, even 2 μ in diameter, when there are only one or two in a cell, and smaller, even barely visible, when they are numerous. They have been seen in red cells of all sizes, shapes and hemoglobin content. Their presence in hypochromic corpuscles suggests that the deficiency in hemoglobin is due to an abnormality in hemoglobin synthesis rather than iron deficiency.

It appears that siderotic granule formation occurs normally in ripening normoblasts except when there is iron de-

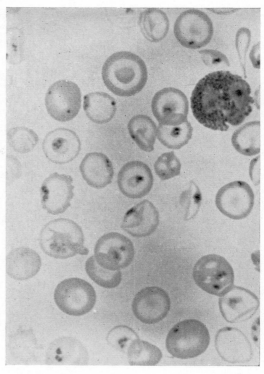

Fig. 2–6.—Siderocytes and target cells in the blood of a splenectomized patient with pyridoxine-responsive anemia. (Wright's stain, counterstained with Prussian blue, $\times$ 1220).

ficiency.[2c,9a] The phenomenon is probably a normal, though transient one ordinarily demonstrable only in a small proportion of red corpuscles. It appears that the spleen is able to bring about the removal of the iron particles without destroying the red cells containing them (p. 1049). This would explain the abundance of siderocytes in the blood following splenectomy.

Siderocytes are most easily demonstrated by immersing the blood smear, already stained in the usual fashion with Wright's stain, in Prussian blue reagent for 10 minutes, after which the cover glass or slide is washed under a stream of distilled water until a pink color appears.[47] This is then allowed to dry and, if the smear was made on a cover glass, it is mounted with balsam. The Prussian

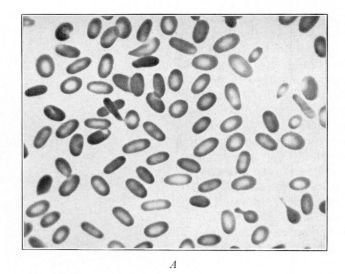

A

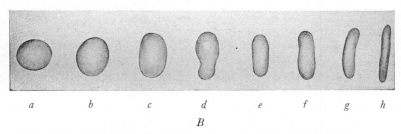

a   b   c   d   e   f   g   h

B

Fig. 2–7.—*A*, Hereditary elliptocytosis. Blood smear, Wright's stain, × 900. *B*, Camera lucida
drawings of erythrocytes found in the blood of persons having the elliptical red corpuscle trait. *a* represents an approximately normal cell; *b*, *c* and *d* represent "oval" forms; *e*, *f*, *g* and *h* represent "rod"
forms. (Florman and Wintrobe, Bull. Johns Hopkins Hosp.)

blue reagent must be made up just before
use and is prepared by adding 25 ml. of
a 2 per cent potassium ferrocyanide
solution to 75 ml. dilute hydrochloric
acid solution (1 ml. concentrated HCl
in 99 ml. distilled water).

Heinz bodies are irregularly shaped,
refractile granules which can be seen in
wet, unstained preparations but are
usually not visible in blood films fixed
with methanol and stained with Romanowsky dyes since the bodies and the
surrounding hemoglobin stain the same
pink color (see p. 624).

ELLIPTICAL RED CORPUSCLES

The red corpuscles of the camel and
those of the non-mammalian vertebrates
are characteristically oval in shape. The
latter are all nucleated but the corpuscles of the camel, like those of man,
are non-nucleated. In man, from 1 to 15
percent of the red corpuscles of most non-
anemic individuals are oval in shape.[12]
As stated earlier (p. 98), such cells
are more common in anemia. In 20
per cent of a series of cases of macrocytic
anemia we found more than 25 per cent
of the erythrocytes to be oval and an equal
number of ovalocytes was found in 6 per
cent of cases of hypochromic microcytic
anemia and in 8 per cent of the simple
microcytic anemias.[12]

Such **"symptomatic ovalocytosis"**
is to be distinguished from an hereditary
anomaly first observed by Dresbach in
1904 and later by Bishop, Huck and

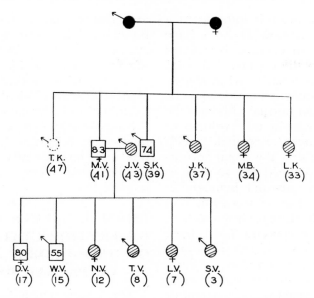

FIG. 2–8.—Family K (negro) showing incidence of elliptical cell trait. The open blocks represent those in whom many elliptical cells were found. The proportion of such cells is given within the block. A hatched circle represents an individual whose red corpuscles were not elliptical, an open circle indicates those not examined, and a black circle refers to those dead. Each individual's age is shown in brackets below the initials. (Florman and Wintrobe, *loc. cit.*)

others. In normal persons and in cases of anemia the great majority of the elliptical cells are of the oval type (Fig. 2–7B, *b, c, d*). In **hereditary elliptocytosis,** on the other hand, rod forms (Fig. 2–7B, *e, f, g, h*) are common and, together with the ovalocytes, may make up 50 to 90 per cent of the red cell population. The demonstration of a family occurrence confirms the diagnosis.

It has been estimated that the incidence of hereditary elliptocytosis in the general population is about 0.04 per cent.[50a] Although especially common in Dutch, German and Italian families, it has also been described in all but the Chinese, Japanese and Hindu.[13b] The trait is transmitted as a simple Mendelian dominant and either sex may be affected (Fig. 2–7). Linkage of the gene for elliptocytosis with the Rh blood type is striking.[37] Elliptocytosis has been observed in association with other hereditary disorders, such as hereditary hemor

rhagic telangiectasia,[41] thalassemia,[8a] sickling and the hemoglobin C trait.[50]

Usually harmless, the condition nevertheless has been found to be associated with evidence of increased blood destruction in about 12 per cent of those carrying the trait.[41] The cases can be divided in three categories: (1) those with no signs of hemolysis; (2) those with hemolysis but no anemia, a state in which increased blood production compensates for the increased blood destruction; and (3) those with hemolytic disease and anemia. Bone changes such as cranial and maxillo-facial-dental abnormalities have been described in patients with hereditary elliptocytosis[37a] as well as splenomegaly[48] and leg ulcers.[19]

Unlike the phenomenon of sickling, with which this anomaly has been confused, in sealed fresh blood preparations these cells do not assume a sickle shape with sharply pointed ends.[12,46] Average ovalocytes have been found to be 8.1 *u* long and 5.3 μ wide, but some as long as 12.2 μ and as narrow as 1.6 μ have been described. In cases of hereditary elliptocytosis even the circular cells may be smaller than normal.[31] As in thalassemia, the erythrocyte counts may be slightly higher than normal although the amount of hemoglobin and volume of packed red cells may be normal.[12] This is due to the fact that the mean corpuscular volume is reduced (50 to 76 c.μ) as is the mean corpuscular hemoglobin (18 to 28 $\gamma\gamma$). The concentration of hemoglobin within the cells is normal.

Elliptical red corpuscles have been found in blood from the visceral blood vessels and in the bone marrow.[44] Their nucleated precursors, however, are round, the anomaly first making its appearance in the reticulocyte stage. Even reticulocytes do not show the degree of ellipticity seen in mature corpuscles.[46] The number of elliptical forms in the blood of a new-born child gradually increases between the ages of twelve days and three or four months, after which their number becomes stabilized.[17a,19]

The factors which determine the anomalous shape of the red corpuscles are unknown. It appears to be a property of the cells themselves and is not due to a peculiar or unique influence of their environment. No abnormalities in their hemoglobin have been discovered.[31a,b] The abnormality persists in various isotonic solutions, in surviving cells in hypotonic saline, in the serum of normal individuals and in the presence of the usual anticoagulants.[46] Although generally normal,[31] osmotic saline fragility has been found to be increased in some instances,[37a] especially after splenectomy.[31a] The reason for the development of increased blood destruction in some cases is obscure. Studies of red cell survival have revealed normal "life span" in some instances and reduced survival in others.[2f,31b,37a] Only in exceptional cases has homozygosity for the trait been associated with hemolytic anemia;[31b,50a] more frequently the trait has been heterozygous in such patients. It has been suggested that combination of the ellipto-cytic trait with another gene not detectable by ordinary clinical and hematologic examination is the cause.[37a]

Splenectomy has been an effective measure in relieving the hemolytic anemia in a number of cases,[2f,31a,b,37a] but poikilocytosis seems to become more marked.[31b]

NORMAL VALUES FOR NUMBER OF ERYTHROCYTES, QUANTITY OF HEMOGLOBIN AND VOLUME OF PACKED RED CELLS

The values which have so long been cited for the normal red cell count in men and women, 5,000,000 and 4,500,000 per c.mm. respectively, are based on determinations made more than a century ago on four subjects. During the past years, the lack of accurate standards has been recognized by workers in the United States, England and the Scandinavian countries. The figures presented in Table 2–1 represent in round numbers the values derived by the author in 1933 from a compilation of the accurate data available up to that time.[77] The data which have been recorded since then, [56b,57d,59,65,74a] are essentially in agreement with those presented. Exceptions[56h] have been rare. The range of normal represents almost the extremes of the observed variations (93 per cent or more) and therefore the blood counts of most healthy adult men and women should fall well within these limits.

"Per Cent" of Hemoglobin.—The habit of expressing hemoglobin values in per cent is an unfortunate custom difficult to overcome. Its unsoundness is obvious when one considers the normal variation in hemoglobin values not only in persons of different ages and sex but also in those of the same sex and age. To be accurate

Table 2–1.—Normal Values for Red Corpuscles at Various Ages

Age	Red cell count (millions per. c.mm.)	Hemoglobin (gm. per 100 ml.)	Vol. packed R.B.C. (ml. per 100 ml.)	Corpuscular values			
				M.C.V. ($c.\mu$)	M.C.H. ($\gamma\gamma$)	M.C.H.C. (%)	M.C.D. (μ)
First day	5.1 ± 1.0	19.5 ± 5.0	54.0 ± 10.0	106	38	36	8.6
2–3 days	5.1	19.0	53.5	105	37	35	
4–8 days	5.1	18.3 ± 4.0	52.5	103	36	35	
9–13 days	5.0	16.5	49.0	98	33	34	
14–60 days	4.7 ± 0.9	14.0 ± 3.3	42.0 ± 7.0	90	30	33	8.1
3–5 months	4.5 ± 0.7	12.2 ± 2.3	36.0	80	27	34	7.7
6–11 months	4.6	11.8	35.5 ± 5.0	77	26	33	7.4
1 year	4.5	11.2	35.0	78	25	32	7.3
2 years	4.6	11.5	35.5	77	25	32	
3 years	4.5	12.5	36.0	80	27	35	7.4
4 years	4.6 ± 0.6	12.6	37.0	80	27	34	
5 years	4.6	12.6	37.0	80	27	34	
6–10 years	4.7	12.9	37.5	80	27	34	7.4
11–15 years	4.8	13.4	39.0	82	28	34	
Adults. Females	4.8 ± 0.6	14.0 ± 2.0	42.0 ± 5.0	87 ± 5	29 ± 2	34 ± 2	7.5 ± 0.3
Males	5.4 ± 0.8	16.0 ± 2.0	47.0 ± 7.0	87 ± 5	29 ± 2	34 ± 2	7.5 ± 0.3

M.C.V. = mean corpuscular volume.
M.C.H. = mean corpuscular hemoglobin.
M.C.H.C. = mean corpuscular hemoglobin concentration.
M.C.D. = mean corpuscular diameter.

one would have to set up an arbitrary normal at least for each sex and for children of various age groups. Obviously this would be an unnecessary complication of a simple subject. Strangely enough, there has never been any attempt made to express red cell count in "per cent" although it is only consistent to do so if we refer to hemoglobin in this manner.

Many hemoglobinometers were standardized in reference to the oxygen capacity of the blood. From the latter the hemoglobin value is calculated on the assumption that 1 gm. of oxyhemoglobin combines with 1.338 ml. of oxygen at normal temperature and pressure (see p. 397). This value is based on the calculation of Hüfner in 1894. Because of the difficulty of obtaining hemoglobin in stable and pure form, Hüfner's observations could not be confirmed. This was offered as a reason for not expressing hemoglobin in grams since by doing so a "false sense of accuracy" would be implied. On the same grounds one should object to expressing hemoglobin in per cent.

While expression of hemoglobin in per cent is thus deplored, for those who continue to use the "color index" it is necessary to establish some figure as the equivalent of 100 per cent. Since 5,000,000 red cells per c.mm. is used as the equivalent of 100 per cent red cells in the calculation of this index, a value for 100 per cent hemoglobin must be chosen which corresponds in the average man and woman to 5,000,000 red corpuscles. On the basis of the data already cited, this **"hemoglobin coefficient"** is 14.5 gm. To convert hemoglobin values to per cent according to this standard, they can simply be multiplied by the factor 6.9 (100/14.5). For the calculation of volume index, the **"volume coefficient"** 43.2 ml. per 100 ml. of blood, has been calculated in the same way as the hemoglobin coefficient. To convert volume of packed red cells to per cent, the volume found should be multiplied by the factor 2.3 (100/43.2).

The necessity in index determinations for retaining per cent values for hemoglobin constitutes in itself an important reason why the indexes should be discarded. It is easier and clearer to dispense with them and to calculate the mean volume and hemoglobin content of the red corpuscles in absolute terms (p. 404).

Physiological Variations. [76]— Healthy individuals differ widely with respect to their blood formulas. These differences are associated to a very small extent with individual differences in body weight, stature and surface area, the red cell count, hemoglobin and volume of packed red cells tending to be higher in heavier and taller individuals. [76]

Diurnal Variations.—Under ordinary circumstances there is a delicately balanced correlation between blood formation and destruction. The blood formula tends to be the same in each individual. During complete inactivity there is little or no diurnal variation in red cell count or hemoglobin. [75] Under normal conditions of activity, variations equivalent to 4 per cent of the mean hemoglobin for the day have been observed. [53b] These occur from hour to hour [74a] but no consistent variations in relation to meals have been observed. Absorption of water in excessively large amounts, or retention of water from other causes, may be followed by an appreciable decrease in hemoglobin concentration whereas dehydration produces the reverse.

Over long periods of time fluctuations may occur [53g] (see p. 109). These can be accounted for in part, perhaps, by variations in fluid intake, exercise and diet.

Muscular Activity.—It has been suggested that exercise is a factor in the maintenance of an efficient hematopoeitic system for, in experiments in animals it has been shown that training may lead to an eventual rise of blood values above the normal. [54,76] Strenuous exercise may lead to accelerated destruction of cells which may, in turn, serve as a stimulus to erythropoiesis. Competitive heavy muscular work has been found to be associated with a decrease in erythrocyte counts, recovery taking place with rest. [57] It is of interest that the average hemoglobin of Olympic athletes was found to be 16 grams and that this mean was the same in those from temperate and from warm climates as well as in the short-distance competitors and in those trained for other types of activities. [53a] However, in these individuals who represented man at his physical optimum, a significant variation, 13.7 to 18.6 grams, was found.

Psychic Factors. — Psychic factors such as excitement or fear, have long been recognized as causing significant increases in the number of red corpuscles. [76] Since abdominal massage and cold baths have the same effect, redistribution of red corpuscles within the vascular system and expulsion of cells sequestered in the spleen and elsewhere have been considered to be the cause of such *"emotional polycythemia."*

A florid appearance and moderate and persistent polycythemia may lead to an erroneous diagnosis of polycythemia vera in individuals in whom none of the characteristic signs of this disease is present. There is no splenomegaly or marked leukocytosis with immature cells in the blood and total red cell mass is normal while the plasma volume is below normal. *"Stress erythrocytosis,"* as this syndrome has been termed, has been observed more often in middle-aged, overweight men than in women and a number of those affected have been mildly psychoneurotic or had some significant anxiety state. [57b]

Sex.—The difference between *males and females* in regard to the erythrocyte

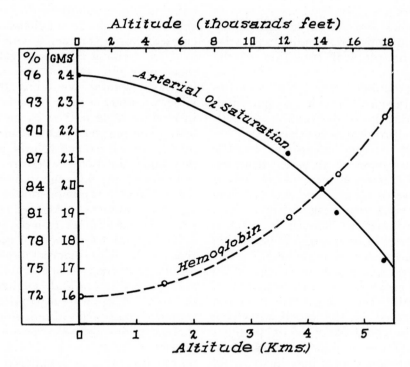

FIG. 2–9.—Relationship between mean arterial oxygen saturation (per cent) and the mean hemoglobin content (Gm. per 100 ml.) in healthy male residents at different altitudes. (Hurtado *et al.*, courtesy Arch. Int. Med.)

formula is well known (Table 2–1). It has not been shown conclusively that there is any correlation between normal menstrual periods and fluctuations in the erythrocytes or hemoglobin[58,71] although a premenstrual decrease has been observed in some women,[53g] possibly as a manifestation of the hydremia which sometimes precedes the onset of menstruation. It is noteworthy that the difference in red corpuscles between males and females does not become manifest until puberty. [56b,57g,74a] Of interest is the reported absence of a significant sex difference among Australian aborigines.[53c] This has been attributed to the scanty loss of blood from menstruation among the women and their high dietary iron intake. In mammals in which menstrual blood loss does not occur, the values for both sexes are the same.[79] The role of sex

hormones in governing erythropoiesis has been discussed already (p. 48).

Low Barometric Pressure.[56g,60,72c] —The anoxemia associated with exposure to low atmospheric pressure, such as occurs at high altitudes, is accompanied by an increase in the erythrocyte count, the quantity of hemoglobin and the volume of packed red cells. The magnitude of the polycythemic response depends on the degree (Fig. 2–9), duration and continuity of the anoxic stimulus but there are wide individual variations in the response. When the period of anoxemia is short, of a few hours' duration, the increase is not constantly found. An increase, when it occurs, is probably the result of hemoconcentration and release of stored blood.[57c] In airplane flight personnel, when exposure to anoxemia is intermittent the occurrence of polycythemia and its level are related to the frequency and intensity of the anoxic stimulus but show great individual variations. The physical condition of the individual may play a part. Thus, following a fatiguing climb to high altitudes the response may be much less than usual, perhaps owing to destruction of cells during the prolonged exertion.

A study of the effects on healthy young adult males of an ascent from sea level to 14,900 feet above sea level showed an increase of plasma and red cell iron turnover rates two hours after arrival. These continued to increase to reach a peak seven to 14 days after the beginning of exposure to the high altitude.[70] The reticulocytes progressively increased in number[60] and the bone marrow appeared hyperplastic[70] but normoblasts have not been observed in the blood nor have changes in the leukocytes or platelets been found under these circumstances. A prompt accompanying increase of intestinal iron absorption was noted.[70] The free erythrocyte protoporphyrin rose and reached a peak at the end of the second month, after which it declined gradually. After six months' residence the iron turnover rate was still elevated.

Native residents of high altitudes showed a red cell iron turnover rate approximately 30 per cent higher than that of healthy subjects at sea level. The amount of free erythrocyte protoporphyrin in their red cells was higher than in residents at sea level.[70] When they were brought down to sea level, the plasma and red cell iron turnover rate decreased progressively for two to five weeks and a marked decrease in erythrocyte protoporphyrin occurred. Red cell life span was not observed to change but the method employed was not adequate to determine if there might be increased destruction during the first week of descent to sea level.

The polycythemia which takes place is absolute in type. The increased circulating blood volume is due to a larger cell mass, with an unchanged or decreased plasma volume.[56g] During ascent or descent changes in blood volume take place only after several weeks. Values for blood volume averaging 100 ml. per kilogram body weight have been found in healthy male natives living at 14,900 feet. The plasma volume averaged only 36 ml. but the red cell volume was 64 ml. per kilogram body weight. In these individuals the average red cell count was 6,150,000, the hemoglobin 20.8 Gm. and the volume of packed red cells 60 ml. per cent. Extremes ranged as high as 7,590,000, 25.4 Gm. and 76 ml., respectively. A slight macrocytosis was also found, the mean corpuscular volume averaging 97.5 c.μ and ranging from 86 to 107. This was attributed to the presence of an excess of reticulocytes even though their number was only slightly greater than at sea level, 1.5 per cent, on the average, as compared with 0.5 per cent. Mean corpuscular hemoglobin concentration was not found to be altered from the normal.

It appears, then, that an increase in production of red cells occurs quite soon in compensation for hypoxia. On descent to sea level there is a temporary diminution or inhibition of erythropoiesis, probably together with greater blood destruction. When natives of high altitudes come down to sea level their blood acquires, after a certain time, the same morphologic characteristics as those found in persons who have always resided there. Thus, chronic anoxemia, even when present at birth, does not modify permanently the activity of the hemopoietic organs. The physical changes often found in natives of high altitudes, such as an increase in the width of the chest in proportion to the height and a lessened rib slope,[76] do not, of course, change. The reduction in the blood levels to those normal at sea level is slower in natives than in subjects coming from sea level made polycythemic by a temporary stay at high altitude. The latter regain their original blood values within 15 to 30 days after their return to sea level.[60]

There appears to be a limit to the capacity for compensatory adjustment. Hurtado[56g] observed that when the arterial oxygen saturation reached a value of about 60 to 70 per cent a decrease, rather than a further increase, in the hemoglobin and red cell count occurred. The hematologic adjustment ceased to be effective at a degree of anoxemia corresponding to an altitude of 20,000 feet. An increasing degree of anoxemia tended to lower the hemoglobin concentration of the erythrocytes, a finding which led to the suggestion that anoxemia ultimately interferes with the production of hemoglobin. Similar observations were made in a Himalayan expedition.[3b]

In normal subjects who are temporarily or permanently exposed to an atmosphere of low barometric pressure, the *excretion* of fecal urobilinogen does not exceed the limits considered normal at sea level but increases with relation to the larger circulatory mass; the normal hemolytic index is maintained[60] and red cell life span is normal.[69] This finding is contradictory to that of Heilmeyer who reported decreased destruction of cells at high altitudes.[56c] The hyperbilirubinemia very frequently found in the natives and in those resident for a long time at high altitudes appears to be related to a lesser excretion of this pigment by the liver, probably on the basis of the anoxic state.[60] The red cell life span in Peruvian natives born and living at an altitude of 12,000 feet has been found to be normal.[52a]

The ascent to high altitudes is accompanied in some persons by symptoms which pass off in a short time or may persist. In other individuals a serious disorder known as chronic mountain sickness develops. This subject will be discussed elsewhere (p. 790).

Even within the ranges of altitude in which large communities are to be found in the United States, differences can be detected in blood values as compared with those found at sea level (p. 104). Thus in 30 males and in an equal number of adult females in Salt Lake City, at an altitude of 4,250 feet above sea level, the mean volumes of packed red cells, respectively, were 49.7 ml. and 44.5 ml. per 100 ml. The standard deviation was 2.3 and 95 per cent of the observations ranged from 45 to 54 ml. in the males and 40 to 49 in the females.

Climate, Temperature and Season.—A seasonal difference in volume of packed red cells has been described, lower values being observed during the warmer periods.[75b] On the other hand, low values for hemoglobin have been recorded in members of an Arctic expedition.[53d] As a whole, however, the available data purporting to show that climate, temperature and season have a significant effect on the blood formula[55b] are not convincing. The contrary seems more probable.[74,75d] Disease and malnutrition may well explain lower values as compared with those recorded as "normal," in Japanese[72a,73a] and other groups. Almost identical values have been found in healthy subjects in this country and in East Africa[57d] and Malaya.[74] The absence of the fresh color of the cheeks and the "picture of health" in individuals residing in tropical and subtropical regions, once led to the impression that a tropical climate causes a "physiological" anemia. This conception has been shown to be quite incorrect, for the blood of healthy persons in such climates contains as many or more red corpuscles and corresponding amounts of hemoglobin as does that of residents of temperate zones.[59a,76]

Age.—The most striking variation in the erythrocytic formula is that related

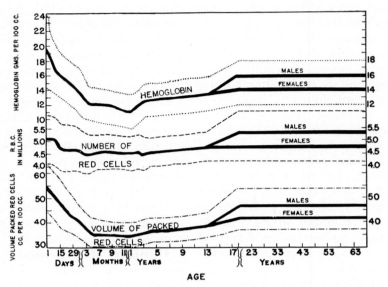

FIG. 2–10.—Normal curve for hemoglobin, red cells and volumes of packed red cells, from birth to old age. The mean values are heavily outlined. The range of variation is indicated by dotted lines for hemoglobin, interrupted lines for red cell count and dotted interrupted lines for volume of packed red cells. The scales for hemoglobin, red cell count and volume of packed red cells are similar and therefore the relative changes in these three values are apparent on inspection. The scale for age, however, is progressively altered. (Derived from the data of Williamson, Appleton, Haden and Neff,[76] Merritt and Davidson,[61] Poncher, Guest, Osgood and Baker,[65] Kato, Mugrage and Andresen[63] and the author.[77])

to age. *At birth* the values for hemoglobin and volume of packed red cells are usually very high, averaging 19.5 gm. and 54 ml. respectively. The recorded data show considerable variation (25 per cent) about these averages[53f,55f,56] and values as high as 27 gm. and 68 ml. respectively, have been reported. Erythrocyte counts as high as 6,800,000[61]—even 9,670,000[56d] have been noted, but the average erythrocyte count at birth is usually in the neighborhood of 4.8 million cells with a variation of about 0.5 to 1.0 million on either side of this mean. The recorded differences in findings can be accounted for, in part, by the fact that values as much as 15 per cent higher are found when the umbilical cord of the newborn is not clamped until the placenta has separated as compared with those obtained from infants whose cords are clamped immediately at birth; and in part by the fact that blood obtained from

the peripheral capillaries, as by puncturing the heel, yields significantly higher values than venous blood.[54a] An important factor is the shift of fluid from the vascular compartment to the tissues immediately after birth.[55d]

As shown in Figure 2–9 and in Table 2–1 the initial high values begin to fall after a week or more. At the end of four weeks a substantial change is usually evident.[55d] The decrease in hemoglobin and in volume of packed red cells is much more rapid than the fall in red cell count. This is due to the appearance of smaller corpuscles. These changes continue at a slower rate for the succeeding two or three months and even more slowly after that. There is some disagreement regarding the time at which the lowest blood values are reached, some observers placing this point at the end of two or three months,[55f,75a] and others at about five months. The determining factor probably is the time at which the milk diet of the infant is supplemented with iron containing foods. At eighteen months the average red cell count is 4,500,000, the hemoglobin 11.5 gm. and the volume of packed red cells 35 ml. Variations of 10 per cent above or below these values are common and still greater differences are sometimes seen in apparently healthy-children.[56,57f,74a]

The high values found in the blood at birth have been attributed to alterations in oxygen tension. Studies of the oxygen content and oxygen saturation of the blood in the umbilical cord of the normal human fetus have shown a gradual fall in both these values as term approaches.[73b] It is not generally appreciated that the high values for hemoglobin and volume of packed red cells which are found at birth are somewhat misleading in giving the impression that polycythemia is present at that time. As will be described later (p. 112), the cells of the newborn are larger than normal adult corpuscles and their hemoglobin content is correspondingly greater. This macrocytosis is, in fact, like that of the fetus (p. 34) but less in degree. The changes which take place after birth are probably attributable in part to a shorter corpuscular life span as compared with that of adult-red cells[56f] but this difference probably is not sufficient to account for all the changes which occur in erythropoiesis in infants. Atrophy of erythropoietic tissue in the liver has been proposed as one additional factor,[57a] the replacement of the fetal macrocytes by post-natal normocytes is another but the altered oxygen saturation of the blood after birth and the demands on the hemopoietic system introduced by rapid growth are probably the most important factors.[55d]

During the *second, third and fourth years of life* there is a gradual increase in the blood values[74a] and during the succeeding years an even more gradual change occurs until at puberty the values in boys and girls are almost equal to those found in adult women.[56b,74a] From this time on, changes in the blood of girls are slight[57e] but the red cell count, hemoglobin and volume of packed red cells of boys rise rapidly to attain the figures characteristic of the adult male.

After the sixth decade of life many workers have found a gradual decrease in the values for red cell count, hemoglobin and volume of packed red cells in men and women,[56b,64b] However, this has not been true in all the groups which have been studied.[55e] The fact that males living alone were found to have lower hemoglobin levels than those living with their wives in their own homes[56e] suggests that malnutrition may be one factor responsible for the declining values found in old age. This probably explains the very low values reported in studies carried out in institutions.[64]

NORMAL VALUES FOR THE SIZE AND HEMOGLOBIN CONTENT OF THE RED CORPUSCLE

The data in Table 2–1 for **mean corpuscular volume, hemoglobin** and **hemoglobin concentration** in normal adults are based on an earlier analysis of values for nearly 700 individuals.[78] Reports made since that time are either in exact agreement with those given or differ so slightly that the mean values remain the same when these additional data are used.[53,58a,59,71] The normal range of variation has been determined statistically and represents the values found in 85 to 88 per cent of normal persons.

The same data[78] make it possible to define **microcytosis, macrocytosis** and **hypochromia.** The probability that a mean corpuscular volume of 79 c. μ, when determined by the methods described elsewhere (p. 408), represents an abnormally low value (microcytosis), or that a volume of 95 c.μ represents an abnormally high value (macrocytosis), is 49:1, and values of 75 and 99 c.μ respectively, are certainly indicative (1999:1) of microcytosis or macrocytosis. Likewise the probability that a mean corpuscular hemoglobin concentration of 31 per cent is abnormally reduced is 37:1 and the probability for a concentration of 30 per cent is 332:1.

It cannot be emphasized too often that these statistics are valid only when scrupulous care is taken in carrying out the red cell count and in determining the hemoglobin and volume of packed red cells on which the corpuscular constants are based. Unless such measurements are made with care, they are better not done at all. The principles and technic of blood examinations and the errors inherent in the various methods are discussed in Chapter 8. It remains to be seen whether the introduction of machines for counting red corpuscles (p. 390) will give different normal values from those cited above. In our own laboratory no differences have been found.

The normal **mean diameter** of red cells, measured after drying and staining, is variously given as 7.2 to 7.9 μ[42,55,76] Means as low as 6.9[67] and 6.5 μ[55] have been found in normal persons. In individual preparations, cells as small as 4.75 μ and as large as 9.5 μ may be found[67] but generally the greatest variation in the diameters of the cells is 3.5 μ[55]. Diameters measured in wet films are 0.8 to 1 μ greater than those mentioned above.

The normal **mean corpuscular thickness** has been given as 2.14 μ,[67] 2.05 μ or 1.84 μ.[76]

Physiological Variations.—Generally speaking, when technical factors are considered, the size and hemoglobin content of the red corpuscles are quite constant during health. Several observers have recorded differences between the **sexes** in regard to mean diameter

and mean corpuscular volume.[52,76] Were it not for the fact that the difference in each case has been in the same direction,[51,65,78] namely in indicating that the cells of females are slightly larger, this observation might be entirely disregarded for the differences noted have been only slight (0.14 μ in diameter and 2 to 4 c.μ in volume). In any event, the difference is too small to be of clinical significance.

Diurnal variations in the size of cells have been described,[67] but none of the observed changes have been significantly greater than those which might be attributed to variations inherent in the technic. There may be a slight variation from day to day but this does not exceed 4.5 per cent.[78]

The evidence regarding the effects of **exercise** is conflicting. Some writers have described an increase in the size of the cells,[67] while others have denied this. Smith,[72] in carefully controlled observations, reported that strenuous exercise for two minutes was followed by an average *decrease* in mean corpuscular volume from 90 to 82 c.μ and a corresponding decrease in mean corpuscular hemoglobin.

Conflicting reports have been made regarding the effects of alterations in the hydrogen-ion concentration of the blood.[66,76]

Low barometric pressure has been reported as causing an increase in the mean size of the cells,[56g,73] and has been attributed to increased hemopoietic activity. At altitudes up to 8720 feet, however, Lewis and his associates[58b] could find no definite trend in any of the corpuscular constants.

Quite different from the variations mentioned above are the **changes** which occur in the size and hemoglobin content of the red corpuscles **from** the time of **birth until adult life** is reached (Table 2–1). These are regularly encountered and are of such magnitude that they are readily appreciated. At birth the mean corpuscular volume is usually about 106 to 115 c.μ but differences of 10 per cent on either side of this range may be observed.[56] A corresponding increase in mean corpuscular hemoglobin (35 to 38 $\gamma\gamma$) is found while the mean corpuscular hemoglobin concentration is the same as in adults. Mean diameters of 8.25 to 8.63 μ have been reported.[76]

The macrocytosis persists for several weeks but at the end of two weeks a substantial decrease in the mean size of the cells is usually evident.[56,75c] At the end of about two months adult values are reached. The decrease in the size and hemoglobin content of the cells continues, however, and an upward rise of the curve does not begin until the age of one year or eighteen months.[52] During this period the mean corpuscular volume may be as low as 65 c.μ or as high as 85 c.μ.[63] The mean corpuscular hemoglobin ranges from 20 to 27 $\gamma\gamma$ and even mean corpuscular hemoglobin concentration may be slightly reduced (31 to 32 per cent).[56]

The erythrocytes in children of all ages characteristically remain smaller than those of adults and it is not until puberty or later that cells of the size and hemoglobin content of those of adults are found. The mean corpuscular diameter in the aged has been found to be significantly greater than in adult life.[72b]

It is of interest that, in spite of these marked changes in the size and hemoglobin content of the red corpuscles, the mean corpuscular hemoglobin concentration changes little or not at all. The ratio of hemoglobin to volume of packed red cells, which this constant expresses, tends in fact, to remain the same not only under different conditions in normal man, but in the blood of other vertebrates as well.[49] The *mean corpuscular weight* has been found to be 96.8 micromicrograms.[53e]

8

THE RESPONSE TO INCREASED DEMANDS FOR HEMOGLOBIN AND RED CORPUSCLES

The daily breakdown of cells damaged during their interminable passage through the blood vessels acts as a continuous stimulus to blood formation. The passage of new cells into the circulation is manifested by the presence of reticulocytes in normal blood. Other immature forms, however, are usually absent.

When the need for new cells is increased, it can be met by two means:

(*a*) **Role of the Spleen.**—According to Barcroft[1d] in the dog, cat and horse the spleen acts as a "kind of fine adjustment" for varying temporary demands. It is a reservoir for red corpuscles which can be called upon in emergency. During life it is two to four times larger than after death and this difference in size is chiefly made up by the content of red corpuscles. Stimuli such as severe exercise, sudden loss of blood, and diminished oxygen supply (asphyxia, carbon monoxide poisoning, diminished atmospheric pressure) cause the spleen to contract and deliver corpuscles to the circulation.

More recent studies have modified somewhat the concept drawn from Barcroft's experiments. Emotional stimuli, epinephrine and drugs stimulating the sympathetic nervous system (eesrine) have been found, in adult intact dogs, to cause a rise in the venous hematocrit, without an increase in the circulating cell mass. Following sodium pentobarbital anesthesia, however, red cells appear to be sequestered from the circulation and then administration of epinephrine produces an increment in circulating cells as great as 37 per cent of the total cell mass.[56a] In splenectomized animals a similar effect is produced but the increased mass of circulating cells is only about half as great as that obtained in the intact dog.

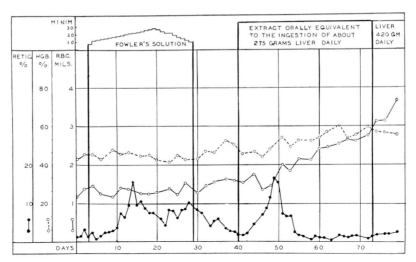

FIG. 2–11.—Effect of the daily administration in pernicious anemia of Fowler's solution (potassium arsenite) followed in a subsequent period by liver extract. The reticulocyte response to Fowler's solution, although irregularly maintained for over twenty days, was not associated with a significant increase of the red blood cells or of the hemoglobin. The subsequent orderly reticulocyte response to liver extract is typical in time of onset and duration, and was followed by a rapid rise of the red blood cell count characteristically exceeding the rate of hemoglobin production. (Minot and Castle, courtesy of Lancet.[36])

In man the rôle of the spleen as a reservoir has not been found to be as important or as specialized as was assumed on the basis of Barcroft's experiments.[64a] Thus exercise and epinephrine have been observed to cause an increase in hemoglobin and volume of packed red cells even in splenectomized subjects. This is accompanied by a decrease in plasma volume.[55a]

(b) **Increased Activity of the Hematopoietic System.**—The same stimuli, as well as blood destruction and other factors which are not well understood, and also the administration of essential hemopoietic factors such as vitamin B_{12} and iron when these substances are lacking, call forth an increased activity of the hematopoietic system. This can be recognized by examination of the blood.

1. **Reticulocytes.**—An increase in the number of reticulocytes in the circulation is the surest index of accelerated hematopoiesis. In response to an appropriate stimulus the percentage of these cells rises, usually within two to ten days and, increasing rapidly, their number reaches a maximum within a period of three to ten days thereafter (Fig. 2–11.) This rise is a steady and progressive one and is followed by a slower and somewhat less regular decline. The first reticulocytes which appear are "young," with large amounts of reticulum, while later the cells contain less and less reticulum—presumably older forms. Up to the peak of the reticulocyte curve, the increase in the total red cell count is only such as can be accounted for by the increment of reticulocytes. The decline of the reticulocyte curve to normal values is followed, if adequate material for blood formation continues to be available, by a rise in the quantity of mature corpuscles. These cells tend to be more and more of normal size and hemoglobin content. Thus all of the morphological changes which occur are in the direction of the restoration of normal conditions with mature red corpuscles replacing the young and probably less efficient forms (see Fig. 2–2, p. 91).

The reticulocyte curve described above can be observed not only in response to adequate therapy in pernicious anemia, as is now universally known, but also when iron is given in conditions of iron deficiency, as well as following such stimuli as acute blood loss when adequate blood building material is available and the hemorrhage has ceased.[36] From a diagnostic standpoint, the reticulocyte reaction is very valuable for if, in the last-mentioned instance, bleeding is continuing, the reticulocyte percentage will remain elevated as long as blood building material is available. Only in cases of chronic blood loss in which iron deficiency has developed, does the proportion of reticulocytes fall and even in such cases a suddenly increased loss of blood may cause a reticulocytosis. In cases of chronic blood destruction, as in hereditary spherocytosis or in sickle cell anemia, the stimulus to hematopoiesis persists while materials for cell building are probably in large measure preserved. In such cases the reticulocytes remain at a continuously high level (15 to 40 per cent) for many years.

Factors Governing the Magnitude of Reticulocyte Response.—The magnitude of the reticulocyte response depends on the size of the stimulus, the quantity of blood building material available and the reactive state of the bone marrow. Under the first head may be included the seriousness of the need for new cells as indicated by the degree of anemia and as controlled by the extent of blood loss or blood destruction, or the degree of deficiency as the case may be. The more severe the anemia the greater the reticulocyte response, other things being equal.

Under the second head may be added, in reference to the deficiency anemias, the amount of active material given, the portal of entry and the rate at which it is given. As will be considered in greater detail in the discussion of these anemias,

there is a direct relationship up to a certain maximal point between the amount of material given and the peak of the rise in reticulocytes. Again, the daily administration of small doses of active material tends to produce a prolonged low reticulocyte curve with a delayed and not very acute apex, whereas a single massive dose produces a relatively early and high peak. It is of interest in this respect, however, that given the same conditions, differing only in route of administration of maximally effective amounts of material, the absolute numbers of reticulocytes poured forth are practically equal.

The reactive state of the bone marrow is affected by the general condition of of the patient. Thus the presence of arteriosclerosis, severe damage to various internal organs, toxic factors such as those associated with nitrogen retention, intercurrent infection, and faulty absorption of orally administered material, all have a significant depressing effect on the reticulocyte response and the subsequent rise in erythrocyte count.

An increase in the number of reticulocytes does not, however, necessarily mean a physiological and orderly response to specific stimuli. In various types of myelophthisic anemia, as in that associated with metastatic carcinoma, in leukemia and following the administration of various drugs (e.g., potassium arsenite, Fig. 2–11) and other substances (especially when given parenterally), reticulocytosis may occur which is not the prognostically favorable reaction which has been discussed heretofore. The mechanism underlying the release of the cells in such instances is not understood. It is generally thought that abnormal cells in the bone marrow, or excessive numbers of relatively normal cells, act either as "irritants" to the erythroblastic tissue or through excessive multiplication of cells in a limited space, cause crowding out of reticulocytes and other immature cells.

In such cases the reticulocyte curve tends to be irregular, and frequently it is maintained for several weeks. The progressive alteration of the age of the reticulocyte towards the more mature forms is lacking and the young reticulocytes are accompanied by many other immature erythrocytes, particularly nucleated red cells. Furthermore, the erythrocyte count usually fails to rise.

2. **Other Morphological Changes in the Red Corpuscles.**—Of much less significance are other changes in the morphology of the red corpuscles. New cells which are being liberated into the circulation tend to be larger than their fellows. Macrocytes and, to a lesser extent, polychromatophilia are, like reticulocytosis, manifestations of orderly, and probably efficient new blood formation. Nucleated red corpuscles, although they usually reflect increased activity, do not represent orderly maturation in the same sense as reticulocytosis. They find their way into the circulation probably because they have been swept out of suddenly opened capillaries. Their presence in the blood, in fact, is an unfavorable sign, especially in congestive heart failure.[55e]

3. **Thrombocytosis and Leukocytosis.**—The morphological changes in the red corpuscles which occur in response to a suddenly increased demand for new cells are frequently accompanied by an *increase in the numbers of platelets* and in the numbers of those forms of the *leukocytes* which are produced in the bone marrow. The thrombocytosis may appear before an increase in reticulocytes is found. The leukocyte count may rise even as high as 60,000 per c.mm. (in acute hemolytic anemia), and this is accompanied by a "shift to the left."

In the chapter which follows, the chemical structure of the red corpuscle will be considered together with what is known regarding the substances needed for its production. The fate of the red corpuscle, its breakdown and the disturbances which may occur in pigment metabolism, as well as hemagglutination and hemolysis will also be discussed.

BIBLIOGRAPHY

Development, Morphology, Structure, Function and Shape of the Erythrocyte

1. AHERNE, W. A.: The "Burr" Red Cell and Azotaemia, J. Clin. Path., *10*, 252, 1957.
1a. ALPEN, E. L. and CRANMORE, DORIS: Observations on the Regulation of Erythropoiesis and on Cellular Dynamics by Fe^{59} Autoradiography, *in The Kinetics of Cellular Proliferation*, edited by F. Stohlman, Jr., New York, Grune and Stratton, 1959, p. 290.
1b. ANDERSON, HELEN M. and TURNER, J. C.: Relation of Hemoglobin to the Red Cell Membrane, J. Clin. Invest., *39*, 1, 1960.
1c. BARCROFT, J.: The Significance of Hemoglobin, Physiol. Rev., *4*, 329, 1924.
1d. ———— Alterations in the Volume of the Normal Spleen and Their Significance, Am. J. M. Sc., *179*, 1, 1930.
2. BELCHER, E. H. and COURTENAY, V. DOREEN: Studies of Fe^{59} Uptake by Rat Reticulocytes *in vitro*, Brit. J. Haemat., *5*, 268, 1959.
2a. BERMAN, L.: The Clinical Significance of Cellular Gigantism in Human Erythropoiesis, J. Lab. & Clin. Med., *32*, 793, 1947.
2b. BERNARDELLI, E., RONDANELLI, E. G. and GORINI, P.: Ricerche Citometriche Sull' Eritroblasto Embrionario, Haematologica, *37*, 1, 1953.
2c. BESSIS, M. and BRETON-GORIUS, J.: Étude au microscope électronique des granulations férrugineuses des érythrocytes normaux et pathologiques, Rev. hémat., *12*, 43, 1957; Compt. rend. Acad. d. sc., *244*, 2846, 1957.
2d. BILGER, R. and TETZNER, K. H.: Uber siderophile Einschlusskorperchen in den Zellen des erythropoetischen Systems, Acta haemat., *9*, 137, 1953.
2e. BJORKMAN, S. E.: Method for Determining Absolute Reticulocyte Count, Scandinav. J. Clin. & Lab. Invest., *10*, 435, 1958.
2f. BLACKBURN, E. K. *et al.*: Hereditary Elliptocytic Haemolytic Anaemia, J. Clin. Path., *11*, 316, 1958.
2g. BOND, V. P. *et al.*: Cell Turnover *in* Blood and Blood-forming Tissues Studied with Tritiated Thymidine, *in The Kinetics of Cellular Proliferation*, edited by F. Stohlman, Jr., New York, Grune and Stratton, 1959, p. 188.

3. Brecher, G.: New Methylene Blue as a Reticulocyte Stain, Am. J. Clin. Path., *19*, 895, 1949.

3a. Brecher, G. and Schneiderman, M.: A Time-Saving Device for the Counting of Reticulocytes, Am. J. Clin. Path., *20*, 1079, 1950.

3b. Brendel, W.: Anpassung von Atmung, Hämoglobin, Körpertemperatur und Kreislauf bei langfristigem Aufenthalt in grossen Höhen (Himalaya), Arch. f. d. ges. Physiol., *263*, 227, 1956.

4. Committee for Clarification of the Nomenclature of Cells and Diseases of the Blood and Blood-forming Organs, Second Report, Am. J. Clin. Path., *19*, 56, 1949.

4a. Cuadra, M.: Selenoid (Crescent) Bodies, Blood, *13*, 258, 1958.

5. Dacie, J. V. and Doniach, I.: The Basophilic Property of the Iron-Containing Granules in Siderocytes, J. Path. & Bact., *59*, 684, 1947.

5a. ——— and White, J. C.: Erythopoiesis, J. Clin. Path., *2*, 1, 1949.

6. Daland, G. A. and Zetzel, L.: The Resistance of Reticulocytes to Hypotonic Solutions of Sodium Chloride and of Plasma, Am. J. Med. Sc., *191*, 467, 1936.

8. Davidson, L. S. P.: The Basophilic Substance of the Erythrocyte, Edinburgh Med. J., *37*, 425, 1930.

8a. de Vries, S. I., de Jong, J. and Frenkel, M.: Anémie elliptocytaire hémolytique, Schweiz. med. Wchnschr., *89*, 1078, 1959.

9. Doniach, I., Grüneberg, H. and Pearson, J. E. G.: The Occurrence of Siderocytes in Adult Human Blood, J. Path. & Bact., *55*, 23, 1943.

9a. Douglas, A. S. and Dacie, J. V.: The Incidence and Significance of Iron-containing Granules in Human Erythrocytes and Their Precursors, J. Clin. Path., *6*, 307, 1953.

9b. Downey, H.: The Megaloblast-normoblast Problem, J. Lab. & Clin. Med., *39*, 837, 1952.

9c. Druez, G.: Un nouveau cas d'acanthocytose, Rev. hémat., *14*, 3, 1959.

9d. Engelbreth-Holm, J. and Plum, C. M.: Production of Stippled Erythrocytes *in vitro*, Nature, *166*, 990, 1950.

10. Falconer, E. H.: The Clinical Significance of Punctate Basophilia in the Erythrocyte, Ann. Int. Med., *12*, 1429, 1939.

11. Fieschi, A. and Astaldi, G.: La cultura in vitro del midollo osseo: Problemi di fisiopatologia ematologica studiati con la tecnica della cultura dei tessuti, Pavia, Tipografia del Libro, 1946, 309 pp.

11a. Finch, C. A.: Some Quantitative Aspects of Erythropoiesis, Ann. New York Acad. Sc., *77*, 410, 1959.

12. Florman, A. L. and Wintrobe, M. M.: Human Elliptical Red Corpuscles, Bull. Johns Hopkins Hosp., *63*, 209, 1938.

13. Friedlander, A. and Wiedemer, C.: The Reticulocyte Count in Normal and in Abnormal Conditions, Arch. Int. Med., *44*, 207, 1929.

13a. Fudenberg, H. and Estren, S.: The Intermediate Megaloblast in the Differential Diagnosis of Pernicious and Related Anemias, Am. J. Med., *25*, 198, 1958.

13b. Garrido-Lecca, G., Merino, C. and Lunga, G., Jr.: Hereditary Elliptocytosis in a Peruvian Family, New England J. Med., *256*, 311, 1957.

14. Haden, R. L.: The Red Blood Cell of Man, Internat. Clin., *1*, 68, 1935.

15. Hartridge, H.: Shape of Red Blood Corpuscles, J. Physiol., *81*, 53, 1920.

15a. Hayhoe, F. G. J. and Hynes, M.: An Abnormality of Erythroblastic Karyokinesis, J. Path. & Bact., *63*, 403, 1951.

16. Heath, C. W. and Daland, G. A.: The Life of Reticulocytes, Arch. Int. Med., *46*, 533, 1930.

17. ——— Staining of Reticulocytes by Brilliant Cresyl Blue, Arch. Int. Med., *48*, 133, 1931.

17a. Helz, M. K. and Menten, M. L.: Elliptocytosis, J. Lab. & Clin. Med., *29*, 185, 1944.

17b. Hillier, J. and Hoffman, J. F.: On the Ultrastructure of the Plasma Membrane as Determined by the Electron Microscope, J. Cell. & Comp. Physiol., *42*, 203, 1953.

18. Howell, W. H.: The Life History of the Formed Elements of the Blood: Especially the Red Corpuscles, J. Morphol., *4*, 57, 1890.

19. Hunter, W. C.: A Further Study of a White Family Showing Elliptical Erythrocytes, Ann. Int. Med., *6*, 775, 1932.

19a. Hutchison, H. E. and Ferguson-Smith, M. A.: The Significance of Howell-Jolly Bodies in Red Cell Precursors, J. Clin. Path., *12*, 451, 1959.

20. Isaacs, R.: The Refractive Granule Red Blood Corpuscle: Its Behavior and Significance, Anat. Rec., *29*, 299, 1925.

21. ——— Formation and Destruction of Red Blood Cells, Physiol. Rev., *17*, 291, 1937 (Bibliography).

22. Israëls, M. C. G.: The Pathological Significance of the Megaloblast, J. Path. & Bact., *49*, 231, 1939; *ibid.*, *52*, 361, 1941.

23. Jandl, J. H., Inman, J. K., Simmons, R. L. and Allen, D. W.: Transfer of Iron from Serum Iron-Binding Protein to Human

Reticulocytes, J. Clin. Invest., *38*, 161, 1959; Blood, *15*, 71, 1960.

24. JONES, O. P.: The Origin of Megaloblasts and Normoblasts in Biopsied Human Marrow and the Difference Between the Two Series, Anat. Rec. (Suppl.), *58*, 23, 1934; Folia haemat., *55*, 195, 1936; Downey's *Handbook of Hematology*, New York, Paul B. Hoeber, Inc., *3*, 2045, 1938; Arch. Path., *35*, 752, 1943.

24a. KAPLAN, E., ZUELZER, W. W. and MOURIQUAND, C.: Sideroblasts. A Study of Stainable Nonhemoglobin Iron in Marrow Normoblasts, Blood, *9*, 203, 1954.

25. KATO, K.: Physiological Variation of Reticulocytes in the Newborn, Folia hæmatol., *46*, 377, 1932.

26. KEMPNER, W.: The Metabolism of Human Erythroblasts, J. Clin. Invest., *15*, 679, 1936.

27. KEY, J. A.: Studies of Erythrocytes With Special Reference to Reticulum, Polychromatophilia and Mitochondria, Arch. Int. Med., *28*, 511, 1921.

29. KRUH, J. and BORSOOK, H.: Hemoglobin Synthesis in Rabbit Reticulocytes *in vitro*, J. Biol. Chem., *220*, 905, 1956.

30. KRUMBHAAR, E. B.: The Erythrocyte, *in* E. V. Cowdry, *Special Cytology*, New York, Paul B. Hoeber, Inc., *2*, 533, 1932.

30a. LAJTHA, L. G.: Culture of Human Bone Marrow *in vitro*, J. Clin. Path. *5*, 67, 1952.

31. LEITNER, S. J.: Die familiäre Elliptozytose als vererbbare Anomalie der Erythrozyten, Deutsch. Arch. klin. Med., *183*, 607, 1939.

31a. LETMAN, H.: Hereditary Haemolytic Elliptocytosis, Acta med. scandinav., *151*, 41, 1955.

31b. LIPTON, E. L.: Elliptocytosis with Hemolytic Anemia: The Effects of Splenectomy, Pediatrics, *15*, 67, 1955.

32. MARCUSSEN, P. V.: The Counting of Reticulocytes, With Special Reference to the Accuracy of the Method, Folia haemat., *61*, 49, 1938.

33. MICHELS, N. A.: Erythropoiesis, Folia haemat., *45*, 75, 1931 (Bibliography).

34. ——— The Erythrocyte, Hæmatologica, *2*, 101, 1931 (Bibliography).

35. MIER, M., SCHWARTZ, S. O. and BOSHES, B.: Acanthrocytosis, Pigmentary Degeneration of the Retina and Ataxic Neuropathy: a Genetically Determined Syndrome with Associated Metabolic Disorder, Blood, *16*, 1586, 1960.

36. MINOT, G. R. and CASTLE, W. B.: The Interpretation of Reticulocyte Reactions, Lancet, *2*, 319, 1935.

37. MORTON, N. E.: The Detection and Estimation of Linkage between the Genes for Elliptocytosis and the Rh Blood Type, Am. J. Human Genet., *8*, 80, 1956.

37a. MOTULSKY, A. G., SINGER, K., CROSBY, W. H. and SMITH, V.: The Life Span of the Elliptocyte, Blood, *9*, 57, 1953.

37b. MUIR, A. R. and KERR, D. N. S.: Erythropoiesis: an Electron Microscopical Study, Quart. J. Exper. Physiol., *43*, 106, 1958.

38. NITTIS, S.: The Nature and the Mechanism of Staining of the Erythrocytic Reticulum, Am. J. M. Sc., *196*, 177, 1938.

39. ORTEN, J. M.: The Properties and Significance of the Reticulocyte, Yale J. Biol. & Med., *6*, 519, 1934.

40. PEARLMAN, M. D. and LIMARZI, L. R.: Correlation Studies of Basophilic Aggregation and Reticulocytes in Various Clinical Conditions, Am. J. Clin. Path., *8*, 608, 1938.

40a. PEDERSEN, J., LUND, J., OHLSEN, A. S. and KRISTENSEN, H. P. O.: Partial Megaloblastic Erythropoiesis, Lancet, *1*, 448, 1957.

40b. PENDL, I. and FRANZ, W.: Transformation of Megaloblasts to Normoblasts by Cultivating Human Bone Marrow in Presence of Vitamin B_{12} and Vitamin B_{12}-binding Protein, Nature, *181*, 488, 1958.

41. PENFOLD, J. B. and LIPSCOMB, J. M.: Elliptocytosis in Man Associated With Hereditary Haemorrhagic Telangiectasia, Quart. J. Med., *12*, 157, 1943.

41a. PERUTZ, M. F.: Submicroscopic Structure of the Red Cell, Nature, *161*, 204, 1948.

42. PONDER, E.: *Hemolysis and Related Phenomena*, 1948, Grune and Stratton, New York; Faraday Society Discussion, *6*, 152, 1949.

42a. PONDER, E.: Present Concepts of the Structure of the Mammalian Red Cell, Blood, *9*, 227, 1954; J. Gen. Physiol., *39*, 319, 1956.

43. RAMSEY, R. and WARREN, C. O., JR.: The Rate of Respiration in Erythrocytes, Quart. J. Exper. Physiol., *20*, 213, 1930; *ibid.*, *22*, 49, 1932.

43a. REBUCK, J. W. and WOODS, H. L.: Electron Microscope Studies of Blood Cells, Blood, *3*, 175, 1948.

43b. REIFF, R. H., NUTTER, JANET Y., DONOHUE, D. M. and FINCH, C. A.: The Relative Number of Marrow Reticulocytes, Am. J. Clin. Path., *30*, 199, 1958.

43c. RIND, H.: Kinetik der Erythroblastenentkernung, Folia haemat., *74*, 262, 1956; *ibid.*, *76*, 293, 1959.

44. SCHARTUM-HANSEN, H.: Genesis of Oval Erythrocytes, Acta med. scandinav., *86*, 348, 1935.

45a. SCHLEICHER, E. M.: The Origin and Nature of the Cabot Ring Bodies of Erythrocytes, J. Lab. & Clin. Med., *27*, 983, 1942.

45b.——— Giant Orthochromatic Erythroblasts, J. Lab. & Clin. Med., 29, 127, 1944.

45c.Schwartz, S. O. and Motto, S. A.: The Diagnostic Significance of "Burr" Red Blood Cells, Am. J. M. Sc., 218, 563, 1949.

45d.Seno, S., et al.: Cytochemical Studies of the Hemoglobin Synthesis of Erythroblasts, Acta Med. Okayama, 11, 300, 1957; Folia haemat., 2, 269, 1958; Acta haemat. japonica (supp. 2), 21, 351, 1958; Science, 129, 275, 1959.

45e.Singer, K., Fisher, B. and Perlstein, M. A.: Acanthrocytosis, Blood, 7, 577, 1952.

46. Stephens, D. J. and Tatelbaum, A. J.: Elliptical Human Erythrocytes, J. Lab. & Clin. Med., 20, 375, 1935.

47. Sundberg, R. Dorothy and Broman, H.: The Application of the Prussian Blue Stain to Previously Stained Films of Blood and Bone Marrow, Blood, 10, 160, 1955.

47a.Tasker, P. W. G.: The Direct Action of Folic Acid, Folinic Acid and Vitamin B_{12} on Megaloblasts in vivo, Brit. J. Haemat., 2, 205, 1956.

47b.Valentine, W. N. and Neel, J. V.: The Artificial Production and Significance of Target Cells, Am. J. M. Sc., 209, 741, 1945.

47c.Weicker, H. and Scharfenberger, H.: Das Megaloblasten-Erythroblastenproblem unter karyo- und cytometrischen Gesichtspunkten, Deutsches Arch. klin. Med., 202, 133, 1955.

47d.Weicker, H.: Die hemi-homoplastische Teilung des Proerythroblasten—die Lösung des Stammzellproblems der Erythropoese, Folia haemat., 74, 49, 1956; Schweiz. med. Wchnschr., 87, 1210, 1957; Klin. Wchnschr., 36, 1132, 1958; Folia haemat., 4, 77, 1959.

47e.Weicker, H., Kujath, I. and Fichsel, H.: Achromocyten und Achromoreticulocyten, Acta haemat., 21, 329, 1959.

48. Wilson, H. E. and Long, M. J.: Hereditary Ovalocytosis (Elliptocytosis) with Hypersplenism, Arch. Int. Med., 95, 438, 1955.

49. Wintrobe, M. M.: Variations in the Size and Hemoglobin Content of Erythrocytes in the Blood of Various Vertebrates, Folia haemat., 51, 32, 1933.

49a.——— Relation of Variation in Mean Corpuscular Volume to Number of Reticulocytes in Pernicious Anemia, J. Clin. Invest., 13, 669, 1934.

50. Wolman, I. J. and Ozge, A.: Studies on Elliptocytosis, Am. J. M. Sc., 234, 702, 1957.

50a.Wyandt, H., Bancroft, P. M. and Winship, T. O.: Elliptic Erythrocytes in Man, Arch. Int. Med., 68, 1043, 1941.

50b.Young, L. E. and Lawrence, J. S.: Matura-tion and Destruction of Transfused Human Reticulocytes, J. Clin. Invest., 24, 554, 1945.

Normal Values and Physiologic Variations

51. Andresen, M. I. and Mugrage, E. R.: Red Blood Cell Values for Normal Men and Women, Arch. Int. Med., 58, 136, 1936.

52. ——— Diameter and Volume of Red Blood Cells in Infants and Small Children, Folia hæmat., 61, 201, 1938.

52a.Berlin, N. I., Reynafarje, C. and Lawrence, J. H.: Red Cell Life Span in the Polycythemia of High Altitude, J. Appl. Physiol., 7, 271, 1954.

53. Belk, P., Curtis, E. and Wilson, K.: Erythrocyte Counts, Hemoglobin and Erythrocyte Volume in Normal Young Men and Women Residing in the Eastern United States, Am. J. Clin. Path., 6, 487, 1936.

53a.Berry, W. T. C. et al.: The Diet, Hæmoglobin Values, and Blood Pressures of Olympic Athletes, Brit. M. J., 1, 300, 1949.

53b.Brown, A. and Goodall, A. L.: Normal Variations in Blood Hæmoglobin Concentration, J. Physiol., 104, 404, 1946.

53c.Casley-Smith, J. R.: The Haematology of the Central Australian Aborigine, Australian J. Exper. Biol. & M. Sc., 36, 23, 1958.

53d.Christie, R. W.: Arctic Anemia, New England J. Med., 259, 605, 1958.

53e.Chen-Ting, C.: Determination of Normal Mean Corpuscular Weight, J. Lab. & Clin. Med., 32, 66, 1947.

53f. Chuinard, E. G., Osgood, E. E. and Ellis, D. M.: Hematologic Standards for Healthy Newborn Infants, Am. J. Dis. Child., 62, 1188, 1941.

53g.Cotter, H., Lancaster, H. O. and Walsh R. J.: The Variation from Day to Day in the Haemoglobin Value of Young Women, Australasian Ann. Med., 2, 99, 1953; ibid., 8, 109, 1959.

54. Davis, J. E. and Brewer, N.: Effect of Physical Training on Blood Volume, Hemoglobin, Alkali Reserve and Osmotic Resistance of Erythrocytes, Am. J. Physiol., 113, 586, 1935.

54a.DeMarsh, Q. B., Alt, H. L. and Windle, W. F.: Factors Influencing the Blood Picture of the Newborn, Am. J. Dis. Child., 75, 860, 1948.

55. Donelson, E. G., Leichsenring, J. M. and Wall, L. M.: The Diameter of Red Blood Cells in Healthy Young Women, Am. J. Physiol., 128, 382, 1940.

55a.Ebert, R. V. and Stead, E. A., Jr.: Demonstration that in Normal Man no Reserves of Blood are Mobilized by Exercise, Epinephrine and Hemorrhage, Am. J. M. Sc., *201*, 655, 1941.

55*b*.ENGELBRETH-HOLM, J. and VIDEBAEK, A.: Normal Blood Counts in Different Seasons, Blood, *3*, 612, 1948.

55*c*.FRUMIN, A. M., MENDELL, T. H., MINTZ, S. S., NOVACK, P. and FAULK, A. T.: Nucleated Red Blood Cells in Congestive Heart Failure, Circulation, *20*, 367, 1959.

55*d*.GAIRDNER, D., MARKS, J. and ROSCOE, J. D.: Blood Formation in Infancy, Arch. Dis. Childhood, *27*, 214, 1952; ibid., *33*, 489, 1958.

55*e*. GILLUM, H. L. and MORGAN, A. F.: Nutritional Status of the Aging, J. Nutrition, *55*, 265, 1955.

55*f*. GLASER, K., LIMARZI, L. R. and PONCHER, H. G.: Cellular Composition of the Bone Marrow in Normal Infants and Children, Pediatrics, *6*, 789, 1950.

56. GUEST, G. M. and BROWN, ESTELLE W.: Erythrocytes and Hemoglobin of the Blood in Infancy and Childhood, A. M. A. J. Dis. Child., *93*, 486, 1957.

56*a*.HAHN, P. F., BALE, W. F. and BONNER, J. F., JR.: Removal of Red Cells from the Active Circulation by Sodium Pentobarbital, Am. J. Physiol., *138*, 415, 1943.

56*b*.HAWKINS, W. W., SPECK, E. and LEONARD, V. G.: Variation of the Hemoglobin Level with Age and Sex, Blood, *9*, 999, 1954; Metabolism, *5*, 70, 1956; J. Am. Geriat. Soc., *4*, 24, 1956.

56*c*. HEILMEYER, L., RECKNAGEL, K. and ALBUS, L.: Blutbestand, Blutzusammensetzung, Blutumsatz und Leberfunktion im Höhenklima, Ztschr. ges. exper. Med., *90*, 573, 1933.

56*d*.HICKS, J. D.: Hæmoglobin Values in the Blood of Newborn Infants, Med. J. Australia, *2*, 117, 1942.

56*e*. HOBSON, W. and BLACKBURN, E. K.: Haemoglobin Levels in a Group of Elderly Persons Living at Home Alone or with Spouse, Brit. M. J., *1*, 647, 1953.

56*f*. HOLLINGSWORTH, J. W.: Lifespan of Fetal Erythrocytes, J. Lab. & Clin. Med., *45*, 469, 1955.

56*g*.HURTADO, A., MERINO, C. and DELGADO, E.: Influence of Anoxemia on the Hemopoietic Activity, Arch. Int. Med., *75*, 284, 1945.

56*h*.JUDY, HARRIET E. and PRICE, NOREEN B.: Hemoglobin Level and Red Blood Cell Count Findings in Normal Women, J. A. M. A., *167*, 563, 1958.

57. KARVONEN, M. J. and KUNNAS, M.: Erythrocyte and Haemoglobin Changes during Protracted Heavy Muscular Work, Ann.

med. exper. et biol. Fenniae, *30*, 180, 1952.

57*a*.LANGLEY, F. A.: Hæmopoiesis and Siderosis in the Foetus and Newborn, Arch. Dis. Child., *26*, 64, 1951.

57*b*.LAWRENCE, J. H. and BERLIN, N. I.: Relative Polycythemia—The Polycythemia of Stress, Yale J. Biol. & Med., *24*, 498, 1952.

57*c*. LAWRENCE, J. H., HUFF, R. L., SIRI, W., WASSERMAN, L. R. and HENNESSY, T. G.: A Physiological Study in the Peruvian Andes, Acta med. scandinav., *142*, 117, 1952.

57*d*.LEHMANN, H.: Hæmogram, Serum Protein and Plasma Volume of Healthy, Well-Nourished East Africans in Uganda, Nature, *164*, 954, 1949.

57*e*.LEICHSENRING, J. M., DONELSON, E. G. and WALL, L. M.: Studies of Blood of High School Girls, Am. J. Dis. Child., *62*, 262, 1941.

57*f*.LEICHSENRING, J. M., NORRIS, L. M., and HALBERT, M. L.: Hemoglobin, Red Cell Count, and Mean Corpuscular Hemoglobin of Healthy Infants, Am. J. Dis. Child., *84*, 27, 1952.

57*g*.LEICHSENRING, J. M., NORRIS, L. M. LAMISON, S. A. and HALBERT, M. L.: Blood Cell Values for Healthy Adolescents, Am. J. Dis. Child., *90*, 159, 1955.

58. LEVERTON, R. and ROBERTS, L.: Hemoglobin and Red Cell Content of the Blood of Normal Women, J. A. M. A., *106*, 1459, 1936.

58*a*.LEWIS, G. K., OHLSON, M. A., CEDERQUIST, D. and DONELSON, E G.: Corpuscular Constants of College Women of the North Central States, J. Lab. & Clin. Med., *32*, 419, 1947.

58*b*.LEWIS, R. C., KINSMAN, G. M., ILIFF, A. and DUVAL, A. M.: The Effect of Change of Altitude on the Corpuscular Constants of Wintrobe, Am. J. Clin. Path., *13*, 208, 1943.

59. LINNEBERG, L. L. and SCHARTUM-HANSEN, H.: Hemoglobin Content of Blood and Number and Volume of Red Blood Corpuscles in Healthy Men and Women, Norsk mag. f. lægevidensk., *96*, 832, 1935.

59*a*.MACGREGOR, R. G. S. and LOH, G. L.: The Comparison of Basal Physiological Values in Racial Groups, Part 2, J. Malaya Branch, Brit. M. A., *4*, 385, 1941.

60. MERINO, C. F.: Studies on Blood Formation and Destruction in the Polycythemia of High Altitude, Blood, *5*, 1, 1950.

61. MERRITT, K. K. and DAVIDSON, L. T.: The Blood During the First Year of Life, Am. J. Dis. Child., *46*, 990, 1933.

63. MUGRAGE, E. and ANDRESEN, M. I.: Values for Red Blood Cells of Average Infants and

Children, Am. J. Dis. Child., *51*, 775, 1936; *ibid.*, *56*, 997, 1938.

64. NEWMAN, B. and GITLOW, S.: Blood Studies in the Aged, Am. J. M. Sc., *205*, 677, 1943.

64a. NYLIN, G.: The Effect of Heavy Muscular Work on the Volume of Circulating Red Corpuscles in Man, Am. J. Physiol., *149*, 180, 1947.

65. OSGOOD, E. E.: Normal Hematologic Standards, Arch. Int. Med., *56*, 847, 1935.

66. PAXTON, W. T. W.: The Red Corpuscles in Acidosis and Alkalosis, Arch. Dis. Childhood, *10*, 115, 1935.

67. PRICE-JONES, C.: *Red Blood Cell Diameters*, London, Oxford Medical Publications, 1933.

69. REYNAFARJE, C., BERLIN, N. I. and LAWRENCE, J. H.: Red Cell Life Span in Acclimitization to Altitude, Proc. Soc. Exper. Biol. & Med., *87*, 101, 1954.

70. REYNAFARJE, C., LOZANO, R. and VALDIVIESO, J.: The Polycythemia of High Altitudes: Iron Metabolism and Related Aspects, Blood, *14*, 433, 1959.

71. SMITH, C.: Daily Erythrocyte Counts in Menstrual and Intermenstrual Periods, Am. J. Physiol., *114*, 452, 1936.

72. SMITH, C. and KUMPF, K. F.: The Effect of Exercise on Human Erythrocytes, Am. J. M. Sc., *184*, 537, 1932.

72a. SNELL, F. M.: Observations on the Hematologic Values of the Japanese, Blood, *5*, 89, 1950.

72b. SPRIGGS, A. I. and SLADDEN, R. A.: The Influence of Age on Red Cell Diameter, J. Clin. Path., *11*, 53, 1958.

72c. STICKNEY, J. C. and VAN LIERE, E. J.: Acclimitization to Low Oxygen Tension, Physiol. Rev., *33*, 13, 1953.

73. TALBOTT, J. H. and DILL, B. D.: Clinical Observations at High Altitude: Observations on Six Healthy Persons Living at 17,500 Feet and a Report of One Case of Chronic Mountain Sickness, Am. J. M. Sc., *192*, 626, 1936.

73a. TSUKAMOTO, H.: Normal Values of Blood Cell Counts in Japan, Acta haemat. japonica, *21*, 854, 1958.

73b. WALKER, J. and TURNBULL, E. P. N.: Haemoglobin and Red Cells in the Human Foetus, Lancet, *2*, 312, 1953; Arch. Dis. Childhood, *30*, 102, 1955.

74. WADSWORTH, G. R.: Packed Red-cell Volume in the Tropics, Nature, *170*, 851, 1952; Brit. M. J., *2*, 910, 1954.

74a. WALSH, R. J., *et al.*: A Study of Haemoglobin Values in New South Wales, with Observations on Haematocrit and Sedimentation Rate Values, Special Report Series No. 5, The National Health and Medical Research Council, Canberra, 1953.

75. WALTERS, O. S.: The Variation of Erythrocytes and Hemoglobin in Man during Inactivity, Folia haemat., *56*, 343, 1937.

75a. WASHBURN, A. H.: Blood Cells in Healthy Young Infants, Am. J. Dis. Child., *62*, 530, 1941.

75b. WATANABE, G.-I.: Climatic Effect on the Packed Red-Cell Volume, Brit. J. Haemat., *4*, 108, 1958.

75c. WEICKER, H., *et al.*: Der Erythrocytendurchmesser des Kindes, Acta haemat., *10*, 50, 1953.

75d. WILSON, O.: Physiological Changes in Blood in the Antarctic, Brit. M. J., *2*, 1425, 1953.

76. WINTROBE, M. M.: Erythrocyte in Man, Medicine, *9*, 195, 1930 (Bibliography).

77. ——— Blood of Normal Men and Women, Bull. Johns Hopkins Hosp., *53*, 118, 1933.

78. ——— Anemia, Arch. Int. Med., *54*, 256, 1934.

79. WINTROBE, M. M., SHUMACKER, H. B., JR. and SCHMIDT, W. J.: Values for Number, Size and Hemoglobin Content of Erythrocytes in Normal Dogs, Rabbits and Rats, Am. J. Physiol., *114*, 502, 1936.

Chapter 3

The Erythrocyte (*Continued*)

BIOCHEMICAL CONSIDERATIONS AND KINETICS
PORPHYRIAS AND DISORDERS USUALLY ACCOMPANIED BY CYANOSIS

Introduction.—For many years the mature red corpuscle was thought to be an inert protoplasmic particle consisting essentially of water (64 per cent) and hemoglobin. This was not an improbable assumption since there is but feeble respiration in red corpuscles (p. 125) and in view of the fact that hemoglobin forms 95 per cent of the dry substance of the erythrocyte and is concerned solely with the transport of oxygen. Subsequently, stimulated largely by the need to find better means for the preservation of red corpuscles, investigators found that the red cell is by no means an inert mechanical contrivance but is, instead, a "dynamo of activity."[4] The erythrocyte is now regarded as a living cell in the sense that it exists in a dynamic state, does work and requires sustenance to maintain its energy metabolism. The loss of viability during storage is due to a running down of the energetics of the cell.[11a] Within its one hundred and twenty-day life span and during its 100 miles of shuttling between the heart and various tissues, energy is needed to maintain the

optimum osmotic conditions against a steep ionic gradient, to preserve the discoidal form of the cell against forces that tend to make it spherical and to make possible the transport of glucose and ions across the red cell membrane. In addition, and perhaps most important of all, energy is required to provide a reducing system capable of reconverting methemoglobin to the ferrous state.

This chapter will deal with the internal metabolism of the red corpuscle, the materials needed for red cell production, the various aspects of iron metabolism and the biosynthesis of hemoglobin. The fate of the red corpuscle and quantitative aspects of hemoglobin production and destruction (erythrokinetics) also will be considered and, in addition, the recognized abnormalities of hemoglobin will be discussed. The metabolic aspects of the cells normally found in the bone marrow were reviewed earlier (p. 42), as were the various stages in the development of the red cells, from erythroblast to mature red corpuscle (p. 85). The structure and functions of the red corpuscles were also described earlier (p. 95).

CHEMICAL COMPOSITION AND METABOLISM OF THE RED CORPUSCLE

Although the components of the red corpuscle other than hemoglobin represent a very small fraction of its substance, they are fundamental to its function and survival. These components include those which are concerned with the surface structure of the erythrocyte (membrane), those which govern the passage of substances into and out of the red corpuscle, those involved in maintaining hemoglobin in the functional reduced state, those concerned in supplying the energy required for the various activities which go on in the red corpuscle and, in addition, a number of other substances whose function is unknown. Of special interest to the clinician is the fact that deficiencies of some of these reactions have been shown to occur as heritable abnormalities and are the cause of certain disorders characterized by anemia. In other instances biochemical defects in the red corpuscle may be acquired or may develop as the red cells age.

The insoluble material which remains when red corpuscles are hemolyzed is known as the **stroma.** This constitutes about 2 to 5 per cent of the wet weight of the red corpuscle (Table 3–1). Some 40 to 60 per cent of this is protein and 10 to 12 per cent lipid.[5] Three lipid-containing protein fractions have been separated from stroma by electrophoresis.[29] The stroma proteins include "stromatin," a fibrous or structural protein, and "elinin."[17] The blood group substances A, B and O are present in the slowly moving electrophoretic fraction in high concentration.[29] They were found to be in four or five times greater concentration in the "elinin" fraction than in whole stroma. The Rh antigen was found to be present solely in the "elinin" fraction.[9]

The lipid material of the stroma[5a] consists of the phospholipid (65 per cent), cholesterol (23 per cent), cholesterol esters, glycerides and free fatty acids (2 per cent), and other lipids, primarily glycolipid (10 per cent).[29a] The phospholipids include lecithin (30 per cent), sphingomyelin (22 per cent), phosphatidyl serine (15 per cent) and phosphatidyl ethanolamine (25 per cent).[3,29a] Lysolecithin constitutes about 2 per cent of the total lipid phosphorus and plasmalogen is present as well.[26a] The lipids are in a highly dynamic state but there is no agreement as to whether or not lipid biosynthesis is accomplished in the mature red corpuscle.[21,27a,37] It is known that the cholesterol of red corpuscles is in exchange with the cholesterol in the plasma[21] and the same may be true of the erythrocyte phospholipids.[29a] The exchange of cholesterol and other labile stroma components is probably of great importance in maintaining a viable cell, loss of surface lipids being associated with aging and loss of viability.[27a]

The **erythrocyte membrane,** although not a fixed structure, is a dynamic component of the corpuscle and is preserved in a functional state by the energy metabolism of the cell. This maintains the property of semipermeability and the passage of cations against an ionic gradient.[15a] Potassium is transported across the membrane by a dynamic process which depends on energy derived from anaerobic glycolysis and involves adenosine triphosphate (ATP).[39b] Sodium is excluded by the same or a metabolically linked mechanism. There is evidence that pores are present in the membrane which contain an assemblage of positive charges and that these account for differences in the permeability of the membrane to different ions.[35a]

Water soluble constituents of the red corpuscle **other than hemoglobin** include glucose, a number of reducing

Table 3–1.—Approximate Chemical Composition of Red Blood Corpuscles In Man[1a,4,5a,10,13,17,27]

	Gm./100 ml. RBC
Hemoglobin	33.50
Methemoglobin	0.50
Non-Hb protein	0.87
Lipids	0.48
Glucose	0.83
Minerals	0.67
Water	63.15

	mg./100 ml. RBC
Stroma: proteins, total	500
Stromatin	300
Elinin	200
Blood group substances	
Enzymes	
lipids, total	480
Phosphatides—Cephalin	133
Lecithin	106
Sphingomyelin	73
Cholesterol (free)	130
Cholesterol esters	29
Neutral fats, cerebrosides	98
Glycolytic system, total	188
Glucose	74
Reducing substances calculated as glucose (2, 3-diphosphoglycerate, ATP, hexose phosphates, DPN, TPN)	114
Water-soluble constituents other than proteins	
Glutathione	70
Ergothioneine	3.3
Elemental composition, total	767
P: Organic acid-soluble P	55
Inorganic P	3
ATP–P	10
Hexose mono + diphosphate–P	15
2, 3-diphosphoglycerate–P	28
S: Neutral–S	6
Inorganic sulfate–S	0.04
Ethereal sulfate–S	0.04
Copper	0.115
Zinc	1.44
Lead	0.057
Tin	0.026
Manganese	0.019
Aluminum	0.007
Silver	trace
K+	420
Na+	45
Ca++	
Mg++	3
Cl−	180

Table 3–1.—Continued

mg./100 ml. RBC

Additional quantitative data	
Vitamins and co-enzymes	
Thiamin	0.008
Cocarboxylase	0.01
Riboflavin	0.022
Flavine-adenine dinucleotide	0.075
Niacin	1.0
Diphosphopyridine nucleotide	10
Triphosphopyridine nucleotide	1.2
Pyridoxine	0.005
Pantothenic acid	0.025
Co-enzyme A	0.144
Ascorbic acid	1.0
Adenosine (mono-, di-, tri-phosphate)	62
Compounds related to hemoglobin	
Iron	115
Protoporphyrin (free)	0.031
Coproporphyrin (free)	0.002
Miscellaneous	
Amino acids	30
Total NPN	44
Nucleotide–N	13
Amino-acid-N	7.4
Urea	20
Creatine	2
Creatinine	8
Uric acid, uric acid riboside	

substances, a great number and variety of enzymes,[2] as well as vitamins such as nicotinic acid, riboflavin and ascorbic acid; minerals such as iron, zinc and copper; and a number of cations and anions. The chief cation is potassium, with lesser amounts of sodium, calcium and magnesium, while the major anions are chloride, bicarbonate, hemoglobin, inorganic phosphates and various organic phosphates. A number of the vitamins serve as prosthetic groups for certain enzymes.

Energy Metabolism.—The red corpuscle contains no glycogen. Consequently, for its continued metabolism it must have constant access to glucose. The exact mechanism whereby glucose penetrates the erythrocyte membrane is unknown but most investigators have concluded that this depends on an active transport mechanism rather than on simple diffusion.[20c,39c] Enzyme sites may be located at discontinuities in the lipid outer structure through which glucose phosphate diffuses or is transferred by the action of these enzymes.[4]

Only slight remnants of the citric acid (Krebs) cycle and the cytochrome system remain in the non-nucleated red corpuscle.[11] The metabolic breakdown of glucose depends on the reactions of the Embden-Meyerhof glycolytic pathway whereby glucose is broken down anaerobically through a series of phosphorylated intermediates to lactic acid (Fig. 3–1, reactions 1 to 10). An alternative pathway for the metabolism of glucose is via the "hexose monophosphate shunt" (phosphogluconate oxidative pathway) (reactions 11 to 13) through which the sugar is oxidized with the formation of pentose and triose phosphates.[27] All the intermediate compounds of glycolysis have been isolated and chromatography has

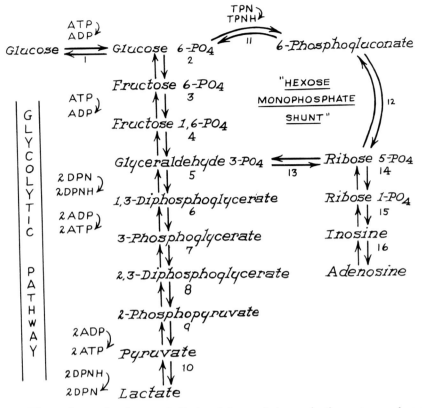

Fig. 3–1.—The pathways for the metabolic breakdown of glucose in the mature red corpuscle.
(Diagram prepared by Dr. G. E. Cartwright).

permitted accurate estimation of the quantities of many of them.[4]

2,3-diphosphoglycerate (DPG), one of the triose phosphates, makes up as much as 50 per cent of the total acid-soluble organic phosphate of the red corpuscle[19a] and is an important store of energy. The red corpuscle contains diphosphopyridine (DPN) and triphosphopyridine nucleotide (TPN) and a large quantity of ATP[19a] and hexose phosphates. Under normal conditions the rate of glycolysis by the red corpuscle of man is 0.3 to 0.4 mg. per 100 ml. of cells per hour.[4]

Certain enzymes important in erythrocyte glucose metabolism, such as glucose-6-phosphate dehydrogenase (G6PD), 6-phosphogluconic dehydrogenase (6PGD) and phosphohexose isomerase, are pres-ent in relatively large amounts in young erythrocytes and decrease with the aging of the red corpuscle, in vivo.[6,22] This is not true of all erythrocyte enzymes[22] but suffices to produce alterations in glucose metabolism and ultimately causes a reduction in available ATP[20d] since ATP is generated during the series of reactions of the Embden-Meyerhof cycle (see Fig. 3–1). Because ATP is an important source of energy for a number of steps essential for the maintenance of the structural integrity of the erythrocyte, the transport of glucose and cations and, probably, lipid synthesis become impaired as less ATP becomes available. This results ultimately in the breakdown of the red corpuscle.

The preservation of the red corpuscle

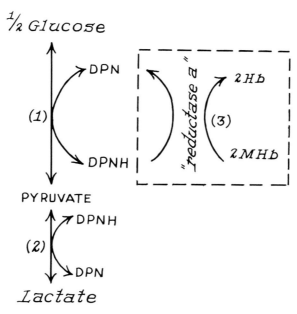

FIG. 3–2.—The maintenance of hemoglobin in the reduced state depends on the action of methemoglobin reductase and requires the generation of DPNH (Diagram supplied by Dr. E. R. Simon).

in vitro can be enhanced by the addition of purine ribosides, particularly adenosine and inosine.[14] This effect probably depends on the entry of the purine riboside into the red corpuscle, where it is phosphorylytically cleaved by a purine nucleoside phosphorylase with the formation of ribose-1-phosphate[21] (Fig. 3–1, reactions *16, 15*). The latter is converted to ribose-5-phosphate (reaction *14*) which can enter the hexose-monophosphate shunt. There it is converted to triosephosphates and ultimately, via the glycolytic pathway, to lactic acid. In this way ATP is generated and the "storage lesion" associated with the storage of blood for transfusion is temporarily healed.

Maintenance of Reduced Hemoglobin.—In the intact red corpuscle hemoglobin is constantly shifting from the functional, reduced state to oxidized, ferric hemoglobin (methemoglobin). The maintenance of reduced hemoglobin depends chiefly on an enzyme ("methemoglobin reductase" of Kiese) which requires

the generation of diphosphopyridine nucleotide (DPNH) in the glycolytic cycle (Fig. 3–1, step *5*, and Fig. 3–2).[18a] In one form of congenital methemoglobinemia such an enzyme, DPN diaphorase, is deficient.[33a,275] Methemoglobin reduction can also be brought about by another methemoglobin reductase which depends on triphosphopyridine nucleotide (TPNH), generated by way of the "hexose monophosphate shunt."[18] This enzyme requires for its activity an added electron carrier and probably normally plays little role in the reduction of methemoglobin. Substitution of this electron carrier by methylene blue may explain the action of this dye in the temporary relief of methemoglobinemia. The effectiveness of ascorbic acid, as well as that of glutathione (GSH) in relieving methemoglobinemia (p. 195) is independent of methemoglobin reductases and depends solely on the fact that these are reducing agents.

Enzymes in Red Corpuscles.—In ad-

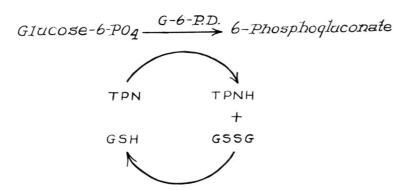

FIG. 3–3.—The key role of glucose-6-phosphate dehydrogenase (G-6-P.D.) in the generation of TPNH, which is required in the reduction of oxidized glutathione (GSSG) to the reduced form (GSH) (Diagram prepared by Dr. G. E. Cartwright).

dition to the enzymes which are involved in the glycolytic cycle and the hexose-monophosphate shunt, 33 of which have been identified and quantitated,[2] red corpuscles contain (1) purine nucleoside phosphorylases specific for nucleosides such as inosine and guanosine;[36] (2) nicotinamide riboside phosphorylase;[17c] (3) malic and lactic dehydrogenase;[39] (4) catalase,[6a] an iron-porphyrin compound which decomposes hydrogen peroxide to water and oxygen and possibly protects hemoglobin against hydrogen peroxide decomposition; (5) carbonic anhydrase,[38] a zinc protein which catalyzes the reversible formation and dissociation of carbonic acid; (6) cholinesterase, a "true" enzyme which differs from the relatively non-specific cholinesterase found in plasma. Cholinesterase is present in far higher concentration in reticulocytes and young red corpuscles than in older ones;[31] (7) proteolytic enzymes[24] and peptidases;[1] (8) arginase,[4,30] glyoxalase,[11a] urease and a thiocyanate oxidase.[16a] The functions of most of these enzymes are unknown.

Other Constitutents of Red Corpuscles. — Water-soluble compounds other than proteins include *ergothioneine*,[19] a substance thought to serve as a co-factor with a nicotinamide riboside phosphorylase;[17c] and the tripeptide, *glutathione* (GSH).[19c] It appears that the con-

stituent amino acids can be conjugated in red corpuscles to form GSH.[20] This compound occurs in the red cell in large amounts but its role is not clear.[27] It is known, however, that GSH in the red cell is in equilibrium with oxidized glutathione (GSSG). The latter is reduced to GSH by a specific enzyme, glutathione reductase. The coenzyme for this reduction is TPNH (Fig. 3–3). Studies of drug induced hemolytic anemia of the "primaquine-sensitive" type (p. 631) have revealed that the erythrocytes of drug-sensitive individuals are markedly deficient in glucose-6-phosphate dehydrogenase (G6PD). This results in failure of TPNH regeneration in the hexose-phosphate metabolic cycle (Fig. 3–1, reaction *11*) with the consequence that GSSG fails to be reduced to GSH. Such cells are vulnerable to hemolysis by a large number of aromatic amino compounds. Whether GSH depletion plays a primary role in such cell death and hemolysis or serves only as a convenient indicator of other, more fundamental changes, is unknown. It has been shown that in the presence of an adequate amount of GSH, glutathione peroxidase protects hemoglobin from oxidative breakdown by catalyzing the destruction of hydrogen peroxide.[23]

Further investigation will undoubtedly

reveal other clinical disorders which depend on the development of a defect in red cell metabolism. It has been shown already that in certain instances of congenital non-spherocytic hemolytic anemia, G6PD activity is absent whereas in another type the activity of this enzyme is increased (p. 651). In hereditary spherocytosis a metabolic defect appears to exist but its nature is obscure (p. 654). Thus, it has been postulated that there is a deficiency of the enzyme enolase, with resulting impaired transport of orthophosphate across the cell boundary.[2] Evidence has also been presented which suggests that energy is utilized inefficiently in maintaining the integrity of the structural lipids of the red corpuscle, "membrane degeneration" resulting as a consequence.[29a] It is possible that coating of the corpuscular surface with isoimmune antibodies, injury by a virus or damage by endogenous metabolites or the products of bacterial metabolism, may interfere with enzyme activities essential for the metabolism of the red corpuscle and thereby lead to its ultimate destruction.

Erythrocuprein, another constituent of red corpuscles, is a copper-protein compound whose function is unknown.[8]

THE REQUIREMENTS FOR RED CELL PRODUCTION

From what is known about the composition of the red cell, it is apparent that a great variety of materials is needed for erythropoiesis. None of these is unique in the sense that it is needed for erythropoiesis alone and not for other tissues of the body. The red corpuscles differ, however, in that they can be examined more readily than many other tissues and shortages of essential materials can therefore be detected more easily because of the development of anemia. Furthermore, in relation to certain essential substances a system of priorities seems

to operate which results in the erythropoietic system being deprived before functional disturbances in other tissues are detected. Thus when iron is in limited supply, hemoglobin production is impaired before detectable deficiencies in certain other iron enzymes occur (p. 740).

In this section it is planned to consider only those substances for which requirement is so critical that without them detectable changes in the blood occur. Of the many other substances required, when they are lacking critical events develop in other tissues long before the hemopoietic system is seriously affected.

Amino Acids and Protein.—Knowledge concerning the substances needed for hemopoiesis was first gained by observing the effects of dietary restrictions. Whipple and his associates pioneered in the field by showing clearly the importance of protein in erythropoiesis.[50,51] They demonstrated that anemia develops in experimental animals fed a diet low in protein and showed that liver, beef muscle and egg products favor hemoglobin production, in this order.

With the possible exception of arginine, all of the ten "essential" amino acids are required for hemopoiesis in the rat, in the following order of decreasing importance: histidine, valine, leucine, isoleucine, lysine, arginine, methionine, tryptophane.[49] Phenylalanine and threonine are also needed, as well as glycine. Peptides are used less efficiently than simple amino acids. Natural amino acids are required.[48] In dogs made anemic by repeated bleeding proline, threonine, glutamic acid, cystine, aspartic acid, histidine, glycine, phenylalanine, methionine, tryptophane, leucine, tyrosine, lysine, valine, isoleucine, alanine, arginine and hydroxyproline when given in amounts of 1 to 2 Gm. daily were found to be effective, in decreasing degree, in producing 34 to 10 Gm. hemoglobin over a two-week period.[51]

9

The specific role of each amino acid in blood formation is yet to be determined. There is no correlation between the quantity of an amino acid found in globin (p. 158) and its effectiveness in hemoglobin regeneration.[44] The feeding of a diet containing acid hydrolyzed casein results in the development of a moderate anemia in rats and severe normocytic, or slightly microcytic anemia, without hypochromia, in swine.[45] This is accompanied by leukopenia, hypoplastic or normal bone marrow and a normal serum iron level and is in all likelihood due to a tryptophane deficiency. The severe anemia which develops in rats maintained on deaminized casein appears to be due to the effects of hexahomoserine which acts as a lysine antagonist.[47]

The B Vitamins.—The standard salmon-bread ration which Whipple fed dogs made anemic by bleeding[51] was deficient in a number of respects. It can now be recognized that some of the beneficial effects of the foods tested in his experiments were due to the vitamins they contained. Thus the striking effect of liver therapy in pernicious anemia is attributable to its content of vitamin B_{12} (p. 443). Later it was shown that the anemia, leukopenia and granulocytopenia produced experimentally in monkeys by feeding them a diet comparable to that taken by natives in India,[214] as well as the "tropical macrocytic anemia" of these natives (p. 508) could be cured by giving autolyzed yeast, a recognized source of "vitamin B." This was followed by demonstration of the antianemic effectiveness of brewers yeast in pernicious anemia.[215] With the isolation of the different B vitamins in pure form it became possible to describe the effects of deficiencies of each of them. It is now clear that deficiencies of vitamin B_{12}, folic (pteroylglutamic) acid and pyridoxine are associated with striking changes in the hemopoietic system and that

pantothenic acid, through its relation to coenzyme A (p. 153), nicotinic acid, riboflavin, thiamin[193,217a] and biotin,[194] by their participation in various metabolic processes, play a role in hemopoiesis.

Folic Acid, Vitamin B_{12} and Related Substances.—Earlier literature on nutrition contains the names of a variety of "B vitamins," in addition to those already mentioned, which were shown to be related to blood formation.[172] These include *vitamin B_6* which was found to relieve macrocytic anemia, leukopenia and thrombocytopenia developing in chicks on a synthetic diet; *vitamin M*, a factor which relieved the anemia and leukopenia occurring in monkeys receiving a deficient diet;[157] *vitamins B_{10} and B_{11}*, water-soluble substances needed by the chick for the maintenance of normal hemoglobin values; and other substances such as "norite eluate factor," factor U and xanthopterin. The last is a yellow pigment obtained from the wings of butterflies which has hemopoietic activity in Chinook salmon with nutritional anemia. The name *"folic acid"* was given to a substance obtained in nearly pure form from spinach[184] which was found to support the growth of two organisms commonly used for microbiological assay: *Lactobacillus casei* and *Streptococcus faecalis* (*S. lactis R*). Substances with similar growth-stimulating properties were isolated from liver, kidney, yeast, milk, casein and fresh green vegetables.

The successful synthesis[146] of *pteroylglutamic acid* ("folic acid"), a compound consisting of pteridine, *p*-aminobenzoic acid and glutamic acid, made it possible to show that the various effects described were due to the action of pteroylglutamic acid or of one of its conjugates. It was demonstrated that the same substance is effective in relieving the megaloblastic bone marrow changes and macrocytic anemia seen in pernicious anemia,[185,206] sprue,[155a,185] macrocytic anemia of preg-

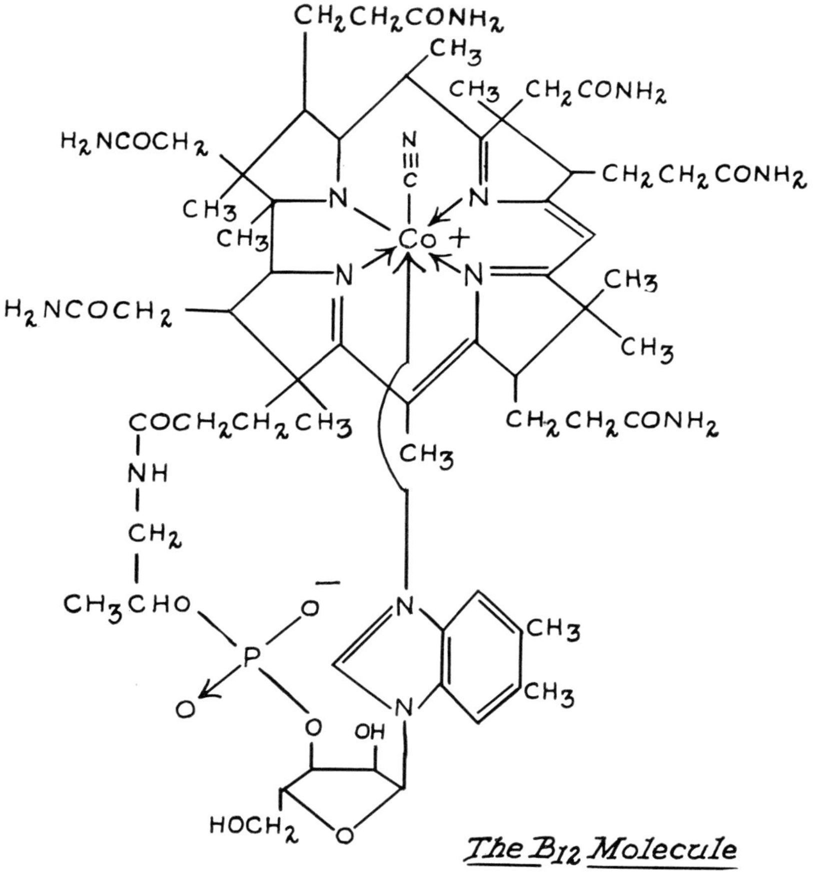

The B_{12} Molecule

Fig. 3-4.—Structure of cyanocobalamin the official form of vitamin B_{12}. There are six primary amide groups and one secondary amide joining the aminopropanol residue to the propionic acid group in ring D. Cyanocobalamin is formulated as a diester of phosphoric acid, the free acid group of the phosphate being neutralized by a positive charge on the cobalt atom. The coenzyme B_{12} differs from the vitamin mainly in the adsence of cyanide and the presence of an adenine nucleoside (Barker et al., J. Biol. Chem., *235*, 480, 1960; *ibid.*, *236*, 3097, 1961).

nancy,[185] tropical macrocytic anemia and related disorders[206] (p. 450). This response was observed when daily amounts of 5 to 50 mg. were given orally or when the synthetic material was administered intramuscularly or intravenously. The leukopenia and thrombocytopenia which accompany pernicious anemia were also relieved However, it soon became clear that folic acid cannot function completely in the place of the anti-pernicious anemia factor, either in human disorders[197] or in animal nutrition. The existence of at least one more hemopoietic factor thus became apparent.

Experimental studies with hens and chicks indicated the need for an *animal protein factor* obtained from meat scraps, fish meal and other animal sources, to permit good growth of chicks and hatchability of eggs on a synthetic medium. Dried *cow manure* was also found to supply a factor promoting growth in chicks. The relation of these and other factors ("zoopherin," "factor X") to human disease was demonstrated by the good hemopoietic response observed in cases of pernicious anemia and related megaloblastic anemias when animal protein factor was given intramuscularly.[205]

With the discovery of a microbiological assay procedure which utilized *Lactobacillus lactis* Dorner, it became possible for Rickes *et al.*[192] to isolate a crystalline compound, vitamin B_{12}, from liver. Independently, Lester Smith[199] obtained this vitamin by means of partition chromatography and human assay procedures. This red substance possesses an atom of cobalt. Since it contains a cyano group bound coordinatively to the cobalt atom, it was named *cyanocobalamin*. On the basis of crystallographic studies[170] as well as from chemical evidence[147b] the structure illustrated in Figure 3–4 was proposed ($C_{63}H_{90}O_{14}N_{14}PCo$). This represented the first time cobalt had been found in a pure substance of biological origin. Vitamin B_{12} was shown to produce positive hemopoietic responses in patients with pernicious anemia in microgram quantities,[212] amounts so small that only such poisons as plutonium and botulinus toxin are known to be physiologically active in any smaller quantities.

Vitamin B_{12} is synthesized chiefly, if not solely, by certain bacteria and by actinomycetes. Its occurrence in animal tissues, such as glandular meats, muscle tissue, eggs and, to a lesser extent, in cheese and milk,[174,178] is explained by the widespread distribution in nature of these microorganisms. Plant materials show no vitamin B_{12} activity but many contain folic acid and its conjugates. A number of vitamin B_{12} analogues have been discovered which arise from rumen or intestinal synthesis. Some, such as nitro-cobalamin (B_{12c}) possess antipernicious anemia activity but most of the compounds appear to be of use neither to man[168a] nor beast.[199]

It is not yet clear whether folic acid and its conjugates together with vitamin B_{12} can account for all the biological activities of the "animal protein factors."[207b] In very rare cases of megaloblastic anemia neither folic acid nor vitamin B_{12} seems to supply all the needs for adequate hematopoiesis.[171] The "Wills factor" (p. 508) present in crude yeast and liver preparations and required in certain cases of nutritional macrocytic anemia is not vitamin B_{12} and has not been conclusively identified with folic acid.

It is now apparent, however, that vitamin B_{12} is the same as the "extrinsic factor"[146a] which Castle postulated as requiring "intrinsic factor" for its absorption (p. 522). It is also the same as the "antipernicious anemia principle," lack of which results in the manifestations of pernicious anemia.

Vitamin B_{12} is unique in that, except when massive doses (50 to 300 micrograms) are supplied, little or no absorption takes place in the absence of a specific protein substance, "intrinsic factor." Since the large quantities mentioned above are unphysiological, it may be assumed that the physiological mode of absorption is mediated by intrinsic factor.[159a] Folic acid, on the other hand, is water soluble and is readily absorbed from the alimentary tract.

The chemical nature of intrinsic factor is not known.[160] It is thought to be a mucoprotein.[177] In man, the glandular structure of the fundus and cardiac portions of the stomach is the site of intrinsic factor secretion. The latter is independent of the production of acid or pepsin.[191a] The site of absorption of vitamin B_{12} is the small intestine, probably the distal portion.[148] The manner of absorption is uncertain but it seems probable that the vitamin is bound by intrinsic factor and that the intrinsic factor, in turn, is bound by receptors in the intestine in the presence of calcium.[145a,169] A binding protein, possibly similar to intrinsic factor, is present in plasma[211] and may be concerned in the selective deposition of vitamin B_{12} in the liver.[169,191] A cobalamin-polypeptide complex has been isolated from ox liver.[168b]

As measured by microbiological assay using *Euglena gracilis* as the test organism, the mean level of vitamin B_{12} in the plasma of normal subjects 15 to 60 years of age was found to be 390 $\mu\mu$g. per ml., with a range of 130 to 750 $\mu\mu$g.[198] No significant difference was found with age but a daily variation of as much as 100 $\mu\mu$g. per ml. was observed. Slightly higher values (means, 450 and 470 $\mu\mu$g. per ml.) were found in other studies with *L. leishmanii* as the test organism.[166,207] Excretion of vitamin B_{12} normally is quite low. It has been estimated that about 0.19 per cent of the whole body B_{12} is excreted per day.[191b] When a large amount of vitamin B_{12} is given, it is excreted in the urine but loss through the bile occurs as well. There is evidence for an enterohepatic circulation of B_{12}, more being found in the bile than in the feces. The minimal daily dietary need for vitamin B_{12} may be of the order of 0.6 to 2.8 μg.[155]

In patients with pernicious anemia in relapse, vitamin B_{12} serum levels have been found to be low (100 $\mu\mu$g. per ml., or less) as a rule, and this has been true also of cases of subacute combined degeneration of the spinal cord and to some degree in cases of megaloblastic anemia associated with pregnancy, partial or total gastrectomy, blind loops following surgery and other "malabsorption syndromes," as well as in instances associated with anticonvulsant therapy.[207] Abnormally high values have been found in patients with chronic myelocytic leukemia and in liver disease.[166]

Although in therapeutics the term folic acid refers to synthetic pteroylglutamic acid, the name also is applied to a group of naturally occurring substances which have folic acid activity. They are found in fresh green vegetables, as well as in parenchymatous organs, such as liver and kidney. The active coenzyme form of folic acid is the N^{10}-formyl derivative of tetrahydrofolic acid.[164] Folic acid is probably reduced to tetrahydrofolic acid in the gastrointestinal tract but reduced and formylated compounds, known as folinic acids and citrovorum factors, occur in nature. It has been postulated that when there is deficiency of tetrahydrofolic acid the catabolism of formiminoglutamic acid (FIGLU) is impaired, resulting in its accumulation and ultimate excretion in the urine. A test for folic acid deficiency depends on the microbiologic assay of FIGLU in the urine.[148a] Another test employs tritium-labelled folic acid.[148b]

The *experimental production* of folic acid deficiency leads to the development of anemia and other changes which have been more clearly characterized in swine [149] than in other experimental animals. The anemia is severe and macrocytic and is accompanied by leukopenia, bone marrow hyperplasia and some thrombocytopenia (Table 3–2). The immature erythroid cells in the bone marrow resemble but are not entirely identical with pernicious anemia megaloblasts. As in pernicious anemia, the plasma iron is increased, the free erythrocyte protoporphyrin is relatively low and the serum copper is normal but, unlike the human disorder, no alterations in gastric secretion or in the nervous system have been observed. This syndrome was produced by feeding a purified diet composed of vitamin-free, extrinsic factor-poor casein together with lard and sucrose, minerals, the fat-soluble vitamins and all the B vitamins except pteroylglutamic acid, as well as succinylsulfathiazole and a crude folic acid antagonist. The anemia can be relieved promptly by the administration of folic acid, but responds poorly if at all to anti-pernicious anemia liver extract, vitamin B_{12}, thymine and other substances.

The replacement of casein in the diet by soybean alpha protein in an attempt to produce vitamin B_{12} deficiency resulted in marked impairment in growth,

Table 3-2.—Hematologic Characteristics of Experimental Nutritional Deficiencies in Swine

Deficiency	Anemia		Leukopenia	Plasma Iron	Copper Serum	E.P.	Bone Marrow Morphology
	Type	Severity					
Protein	N	+	None	Normal	Low	Normal	Normoblastic
Lysine	N	+	None	Normal	Normal	—	Normoblastic
Tryptophane	N	++	Present	Normal	—	Normal	Normoblastic
Iron	MH	++++	None	Low	Normal	Normal	Normoblastic
Copper	MH	++++	Present	Low	Low	Normal	Normoblastic
Pyridoxine	Mi	++++	None	High	Normal	Low	Normoblastic
Niacin plus protein	N	++	None	Normal	Low	Normal	Normoblastic
Riboflavin	N	+	None	—	—	—	Normoblastic
Pantothenic acid	N	++	None	—	—	—	Normoblastic
PGA	Ma	++++	Present	High	Normal	Low	Macronormoblastic
B$_{12}$	N	+	None	—	—	—	Normoblastic
PGA plus B$_{12}$	Ma	++++	Present	—	—	—	Macronormoblastic with a few megaloblasts

Types of Anemia: N indicates normocytic, MH microcytic hypochromic, Mi microcytic and Ma macrocytic. E.P. refers to free erythrocyte protoporphyrin; PGA is pteroylglutamic (folic) acid.

only moderate normocytic anemia, moderately severe neutropenia, and no remarkable alterations in the bone marrow. A combined deficiency of vitamin B_{12} and folic acid, produced by feeding soybean protein instead of casein, omitting both vitamin B_{12} and folic acid from the vitamin supplement and adding succinyl-sulfathiazole and a folic acid antagonist, was marked by the characteristics of folic acid deficiency with the additional feature that the bone marrow contained cells more closely resembling megaloblasts than those seen when simple folic acid deficiency was produced. This anemia responded rapidly and completely to the administration of both vitamin B_{12} and folic acid. Folic acid alone produced an immediate return of the blood and bone marrow to normal but after several months a partial hematologic relapse took place in spite of continued administration of the vitamin. If folic acid was not given, the administration of vitamin B_{12} relieved the anemia only partially and the bone marrow picture did not improve to an impressive degree. No changes in the nervous system were observed.

Thus it has not been possible to produce in experimental animals a disorder which, *in every respect*, is identical with pernicious anemia.

The metabolic functions of vitamin B_{12} and folic acid are, in the main, closely related but they are by no means fully understood. They are both concerned in metabolic reactions which involve one-carbon fragments.[159] Folic acid[163a] controls the movement of preformed labile methyl groups from one acceptor to another (transmethylation) whereas vitamin B_{12} is concerned with the *de novo* synthesis of labile methyl groups from various one-carbon precursors, including serine, glycine, formate and formaldehyde.[199,209] The one-carbon compounds serve as building blocks in the biosynthesis of purines, pyrimidines and certain amino acids. This probably explains such observations as the replacement of folic acid by thymine, a pyrimidine base, in the growth requirement of *L. casei*; the hemopoietic response in pernicious anemia produced by massive doses of thymine;[190,204] and the partial remissions in patients with pernicious anemia produced by the oral administration of orotic acid, a pyrimidine precursor.[195] It is noteworthy that the report of hemopoietic response following intramuscular injections of thymidine has not been confirmed.[207a]

Many other functions have been attributed to vitamin B_{12} but most of them must be indirect; *e.g.* in carbohydrate metabolism through an effect on sulfhydryl synthesis.[179] The widely held assumption that vitamin B_{12} is concerned in the synthesis of deoxyribonucleic acids,[147a] and possibly of ribonucleic acids also, has not found adequate support.[199] Best supported is the evidence that vitamin B_{12} functions in the incorporation of amino acids into protein.[209]

Evidence has been offered which suggests that vitamin B_{12} influences folic acid metabolism by releasing folinic acid from its tissue conjugates, by facilitating the reduction of folic acid to folinic acid or by promoting the formation of the active form of folic acid. Ascorbic acid has also been reported to augment the conversion of folic acid to folinic acid.[189] Both ascorbic acid and vitamin B_{12} were found to stimulate the synthesis of folic acid *in vivo*.[158] That these relationships may be important in man is indicated by the observations that ascorbic acid deficiency plays a part in the development of megaloblastic anemia in infancy (p. 768) and that in certain instances of pernicious anemia a response to liver extract would not take place until ascorbic acid was given (p. 448).

Vitamin B_6 (Pyridoxine).—In dogs,[162] cats[163] and swine[217] a severe and markedly microcytic, somewhat hypochromic anemia develops when the animals are fed a diet lacking in pyridoxine. The anemia may be less consistent or severe in monkeys,[193a] mice[183] and rats.[176] In swine[217] the anemia is accompanied by moderate but irregular reticulocytosis, polychromatophilia and normoblasts in the circulating blood, and the bone marrow is hyperplastic. There is no evidence of increased blood destruction[151] but the plasma iron is elevated even to four times the normal level.[151,162,181,217] The spleen, liver and bone marrow and to a lesser extent the kidneys, are laden with deposited iron. The administration of pyridoxine is followed by a well defined reticulocyte response which is proportional to the dose given, the route of administration and the degree of anemia. There is a very rapid fall in the plasma iron, a rapid rise in the red cell count, hemoglobin and volume of packed red cells and restoration of normal red cell morphology. At the same time the marrow hyperplasia disappears and the deposited iron is removed from the tissues.[217] It appears, however, that some type of deficiency remains, for the hemoglobin does not return entirely to normal[181] or cannot be maintained there unless brewers' yeast or liver is furnished.[200]

Vitamin B_6 is a co-enzyme required in the biosynthesis of hemoglobin, as shown in Figure 3–9. In its absence porphobilinogen cannot be formed and iron is consequently not utilized for erythropoiesis. The position of this vitamin in the formation of porphobilinogen explains the low levels of free erythrocyte protoporphyrin (E.P.) in pyridoxine deficiency and the prompt rise in E. P. following its administration.[151,217]

Vitamin B_6 is a class name for several naturally occurring free forms, including pyridoxine, pyridoxal and pyridoxamine. This vitamin is concerned with the activity of a wide variety of enzyme systems involved in intermediary metabolism. The co-enzyme is the 5-phosphate of pyridoxal. The chemical reactions catalyzed by vitamin B_6 have little in common, except that for the most part they involve action of one sort or another upon amino acids. Thus pyridoxal-5-phosphate serves as a co-enzyme for amino acid decarboxylases, transaminases, desulfurases and racemases.[201] Vitamin B_6 is also essential for the metabolic conversion of tryptophane to quinoline derivatives and nicotinic acid. When there is a deficiency of vitamin B_6 the conversion of tryptophane to the pyridine co-enzymes and N'-methylnicotinamide is restricted and intermediary metabolites of tryptophane, such as xanthurenic acid, are excreted in the urine.[151] Pyridoxine may also be required for the synthesis of the more highly unsaturated fatty acids. The important role of vitamin B_6 in intermediary metabolism explains the variety of manifestations observed in vitamin B_6 deficiency in experimental animals. In addition to impaired growth and the anemia, already described, epileptiform convulsions and sensory neuron degeneration have been observed in swine,[217] symmetrical dermatitis in rats[176] and changes resembling arteriosclerosis in monkeys.[193a]

A need for pyridoxine has been encountered in man in several different circumstances: (1) in infants fed a milk formula which provided an inadequate quantity of vitamin B_6.[146b] Convulsive seizures were the chief manifestations of this deficiency and administration of the vitamin relieved the deficiency. "Rum fits" in alcoholics[177a] may similarly be due to a deficiency of vitamin B_6; (2) in patients receiving large doses of isoniazid. In such persons peripheral neuropathy, characterized by symmetrical numbness and tingling, may be followed by paresthesia, pain and aching in muscle and bone, exaggeration or reduction of tendon reflexes and ataxia.[210a] This is apparently due to the combination of isoniazid and pyridoxine to form a hydrazone and can be prevented by the administration of an excess of pyridoxine; (3) as the consequence of an inborn or acquired need for vitamin B_6 which is above normal. Thus several infants fed adequate diets have been observed who had convulsive seizures which could be relieved by the administration of pyridoxine.[146b] Again, in pregnancy there may be a metabolic defect which increases the need for this vitamin.[208a,210a] Finally, a pyridoxine-responsive anemia has been observed in several instances which could not be attributed to dietary deficiency of the vitamin (see below). In addition to these circumstances, pyridoxine deficiency has been deliberately produced (1) in two hydrocephalic infants by the administration of a deficient diet.[202] In one of these convulsions developed whereas in the other microcytic hypochromic anemia occurred; (2) in human subjects given the pyridoxine antagonist, 4-deoxypyridoxine.[187] In the latter no anemia was produced but lymphopenia, seborrhic dermatitis, glossitis and irritability were common and glossitis, cheilosis, angular stomatitis and peripheral neuritis were observed in a few.

Pyridoxine-responsive anemia has been reported in seven men, 26 to 52 years of age, all of whom had had refractory anemia for many years.[145c,147,148b, 161,162b,168,208] Microcytic, hypochromic anemia was marked in six of these men and moderate in the seventh. Marked anisocytosis, target cells and frequent bizarre forms of erythrocytes were described. Hyperferremia and nearly saturated iron-binding capacity of the serum were reported in six cases.[145c,148b, 162b,168,208] Splenomegaly and hepatomegaly in one patient, previously reported as a member of a family with "hereditary sex-linked (?) anemia" (p. 711), were associated with leukopenia and hemosiderosis of the bone marrow, as well as cardiac deterioration.[147] He had received many blood transfusions. The leukocyte count was elevated (13,000 to 25,000 per c.mm.) in one patient.[168] Abnormal urinary excretion of the metabolites of *l*-tryptophane following oral loading tests were demonstrated in three cases[161,162b,168] but were negative in two.[161,147,208] In all seven the administration of pyridoxine in large quantities (10 to 100 mg. parenterally, 200 mg. orally) was associated with reticulocytosis and relief of anemia, although this was incomplete in at least four cases.[147,148b,161,168] No true dietary deficiency of pyridoxine could be postulated in any of the cases. An instance of pyridoxine responsive hypochromic anemia has also been described in a well nourished male African.[162a]

The writer has seen a similar (unreported) case in Australia and he and his associates have studied two additional cases, one in a boy of 8 years and the other in a man of 43 years of age. Both patients have microcytic, hypochromic anemia, hyperferremia and hyperplastic bone marrow. As in another case,[208] siderocytes are prominent (Fig. 2–6, p. 101). Splenomegaly, hepatomegaly and skin pigmentation are present in both but each had received many blood transfusions. In neither case has it been possible to relieve the anemia completely by the administration of pyridoxine. It is of interest that all of the reported cases, as well as our own, have been in male subjects. Two at least began in early childhood. No familial incidence has been demonstrated as yet.

In marked contrast to the above cases, the patient reported by Maier was a women of 67 years who had refractory macrocytic anemia, megaloblastic marrow, hemochromatosis and mild diabetes. The anemia was partially relieved by the administration of pyridoxine.[180]

Pantothenic Acid.—In spite of its important role in the biosynthesis of hemoglobin (p. 153), deficiency of pantothenic acid, experimentally induced in swine, was associated with the development of only a moderate normocytic anemia.[216a] In these animals, severe sensory neuron degeneration was induced (p. 526) as well as extensive colitis. In rats anemia and granulocytopenia have been reported.[154] In man, experimentally induced pantothenic acid deficiency was found to be associated with fatigue, headache, weakness, emotional lability, impaired motor coordination, paresthesias, muscle cramps, gastrointestinal disturbances and eosinopenia, but anemia did not develop.[169a]

Riboflavin.—Anemia or impaired hemoglobin production following removal of blood has been observed in several species of animals receiving a riboflavin deficient diet. In swine[216] and in dogs[203] the anemia is moderate in degree and gradual in progress. In monkeys[210] a more rapidly developing anemia, sometimes of great severity, has been observed. Morphological studies in swine (Table 3–2) indicated that the anemia is normocytic in type, whereas hypochromic microcytic anemia has been reported in dogs. When the demand for hemoglobin formation was made more severe by phlebotomy, a decreased capacity for hemoglobin formation was demonstrated in dogs,[165,203] which could be corrected by as little as 30 μgm. riboflavin per kilogram body weight daily. Similar observations have been made in rats.[176a,184a] In nutritionally deficient persons with clinical signs attributed to riboflavin deficiency, anemia has not been recorded but in deficiency induced by the administration of the riboflavin antagonist, galactoflavin, together with a riboflavin restricted diet, reticulocytopenia and severe anemia were observed in three subjects after 21 to 30 days.[176b] Seborrheic dermatitis of the face, ears and scrotum, angular stomatitis and cheilosis developed as well. Reticulocytosis occurred promptly upon supplementation with riboflavin. It has been suggested that riboflavin may be concerned in the metabolism and arrangement of the amino acids of the protein of the hemoglobin molecule.[203]

Nicotinic Acid (Niacin).—The significance of nicotinic acid in hematopoiesis has been obscure even though a role for this vitamin has been suspected since the importance of nicotinic acid in pellagra and in acute black-tongue in dogs was first demonstrated. In the latter condition the hemoglobin may not be reduced but may even be increased when the manifestations of the disorder are at their peak. It was shown, however, that the acute symptoms could be alleviated by the parenteral administration of normal saline solution. When this was done a profound anemia made its appearance.[167] This was found to be macrocytic hypochromic and normocytic normochromic in type when two different nicotinic acid deficient diets were fed. The anemia was not associated with evidence of exaggerated blood destruction but was of great severity. Following the administration of nicotinic acid there was an immediate reticulocyte response followed by restoration of normal red cell production. In swine maintained on a low-protein, niacin-deficient diet normocytic anemia developed which responded to either protein or niacin therapy.[150] The anemia occurring in pellagra will be discussed elsewhere (p. 509). Since nicotinic acid is concerned in the synthesis of pyridine nucleotide and thus in cell respiration, lack of this vitamin may interfere with the respiration of immature red cells.

Ascorbic Acid.—Reference was made earlier to observations which indicate that ascorbic acid augments the conversion of folic acid to folinic acid (p. 135). The interrelationship of these substances is also exemplified by experiments in monkeys in which megaloblastic anemia was produced regularly by feeding milk diets deficient in ascorbic acid.[224] The experimental megaloblastosis could be eliminated or prevented by giving folic acid or folinic acid without the addition of ascorbic acid and could be cured by giving ascorbic acid alone. Vitamin B_{12} had no influence on the deficiency. If supplementary folic acid was given, when scurvy appeared the anemia was normoblastic rather than megaloblastic. As scurvy progressed, hemorrhage occurred and iron deficiency ensued. These experiments were interpreted as indicating that ascorbic acid serves no specific function in hematopoiesis but that the requirements for folic acid and for iron are increased in scurvy.

This conclusion is consistent with observations in a normal man in whom ascorbic acid deficiency was induced.[220] Manifest scurvy developed but no anemia occurred in spite of blood loss by venesection over a period of several months totaling 6000 ml. In another well controlled study of human vitamin C deficiency, hemoglobin regeneration took place spontaneously or in response to iron therapy without the addition of ascorbic acid.[223]

In naturally occurring scurvy in man, anemia is usually present and is generally normocytic.[219] It may be slightly macrocytic.[219a] Hypochromic microcytic anemia is sometimes encountered. Persistent reticulocytosis, moderate leukopenia and thrombocytopenia occur frequently and moderate icterus of the hemolytic type is common.[227] The bone marrow is usually quite cellular, with a relative increase of normoblasts[227] but occasional megaloblasts have been reported.[219] The survival time of red cells transfused in patients with scurvy has been found to be shortened,[225] suggesting thereby the existence of a hemolytic process. While this may be true, it must be recognized that some of the increased excretion of pigment which may be encountered in scurvy is attributable to extravascular

hemolysis in the hematomata. That the changes which take place in human scurvy can be similar to those produced in the monkey is suggested by the observation that the urinary excretion of citrovorum factor was found to be reduced in two men with scurvy and this increased to normal levels when ascorbic acid was given.[221] It was also found that hematologic responses to folic acid could be demonstrated in such patients, suggesting that ascorbic acid is necessary for erythropoiesis in man through potentiation of the hematologic effect of folic acid.

Ascorbic acid deficiency develops in man because he does not possess the enzyme system required for the formation of L-ascorbic acid from glucose.[219b] The deficiency, if sufficiently severe and maintained for a sufficiently long period of time, may closely simulate the experimental ascorbic acid deficiency described in monkeys. However, scurvy, the clinical disorder, usually represents a multiple deficiency state in which lack of vitamin C predominates. Iron deficiency may be associated or may result and other deficiencies may complicate the picture.

Pyrrol-containing pigments play no part in blood formation in man, in spite of the close structural relationship between chlorophyll and the prosthetic group of hemoglobin.[222,226]

Minerals.—As a constituent of hemoglobin, iron is essential for erythropoiesis. Iron metabolism will be discussed below (p. 143). Many other minerals have been attributed a role in erythropoiesis but of these only copper and cobalt deserve serious consideration. Thus, no adequate evidence has been offered to show that manganese,[131a] germanium, molybdenum, nickel, vanadium or zinc have erythropoietic activity.[122] The zinc in red corpuscles is mainly attributable to their carbonic anhydrase content.[144a] Calcium and phosphorus influence erythropoiesis only insofar as they affect iron assimilation (p. 144). It is noteworthy that commercial iron preparations contain, as contaminants, small amounts of manganese, copper[125] and even cobalt.[144]

Copper.—Copper Metabolism.—The average diet furnishes 1.7 to 4.2 mg. copper per day. In the adult, positive copper balance is maintained if the dietary intake is approximately 2 mg. per day or greater.[110] It has been estimated that the dietary requirement for children may be about 80 μg. per kilogram of body weight per day. Since fetal stores are high, the requirement in pregnancy may be increased.

Copper is absorbed by the small intestine and transported by the blood.[122] Following oral administration of copper sulfate[121] or after ingestion of radioactive copper,[128] the element appears quickly in the plasma, the concentration reaching its peak in from two to five hours, after which it falls abruptly. This is bound loosely to protein, principally the albumin fraction, but the iron-binding protein (p. 146) is also capable of uniting reversibly with copper. However, only a negligible quantity of the copper normally in plasma represents transport copper. Approximately 96 per cent of it is bound to an α_2 globulin, ceruloplasmin.[115] Radioactive copper also appears rapidly in the circulating red cells but its concentration continues to increase for two days.[123] Within the same period the metal can be demonstrated in the liver.

The copper content of *whole blood* in 40 normal male subjects was found to be 96 $\pm$ 13 μg. per 100 ml. blood and in 23 females it was 100 $\pm$ 11 μg. The *plasma copper* in normal males and females was 105 $\pm$ 16 μg. and 116 μg. $\pm$ 16 μg. per 100 ml. plasma, respectively, whereas the copper content of the red corpuscles was 100 $\pm$ 16 μg. and 122 $\pm$ 29 μg. per 100 ml. red cells, respectively. The calculated amount of copper in the average red corpuscle (mean corpuscular copper) is approximately 100 $\mu\mu$g.[118] At least 80 per cent of the copper in erythrocytes is in the form of a colorless compound, erythrocuprein, which has a molecular weight of 35,000 and contains 0.32 to 0.34 per cent copper in the form of 2 atoms of copper per molecule.[119a] Ceruloplasmin, in contrast, is a blue compound.

Copper is present in all animal tissues and is probably a functional constituent of all living cells.[120] The highest concentrations are found in the liver, brain, heart, lung, and spleen. In newborn animals the liver is particularly rich in copper. Excretion of copper occurs chiefly via the bile ducts into the bowel, but the kidneys take part as well.[124]

Variations in blood copper occur in different clinical conditions.[118] Whole blood and plasma copper are increased in pregnancy, in various subacute and chronic infections and in a variety of diseases, including Hodgkin's disease, acute leukemia, aplastic anemia, hyperthyroidism and hemochromatosis. Less consistently, hypercupremia is found in chronic leukemia, lymphosarcoma, pernicious and iron deficiency anemias, hypothyroidism and collagen disorders. Hypocupremia, on the other hand, is rare, having been found only in the newborn, in nephrosis, in hepatolenticular degeneration, and in some cases of sprue as well as in a syndrome in infants which will be described below.[109] Significantly increased mean corpuscular copper has been observed only in pernicious anemia, while high values for total red cell copper have been found only in infants with iron deficiency anemia. Significantly low total red cell copper values have been encountered only in hyperthyroidism.

The functions of copper can be inferred from the nature of the compounds in which it is found and from the manifestations of copper deficiency. Copper is a constituent of a number of enzymes, such as butyryl coenzyme A dehydrogenase,[110] tyrosinase and, in plants, the polyphenyl-oxidases, laccase and ascorbic acid oxidase.[120] Copper was first shown to be concerned in erythropoiesis when anemia in weanling rats, fed a diet of milk, which is deficient in both iron and copper, failed to respond to iron therapy unless copper was added.[112] Copper deficiency has been observed in ruminants feeding on copper deficient soils in Holland, Great Britain and Ireland, the Scandinavian countries, Florida, Australia and New Zealand. Signs of the deficiency include unthriftiness of the hair, achromotrichia, in sheep loss of crimp in the wool, cachexia, bone changes and, in lambs, ataxia. A neurological disorder due to extensive demyelination of the central nervous system occurs in sheep and is known as "enzoötic ataxia" and "sway-back."[115a] In rats and swine, hypochromic anemia accompanies the copper deficiency and is progressive.[120] These observations suggest, therefore, that copper is involved in the normal process of pigmentation, in keratinization, in maintaining the integrity of the nervous system, in osteogenesis and in hemopoiesis, as well as in a number of other physiological processes.

Role in Erythropoiesis.—Anemia due to copper deficiency in young swine is hypochromic and microcytic in type, as in iron deficiency, and is accompanied by hypoferremia as well as hypocupremia.[117] Experimental copper deficiency in rats also produces hypochromic microcytic anemia, which is accompanied by reticulocytosis.[126] In dogs[107,119] the anemia seems to be normocytic.

A number of studies have indicated that copper is concerned in iron metabolism.[127] That it plays a role in the absorption of iron is suggested by several observations. Thus, the total iron content in the blood, liver, kidneys, spleen and heart of copper deficient swine fed the same amount of iron for the same period of time as litter mate controls was found to be reduced to levels comparable to those seen in iron deficient swine. Again, the total amount of radioactive iron found in the tissues of copper deficient swine following the oral administration of radioactive iron was significantly less than in control animals. Furthermore, copper deficient swine responded to the administration of copper only when iron was included in the diet, suggesting thereby that the tissues did not contain sufficient iron for hemoglobin formation. It is possible that a copper protein may be involved in some manner in the absorption of iron from the gastrointestinal tract.

It is clear, however, that copper does not exert its influence on erythropoiesis by virtue of its effect on iron absorption; the anemia of copper deficiency could neither be prevented nor alleviated by the intravenous administration of iron. Studies of the daily turnover rate of iron through the plasma and the incorporation of iron into the red cells showed this to be increased above the normal in copper-deficient swine.[108] Thus it would appear that movement of iron within the body is not curtailed. It was also found that the life span of the erythrocyte is shortened. Comparison with blood production in animals in which hemolytic anemia was produced by the administration of phenylhydrazine indicated that production of red cells in the presence of copper deficiency is not as active as is possible when copper is available. It would seem, therefore, that the relation of copper to iron metabolism must in some way be concerned with the role of copper in red cell synthesis. Anemia may develop in the absence of copper because of limitation of the capacity of the marrow to produce cells and because of a shortened erythrocyte survival time.

A naturally occurring copper deficiency in man would not be expected since copper is present in a variety of foods and is present even as a contaminant of water.[110] Cow's milk, however, is relatively poor in copper, as well as iron. Consequently it would seem possible for copper deficiency to occur in infants under certain circumstances. Actually in infants with nutritional anemia, an accelerated or a more continued response to iron was observed when copper was added than when iron was given alone.[113,116] The livers of anemic infants were found to contain less copper than those of non-anemic ones.[111] In older children and in adults, on the other hand, several studies failed entirely to indicate a need for copper in the treatment of anemia.[114] It is noteworthy that impurities of copper may be found in various iron salts used therapeutically.[125] In kwashiorkor low plasma copper, iron and total protein levels have been reported.[120a] Nevertheless, the serum copper of infants with nutritional anemia has been found to be normal or increased[127] and attempts to produce copper deficiency, even in premature infants, have been unsuccessful.[126a]

These observations make all the more mystifying a **syndrome** which has been observed in more than 50 infants which is characterized by **hypocupremia,** hypoferremia and hypoproteinemia.[121a] These cases, though varying considerably one from another, form two general groups; namely (1) infants who have subsisted on almost nothing but milk and (2) others who have eaten a more varied diet. Edema and hypoalbuminemia were conspicuous in the majority but either inconspicuous or lacking in others. Study of a large number of infants with iron deficiency revealed a spectrum of deficiencies, ranging from iron deficiency alone to such deficiency accompanied by hypoproteinemia and hypocupremia. It is possible that iron deficiency is the primary defect in these cases and leads to hypoproteinemia and, ultimately, to impaired copper retention.

Cobalt.—That cobalt plays an important *role in animal nutrition* became apparent from the study of a malady of ruminants known variously as pining, coast disease, enzoötic marasmus, bush disease and salt sickness which has been encountered in the British Isles, Australia, New Zealand and Florida.[120] The condition is characterized by unthriftiness, progressive wasting and profound macrocytic[120] or normocytic[143a] anemia as well as hemosiderosis[144] but is not accompanied by neurologic changes. It was observed that the disorder could be relieved when cobalt was administered orally but not when it was given intravenously. The significance of these findings was clarified by the discovery that cobalt is an essential constituent of vitamin B_{12} and that it is incorporated into this vitamin in the rumen. It appears that the only physiologic hemopoietic function of cobalt is as a constituent of vitamin B_{12}.

The experimental production of *cobalt deficiency*[134] is made difficult by the low requirement for cobalt, at least in nonruminants. Cobalt deficiency does not seem to occur naturally except in ruminants. It is noteworthy that nonruminant, herbivorous animals confined to pastures on which cattle and sheep developed enzoötic marasmus remained healthy.[120] It is also perhaps significant that the livers of ruminants are a more potent source of vitamin B_{12} than those of pigs or rats.[143] Studies of cobalt metabolism with the aid of its radioactive isotope indicate that cobalt is absorbed with comparative efficiency and reaches its highest concentration in the glandular organs. It is in great part eliminated, chiefly in the urine.[136] The accuracy of recorded values for the normal human consumption and excretion of cobalt[138] has been questioned.

Cobalt Polycythemia.—The administration of cobalt in quantities far in excess of the normal dietary requirement results in the production of polycythemia in many species of animals.[122] This is due to a true increase in red cell mass[140] and is accompanied by reticulocytosis, hyperplasia of the bone marrow and increased erythropoietic activity in the liver and spleen.[133] The underlying mechanism is obscure. It was thought that cobalt acts by inhibiting those enzymatic activities that deal with the transport of oxygen and that the resulting tissue anoxia produces polycythemia. The cobaltous ion is known to have a marked inhibitory action *in vitro* on the endogeneous respiration of a number of tissues. It was pointed out that the influence of cobalt in producing polycythemia can be lessened materially by the inclusion in the diet of sufficient sulfur-containing amino acids.[137] These substances, especially cysteine,[140] are known to chelate with cobalt. Thus the effect of cobalt might be due to the fixation of thiol groups. Other evidence indicated that cobalt inhibits heme synthesis.[139a] More recent studies suggest that cobalt stimulates the formation of erythropoietin (p. 50). This seems to be the mechanism whereby cobalt overcomes the anemia induced in animals by hypophysectomy[132] and possibly that of protein deficiency.[140]

The simultaneous administration of cobalt, in large amounts, was found to prevent the development of anemia resulting from experimentally induced ininflammation.[145] Likewise in patients with various types of anemia refractory to other forms of antianemic therapy, such as anemia associated with infection,[130] renal disease[135] and cancer,[142] the daily oral administration of 20 to 300 mg., but more usually 60 to 150 mg., of cobaltous chloride is associated with reticulocyte increases and some relief of the anemia. Claims that hemoglobin regeneration in patients with iron deficiency anemia is more rapid when cobalt-iron mixtures are given than that resulting from iron therapy alone are not convincing. Thus reports that cobalt

improves iron utilization in the anemia of prematurity[132,141] fail to offer any observations on the effects of iron therapy as compared with iron-cobalt therapy in parallel series of infants. Cobalt therapy relieved the anemia in a case of "acquired erythrocytic hypoplasia"[141a] but a significant effect in hypoplastic or aplastic anemia seems to be the exception[130] rather than the rule.

The prolonged administration of cobaltous chloride in the doses cited may be associated with anorexia, nausea and vomiting. Less frequent ill effects include flushing of the face and extremities, skin rash, tinnitus and nerve deafness, substernal pain and even thyroid hyperplasia associated with thyroid hypofunction.[139] Furthermore, in cases of anemia associated with infection and cancer and treated with cobalt the patients seemed to derive no real benefit even though the anemia was less severe. In the cases of renal anemia[135] cobalt therapy was associated with improved appetite and greater tolerance for medications necessary to correct electrolyte abnormalities. However, the increased blood values promptly declined to pretreatment levels when the drug was discontinued. It appears, therefore, that the uses of cobalt as a therapeutic agent are very limited and the indiscriminate administration of cobalt-iron preparations in the treatment of anemia finds no justification.

IRON METABOLISM

The total body iron of an adult man amounts to 4 to 5 grams. Only a minute proportion is in the form of free ferrous ions. These, together with iron in transport in the plasma, where it is carried in bond with a β_1 serum globulin (transferrin), make up only 0.1 per cent of the total body iron. The remainder is either bound in a porphyrin ring, as a part of blood or muscle hemoglobin or as one of

Table 3–3.—*Approximate Composition of the Iron-containing Compounds in the Human (70-Kilo Man) (after Drabkin)*[58]

Compound	Total Amt. gm.	Iron Content gm.	Per Cent of Total Fe
Iron porphyrin (heme) compounds:			
Blood hemoglobin	900	3.06	72.9
Muscle hemoglobin (myoglobin)	40	0.14	3.3
Heme enzymes:			
Cytochrome c	0.8	0.0034	0.08
Catalase	5.0	0.0045	0.11
Cytochrome a, a_3, b	—	—	—
Peroxidase	—	—	—
Non-iron porphyrin compounds:			
Transferrin (siderophilin)	7.5	0.003	0.07
Ferritin	3.0	0.69	16.4
Hemosiderin	—	—	—
Total available iron stores	—	1.2–1.5	—
Total iron	—	4.2	100

the heme enzymes (Table 3–3), or is laid aside as storage iron. The storage forms of iron, ferritin and hemosiderin, constitute normally about 16 per cent of the body iron and are in the form of ferric hydroxide units.[67] The total iron store in man which is available for blood formation is approximately 1.2 to 1.5 grams.[78] The metabolism of iron is presented schematically in Figure 3–5.

Absorption of Iron.—The earlier literature concerning the availability of iron in various foods is not wholly reliable[89] because the technical difficulties involved in such measurements were not fully appreciated. Thus iron in food of both plant and animal origin must be released from its conjugates before it can be absorbed from the gastrointestinal tract. It is mainly in the ferric state, much of it as ferric hydroxide and as iron bound loosely to organic molecules such as citrate, lactate and amino acids. Only ionic iron can be absorbed and, in man, ferrous ions are more readily absorbed than the trivalent form.[90a] However, the α,α'-dipyridyl test[53] which depends on reaction with ionizable, ferrous iron and was used for a long time as an index of the value of different foods as a source of

iron, has not been found reliable when comparison has been made with physiological activity. Again, tests of the utilization of food iron which depend on hemoglobin regeneration[105] are reliable as a measure of iron absorption only if the anemia is solely due to iron deficiency.

Many factors influence the absorption of iron. Iron readily forms insoluble compounds with various constituents of the diet, especially in a medium which is not strongly acid. Phytates, which are present in various cereals, are among such compounds.[98] Iron phosphates are practically insoluble and consequently a high phosphorus content in the diet could interfere with iron absorption[79] unless other factors counteracted this. A high level of calcium in the diet diminishes the formation of insoluble iron phosphates but excess calcium inhibited iron assimilation.[52] Experimentally a diet very low in phosphate was found to produce a progressive increase in body iron stores.[79] In rats, antacids such as calcium carbonate, aluminum hydroxide and magnesium trisilicate reduced iron retention.[65] To what extent observations such as these are applicable to man is uncertain, however.

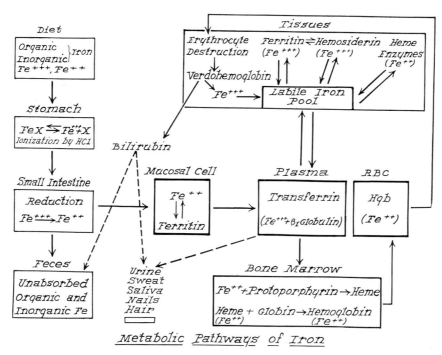

Metabolic Pathways of Iron

Fig. 3–5.—Schematic outline of iron metabolism.
(Prepared by Dr. G. E. Cartwright.)

Concerning the relative value of different foods, there is comparatively little dependable information. In one of the few significant earlier studies, it was found that 11 to 14 per cent of the iron in spinach and in mixed diets is absorbed and as much as 21 per cent of that in beef.[87] The long held concept that iron present in food in the form of heme compounds is not available for absorption, has been found erroneous, as much as 11 per cent being absorbed in normal subjects.[55] Valuable information has been obtained by incorporating radioactive iron in poultry products and vegetables by injection into hens and by its addition to the nutrient solutions in which vegetables were grown.[89] As judged by the amount of radioiron incorporated into circulating hemoglobin and the quantity recovered in the feces and presumably unabsorbed, it appears that the amount of iron absorbed from foods

by normal subjects is 10 per cent or less. Greater assimilation was not achieved on mixture of the test foods with other foods except with relatively large amounts (200 to 250 ml.) of citrus fruit juices. Ascorbic acid and reducing substances such as cysteine had a similar effect but organic acids, such as citric and lactic acid were without effect. The influence of ascorbic acid can probably be attributed to the reduction of ferric iron in food to the ferrous form. In other studies, normal children were found to absorb an average of about 10 per cent of the naturally occurring iron in milk, eggs and chicken liver, as well as the iron supplements added to commercially prepared infant cereals.[97] The iron added to bread in the food fortification program is a significant source of iron in human nutrition.[100] In general it can be stated that inorganic iron supplementation is a more effective way of increasing iron retention than the giving of iron in the form of vegetables.[83]

Peptic digestion of cooked foods is probably important. The role of other enzymes in the gastrointestinal tract has not been investigated. Although the absorption of iron may take place all along the gastrointestinal tract,[73] it probably is absorbed chiefly in the duodenal region because the actively absorptive surface there is abetted by the relatively low pH which prevents the auto-oxidizable ferrous iron from being converted to ferric hydroxide.[67]

The importance of the hydrochloric acid of the gastric juice has long been the subject of debate. Clinical experience shows that iron deficiency is commonly associated with achlorhydria (p. 746) and early studies revealed that an iron-rich diet had practically no effect on hemoglobin formation during periods of alkalinization as carried out with a modified Sippy regimen, in contrast to the evidence of hemoglobin regeneration when the regimen was withdrawn.[84] On the other hand, studies with food containing radioiron failed to show increased absorption of iron as the consequence of addition of hydrochloric acid to cooked eggs.[89] Yet, in partially gastrectomized subjects, absorption of radioiron from a test meal was found to be below the average normal in six out of eight subjects.[101] These conflicting observations can be resolved if one assumes that the facilitation of iron absorption attributed to the normal acid secretion of the stomach is real but, nevertheless, relatively unimportant under normal circumstances. However, when the requirement for iron becomes relatively high, the presence of free hydrochloric acid may be important in making additional dietary iron available for absorption.

Regulation of Iron Absorption.—For many years it was assumed that a mechanism exists for the regulation of iron absorption, a "mucosal block" serving to prevent absorption when iron is not needed. Thus it was found that considerably more radioactive iron was present in the tissues of dogs made anemic by repeated bleeding as compared with those of normal dogs given similar amounts of radioiron by mouth.[73] Similarly, in humans during pregnancy and following repeated blood loss, a high percentage of fed radioactive iron was found in the red corpuscles. However, in disease states such as pernicious anemia and familial icterus where it is known that iron stores are very abundant, very little iron appeared in the red cells.[54] Unfortunately, in these experiments the factor of iron utilization was overlooked. Failure of iron to appear in red corpuscles is not necessarily due to failure of absorption; for example, in pernicious anemia in relapse erythropoiesis is impaired and administered radioiron cannot be used.[62]

It was shown in our laboratory that, unless it is withheld from the diet, iron continues to be absorbed by pyridoxine deficient pigs even though the plasma iron is greatly elevated and the tissues are laden with deposited iron.[151] Later it was found, by measuring the quantity of unabsorbed isotope in the feces, that patients with pernicious anemia or other conditions actually absorb more iron than they utilize for hemoglobin synthesis.[59] With alterations of diet and administration of large amounts of iron, increased absorption of iron was observed in rats in the absence of anemia.[63] Increased iron absorption was also demonstrated in experimentally induced hemolytic anemia.[102] Many investigators have finally come to question the theory of "intestinal intelligence."

There is evidence that in the intestinal mucosa an "iron acceptor" compound exists. Iron absorbed into the mucosal cells[91] in the ferrous form probably combines there with a protein, apoferritin, to form ferritin.[67] In the cell there may be an equilibrium between ferrous iron and the ferric iron stored in ferritin. It is thought that the iron acceptor compound is concerned with the transport of iron across the mucosal barrier and into the blood stream.

Significant studies continue to indicate, however, that iron absorption can be influenced. Thus, iron absorption appeared to be increased above the normal in iron deficient subjects[83] and other investigators noted that iron absorption was accelerated when erythropoiesis was active, and depressed when iron stores were large.[54b] Yet, if there is a regulatory mechanism, its nature is obscure[90] and its operation imperfect. Possibly the plasma iron transport mechanism, described below, mediates the iron demand of the body to the absorptive area.[76a]

Iron Transport.—A schematic outline of iron metabolism is presented in Figure 3–5. Upon absorption by intestinal mucosal cells, iron is enveloped within ferritin molecules.[67] In the presence of reducing agents, ferritin iron is released to the surfaces of the ferritin molecules[86] and is then bound by a specialized transport protein of the plasma ("*transferrin*," "*siderophilin*"). This is a β_1 globulin of 90,000 molecular weight. Each molecule binds two iron atoms to form a colored complex.[96] The iron is in the ferric state.[85] Three transferrins have been identified, these being genetically controlled at a single locus.[99] In the blood stream transferrin is normally only about one-third saturated with iron.[95] In three different series, the mean value for the total **iron-binding capacity of serum**[96] was 300,[95] 315,[85] and 359[56] μgm. per cent. The standard deviation in the last group was 30.8 μgm. per cent. These values correspond to 0.24 to 0.28 Gm. transferrin per 100 ml. serum. Measurements by means of the quantitative precipitin reaction gave a similar figure (0.27 Gm.).[81]

The **normal content of iron in plasma** has been found in various studies to be between 50 and 180 μgm. per cent.[91] Powell[93] found average values of 143 and 117 μgm. per cent in men and women, respectively, with standard deviations of 24 and 26.5 μgm., respectively, but our own observations[10] revealed no significant difference between the sexes. The mean $\pm$ standard error of the mean was 104.7 $\pm$ 3.4 μgm. %. The standard deviation was $\pm$ 32.8. A diurnal variation in plasma iron level has been observed,[77] hypoferremia occurring in the evening.[92]

The serum iron of umbilical cord blood at parturition is high (173 to 193 μgm. per cent[71,103]) but in twelve hours hypoferremia is found.[103] Until two months of age a normal[103] or increased[71] plasma iron level is present but after this time hypoferremia of varying degree develops. Values in older children successively approach adult levels.

The plasma iron reflects the balance between the iron absorbed from the bowel, that coming from hemoglobin catabolism, that going to and from the stores and tissues and that going to the bone marrow for hemoglobin synthesis. Approximately 27 mg. of iron enter and leave the blood plasma each day in a normal adult. Of this amount, about 21 mg. is derived more or less directly from the catabolism of the red corpuscles and the remainder comes primarily from storage iron, with a small per cent coming from ingested iron. Following the administration of iron salts an increase in plasma iron is apparent within the first half hour, the quantity of iron reaches a maximum within two and a half to five hours, and falls to the basal level in 12 to 18 hours.[90] Radioactive iron has been detected in red corpuscles four hours after it has been fed and has been found to be entirely converted to hemoglobin in four to seven days.[76] There seems to be no direct interchange between the plasma iron and that present in red cells as hemoglobin.[75] The plasma iron is reduced in iron deficiency anemias and in infection (p. 578) as well as in periods of active hemopoiesis and is elevated above normal in untreated pernicious anemia, hemolytic anemias and hypoplastic anemias. Pronounced increases in plasma iron, together with normal or reduced iron-binding capacity, have been observed in viral hepatitis in contrast to the normal values found in jaundice due to extrahepatic biliary obstruction.[57,106] The plasma iron is always increased in transfusion siderosis and in hemochromatosis, unless infection or neoplastic disease is present, and the iron-binding capacity is usually saturated.[63]

The capacity of the plasma to bind iron is increased in acute and chronic blood loss[56] and in pregnancy[85] while in acute and chronic infections, pernicious anemia, hemolytic anemia, cirrhosis of the liver, uremia and malignancy the capacity is diminished.[85] It has been suggested that transferrin exists in two phases: one circulating in the plasma and the other sequestered at cellular sites.[88a] Sequestration may result from orientation of iron-laden transferrin to iron receptors at cellular sites during the transfer of the iron to the cells. Possibly when the iron stores are heavily laden, iron is not readily unloaded, the sequestered transferrin tends to remain there and the iron-binding capacity of the plasma is low, as a consequence. One result of such reduced plasma iron-binding capacity may be decreased iron absorption at the level of the intestinal mucosa.

If iron is introduced intravenously in excess of the iron-binding capacity of the plasma, the concentration of plasma iron is found to be lower than would be expected on the basis of the quantity injected.[104] This has been called a "braking effect" but in reality is due to the fact that the excess iron is rapidly eliminated from the circulation. It is such infusions, in excess of the amount which can be bound, which produce toxic symptoms.

Iron is carried via the plasma to the bone marrow, liver and other tissues. Electron microscope studies of immature red cells suggest that erythroblasts obtain iron for hemoglobin synthesis by removing iron particles from contiguous macrophages.[54a] In the center of islands of erythroblasts one or two reticulum cells can be seen which give up their ferritin molecules to the erythroblasts by a phenomenon closely related to pinocytosis ("ropheocytosis"). Another mechanism, and perhaps the more usual one, consists in the direct transfer of iron from transferrin to the immature red cell. It has been shown that iron can be transferred directly to iron-binding receptors on the reticulocyte membrane without existing in a free form.[82] The transfer of the iron is accelerated by glucose and oxygen. Iron is then incorporated into hemoglobin, presumably under the control of the microsomes and mitochondria of the cytoplasmic reticulum.

The transfer of iron from plasma to liver has been studied with liver slices.[86] Mazur et al. concluded that the incorporation of iron into ferritin depends on energy produced during oxidative metabolic reactions and requires the synthesis of adenosine triphosphate (ATP). Ascorbic acid is also required. They believe that the plasma-bound ferric iron is reduced to the ferrous state, thus releasing it from its bond to the protein and making it available for incorporation into ferritin. The reverse process, the release of ferritin iron in the liver to the plasma, was found to involve the participation of the enzyme, xanthine oxidase, and was influenced by liver hypoxia as, for example, following extensive blood loss.[86] Saltman,[95b] on the other hand, found that oxidative metabolism of the liver cell was not concerned and believes that the process is diffusion controlled.

Excretion of Iron.—Once absorbed, iron is conserved tenaciously. However, some is inevitably lost since iron is present in all cells. Injected radioiron appears in sweat but it is difficult to determine whether this is by a process of true excretion or from desquamated epithelial cells. Under normal conditions the total iron lost from dermal surfaces is less than 1 mg. per day.[89] Whether or not very large amounts are lost when sweating is profuse[64,88] has yet to be answered conclusively.[63] Iron is also shed in the hair and nails. Fecal loss, whether by true excretion in the bile or in desquamated epithelial cells is normally of the order of 0.3 to 0.5 mg. per day.[61] Extremely small amounts are found in the urine.[72] The total loss in a normal adult per day is estimated to be between 0.5 and 1.5 mg. For the normally menstruating female an additional average loss of 0.5 to 1 mg. per day may be added.

Iron Storage.—Reserve iron is to be found in the liver, spleen, bone marrow and elsewhere. It seems to be in part very easily mobilized ("labile iron pool")[69] and, in the main, is held in a somewhat less mobile state.[91b] Two forms of iron have been recognized but it is doubtful whether there is any fundamental difference between them.[63] Iron is stored chiefly as ferritin. The ferritin molecule consists of a central nucleus of high iron content surrounded by a shell of protein approximately spherical in shape.[91a] By electron microscopy it appears that the iron is held in six micelles of ferric hydroxide[67] arranged at the corners of a regular octahedron. Ferritin is not detectable with iron stains because it is too diffusely scattered in the cells. The term *hemosiderin*[66] refers to clusters of iron visible in the optical microscope.[95a] Among such clusters ferritin molecules and other substances, not yet defined, have been observed by electron microscopy.[54a]

A method for staining hemosiderin in aspirated marrow is described elsewhere (p. 60).

Iron Requirements.—The amount of iron required by man depends on a number of factors, of which age and sex are the most important. The iron derived from destruction of red corpuscles is used repeatedly for blood formation and most or all of the stored iron is available. Some 20 mg. of iron are derived from the catabolism of red cells each day in the average adult. As already indicated, up to 1.5 mg. Fe is needed daily to make up for normal losses in the male and another 1 mg. in the normal female. The amount of iron furnished in the average normal diet is 12 to 15 mg. per day.[67] If but 10 per cent of the iron is normally absorbed, it follows that the adult male maintains a positive balance rather easily but the adult woman during the childbearing period is in a more precarious state as far as iron balance is concerned. Childbearing represents approximately a drain of 725 mg. iron, 400 mg. being contributed to the fetus, 150 mg. to the placenta and 175 mg. in blood loss. This amounts to an average requirement of 2.7 mg. per day throughout pregnancy.[80] Allowing for conservation of iron resulting from amenorrhea, there is a deficit of about 400 mg. during pregnancy or about 1 mg. per day. During lactation the extra need is less than in pregnancy, perhaps 0.5 mg. per day. The daily need of normal women for iron thus is somewhat in excess of 2 mg. and increases during pregnancy to 3 mg. or more.

Growth, because it presents a demand for an increased blood volume, increasing muscle (myoglobin) mass and respiratory enzymes, augments the need for iron. Estimated iron requirements at different ages are presented in Figure 14–2 (p. 733). Since the body of an infant contains about 0.5 gram Fe and that of an adult 4 to 5 grams, there must be a net gain during the first 20 years of life of

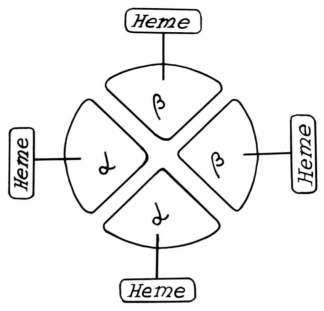

Fig. 3–6.—Diagrammatic representation of hemoglobin. The four polypeptide chains of globin are labelled α and β.

3.5 to 4.5 grams. This averages 0.18 to 0.22 gram per year or about 0.4 to 0.6 mg. per day. If excessively rapid growth occurs, and in the premature infant, the need is greater. It has been estimated that a daily dietary allowance of 1.0 to 1.5 mg./Kg./day is desirable to achieve optimal iron nutrition for the infant.

HEMOGLOBIN

Introduction.—Hemoglobin is a conjugated protein of approximately 67,000 molecular weight which contains four heme groups and globin. The latter consists of two (α,β) pairs of polypeptide chains. According to X-ray crystallography of horse hemoglobin, four subunits are arranged in a tetrahedral array, the four heme groups lying in separate pockets on the surface of the molecule (Fig. 3–6).[26] The various chains are held together by noncovalent forces to form a three dimensional, globular protein. These forces probably involve hydrogen bonds, ionic or salt linkages and hydrophobic interactions.

Hemoglobin, as a readily available protein, has been the subject of intense investigation. It is very widely distributed in nature and, wherever found, has the same fundamental property of reversible oxygenation and possesses the same heme nucleus as the prosthetic group. Nevertheless, the hemoglobins found in various species of animals and in certain protozoa, yeasts, molds and plants differ greatly in their biological, chemical and physical properties. What is more, different hemoglobins have been found within the same species of animals and even in the same individual. This is of importance from the clinical standpoint and is proving to be of value from the viewpoint of human genetics and in relation to an understanding of the migrations of mankind in the imperfectly documented past. In the latter studies, whole hemoglobin has been the primary material used in analysis but there is no evidence that the observed differences are related to the heme component of hemoglobin.[237] Consequently, the globin portion of the hemoglobin molecule has received special attention.

It will be convenient to discuss heme and globin separately since certain clinical states are related to one or the other and also because, from the standpoint of hemoglobin biosynthesis and catabolism, knowledge and interest center about the heme moiety rather than the globin. The amino acids of globin form a part of the body protein pool, coming therefrom and returning thereto, and no way has been found so far whereby the tracing of these steps might be helpful in the study of disorders of the blood.

The Heme Moiety of Hemoglobin

Heme, which constitutes about 4 per cent of the weight of the molecule, is a metal complex consisting of an iron atom in the center of a porphyrin structure (Fig. 3–7). The hemes impart to hemoglobin its red color.

For an understanding of hemoglobin biosynthesis and catabolism and also in relation to the porphyrias, the *terminology applied to the porphyrins* must be appreciated. Porphyrins are tetra-pyrroles. The four pyrrole rings are united by four methene ($_=\overset{H}{C}_-$) bridges, thus forming the porphin nucleus. This tetra-pyrrole, shown diagrammatically in Figure 3–8, is found in nature or can be prepared synthetically only when the eight hydrogen atoms have been replaced by certain substituent groups; namely methyl ($-CH_3$), vinyl ($-CH=CH_2$), acetic ($-CH_2-COOH$) or propionic acid ($-CH_2-CH_2-COOH$), the last two of which, it will be noted, contain carboxyl groups. The porphyrin in hemoglobin is a protoporphyrin and has only two carboxyl groups. It consists of a porphin nucleus in which the hydrogen atoms are replaced by 4 methyl, 2 vinyl and 2 pro-

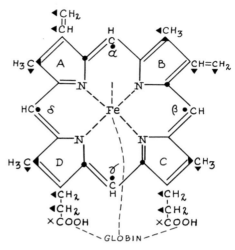

Fig. 3–7.—Chemical structure of heme and its manner of union with globin to form hemoglobin. The carbon atoms derived from the alpha carbon of glycine are represented by •, those supplied from the methyl carbon of acetate by ▲, those derived from the carboxyl group of acetate by x. The unmarked carbons are those which are derived from either the methyl carbon atom of acetate or from the carboxyl atom. (Prepared by Dr. G. E. Cartwright.)

pionic acid groups. Normal feces contains small amounts of a tetra-carboxylated porphyrin which Fischer called coproporphyrin. This is soluble in ether, as is protoporphyrin. The third important porphyrin compound is uroporphyrin, so-named because it was first isolated from urine. Uroporphyrin differs from coproporphyrin in that the four methyl groups are replaced by acetic acid side chains (Fig. 3–8). This octa-carboxylated acid is insoluble in ether and in most organic solvents.

The classification of the porphyrins is based upon four isomeric etioporphyrins which have been prepared by synthetic means and have been termed types I, II, III and IV. However, only types I and III are found in nature. The simultaneous formation along two isomeric lines is spoken of as the "dualism" of the porphyrins. In type I the substituent groups alternate regularly, in type III one pair

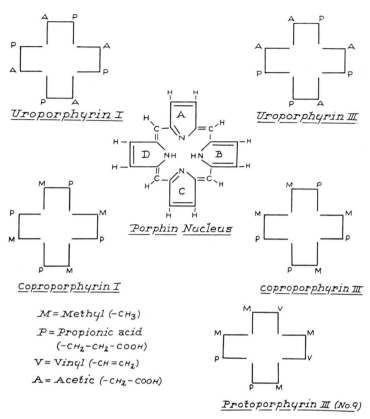

FIG. 3–8.—Structural formula of the porphin nucleus and diagrammatic representation of some naturally occurring porphyrins. (Prepared by Dr. G. E. Cartwright.)

is asymmetrical. When three types of side chains are present, as in protoporphyrin, the number of possible isomers is 15. The protoporphyrin of hemoglobin is classified as protoporphyrin 9, type III.

The propionic acid side chains of protoporphyrin, as mentioned earlier, may possibly function in the ionized form to orient the heme and help attach it to globin. The methyl groups protect the positions at which they are attached. The vinyl groups are required to make possible the insertion of iron into the porphyrin ring.[17]

The *iron* content of hemoglobin is 0.338 per cent. The iron has a coordination valence of six. Of these, four lie in one plane and link the iron to the nitrogen atoms of the pyrrole rings of heme whereas the remaining two valencies, one on each side of the flat heme molecule, have been believed to be linked to imidazole groups of two histidine residues of globin. Combination of hemoglobin with oxygen involves displacement of imidazole and leads to an iron-oxygen bond.[43]

The manner of linkage between heme and globin is uncertain, however, and a number of possibilities have been suggested.[20] Perhaps the best evidence supports the imidazole nature of the heme-binding group. There is some evidence that the carboxyl groups of the propionic acid side chains of heme interact with globin and add further stability to the linkage.[25b]

Biosynthesis of Hemoglobin (Fig. 3–9).—Incubation of labelled precursors

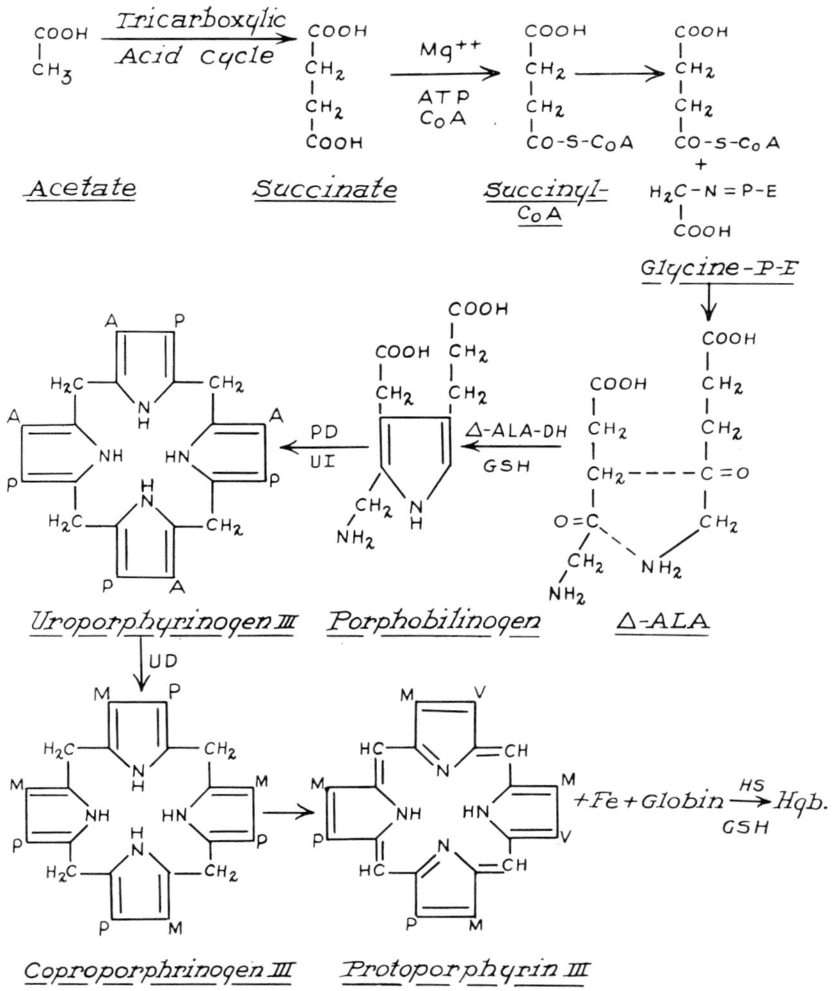

FIG. 3–9.—Chemical steps in the biosynthesis of hemoglobin (prepared by Dr. G. E. Cartwright). For abbreviations see text.

with duck and chicken erythrocytes,[34] rabbit reticulocytes and other sources of metabolically active cells,[2a] as well as evidence derived from isotope studies *in vivo*,[41] clarified the steps which take place in the natural synthesis of hemoglobin. These investigations showed that acetate, transformed into succinate via the tricarboxylic acid cycle[35] gives rise in the presence of $Mg++$, ATP and coenzyme A(CoA), to "active" succinate (succinyl-CoA). Since pantothenic acid is a component of CoA, this is at least one of the sites in which this vitamin functions in erythropoiesis (p. 137).

The activated form of succinate condenses with a pyridoxal phosphate-glycine-enzyme complex (glycine-P-E) to form delta-aminolevulinic acid ($\triangle$-ALA) and carbon dioxide,[15,17a,20b,31a] via several intermediate compounds.[35]

Two molecules of delta-aminolevulinic acid, in the presence of glutathione (GSH) and an enzyme, delta-aminolevulinic acid dehydrase ($\triangle$-ALA-DH),[15] condense to form a mono-pyrrole, por-

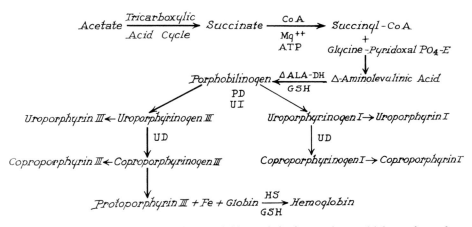

FIG. 3–10.—The biosynthesis of hemoglobin and the by-products which are formed
(prepared by Dr. G. E. Cartwright).

phobilinogen, which contains acetic acid and propionic acid side chains.[17a]

In the next step, four molecules of porphobilinogen condense to form the tetrapyrrolic structure, uroporphyrinogen. This step is catalyzed by at least two enzymes, porphobilinogen deaminase (PD) and uroporphyrin isomerase (UI).[7,17a] Details of the action of the enzymes and the sequence of reactions leading from porphobilinogen to uroporphyrinogen types I and III are not known. Shemin *et al.*[35] suggested that three moles of porphobilinogen may condense to form a tripyrrylmethane intermediate which breaks down to form a dipyrrylmethane and a monopyrrole. Condensation of two dipyrrylmethane molecules would then result in the synthesis of uroporphyrinogen I or III. Wittenberg,[40] on the other hand, suggested that porphobilinogen deaminase converts porphobilinogen to two linear tetrapyrroles (bile pigments). Under the influence of uroporphyrinogen isomerase, two molecules of the tetrapyrrole are condensed to form a cyclic octapyrrole. The cyclic octapyrrole then undergoes rearrangement, either spontaneously or under the further action of the uroporphyrinogen isomerase, to preferentially yield two molecules of uroporphyrinogen

III. This theory is particularly interesting because it might explain the early appearance of labelled bile pigment in the stool following the administration of labelled glycine (p. 175).

It was formerly assumed that uroporphyrin III is in the direct pathway of heme synthesis. It is now recognized that uroporphyrinogen III (reduced uroporphyrin) is the compound which is converted to coproporphyrinogen[25] by the enzyme, uroporphyrinogen decarboxylase (UD),[17a] uroporphyrin III being only a byproduct. Coproporphyrinogen III is next converted to protoporphyrin III.[17a] Coproporphyrin III is a byproduct. Protoporphyrin III is then converted to hemoglobin in the presence of iron, glutathione,[16,19b,20a] globin and an enzyme, heme synthetase (HS).[19b,20a,33] The intermediate steps between protoporphyrin and hemoglobin have not been identified. It is not known whether iron is first joined to protoporphyrin to form heme, or whether a porphyrin-globin compound is an intermediate in this reaction. The synthesis of heme and globin is simultaneous.[25a]

The pathway of hemoglobin synthesis is represented diagrammatically in Figure 3–10. Details of the steps in the synthesis of globin are unknown but, as will be discussed below (p. 163), it is clear that the formation of the four polypeptide chains of which it is composed is under genetic control.

The natural porphyrins can be found in red corpuscles and in the urine and stools. They are usually identified by their solubility in ether, their spectroscopic characteristics, and the crystal form and melting point of their esters. They all show a strong fluorescence in Wood's light (ultraviolet rays).

Porphyrins in Red Corpuscles, Urine and Stools.—In *red corpuscles*, in addition to the protoporphyrin which is incorporated in heme, *free protoporphyrin* (E.P.) and free coproporphyrin (E.C.P.) are found.[253] Normally less than 40 μg. E.P. (20 to 38 μg., mean 31 μg.)[10] is present per 100 ml. erythrocytes. However, in the first year of life, especially in the first four months, higher values are found.[25b] In iron deficiency anemia and in anemia due to heavy metal intoxication the quantity is greatly increased (50 to 600 μg.). A marked increase is also associated with the anemia of chronic infection (p. 578). Moderate increases (30 to 150 μg.) have been observed in hemolytic and in refractory or hyporegenerative anemias as well as in leukemia, Hodgkin's disease and multiple myeloma. In untreated pernicious anemia, low normal values (15 to 30 μg.) have been found. The concentration of E.P. correlates well with the number of "fluorescytes," red blood cells exhibiting fluorescence in ultraviolet light.[33b]

Under normal circumstances the amount of free *coproporphyrin in erythrocytes* does not exceed 2 μg. per 100 ml. red blood cells.[253] Although reticulocytes are rich in both E.P. and E.C.P., changes in their number have been found to be more closely correlated with changes in E.C.P. than in E.P.[39a] In pernicious anemia in relapse E.C.P. is negligible or absent but increases during the response to therapy. In iron deficiency there is slight or no increase in E.C.P., in contrast to the high levels of E.P. In hemolytic anemias a relatively marked increase of E.C.P. occurs although the quantity of E.P. is only moderately elevated.[39a]

Uroporphyrin and *coproporphyrin*, formed as byproducts in the biosynthesis of hemoglobin (Fig. 3–10), are found in the urine and stools. Coproporphyrin is normally the predominant porphyrin in urine and in feces. Approximately one-half of the freshly passed *urinary coproporphyrin* is excreted as a non-fluorescent precursor compound which is convertible to the fluorescent coproporphyrin by air, ultraviolet light, iodine or peroxide. Normal males excrete 100 to 300 μg. per day, females 75 to 257 μg.[257] Increased erythropoiesis is generally associated with increased coproporphyrin excretion (up to 400 μg. per day). In association with liver damage 300 to 800 μg. is excreted. Excretion of coproporphyrin in excessive amounts has also been observed in Hodgkin's disease (200 to 1000 μg.) and very high values (500 to 3000 μg.) are found in lead poisoning. The increased pigment is the type III isomer.[254] This type has also been found to predominate in alcoholic cirrhosis whereas the type I isomer has been found in non-alcoholic cirrhosis.[255]

Coproporphyrin is the predominant porphyrin in the feces. Normally 150 to 400 μg. porphyrin is excreted per day.[237] Values for infants have been reported.[251a] Fecal coproporphyrin is increased in patients with hemolytic anemia and is depressed in those with liver disease. The ratio of urinary to fecal excretion of porphyrin is thought to depend on the patency of the bile passages and the efficiency of the liver.

Approximately 5 to 10 μg. of *uroporphyrin* are excreted per day in normal urine and, in addition, small amounts of porphyrins with five, six and seven carboxyl groups are found.[262] Ordinary

quantities of uroporphyrin and coproporphyrin in the urine do not produce
obvious changes in its color. When they
are present in pathologic quantities, the
color of the urine may vary from Burgundy red to almost black. When urine
containing large amounts of porphyrin
is exposed to filtered ultraviolet rays
(Wood's light), a pink fluorescence is
detected.

What is known concerning the catabolism of hemoglobin is concerned essentially with its heme moiety. This will be
discussed later, as part of the consideration of the fate of the red corpuscle
(p. 173). Certain disorders which involve heme, in particular, such as the
porphyrias, and conditions usually accompanied by cyanosis, will also be discussed later in this chapter (p. 187).

The Chemical Structure of Normal and Abnormal Globins

Among the most interesting of recent
advances in human biology is the knowledge which has been gained concerning
differences in hemoglobin between individuals, and even in the same individual. Although the earliest investigations of differences in hemoglobins
were carried out by studies of crystallization and of antigenic specificity, as well
as by amino acid analysis, it was the
development of the moving-boundary
technic of electrophoresis by Tiselius
in 1937 which provided impetus to the
field. The value of this technic became especially evident when Pauling
and his associates in 1949 demonstrated
a clear difference between normal and
sickle cell hemoglobin.[350] From these
studies the concept of "molecular disease" developed; namely, that variation
in a normal protein at the molecular
level can be the underlying defect which
results in the whole chain of clinical and
laboratory abnormalities which characterize a disease. The applications of

this concept are extremely broad. Insofar as the present discussion is concerned,
its validity was proved by Ingram in
1956 through the discovery of a precise
chemical difference between adult and
sickle cell hemoglobins.[341]

**Methods for the Study of Normal
and Abnormal Hemoglobins.**—Before discussing the chemical structure
of normal and abnormal globins, it will be
useful to consider some of the technics
which have been employed. Some of the
procedures have direct bearing on the
study of patients. Others are only research tools. Here only the principles of
the various methods will be presented.
Certain simple technics which can be used
in clinical laboratories will be described
in a later chapter (p. 717).

Electrophoresis.—The iso-electric points
of mammalian hemoglobin are usually
just on the acid side of 7. Slight variations in the iso-electric points of the
various human hemoglobins provide the
basis for their recognition by electrophoresis. The "free" or gravitationally
stabilized, moving-boundary method of
Tiselius permits the optical demonstration of differences in movement and
allows separation of boundaries between
overlapping components of different mobility. Satisfactory separation of some
components with very similar mobilities
is achieved. In zone electrophoresis, on
the other hand, components migrate as
separate zones and are stabilized against
convection by the supporting medium,
which may be filter paper or starch gel
or starch grain block preparations. Although the zone technics are generally
not as precise as the moving-boundary
procedure, they have great utility, not
only because of simplicity of operation
and the small amount of hemoglobin
required for a single analysis, but also
because they can be used for screening
a large number of hemoglobin samples in
a short period of time. The zone technic has permitted the rapid identifica-

tion of several previously unrecognized hemoglobins. This has been possible because some zone techniques, such as starch block,[332] readily allow elution of the separated hemoglobins from the supporting medium, thus providing useful quantities of material for further analysis even though the hemoglobin so obtained may be heterogeneous.

As valuable as these procedures are, however, additional methods are needed to distinguish between certain hemoglobins which are electrophoretically similar; for example, the various G hemoglobins and P and Q; D_α, D_β and D_γ.[333]

Chromatography.—Ion exchange chromatography,[337] especially the column chromatographic system[32] best demonstrates the heterogeneity of normal adult and fetal hemoglobins (see below) and also provides useful methods for separating abnormal hemoglobins. The method depends on the observation that under certain experimental conditions the absorption rates of some hemoglobins on a cation exchanger are different. The carboxylic acid resin, IRC-50, has been used at 5° C. in conjunction with sodium phosphate buffers between pH 6.8 and 7.2.[32] Another technic employs carboxymethylcellulose as the cation exchanger.[337]

Alkali Denaturation.—The characteristic property of hemoglobin of reversible combination with oxygen is lost when the globin moiety is denatured. It was noted almost a century ago that human fetal hemoglobin is much more resistant to denaturation by alkali than adult hemoglobin. The reaction rates for Hb A and Hb F differ so markedly that it is possible to select a reaction period during which only Hb A has been completely denatured. For a pH of about 12.7 (N/12 KOH) and temperature of 20° C., a period of one minute is convenient.[357] Because of its simplicity the alkali denaturation procedure has provided a useful means for the estimation of fetal hemoglobin (F). However, it is not sensitive for amounts less than 2 or perhaps 5 per cent. The technic is described on page 719.

Solubility.[343a]—The fact that proteins are very sensitive to such factors as the concentration of neutral salts and pH has made it possible to distinguish fetal hemoglobin from the adult type because it is more soluble in strong phosphate buffer. Again, Hb D, which manifests electrophoretic mobility resembling Hb S, can be distinguished from the latter because of its normal solubility when reduced. Hb S, on the other hand, when reduced is only about one-hundredth as soluble as the oxy-compound. As a consequence sickling of the erythrocytes occurs when the hemoglobin is reduced.

Immunologic Procedures.—Human hemoglobin is only weakly antigenic. Nevertheless it can induce the formation of specific antibodies in a number of species. Technical advances which permit better separation of hemoglobins have provided purer materials for the employment of immunologic technics, which themselves have also been advanced. Normal and fetal hemoglobins can be differentiated by immunologic methods but no immunologic specificity among the other forms of human hemoglobin has been demonstrated.[334]

Amino Acid Composition.—The amino acids in globin have been completely identified (Table 3–4).

Combination and Sequence of Amino Acids. —Fundamental advances in our understanding of the differences in the various types of hemoglobin, as well as highly significant gains in our knowledge of human genetics have come from the study of the sequence of the amino acids in hemoglobin. It is well established that the peptide bond is the primary mode of linkage of the amino acids, these being joined in chains. It is also known that proteins possess free amino groups and methods have been developed, such

Table 3–4.—Amino Acid Composition of Human Hemoglobins*

Amino Acid	Hemoglobin, Residues per Mole		Polypeptide Chains		
	Adult	Fetal	α	β	γ
Alanine	68	62	20	14	11
Arginine	12	12	3	3	3
Aspartic acid	50	50	12	13	13
Cysteine	6	4	1	2	1
Glutamic acid	30	32	5	10	11
Glycine	34	40	7	10	13
Histidine	38	34	10	9	7
Isoleucine	0	8	0	0	4
Leucine	72	68	17	19	17
Lysine	44	46	11	11	12
Methionine	6	8	2	1	2
Phenylalanine	30	28	7	8	7
Proline	28	22	7	7	4
Serine	30	40	10	5	10
Threonine	30	36	8	7	10
Tryptophan	6	10	1	2	4
Tyrosine	12	12	3	3	3
Valine	60	50	12	18	13
Total Residues	556	562	136	142	145

*These are tentative estimates, pending final and complete analysis of the structure of the three polypeptides. Values are given in residues per mole. Assumed molecular weight: α and β chains, 17,000; Hb A and Hb F, 68,000. Calculated from Schroeder[32] and from Stein et al. (Biochim. et biophys. acta, 24, 640, 1957) and Hill and Craig (J. Am. Chem. Soc., 81, 2272, 1959). Prepared by Dr. Robert L. Hill.

as those of Sanger and of Edman, whereby a reagent reacts with the terminal α-amino groups ("N-terminal") of proteins in a way which prevents their removal by subsequent hydrolytic procedures. This is the basis of Sanger's classic dinitrofluorobenzene procedure. The technic has provided a means for identifying the amino terminal residue in a protein and the identification of more than one free α-amino group in a protein has made it possible to recognize multiple polypeptide chains. Thus it was discovered that human adult hemoglobin consists of four polypeptide chains.[351] By the use of another reagent the amino-terminal residues can be liberated, stepwise, and identified without hydrolysis of the remainder of the polypeptide chain. The application of these methods, together with the use of the countercurrent distribution technic and chromatography,

has permitted differentiation of the polypeptide chains of adult and fetal hemoglobin. Studies of the carboxyl-terminal ("C-terminal") of the polypeptide chain have also been fruitful.[334b]

Proteins, such as hemoglobin, can be partially characterized by digestion of the protein by trypsin or other enzymes with subsequent analysis of the liberated peptides. Here a two-dimensional combination of paper electrophoresis and paper chromatography has proved extremely valuable. The resulting chromatogram is known as a "fingerprint" of hemoglobin[343] (Fig. 3–11). The various peptides derived from tryptic hydrolysis are given arbitrary numbers and, by elution technics, they can be separated and their amino acid composition determined.[333a] By this technic it was found that certain peptides are absent in particular hemoglobins.

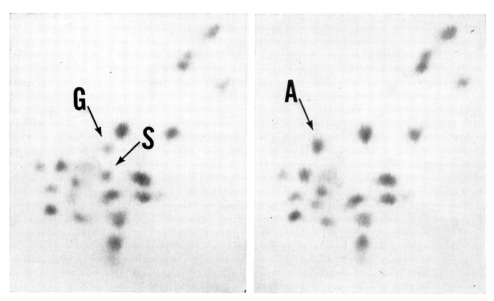

Fig. 3–11.—Peptide pattern ("fingerprint") of tryptic digests of an equal mixture of Hb G$_{San\ Jose}$ and Hb S (left) compared with that of normal hemoglobin (A) (right). The peptide from A (indicated by the arrow) is absent from the pattern of G and S and is replaced by two abnormal peptides (indicated by arrows), one from G and the other from S. The amino acid sequences of these peptides are given in Table 3–6. (Prepared by Dr. Robert L. Hill.[335])

The above technics naturally are not without limitations, which the investigator must take into consideration.[332,335] Other methods are being developed and employed, such as high voltage paper electrophoresis under conditions for cooling the paper during the procedure, the use of spray reagents to detect specific amino acids in the peptides and the production of hybrid molecules through the dissociation of hemoglobins at an acid pH and their reassociation at neutrality. By hybridization of hemoglobins with C[14]-leucine-labelled compounds, it was possible to localize aberrant polypeptide chains by measuring the radioactivity in each of the chains.[344,345,360]

Composition of Normal Globin.— It is now clear that globin derived from adult hemoglobin is composed mainly of two pairs of polypeptide chains. These have been designated, respectively, α and β. In fetal hemoglobin the second pair of chains differs from the β chains of Hb A and have therefore been designated γ.[356] Almost the entire amino acid sequence of the α and β chains has been disclosed, as well as a large proportion of the γ chain.[333a,334d,356] Each polypeptide chain consists of almost 150 amino acids. Isoleucine is absent in adult hemoglobin whereas four residues are found in each gamma chain of fetal hemoglobin. Other differences are indicated in Table 3–4. It is of interest that hemoglobin has a very high content of the aliphatic amino acids valine, leucine and alanine, in addition to a high histidine content. The sulfur content of hemoglobin is rather low, there being six residues of cysteine and six of methionine per mole. No cystine has been identified.

The first three amino acids of the amino terminal residues of the three normal polypeptides are as follows:

Table 3–5—Designation and Polypeptide and Amino Acid Composition of Some Normal and Abnormal Hemoglobins

Hemoglobin	Abnormal Chain	Designation	Abnormality	Reference
A		$\alpha_2^A\,\beta_2^A$	none	336, 342
A$_2$		$\alpha_2^A\,\delta_2^{A_2}$	normal δ chains in place of β	358
C	β	$\alpha_2^A\,\beta_2^{6\ lys}$	lys replaces glu in residue no. 6	338
D$_{Punjab}$ . . .	β	$\alpha_2^A\,\beta_2^{T-13}$		333
E	β	$\alpha_2^A\,\beta_2^{26\ lys}$	lys replaces glu in residue no. 26	340
F		$\alpha_2^A\,\gamma_2^F$	none	337a, 346a, 354
G$_{San\ Jose}$ . . .	β	$\alpha_2^A\,\beta_2^{7\ gly}$	gly replaces glu in residue no. 7	336
G$_{Philadelphia}$ . .	α	$\alpha_2^{68\ lys}\,\beta_2$	lys replaces asp-NH$_2$ in residue no. 68	331a
G$_{Honolulu}$ . . .	α	$\alpha_2^{27\ glu\ NH_2}\,\beta_2$	glu-NH$_2$ replaces glu in residue no. 27	335a
H		β_4^A	α chains absent	346
I	α	$\alpha_2^{16\ asp}\,\beta_2^A$	asp replaces lys in residue no. 16	349
M$_{Boston}$ . . .	α	$\alpha_2^{58-tyr}\,\beta_2^A$	tyr replaces his in residue no. 58	334b
M$_{Emory}$ . . .	β	$\alpha_2^A\,\beta_2^{63-tyr}$	tyr replaces his in residue no. 63	334b
M$_{Milwaukee-1}$ . .	β	$\alpha_2^A\,\beta_2^{67-glu}$	glu replaces val in residue no. 67	334b
S	β	$\alpha_2^A\,\beta_2^{6\ val}$	val replaces glu in residue no. 6	336, 342
Norfolk . . .	α	$\alpha_2^{57\ asp}\,\beta_2^A$	asp replaces gly in residue no. 57	331a
Bart's		γ_4^F	α and β chains absent	340a
Lepore . . .	δ	$\alpha_2^A\,\delta_2^{Lepore}$		334b

The abnormality in the following hemoglobins is thought to be in the α chain:
  G$_{Ibadan}$, G$_{Bristol}$, K, M$_{Iwate}$, Q[345a], Hopkins-1.
The abnormality in the following is in the β chain:
  D$_{Hollywood}$,[345a] G$_{Accra}$, J, L,[345a] M$_{Milwaukee-2}$, N, O, P.
The designation for the above hemoglobins consequently is at present incomplete; for example,
  Hb G$_{Accra}$ is $\alpha_2^A\,\beta_2^{G\,Accra}$; Hb J is $\alpha_2^A\,\beta_2^J$.

α chain: val.leu.ser.

β chain: val.his.leu.

γ chain: gly.his.phe.

The carboxyl-terminal residues of the α chains are ser.lys.tyr.arg. and for the β chains ala.his.lys.tyr.his.[334b] The abbreviations are those currently used for the various amino acids.

Heterogeneity of Normal Adult and Fetal Hemoglobins.—Originally suggested by alkali denaturation, immunologic and salting-out experiments, the application of starch block electrophoresis by Kunkel[347] clearly showed a slowly moving component in normal adult hemoglobin which he designated as A$_2$. Column chromatography revealed a still more complex picture with at least eight different hemoglobins (Fig. 3–12).[32,331] In this the main component is designated A$_{II}$. The A$_{IIIb}$ compound corresponds to Kunkel's A$_2$. This component is not an artifact of preparation or electrophoresis; in fact, there is good evidence that this hemoglobin is a normal constituent of adult hemoglobin and is made up of two α chains similar to those of Hb A and Hb F together with two chains which differ sufficiently from the β chains

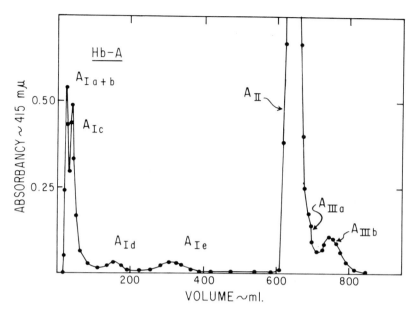

FIG. 3–12.—Column chromatography of hemoglobin A on IRC-50 (method of Clegg and Schroeder, Developer No. 5 used; courtesy of Dr. Robert L. Hill).

that they have been designated as δ chains.[358] In contrast to A_{II}, isoleucine has been found in A_{IIIb}.[352]

The origin of the several components designated as A_I is uncertain. It has been suggested that they may be precursors of hemoglobin, or are non-hemoglobin enzymes or degradation products of the main component (A_{II}). It is not known that they are genetically determined.

Fetal hemoglobin is also chromatographically heterogeneous.[331]

The Abnormal Hemoglobins. — The abnormalities which have been discovered to date have been essentially of two varieties; namely (1) the absence of one or both normal adult polypeptide chains; or (2) abnormality in the amino acid sequence of one of the peptides separated from the polypeptide chain. Thus, in Hb H, only β chains are present but these seem to be normal.[346] Again, Hb Bart's is composed of only γ chains.[340a]

The clinical manifestations and other details of the abnormal hemoglobin-opathies and of thalassemia will be considered in a later chapter (p. 668) but certain general implications may be discussed here.

Nomenclature of the Hemoglobins.—Normal adult hemoglobin has been known as Hb A, fetal hemoglobin as Hb F. When sickle cell hemoglobin was discovered it was at first briefly called "b" but soon the letter S was assigned to it. As other hemoglobins were discovered they were given other letters of the alphabet. It has become apparent, however, that this system will not suffice. Attempts are being made to design a more satisfactory nomenclature. Some of these proposals have been published,[349a] others are pending. Essentially, it has been suggested that capital letter designations be used for the positions taken by the abnormal hemoglobins on the paper electrophoretic pattern (Fig. 13–27 p. 718). If more than one hemoglobin takes the same position, this should be indicated by stating the geographical area where the abnormal hemoglobin

11

Table 3–6.—Amino Acid Sequences of Some Normal and Abnormal Hemoglobins

Hb	*β Chain*
A	Val.His.Leu.Thr.Pro.Glu.Glu.Lys. . . . .
	1 2 3 4 5 6 7 8
S	Val.His.Leu.Thr.Pro.*Val*.Glu.Lys.. . . . .
C	Val.His.Leu.Thr.Pro.*Lys*.Glu.Lys. . . . .
G_{San Jose}	Val.His.Leu.Thr.Pro.Glu.*Gly*.Lys. . . . .

	β Chain
A	. . . Val.Asp.Val.Asp.Glu.Val.Gly.Gly.Glu.Ala.Leu.Gly.Arg. . . .
	18 19 20 21 22 23 24 25 25 27 28 29 30
E	. . . Val.Asp.Val.Asp.Glu.Val.Gly.Gly.*Lys*.Ala.Leu.Gly.Arg. . . .

	δ Chain
A$_2$	. . . Val.Asp.Val.Asp.*Ala*.Val.Gly.Gly.Glu.Ala.Leu.Gly.Arg. . . .
	18 19 20 21 22 23 24 25 26 27 28 29 30

	α Chain
A	. . . Try.Gly.Lys.Val.Gly.Ala.His.Ala.Gly.Glu.Tyr. . . . . .
	14 15 16 17 18 19 20 21 22 23 24
I	. . . Try.Gly.*Asp*.Val.Gly.Ala.His.Ala.Gly.Glu.Tyr. . . . . .

The amino acids are numbered in orderly sequence, beginning with the amino (NH₂) terminal, but only that segment of the chain is shown in which a variant amino acid is present. The variant amino acids are italicized.

Val refers to valine; His, histidine; Leu, leucine; Thr, threonine; Pro, proline; Glu, glutamic acid; Lys, lysine; Gly, glycine; Asp, aspartic acid; Ala, alanine; Arg, arginine; Try, tryptophan; Tyr, tyrosine

was first found; thus Hb G$_{San Jose}$, Hb G$_{Philadelphia}$, etc. This is necessary because there may be nine varieties of Hb D (p. 694) and as many forms of Hb G (p. 695). In addition, when known, the kinds of chains present are indicated, as well as their number and, if it is known which chain is aberrant, this is indicated. Thus Hb A is represented as $\alpha_2\beta_2$ and Hb F is $\alpha_2\gamma_2$. The subscripts denote the number of chains per mole. When an abnormal chain is present, this is indicated by adding the letter designation of the abnormal hemoglobin in superscript; thus, Hb G$_{Accra}$ is $\alpha_2^A \beta_2^{G\,Accra}$ to indicate that the abnormality has been shown to be present in the beta chains. However, when analysis has revealed the location of the abnormality in that chain, this is denoted by giving the number of the abnormal tryptic peptide or, still better when possible, the number of the altered amino acid

and the nature of the replacement. In the following an attempt will be made to follow the recommendations proposed (Table 3–5).

Significance of Abnormal Hemoglobins.—The study of the biochemical aberrations of hemoglobin has great importance from the standpoints of human genetics and of anthropology.[333b] A generally held working hypothesis is that the gene can be represented as a molecule of deoxyribonucleic acid and that the linear sequence of base pairs in this double-stranded, helical molecule determines the linear sequence of amino acids in the primary structure of the protein controlled by the gene. From this it is inferred that the presence of a different sequence of amino acids in an abnormal hemoglobin is the result of a mutation in the gene which controls the amino acid sequence in the hemoglobin.

The characterization of the abnormal

hemoglobins should be of great importance in determining the validity of this hypothesis. At the same time the study of hemoglobinopathic families becomes important, especially the study of those in which two or more of the genes responsible for abnormalities in the structure of hemoglobin are present together. Such investigations have led to the suggestion that two non-allelic genes control hemoglobin production, one being responsible for each normal chain, α and β. This was suggested by investigation of the pattern of inheritance of Hb S and Hb G[355] as well as in a study involving "Hopkins-2" (p. 699). Hybridization studies give support to this hypothesis.[345]

The genes involved in the development of the hemoglobinopathies are, in certain instances, quite common. Thus, in parts of Africa 46 per cent of the population are heterozygous for Hb S (p. 669) and, in other parts, 28 per cent for the Hb C gene (p. 690). Heterozygotes for the Hb E gene make up 13.6 per cent of the population of Thailand and an incidence of 35 per cent was reported among Cambodians (p. 695). In parts of Italy, thalassemia minor frequencies of 20 per cent are known (p. 701). It has been pointed out that gene frequencies of this magnitude do not arise by chance. It follows that the genes in question may make some positive contribution to the fitness of the population by offering a protective factor. The most thoroughly studied aspect of this problem is the observed relative immunity of individuals possessing the Hb S trait to *P. falciparum* malaria (p. 670). This is but one example of the manner in which investigation of the hemoglobinopathies may be expected to contribute in an important way to the study of population genetics. Together with exploration of the distribution of the blood groups and of other inherited blood factors, such as the haptoglobins, the discovery of abnormal hemoglobins may be expected to add to our knowledge of the migration of races and of anthropology.

FATE OF THE RED CORPUSCLE

Although the red corpuscle is no longer regarded as being a completely inert protoplasmic particle, it is nevertheless a highly specialized structure which bears the well known biological stigma that, with increased specialization, adaptability and durability are more or less proportionately diminished. This biological device, which loads, transports and unloads oxygen with such speed and yet consumes so little of the gas itself, is not capable of much repair and is ultimately destroyed. The continuous excretion of bile pigment gives evidence of the continuity of the process of red cell destruction.

Life Span of Red Corpuscles.— Considerable evidence indicates that the normal red corpuscle has a finite life span due to aging but, in addition, there is a variable degree of random destruction.[229] Factors concerned in the aging of red corpuscles were discussed earlier (p. 126). It is possible, furthermore, that there may be more than one population of red cells, with either population having either predominantly a finite life span or being randomly destroyed. Better methods for the separation of red cells as a function of age would allow a clearer understanding of the physiology of the erythrocyte.

A number of *methods* have been used in attempts to measure the life span of the erythrocyte.[229] The most important are the differential agglutination (Ashby) technic and the isotopic, Cr[51], method. Estimates based on measurements of total pigment excretion are unsatisfactory, as will be discussed below.

The method of *differential agglutination* [228,233] involves the transfusion of compatible but immunologically identifiable blood. Periodically the donor red cells are enumerated following agglutination of the recipient's cells by appropriate antisera. The ABO or the MN blood group system has been utilized as a rule although it is also possible to use the Rh blood groups and antisera.[229] The original technic has been modified and improved in many ways, including the development of hemolytic anti-A and anti-B sera to eliminate errors due to trapping of O cells in the A or B agglutinates.[235]

The principle of "mixed agglutination" has been applied in the detection of minor populations of erythrocytes in mixtures in which the minor component is identifiable by means of one or another of the blood group iso-antigens.[236]

Isotopic methods include the use of N^{15}, C^{14}, Fe^{55}, and Fe^{59}, Cr^{51} or DFP^{32}. The use of glycine labelled with N^{15} or C^{14} has the important advantage that these elements are incorporated metabolically into red cells at a particular stage of their formation. However, the need for special equipment not available in many laboratories reduces the applicability of an otherwise satisfactory method. Radio-iron procedures involve problems of reutilization and complex methods of analysis which seriously limit the utility of the method (p. 184). The use of diisopropylfluorophosphate labelled with P^{32} (DFP^{32}) depends on the inhibition of cholinesterase activity of the red cell and the fixation of P^{32} in red cells thereby. The method has serious limitations.[231]

With the discovery by Gray and Sterling that sodium chromate will penetrate and become fixed in the red cell, a very useful and practical method for estimation of red cell survival was introduced.[239] Red cells are labelled *in vitro* with Cr^{51}-*labelled sodium chromate*, they are given to a recipient and the rate of change of Cr^{51} concentration per ml. of red blood cells is determined. There appears to be no reutilization of isotope released from cells. This is important because part of the decrease in radioactivity is attributable

to elution of the metal from intact red cells. Problems of elution, physical decay of the isotope, which has a half-life of 28 days, and limitation as to the quantity of chromium that will not adversely affect the red cell have led to the introduction of a multiplicity of methods for analysis of the data in order to avoid the necessity of following the isotope content of the circulating red cells to the end of the life span.

Method.—Approximately 100 μc. (microcuries) of Cr^{51} in the form of a sterile, isotonic solution of sodium chromate ($Na_2Cr^{51}O_4$) is injected into a sterile siliconized blood collection bottle containing 10 ml. ACD solution (p. 356). Approximately 40 ml. blood is removed from the patient and injected into the bottle. The sample is incubated at 37°C for 45 to 60 minutes and is occasionally gently shaken during this time. No more than 25 μg. (micrograms) of chromium per ml. red cells should be used since larger amounts produce abnormal survival curves.[233a] Material with a specific activity of 10 mc./mg., or better, is suitable. If material of this specific activity is used, 100 μc. will contain only 10 μg. of chromium. More than 90 per cent of the Cr^{51} is taken up by the cells within this period. Ascorbic acid (50 to 200 mg. "intravenous solution") is added as a reducing agent to prevent further transfer of plasma activity to red cells. The cells may then be injected into the patient or, if preferred,[238a,239] they are washed twice in saline and resuspended in a final volume of about 50 ml., 40 ml. of which is injected from a calibrated syringe. A standard is prepared from the remaining suspension.

To define the disappearance curve, blood samples are taken from the recipient 30 minutes after injection and thereafter at suitable intervals. Samples are lysed and counted in a scintillation counter. When it can be assumed that the total circulating red cell volume

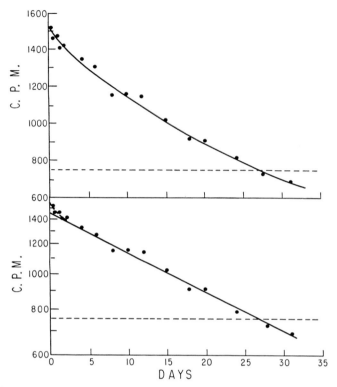

Fig. 3–13.—Cr⁵¹ erythrocyte survival curve in a normal male adult. The net counts per minute (c.p.m.) are shown on an arithmetic (above) and a semi-log scale (below), plotted against time in days. Fifty per cent of the radioactivity at 24 hours (T½) was reached at 28 days.

remains constant, the counts in whole blood samples are divided by the proportion of red cells in the sample (hematocrit) and expressed as counts/min./ml. of red cells. The Cr⁵¹ method can also be used, if desired, to measure the red cell volume (p. 318).

The survival of normal donor cells as measured by the Cr⁵¹ method is represented by a complex curve which is neither logarithmic or linear[234a] but its end point coincides with the total disappearance of inagglutinable cells (Ashby method). Approximately 10 per cent of the chromium is removed rapidly (half-time 1.5 days) whereas the remainder disappears much more slowly. The early loss is unexplained.[238a] The later disappearance is due to elution of chromium from surviving cells as well as to loss of

cells by aging. When the logarithm of the specific activity of the red cells is plotted as a function of time, and if the early loss phase is ignored, the points for the first 40 or 50 days can be fitted satisfactorily by a straight line.[238a] In other words, when the first 24 hours are excluded, Cr⁵¹ measurements indicate a simple exponential disappearance rate over the first 40 or 50 days.[233a] Since it is useful to provide a quantitative expression of red cell destruction, the time required for the specific activity to decrease to one-half (T½) is customarily determined and the findings are compared with the normal. The presence of 48 to 54 per cent of the Cr⁵¹ at 26 to 29 days is taken to indicate normal survival.

Loss of chromium by elution (i.e. biologic decay) has been calculated on the basis of changes in the ratio of cell survival determined by Cr[51] counts and the corresponding values based on selective agglutination counts. The mean half-life of chromium elution has been found by different workers to be 46[233a] to 77[234a] days. In calculations of red cell survival a correction factor for chromium elution can be introduced. The true survival can be approximated by adding the amount lost by elution to the apparent survival from Cr[51] data. A table for this purpose has been provided.[233a]

Comparison of Ashby and Cr[51] Methods.— A basic assumption of the Ashby technic is that the infused red cells have at least as long a life span in a normal recipient as in the donor. This is not always true. Furthermore, selective destruction of transfused cells can occur without demonstrable antibodies, making interpretation of Ashby survival curves difficult.[238a] The Ashby procedure also suffers from the basic defect of not measuring red cell survival in its natural environment. There are a number of other disadvantages, such as limitation by the blood groups of the donor and recipient, the need to transfuse or to remove relatively large volumes of blood, the need for exceptionally potent antisera and the necessity that many hours of labor be expended.[234] Nevertheless the method has yielded valuable information.

Some of the limitations of the Cr[51] method have been mentioned in the discussion of the procedure. However, in spite of the assumptions concerning elution of the label which have to be made, the Cr[51] method has the distinct advantage that it can be carried out very readily and yields reproducible results. A steady state, unmodified by transfusions or hemorrhage is essential for its application. However, it is possible to measure the amount of Cr[51] loss in the stools.[238a] Furthermore, since Cr[51] emits gamma rays, useful information can be obtained about its distribution in the body by scanning the body surface with a scintillation counter.

It is significant that, as measured by many of the procedures employed, the *life span of the normal erythrocyte* is essentially the same; namely 117 (110–135) days by the Ashby method, 113 (108–120) days when the Cr[51] label was measured to extinction, 118 (109–127) days with N[15] glycine, and 124 days with DFP[32]. The $T\frac{1}{2}$ by the Cr[51] procedure is 29 (25–40) days.[229] Thus it appears that approximately 0.83 per cent of the blood, or 50 ml. in the average male adult, is replaced each day.

Measurements of erythrocyte life span make it possible to plot curves of disappearance of tagged cells, which indicate whether normal senescence or random destruction is taking place. Normally the rate of elimination of red corpuscles from the recipient's circulation is slow and uniform and when the results are plotted on arithmetic graph paper the course of elimination is almost straight, that is, "*linear.*" In the acquired hemolytic anemias the rate of elimination is greatly accelerated; in addition, the course of elimination is different. When plotted on an arithmetic scale the disappearance of the corpuscles is at first rapid and then gradually slows ("*exponential*"). This indicates random destruction in which the age of the corpuscles is unimportant.

In considering erythrocyte life span, *potential life span* and *survival time* must be differentiated. The former refers to the length of life of a corpuscle whose ultimate loss depends on senescence and is in all likelihood a characteristic of the cell itself; the latter refers to the actual life span under the given conditions. Congenitally abnormal cells may only have a potential life span which is considerably shorter than is normal. Even so, their actual survival depends upon various factors; as, for example, the presence or absence of the spleen in a case of hereditary spherocytosis.

Findings in various pathological states will be discussed as these are considered. Data for various animals will be found in the review by Berlin et al.[229] The employment of measurements of red cell life span in the evaluation of erythrokinetics will be considered shortly.

Manner of Destruction.—The manner in which the destruction of red corpuscles takes place in the normal individual is not fully understood. It is obvious enough that hemolysis occurs and hemoglobinemia and hemoglobinuria are found when incompatible red cells are injected by transfusion. Toxic symptoms develop as well. Since these findings are absent under normal conditions, it is plausible to assume, although it does not necessarily follow, that hemolysis is not the customary way in which red cells are destroyed.

It is known that certain large endothelial cells, found especially in the spleen, take up red corpuscles and destroy them. Yet phagocytosis does not suffice as a general explanation of normal blood destruction. Rous and Robertson[241] searched the body, organ by organ, for disintegrating red corpuscles, and found phagocytosis slight in man, shadows of red cells were not present, and no hemolyzing cells were found. They suggested that the chief means of erythrocyte destruction is by *fragmentation*. In the circulation the red corpuscles are buffeted about, eventually become distorted and portions are broken off. In the opinion of these investigators, poikilocytosis and microcytes are morphological evidences of blood destruction. Fragmentation goes on until finally a fine, hemoglobin-containing dust is formed. This is removed chiefly by the spleen.

Support for this hypothesis is found in the observations that red corpuscles can be torn in pieces by microdissection without hemoglobin loss; that poikilo-cytes are absent at the site of blood formation, namely, the bone marrow; and that signs of hemolysis and of phagocytosis are not found in the normal individual.

Although the changes occurring in the erythrocyte or at its surface which permit fragmentation are obscure, it is reasonable to suppose that they are associated with a wearing out of the enzyme systems which control its metabolic activities (p. 126). It is probable also that influences outside the cells play a part in limiting the life span of the normal erythrocyte. These include stagnation of the blood stream and the action of tissue lysins. Elsewhere (p. 636) the changes which take place in red corpuscles sequestered in the spleen will be discussed. Among these are increased spheroidicity and fragility and intracorpuscular degradation of their hemoglobin. The spherical shape assumed by erythrocytes on incubation has been attributed to the action of a lysolecithin.[325] It has been suggested that there exists in the animal body an enzyme capable of destroying red cells and that blood serum and the tissues themselves carry an inhibitor of such lysis. In certain tissues (lung, liver, kidney, spleen, bone marrow and muscle) a species specific lytic agent has been found.[238]

The final breaking up of effete erythrocytes occurs in the cells of the *"reticulo-endothelial system"* (Chapter 1, p. 33). These cells possess in common one important functional characteristic, namely, an extreme avidity for particulate matter. When India ink, carmine particles or colloidal dyes such as pyrrole blue are injected into the blood stream, they are immediately taken up by the cells of the reticulo-endothelial system. In the same way, these cells engulf fragmented erythrocytes.

For many years, especially as the result of the experiments of Minkowski and Naunyn, it was considered that the liver plays the major rôle in the breakdown of the red corpuscles. This theory arose because their experiments were conducted in ducks and geese, in which animals the bulk of the reticulo-endothelial system is made up of the Kupffer cells in the liver. In man the cells of the reticulo-endothelial system are more widely distributed and consequently other organs, particularly the bone marrow and the spleen play major roles in pigment metabolism and other tissues participate as well. Thus, even in contused wounds or in subcutaneous tissue into which erythrocytes have been injected, erythrocyte breakdown can occur.[240] In view of the size of the bone marrow compartment and its rich content of phagocytic cells, and since the life span of red corpuscles before and after splenectomy in normal subjects is the same,[243] it can be assumed that the bone marrow is the most important organ in physiologic erythroclasis in man.

Should free hemoglobin reach the blood plasma, it is bound and removed from the circulation. This is the property of the **haptoglobins,**[240a] proteins first recognized by Polonovski and Jayle, which migrate with the α_2 fraction on filter paper or moving boundary electrophoresis. Normally the haptoglobin concentration is 128 ± 25 mg. per 100 ml.[236a] A simple method for the measurement of haptoglobin has been described.[240c] The amount rises in association with inflammatory reactions and in other conditions, and in many respects varies as does the erythrocyte sedimentation rate. Electrophoresis in starch gel has shown that at least three types of haptoglobins[244] can be distinguished in different individuals, these being genetically controlled by a pair of autosomal alleles, Hp^1 and Hp^2. The homozygote Hp^1/Hp^1 shows a single haptoglobin component on electrophoresis whereas the other homozygote Hp^2/Hp^2 shows many components. The heterozygote Hp^2/Hp^1 also

shows several haptoglobin components. It is likely that unusual or modifying genes also occur. Complete absence of haptoglobin has been encountered in Nigeria.[227a] There is evidence[234c] also of a third allele, Hp^{2m}.

In addition to haptoglobin two other serum proteins are capable of carrying appreciable amounts of hemoglobin or its naturally occurring heme-containing metabolites.[240b] These are a heme-binding globulin which, *in vitro*, could be demonstrated in sera whose haptoglobins were not saturated; and albumin which, by union with the ferric complex of protoporphyrin, forms methemalbumin (p. 176). When intravascular hemolysis takes place these compounds and, in particular, the haptoglobin bind the liberated hemoglobin and the complexes which are formed are eliminated from the plasma without being excreted in the urine. Hemoglobinuria does not appear until the amount of hemoglobin in the plasma exceeds the capacity of the binding proteins.[236a,236b]

Hemoglobin is probably normally present in the plasma in small amounts, approximately 0.42 mg. per 100 ml. It has been calculated that a total of about 0.8 Gm. of hemoglobin normally flows in and out of the plasma compartment each day, an amount which corresponds to only slightly more than 10 per cent of the overall red cell hemoglobin breakdown. The liver, spleen and bone marrow remove most of the haptoglobin complex.[234b] Free hemoglobin was found to be cleared from the plasma at a glomerular clearance rate of 5 ml. per minute per 1.73 sq.m. of body surface area.[236a] No conclusive evidence of tubular reabsorption was obtained.

Agglutination and Hemolysis of Red Corpuscles.—Although they do not appear to be concerned in the physiological process of red cell breakdown, both agglutination and hemolysis of red cells occur under abnormal conditions and in disease.

True agglutination must be distinguished from *pseudoagglutination*. The latter is in actuality rouleau formation and is seen in pronounced degree in multiple myeloma, but it is also met with in other conditions in which the globulin or fibrinogen content of the plasma is high. This is the underlying process which results in an increased erythrocyte sedimentation rate (p. 326). Pseudoagglutination occurs most readily at 37°C. but also occurs in the cold. It is decreased when spherocytosis of the erythrocytes is present, disappears on slight dilution of the plasma and is inhibited by the presence of lecithin. The pseudoagglutinating properties of a plasma cannot be exhausted by repeated absorption with erythrocytes.[326]

Isoagglutination refers to the agglutination of the erythrocytes of one individual by the serum of another and depends on the various blood groups. These will be discussed subsequently (p. 338). *Autoagglutination* refers to the agglutination of the red cells of the individual by his own serum and is a rare phenomenon except in one form, cold agglutination. The role of "warm" and "cold" auto-antibodies in acquired hemolytic anemias and in paroxysmal cold hemoglobinuria will be considered in a later chapter (p. 633).

Cold hemagglutination[326] is the term applied to a phenomenon in which a mixture of red corpuscles and serum from the same individual exhibits agglutination in the cold (0° to 5° C.). This phenomenon can be reversed by warming to temperatures above 20° or 30° C. and can be restored by cooling below 10° or 20° C. The antibody in such a serum agglutinates all human red cells regardless of group and is also active in varying degree against the erythrocytes of many unrelated species. Appropriate adsorption with erythro-

cytes in the cold can exhaust the cold hemagglutinins from the serum.

Cold hemagglutination is often first discovered in the counting chamber while a red cell count is being made (p. 386) and clumping may be visible on the stained smear. If the phenomenon is due to cold hemagglutinins rather than to rouleau formation (pseudoagglutination) slight warming of the reagents and apparatus will either prevent clumping or will disrupt clumps which are present. The same phenomenon should be suspected when unexpected results are obtained in blood group determinations.

Cold hemagglutinins were found in titers of 40 or higher in 68.5 per cent of 200 cases of primary atypical pneumonia and have also been found in certain cases of acquired hemolytic anemia (p. 615). In only 1.2 per cent of 851 other cases, which included a great variety of conditions, were cold hemagglutinins demonstrated in similar titer.[314] Cold hemagglutinins are also found in trypanosomiasis (human and animal) and in spirillosis (animal), as well as in some cases of cirrhosis of the liver.[326]

Cold auto-antibodies are sometimes classed as natural or abnormal. The former react within a temperature range not exceeding 5° C. "Incomplete" cold antibodies have been described which can be brought out when normal human red cells are left in their own serum at 2° to 5° C. for two hours and are then washed in warm saline solution. These can be found in most sera from apparently healthy persons and have anti-H specificity (p. 339).[310] The abnormal variety of cold hemagglutinins have a greater thermal amplitude than the natural ones and are probably produced by immunization of one kind or another. They will be discussed in the chapter on hemolytic anemias (p. 615).

In those rare individuals in whom cold hemagglutinins are present in high titer, cyanosis of the digits and other parts may develop on exposure to cold and even gangrene may supervene. Reversible intravascular hemagglutination with cessation of blood flow has been observed in their conjunctival vessels and it appears that similar events, aided by the normal degree of vasoconstriction which occurs on exposure to cold, are the cause of their Raynaud-like symptoms.[321] Severe hemolytic anemia and attacks of hemoglobinuria may occur as well (p. 602), although not invariably. These events may be the consequence of the greater mechanical fragility of agglutinated red corpuscles.

Cryoglobulinemia,[306] a phenomenon which refers to the presence of a cold precipitable protein in the plasma, differs from the phenomenon of cold hemagglutination but the clinical manifestations may be similar. Cryoglobulins have been observed most often in association with multiple myeloma (p. 1072) but have been encountered also in chronic lymphocytic leukemia, kala-azar and other disorders.

Polyagglutination refers to the tendency of certain red cells to be agglutinated by all human sera, irrespective of the ABO groups involved. This may be acquired through aging *in vitro* (panagglutination, p. 352) but has also been found to occur spontaneously in patients with infections and, in one case, with hemolytic anemia (p. 617).

Hemolysis, as already mentioned, may occur under certain abnormal conditions. Hemolysis may or may not be associated with or preceded by agglutination of red corpuscles. Certain animal and bacterial poisons, such as snake venoms and substances extracted from many microörganisms, have hemolytic properties (p. 612). Certain drugs, such as phenylhydrazine, are given with the object of causing hemolysis (p. 804). The transfusion of incompatible blood is followed by hemolysis, and in paroxysmal cold hemoglobinuria an autohemolysin is produced by exposure to cold. It is possible to produce serums which have a high titer of hemolysins and it has been shown that the erythrocytes of normal persons are rendered more susceptible to hypotonic hemolysis by exposure to lipemic serum.[320,328] *In vitro*, physical as well as chemical agents may cause destruction of red cells. These include rapid freezing and thawing, increase of temperature above 64° C., saponin, ammonium salts, lipoidal solvents such as ether, chloroform and bile salts[323] and diethylstilbesterol and progesterone.[329] When blood contains many spherocytes, in paroxysmal nocturnal hemoglobinuria and in poisoning with phenylhydrazine spontaneous *autohemolysis* takes place.

In vivo, however, many factors counteract the effects of hemolytic agents, and substances which are known to be hemolytic *in vitro* often have little or no effect. Thus, considerable quantities of water must be injected into the blood stream before any appreciable hemolysis can be produced (p. 610), the cells being protected by the passage of salts from the tissues in an attempt to maintain a uniform osmotic pressure. Likewise, hypotonic and hypertonic solutions have little or no hemolytic action *in vivo*. The circuitous course *via* the lymphatics which is taken by fatty acids in their passage from the intestine to the blood stream and their conversion to neutral fats probably serves to protect red corpuscles by permitting dilution of these hemolytic substances.[320] The normal red corpuscle is in osmotic equilibrium with its surrounding fluid and this equilibrium is maintained over a wide range of concentrations.[330a]

Extensive studies have been made of the physical and chemical laws of hemolysis in the test tube,[309,318] but little is known concerning the process in the body. The possible modes of action of various drugs in producing hemolytic anemia will be discussed in a later chapter (p. 631).

In clinical work, study of erythrocyte hemolysis was until recently chiefly concerned with observation of the resistance of these cells to hemolysis in decreasing strengths of hypotonic saline solutions. It has been shown that the swelling of normal human erythrocytes suspended in hypotonic salt solutions follows closely that expected of perfect osmometers.[316] The **erythrocyte fragility test,** first proposed by Hamburger (1883), has been modified many times. A simple presumptive test may be carried out first. If positive, a quantitative test should be performed. For these tests a stock solution of buffered sodium chloride should be available. To prepare this, a reagent grade of sodium chloride must be used and should be dried for 24 hours in a desiccator over calcium chloride. The stock solution, osmotically equivalent to 10 per cent NaCl is prepared from NaCl 180 Gm., dibasic sodium phosphate (Na$_2$HPO$_4$) 27.31 Gm., monobasic sodium phosphate (NaH$_2$PO$_4$:2H$_2$O) 4.86 Gm. and distilled water to make 2 liters. In a glass-stoppered, tightly closed bottle this solution will keep for months. A 1 per cent working solution is made from this.

Screening Test.—0.1 ml. of venous blood, collected in the usual manner (p. 377) is pipetted into each of three test tubes. To these is added, respectively, 1.0 ml. of 0.85 per cent, 0.50 per cent and 0.25 per cent sodium chloride, made up from the 1 per cent working solution. The blood and saline solution in each tube is mixed and then centrifuged. Normally there should be hemolysis only in the tube containing 0.25 per cent saline. If the erythrocyte osmotic fragility is increased, hemolysis will probably be evident in 0.50 per cent saline. If there is hemolysis in all three tubes, the saline solutions are incorrect or some other error has been made.

Quantitative Test.—15 to 20 ml. blood is drawn under aseptic conditions and placed in a sterile Erlenmeyer flask containing 15 small glass beads (3–4 mm. diameter) and rotated gently until the hum of the beads on the glass is no longer audible. Approximately 2 ml. of blood is then pipetted under sterile conditions into each of four sterile screw-capped vials and set aside for the incubated osmotic fragility and for the autohemolysis test (p. 620). The remainder of the blood is used for the determination of the osmotic fragility prior to incubation. If osmotic fragility and autohemolysis after incubation are not to be determined, a smaller volume of blood may be drawn and aseptic precautions need not be observed. However, it is frequently desirable to determine the osmotic fragility both before and after incubation and also to do the autohemolysis test.

Five ml. of each of the following solutions is placed in a tube: 0.85, 0.75, 0.65 0.60, 0.55, 0.50, 0.45, 0.40, 0.35, 0.30, 0.20 and 0.10 per cent sodium chloride. Five ml. of distilled water is placed in an additional tube. Intermediate concentrations of saline such as 0.475 and 0.525 per cent may be helpful for critical work.

To each tube 0.05 ml. defibrinated blood is added. The solutions are then mixed and allowed to stand at room temperature (20° C.) for 30 minutes. Following this, the solutions are shaken gently again and centrifuged for five minutes at 2000 r.p.m.

Hemolysis can be read visually and recorded as the point of beginning and complete hemolysis. The slightest trace of red color in the supernatant fluid indicates the destruction of the least resistant cells. Complete hemolysis is indicated by a clear red solution and the absence of a residue in the bottom of the tube or of any cloudiness on gently shaking the tube. For more quantitative work, the supernatant solutions are pipitted off and read in a photoelectric colorimeter. This is done by making an appropriate dilution (1:2 or 1:5) of the supernatant solutions. The amount of hemoglobin present is determined by the routine method in use in the laboratory. The supernatant solution from the 0.85 per cent sodium chloride tube is used as a blank. The hemoglobin value in the tube containing no saline is taken to represent 100 per cent hemolysis and the per cent hemolysis in each of the other tubes is calculated by dividing the hemoglobin value by the value in the tube containing no saline ($\times$ 100).

The osmotic fragility after incubation of the blood at 37 C. for 24 hours is determined in the same manner as outlined above. However, since the fragility may be markedly increased it is desirable to set up additional saline solutions containing 1.2, 0.90, 0.80 and 0.70 per cent sodium chloride. The 1.2 per cent solution is then used as the blank in the photoelectric estimation of hemoglobin.

It is always desirable to perform the test on normal blood at the same time. Various other technics have been described.[315,317a,318,330] The results of the test are plotted as a "fragility curve" on graph paper, the percentage of hemolysis in each tube being plotted against the corresponding concentration of salt solution. In normal subjects an almost symmetrical curve of sigmoid shape is obtained[318] (see p. 622). An alternative method of plotting the results is as increments of increasing hemolysis.[308] A photographic method for recording hemolysis has also been described.[319]

It is important to bear in mind that temperature,[322] the anticoagulant used, the pH of the hemolytic solution,[312] the amount of bile pigment present in the plasma, and the presence of hemolytic organisms, will affect the result.[318] Another factor which is sometimes overlooked is the degree of anemia in the blood examined, significantly fewer cells being available for destruction in severely anemic cases. These factors can be controlled by washing the red corpuscles of the specimen to be examined and of the control blood in physiological saline solution and resuspending them so that the ratio of cells to the medium is the same in both.[313,330]

Normal blood shows slight hemolysis at 0.45 to 0.39 per cent; it becomes well marked in the next one or two tubes (0.42 to 0.36 per cent); complete hemolysis occurs at 0.33 to 0.30 per cent. The fragility of cells from venous blood which has not been thoroughly oxygenated is said to be greater than that of cells from arterial blood.[330] The corpuscles of newborn children are somewhat more fragile than those of adults.[330] Young mature red corpuscles of man are more resistant to hemolysis in hypotonic media than old cells[320a] but in the dog the reverse may be true.[327] The resistance of red cells can be enhanced by incubation with purine ribosides.[319a] The metabolism of these substances probably provides the energy required for the maintenance of the structural integrity of the erythrocyte.

In *hereditary spherocytosis* (p. 649) the fragility of the red corpuscles usually is markedly increased. This has been attributed to the fact that the erythrocytes in these cases are smaller in diameter and thicker than normal corpuscles, the assumption being made that, when placed in hypotonic salt solutions, normal erythrocytes become progressively more globular; consequently, the spherocytes of hereditary spherocytosis are nearer the hemolyzing point than are normal corpuscles.[317] It is noteworthy that, in the various mammals, the fragility of the red corpuscles is greater the more globular the shape of the cells.[317] Following splenectomy in cases of hereditary spherocytosis, the fragility of the red corpuscles may decrease, remain unchanged or even increase slightly.

In other conditions, no striking increases in corpuscular fragility have been noted. *Increased maximum resistance* has been observed in the presence of jaundice and in cases of hypochromic anemia, thalassemia, sickle cell anemia (p. 680) and polycythemia vera. In thalassemia (p. 707) the increased resistance may be so great that a residue of cells may remain in 0.03 per cent saline or even in distilled water. Furthermore, well-marked hemolysis, instead of appearing in the first one or two tubes following that in which hemolysis commences, may be found to begin only in 0.30 per cent saline.

The **mechanical fragility** of the red corpuscles can be measured by shaking blood in a flask containing glass beads.[327] This test was introduced as more nearly representing the traumatic conditions to which erythrocytes are subjected in the circulation than other tests of fragility. Various conditioning factors influence the results of the test.[324] Senescent cells have been shown to have increased mechanical fragility. In general, mechanical fragility is increased when osmotic fragility is increased, but in some instances it has been found to be increased when osmotic fragility was normal or actually decreased. Spherocytes, sickled cells and agglutinated corpuscles have been shown to have an increased susceptibility to mechanical trauma but poikilocytes do not seem to be especially fragile.

The resistance of erythrocytes to solutions of *lysolecithin* has been reported to be diminished in cases of hereditary spherocytosis whereas it was normal in acquired forms of hemolytic anemia even when osmotic resistance was diminished.[325] The use of these and other technics in the study of hemolytic anemias will be discussed in the chapter dealing with that subject (p. 620).

Catabolism of Hemoglobin.— There is still some uncertainty about the exact nature and sequence of the individual steps in hemoglobin catabolism.

There is some evidence that the first step is the splitting of the iron-protoporphyrin complex from globin to produce hematin.[252,256] However, it is more generally held that the protoporphyrin ring is opened by an oxidative removal of the α-methene bridge, the iron remaining and the union with globin persisting to form a green iron-protein compound, *choleglobin* or verdohemoglobin[237] (Fig. 3–14). How the cleavage is achieved is not clear. Nor is it understood how iron is split off and globin liberated to yield the bile pigment, biliverdin. It is known, however, that this takes place in the reticuloendothelial system and that the liberated iron is bound to protein in the tissues and then is transported via the plasma iron-binding proteins to be used again (p. 148). The liberated globin is degraded and is returned to the body pool of amino acids.

Biliverdin, the predominant pigment of many species of amphibia and of birds, is apparently rapidly reduced in man to bilirubin. In the plasma, bilirubin, which is insoluble in water, is transported from the site of hemoglobin breakdown to the liver as a protein complex, bound to albumin chiefly but also to α- and β-globulins.[248]

In the liver, bilirubin is converted into water-soluble forms. This is achieved by conjugation with hydrophilic compounds of which glucuronic acid is the most important.[248] Bilirubin diglucuronide is derived by a dehydrogenase reaction with uridine nucleotide as the substrate. Some bilirubin may also be present in bile as a monoglucuronide, and a small fraction is in the form of a sulfate.[247] The difference in solubility of bilirubin and bilirubin glucuronide probably accounts for the indirect and direct reactions of the Van den Bergh test (p. 177).

The mechanisms responsible for the transport of bilirubin into the liver cells are obscure. It is not known whether the retention of non-conjugated bilirubin

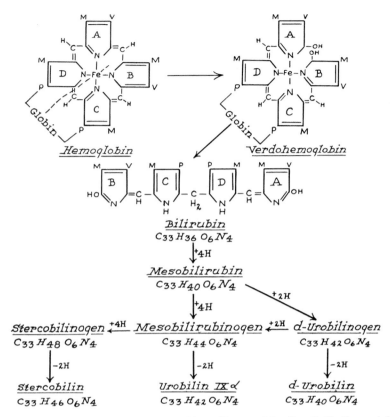

Fig. 3–14.—The breakdown of hemoglobin. (Prepared by Dr. G. E. Cartwright.)

associated with the excessive production of bilirubin in hemolytic anemia is attributable to limitations in the passage of the pigment into the liver cells or is caused by a rate-limiting factor in the conjugating enzyme system.

In the intestine, probably through the activity of the bacterial flora, bilirubin is converted to "urobilinogen." "Urobilinogen" consists of three colorless chromogens all of which are characterized by a strong Ehrlich aldehyde reaction, as well as by instability and ease of oxidation to three corresponding orange-yellow pigments which compose the "urobilin" group.[256a] The transition to urobilin can be hastened by mild oxidizing agents, such as iodine, and this is the basis of the Schlesinger (alcoholic zinc acetate) qualitative test for urobilin. Of the uro-

bilinogen group, stercobilinogen is normally preponderant in the feces and urine. The remaining two substances are mesobilirubinogen and d-urobilinogen. Mesobilirubinogen is converted to stercobilinogen.[249] d-Urobilinogen may be a precursor of mesobilirubinogen.

Although some investigators have maintained that the urobilinogens in urine come directly from bilirubin in the plasma, it is more generally held that they are derived from pigments absorbed from the colon into the portal circulation and returned to the liver. The *amount of urobilinogen excreted* in the urine in 24 hours (U.U.) by the normal adult is 0 to 3.5 mg., most frequently 0.5 to 1.5 mg. The normal range for *fecal urobilinogen* (F.U.), as calculated from a four-day period of collection is 40 to 280 mg. per day, usually 100 to 200 mg.[256] Lower values are found in young children.[251] Mean values have been found to increase with age. The oral administration of aureomycin causes a marked decrease in the concentration of fecal urobilinogen but this can be counteracted by the administration of aluminum hydroxide gel.[294]

The measurement of fecal and urinary urobilinogen excretion is a very imperfect *index of hemoglobin breakdown*. In addition to obvious sources of error such as incomplete evacuation from the bowel and variations in the degree of reabsorption of urobilinogen therefrom, there are other difficulties. On the one hand, worn out red corpuscles are not the only sources of bile pigment. It has been found in studies of the fate of glycine tagged with isotopic nitrogen that a significant portion, at least 11 per cent of bile pigment and possibly as much as 30 per cent, is derived from one or more sources other than the hemoglobin of mature circulating erythrocytes,[249] possibly from heme produced in the liver which has not been utilized for hemoglobin formation.[17] Again, muscle hemoglobin and other porphyrin pigments of endogenous origin probably contribute to the fecal urobilinogen.[237,252] Exogenous (dietary) porphyrins do not do so since iron porphyrins cannot be split in the gut.[67] On the other hand, the fecal and urinary urobilinogen will be lower than may be expected because other oxidation products of heme than urobilinogen, such as dipyrroles, propentdyopent,[230] the mesobilifuscins and urochromes, are not included in the measurement. An occasional factor leading to reduction in fecal and urinary urobilinogen is the use of an antibiotic, as mentioned already.

The employment of bile pigment excretion as a measure of hemoglobin breakdown will be discussed further in a later section (p. 180).

Evidence of Exaggerated Red Cell Destruction.—The *normal breakdown* of red corpuscles which goes on continuously is indicated by the presence of bilirubin in the blood plasma and the finding of urobilinogen, or its oxidation product, urobilin in the stools and urine. Normally 0.5 to 0.8 mg. of bilirubin are found in 100 ml. of blood (mean 0.54 mg., range 0.2 to 1.7 mg., with 93 per cent of the values less than 0.8 mg.[299]). "One-minute" or "direct" bilirubin (see below) is less than 0.2 mg. in normal persons.[293] Normal values for fecal (F.U.) and urinary urobilinogen (U.U.) have been given already (p. 174).

A marked *increase in blood destruction* is manifested by an increase in *bilirubinemia* and in the quantity of *urobilinogen in the urine and stools*. In frank hemolytic disease the F.U. ranges from 300 to 4000 mg. per day, usually 600 to 2000 mg., and the U.U. varies from 1 to 200 mg. per day, usually 5 to 30 mg.[256] At the same time, unless destruction is completely balanced by increased blood formation, anemia develops. However, high values for urobilinogen may be found in the face of little anemia and modest increases in blood destruction accompanied by anemia may occur without significant increases in fecal urobilinogen being demonstrable. One may also encounter a marked increase in the fecal urobilinogen with but little increase or a normal amount in the urine.

Morphological evidence of red cell destruction such as poikilocytosis and spherocytosis may appear, but the more striking morphological changes in the blood may be those indicative of increased red cell formation. Thus reticulocytes are usually greatly increased in number, polychromatophilia is evident and nucleated red cells may be seen, sometimes in very large numbers. Often, if the blood destruction is rapid, so many macrocytes are produced that the anemia becomes macrocytic in type. The blood picture in hemolytic anemia will be discussed more fully in a later chapter (p. 603).

Hemoglobinemia, which refers to the presence of extracorpuscular circulating hemoglobin in the plasma, is rarely apparent when blood destruction is increased and is seen only in those types of hemolytic disease characterized by hemoglobinuria and when there is sudden and extensive hemolysis, as in the hemolytic crisis of hereditary spherocytosis. Small, invisible quantities of free hemoglobin, detectable by the use of benzidine,[295] are found more often. The upper limit of hemochromogens in normal plasma giving this reaction is 5 mg., or even only 3 mg. per 100 ml.[292] Slight increases above normal have been observed in hemoglobin-C disease and in sickle cell-thalassemia. Moderate elevations (10 to 25 mg.) have been encountered in sickle cell anemia, sickle cell-hemoglobin C disease, thalassemia major, and in severe, auto-immune hemolytic anemia. High levels are found only in association with hemoglobinuria.

As indicated earlier (p. 168), hemoglobin released by intravascular hemolysis is bound by the plasma haptoglobin to the extent of its capacity. Some is joined with albumin to form methemalbumin and the excess above these amounts is lost in the urine. **Methemalbumin**[266] is produced by the union of hematin, the ferric complex of protoporphyrin, with albumin, formation of the complex serving to remove free hematin from the plasma and providing a mechanism for its transport in the blood stream. This brownish pigment is distinct from methemoglobin and has a faint absorption band at 624 mμ. It is more readily demonstrated by covering the serum or plasma with ether and then adding a one-tenth volume of concentrated ammonium sulfide. This results in the formation of a hemochromogen with a relatively intense, sharply defined α absorption band at 558 mμ (*Schumm's test*). First described in blackwater fever (p. 607), methemalbumin is now recognized as a reliable indication of intravascular hemolysis due to any cause. Contrary to previous views, hematin, like other derivatives of hemoglobin, can be converted to bile pigment and contributes to the fecal urobilinogen.[273a]

Although little free hemoglobin is necessary to produce hemoglobinemia, a large amount, several times the amount normally produced, is necessary to maintain hemoglobinemia because of the efficiency of the removal mechanism. The tubular epithelium removes and degrades unbound hemoglobin entering the glomerular filtrate. Some of this hemoglobin iron finds its way into the urine where it may be detected as **hemosiderin.** Particularly marked and persistent hemosiderinuria occurs in paroxysmal nocturnal hemoglobinuria but it is found in the urine of every patient whose plasma continuously contains abnormal amounts of hemoglobin. It is demonstrated by centrifuging a specimen of urine, placing one drop of the sediment on a glass slide, adding a drop of 30 per cent aqueous ammonium sulfide solution and mixing the two drops together. The iron in the hemosiderin reacts with ammonium sulfide to form black granules of ferric sulfide of varying sizes which will be seen separately or within epithelial cells or casts. Other staining technics will be described later (p. 641).

When increased blood destruction occurs in a chronic form, there may be no clinical signs whatever; or jaundice, anemia and other signs may be found. When destruction is very rapid, toxic symptoms develop. These will be considered in the chapter on hemolytic anemia (p. 602).

The tests employed for the demonstration of the products of blood destruction may be described at this point.

Icterus Index (Meulengracht

Test).—In this test the degree of yellow color in the plasma or serum is measured by comparing it with the color of standard solutions of potassium dichromate. These are generally made up in a series of tubes numbered according to the quantity of dichromate in 10,000 parts of water; thus 1 unit is 1:10,000, 5 is 5:10,000 and so on.

The simplest procedure is to compare the color of the plasma, as seen in the hematocrit after it has been centrifuged, with that of a series of standards in tubes of glass of the same thickness and bore as the hematocrit (Fig. 3–15, and Frontispiece). Tubes corresponding to 1, 3, 5, 7.5, 10, 15, 25, 50 and 100 units may be obtained. If the icterus index is greater than 100, the plasma may be diluted until a match is obtained.

The icterus index is a useful, simple and rapid test. When the icterus index value is normal (4 to 7 units) it can be assumed that there is no increase in the bilirubin content of the blood stream. The test is important in calling attention during a routine blood examination to the presence of unsuspected hyperbilirubinemia. Yet it must be borne in mind that *the test is not specific* and that substances other than bilirubin may cause an increase in the yellow color. Of these, the lipochromes (carotin, lutein, *etc.*) are the most important, while the drugs dinitrophenol and atabrine may occasionally be sufficiently concentrated in the blood to cause an elevation in the icterus index. Thus, in vegetarians, diabetics and infants there may be an increased icterus index which is not the result of hyperbilirubinemia.

Another source of error is hemolysis. The accuracy of the icterus index test is increased by mixing the plasma with one or more parts of redistilled, colorless acetone. This produces a white, flocculent precipitate of protein which includes any hemoglobin free in the plasma. When this is centrifuged, clear plasma

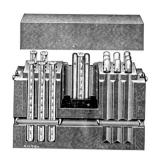

Fig. 3–15.—Icterus index and blood sedimentation apparatus for use in conjunction with hematocrit. The standard icterus index tubes are shown on the right. The unknown is matched against the standards in the central portion of the block. The section at the front of the block is for holding hematocrits vertically during sedimentation. (Courtesy of Arthur H. Thomas Company.)

containing most of the bilirubin originally present in the plasma remains; the quantity carried down with the proteins does not produce a significant difference in the result. This procedure may be incorporated as a part of the usual hematocrit technic by drawing off a column of plasma 2.5 cm. high with a capillary pipet such as is used in filling the hematocrit, placing this in another hematocrit and then adding acetone until the column of fluid reaches the 5 cm. mark. The tube is then centrifuged and the color of the clarified plasma is matched with that of the standards. The correct icterus index is obtained by multiplying the number on the tube with which the plasma matches by two in order to make up for the dilution of the plasma.

The acetone procedure is cumbersome and need not be used unless for some reason a sample of blood free of hemolysis cannot be obtained.

Van den Bergh Test.—This, as distinguished from the icterus index, is a specific test for bilirubin. The test is based on Ehrlich's discovery that a mixture of sulfanilic acid, hydrochloric acid and sodium nitrite (diazo reagent) yields a reddish-violet color when added to solutions containing bilirubin, such as blood plasma. The color may appear and reach its maximum intensity at once ("direct" reaction); if no color develops in one minute, alcohol is added. If the reddish-violet color now appears, the reaction is called "indirect." As mentioned earlier (p. 173), the "direct" and "indirect" reactions depend on differences in the solubility of bilirubin and bilirubin glucuronide. The latter, being water-soluble, gives a direct reaction; that is, the coupling with the reagent occurs without prior addition of alcohol. Free bilirubin, on the other hand, cannot couple until alcohol has been added to bring it into solution; thus, an "indirect" van den Bergh reaction is obtained. It should be borne in mind that because of the kinetics of the van den Bergh reaction and the presence of solubilizing substances in the plasma, the direct and indirect test yields only approximations of the respective concentrations of bilirubin glucuronide and of bilirubin.

When there is increased blood destruction, the direct-reacting fraction usually constitutes less than 15 per cent of the total serum bilirubin and rarely exceeds 1.2 mg. per cent unless there is accompanying hepatic dysfunction. The larger proportion of this is probably attributable to bilirubin glucuronide regurgitated from the bile. Its quantity is related to the amount of bilirubin excreted in the bile, increasing as the latter increases.[298] These findings explain the bilirubinuria seen occasionally in patients with hemolytic jaundice in the absence of complicating hepatic disease.

The technic of the van den Bergh test is described in standard works on clinical chemistry.

Tests for Urobilinogen and Urobilin.—*Qualitative procedures.*— (a) *Fluorescence in the Presence of Zinc Salts.*—Bile pigments, if present, are first removed by adding to 10 ml. of urine (or aqueous suspension of feces) 2 ml. of 10 per cent calcium chloride and filtering. Any urobilinogen which has not yet been converted to urobilin is oxidized by adding 1 or 2 drops of Lugol's solution to the filtrate. Ten ml. of Schlesinger's reagent is added next, the preparation then being filtered and allowed to stand one or two hours. (Schlesinger's reagent is made by placing 4 gm. of zinc acetate in a 100 ml. bottle and filling it with 95 per cent ethyl alcohol. This must be shaken occasionally. The supernatant fluid is used.)

The presence of urobilin is indicated by a green fluorescence which may be seen by viewing the tube in a bright light against a dark background. The specimen can be examined spectroscopically and the test can be made roughly quantitative by noting at what dilution of the specimen the absorption bands for the urobilin disappear. Normally a dilution of 1:1000 is required for elimination of the absorption band.[303]

(b) *Ehrlich's Aldehyde Reaction.*—The aldehyde reagent is made up of 1.7 Gm. paradimethylaminobenzaldehyde, 150 ml. concentrated hydrochloric acid and 100 ml. distilled water. A series of dilutions of urine is made by adding to 1 ml. 10, 20, 30 *etc.*, ml. of water. Ten ml. of each dilution is placed in test tubes and 1 ml. of Ehrlich's aldehyde reagent is added. When urobilinogen is present, a pink color appears promptly or within five minutes. The color is best seen by looking through the mouths of the tubes. The dilution at which the pink color is still perceptible is noted. Normally this does not exceed the 1:20 dilution. Because urobilinogen is readily oxidized to urobilin on exposure to air, fresh urine is required for this test.

Semi-quantitative procedures which are of practical value have been devised by Watson *et al.*[302] For serial observations of urine urobilinogen, a two-hour sample is collected between 2 and 4 P.M. following emptying of the bladder and drinking one glass of water. During this period of the day the peak excretion of urobilinogen usually occurs. The sample is cooled to room temperature and examined within 30 minutes after voiding.   2.5 ml. of urine are pipetted into each of two colorimeter tubes. If the urine contains large amounts of urobilinogen a 1:10 dilution should be made first.   To the first tube are added 2.5 ml. of a modified Ehrlich's reagent (0.7 gm. paradimethyl aminobenzaldehyde, 150 ml. conc. HCl, 100 ml. distilled H_2O).   The contents are mixed and immediately 5 ml. of a saturated aqueous solution of sodium acetate are added

of the difference between the spectral and visual color characteristics of the dye, a dilution of 1 part in 4.9 of 0.5 per cent acetic acid is made by adding 20.5 ml. of the stock dye solution to 100 ml. of the acetic acid.   This will give a Pontacyl dye mixture of 2.04 mg. in 100 ml. and has a color intensity equivalent to that of a urobilinogen aldehyde solution containing 0.6 mg. of urobilinogen per 100 ml.   Further dilutions are made for the various standards in the comparator block or for the calibration curve.[302]

The total amount of urobilinogen for the two-hour period is calculated as follows:

$$\left.\begin{array}{l}\text{Conc. of final solution} \\ \text{in terms of mg. urobilinogen} \\ \text{per 100 ml.}\end{array}\right\} \times 4 \times \dfrac{\text{urine volume}}{100 \text{ ml.}} = \begin{array}{l}\text{Ehrlich} \\ \text{units per} \\ \text{two hours}\end{array}$$

and thoroughly mixed.   To the other tube, which is to serve as a blank, the reagents are added in reverse order to prevent color development.   First the 5 ml. of saturated sodium acetate are added and the contents mixed thoroughly; then the 2.5 ml. of Ehrlich's reagent are added and the contents are again mixed.   The first tube is then read on a photoelectric colorimeter at 565 mμ, using the second tube as a blank for the center setting.   If a photoelectric instrument is not available the readings may be made on a comparator block which is available commercially.[304]

A mixture of Pontacyl dyes (DuPont) serves for making a calibration curve for the photoelectric colorimeter or to prepare standards for the comparator block. The initial stock standard solution consists of a mixture of 5 mg. of Pontacyl Carmine 2B and 95 mg. of Pontacyl Violet 6R 150 per cent, dissolved in 1000 ml. of 0.5 per cent acetic acid.   For the comparator blocks an initial dilution of 1 part in 6 of 0.5 per cent acetic acid is made.   For the photoelectric colorimeter calibration curve, however, because

Normal values are below one unit for the two-hour period.   The results are expressed in units because the method is not specific for urobilinogen and other Ehrlich-reacting substances are measured as well.   The increase of the latter has been found to be roughly proportional to that of the former and the test is consequently useful for serial observations.   The test has been found to give false-negative results in about 15 per cent of patients with significant degrees of hyperurobilinogenuria.[300]

For semi-quantitative measurements of urobilinogen in *feces*, 10 gm. of a random sample are weighed out into a small evaporating dish.   This amount is thoroughly ground with repeated small amounts of water up to a total of 90 ml. The supernatant suspension obtained in all these washings is added to a 500 ml. Erlenmeyer flask containing 100 ml. of a 20 per cent ferrous sulfate ($FeSO_4 \cdot 7H_2O$) solution (20 gm. of ground crystals plus 92 ml. of distilled water).   An additional 100 ml. of distilled water is added to the residue of feces in the evaporating dish and mixed with it, though this may be omitted if the specimen is acholic; finally the residue is washed out with 100 ml. of 10 per cent NaOH. All of the suspensions of feces are added to the Erlenmeyer flask which finally is corked, mixed and set aside in the dark for at least one hour. The supernatant fluid should be almost colorless or at most a pale yellow at the end of this period; otherwise the reduction should be continued for another hour or two. A small amount is then filtered, diluted 1 to 10 or more (unless the stool is acholic), and this solution is treated in exactly the same manner as the urine specimen. The calculation is as follows:

man weighing 70 Kg. who destroys 6.25 Gm. hemoglobin daily. The reasons for considering urobilinogen excretion an imperfect index of hemoglobin breakdown were given earlier (p. 175). It has been found empirically that the recovery of bile pigment, as urobilinogen, in the stool ranges from 20 to 100 per cent of the actual production and often is of the order of 30 to 50 per cent. An additional variable which must be taken into account in the interpretation of the fecal urobilinogen value is the quantity of circulating hemoglobin.

The *hemolytic index*[297] was devised to take into account both the relation of

$$\left.\begin{array}{l}\text{Conc. of final solution}\\\text{in terms of mg. urobi-}\\\text{linogen per 100 ml.}\end{array}\right\} \times 4 \times \frac{400 \text{ (or 300)}}{10} \text{ dilution of filtrate} = \begin{array}{l}\text{Ehrlich units}\\\text{per 100 gm.}\\\text{feces}\end{array}$$

The upper limit of normal per 100 gm. feces is about 350 Ehrlich units.

Quantitative procedures entail a four-day collection of feces, the average per diem amount of urobilinogen for this

urobilinogen to the total mass of circulating hemoglobin and the fact that less than the amount expected on stoichiometric grounds is actually found in the stools. It is calculated as follows:

$$\frac{\text{Daily fecal urobilinogen (average of four days) mg.} \times 100}{\text{Hemoglobin (Gm. per 100 ml.)} \times \text{total blood volume}/100}$$

The normal index is 11 to 21.

period being determined. Preformed fecal urobilin is reduced to urobilinogen by means of ferrous hydroxide and the Ehrlich reaction is then employed. Quantitative studies of urinary urobilinogen require the collection of a 24-hour specimen which must be collected in a special manner.[301] The use of these procedures is based on the fact that the porphyrin moiety of hemoglobin, exclusive of iron, makes up 3.5 per cent by weight of the hemoglobin molecule. Since protoporphyrin and bilirubin have practically the same molecular weight, it follows that the destruction of 1 gram of hemoglobin should make available 35 mg. of bilirubin. On this basis, 220 mg. bilirubin should be formed each day in a

QUANTITATIVE ASPECTS OF HEMOGLOBIN PRODUCTION AND DESTRUCTION

A normal, average man weighing 70 Kg., possesses about 3000 Gm. of bone marrow (3.4 to 5.9 per cent of the body weight). This maintains a circulating erythrocyte population of some 25 million millions (25×10^{12}) (Fig. 3–16) which is equivalent to approximately 750 Gm. of hemoglobin. Since the average potential erythrocyte life span is 120 days, this requires the production of 6.25 Gm. hemoglobin each day. In the normal individual, erythrocyte destruction balances red cell production. In maintaining the equilibrium, therefore, the same

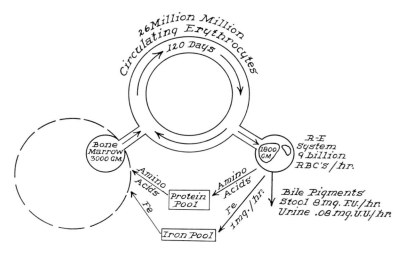

Fig. 3–16.—The erythron.

quantity of hemoglobin is destroyed and from this about 21 mg. iron and 220 mg. of bilirubin are derived. (From each gram of hemoglobin 3.35 mg. iron and 35 mg. bilirubin are obtained.) The iron is re-utilized but the bilirubin is a waste product, the excretion of which can be measured as described already (p. 175).

An increase in output of red corpuscles and hemoglobin can be achieved by increasing the concentration of red cell precursors in the bone marrow and by expanding the volume of active marrow. Normally but a fifth of the nucleated cells in bone marrow are erythroid. As is often seen in hemolytic anemias, this proportion of normoblasts can increase so that their number equals the number of leukocytes. Furthermore, ordinarily but a half of the red marrow is occupied by cells and, in the adult, only 50 per cent of the marrow is red. On demand the activity of the red marrow can be increased and the fatty marrow can be invaded by hemopoietic tissue. By calculation, therefore, one might estimate that it would be possible to increase erythropoiesis perhaps tenfold. Actual measurements have shown that the erythropoietic capacity of the

bone marrow can increase six to eight times.[292] However, the extent to which erythropoiesis does increase depends on various factors. These will be considered further, below (p. 186).

Production of red corpuscles increases whenever required, provided the necessary materials for blood formation are available and the synthetic mechanisms are intact. Depending on the extent of the demand, it is possible for production to increase so that no anemia develops. This can occur in response to blood loss, although ultimately anemia ensues. The critical factor in this situation is depletion of iron stores since the stores of other essentials are exhausted much less readily. In hemolytic disease, on the other hand, since there is no loss of essential building materials, it is possible for blood production to increase and keep pace with the shortened survival of the red corpuscles, with the result that no anemia may result, whatever. Thus, if the erythrocyte survival time is reduced to thirty days (one-fourth normal), an increase in hemoglobin production to 25 grams per day (four times normal) will maintain normal blood value. On the other hand, if the erythrocyte survival time is reduced to 10 days (one-twelfth normal) and the marrow production capacity can only expand sevenfold, anemia must develop. Nevertheless, unless production is inhibited for some reason, a new equilibrium is achieved. The new equilibrium level is represented by the maximal marrow hemoglobin production capacity (7 × 6.25 Gm.) divided by the demand (12 × 6.25 Gm.). Thus the new level will be, in this case, seven-twelfths of normal (58 per cent) and the quantity of hemoglobin per 100 ml. blood will be this proportion of the normal, providing no change in plasma volume has taken place.

In the preceding chapters the alterations in the bone marrow and the morphologic manifestations in the blood which occur in response to increased

it to combine with the iron-binding globulin and this is then injected intravenously. If blood samples are taken at approximately hourly intervals for radio-iron analysis, and if the total plasma iron content and the plasma volume have been determined, the quantity of iron entering or leaving the plasma per unit of time can be calculated, if one assumes that the plasma iron level remains relatively stable during the experimental period. Thus, the values for Fe^{59} concentration in the plasma are plotted as a function of time on semi-log paper. The time at which half of the radioactivity $(T\frac{1}{2})$ has disappeared is determined. The number of milligrams of iron entering and leaving the plasma per unit of time, the *"plasma iron turnover rate"* (PITR), is calculated as follows:

$$\frac{0.693}{Fe^{59}\ T\frac{1}{2}\ (hrs.)} \times mg.\ Fe/ml.\ plasma \times total\ plasma\ vol.\ (ml.) \times 24\ hr.$$

$$= PITR\ mg./day$$

demands for hemoglobin and red corpuscles were described. Unfortunately, an increased percentage of reticulocytes, or a reduced myeloid:erythroid (M:E) ratio in the bone marrow, while reflecting increased erythropoiesis, does not offer a quantitative measure of the increase in red cell production; neither does a rising red cell count, since this is the resultant of changes in destruction or blood loss and in total plasma volume as well as changes in production. Consequently attempts have been made to develop quantitative methods for the measurement of total production and destruction within the erythron.

Ferrokinetics.[79a,92a]—From measurements of iron kinetics it is possible to estimate the rates and sites of red cell formation and destruction, mean erythrocyte life span and plasma-storage iron exchange. Fe^{59} is incubated in the subject's plasma for 20 minutes to allow

(The number 0.693, the natural log of 2, is chosen because of the time unit used, that is, the half-period.)

Since the PITR does not differentiate between iron turnover as the result of incorporation into red cells or exchange elsewhere, it is useful to measure radioactivity in samples of hemolyzed blood, thereby measuring radioactivity in the red corpuscles. This will reveal the rate at which the administered Fe^{59} is being incorporated in new red cells. Such measurements are repeated daily until the activity in the red corpuscles ceases to increase. As a rule measurements are made daily for the first six or seven days and then less frequently for another week. The maximum concentration (MC) attained is noted. Normally this is in the range of 75 per cent. A close approximation of the *red cell iron turnover rate* (RBC ITR) can be computed from the product of the PITR and the per

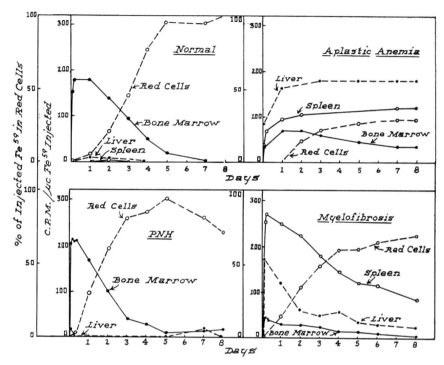

Fig. 3–17.—Uptake of Fe^{59} into red corpuscles and various tissues in a normal subject and in various disorders. The actual data are presented in Table 3–7. The iron found in the red corpuscles is expressed as a proportion of the amount injected; the iron in the bone marrow, liver and spleen is expressed as counts per minute (CPM) in proportion to the number of microcuries injected. (Prepared by Dr. James A. Bush.)

cent of the tracer iron present in red cells at maximum concentration; thus, PITR (mg./day) × MC (%) = RBC ITR mg./day.

If the red cell mass is known (p. 317) and from the estimated total red cell iron (1 ml. packed red cells = 1 mg. iron), the *fraction of red cell iron renewed each day* (RBC IRF) can be calculated; thus,

$$\frac{\text{RBC ITR}}{\text{mg.Fe/ml. packed cells} \times \text{RBC mass (ml.)}} = \text{RBC IRF}$$

The reciprocal of this is the *red cell life span*; thus, $\dfrac{100}{\text{RBC IRF}}$

Examples of the types of data obtainable are presented in Table 3–7.

A mobile scintillation counter makes it possible to note the entry of Fe^{59} into various areas where erythropoiesis may be taking place or blood destruction is going on, such as the bone marrow, liver and spleen. (The use of Cr^{51} for this purpose is described on page 630). In Figure 3–17 is shown the uptake of radioactive iron into red corpuscles following the injection of 5 microcuries in 5 μg. Fe^{59}, as carried out in our laboratory in several different types of disorders. By measuring gamma-ray emission of radio-iron over the sacrum (marrow), liver (representing tissue iron

Table 3–7.—Data for Cases Presented in Figure 3–17

	$T\frac{1}{2}/hrs.$	PITR		RBC ITR		RBC Iron Renewed fraction /day	RBC Life Span /days
		mg. /day	mg./kg. /day	mg. /day	mg./kg. /day		
Normal	1.40	38.0	0.47	38.0	0.47	.01	100
Aplastic anemia	5.52	29.2	0.32	8.5	0.09	.01	100
Paroxysmal nocturnal hemoglobinuria (post-splenectomy)	0.37	83.3	1.28	78.3	1.20	.08	12
Myelofibrosis with myeloid metaplasia in spleen	1.20	90.7	1.16	71.6	0.92	.03	33

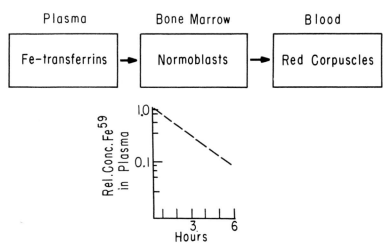

Fig. 3–18.—A simple model of iron kinetics and curve to show fall in Fe[59] radioactivity in the plasma of a normal adult following the intravenous injection of radioiron.

stores) and spleen, it was possible to show that when erythropoiesis was reduced, there was decreased uptake of iron in the bone marrow and, instead, uptake in tissue stores (aplastic anemia) and in sites of extramedullary hemopoiesis (myelofibrosis). On the other hand, when erythropoiesis was accelerated, uptake into marrow was active and appearance of Fe[59] in circulating red cells was prompt. However, when there was increased blood destruction, as in the case of paroxysmal nocturnal hemoglobinuria (PNH), the curve of radioactivity in circulating red cells, instead of remaining straight, fell off as the red cells were destroyed.

Normally, the disappearance of Fe[59] from the plasma following its intravenous injection is rapid and constant. Huff injected 4 μc. Fe[59] in 4 to 80 μg. iron and found that half the labelled iron in the plasma ($T\frac{1}{2}$) disappeared in 80 to 100 minutes.[79a] Using iron of higher specific activity (1 to 15 μc./μg.) Pollycove observed that, following the initial rapid decrease in plasma radio-iron, after approximately two days a second, much slower constant rate of radio-iron decrease appeared which persisted for the next eight to twelve days.[92a] This pattern he interpreted as indicating continuous feedback of radioactive iron from another iron pool into the plasma. This pool was

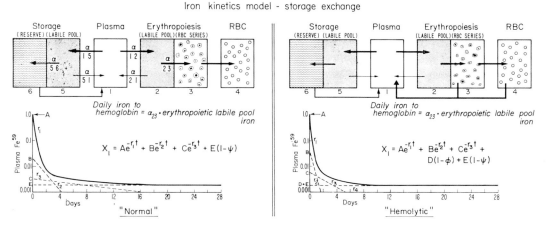

Iron kinetics model - storage exchange

FIG. 3–19.—Iron kinetics, as postulated by Pollycove,[92a] in a normal subject and in hemolytic anemia. "Erythropoiesis" refers to the bone marrow, where nucleated red cells as a source of iron, as well as a "labile pool" of iron are assumed to be present. In addition, there are tissue pools, labile and reserve. Solutions of the differential equations are indicated.

The concept postulates that, in the absence of hemolysis, injected radioiron after two weeks slowly equilibrates (α 51) with the labile storage pool (5). When there is increased breakdown of the erythrocyte precursors in the marrow and increased destruction of red corpuscles, rapid feedback of radioiron to plasma occurs and there is earlier equilibration of plasma radioiron than in the absence of hemolysis.

designated "labile" and was assumed to exist in the marrow, since virtually all plasma radio-iron transfers initially to marrow. He assumed that this was not derived from storage depots and from destroyed circulating erythrocytes since re-entry of radio-iron from these sources is usually delayed and would therefore have no influence on plasma radio-iron during a two week period of measurement.

Figure 3–19 illustrates Pollycove's complete model of iron kinetics both in a normal individual and in a case in which increased blood destruction is occurring. In this the postulated bone marrow "labile" iron pool as well as storage pools are shown. When there is negligible storage of iron, pools 5 and 6 are omitted. When there is increased blood destruction, the return of iron from destroyed red cells to plasma and labile and reserve pools is included in the analysis. Simultaneous differential equations have been devised for the purpose of determining the intercompartmental rate constants

and the amounts of iron in the various pools and in red corpuscles.[92a]

The validity of Pollycove's theoretical and mathematical formulations remains to be proved. Huff's model (Fig. 3–18) has the merit of simplicity and has made it possible to secure roughly quantitative data which have proved useful, as will be discussed further below.

Erythrokinetics.—A roughly quantitative estimate of erythrocyte production and destruction can be made by the use of ferrokinetic studies, if carried out in conjunction with measurements of red cell life span (p. 164), absolute reticulocyte counts (p. 90), myeloid-erythroid ratio of the cells in the bone marrow (p. 66), total red cell mass (p. 317) and fecal urobilinogen (p. 180).[66a] Although there is considerable variation in the results of such measurement from one normal individual to another, a range of normal values can be established for daily turnover of red cells, hemoglobin, iron and urobilinogen which provide a reference point for comparison with the changes occurring in disease. Finch and his associates attempted to evaluate marrow response and hemolytic rate in patients with anemia by calculating an erythropoietic index and a hemolytic index on the basis of measures of red cell production and destruction as compared with the normal.[66a] With reference to ferrokinetic data, for example, they observed, as had others, that the PITR is increased when the bone marrow is inactive and is greatly accelerated in conditions of hyperactivity, as in hemolytic anemias. It was increased in polycythemias, especially erythremia, in the leukemias and in pernicious anemia. In hemolytic anemias RBC ITR was increased, whereas in aplastic anemia it was decreased below normal. When total production was estimated it was observed that the bone marrow in some hemolytic states is capable of increasing production eight to ten times normal. However, these great increases were noted only in the congenital disorders, suggesting that time is an important factor in achieving maximal compensation. With anemia of short duration, whether due to blood loss or blood destruction, blood production reached two to three times normal.

Two important concepts arise from these and similar studies. One concerns the *balance between production and destruction*. Both in the normal individual and in "compensated hemolytic disease" these are in equilibrium and no anemia is found. Likewise in many patients with chronic anemia a similar equilibrium can be detected. Thus, in leukemia, uremia, arthritis and in many other conditions a shortened red cell life span has been demonstrated. The reduction is often of small degree and a normal marrow would be easily capable of increasing production to meet this charge. However, in these same conditions production is impaired; in fact, it may be impaired production which results in the formation

of red cells with a shortened life span. As a consequence of the failure of production to make up for increased destruction, anemia develops. A new equilibrium is usually reached at a level ranging from just under normal in the mild chronic anemias to a very low level, as in many cases of uremia. The balance between production and destruction can be altered favorably in many ways; *e.g.* interruption of blood loss or of blood destruction, the supplying of an essential substance which is lacking (iron, vitamin B_{12}) or treatment of the underlying disease (leukemia, arthritis); or, to the disadvantage of the patient by, for example, a sudden increase in blood loss or by temporary cessation of erythropoiesis, as in the crises which occur in certain congenital hemolytic anemias.

Erythrokinetic studies have shown, furthermore, that a distinction must be drawn between *total* erythropoiesis and *effective* erythropoiesis.[66a] When the production of erythrocytes which had a measurable life span in the circulating blood (effective erythropoiesis) was estimated from the red cell life span, reticulocyte count and red cell utilization of radio-iron, it was found that in certain disease states a large gap could be demonstrated between the effort of the marrow and the red cells which reached the circulation. The former was calculated from the myeloid-erythroid ratio of the bone marrow, the plasma iron turnover and urobilinogen excretion. In certain pathological states it appeared that red cell proliferation and hemoglobin synthesis took place which did not result in the production of viable circulating erythrocytes. Such "shunts" were observed in thalassemia, in pernicious anemia and in patients with bone marrow failure. Thus, it was found that there was normoblastic hyperplasia with increased mitotic activity, increased production of urobilinogen and a roughly comparable increase in serum radio-iron turnover;

yet the red cell uptake of radio-iron was low and the absolute number of reticulocytes was normal. These findings were interpreted as indicating that, in certain states of dyspoiesis, qualitatively defective red cells are formed in the marrow and destroyed there without reaching the circulation.

It is very useful to give thought to both of these concepts in any case of anemia, even if the opportunity does not exist to make all the measurements which have been discussed. Anemia, in essence, is the result of (1) a hemorrhagic or hemolytic process of sufficient severity to exceed the maximal compensatory capacity of the normal marrow; (2) impairment of total production by the marrow; or (3) ineffective erythropoiesis. Life span measurements, reticulocyte counts and red cell utilization of radio-iron indicate effective erythropoiesis. The M:E ratio, PITR and stool urobilinogen refer to total erythropoiesis.

THE PORPHYRIAS[287,288]

The term porphyria refers to an uncommon disorder of pyrrole metabolism and should not be confused with porphyrinuria, which refers to the urinary excretion of porphyrins in excessive amounts and, as discussed above, may occur under a variety of circumstances. Understanding of the porphyrias has come from an extension of the classical studies of Hans Fischer. There are several varieties but their classification is unsettled.

Porphyria erythropoietica (Congenital porphyria)[283] is one of the rarest of human diseases. This inborn error of metabolism makes its appearance in early infancy and may be first noticed because the child's diapers are colored by the urine. The urine is Burgundy red in color and contains uroporphyrin and some coproporphyrin, mainly type I. No porphobilinogen is present. Both the urine and the feces darken on exposure to light, the latter turning almost black, even though it may appear dark reddish brown when fresh.

Another symptom which calls attention to the disease is the development of bullous or erythematous lesions of the skin following exposure to light (hydroa aestivale).[285b] Epidermolysis bullosa may be simulated because slight trauma may appear to be the precipitating factor.[290] Round vesicles appear over the affected areas, central necrosis occurs and this is followed by the development of pustules and, subsequently, deep scarring. Mutilation may become so severe as to produce loss of the fingers, nose or ears and leprosy may be suspected. Hypertrichosis is often present. The teeth may appear bright red and range from this color to brown or yellowish. Examination with ultraviolet light has demonstrated considerable deposition of porphyrin in the dentin. The bones of the skeleton are also discolored, being chocolate brown from impregnation with uroporphyrin I.

Anemia, associated with the presence in the blood of punctate basophilia, polychromatophilia and erythroblasts, as well as other signs of hemolytic disease, may be present, in addition to splenomegaly.[288] The anemia is usually mild and evidence of increased blood destruction is not always present.[277a] Needle-like structures, thought to consist of porphyrins, have been observed in some of the abnormal normoblasts and erythrocytes.[286]

Fluorescence microscopy of the bone marrow of these patients has revealed an abnormal variety of normoblasts which exhibit intense red fluorescence, localized chiefly in their nuclei. These cells can be distinguished in stained preparations of bone marrow from normal cells, which do not fluoresce, by the presence of nuclear inclusion bodies containing hemoglobin. The increased porphyrin formation in this form of porphyria has been

Table 3–8—Distinguishing Characteristics of Porphyrias

	Porphyria Erythropoietica	Porphyria Hepatica		
		Acute Intermittent	Cutanea Tarda Hereditaria	Cutanea Tarda Symptomatica
Inheritance	Recessive (?)	Dominant	Dominant (?)	Acquired
Age at onset, years	Infancy	15–40	15–30	±30–50
		Latent　Acute	Latent　Acute	
Cutaneous lesions and photosensitivity	++++	0　　　0	0　　　±	+
Abdominal, psychic and/or neurologic symptoms	0	0　　　+++	0　　　++	0
Urine: Color	Red	N*　　Brownish red*	N　　N* or red	Red
Porphobilinogen	N	++　　++++	0　　　++	N
Uroporphyrin	++++	++　　++	N　　　++	+++
Coproporphyrin	++	++　　++	N　　　+++	++
Feces: Porphyrins	++	N　　　+	++++　+++	N

*Freshly voided urine may be normal but, on standing, becomes deep brownish red or even black. N indicates "normal," 0 "absent." The plus signs indicate increases of various degrees.

attributed to these abnormal cells which, it is postulated, release the porphyrins into the plasma.[283] The observation that splenectomy has been followed not only by marked clinical improvement but also a decrease in the concentration of uro- and coproporphyrin in the erythrocytes, marrow and urine,[276,286] suggests that increased blood destruction in these cases results in increased erythropoietic activity and excessive formation and excretion of porphyrin. Whether the skin photosensitivity is related directly to the concentration of porphyrin in the body or is due to other causes, is unknown. The erythrodontia and pigmentation of the bones is no doubt related to deposition of porphyrin in the growing bones.

It has been suggested that congenital porphyria is due to a disordered pigment metabolism in which the normal ratio between the formation of type I and type III porphyrins is disturbed, giving a disproportionate or disorderly type of synthesis in favor of type I. Studies with isotopically labelled glycine showed that the formation and degradation of uroporphyrin I and of coproporphyrin I are rapid. This condition has never been observed in succeeding generations and its mode of inheritance is uncertain. However, a very similar disorder which occurs in cattle[282,288b] is inherited as a recessive Mendelian character.[276a] Such a disorder has also been reported in pigs.[279a]

The victims of this disease must be protected against light. Splenectomy may be helpful, as indicated above. The abdominal and neurological symptoms which trouble patients with acute intermittent porphyria do not occur.

Porphyria hepatica is the term suggested by Watson for the remaining forms of porphyria since in these, in contrast to porphyria erythropoietica, the amounts of porphyrin and porphyrin precursors are found greatly increased in the liver rather than in the bone marrow.[283]

Acute intermittent porphyria,[287] in contrast to congenital porphyria, is not extremely rare but it is often overlooked.

Although the presenting complaints are often sudden in onset, this disorder, like congenital porphyria, appears to be inborn and the metabolic disturbance is found even in the absence of the acute symptoms. These patients manifest no light sensitivity and a porphyrin precursor, porphobilinogen, rather than uroporphyrin type I is excreted in large amounts. The disease is familial. Waldenström's thorough studies in Sweden showed that the disorder is inherited as a Mendelian dominant.[287] It is somewhat more common in women than in men. Symptoms first appear some time after puberty, most often in the third and fourth decades.

The classical symptoms are of three types and these may appear independently or together. The *abdominal* symptoms are marked by extremely severe, cramp-like pains, vomiting and pronounced constipation. The pain is usually centered about the umbilical area and often radiates into the back, the chest and the thighs. The abdomen may be soft, tenderness is minimal and rebound tenderness is absent. There is little or no distention and usually no visible peristalsis. *X*-ray examination reveals areas both of spasm and of gaseous distention. Slight fever, hypertension and tachycardia may be associated. The skin may show a diffuse or spotted pigmentation. Leukocytosis usually accompanies an acute episode. The acute symptoms together with the leukocytosis have often led to an erroneous diagnosis of acute surgical abdomen and to surgical intervention. After a variable period of time the abdominal symptoms may subside. In other cases, neurological symptoms appear and dominate the clinical picture.

Neurologic disturbances are common and consist of paralysis of skeletal muscles. The pareses are scattered irregularly and may develop as slight feebleness, often accompanied by aching and tenderness in the muscles. These signs may be transitory or widespread paralysis may occur and cranial muscles may be involved. Respiration may become very shallow and death usually occurs from respiratory paralysis.

In contrast, there are few symptoms implicating the sensory nervous system other than pain (neuralgia, headache). Cutaneous senses are usually not impaired. Sudden, transient amblyopia may occur, as well as epileptic fits.

Psychic symptoms, often of a psychotic nature, are common and as a result a number of these patients have been heavily sedated as instances of acute delirium or hysteria, or have been transferred to mental institutions. Mental confusion may be associated with abdominal colic and a comatose state may develop.

The course of the disease is extraordinarily variable. Spontaneous remissions from the acute attack occur commonly and may be dramatic in their extent. It is not unusual to find in one parent or in several siblings of a patient with porphyria that porphobilinogen is present in the urine even though active symptoms of the disease have never developed. This is known as *latent porphyria*. However, once symptoms have developed, they are likely to recur and eventually lead to death. The most common age of death is between 20 and 45 years.[287] In cases with severe abdominal complaints the mortality has been as high as 50 per cent and, when nervous symptoms have supervened, the incidence of death has been even higher.

The mechanism whereby the latent state is converted to active disease is unknown. It is clear, however, that certain conditions may precipitate attacks. These include pregnancy, the early puerperium, infections and, *particularly*, barbiturates.[280a] Other drugs which seem to have precipitated attacks include sulfonmethane (Sulfonal®), sulfonethylmethane (Trional), alcohol, allylisopropylacetylcarbamide (Sedormid), chloroquine,[277c] progesterone[281b] and lead.[279b]

The characteristic abnormality is the excretion of *porphobilinogen*,[287] a colorless substance which is derived from δ-aminolevulinic acid (p. 153). The freshly voided urine is frequently normal in color but, on standing, it turns to a Burgundy wine color or even black. Sunlight is the most effective agent in causing the urine to change in color but oxidizing agents such as permanganate or Lugol's solution, or the addition of a weak acid and heating will do the same. When porphobilinogen is heated in an acid medium, non-enzymic formation of uroporphyrin, a red compound, takes place. In addition, a number of other pigments are formed from the porphobilinogen but their nature has been disputed.[282, 288a] They include type I and type III porphyrins and make up what has come to be called the Waldenström porphyrin complex. In the feces coproporphyrins types I and III have both been found and uroporphyrin has also been identified.

A simple test for porphobilinogen consists in mixing 5 ml. of Ehrlich's reagent (p. 178) with 5 ml. urine and then adding 10 ml. saturated aqueous solution of chemically pure sodium acetate.[289] If any pinkish or reddish color appears, 3 to 5 ml. of chloroform are added and the mixture is shaken vigorously in a stoppered tube. If porphobilinogen is present it will remain in the aqueous (upper) fraction. Urobilinogen, which also forms a red aldehyde compound with Ehrlich's reagent, is soluble in chloroform and, if also present in the urine, will remain in the lower layer.

Quantitative urine measurements have shown that all patients with latent or manifest acute intermittent porphyria excrete pathologically increased amounts of porphobilinogen in the urine.[281] In two-thirds of those examined the excretion of δ-aminolevulinic acid was also found to be increased. These compounds were found in the urine in abnormal amounts even in the apparently healthy carriers of the disease.

Examination of the tissues of patients who have died of acute intermittent porphyria, in contrast to porphyria erythropoietica, has shown that the porphyrin content of the bone marrow is normal. The liver, on the other hand, exhibits increased quantities of porphyrin and porphyrin precursors. The symptoms of this disorder are thought to be the consequence of a disturbance in pyrrole metabolism in the nervous system.[280a] Patchy demyelination has been demonstrated. Abdominal pain may be the result of disturbed motility of the bowel arising from the irregular alterations in its motor innervation.[280]

Treatment consists first in the avoidance of barbiturates and other drugs which may precipitate or aggravate the attacks, chlorpromazine being used, is needed, instead. Opiates may be used, although they are best avoided in a disorder of this kind. Ganglionic blocking agents are sometimes helpful if pain is severe. Fluids should be forced parenterally, if necessary, since oliguria and azotemia may ensue. Electrolyte balance must be watched. Severe constipation should be treated with enemas. Steroid therapy[280a] and chelating agents such as BAL[281d] have been claimed to be of value but their evaluation is difficult in a disease of intermittent character.

Porphyria cutanea tarda has often been confused with erythropoietic or congenital porphyria because photosensitivity and sensitivity to trauma are present, as well as brownish or violaceous skin pigmentation. The original concept of this disorder as a single entity appearing late in life has been revised. Several types can be distinguished.[287]

(1) *Porphyria cutanea tarda hereditaria*[287] refers to cases in which blisters occur in the skin comparatively early in life, that

is between the ages of 15 to 30 years. The characteristic biochemical feature of this disease is the presence of both copro- and protoporphyrins in large quantities in the feces at all times in the course of the disease. In addition, uroporphyrin may sometimes be identified in the urine. A simple screening test may be carried out by obtaining a small specimen of stool. The specimen is extracted with about 2 ml. of solvent containing equal parts of glacial acetic acid, amyl alcohol and ether. The supernatant fluid is then decanted and viewed in Wood's light. Negative specimens show a green or gray fluorescence. A positive specimen is brilliant pink. A false positive result may be given by excess chlorophyll.

During exacerbations of the disease the feces contain less porphyrin whereas the urinary output increases.[282] Probably inherited as a dominant trait,[281a] the condition may be completely symptomless. Unlike other forms of porphyria cutanea tarda, porphobilinogen may appear in the urine but this occurs only when porphyrin metabolism is severely disturbed.[287] Then, as in acute porphyria, colic and paralysis have been noted. It has been suggested that the disease remains asymptomatic as long as the liver is capable of excreting the porphyrins in the bile. When this is impaired, bilirubinemia, porphyrinemia, porphyrinuria and cutaneous lesions appear and thus the latent phase changes to the cutaneous stage. When porphyrin metabolism is greatly disturbed, δ-aminolevulinic acid and porphobilinogen appear in the urine and all of the manifestations of acute intermittent porphyria develop.

Porphyria variegata[279] is the name proposed for a form of porphyria studied in Caucasians in South Africa which is characterized both by acute attacks like those in acute intermittent porphyria and by cutaneous lesions. The latter are

commoner
acute epis
women.
Mendelia
is excrete
attacks b
the patie
porphyri
even du
cases w
Thus th
resembl
phyria
The te
posed
signs
porphyria cu

(2) *Porphyria cutanea tarda symptomatica* is seen in chronic alcoholics, is more common in males and signs of disturbed liver function are usually present. The usual age of onset is in the fourth and fifth decades. The photosensitivity is not as marked as in porphyria congenita. The lesions are found on exposed skin areas and mechanical factors are of great importance in the production of blisters, which may later ulcerate and lead to scar formation. Intense pigmentation is characteristic, as is also the occurrence of hypertrichosis on the face. There are no abdominal or neurological manifestations as in acute porphyria and porphobilinogen is not found in the urine. In the liver, preformed porphyrin rather than porphobilinogen has been found.[283] The urine is red and contains uroporphyrins (I, III) and coproporphyrin, and the feces contain uro-, copro- and, sometimes predominantly, protoporphyrin.[277]

Porphyria cutanea tarda has also been described in the *Bantu of South Africa*[276b] and in many ways resembles the symptomatic form described above. Hepatic disease, developing in livers originally damaged by infantile malnutrition, as well as by the toxic concoctions and home-brewed fermented drinks which these people habitually consume, may serve as precipitating factors. No conclusive evidence of a hereditary factor has been found.

In association with the presence of *liver cell adenoma* several cases of symptomatic porphyria cutanea tarda have been reported.[285a] In these cases considerable amounts of uroporphyrin and smaller amounts of protoporphyrin and coproporphyrin were found in the urine. These disappeared when the tumor was removed and the skin became normal. The cytoplasm of the tumor cells contained large quantities of porphyrins, as did the bile ducts. A similar case of ovarian teratoma has been reported.[287]

An outbreak of cutaneous porphyria in Turkey has been attributed to the ingestion of the fungicide, hexachlorobenzene.

The excretion of porphyrin only when the patient was recumbent has been described.[285]

Some of the distinguishing features of the porphyrias are presented in Table 3–8.

As yet the relationship of the various forms of porphyria to one another and the pathogenesis of their intriguing array of manifestations are obscure. The photosensitivity in cases of congenital or later forms of porphyria appears to be due to the presence of porphyrins in the skin.[277b,281c] Possibly experimental studies will furnish some answers. Porphyria is not confined to the human species. Congenital porphyria has been observed in cattle[282] and has been recognized under the misleading term "ochronosis" in slaughter-house animals.[12] Uroporphyrin I has been isolated from the bones of swine with porphyria[12] and from the urine of the ground or fox squirrel, *Sciurus niger*. The latter normally has brownish bones and teeth which exhibit a lively fluorescence in ultra-violet light.[285c] The administration to rats, rabbits or chickens of lead, phenylhydrazine or the dye, rose bengal, or excessive exposure to sunlight has produced a condition resembling in many respects the porphyria erythropoietica of man. A temporary condition similar to porphyria hepatica of the acute intermittent type has been produced in animals and in chicken embryos by the administration of allisopropylacetylcarbamide ("Sedormid").[284]

DISORDERS USUALLY ACCOMPANIED BY CYANOSIS

Van den Bergh in 1905 first recognized abnormal pigments in the blood when he introduced spectroscopy in clinical work. Most of the disorders which will be discussed below are related to the heme moiety of hemoglobin. This is not invariably true, however, since it is now known that one variety of hereditary methemoglobinemia is due to the inheritance of a defect in the globin portion of the hemoglobin molecule. Again, sulfhemoglobinemia does not represent a defect in heme. However, these disorders possess two features in common; namely all can be recognized by spectroscopy and cyanosis is a common finding.

The cyanosis occurring in cardiac or pulmonary disease is due to the presence of increased amounts of reduced hemoglobin. It is often less striking than that caused by the presence of abnormal pigments but is more frequently accompanied by symptoms such as dyspnea. Patients with cyanosis due to methemoglobinemia or sulfhemoglobinemia are more startling to see than they are themselves disturbed by the presence of the abnormal pigments in the blood. The relative capacity of each of these pigments to produce cyanosis can be appreciated from the fact that about 5 Gm. of reduced hemoglobin per 100 ml. of blood is required to produce recognizable cyanosis, whereas 1.5 Gm. of methemoglobin and less than 0.5 Gm. of sulfhemoglobin have comparable effects.

The cyanosis of carbon monoxide

poisoning is unique in two respects. Since carboxyhemoglobin is bright red in color, the poisoned subject is found to have a "cherry-red" cyanosis. However, after the subject's removal from the polluted atmosphere, if he is still breathing, both the characteristic cyanosis and the concentration of the carboxyhemoglobin in the blood will disappear within a few hours since carboxyhemoglobin is a readily dissociable compound. Depending on the cause, methemoglobinemia and sulfhemoglobinemia produce cyanosis of much longer duration.

Other than the effects on the hemoglobin, substances which cause methemoglobinemia and sulfhemoglobinemia may also produce polycythemia or anemia. Whereas no significant alterations of this type are observed in carbon monoxide poisoning, where the effects are lethal or recovery takes place in a short time, in the case of methemoglobinemia and sulfhemoglobinemia the chronic character of the disorder permits compensatory polycythemia to take place. Furthermore, some of the agents producing the changes in the hemoglobin cause blood destruction as well, with the result that the manifestations of hemolytic anemia will be found.

The search for abnormal pigments in the red cell requires careful collection of the blood, as described elsewhere (p. 399), and separation of cells and plasma. If the plasma is clear, hemolysis and abnormal plasma pigments can be ruled out. The whole blood can then be shaken in air for 15 minutes. Normally, the blood will become bright red as all the reduced hemoglobin is converted to oxyhemoglobin. If it remains dark, abnormal intracellular pigments must be present. When carboxyhemoglobin is the abnormal pigment, the color of the blood is cherry-red. Methemoglobin produces a chocolate-brown appearance and sulfhemoglobin a mauve-lavender color. These changes can be recognized,

however, only when the concentration of the pigment is very great so that it is not masked by the color of oxyhemoglobin. Lesser concentrations, and quantitative determinations, require spectroscopic examination, which is taken up in a later chapter (p. 399). In addition to these examinations, appropriate studies should be made to demonstrate or rule out the presence of polycythemia, anemia, Heinz bodies (p. 624), hemoglobinuria and increased urobilinogen excretion.

Carboxyhemoglobin (HbCO)[270] is produced by the combination of hemoglobin and carbon monoxide, a gas resulting from incomplete combustion of organic matter and found, for example, in coal gas and water gas, and in the exhaust from automobiles.[260] Although carboxyhemoglobin is a dissociable compound, the affinity of carbon monoxide for human hemoglobin is 210 times that of oxygen with the result that as little as 0.1 per cent concentration of carbon monoxide in the inspired air is sufficient to produce equal amounts of carboxy- and oxyhemoglobin. Hemoglobin in the form of carboxyhemoglobin is unavailable for the carriage of oxygen. The toxic reactions following the inhalation of carbon monoxide are solely the result of tissue anoxia but this may cause tissue changes such as edema, small hemorrhages and perivascular infiltration with focal necrosis. Consequently, although the administration of oxygen relieves the immediate ill effects of carbon monoxide inhalation, this gas can also produce permanent damage, especially to the central nervous system and the heart.[260]

Methemoglobin (HbFe^{+++}OH)[267] is a derivative of hemoglobin in which the ferrous porphyrin complex is converted to the ferric form. It does not combine with oxygen and is, therefore, of no value in respiration. It can be reduced, however, to hemoglobin through the action of reducing agents such as those normally found in the blood (ascorbic

13

acid, glutathione) or by the administration of methylene blue. It was pointed out earlier (p. 127) that, in the intact red corpuscle, methemoglobin is formed continuously and is also promptly reduced to the functional ferrous form. It has been stated that the methemoglobin concentration of normal blood is 1.7 per cent or less.[237]

Various chemical compounds used in industry or as therapeutic agents can cause methemoglobinemia and a congenital or familial form of methemoglobinemia occurs as well. The chemical compounds which convert hemoglobin to methemoglobin preferentially oxidize hemoglobin and, in sufficient amounts, overcome the normal reducing mechanisms. The *toxic agents* include anilin, phenacetin, acetanilid (p. 609) sulfonamides (sulfanilamide, sulfapyridine, sulfathiazole), nitrobenzene, various nitrites (sodium, amyl, ethyl), nitroglycerin, bismuth subnitrate and ammonium nitrate.[267] Exposure to these agents occurs not only when they are used therapeutically (bismuth subnitrate in the treatment of diarrhea, ammonium nitrate used as a diuretic or amyl nitrite or nitroglycerin) but also in arc welders (inhalation of nitrous gases), or through contact with dyed blankets, laundry marks on diapers and freshly dyed shoes.

Food high in nitrates,[272b] or nitrates ingested for therapeutic purposes, may be converted to nitrites by intestinal bacteria and cases have been reported in *infants drinking well water* containing high concentrations of nitrates.[269] Cases of methemoglobinemia have also been described in children swallowing red wax crayons containing *p*-nitroaniline. The susceptibility of infants to methemoglobinemia has been attributed to transient deficiency of the methemoglobin reductase (p. 127) responsible for the generation of DPNH in the erythrocyte.[274a]

The rapidity of methemoglobin production depends on the metabolism of the offending chemical compound within the body and on its excretion. Thus, the effect of nitrite introduced intravenously is expended within an hour while nitrobenzene does not produce its maximum effect for 12 to 15 hours. *Symptoms* vary in intensity but are often mild. In addition to the blue cyanosis that is produced, headaches, vertigo, mental confusion and a desire to sleep may develop, Heinz bodies may be formed in the red corpuscles and, as already mentioned, hemolytic anemia may occur as well (p. 609).

The signs of toxicity in both carbon monoxide poisoning and in conditions leading to the production of methemoglobinemia are much greater than those produced by the same amount of anemia. Consequently, some further action besides the lowering of the oxygen carrying power of the blood has been suspected. It has been observed that when part of the hemoglobin of the blood is combined with CO, the oxygen dissociation curve of the remaining hemoglobin is shifted, with the result that the unloading of oxygen from the blood to the tissues is hindered. In cases of methemoglobinemia it has been assumed that the toxic symptoms not accounted for by the lowered amount of available oxyhemoglobin, are due to the effect of the methemoglobin-producing agent on the tissues. It has been found, however, that a definite and reversible shift of the dissociation curve occurs also, as in the presence of carboxyhemoglobin.[263] This means that in methemoglobinemia the tissues are liable to anoxemia, not only from loss of the oxygen capacity of the blood, but also from increasing difficulty in unloading from the blood such oxygen as is available. The mechanism of this effect has been attributed to the formation of compounds intermediate between reduced hemoglobin, which is wholly ferrous, and methemoglobin, which is wholly ferric, the conversion of one or more of the four ferrous atoms in the hemoglobin molecule to ferric leading to an increased affinity of the remaining ferrous atoms for oxygen.

No *therapy* other than prohibition of the offending chemical agent is needed if the methemoglobinemia is sufficiently mild, since reduction of the methemoglobin will occur rapidly as the result of the intact normal reconversion mechanism. If symptoms are sufficiently pronounced, methylene blue, 1 mg. per Kg. body weight in a 1 per cent solution, slowly given intravenously over a period of five minutes, is the agent of choice. In infants twice this dose is used. In either age group, if cyanosis has not disappeared within an hour, a second dose of 2 mg. per Kg. body weight should be given. Dosages should not exceed 7 mg. per Kg. since toxic effects such as dyspnea, precordial pain, restlessness and apprehension, a sense of oppression, fibrillar tremors and even persisting cyanosis and hemolytic anemia[268a] may develop. Methylene blue may also be given orally in doses of 3 to 5 mg. per Kg. Ascorbic acid has been given in doses of 100 to 500 mg. per day by mouth[259] but methylene blue is more useful since it brings about reversion of methemoglobin by activating the hexose monophosphate shunt (p. 127) rather than by non-enzymatic reduction, a process which is slower than the normal cell conversion system.

Several different types of *methemoglobinemia* have now been found to be **congenital and hereditary** in nature. Under the title of *hereditary methemoglobinemic cyanosis* a condition has been described in Greece[261] and elsewhere[258,264,265,267, 272a] which is transmitted as a non-sex-linked Mendelian dominant.[261] Manifest often at birth, the disorder is characterized by cyanosis, which differs in degree with each patient and may be slight, medium or marked. The hue is violet, sometimes even brownish and is usually dichromatic between blue and red or violet blue and brown. It is generalized over the whole body but is particularly noticeable in the lips, the mucous membranes of the mouth, the tongue, the palate and the nose, in the cheek bones and ears, and at the extremities of the fingers and toes, especially under the nails. There is no associated clubbing of the fingers.

In the light forms there are no symptoms other than the cyanosis but in those of greater severity symptoms attributable to anoxemia may be present. These include headaches, dizziness, dyspnea, tachycardia and sometimes even physical weakness. Quantitative measurements of methemoglobin have given values from 10 to 52.5 per cent. However, even strenuous exercise has been possible with levels as high as 40 per cent.[267]

The nature of the disorder in the above cases has not been clarified and it may well be that, among the more than 100 reported cases, more than one variety of hereditary methemoglobinemia will be found to have been included. It is now known that there are at least two distinct forms of hereditary methemoglobinemia. In one, discovered to be prevalent in Alaskan Eskimos and Indians,[275] the methemoglobinemia was associated with absence of *diphosphopyridine nucleotide diaphorase* activity. This enzyme may be the "methemoglobin reductase" of Kiese (p. 127). The condition is transmitted as an autosomal recessive trait. The red cells of parents of affected children were found to have about half the normal level of erythrocyte diaphorase and no methemoglobin was detected in their red cells. In the homozygotes 5 to 60 per cent of the hemoglobin was present as methemoglobin. Since the disease has been described only in infants, children and adolescents, it is possible that the condition is associated with early mortality or that the methemoglobinemia disappears with age. A curious observation is the fact that the amount of methemoglobinemia both in the cases reported from Greece and in those from Alaska was variable. It has been postulated that these variations are related to plasma ascorbic acid levels. In the Greek patients the plasma ascorbic acid was low despite adequate diets. In Alaska it was noted that the dietary intake of ascorbic acid was low.

The second type of hereditary methemoglobinemia is due to the inheritance of an abnormal hemoglobin, *hemoglobin M*. First recognized in a German family by Hörlein and Weber[268b] the defect was shown to be present in the globin portion of the molecule. Here methemoglobinemia is due to abnormal sensitivity of Hb M to oxidation rather than because of a slow rate of methemoglobin reduction. The abnormal hemoglobin crystallizes in the ferric form.[274b] On the basis of differences in absorption spectra, three distinct varieties of Hb M were identified, named respectively M_B (Boston),[268] M_M (Milwaukee)[273] and M_S (Saskatoon).[268] Hb M was found to comprise approximately 30 per cent of the total hemoglobin, the remainder being Hb A. Cyanosis is the only clinical manifestation and the appearance of the cyanosis may be delayed in infancy pending the disappearance of fetal hemoglobin.[273] A dominant hereditary pattern has been observed. Further investigation has revealed those varieties of Hb M, a second from Milwaukee, one from Germany (M_L)[260a] and M_{Japan}. In the last the abnormality is present in tryptic peptide number 9 of the α chain.[335a] In Hb M_{Boston} the defect is present in the seventh tryptic peptide of the same chain, histidine being replaced by tyrosine, whereas in Hb M_{Emory} a similar alteration has been found in tryptic peptide 7 of the β chain.[334b] In Hb $M_{Milwaukee\ 1}$ valine is replaced by glutamic acid in tryptic peptide 9 of the β chain.[334b]

Sulfhemoglobin[271] is a compound formed by the reaction of hemoglobin with soluble inorganic sulfides and hydrogen peroxide. It is thought that the formation of sulfhemoglobin involves the introduction of one atom of relatively labile sulfur into the hemoglobin molecule and also a change in the mode of linkage of globin to the heme. Unlike carboxy- and methemoglobin, sulfhemoglobin cannot be converted into hemoglobin without splitting the molecule into its constituent groups. Consequently treatment consists only in avoidance of the offending agent. Sulfhemoglobinemia has been observed to be a common result of chronic acetanilid use,[274] often in the form of Bromo-seltzer, but phenacetin (A.P.C., Empirin, Anacin, Stanback) is also a common offender. Anemia and hepatosplenomegaly, both of unknown cause, have been observed in a number of cases. A case of congenital sulfhemoglobinemia has been reported.[272]

Since the reaction between hemoglobin and sulfide to produce sulfhemoglobinemia is a slow one and since hydrogen sulfide is rapidly excreted, one would not expect sulfhemoglobin to be formed unless sulfide were continuously available. Furthermore, it has been noted that sulfhemoglobinemia is relatively uncommon despite the widespread use of drugs such as phenacetin. Some factor peculiar to the individual other than drugs appears to be required for the development of this disorder. For a long time constipation was assumed to provide the required continuous supply of hydrogen sulfide but there has been no convincing evidence for this claim. In several cases of sulfhemoglobinemia the erythrocyte GSH concentration was found to be increased; it was suggested that the erythrocyte itself rather than the bowel may be the source of hydrogen sulfide.[270a]

"Enterogenous cyanosis" refers to methemoglobinemia and sulfhemoglobinemia of unknown origin but it is attributed to absorption of nitrites and sulfides from the intestine, perhaps as the result of disturbed bowel function.[267] The pa-

tients usually have abdominal pain with diarrhea or constipation. There are attacks of slate-blue cyanosis accompanied by headache, often shortness of breath, dizziness, collapse and syncope. Anemia is frequently present and indicanuria is found. Enterogenous methemoglobinemia clears in a few hours but enterogenous sulfhemoglobinemia disappears only gradually in the course of three to four months.

BIBLIOGRAPHY

Chemical Composition and Metabolism of the Red Corpuscle

1. ADAMS, E., McFADDEN, M. and SMITH, E. L.: Peptidases of Erythrocytes, J. Biol. Chem., *198*, 663 and 671, 1952; *Ibid.*, *199*, 845, 1952.

1a. ALBRITTON, E. C., Ed.: Standard Values in Blood, Committee on the Handbook of Biological Data, National Res. Council, A. F. Tech. Rpt., 6039, Wright Air Development Center, Dayton, Ohio, 1952.

2. ALTMAN, K. I.: Some Enzymologic Aspects of the Human Erythrocyte, Am. J. Med., *27*, 936, 1959.

2a. ALTMAN, K. I. and SALOMON, K.: Hemin Synthesis in Spleen Homogenates, Science, *3*, 117, 1950; J. Biol. Chem., *196*, 463, 1952.

3. AXELROD, J., REICHENTHAL, J. and BRODIE, B. B.: The Direct Determination of Phosphatidyl Ethanolamine and Phosphatidyl Serine in Plasma and Red Blood Cells, J. Biol. Chem., *204*, 903, 1953.

4. BARTLETT, G. R. and MARLOW, A. A.: Enzyme Systems in the Red Blood Cell, Bull. Scripps Metabolic Clin., *2*, 1, 1951; J. Appl. Physiol., *6*, 51, 1953; J. Lab. & Clin. Med., *42*, 178 and 188, 1953; Ann. New York Acad. Sc., *75*, 110, 1958; J. Clin. Invest., *39*, 56, 1960.

5. BEACH, E. F., ERICKSON, B. N., BERNSTEIN, S. S., WILLIAMS, H. H. and MACY, I. G.: The Amino Acid Composition of Erythrocyte Posthemolytic Residue of Five Mammalian Species, J. Biol. Chem., *128*, 339, 1939.

5a. BEHRENDT, H.: *Chemistry of Erythrocytes*, Springfield, Ill., C. C Thomas, 1957, 227 pp.

6. BERNSTEIN, R. E.: Alterations in Metabolic Energetics and Cation Transport during Aging of Red Cells, J. Clin. Invest., *38*, 1572, 1959.

6a. BEUTLER, E. and BLAISDELL, R. K.: Iron Enzymes in Iron Deficiency, J. Clin. Invest., *37*, 833, 1958.

7. BOGORAD, L.: The Enzymatic Synthesis of Porphyrins from Porphobilinogen, J. Biol. Chem., *233*, 501, 510 and 516, 1958.

8. BUSH, J. A., MAHONEY, J. P., GUBLER, C. J., CARTWRIGHT, G. E. and WINTROBE, M. M.: Studies on Copper Metabolism. XXI. The Transfer of Radiocopper between Erythrocytes and Plasma, J. Lab. & Clin. Med., *47*, 898, 1956.

9. CALVIN, M., EVANS, R., BEHRENDT, V. and CALVIN, G.: Rh Antigen and Hapten-Antigen and Its Isolation from Erythrocyte Stroma, Proc. Soc. Exper. Biol. & Med., *61*, 416, 1946; J. Immunol., *65*, 383, 1950; J. Am. Chem. Soc., *72*, 5587, 1950.

10. CARTWRIGHT, G. E., HUGULEY, C. M., JR., ASHENBRUCKER, H., FAY, J. and WINTROBE, M. M.: Studies on Free Erythrocyte Protoporphyrin, Plasma Iron and Plasma Copper in Normal and Anemic Subjects, Blood, *3*, 501, 1948.

11. DAJANI, R. M. and ORTEN, J. M.: A Study of the Citric Acid Cycle in Erythrocytes, J. Biol. Chem., *231*, 913, 1958.

11a. DENSTEDT, O. F.: The Enzymology of the Erythrocyte, *in Blood Cells and Plasma Proteins*, James L. Tullis, Ed., New York, Academic Press, Inc., 1953, pp. 223–253.

12. DOBRINER, K. and RHOADS, C. P.: The Porphyrins in Health and Disease, Physiol. Rev., *20*, 416, 1940.

13. ERICKSON, B. N., WILLIAMS, H. H., BERNSTEIN, S. S., AVRIN, I., JONES, R. L. and MACY, I. G.: The Lipid Distribution of Posthemolytic Residue or Stroma of Erythrocytes, J. Biol. Chem., *122*, 515, 1938.

14. GABRIO, B. W. and FINCH, C. A.: Erythrocyte Preservation, J. Clin. Investigation, *33*, 242, 247, 252 and 932, 1954; J. Biol. Chem., *215*, 357, 1955; Blood, *11*, 103, 1956; J. Clin. Invest., *36*, 429, 1957; *ibid.*, *37*, 1485, 1958.

15. GIBSON, K. D., NEUBERGER, A. and SCOTT, J. J.: The Purification and Properties of δ-Aminolaevulic Acid Dehydrase, Biochem. J., *61*, 618, 1955; *ibid.*, *70*, 4 and 71, 1958.

15a. GLYNN, I. M.: Sodium and Potassium Movements in Human Red Cells, J. Physiol., *134*, 278, 1956.

16. GOLDBERG, A., ASHENBRUCKER, HELEN, CARTWRIGHT, G. E. and WINTROBE, M. M.: Studies on the Biosynthesis of Heme

In Vitro by Avian Erythrocytes, Blood, *11*, 821, 1956; Brit. J. Haemat., *5*, 150, 1959; Lancet, *2*, 271, 1959.

16a.GOLDSTEIN, F. and RIEDERS, F.: Conversion of Thiocyanate to Cyanide by an Erythrocytic Enzyme, Am. J. Physiol., *173*, 287, 1953.

17. GRANICK, S.: The Chemistry and Functioning of the Mammalian Erythrocyte, Blood, *4*, 404, 1949 (Bibliography); *see also*, The Harvey Lectures, 1948–49, Series 44, p. 220, Springfield, Ill., Charles C Thomas; Proc. Soc. Exper. Biol. & Med., *88*, 270, 1955.

17a.GRANICK, S. *et al.*: The Occurrence and Determination of δ-Aminolevulinic Acid and Porphobilinogen in Urine, J. Biol. Chem., *219*, 435, 1956; *ibid.*, *232*, 1101, 1119 and 1141, 1958.

17c.GROSSMAN, L. and KAPLAN, N. O.: Nicotinamide Riboside Phosphorylase from Human Erythrocytes, J. Biol. Chem., *231*, 717 and 727, 1958.

18. HUENNEKENS, F. M., CAFFREY, RUTH WADE, BASFORD, R. E. and GABRIO, BEVERLY W.: Erythrocyte Metabolism, J. Biol. Chem., *227*, 261, 1957; Ann. New York Acad. Sc., *75*, 167, 1958.

18a.JAFFÉ, E. R.: The Reduction of Methemoglobin in Human Erythrocytes Incubated with Purine Nucleosides, J. Clin. Invest., *38*, 1555, 1959.

19. JOCELYN, P. C.: The Distribution of Ergothioneine in Blood as Determined by a New Method of Estimation, Biochem. J., *70*, 656, 1958.

19a.JONES, N. C. H. and ROBINSON, MARGARET A.: Estimation of Nucleotide Content of Red Cells, J. Clin. Path., *10*, 191, 1957.

19b.KAGAWA, Y., MINAKAMI, S. and YONEYAMA, Y.: Heme Synthesis in the Soluble Preparation from Avian Erythrocytes, J. Biochem., *46*, 771, 1959.

19c.KASBEKAR, D. K. and SREENIVASAN, A.: Biosynthesis of Glutathione by Rat Erythrocytes, Biochem. J., *72*, 389, 1959.

20. KEILIN, JOAN: Nature of the Haem-Binding Groups in Native and Denatured Haemoglobin and Myoglobin, Nature, *187*, 365, 1960.

20a.KRUEGER, R. C., MELNICK, I. and KLEIN, J. R.: Formation of Heme by Broken-Cell Preparations of Duck Erythrocytes, Arch. Biochem. & Biophys., *64*, 302, 1956,

20b.LASCELLES, J.: Synthesis of Porphyrins by Cell Suspensions of *Tetrahymena vorax:* Effect of Members of the Vitamin B Group, Biochem. J., *66*, 65, 1957.

20c.LEFEVRE, P. G. and MARSHALL, J. K.: Conformational Specificity in a Biological Sugar Transport System, Am. J. Physiol., *194*, 333, 1958; J. Biol. Chem., *234*, 3022, 1959.

20d.LÖHR, G. W. *et al.*: Zur Biochemie der Alterung menschlicher Erythrocyten, Klin. Wchnschr., *21*, 1008, 1958.

21. LONDON, I. M. and SCHWARZ, H.: Erythrocyte Metabolism. The Metabolic Behavior of the Cholesterol of Human Erythrocytes, J. Clin. Invest., *32*, 1248, 1953; Bull. New York Acad. Med., *36*, 79, 1960.

22. MARKS, P. A., JOHNSON, ANNE B., HIRSCHBERG, E. and BANKS, JULIA: Studies on the Mechanism of Aging of Human Red Blood Cells, Ann. New York Acad. Sc., *75*, 95, 1958.

23. MILLS, G. C.: Hemoglobin Catabolism, J. Biol. Chem., *229*, 189, 1957; *ibid.*, *232*, 589, 1958; *ibid.*, *234*, 502, 1959.

24. MORRISON, W. L. and NEURATH, H.: Proteolytic Enzymes of the Formed Elements of Human Blood, J. Biol. Chem., *200*, 39, 1953.

24a.MUNN, J. I.: Studies of Lipids in Human Red Cells, Brit. J. Haemat., *4*, 344, 1958.

25. NEVE, R. A., LABBE, R. F. and ALDRICH, R. A.: Reduced Uroporphyrin III in the Biosynthesis of Heme, J. Am. Chem. Soc., *78*, 691, 1956.

25a.NIZET, A.: Recherches sur les relations entre les biosynthèses de l'hème et de la globine, Bull. Soc. chim. biol., *39*, 265, 1957.

25b.O'HOGAN, J. E.: The Haem-Globin Linkage, Biochem. J., *74*, 417, 1960.

26. PERUTZ, M. F., ROSSMANN, M. G., CULLIS, ANN F., MUIRHEAD, H., WILL, G. and NORTH, A. C. T.: Structure of Haemoglobin, Nature, *185*, 416, 1960.

26a.PHILLIPS, G. B. and ROOME, N. S.: Phospholipids of Human Red Blood Cells, Proc. Soc. Exper. Biol. & Med., *100*, 489, 1959.

27. PRANKERD, T. A. J.: The Metabolism of the Human Erythrocyte: A Review, Brit. J. Haemat., *1*, 131, 1955; Internat. Rev. Cytol., *5*, 279, 1956.

27a.PRANKERD, T. A. J.: The Ageing of Red Cells, J. Physiol., *143*, 325, 1958.

28. PRANKERD, T. A. J. and ALTMAN, K. I.: A Study of the Metabolism of Phosphorus in Mammalian Red Cells, Biochem. J., *58*, 622, 1954.

29. PRANKERD, T. A. J., ALTMAN, K. I. and ANDERSON, J. R.: Electrophoresis of Human Red-cell Stroma, Nature, *174*, 1146, 1954.

29a. REED, C. F., SWISHER, S. N., MARINETTI, G. V. and EDEN, EVA G.: Studies of the Lipids of the Erythrocyte, J. Lab. & Clin. Med., *56*, 281, 1960.

30. REYNOLDS, J., FOLLETTE, J. H. and VALENTINE, W. N.: The Arginase Activity of Erythrocytes and Leukocytes with Particular Reference to Pernicious Anemia and Thalassemia Major, J. Lab. & Clin. Med., *50*, 78, 1957.

31. SABINE, J. C.: Erythrocyte Cholinesterase Titers in Hematologic Disease States, Am. J. Med., *27*, 81, 1959.

31a. SCHULMAN, M. P. and RICHERT, D. A.: Heme Synthesis in Vitamin B₆ and Pantothenic Acid Deficiencies, J. Biol. Chem., *226*, 181, 1957; Am. J. Clin. Nutrition, *7*, 416, 1959.

32. SCHROEDER, W. A.: The Chemical Structure of the Normal Human Hemoglobins, *in Progress in the Chemistry of Organic Natural Products*, L. Zechmeister, Ed., Vienna, Springer-Verlag, 1959, p. 322.

33. SCHWARTZ, H. C., CARTWRIGHT, G. E., SMITH, E. L. and WINTROBE, M. M.: Studies on the Biosynthesis of Heme from Iron and Protoporphyrin, Blood, *14*, 486, 1959; Biochim. et biophys. acta, *36*, 567, 1959, J. Clin. Invest., *40*, 188, 1961.

33a. SCOTT, E. M. and GRIFFITH, ISABELLE V.: The Enzymic Defect of Hereditary Methemoglobinemia: Diaphorase, Biochim. et biophys. acta, *34*, 584, 1959.

33b. SEGGEL, K. A.: Uber das Vorkommen fluoreszierender Erythrozyten, Fol. hæmat., *52*, 250, 1934; Ergebn. d. inn. Med. u. Kinderh., *58*, 582, 1940.

34. SHEMIN, D., LONDON, I. M. and RITTENBERG, D.: The In Vitro Synthesis of Heme from Glycine by the Nucleated Red Blood Cell, J. Biol. Chem., *173*, 799, 1948; *ibid.*, *183*, 749 and 757, *184*, 745 and 755, 1950; *ibid.*, *185*, 103, 1950; *ibid.*, *192*, 315 1951; *ibid.*, *198*, 827, 1952; J. Am. Chem. Soc., *75*, 4873, 1953; *ibid.*, *76*, 1204, 1954.

35. SHEMIN, D., RUSSELL, CHARLOTTE, S. and ABRAMSKY, TESSA: The Succinate-Glycine Cycle, J. Biol. Chem., *215*, 603 and 613, 1955; *ibid.*, *233*, 1214, 1958; Fed. Proc., *18*, 259, 1959.

35a. SOLOMON, A. K.: Red Cell Membrane Structure and Ion Transport, J. Gen. Physiol., *43* (Suppl. Part 2 of vol. 43), 1, 1960.

36. TSUBOI, K. K. and HUDSON, P. B.: Enzymes of the Human Erythrocyte, J. Biol. Chem., *224*, 879 and 889, 1957.

37. TURNER, J. C.: Red Cell Lipids, A.M.A. Arch. Int. Med., *101*, 310, 1958.

38. VALLEE, B. L. and ALTSCHULE, M. D.: Zinc in the Mammalian Organism, with Particular Reference to Carbonic Anhydrase, Physiol. Rev., *29*, 370, 1949.

39. VESELL, E. S. and BEARN, A. G.: Observations on the Heterogeneity of Malic and Lactic Dehydrogenase in Human Serum and Red Blood Cells, J. Clin. Invest., *37*, 672, 1958.

39a. WATSON, C. J.: The Erythrocyte Coproporphyrin and Its Variations in Respect to Protoporphyrin and Reticulocytes in Certain of the Anemias, Arch. Int. Med., *86*, 797, 1950.

39b. WHITTAM, R.: Potassium Movements and ATP in Human Red Cells, J. Physiol., *140*, 479, 1958.

39c. WIDDAS, W. F.: Facilitated Transfer of Hexoses across the Human Erythrocyte Membrane, J. Physiol., *125*, 163, 1954; J. Physiol., *141*, 219, 1958.

40. WITTENBERG, J. B.: Formation of the Porphyrin Ring, Nature, *184*, 876, 1959.

41. WITTENBERG, J. and SHEMIN, D.: The Utilization of Glycine for the Biosynthesis of Both Types of Pyrroles in Protoporphyrin, Biol. Chem., *178*, 47, 1949.

43. WYMAN, J., JR.: Heme Proteins *in Advances in Protein Chemistry*. IV, p. 410, 1948, Academic Press, N. Y.

Amino Acids and Protein

44. CARTWRIGHT, G. E.: Dietary Factors Concerned in Erythropoiesis, Blood, *2*, 111 and 256, 1947 (Bibliography).

45. CARTWRIGHT, G. E., WINTROBE, M. M., BUSCHKE, W. H., FOLLIS, R. H., JR., SUKSTA, A. and HUMPHREYS, S.: Anemia, Hypoproteinemia, and Cataracts in Swine Fed Casein Hydrolysate or Zein, Comparison with Pyridoxine Deficiency Anemia, J. Clin. Invest., *24*, 268, 1945.

47. MERTZ, E. T., BEESON, W. M., WALTZ, R. H., JR. and GAUDRY, R.: Effect of the Amino Acid Hexahomoserine on Growth and Hematopoiesis in Swine, Proc. Soc. Exper. Biol. & Med., *69*, 609, 1948; *Ibid.*, *73*, 75, 1950.

48. NIZET, A. and LAMBERT, S.: Utilisation de di- et tripeptides pour la synthése de l'hémoglobine, étudié a l'aide du carbon radioactif, Bull. Soc. chim. biol., *36*, 307, 1954.

49. SEBRELL, W. H. JR., and McDANIEL, E. G.: Amino Acids in the Production of Blood Constituents in Rats, J. Nutrition, *47*, 477, 1952.

50. WHIPPLE, G. H. and MADDEN, S. C.: Hemo-

globin, Plasma Protein and Cell Protein—
Their Interchange and Construction in
Emergencies, Medicine, 23, 215, 1944;
Jour. Exper. Med., 85, 277, 1947.

51. WHIPPLE, G. H. and ROBSCHEIT-ROBBINS,
F. S.: Amino Acids and Hemoglobin
Production in Anemia, J. Exper. Med.,
71, 569, 1940; ibid., 85, 243 and 267, 1947;
ibid., 89, 339, 1949.

Iron

52. ANDERSON, H. D., McDONOUGH, K. B. and
ELVEHJEM, C. A.: Relation of the Dietary
Calcium-Phosphorus Ratio to Iron Assimi-
lation, J. Lab. & Clin. Med., 25, 464, 1940.

53. ASCHAM, L., SPEIRS, M. and MADDOX, D.:
The Availability of Iron in Various Foods,
J. Nutr., 16, 425, 1938.

54. BALFOUR, W. M., HAHN, P. F., BALE, W. F.,
POMMERENKE, W. T. and WHIPPLE, G. H.:
Radioactive Iron Absorption in Clinical
Conditions: Normal Pregnancy, Anemia,
and Hemochromatosis, J. Exper. Med., 76,
15, 1942.

54a. BESSIS, M. C. and BRETON-GORIUS, J.: Ferritin
and Ferruginous Micelles in Normal
Erythroblasts and Hypochromic Hyper-
sideremic Anemias, Blood, 14, 423, 1959;
Rev. hémat., 14, 165, 1959.

54b. BOTHWELL, T. H., PIRZIO-BIROLI, G., FINCH,
C. A., LODEN, B. and MELLY, A.: Iron
Absorption, J. Lab. & Clin. Med., 51, 24,
1958; ibid., 55, 216, 1960.

55. CALLENDER, SHEILA T., MALLETT, BARBARA
J. and SMITH, MARY D.: Absorption of
Haemoglobin Iron, Brit. J. Haemat., 3,
186, 1957.

56. CARTWRIGHT, G. E. and WINTROBE, M. M.:
The Anemia of Infection. Studies of the
Iron-Binding Capacity of Serum, J. Clin.
Invest., 28, 86, 1949.

57. CHRISTIAN, E. R.: Behavior of Serum Iron
in Various Diseases of Liver, Arch. Int.
Med., 94, 22, 1954.

58. DRABKIN, D. L.: Metabolism of the Hemin
Chromoproteins, Physiol. Rev., 31, 245,
1951.

59. DUBACH, R., CALLENDER, S. T. E. and
MOORE, C. V.: Absorption of Radioactive
Iron in Patients with Fever and with
Anemias of Varied Etiology, Blood, 3,
526, 1948.

61. DUBACH, R., MOORE, C. V. and CALLENDER,
S.: Studies in Iron Transportation and
Metabolism. IX. The Excretion of Iron
as Measured by the Isotope Technique,
J. Lab. & Clin. Med., 45, 599, 1955.

62. FINCH, C. A., GIBSON, J. G., II, PEACOCK,

W. C. and FLUHARTY, R. G.: Iron Metabolism, Blood, 4, 905, 1949; J. Lab. &
Clin. Med., 34, 1480, 1949.

63. FINCH, C. A., HEGSTED, M., KINNEY, T. D.,
THOMAS, E. D., RATH, C. E., HASKINS,
D., FINCH, S. and FLUHARTY, R. G.: Iron
Metabolism, the Pathophysiology of Iron
Storage, Blood, 5, 983, 1950; J. Biol.
Chem., 204, 823, 1953; Medicine, 34,
381, 1955.

64. FOY, H. and KONDI, ATHENA: Anaemias of
the Tropics, J. Trop: Med., 60, 105, 1957.

65. FREEMAN, S. and IVY, A. C.: The Influence
of Antacids upon Iron Retention by the
Anemic Rat, Am. J. Physiol., 137, 706,
1942.

66. GEDIGK, P. and STRAUSS, G.: Zur Histo-
chemie des Hämosiderins, Virchows Arch.,
324, 373, 1953.

66a. GIBLETT, ELOISE R. et al.: Erythrokinetics:
Quantitative Measurements of Red Cell
Production and Destruction in Normal
Subjects and Patients with Anemia, Blood,
11, 291, 1956.

67. GRANICK, S.: Iron Metabolism, Bull. New
York Acad. Med., 30, 81, 1954.

69. GREENBERG, G. R. and WINTROBE, M. M.:
A Labile Iron Pool, J. Biol. Chem., 165,
397, 1946.

70. GRINSTEIN, M. and MOORE, C. V.: Evidence
Obtained with Radioactive Iron that
"Easily Split-Off" Blood Iron is an Arti-
fact, J. Clin. Invest., 28, 505, 1949.

71. HAGBERG, B.: Studies on the Plasma Transport of Iron, Acta paediat., Supp. 93,
1953.

72. HAHN, P. F., BALE, W. F., HETTIG, R. A.,
KAMEN, M. D. and WHIPPLE, G. H.:
Radioactive Iron and Its Excretion in
Urine, Bile and Feces, J. Exper. Med., 70,
433, 1939.

73. HAHN, P. F., BALE, W. F., LAWRENCE, E. O.
and WHIPPLE, G. H.: Radioactive Iron
and Its Metabolism in Anemia, J. Exper.
Med., 69, 739, 1939; ibid., 70, 443, 1939;
ibid., 74, 197, 1941.

75. HAHN, P. F., BALE, W. F., ROSS, J. F.,
HETTIG, R. A. and WHIPPLE, G. H.: Radio
Iron in Plasma Does Not Exchange with
Hemoglobin in Red Cells, Science, 92,
131, 1940.

76. HAHN, P. F., ROSS, J. F., BALE, W. F. and
WHIPPLE, G. H.: The Utilization of Iron
and the Rapidity of Hemoglobin Formation in Anemia Due to Blood Loss, J.
Exper. Med., 71, 731, 1940.

76a. HALLBERG, L. and SÖLVELL, L.: Iron Absorption Studies, Acta Med. scandinav., 168,
(Suppl. 358), 1, 1960.

77. HAMILTON, L. D., GUBLER, C. J., CART-
WRIGHT, G. E. and WINTROBE, M. M.:
Diurnal Variation in the Plasma Iron
Level of Man, Proc. Soc. Exper. Biol. &
Med., 75, 65, 1950.

78. HASKINS, D., STEVENS, A. R., JR., FINCH, S.
and FINCH, C. A.: Iron Metabolism. Iron
Stores in Man as Measured by Phlebotomy, J. Clin. Invest., 31, 543, 1952.

79. HEGSTED, D. M., FINCH, C. A. and KINNEY,
T. D.: The Influence of Diet on Iron
Absorption, J. Exper. Med., 90, 147,
1949; ibid., 96, 115, 1952.

79a.HUFF, R. L., HENNESSY, T. G., AUSTIN, R. E.,
GARCIA, J. F., ROBERTS, B. M. and LAW-
RENCE, J. H.: Plasma and Red Cell Iron
Turnover in Normal Subjects and in
Patients Having Various Hematopoietic
Disorders, J. Clin. Invest., 29, 1041, 1950;
ibid., 30, 1512, 1951; Acta haematol.,
7, 129, 1952; ibid., 9, 73, 1953.

80. HYNES, M.: Iron Metabolism, J. Clin. Path.,
1, 57, 1948.

81. JAGER, B. V.: Immunological Studies of an
Iron-Binding Protein in Human Serum,
J. Clin. Invest., 28, 792, 1949.

82. JANDL, J. H., INMAN, J. K., SIMMONS, R. L.
and ALLEN, D. W.: Transfer of Iron from
Serum Iron-Binding Protein to Human
Reticulocytes, J. Clin. Invest., 38, 161,
1959.

83. JOSEPHS, H. W.: Absorption of Iron as a
Problem in Human Physiology, Blood, 13,
1, 1958.

84. KELLOGG, F. and METTIER, S. R.: Effect of
Alkaline Therapy for Peptic Ulcer on
Utilization of Dietary Iron in the Regeneration of Hemoglobin, Arch. Int. Med.,
58, 278, 1936.

85. LAURELL, C. B.: Studies on the Transportation and Metabolism of Iron in the Body,
Acta physiol. scandinav., 14, suppl. 46,
1947; Blood, 6, 183, 1951; Scandinav. J.
Clin. & Lab. Invest., 5, 118, 1953.

86. MAZUR, A., GREEN, S., SAHA, A. and
CARLETON, A.: Mechanism of Release of
Ferritin Iron in vivo by Xanthine Oxidase,
J. Clin. Invest., 37, 1809, 1958; J. Biol.
Chem., 235, 595, 1960, ibid., 236, 1109,
1961.

87. McMILLAN, T. J. and JOHNSTON, F. A.: The
Absorption of Iron from Spinach by Six
Young Women, and the Effect of Beef
upon the Absorption, J. Nutrition, 44,
383, 1951.

88. MITCHELL, H. H. and HAMILTON, T. S.:
The Dermal Excretion under Controlled
Environmental Conditions of Nitrogen and

Minerals in Human Subjects, J. Biol.
Chem., 178, 345, 1949.

88a.MITCHELL, J. et al.: Lowering of Transferrin
during Iron Absorption in Iron Deficiency,
J. Lab. & Clin. Med., 56, 555, 1960.

88b.MITCHELL, T. G., SPENCER, R. P. and
KING, E. R.: The Use of Radioisotopes in
Diagnostic Hematologic Procedures, Am.
J. Clin. Path., 28, 461, 1957.

89. MOORE, C. V.: The Importance of Nu-
tritional Factors in the Pathogenesis of
Iron-Deficiency Anemia, Am. J. Clin.
Nutrition, 3, 3, 1955; Scandinav. J. Clin.
& Lab. Invest., 9, 292, 1957.

90. MOORE, C. V., ARROWSMITH, W. R., WELCH,
J. and MINNICH, V.: Studies in Iron Transportation and Metabolism, J. Clin. Invest.,
18, 553, 1939; J. Lab. & Clin. Med., 52,
335, 1958.

90a.MOORE, C. V., DUBACH, R., MINNICH, V.
and ROBERTS, H. K.: Absorption of
Ferrous and Ferric Radioactive Iron by
Human Subjects and by Dogs, J. Clin.
Invest., 23, 755, 1944.

91. MOURIQUAND, C.: Villosité intestinale et
métabolisme du fer, Rev. hemat., 15, 472,
1960.

91a.MUIR, A. R.: The Molecular Structure of
Isolated and Intracellular Ferritin, Quart.
J. Exper. Physiol., 45, 192, 1960.

91b.NOYES, W. D., BOTHWELL, T. H. and FINCH,
C. A.: The Role of the Reticulo-Endo-
thelial Cell in Iron Metabolism, Brit. J.
Haemat., 6, 43, 1960.

92. PATERSON, J. C. S., MARRACK, D. and
WIGGINS, H. W.: Hypoferraemia in the
Human Subject: The Importance of Diurnal Hypoferraemia, Clin. Sci., 11, 417,
1952.

92a.POLLYCOVE, M. and MORTIMER, R.: The
Quantitative Determination of Iron Kinetics and Hemoglobin Synthesis in Human Subjects, J. Clin. Invest., 40, 753,
1961.

93. POWELL, J. F.: Serum-Iron in Health and
Disease, Quart. J. Med., 13, 19, 1944.

94. RATH, C. E. and FINCH, C. A.: Sternal Marrow Hemosiderin, J. Lab. & Clin. Med.,
33, 81, 1948; Ann. Int. Med., 38, 199,
1953.

95. ————: Serum Iron Transport Measurement of Iron Binding Capacity of Serum
in Man, J. Clin. Invest., 28, 79, 1949.

95a.RICHTER, G. W.: The Cellular Transformation of Injected Colloidal Iron Complexes
into Ferritin and Hemosiderin in Experimental Animals, J. Exper. Med., 109, 197,
1959.

95b. SALTMAN, P., FRISCH, H. L., FISKIN, R. D. and ALEX, T.: The Kinetics of Iron Metabolism in Rat Liver Slices, J. Biol. Chem., *221*, 777, 1956; Exper. Cell Res., *18*, 560, 1959; Arch. Biochem. & Biophys., *86*, 169, 1960.

96. SCHADE, A. L., OYAMA, J., REINHART, R. W. and MILLER, J. R.: Bound Iron and Unsaturated Iron-Binding Capacity of Serum; Rapid and Reliable Quantitative Determination, Proc. Soc. Exper. Biol. & Med., *87*, 443, 1954.

97. SCHULZ, JEANETTE and SMITH, N. J.: A Quantitative Study of the Absorption of Food Iron in Infants and Children, A. M. A. J. Dis. Child., *95*, 109, 1958.

98. SHARPE, L. M., PEACOCK, W. C., COOKE, R. and HARRIS, R. S.: The Effect of Phytate and Other Food Factors on Iron Absorption, J. Nutrition, *41*, 433, 1950.

99. SMITHIES, O. and HILLER, O.: The Genetic Control of Transferrins in Humans, Biochem. J., *72*, 121, 1959; Nature, *183*, 1589, 1959.

100. STEINKAMP, R., DUBACH, R. and MOORE, C. V.: Studies in Iron Transportation and Metabolism. VIII. Absorption of Radioiron from Iron-Enriched Bread, Arch. Int. Med., *95*, 181, 1955.

101. STEVENS, A. R., JR., PIRZIO-BIROLI, G., HARKINS, H. N., NYHUS, L. M. and FINCH, C. A.: Iron Metabolism in Patients after Partial Gastrectomy, Ann. Surg., *149*, 534, 1959.

102. STEWART, W. B., VASSAR, P. S. and STONE, R. S.: Iron Absorption in Dogs during Anemia due to Acetylphenylhydrazine, J. Clin. Invest., *32*, 1225, 1953.

103. STURGEON, P.: Studies of Iron Requirements in Infants and Children, Pediatrics, *13*, 107, 1954.

104. WALDENSTRÖM, J.: Järnbelastningar Och Vad De Lära Oss Om Jarnomsättningen, Ferrosan, Malmö, 1944.

105. WHIPPLE, G. H. and ROBSCHEIT-ROBBINS, F. S.: Iron and Its Utilization in Experimental Anemia, Am. Jour. Med. Sci., *191*, 11, 1936; *Ibid.*, *134*, 263, 1941.

106. WUHRMANN, F. and JASINSKI, B.: Untersuchungen über die Bindung des Eisens an das Serumglobin B_1 mit Hilfe des Radioeisens 59Fe und dessen klinische Bedeutung, Schweiz. med. Wchnschr., *83*, 661, 1953.

Copper

107. BAXTER, J. H. and VAN WYK, J. J.: A Bone Disorder Associated with Copper Deficiency, Bull. Johns Hopkins Hosp., *93*, 1, 25 and 41, 1953.

108. BUSH, J. A., JENSEN, W. N., ATHENS, J. W., ASHENBRUCKER, HELEN E., CARTWRIGHT, G. E. and WINTROBE, M. M.: Studies on Copper Metabolism, J. Exper. Med., *103*, 701, 1956.

109. CARTWRIGHT, G. E.: The Relationship of Copper, Cobalt and Other Trace Elements to Hemopoiesis, Am. J. Clin. Nutrition, *3*, 11, 1955.

110. CARTWRIGHT, G. E.: Copper Metabolism in Human Subjects, *in Copper Metabolism:* A Symposium on Animal, Plant and Soil Relationships, W. D. Elroy, Ed., Baltimore, Johns Hopkins University Press, 1950.

111. CHOU, T. P. and ADOLPH, W. H.: Living Copper Metabolism in Man, Biochem. J., *29*, 476, 1935.

112. ELVEHJEM, C. A.: The Biological Significance of Copper and Its Relation to Iron Metabolism, Physiol. Rev., *15*, 471, 1935.

113. ELVEHJEM, C. A., DUCKLES, D. and MENDENHALL, D. R.: Iron *versus* Iron and Copper in the Treatment of Anemia in Infants, Am. J. Dis. Child., *53*, 785, 1937.

114. FOWLER, W. M. and BARER, A. P.: The Effect of Copper and Iron on Hemoglobin Regeneration, J. Lab. & Clin. Med., *26*, 832, 1941.

115. HOLMBERG, C. G. and LAURELL, C. B.: Investigations in Serum Copper, Acta Chem. Scandinav., *1*, 944, 1947; *ibid.*, *2*, 550, 1948; Nature, *161*, 236, 1948.

115a. HOWELL, J. McC. and DAVISON, A. N.: The Copper Content and Cytochrome Oxidase Activity of Tissues from Normal and Swayback Lambs, Biochem. J., *72*, 365, 1959.

116. HUTCHISON, J. H.: The Rôle of Copper in Iron-Deficiency Anaemia in Infancy, Quart. J. Med., *7*, 397, 1938.

117. LAHEY, M. E., GUBLER, C. J., CHASE, M. S., CARTWRIGHT, G. E. and WINTROBE, M. M.: Studies on Copper Metabolism. II. Hematologic Manifestations of Copper Deficiency in Swine, Blood, *7*, 1053 and 1075, 1952; Blood, *11*, 143, 1956.

118. ————: Studies on Copper Metabolism. VI. Blood Copper in Normal Human Subjects, J. Clin. Invest., *32*, 322 and 329, 1953.

119. MAASS, A. R., MICHAUD, L., SPECTOR, H., ELVEHJEM, C. A. and HART, E. B.: The Relationship of Copper to Hematopoiesis in Experimental Hemorrhagic Anemia, Am. J. Physiol., *141*, 322, 1944.

119a. MARKOWITZ, H., CARTWRIGHT, G. E. and WINTROBE, M. M.: Erythrocuprein, (to be published).

120. MARSTON, H. R.: Cobalt, Copper and Molybdenum in the Nutrition of Animals and Plants, Physiol. Rev., *32*, 66, 1952; Med. J. Australia, *2*, 105, 1959.

120a. REIFF, B. and SCHNIEDEN, H.: Plasma Copper and Iron Levels and Plasma Paraphenylene Diamine Oxidase Activity (Plasma Copper Oxidase Activity) in Kwashiorkor, Blood, *14*, 967, 1959.

121. SACHS, A., LEVINE, V. E., HILL, F. C. and HUGHES, R.: Copper and Iron in Human Blood, Arch. Int. Med., *71*, 489, 1943.

121a. SCHUBERT, W. K. and LAHEY, M. E.: Copper and Protein Depletion Complicating Hypoferric Anemia of Infancy, Pediatrics, *24*, 710, 1959.

122. SCHULTZE, M. O.: Metallic Elements and Blood Formation, Physiol. Rev., *20*, 37, 1940 (Bibliography).

123. SCHULTZE, M. O. and SIMMONS, S. J.: The Use of Radioactive Copper in Studies on Nutritional Anemia of Rats, J. Biol. Chem., *142*, 97, 1942.

124. SCOULAR, F. I.: A Quantitative Study, by Means of Spectrographic Analysis, of Copper in Nutrition, J. Nutrition, *16*, 437, 1938.

125. SHELDON, J. H. and RAMAGE, H.: On the Occurrence of Copper and Manganese in Preparations of Iron, Quart. J. Med., *1*, 135, 1932.

126. SMITH, S. E. and MEDLICOTT, M.: The Blood Picture of Iron and Copper Deficiency Anemias in the Rat, Am. J. Physiol., *141*, 354, 1944.

126a. WILSON, J. F. and LAHEY, M. E.: Failure to Induce Dietary Deficiency of Copper in Premature Infants, Pediatrics, *25*, 40, 1960.

127. WINTROBE, M. M., CARTWRIGHT, G. E. and GUBLER, C. J.: Studies on the Function and Metabolism of Copper, J. Nutrition, *50*, 395, 1953.

128. YOSHIKAWA, H., HAHN, P. F. and BALE, W. F.: Red Cell and Plasma Radioactive Copper in Normal and Anemic Dogs, J. Exper. Med., *75*, 489, 1942.

Cobalt and Miscellaneous Minerals

130. BERK, L., BURCHENAL, J. H. and CASTLE, W. B.: Erythropoietic Effect of Cobalt in Patients with or without Anemia, New England J. Med., *240*, 754, 1949.

131. COLES, B. L. and JAMES, U.: The Effect of Cobalt and Iron Salts on the Anaemia of Prematurity, Arch. Dis. Childhood, *29*, 85, 1954.

131a. COTZIAS, G. C.: Manganese in Health and Disease, Physiol. Rev., *38*, 503, 1958; Nature, *182*, 1677, 1958.

132. CRAFTS, R. C., TURNBULL, D. S. and WEBER, P. R.: The Effects of Cobalt, Liver Extract and Vitamin B$_{12}$ on the Anemia Induced by Hypophysectomy in Adult Female Rats, Blood, *7*, 863, 1952.

133. DORRANCE, S. S., THORN, G. W., CLINTON, M., JR., EDMONDS, H. W. and FARBER, S.: Effect of Cobalt on Work Performance under Conditions of Anoxia, Am. J. Physiol., *139*, 399, 1943.

134. FROST, D. V.: A Study of the Need for Cobalt in Dogs on Milk Diets, J. Nutrition, *21*, 93, 1941.

135. GARDNER, F. H.: The Use of Cobaltous Chloride in the Anemia Associated with Chronic Renal Disease, J. Lab. & Clin. Med., *41*, 56, 1953.

136. GREENBERG, D. M., COPP, D. H. and CUTHBERTSON, D. H.: Studies in Mineral Metabolism with the Aid of Artificial Radioactive Isotopes, J. Biol. Chem., *147*, 749, 1943.

137. GRIFFITH, W. H., PAVCEK, P. P. and MULFORD, D. J.: The Relation of the Sulfur Amino Acids to the Toxicity of Cobalt and Nickel in the Rat, J. Nutrition, *23*, 603, 1942.

138. HARP, M. J. and SCOULAR, F. I.: Cobalt Metabolism of Young College Women on Self-Selected Diets, J. Nutrition, *47*, 67, 1952.

139. KRISS, J. P., CARNES, W. H. and GROSS, R. T.: Hypothyroidism and Thyroid Hyperplasia in Patients Treated with Cobalt, J. A. M. A., *157*, 117, 1955.

139a. LAFORET, M. T. and THOMAS, E. D.: The Effect of Cobalt on Heme Synthesis by Bone Marrow *in Vitro*, J. Biol. Chem., *218*, 595, 1956.

140. ORTEN, J. M., UNDERHILL, F. A., MUGRAGE, E. R. and LEWIS, R. C.: Blood Volume Studies in Cobalt Polycythemia, J. Biol. Chem., *99*, 457, 1933; Am. J. Physiol., *144*, 464, 1945; J. Biol. Chem., *176*, 961, 1948; J. Nutrition, *45*, 487, 1951.

141. QUILLIGAN, J. J., JR.: Effect of a Cobalt-Iron Mixture on the Anemia of Prematurity, Texas State J. Med., *50*, 294, 1954.

141a. SEAMAN, A. J. and KOLER, R. D.: Acquired Erythrocytic Hypoplasia: A Recovery during Cobalt Therapy, Acta haemat., *9*, 153, 1953.

142. SHEN, S. C. and HOMBURGER, F.: The Anemia of Cancer Patients and Its Relation to Metastases to the Bone Marrow, J. Lab. & Clin. Med., *37*, 182, 1951.

143. SHENOY, K. G. and RAMASARMA, G. B.: Extraction Procedure and Determination of the Vitamin B_{12} Content of Some Animal Livers, Arch. Biochem., *51*, 371, 1954.

143a.SMITH, S. E. and LOOSLI, J. K.: Cobalt and Vitamin B_{12} in Ruminant Nutrition, J. Dairy Sc., *40*, 1215, 1957.

144. UNDERWOOD, E. J.: The Significance of the "Trace Elements" in Nutrition, Nutr. Abstr. and Rev., *9*, 515, 1940.

144a.VALLEE, B. L.: Biochemistry, Physiology and Pathology of Zinc, Physiol. Rev., *39*, 443, 1959.

145. WINTROBE, M. M., GRINSTEIN, M., DUBASH, J. J., HUMPHREYS, S. R., ASHENBRUCKER, H. and WORTH, W.: The Influence of Cobalt on the Anemia Associated with Inflammation, Blood, *2*, 323, 1947.

The B Vitamins and Related Substances

145a.ABELS, J., VEGTER, J. J. M., WOLDRING, M. G., JANS, J. H. and NIEWEG, H. O.: The Physiologic Mechanism of Vitamin B_{12} Absorption, Acta med. scandinav., *165*, 105, 1959.

145b.ANDERSON, BARBARA *et al.:* The Urinary and Faecal Excretion of Radioactivity after Oral Doses of H-Folic Acid, Brit. J. Haemat., *6*, 439, 1960.

145c.ANDRÉ, R., JACOB, S., MALASSENET, R. and CAROLI, J.: Anémie hypochrome avec hémochromatose. Normalisation du tableau hématologique par la pyridoxine, Nouv. rev. fr. d'hémat., *1*, 270, 1961.

146. ANGIER, R. B., *et al.:* Synthesis of a Compound Identical with the *L. casei* Factor Isolated from Liver, Science, *102*, 227, 1945; *Ibid.*, *103*, 667, 1946.

146a.BERK, L., CASTLE, W. B., WELCH, A. D., HEINLE, R. W., ANKER, R. and EPSTEIN, M.: Observations on the Etiologic Relationship of Achylia Gastrica to Pernicious Anemia. X. Activity of Vitamin B_{12} as Food (Extrinsic) Factor, New England J. Med., *239*, 911, 1948.

146b.BESSEY, O. A., ADAM, DORIS, J. D., and HANSEN, A. E.: Intake of Vitamin B_6 and Infantile Convulsions: a First Approximation of Requirements of Pyridoxine in Infants, Pediatrics, *20*, 33, 1957.

147. BISHOP, R. C. and BETHELL, F. H.: Hereditary Hypochromic Anemia with Transfusion Hemosiderosis Treated with Pyridoxine, New England J. Med., *261*, 486, 1959.

147a.BOLINDER, A. and REICHARD, P.: The Biosynthesis of Deoxyribonucleic Acid by the Chick Embryo, J. Biol. Chem., *234*, 2723, 1959.

147b.BONNETT, R., CANNON, J. R., JOHNSON, A. W., SUTHERLAND, I., TODD, A. R. and SMITH, E. L.: The Structure of Vitamin B_{12} and Its Hexacarboxylic Acid Degradation Product, Nature, *176*, 328, 1955.

148. BOOTH, C. C. and MOLLIN, D. L.: The Site of Absorption of Vitamin B_{12} in Man, Lancet, *1*, 18, 1959.

148a.BROQUIST, H. P. and LUHBY, A. L.: Detection and Isolation of Formiminoglutamic Acid Deficiency in Humans, Proc. Soc. Exper. Biol. & Med., *100*, 349, 1959.

148b.CAROLI, J. *et al.:* Hémochromatose avec anémie hypochrome et absence d'hémoglobine anormale. Etude au microscope électronique, Presse méd., *65*, 1991, 1957; Rev. hémat., *15*, 318, 1960.

149. CARTWRIGHT, G. E., TATTING, B., ASHENBRUCKER, H. and WINTROBE, M. M.: Experimental Production of a Nutritional Macrocytic Anemia in Swine, Blood, *4*, 301, 1949; J. Lab. & Clin. Med., *36*, 675, 1950; Blood, *6*, 867, 1951; *ibid.*, *7*, 992, 1952.

150. CARTWRIGHT, G. E., TATTING, B. and WINTROBE, M. M.: Niacin Deficiency Anemia in Swine, Arch. Biochem., *19*, 109, 1948.

151. CARTWRIGHT, G. E., WINTROBE, M. M. and HUMPHREYS, S.: Studies on Anemia in Swine due to Pyridoxine Deficiency, Together with Data on Phenylhydrazine Anemia, J. Biol Chem., *153*, 171, 1944.

154. DAFT, F. S., KORNBERG, A., ASHBURN, L. L. and SEBRELL, W. H.: Anemia and Granulocytopenia in Rats Fed a Diet Low in Pantothenic Acid, Pub. Health Rep., *60*, 1201, 1945; Blood, *2*, 451, 1947.

155. DARBY, W. J. *et al.:* Vitamin B_{12} Requirement of Adult Man, Am. J. Med., *25*, 726, 1958.

155a.DARBY, W. J. and JONES, E.: Treatment of Sprue with Synthetic *L. casei* Factor (Folic Acid, Vitamin M), Proc. Soc. Exper. Biol. and Med., *60*, 259, 1945.

157. DAY, P. L., LANGSTON, W. C., DARBY, W. J., WAHLIN, J. G. and MIMS, V.: Nutritional Cytopenia in Monkeys Receiving the Goldberger Diet, J. Exper. Med., *72*, 463, 1940; J. Biol. Chem., *152*, 147, 1944; *ibid.*, *161*, 45, 1945.

158. DIETRICH, L. S., NICHOL, C. A., MONSTON, W. J. and ELVEHJEM, C. A.: Observations on the Interrelation of Vitamin B_{12}, Folic Acid, and Vitamin C in the Chick, J. Biol. Chem., *181*, 915, 1949.

159. DINNING, J. S. and YOUNG, RUTH S.: Further Studies on Vitamin B_{12} and Thymine Biosynthesis, J. Biol. Chem., *234*, 3241, 1959.

159a.DOSCHERHOLMEN, A., HAGEN, P. S., LIU, MARGARET and OLIN, LOIS: A Dual Mechanism of Vitamin B$_{12}$ Plasma Absorption, J. Clin. Invest., *36*, 1551, 1957; J. Lab. & Clin. Med., *54*, 434, 1959.

160. ELLENBOGEN, L., BURSON, S. L. and WILLIAMS, W. L.: Purification of Intrinsic Factor, Proc. Soc. Exper. Biol. & Med., *97*, 760, 1958.

161. ERSLEV, A. J., LEAR, A. A. and CASTLE, W. B.: Pyridoxine-Responsive Anemia, New England J. Med., *262*, 1209, 1960.

162. FOUTS, P. J., HELMER, O. M. and LEPKOVSKY, S.: Nutritional Microcytic Hypochromic Anemia in Dogs Cured with Crystalline Factor I, Am. J. M. Sc., *199*, 163, 1940.

162a.FOY, H. and KONDI, ATHENA: Hypochromic Anemias of the Tropics Associated with Pyridoxine and Nicotinic Acid Deficiency, Blood, *13*, 1054, 1958.

162b.GEHRMANN, G.: Pyridoxinmangel-Anämie beim Menschen, Folia haemat., *2*, 225, 1958.

163. GERSHOFF, S. N., FARAGALLA, F. F., NELSON, D. A. and ANDRUS, S. B.: Vitamin B$_6$ Deficiency and Oxalate Nephrocalcinosis in the Cat, Am. J. Med., *27*, 72, 1959.

163a.GIRDWOOD, R. H.: *Folic Acid, its Analogs and Antagonists*, 1960, New York, Academic Press, Inc., Vol. 3, p. 235.

164. GREENBERG, G. R.: Role of Folic Acid Derivatives in Purine Biosynthesis, Fed. Proc., *13*, 745, 1954; Biochem. et biophys. acta, *17*, 588, 589, 1955.

165. GYÖRGY, P., ROBSCHEIT-ROBBINS, F. S. and WHIPPLE, G. H.: Lactoflavin Increases Hemoglobin Production in the Anemic Dog, Am. J. Physiol., *122*, 154, 1938.

166. HALSTED, J. A., CARROLL, JEAN and RUBERT, SHIRLEY: Serum and Tissue Concentration of Vitamin B$_{12}$ in Certain Pathologic States, New England J. Med., *260*, 575, 1959.

167. HANDLER, P. and FEATHERSTON, W. P.: The Biochemical Defect in Nicotinic Acid Deficiency, J. Biol. Chem., *151*, 395, 1943.

168. HARRIS, J. W., WHITTINGTON, R. M., WEISMAN, R., JR. and HORRIGAN, D. L.: Pyridoxine Responsive Anemia in the Human Adult, Proc. Soc. Exper. Biol. & Med., *91*, 427, 1956.

168a.HAUSMANN, K., LUDWIG, J. and MULLI, K.: Über die blutbildene Wirkung verschiedener Formen des Vitamin B$_{12}$ aus Kuhmist, Schafmist, Bakterien- und Streptomyces-Kulturen, Acta haemat., *10*, 282, 1953.

168b.HEDBOM, A.: A Native Cobalamin-Polypeptide Complex from Liver: Isolation and Characterization, Biochem. J., *74*, 307, 1960.

169. HERBERT, V.: Mechanism of Intrinsic Factor Action in Everted Sacs of Rat Small Intestine, J. Clin. Invest., *38*, 102, 1959; Am. J. Clin. Nutrition, 7, 433, 1959.

169a.HODGES, R. E., OHLSON, MARGARET A. and BEAN, W. B.: Pantothenic Acid Deficiency in Man, J. Clin. Invest., *37*, 1642, 1958; ibid., *38*, 1421, 1959.

170. HODGKIN, D. C., PICKWORTH, J., ROBERTSON, J. H., TRUEBLOOD, K. N., PROSEN, R. J. and WHITE, J. G.: The Crystal Structure of the Hexacarboxylic Acid Derived from B$_{12}$ and the Molecular Structure of the Vitamin, Nature, *176*, 325, 1955.

171. JONES, E., DARBY, W. and TOTTER, J. R.: Pernicious Anemia and Related Anemias Treated with Vitamin B$_{12}$, Blood, *4*, 827, 1949.

172. JUKES, T. H. and STOKSTAD, E. L. R.: Pteroylglutamic Acid and Related Compounds, Physiol. Rev., *28*, 51, 1948 (Bibliography); *B-Vitamins*, Springfield, Ill., Charles C Thomas, 1952.

174. KARLIN, R.: La vitamine B$_{12}$ dans le lait humain et bovin, Compt. rend. Soc. de Biol., *148*, 371, 1954.

176. KORNBERG, A., TABOR, H. and SEBRELL, W. H.: Blood Regeneration in Pyridoxine-Deficient Rats, Am. J. Physiol., *143*, 434, 1945.

176a.KORNBERG, A., TABOR, H. and SEBRELL, W. H.: Blood Regeneration in Rats Deficient in Biotin, Thiamin or Riboflavin, Am. J. Physiol., *145*, 54, 1945.

176b.LANE, M., MANGEL, C. E. and DOHERTY, DOROTHY J.: Rapid Induction of Isolated Riboflavin Deficiency in Man (abst.), Proc. Am. Soc. Clin. Invest., J. Clin. Invest., *39*, 1004, 1960.

177. LATNER, A. L. and MERRILLS, R. J.: Further Observations Related to the Isolation of Intrinsic Factor Mucoprotein, *in Vitamin B$_{12}$ and Intrinsic Factor*, H. C. Heinrich, Ed., Stuttgart, Germany, Ferdinand Enke Verlag, 1957, p. 201; Brit. M. J., *2*, 278, 1958.

177a.LERNER, A. M., DECARLI, LEONORE M. and DAVIDSON, C. S.: Association of Pyridoxine Deficiency and Convulsions in Alcoholics, Proc. Soc. Exper. Biol. & Med., *98*, 841, 1958.

178. LEWIS, U. J., REGISTER, U. D., THOMPSON, H. T. and ELVEHJEM, C. A.: Distribution of Vitamin B$_{12}$ in Natural Materials, Proc. Soc. Exper. Biol. & Med., *72*, 479, 1949.

179. LING, C. T. and CHOW, B. F.: The Influence of Vitamin B_{12} on Carbohydrate and Lipid Metabolism, J. Biol. Chem., *206*, 797, 1954.

180. MAIER, C.: Megaloblastäre Vitamin-B_6 Mangelanämie bei Hämochromatose, Schweiz. med. Wchnschr., *87*, 1234, 1957.

181. McKIBBIN, J. M., SCHAEFER, A. E., FROST, D. V. and ELVEHJEM, C. A.: Studies on Anemia in Dogs Due to a Pyridoxine Deficiency, J. Biol. Chem., *142*, 77, 1942.

183. MIRONE, LEONORA and JACKSON, CHARLOTTE D.: The Development and Cure of Pyridoxine Deficiency Symptoms in Weanling Mice, J. Nutrition, *67*, 167, 1959.

184. MITCHELL, E. K., SNELL, E. E. and WILLIAMS, R. J.: Folic Acid, J. Am. Chem. Soc., *66*, 267, 1944.

184a. MOOKERJEA, S. and HAWKINS, W. W.: Haematopoiesis in the Rat in Riboflavin Deficiency, Brit. J. Nutrition, *14*, 239, 1960.

185. MOORE, C. V., BIERBAUM, O. S., WELCH, A. D. and WRIGHT, L. D.: The Activity of Synthetic *Lactobacillus casei* Factor ("Folic Acid") as an Antipernicious Anemia Substance, J. Lab. & Clin. Med., *30*, 1056, 1945.

187. MUELLER, J. F. and VILTER, R. W.: Pyridoxine Deficiency in Human Beings Induced with Desoxypyridoxine, J. Clin. Invest., *29*, 193, 1950; J. Lab. & Clin. Med., *42*, 335, 1953; J.A.M.A., *156*, 549, 1954.

189. NICHOL, C. A. and WELCH, A. D.: Synthesis of Citrovorum Factor from Folic Acid by Liver Slices; Augmentation by Ascorbic Acid, Proc. Soc. Exper. Biol. & Med., *74*, 52, 1950; Science, *121*, 275, 1955.

190. PETRIDES, P.: Die Perniciosabehandlung mit Thymin und Folsäure, Deutsches Arch. f. klin. Med., *194*, 661, 1949.

191. PITNEY, W. R., BEARD, M. F. and VAN LOON, E. J.: The Vitamin B_{12} Content of Electrophoretic Fractions of Liver Homogenates, J. Biol. Chem., *212*, 117, 1955.

191a. POLINER, I. J. and SPIRO, H. M.: The Independent Secretion of Acid, Pepsin, and "Intrinsic Factor" by the Human Stomach, Gastroenterology, *34*, 196, 1958.

191b. REIZENSTEIN, P. G.: Excretion, Enterohepatic Circulation, and Retention of Radiovitamin B_{12} in Pernicious Anemia and in Controls, Proc. Soc. Exper. Biol. & Med., *101*, 703, 1959; Acta med. scandinav., *165*, 313 and 467, 1959; *ibid.* (Suppl. 347), *165*, 3, 1959.

192. RICKES, E. L., BRINK, N. G., KONIUSZY, F. R., WOOD, T. R. and FOLKERS, K.: Crystalline Vitamin B_{12}, Science, *107*, 396, 1948; *ibid.*, *112*, 354, 1950.

193. RINEHART, J. F., GREENBERG, L. D. and GINZTON, L. L.: Thiamin Deficiency in the Rhesus Monkey. Clinical, Metabolic and Hematologic Observations, Blood, *3*, 1453, 1948.

193a. RINEHART, J. F. and GREENBERG, L. D.: Vitamin B_6 Deficiency in the Rhesus Monkey, Am. J. Clin. Nutrition, *4*, 318, 1956.

194. RUEGAMER, W. R., MICHAUD, L., ELVEHJEM, C. A. and HART, E. B.: Growth and Hemoglobin Production in Dogs on Purified Rations, Am. J. Physio'., *145*, 23, 1945.

195. RUNDLES, R. W. and BREWER, S. S., Jr.: Hematologic Responses in Pernicious Anemia to Orotic Acid, Blood, *13*, 99, 1958.

197. SCHIEVE, J. F. and RUNDLES, R. W.: Response of Lingual Manifestations of Pernicious Anemia to Pteroylglutamic Acid and Vitamin B_{12}, J. Lab. & Clin. Med., *34*, 439, 1949

198. SHINTON, N. K.: Total Serum Vitamin B_{12} Concentration in Normal Human Adult Serum Assayed by *Euglena gracilis*, Clin. Sc., *18*, 389, 1959.

199. SMITH, E. L.: Purification of Anti-Pernicious Anæmia Factors from Liver, Nature, *161*, 638, 1948; Brit. Med. J., *2*, 1367, 1949; Proc. Royal Soc., B, *136*, 592, 1949; Ann. Rev. Biochem., *23*, 245, 1954; Nature, *181*, 305, 1958.

200. SMITH, S. G., CURRY, R., and HAWFIELD, H.: Vitamin B_6 Deficiency Anemia in the Dog, Science, *98*, 520, 1943.

201. SNELL, E. E.: Summary of Known Metabolic Functions of Nicotinic Acid, Riboflavin and Vitamin B_6, Physiol. Rev., *33*, 509, 1953.

202. SNYDERMAN, S. E., HOLT, L. E., JR., CARRETERO, R. and JACOBS, K.: Pyridoxine Deficiency in the Human Infant, J. Clin. Nutrition, *1*, 200, 1953.

203. SPECTOR, H., MAASS, A. R., MICHAUD, L., ELVEHJEM, C. A. and HART, E. B.: The Rôle of Riboflavin in Blood Regeneration, J. Biol. Chem., *150*, 75, 1943.

204. SPIES, T. D., FROMMEYER, W. B., JR., VILTER, D. F. and ENGLISH, A.: Anti-Anemic Properties of Thymine, Blood, *1*, 185, 1946; Lancet, *2*, 519, 1948.

205. SPIES, T. D., LOPEZ, G. G., MILANES, F., STONE, R. E., TOCA, R. L., ARAMBURU, T. and KARTUS, S.: Observations on the Effect of an Animal Protein Factor Concentrate on Persons with the Macrocytic Anemia of Pernicious Anemia, of Nutritional Macrocytic Anemia and of Sprue,

and on Persons with Nutritional Glossitis, Blood, *4*, 819, 1949.

206. Spies, T. D., Vilter, C. F., Koch, M. B. and Caldwell, M. H.: Observations on the Anti-Anemic Properties of Synthetic Folic Acid, South. Med. J., *38*, 707, 1945; Ibid., *38*, 781, 1945; J.A.M.A., *130*, 474, 1946.

207. Spray, G. H. and Witts, L. J.: Results of Three Years' Experience with Microbiological Assay of Vitamin B₁₂ in Serum, Brit. M. J., *1*, 295, 1958.

207a. Spray, G. H. and Witts, L. J.: Thymidine in Megaloblastic Anaemia, Lancet, *2*, 869, 1958.

207b. Stokstad, E. L. R., Jukes, T. H., Pierce, J., Page, A. C., Jr. and Franklin, A. L.: The Multiple Nature of the Animal Protein Factor, J. Biol. Chem., *180*, 647, 1949.

208. Verloop, M. C. and Rademaker, W.: Anaemia Due to Pyridoxine Deficiency in Man, Brit. J. Haemat., *6*, 66, 1960.

208a. Wachstein, M.: Evidence for Abnormal Vitamin B₆ Metabolism in Pregnancy and Various Disease States, Am. J. Clin. Nutrition, *4*, 369, 1956.

209. Wagle, S. R., Mehta, R. and Johnson, B. C.: Vitamin B₁₂ and Protein Biosynthesis, J. Biol. Chem., *233*, 619, 1958; Am. J. Clin. Nutrition, *6*, 34, 1958.

210. Waisman, H. A.: Production of Riboflavin Deficiency in the Monkey, Proc. Soc. Exper. Biol. & Med., *55*, 69, 1944; J. Nutrition, *30*, 45, 1945.

210a. Wayne, L., Will, J. J., Friedman, B. I., Becker, L. S. and Vilter, R. W.: Vitamin B₆ in Internal Medicine, A. M. A. Arch. Int. Med., *101*, 143, 1958.

211. Weinstein, I. B., Weissman, S. M. and Watkin, D. M.: The Plasma Vitamin B₁₂ Binding Substance, J. Clin. Invest., *38*, 1904, 1959.

212. West, R. and Reisner, E. H., Jr.: Treatment of Pernicious Anemia with Crystalline Vitamin B₁₂, Am. J. Med., *6*, 643, 1949.

213. Will, J. J. et al.: Folic Acid and Vitamin B₁₂ in Pernicious Anemia, J. Lab. & Clin. Med., *53*, 22, 1959.

214. Wills, L. and Bilimoria, H. S.: Production of a Macrocytic Anæmia in Monkeys by Deficient Feeding, Indian J. Med. Res., *20*, 391, 1932.

215. Wintrobe, M. M.: The Antianemic Effect of Yeast in Pernicious Anemia, Am. J. M. Sc., *197*, 286, 1939.

216. Wintrobe, M. M., Buschke, W., Follis, R. H., Jr. and Humphreys, S.: Riboflavin Deficiency in Swine, Bull. Johns Hopkins Hosp., *75*, 102, 1944.

216a. Wintrobe, M. M., Follis, R. H., Jr., Alcayaga, R., Paulson, M. and Humphreys, S.: Pantothenic Acid Deficiency in Swine, Bull. Johns Hopkins Hosp., *73*, 313, 1943.

217. Wintrobe, M. M., Follis, R. H., Jr., Miller, M. H., Stein, H. J., Alcayaga, R., Humphreys, S., Suksta, A. and Cartwright, G. E.: Pyridoxine Deficiency in Swine, Bull. Johns Hopkins Hosp., *72*, 1, 1943; ibid., *75*, 35, 1944.

217a. Wolfe, S. J., Brin, M. and Davidson, C. S.: The Effect of Thiamine Deficiency on Human Erythrocyte Metabolism, J. Clin. Invest., *37*, 1476, 1958.

Ascorbic Acid and Miscellaneous Substances

219. Bronte-Stewart, B.: The Anaemia of Adult Scurvy, Quart. J. Med., *22*, 309, 1953.

219a. Brown, A.: Megaloblastic Anaemia Associated with Adult Scurvy, Brit. J. Haemat., *1*, 345, 1955.

219b. Burns, J. J.: Biosynthesis of L-Ascorbic Acid; Basic Defect in Scurvy, Am. J. Med., *26*, 740, 1959.

220. Crandon, J. H., Lund, C. C. and Dill, D. B.: Experimental Human Scurvy, New England J. Med., *223*, 353, 1940.

221. Gabuzda, G. J., Jr., Phillips, G. B., Schilling, R. F. and Davidson, C. S.: Metabolism of Pteroylglutamic Acid and the Citrovorum Factor in Patients with Scurvy, J. Clin. Invest., *31*, 756, 1952; Proc. Soc. Exper. Biol. & Med., *84*, 452, 1953.

222. Kohler, G. O., Elvehjem, C. A. and Hart, E. B.: The Relation of Pyrrole-Containing Pigments to Hemoglobin Synthesis, J. Biol. Chem., *128*, 501, 1939.

223. Lozner, E. L.: Studies on Hemoglobin Regeneration in Patients with Vitamin C Deficiency, New England J. Med., *224*, 265, 1941.

224. May, C. D., Sundberg, R. D., Schaar, F., Lowe, C. U. and Salmon, R. J.: Experimental Nutritional Megaloblastic Anemia: Relation of Ascorbic Acid and Pteroylglutamic Acid, Am. J. Dis. Child., *82*, 282, 1951; Blood, *7*, 671 and 978, 1952; J. Nutrition, *49*, 121, 1953.

225. Mersky, C.: Survival of Transfused Red Cells in Scurvy, Brit. M. J., *2*, 1353, 1953.

226. Patek, A. J.: Chlorophyll and Regeneration of the Blood, Arch. Int. Med., *57*, 73, 1936.

227. Vilter, R. W., Woolford, R. M. and Spies, T. D.: Severe Scurvy, J. Lab. & Clin. Med., *31*, 609, 1946.

Fate of the Red Corpuscle. Extent and Manner
of Blood Destruction

227a. ALLISON, A. C. and AP REES, W.: The Binding of Haemoglobin by Plasma Proteins (Haptoglobins), Brit. M. J., *2*, 1137, 1957; Nature, *181*, 824, 1958.

228. ASHBY, W.: Determination of Length of Life of Transfused Blood Corpuscles in Man, J. Exper. Med., *29*, 267, 1919; Blood, *3*, 486, 1948.

229. BERLIN, N. I., WALDMANN, T. A. and WEISSMAN, S. M.: Life Span of Red Blood Cell, Physiol. Rev., *39*, 577, 1959.

230. BINGOLD, K.: Uber das Schicksal des Blutfarbstoffes, Artz. Wchnschr., *4*, 225, 1949; Med. Monatschr., *4*, 243, 1949.

231. BOVE, J. R. and EBAUGH, F. G., JR.: The Use of Diisopropylfluorophosphate[32] for the Determination of *In Vivo* Red Cell Survival and Plasma Cholinesterase Turnover Rates, J. Lab. & Clin. Med., *51*, 916, 1958.

233. DEGOWIN, E. L., ELLIS, J. A., SHEETS, R. F., HAMILTON, H. E. and JANNEY, C. D.: Studies with Inagglutinable Erythrocyte Counts. IV. Graphic Analyses of Rates of Production and Destruction of Human Erythrocytes, J. Clin. Invest., *33*, 163, 1954.

233a. DONUHUE, D. M. *et al.*: The Use of Chromium As a Red-Cell Tag, Brit. J. Haemat., *1*, 249, 1955.

234. EADIE, G. S. and BROWN, I. W., JR.: Red Blood Cell Survival Studies, Blood, *8*, 1110, 1953.

234a. EBAUGH, F. G., JR., EMERSON, C. P. and ROSS, J. F.: The Use of Radioactive Chromium 51 as an Erythrocyte Tagging Agent for the Determination of Red Cell Survival *In Vivo*, J. Clin. Invest., *32*, 1260, 1953.

234b. GARBY, L. and NOYES, W. D.: The Kinetic Properties of the Plasma Hemoglobin Pool in Normal Man, J. Clin. Invest., *38*, 1479, 1959; Blut, *6*, 143, 1960.

234c. GIBLETT, ELOISE R. and STEINBERG, A. G.: The Inheritance of Serum Haptoglobin Types in American Negroes: Evidence for a Third Allele Hp[2m], Am. J. Human Genet., *12*, 160, 1960.

235. HURLEY, T. H. and WEISMAN, R., JR.: The Determination of the Survival of Transfused Red Cells by a Method of Differential Hemolysis, J. Clin. Invest., *33*, 835, 1954.

236. JONES, A. R. and SILVER, SHEILA: The Detection of Minor Erythrocyte Populations by Mixed Agglutinates, Blood, *13*, 763, 1958.

236a. LATHEM, W. and WORLEY, W. E.: The Distribution of Extracorpuscular Hemoglobin in Circulating Plasma, J. Clin. Invest., *38*, 474 and 652, 1959.

236b. LAURELL, C-B. and NYMAN, MARGARETA: Studies on the Serum Haptoglobin Level in Hemoglobinemia and Its Influence on Renal Excretion of Hemoglobin, Blood, *12*, 493, 1957.

237. LEMBERG, R. and LEGGE, J. W.: *Hematin Compounds and Bile Pigments*, 1949, New York, Interscience Pub., Inc.

238. MAEGRAITH, B., FINDLAY, G. M. and MARTIN, N. H.: Mechanism of Lysis of Red Blood Cells, Nature, *151*, 252, 1943; Brit. J. Exper. Path., *24*, 58, 1943.

238a. MOLLISON, P. L.: Measurement of Survival and Destruction of Red Cells in Haemolytic Syndromes, Brit. M. Bull., *15*, 59, 1959.

239. MOLLISON, P. L. and VEALL, N.: The Use of the Isotope ^{51}Cr as a Label for Red Cells, Brit. J. Haemat., *1*, 62, 1955; Clin. Sc., *15*, 207, 1956.

240. MUIR, R. and NIVEN, J. S. F.: The Local Formation of Blood Pigments, J. Path. & Bacteriol., *41*, 183, 1935.

240a. NYMAN, MARGARETA: Serum Haptoglobin, Scandinav. J. Clin. & Lab. Invest. (Suppl. 39), *11*, 1, 1959.

240b. NYMAN, N.: On Plasma Proteins with Heme or Hemoglobin Binding Capacity, Scandinav. J. Clin. & Lab. Invest., *12*, 121, 1960.

240c. OWEN, J. A., BETTER, F. C. and HOBAN, J.: A Simple Method for the Determination of Serum Haptoglobins, J. Clin. Path., *13*, 163, 1960.

241. ROUS, P.: Destruction of the Red Blood Cells, Physiol. Rev., *3*, 75, 1923.

242. SHEMIN, D. and RITTENBERG, D.: The Life Span of the Human Red Blood Cell, J. Biol. Chem., *166*, 627, 1946.

243. SINGER, K. and WEISZ, L.: The Life Cycle of the Erythrocyte after Splenectomy and the Problems of Splenic Hemolysis and Target Cell Formation, Am. J. M. Sc., *210*, 301, 1945; J. Lab. & Clin. Med., *30*, 784, 1945.

244. SMITHIES, O.: Zone Electrophoresis in Starch Gels: Group Variations in the Serum Proteins of Normal Human Adults, Biochem. J., *61*, 629, 1955; Nature, *178*, 694, 1956; Biochem. J., *72*, 115, 1959.

246. WILLENEGGER, H.: Fate of Transfused Erythrocytes, Helv. med. acta, *9*, 15, 1942.

The Breakdown of Hemoglobin

247. ISSELBACHER, K. J. and McCARTHY, ELIZABETH A.: Studies on Bilirubin Sulfate and

Other Nonglucuronide Conjugates of Bilirubin, J. Clin. Invest., *38*, 645, 1959.

248. LATHE, G. H.: The Chemical Pathology of Bile Pigments, Biochemical Society Symposia, No. 12, p. 34, 1954; Biochem. J., *65*, 774, 1957; Am. J. Med., *24*, 111, 1958.

249. LONDON, I. M., WEST, R., SHEMIN, D. and RITTENBERG, D.: On the Origin of Bile Pigment in Normal Man, J. Biol. Chem., *184*, 351 and 373, 1950.

250. LOWRY, P. T., ZIEGLER, N. R., CARDINAL, R. and WATSON, C. J.: The Conversion of N^{15} Labeled Mesobilirubinogen to Stercobilinogen by Fecal Bacteria, J. Biol. Chem., *208*, 543, 1954; Trans. Assoc. Am. Phys., *67*, 242, 1954.

251. MILLS, S. D. and MASON, H. L.: Values for Fecal Urobilinogen in Childhood, Am. J. Dis. Childhood, *84*, 322, 1952.

251a. POLITZER, W. M. and KESSEL, I.: Normal Faecal Porphyrin Values in Babies, J. Clin. Path., *11*, 183, 1958.

252. SCHMID, R.: Some Aspects of Bile Pigment Metabolism, Clin. Chem. (Suppl.), *3*, 394, 1957; Bull. New York Acad. Med., *35*, 755, 1959.

253. SCHWARTZ, S. and WIKOFF, H. M.: The Relation of Erythrocyte Coproporphyrin and Protoporphyrin to Erythropoiesis, J. Biol. Chem., *194*, 563, 1952.

254. WATSON, C. J. and LARSON, E. A.: The Urinary Coproporphyrins in Health and Disease, Physiol. Rev., *27*, 478, 1947 (Bibliography).

255. WATSON, C. J., HAWKINSON, V., CAPPS, R. B. and RAPPAPORT, E. M.: Studies of Coproporphyrin I and IV, J. Clin. Invest., *28*, 447, 1949.

256. WATSON, C. J.: The Bile Pigments, New England J. Med., *227*, 665 and 705, 1942; Ann. Int. Med., *47*, 611, 1957.

256a. WATSON, C. J.: Composition of the Urobilin Group in Urine, Bile and Feces, and the Significance of Variations in Health and Disease, J. Lab. & Clin. Med., *54*, 1, 1959.

256b. WRANNE, L.: Free Erythrocyte Copro- and Protoporphyrin, Acta paediat. (Suppl. 124), *49*, 5, 1960.

257. ZIEVE, L., HILL, E., SCHWARTZ, S. and WATSON, C. J.: Normal Limits of Urinary Coproporphyrin Excretion Determined by an Improved Method, J. Lab. & Clin. Med., *41*, 663, 1953.

Disturbances in Pigment Metabolism and Abnormal Pigments

258. BAIKIE, A. G. and VALTIS, D. J.: Gas Transport Function of the Blood in Congenital Familial Methaemoglobinaemia, Brit. M. J., *2*, 73, 1954.

259. BANCROFT, H., GIBSON, Q. H., HARRISON, D. C. and McMURRAY, J.: Familial Idiopathic Methaemoglobinaemia and Its Treatment with Ascorbic Acid. Clin. Sc., *5*, 145, 1945; Biochem. J., *42*, 13, 1948.

260. BECK, H. G., SCHULZE, W. H. and SUTER, G. M.: Carbon Monoxide—A Domestic Hazard, J.A.M.A., *115*, 1, 1940.

260a. BETKE, K., GRÖSCHNER, E. and BOCK, K.: Properties of a Further Variant of Haemoglobin M, Nature, *188*, 864, 1960.

261. CODOUNIS, A., LOUCATOS, G. and LOUTSIDES, E.: Hereditary Methemoglobinemic Cyanosis, Sang, *19*, 65, 1948; *ibid.*, *20*, 195, 1949; Brit. Med. J., *2*, 368, 1952; Sem. d. hôp. Paris, *28*, 3876, 1952; Vie Méd., *37*, 19, 1955; Acta genet. statist. med., *7*, 131, 1957.

262. COMFORT, A., MOORE, H. and WEATHERALL, M.: Normal Human Urinary Porphyrins, Biochem. J., *58*, 177, 1954.

263. DARLING, R. C. and ROUGHTON, F. J. W.: The Effect of Methemoglobin on the Equilibrium Between Oxygen and Hemoglobin, Am. J. Physiol., *137*, 56, 1942.

264. DE GASPERIS, A., DONATELLI, R. and ROVELLI, F.: Congenital Cyanosis Due to Methemoglobinemia, Minerva med., *44*, 664, 1953.

265. DEPREE, H. E. and HICKMAN, M. J.: Familial Congenital Methemoglobinemia, Ann. Int. Med., *51*, 1078, 1959.

266. FAIRLEY, N. H.: Methæmalbumin, Quart. J. Med., *10*, 95, 1941.

267. FINCH, C. A.: Methemoglobinemia and Sulfhemoglobinemia, New England J. Med., *239*, 470, 1948; J. Clin. Invest., *28*, 265, 1949.

268. GERALD, P. S., COOK, C. D. and DIAMOND, L. K.: Hemoglobin M, Science, *126*, 300, 1957; Blood, *13*, 936, 1958; Science, *129*, 393, 1959.

268a. GOLUBOFF, N. and WHEATON, R.: Methylene Blue Induced Cyanosis and Acute Hemolytic Anemia Complicating the Treatment of Methemoglobinemia, J. Pediat., *58*, 86, 1961.

268b. HÖRLEIN, A. and WEBER, G.: Über chronische familiäre Methämoglobinämie und eine neue Modifikation des Methämoglobins, Deutsche med. Wchnschr., *735*, 476, 1948.

269. MARCUS, H. and JOFFE, J. R.: Nitrate Methemoglobinemia, New England J. Med., *240*, 599, 1949.

270. MAYERS, M. R.: Carbon Monoxide Poisoning in Industry and Its Prevention, New York State Department of Labor, Albany, N. Y., 1938, Special Bulletin No. 194.

270a. McCUTCHEON, A. D.: Sulphaemoglobinemia and Glutathione, Lancet, *2*, 240, 1960.

271. MICHEL, H. O.: A Study of Sulfhemoglobin, J. Biol. Chem., *126*, 323, 1938.

272. MILLER, A. A.: Congenital Sulfhemoglobinemia, J. Pediat., *51*, 233, 1957.

272a. NEWCOMBE, C. P. and DAWSON, J.: Two Cases of Congenital Methaemoglobinaemia, Brit. M. J., *1*, 1396, 1958.

272b. ORGERON, J. D. *et al.*: Methemoglobinemia from Eating Meat with High Nitrite Content, Pub. Health Rep., *72*, 189, 1957.

273. PISCIOTTA, A. V., EBBE, SHIRLEY N. and HINZ, JEAN E.: Clinical and Laboratory Features of Two Variants of Methemoglobin M Disease, J. Lab. & Clin. Med., *54*, 73, 1959.

273a. PASS, I. J., SCHWARTZ, S. and WATSON, C. J.: The Conversion of Hematin to Bilirubin Following Intravenous Administration in Human Subjects, J. Clin. Invest., *24*, 283, 1945.

274. REYNOLDS, T. B. and WARE, A. G.: Sulfhemoglobinemia following Habitual Use of Acetanilid, J. A. M. A., *149*, 1538, 1952.

274a. ROSS, JEAN D. and DESFORGES, JANE F.: Reduction of Methemoglobin by Erythrocytes from Cord Blood, Pediatrics, *23*, 718, 1959.

274b. ROSSI-FANELLI, A., ANTONINI, E. and MONDOVI, B.: Ferrihemoglobin Reduction in Normal and Methemoglobinemia Subjects, Clin. chim. acta, *2*, 476, 1957.

275. SCOTT, E. M. and HOSKINS, D. D.: Hereditary Methemoglobinemia in Alaskan Eskimos and Indians, Blood, *13*, 795, 1958; J. Clin. Invest., *39*, 1176, 1960.

The Porphyrias

276. ALDRICH, R. A., HAWKINSON, V., GRINSTEIN, M. and WATSON, C. J.: Photosensitive or Congenital Porphyria with Hemolytic Anemia, Blood, *6*, 685, 1951.

276a. AMOROSO, E. C., LOOSMORE, R. M., RIMINGTON, C. and TOOTH, B. E.: Congenital Porphyria in Bovines: First Living Cases in Britain, Nature, *180*, 230, 1957.

276b. BARNES, H. D.: The Excretion of Porphyrins and Porphyrin Precursors by Bantu Cases of Porphyria, South African M. J., *33*, 274, 1959.

277. BRUNSTING, L. A.: Observations on Porphyria Cutanea Tarda, Arch. Dermat. and Syph., *70*, 551, 1954.

277a. CANIVET, J. and PELNARD-CONSIDÈRE, M.: Etude de l'hémolyse dans deux cas de porphyrie congénitale, Rev. franç. étud. clin. et biol., *3*, 27, 1958.

277b. CORNBLEET, T.: Cutaneous Appearance of Porphyria by Ultraviolet Light, A. M. A. Arch. Dermat., *73*, 34, 1956.

278. DAVIS, M. J. and VANDER PLOEG, D. E.: Acute Porphyria and Coproporphyrinuria following Chloroquine Therapy, A. M. A. Arch. Dermat., *75*, 796, 1957.

279. DEAN, G.: Porphyria, a Familial Disease, South African M. J., *30*, 377, 1956; *ibid.*, *33*, 246, 1959.

279a. DOBRINER, K. and RHOADS, C. P.: The Porphyrins in Health and Disease, Physiol. Rev., *20*, 416, 1940.

279b. GALAMBOS, J. T. and DOWDA, F. W.: Lead Poisoning and Porphyria, Am. J. Med., *27*, 803, 1959.

280. GIBSON, J. B. and GOLDBERG, A.: The Neuropathology of Acute Porphyria, J. Path. & Bact., *71*, 495, 1956.

280a. GOLDBERG, A.: Acute Intermittent Porphyria, Quart. J. Med., *28*, 183, 1959.

281. HAEGER, BIRGITTA: Urinary δ-Aminolaevulic Acid and Porphobilinogen in Different Types of Porphyria, Lancet, *2*, 606, 1958.

281a. HOLTI, G., RIMINGTON, C., TATE, B. C. and THOMAS, G.: An Investigation of 'Porphyria Cutanea Tarda,' Quart. J. Med., *27*, 1, 1958.

281b. LEVIT, EDITHE J., NODINE, J. H. and PERLOFF, W. H.: Progesterone-Induced Porphyria, Am. J. Med., *22*, 831, 1957.

281c. MAGNUS, I. A., PORTER, A. D. and RIMINGTON, C.: The Action Spectrum for Skin Lesions in Porphyria Cutanea Tarda, Lancet, *1*, 912, 1959.

281d. PETERS, H. A., WOODS, S., EICHMAN, P. L. and REESE, H. H.: The Treatment of Porphyria with Chelating Agents, Ann. Int. Med., *47*, 889, 1957.

282. RIMINGTON, C.: Haems and Porphyrins in Health and Disease. II. Acta med. Scandinav., *143*, 177, 1952; Arch. Int. Med., *90*, 483, 1952; Biochem. J., *55*, 109 and 867, 1953.

282a. SCHMID, R.: Cutaneous Porphyria in Turkey, New England J. Med., *263*, 397, 1960.

283. SCHMID, R., SCHWARTZ, S. and WATSON, C. J.: Porphyrin Content of Bone Marrow and Liver in the Various Forms of Porphyria, Arch. Int. Med., *93*, 167, 1954; Blood, *10*, 416, 1955.

284. SCHWARTZ, S., KEPRIOS, M. and SCHMID, R.: Experimental Porphyria, Proc. Soc. Exper. Biol. & Med., *79*, 463, 1952; *ibid.*, *81*, 685, 1952; J. Biol. Chem., *217*, 263, 1955.

285. SMITH, J. A. and FRUMIN, A. M.: Paroxysmal Nocturnal Porphyrinuria, New England J. Med., *255*, 705, 1956.

285a. TIO, T. H., LEIJNSE, B., JARRETT, A. and RIMINGTON, C.: Acquired Porphyria from a Liver Tumour, Clin. Sc., *16*, 517, 1957.

285b. TOWNSEND-COLES, W. F. and BARNES, H. D.: Erythropoietic (Congenital) Porphyria, Lancet, *2*, 271, 1957.

285c. TURNER, W. J.: Studies on Porphyria, J. Biol. Chem., *118*, 519, 1937; Arch. Dermat. & Syphilol., *37*, 549, 1938.

286. VARADI, S.: Haematological Aspects in a Case of Erythropoietic Porphyria, Brit. J. Haemat., *4*, 270, 1958.

287. WALDENSTRÖM, J.: The Porphyrias as Inborn Errors of Metabolism, Am. J. Med., *22*, 758, 1957.

288. WATSON, C. J.: The Problem of Porphyria, New England J. Med., *263*, 1205, 1960.

288a. WATSON, C. J., BERG, M. H., HAWKINSON, V. E. and BOSSENMAIER, IRENE: Studies of the Uroporphyrins, Clin. Chem., *6*, 71, 1960.

288b. WATSON, C. J.: Some Studies of the Comparative Biology of Human and Bovine Porphyria Erythropoietica, Tr. A. Am. Physicians, *71*, 196, 1958.

289. WATSON, C. J. and SCHWARTZ, S.: A Simple Test for Urinary Porphobilinogen, Proc. Soc. Exper. Biol. & Med., *47*, 393, 1941; *see also* J. Lab. & Clin. Med., *33*, 1254, 1948; Arch. Int. Med., *93*, 643, 1954.

290. ZELIGMAN, I. and BAUM, M.: Porphyric Bullous Dermatosis, Arch. Dermat. and Syphilol., *58*, 357, 1948.

Evidences of Exaggerated Red Cell Destruction

292. CROSBY, W. H.: The Metabolism of Hemoglobin and Bile Pigment in Hemolytic Disease, Am. J. Med., *18*, 112, 1955; Blood, *11*, 380, 1956.

293. DUCCI, H. and WATSON, C. J.: The Quantitative Determination of the Serum Bilirubin with Special Reference to the Prompt-Reacting and the Chloroform-Soluble Types, J. Lab. & Clin. Med., *30*, 293, 1945.

294. HAYFORD, W. D. and WAISBREN, B. A.: Effect of Simultaneous Oral Administration of Aureomycin and Aluminum Hydroxide Gel on Fecal Urobilinogen, Surgery, *31*, 361, 1952.

295. JOHNSON, THELMA R.: An Improvement of the Method for Determination of Plasma and Urine Hemoglobin, J. Lab. & Clin. Med., *53*, 495, 1959.

297. MILLER, E. B., SINGER, K. and DAMESHEK, W.: Use of the Daily Fecal Output of Urobilinogen and the Hemolytic Index in the Measurement of Hemolysis, Arch. Int. Med., *70*, 722, 1942.

298. TISDALE, W. A., KLATSKIN, G. and KINSELLA, E. D.: The Significance of the Direct-Reacting Fraction of Serum Bilirubin in Hemolytic Jaundice, Am. J. Med., *26*, 214, 1959.

299. VAUGHAN, J. M. and HASLEWOOD, G. A. D.: The Normal Level of Plasma Bilirubin, Lancet, *1*, 133, 1938.

300. VOEGTLIN, W. L., MOSS, M. H. and MARCH, E.: A Comparison of the Quantitative Urine Urobilinogen Determination with the Urine Ehrlich Test, Gastroenterology, *14*, 538, 1950.

301. WATSON, C. J.: Studies of Urobilinogen, Am. J. Clin. Path., *6*, 458, 1936; Arch. Int. Med., *59*, 196 and 206, 1937; *ibid., 68*, 740, 1941.

302. WATSON, C. J., SCHWARTZ, S., SBOROV, V. and BERTIE, E.: A Simple Method for the Quantitative Recording of the Ehrlich Reaction as Carried Out with Urine and Feces, Am. J. Clin. Path., *14*, 598 and 605, 1944; *ibid., 17*, 108, 1947.

303. WILBUR, R. L. and ADDIS, T.: Urobilin: Its Clinical Significance, Arch. Int. Med., *13*, 235, 1914.

304. YOUNG, L. E., DAVIS, R. W. and HOGESTYN, J.: Simplified Equipment for Determination of Urobilinogen in Urine and Stool, J. Lab. & Clin. Med., *34*, 287, 1949.

Agglutination and Hemolysis of Red Corpuscles

306. BARR, D. P., READER, G. G. and WHEELER, C. H.: Cryoglobulinemia, Ann. Int. Med., *32*, 6, 1950.

308. BOLTON, J. H.: The Distribution Curve of Erythrocyte Fragility, Blood, *4*, 172, 1949.

309. CASTLE, W. B. and DALAND, G. A.: Susceptibility of Mammalian Erythrocytes to Hemolysis with Hypotonic Solutions, Arch. Int. Med., *60*, 949, 1937.

310. CRAWFORD, H., CUTBUSH, M. and MOLLISON, P. L.: Specificity of Incomplete "Cold" Antibody in Human Serum, Lancet, *1*, 566, 1953.

312. DACIE, J. V. and VAUGHAN, J. M.: The Fragility of the Red Blood Cells: Its Measurement and Significance, J. Path. and Bacteriol., *46*, 341, 1938.

313. DALAND, G. and WORTHLEY, K.: The Resistance of Red Blood Cells to Hemolysis in Hypotonic Solutions of Sodium Chloride—Observations in Blood Disorders, J. Lab. & Clin. Med., *20*, 1122, 1935.

314. FINLAND, M., PETERSON, O. L., ALLEN, H. E. and SAMPER, B. A.: Cold Agglutinins, J. Clin. Invest., *24*, 451, 1945.

315. GUEST, G. M. and WING, M.: A Method for the Determination of Erythrocyte Fragility, Using Van Allen Hematocrit Tubes for the Measurement of Changes in Volume of the Cells in Hypotonic Salt Solutions, J. Lab. & Clin. Med., *24*, 850, 1939.

316. ———: Osmometric Behavior of Normal Human Erythrocytes, J. Clin. Invest., *21*, 257, 1942; Blood, *3*, 541, 1948.

317. HADEN, R. L.: The Mechanism of the Increased Fragility of the Erythrocytes in

Congenital Hemolytic Jaundice, Am. J. M. Sc., *188*, 441, 1934.

317a.HAM, T. H.: A Syllabus of Laboratory Examinations in Clinical Diagnosis, Harvard Univ. Press, Cambridge, Mass., 1950, p. 161; Arch. Int. Med., *97*, 1, 1956.

318. HUNTER, F. T.: A Photoelectric Method for the Quantitative Determination of Erythrocyte Fragility, J. Clin. Invest., *19*, 691, 1940.

319. JACOBS, M. H., STEWART, D. R., BROWN, W. J. and KIMMELMAN, L. J.: An Improved Method for the Detection of Osmotic Abnormalities of Erythrocytes, Am. J. M. Sc., *217*, 47, 1949.

319a.JAFFÉ, E. R. *et al.*: The Effects of Nucleosides on the Resistance of Normal Human Erythrocytes to Osmotic Lysis, J. Clin. Invest., *36*, 1498, 1957.

320. JOHNSON, V., FREEMAN, L. W. and LONGINI, J.: Erythrocyte Damage by Lipemic Serum in Normal Man and in Pernicious Anemia, J.A.M.A., *124*, 1250, 1944.

320a.MARKS, PAUL A. and JOHNSON, ANNE B.: Relationship between the Age of Human Erythrocytes and Their Osmotic Resistance; a Basis for Separating Young and Old Erythrocytes, J. Clin. Invest., *37*, 1542, 1958.

321. MARSHALL, R. J., SHEPHERD, J. T. and THOMPSON, I. D.: Vascular Responses in Patients with High Serum Titres of Cold Agglutinins, Clin. Sci., *12*, 255, 1953; Brit. M. J., *2*, 314, 1953.

322. PARPART, A. K., LORENZ, P. B., PARPART, E. R., GREGG, J. R. and CHASE, A. M.: The Osmotic Resistance of Human Red Cells, J. Clin. Invest., *26*, 636, 1947.

323. PONDER, E.: *Hemolysis and Related Phenomena,* 1948, New York, Grune and Stratton.

324. SCHUBOTHE, H. and FOK, F. P.: The Quantitative Estimation of Mechanical Haemolysis for Clinical Application, Brit. J. Haemat., *6*, 350, 1960.

325. SINGER, K.: The Lysolecithin Fragility Test, Am. J. M. Sc., *199*, 466, 1940. *See also* Helv. med. acta, *14*, 470, 1947.

326. STATS, D. and WASSERMAN, L. R.: Cold Hemagglutination, Medicine, *22*, 363, 1943.

327. STEWART, W. B., STEWART, J. M., IZZO, M. J. and YOUNG, L. E.: Age as Affecting the Osmotic and Mechanical Fragility of Dog Erythrocytes Tagged with Radioactive Iron, J. Exper. Med., *91*, 147, 1950.

328. SWANK, R. L. and ROTH, E. S.: Hemolysis and Alimentary Lipemia, Blood, *9*, 348, 1954.

329. TATENO, I. and KILBOURNE, E. D.: Hemo-

lytic Activity of Diethylstilbestrol and Some Steroid Hormones, Proc. Soc. Exper. Biol. & Med., *86*, 168, 1954.

330. WHITBY, L. E. H. and HYNES, M.: The Quantitative Estimation of the Fragility of the Red Corpuscles, J. Path. & Bact., *40*, 219, 1935.

330a.WILLIAMS, T. F., FORDHAM, C. C., III, HOLLANDER, W., JR. and WELT, L. G.: A Study of the Osmotic Behavior of the Human Erythrocyte, J. Clin. Invest., *38*, 1587, 1959.

Abnormal Hemoglobins

331. ALLEN, D. W., SCHROEDER, W. A. and BALOG, JOAN: Observations on the Chromatographic Heterogeneity of Normal Adult and Fetal Human Hemoglobin, J. Am. Chem. Soc., *80*, 1628, 1958.

331a.BAGLIONI, C.: Chemistry of Hemoglobin Norfolk, Fed. Proc., *20*, 254, 1961.

332. BEAVEN, G. H. and GRATZER, W. B.: A Critical Review of Human Haemoglobin Variants, J. Clin. Path., *12*, 1 and 101, 1959.

333. BENZER, S., INGRAM, V. M. and LEHMANN, H.: Three Varieties of Human Haemoglobin D, Nature, *182*, 852, 1958.

333a.BRAUNITZER, G., LIEBOLD, BRIGITTE, MÜLLER, RENATE and RUDLOFF, V.: Der homologe chemische Aufbau der Peptidketten im Humanhämoglobin A, Ztschr. f. physiol. chem., *320*, 170 and 283, 1960; *ibid*, *322*, 96, 1960.

333b.BRENNER, S.: The Mechanism of Gene Action, *in Biochemistry of Human Genetics*, G. E. W. Wolstenholme, Editor, Boston, Little, Brown & Co., 1959.

334. CHERNOFF, A. I.: Immunologic Studies of Hemoglobins, Blood, *8*, 399, 1953; New England J. Med., *253*, 322, 365 and 416, 1955; *in* Conference on Hemoglobin, National Academy of Sciences, National Research Council, Publication No. 557, Washington, 1958, p. 179.

334a.DHERTE, P., LEHMANN, H. and VANDEPITTE, J.: Haemoglobin P in a Family in the Belgian Congo, Nature, *184*, 1133, 1959.

334b.GERALD, P. S. and ETRON, MARY: Personal communication.

334c.GUIDOTTI, G.: The Action of Carboxypeptidases A and B in the Separated α and β Chains of Normal Adult Hemoglobin, Biochim. et biophys. acta, *42*, 177, 1960.

334d.HILL, R. J. and KOENIGSBERG, W.: The Partial Structural Formula of the Alpha Chain of Human Hemoglobin, J. Biol. Chem., *236*, 7 p, 1961.

335. HILL, R. L.: Methods for the Structural

Analysis of the Human Hemoglobins, Lab. Invest. (to be published).

335a.————: Personal communication.

336. HILL, R. L. and SCHWARTZ, H. C.: A Chemical Abnormality in Haemoglobin G, Nature, *184*, 641, 1959; J. Biol. Chem., *235*, 3182, 1960.

337. HUISMAN, T. H. J., MARTIS, E. A. and DOZY, ANDREE: Chromatography of Hemoglobin Types on Carboxymethylcellulose, J. Lab. & Clin. Med., *52*, 312, 1958; Clin. chim. acta, *5*, 103, 1960.

337a.HUNT, J. A.: Identity of the α-Chains of Adult and Foetal Human Haemoglobins, Nature, *183*, 1373, 1959.

338. HUNT, J. A. and INGRAM, V. M.: Allelomorphism and the Chemical Differences of the Human Haemoglobins A, S and C, Nature, *181*, 1062, 1958.

339. HUNT, J. A. and INGRAM, V. M.: A Terminal Peptide Sequence of Human Haemoglobin? Nature, *184*, 640, 1959.

340. HUNT, J. A. and INGRAM, V. M.: Human Haemoglobin E: the Chemical Effect of Gene Mutation, Nature, *184*, 870, 1959.

340a.HUNT, J. A. and LEHMANN, H.: Haemoglobin 'Bart's': a Foetal Haemoglobin without α-Chains, Nature, *184*, 872, 1959.

341. INGRAM, V. M.: A Specific Chemical Difference between the Globins of Normal Human and Sickle-Cell Anemia Hemoglobin, Nature, *178*, 792, 1956.

342. INGRAM, V. M.: Gene Mutations in Human Haemoglobin: the Chemical Difference between Normal and Sickle Cell Haemoglobin, Nature, *180*, 326, 1957.

343. INGRAM, V. M.: Comparison of Normal Human and Sickle Cell Hemoglobins by fingerprinting, Biochim. et biophys. acta, *28*, 539, 1958.

343a.ITANO, H.: Human Hemoglobins, Properties and Genetic Composition, Advances in Protein Chemistry, *12*, 213, 1957.

344. ITANO, H. A. and ROBINSON, ELIZABETH: Formation of Normal and Doubly Abnormal Haemoglobins by Recombination of Haemoglobin I with S and C, Nature, *183*, 1799, 1959.

345. ITANO, H. A. and ROBINSON, ELIZABETH: Properties and Inheritance of Haemoglobin by Asymmetric Recombination, Nature, *184*, 1468, 1959.

345a. JONES, R. T. and SCHROEDER, W. A.: Personal communication.

346. JONES, R. T., SCHROEDER, W. A., BALOG, J. E. and VINOGRAD, J. R.: Gross Structure of Hemoglobin H, J. Am. Chem. Soc., *81*, 3161, 1959.

346a.JONES, R. T., SCHROEDER, W. A. and VINOGRAD, J. R.: Identity of the α Chains of Hemoglobins A and F, J. Am. Chem. Soc., *81*, 4749, 1959.

347. KUNKEL, H. G. and WALLENIUS, G.: New Hemoglobin in Normal Adult Blood, Science, *122*, 288, 1955.

349. MURAYAMA, M. and INGRAM, V. M.: Comparison of Normal Adult Human Haemoglobin with Haemoglobin I by 'Fingerprinting,' Nature, *183*, 1798, 1959; Fed. Proc., *19*, 78, 1960.

349a.Nomenclature of Abnormal Hemoglobins, Report, Blood, *17*, 125, 1961.

350. PAULING, LINUS: Abnormality of Hemoglobin Molecules in Hereditary Hemolytic Anemias, The Harvey Lectures, 1955, New York, Academic Press, Inc., p. 216.

351. RHINESMITH, H. S., SCHROEDER, W. A. and PAULING, L.: The N-Terminal Residues of Normal Adult Human Hemoglobin, J. Am. Chem. Soc., *79*, 609 and 4682, 1957.

352. ROSSI-FANELLI, A., DE MARCO, C., BENEREDETTI, A. S. and GRACCI, L.: Amino Acid Composition of Hemoglobin A₂, Biochim. et biophys. acta, *38*, 380, 1960.

354. SCHROEDER, W. A. and MATSUDA, GENJI: N-Terminal Residues of Human Fetal Hemoglobin, J. Am. Chem. Soc., *80*, 1521, 1958.

355. SCHWARTZ, H. C. *et al.*: Combinations of Hemoglobin G, Hemoglobin S and Thalassemia Occurring in One Family, Blood, *12*, 238, 1957.

356. SHELTON, J. E. and SCHROEDER, W. A.: Further N-Terminal Sequences in Human Hemoglobins A, S and F by Edman's Phenylthiohydantoin Method, J. Am. Chem. Soc., *82*, 3342, 1960.

357. SINGER, K., CHERNOFF, A. I. and SINGER, L.: Studies on Abnormal Hemoglobins. I. Their Demonstration in Sickle Cell Anemia and Other Hematologic Disorders by Means of Alkali Denaturation, Blood, *6*, 413 and 429, 1951; *in* Conference on Hemoglobin, National Academy of Sciences, National Research Council, Washington, Publication No. 557, 1958, p. 172.

358. STRETTON, A. O. W. and INGRAM, V. M.: An Amino Acid Difference between Human Hemoglobins A and A₂, Fed. Proc., *19*, 343, 1960.

360. VINOGRAD, J. R., HUTCHINSON, W. D. and SCHROEDER, W. A.: C¹⁴-Hybrids of Human Hemoglobins, J. Am. Chem. Soc., *81*, 3168, 1959.

Chapter 4

The Leukocytes

DESCRIPTION OF THE LEUKOCYTES

THE various theories concerning the origin and relationship of the cells of the blood have been discussed already in Chapter 1. Whatever views may be held concerning the interrelationship of the lymphocytes, the myeloid or granular leukocytes and the monocytes, it is clear that at least the more mature forms of these three series of cells can be distinguished readily from one another in the circulating blood. In the following pages these cells will be described and their significance considered.

The Myeloid Series

The Myeloblast.—The term myeloblast is applied to an immature cell not normally found in the circulating blood which gives rise to myelocytes and granulocytes and, according to certain hematologists, to other types of cells as well. Sabin and her school use the term in the restricted sense (Fig. 1–4, p. 38). Downey[12] and others regard the myeloblast as giving rise to monocytes, normoblasts, and megakaryocytes as well as to myelocytes and, under pathological conditions, even lymphocytes (Fig. 1–3, p. 37). In the latter sense the myeloblast corresponds to the **lymphoidocyte of Pappenheim** and the **hemocytoblast of Ferrata.**[12] It differs, however, from the **hemocytoblast of Maximow, Bloom** and **Jordan.**[42a]

The myeloblast (Plate V, 1, and Fig. 4–1, 1 to 4) possesses a relatively large nucleus, round or slightly oval in shape, and a small amount of cytoplasm. In preparations stained with Wright's stain, the nuclear membrane is smooth and even in outline and exceedingly thin, with no condensation of chromatin near its inner surface as in lymphoblasts. The chromatin shows an even, diffuse distribution with no aggregation into larger masses, although there may be some condensation about the nucleoli. The chromatin may appear in the form of very fine strands, thus giving the nucleus a sieve-like appearance; or it may be in the form of fine dust-like granules, producing a uniform stippled effect. There are, generally, from two to five nucleoli, pale sky-blue in color. It has been claimed that a large number of nucleoli favors the myeloblast as against the lymphoblast, but this has been disputed. The cytoplasm is basophilic (blue) and generally, although not invariably, there is no clear zone about the nucleus. Sometimes the cytoplasm is reticular, spongy or foamy. Sabin restricted the term "myeloblast" to cells without granulation but others extend the name to what may be slightly more mature forms, namely, those with several, rather large, angular, irregular and dark-staining azurophilic granules in the cytoplasm.

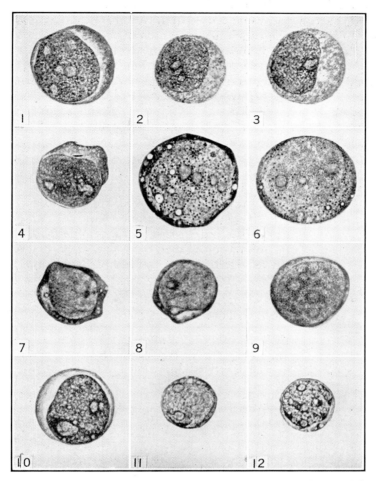

Fig. 4–1.—Myeloblasts, myelocytes, and lymphoblasts. From Pappenheim's Atlas, and Downey. Photographs of colored drawings. *1, 2, 3* and *4* are myeloblasts from cases of myeloblastic leukemia. In *4* there is an Auer body. *5* and *6* are promyelocytes from human marrow. *7* and *8* are very immature lymphoid cells (lymphoblasts) from a lymph node of a newly born rabbit. *9, 10, 11* and *12* are "lymphoblasts" from cases of acute lymphoblastic leukemia. (Cowdry's Special Cytology, courtesy of Paul B. Hoeber, Inc.)

In wet films (Fig. 4–2) these cells appear immobile, with thin, tenacious borders. The cytoplasm is hazy and usually contains no stainable substance except mitochondria. These are extremely fine or slender threads or commas or small spherical bodies staining brilliant blue-green with Janus green and diffusely scattered throughout the cytoplasm.

The failure of myeloblasts to move in supravital preparations is probably caused by the nature of the preparation itself rather than due to immobility of these cells. In motion picture studies of myeloblasts in hanging drop preparations, Rich, Wintrobe and Lewis[37] found that myeloblasts possessed a characteristic snail-like movement which served to distinguish these cells from lymphoblasts (Figs. 4–3 and 4–4). De Bruyn[10], however, questioned the significance of this observation. Studying cells from rabbit lymph nodes and marrow and using only a slightly different technic, he concluded that both lymphocytes and hemocytoblasts (myeloblasts) present the general shape of a "hand mirror" when moving on a flat surface and assume a "worm-like" motion when moving inside the plasma clot. He attributed "constriction rings" in moving leukocytes to external factors in the culture medium.

Since they are in the process of growth and division, myeloblasts vary in size (10 to 20 μ). Mitosis is sometimes observed. Particularly in acute leukemia, the nucleus may show several wide and deep indentations suggesting lobulation. Such myeloblasts are known as **Rieder** cells,[12] which may represent a more rapid maturation on the part of the nucleus as compared with the cytoplasm (asynchronism of Di Guglielmo). In the same condition **Auer bodies** (p. 935) may be found in the cytoplasm of some myeloblasts (Fig. 4–1, *4*). These are large granules, globules or slender rods of azurophilic substance. The **Türk irrita-cell** is one resembling a plasma cell but retaining the nuclear pattern of the myeloblast.[32] It may be added that the terms "Rieder cell" and "Türk cell" have been interpreted in different ways by various workers. Rather than being related to myeloblasts, as implied above, they have been regarded as the result of the atypical maturation of hemocyto-

---

LEGEND FOR PLATE VI.

NORMAL AND ABNORMAL WHITE CORPUSCLES

1 to 13—*Myeloid series.* 1 to 11 are arranged in order of maturity.

1. Myeloblast. The nuclear chromatin is very fine, there is only a faint nuclear membrane, and the nucleus contains 6 nucleoli. The cytoplasm is deeply basophilic and contains no granules.

2 to 6. Myelocytes, in order of maturity. 2, which some writers would call a myeloblast and others a promyelocyte or myelocyte "A," differs from 1 only in that there are a few granules in the cytoplasm; 3 and 4 are also spoken of as promyelocytes, or as myelocytes "B" because their cytoplasm contains a moderate number of granules. In 4 a few granules are seen overlying the nucleus which is becoming less distinct than that of myeloblasts and very young myelocytes. 5 and 6 represent the typical "differentiated" neutrophilic myelocyte or myelocyte "C"—there are many granules in an abundant cytoplasm, and the nucleus is relatively indistinct and has the appearance of lying deep in the cell.

7 and 8. Metamyelocytes, or "juveniles." The nucleus has again become distinct; the basichromatin is more compact than in the younger cells of this series.

9, 10, 11. Polymorphonuclear neutrophils with two, three and nine segments respectively. 11 represents the giant, multilobed neutrophil which is most commonly seen in pernicious anemia in relapse.

12. Basophil. The granules are characteristically very large and bluish-black in color. The nucleus is not readily distinguished.

13. Eosinophil. The granules are numerous, large, uniform in size and brick-red in color.

14. Portion of a megakaryocyte found in the blood.

15. Degenerated nucleus, a so-called "basket-cell."

16 to 21—*Lymphocytes.*

16. Lymphoblast. The nuclear chromatin is fine and somewhat stippled. There is a distinct membrane about the nucleus and around the three nucleoli, and there is more of a tendency for the chromatin to clump than in the myeloblast. The cytoplasm is deeply basophilic.

17 to 21. Mature lymphocytes. The nuclear chromatin is more compact than that of the lymphoblast and there are no nucleoli. There is a fine perinuclear clear zone in some of the cells. The cytoplasm is deeply basophilic in 17 but quite pale in the others. Azurophilic granules are seen in several of the cells. The light areas in the nucleus of 19 should not be confused with nucleoli.

22 to 25—*Monocytes.* The nuclear chromatin is quite fine and strand-like and thus differs from that of the myeloid and lymphocytic series of cells. The cytoplasm is slate gray and contains many fine, lilac or reddish-blue azure granules.

PLATE VI

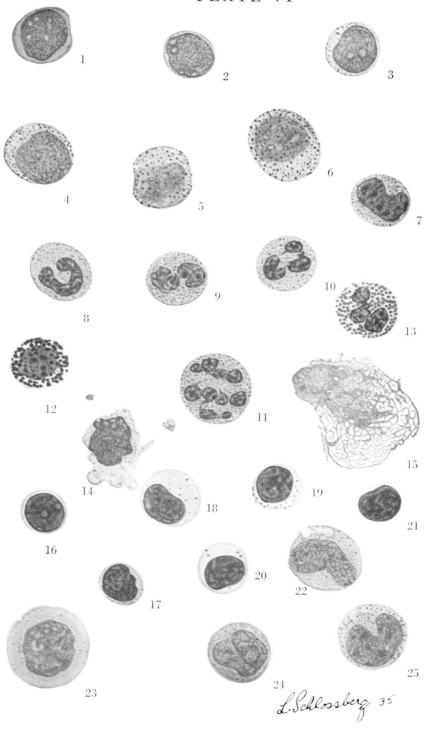

L. Schlossberg 35

NORMAL AND ABNORMAL WHITE CORPUSCLES

(WRIGHT'S STAIN. 1 MM. = 1 μ)

(Wintrobe, Tice Practice of Medicine, courtesy of W. F. Prior Company.)

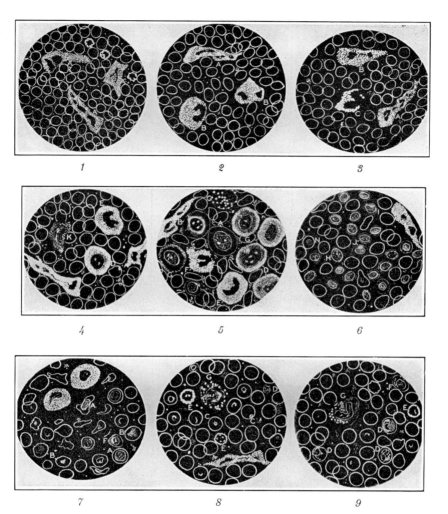

Fig. 4–2.—Camera lucida drawings of fresh (human) blood preparations as seen by dark-ground illumination. In *1, 2* and *3* adult myeloid granulocytes are shown in various phases of motion; *A*, neutrophilic leukocyte; *B*, eosinophil; *C*, basophil. In *4, 5* and *6, A* and *B* are myeloblasts; *C, D*, early myelocytes; *E*, neutrophilic myelocyte; *F*, eosinophilic myelocyte; *G*, basophilic myelocyte; *H*, lymphoblast; *I, J*, lymphocytes; *K*, monocyte; *N*, normoblast. No. *7* is from a case of erythroblastic anemia; *8* and *9* from patients infected with *Plasmodium vivax.* In *7, 8* and *9, A* is a nucleated red cell; *B*, erythrocyte containing nuclear chromatin; *C*, young trophozoites; *D*, ameboid trophozoites; *E*, crenated erythrocytes; *F*, lymphocyte; *G*, monocyte. Magnification approximately × 800. (Hansen-Pruss, courtesy of Am. Jour. Clin. Path.)

blasts (Ferrata) or as pathological forms in the lymphoid series (Heilmeyer).

It is extremely difficult and, some believe, impossible by present staining methods, *to distinguish myeloblasts from lymphoblasts and "monoblasts."* In the lymphoblast the nuclear membrane is described as more dense than that of the myeloblast and the chromatin is more coarse and may show some aggregation. These cells are contrasted in Plate XVI, page 934. There are generally only one or two nucleoli in lymphoblasts and their membrane is usually very clear. The

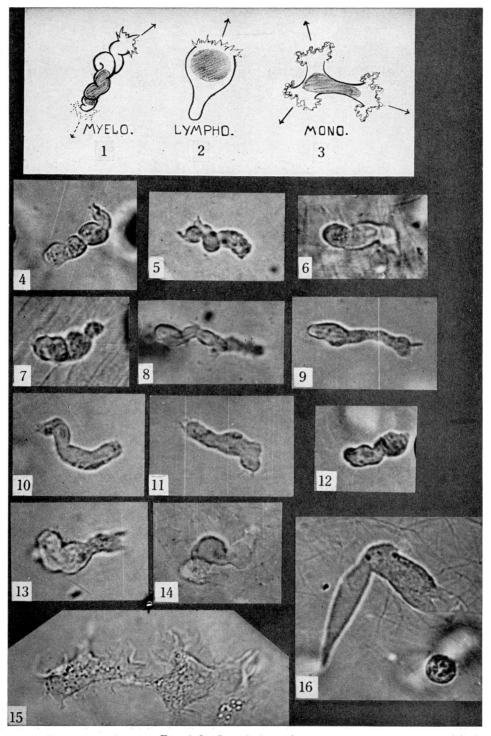

Fig. 4–3—*Legend on opposite page.*

mitochondria in the latter are short and more plump and often assume a position close to the nucleus. The "monoblast" is described as showing characteristics similar to those of the mature monocyte, such as very fine chromatin, pale nucleus, and ground-glass cytoplasm with a fine, irregular border. Further morphological differences will be given below (p. 226), but in spite of these it will often be found that the "blast" cell must be identified by the company it keeps—the more mature and more easily recognized cells about it in sections, or in the same blood smear. In the case of the myeloblast, the demonstration of promyelocytes which show azure granulation in Wright's or similar stains, or positive reaction in peroxidase stains, is strong presumptive evidence for its identification.

Pappenheim gave the name **"leuko-blast"** to a cell transitional between the "lymphoidocyte" (myeloblast of Naegeli and Downey) and the promyelocyte (Fig. 1–3, p. 37). The chromatin network of this cell is more thickened and the nucleoli are less distinct than in the lymphoidocyte. The cytoplasm is polychromatophilic or slightly acidophilic.

Myelocytes. — The developmental stages in the granulocytic series and some of their morphological variations are shown in Plate VI, 2 to 6. Naturally the changes are gradual and modifications in degree of basophilia, in mitochondria, granulation and other morphological characteristics do not parallel one another. It is therefore often difficult in practice to classify cells of the myeloid series into sharply defined categories. The myelocyte may be defined as that stage following the myeloblast in which specific granules are present in the cytoplasm and the nucleus is not yet markedly indented. These cells may be classified, as Sabin did, into the earliest stage (*A*) when there are no more than 10 granules; the second stage (*B*) in which there is a moderate number; and the third stage (*C*) in which the maximum number of granules is attained. The first two periods correspond to the *promyelocyte* stage of Pappenheim, whereas the last type is sometimes referred to as the *differentiated myelocyte* (or, more simply, *myelocyte*) because at this time the granules become definitely neutrophilic, eosinophilic or basophilic. In the promyelocyte ("progranulocyte") some of the granules are azurophilic but others may be the first "specific" granules. The earliest granules which eventually become the neutrophilic or the eosinophilic granules are generally dark and may even appear basophilic. In Wright's stain they are sometimes missed or seen only with difficulty because of the deep basophilia of the cytoplasm at this stage. They are more easily detected in supravital preparations as neutral red bodies and they give a positive peroxidase reaction. As already mentioned, their presence is presumptive evidence for regarding as myeloblasts neighboring non-granular cells otherwise similar in morphology.

The nuclear chromatin becomes some-

FIG. 4–3.—Photographs of living, moving, unstained cells, enlarged from negatives of motion picture films of tissue cultures. The cells are from normal human bone marrow and lymph nodes and from leukemic blood. *1*, Diagram of "worm-like" shape of myeloblast in motion. *2*, Diagram of "hand-mirror" shape of lymphoblast in motion. *3*, Diagram of monocyte (histiocyte) in motion. *4, 5, 6, 7* (× 1000), Myeloblasts from bone marrow of normal rabbits. *8* (× 1000), Myeloblast from normal human bone marrow. *9, 10, 11, 12, 13* (× 1000), Myeloblasts from blood of human acute myeloblastic leukemia. *14* (× 1000), Myeloblast from blood of another case of human acute myeloblastic leukemia. *15* (× 1000), Two monocytes from normal blood. Note broad, ruffle-like pseudopodia. *16* (× 1000), Megakaryocyte from normal rabbit bone marrow. Below is a rounded-up polymorphonuclear leukocyte. (Rich, Wintrobe and Lewis, courtesy of Bull. Johns Hopkins Hosp.)

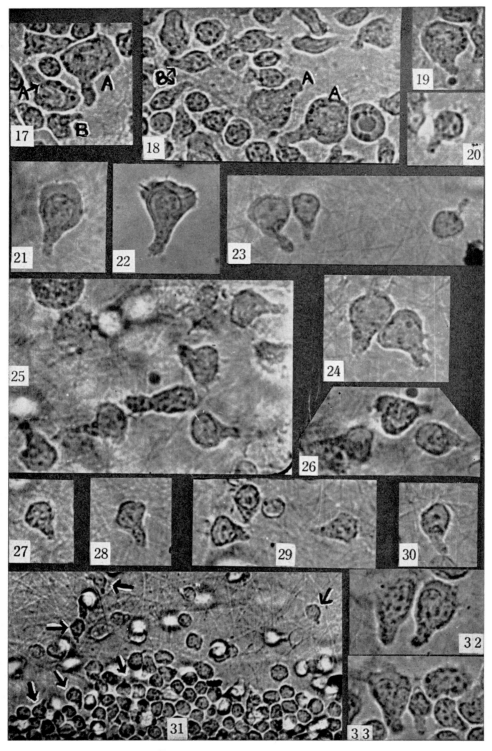

FIG. 4–4—*Legend on opposite page.*

what more coarse as the myelocyte develops, but it continues to stain relatively faintly and lacks a well-defined membrane. Characteristically the nucleus of the differentiated myelocyte appears buried under the granules in the cytoplasm. This is an important point of distinction from the monocyte with which it is often confused. Another point of difference is the more homogeneous character of the chromatin in the myelocyte.

The nucleoli of the promyelocyte are smaller than those of the myeloblast and, in the later stages, may not be visible. The nucleus of the myelocyte tends to become oval and eccentric, and finally is slightly indented. The cytoplasm loses its basophilia and becomes pink.

Like the myeloblast, the myelocyte appears immobile in flat slide and coverslip preparations and only in the last stage may slight locomotion be seen. Even then, streaming of the granules, so characteristic of the mature forms, is lacking. For this reason the cytoplasm has been thought to be in the form of a gel. The cytoplasm appears homogeneous. In *supravital preparations*, 3 to 10 neutral red bodies are seen in the *A* stage. These are generally scattered among the mitochondria which are like those of the myeloblast. The neutral red bodies clump in the region of the centrosphere

only rarely. In the *B* form 30 to 100 or more neutral red bodies are found while the mitochondria are less numerous and may be displaced toward the periphery of the cell. *C* myelocytes are often larger than earlier forms. They may be distinguished as basophilic, neutrophilic or eosinophilic according to the color of the specific bodies in their cytoplasm which take up the neutral red dye and stain deep maroon, red, or bright yellow, respectively.

In hanging drop preparations, where the force exerted by the capillary attraction between cover-slip and slide does not need to be overcome, myelocytes, like myeloblasts, are found to be actively motile.

Metamyelocytes or "Juvenile" Forms.—Indentation of the nucleus (Plate VI, 7) inaugurates the next stage in the myeloid series. This proceeds until the nucleus is horseshoe- (Plate VI, 8) or sausage-shaped, after which it divides into two lobes. Arneth's hypothesis that lobulation continues as the cell ages and that granulocytes with several lobes are more mature than those with only two lobes, has long been accepted although it has been subjected to only limited study.[2d] In the metamyelocyte the nuclear outline becomes well marked once more, and the nuclear chromatin becomes more coarse. The nucleoli are usually

FIG. 4–4.—*17, 18, 19* (× 1000), Cells from lymph node of three weeks' old normal rabbit. There are two moving large lymphoblasts (*A*) in *17*, two (*A*) in *18* and one in *19*. Note the "hand-mirror" shape of the moving small lymphocytes (*B*) in *17* and *18* in comparison with that of the lymphoblasts. *20* (× 1800), Lymphocyte from normal rabbit spleen. *21* and *22* (× 1000), Lymphoblasts from blood of human acute lymphoblastic leukemia (subleukemic state). Case M. P. *23* and *24* (× 1000), Lymphoblasts from blood of human acute lymphoblastic leukemia. Case W. H. *25* and *26* (× 1000), Lymphoblasts from blood of human acute lymphoblastic leukemia. Case V. B. *27, 28, 29* (× 1000), Typical cells from blood of human chronic lymphocytic leukemia. *30* (× 1000), Lymphoblast of moderate size from blood of human acute lymphoblastic leukemia. Case E. L. *31*, Low-power picture showing cells beginning to migrate out from the explant into the clot. Mass of cells at bottom are leukocytes of buffy coat of blood of human acute lymphoblastic leukemia. Note the uniformity of the "hand-mirror" contour of the migrating lymphoblasts, to which the arrows point. *32* and *33* (× 1000), Characteristic large lymphoid cells from blood of case of infectious mononucleosis. Note the lobulated nuclei. *33* shows two small lymphocytes in motion near the large cell. (Rich, Wintrobe and Lewis, courtesy of Bull. Johns Hopkins Hosp.)

no longer visible. In supravital preparations, a slight local shifting of the granules will be seen at this stage. By the time the nucleus is horseshoe-shaped, ameboid movement is apparent even in cover-slip-slide preparations. Mitochrondria are still present but may be difficult to see because of the numerous granules.

Polymorphonuclear Neutrophils. —In this stage of full maturity the granulocytes are of uniform size and granule content. In Wright's stained preparations, the nucleus is found to take a deep purplish-blue color, is sharply distinguished from the cytoplasm and is made up of a rather coarse chromatin network. The lobes are joined by thin strands of chromatin, although these may not be visible if the lobes happen to lie in close apposition. The significance of the number of lobes in indicating the relative ages of these cells has been mentioned already and will be discussed more fully below (Fig. 4–10, p. 247). The cytoplasm is faint pink in color and contains fine pink or violet-pink granules.

In wet films, whether viewed unstained with or without dark-ground illumination (Fig. 4–2, p. 217) or in supravital preparations, the marked activity of these cells is their most pronounced characteristic. They are rarely still if the surrounding temperature is that of the body. A long pseudopod of hyaline ectoplasm is projected and into this the endoplasm with its dancing granules is extended. The cell moves in this ameboid fashion, generally in one direction for a considerable length of time. The nucleus follows passively and may be elongated or compressed into bizarre shapes. Often, as the cell proceeds, it may permit a long strand of cytoplasm to remain stretched out behind it. Finally, this is drawn up but occasionally the tip is broken off. The rate of locomotion has been estimated at 19 μ per minute.[28] In supravitally stained films the granules are seen as tiny, round,

yellowish-pink refractile bodies which completely fill the cytoplasm. In occasional cells one or more large non-refractile, deep red vacuoles may appear.

Sabin[39] described "senile" polymorphonuclear leukocytes which are no longer motile and fail to take up the neutral red stain. Mitochondria are absent and the cells are usually circular in outline. In the rabbit these appeared in cyclic showers throughout the day.

Eosinophils.—Eosinophils exhibit the same maturation phenomena as neutrophils. It is rare, however, to find eosinophils with more than two lobes. A small third lobe may be interposed on the connecting strand of chromatin. The nuclei are usually larger than those of neutrophils and do not stain as deeply. Sometimes neutrophilic granules are deeply stained and may be confused with eosinophils. The granules of the latter are distinguished by their large, uniform size and bright yellowish-red color. Eosinophils are less persistently motile than neutrophils. In supravital preparations the granules are very refractile, uniformly large and bright yellow.

Basophils ("Mast" Leukocytes).— Basophils are distinguished by their large, coarse, metachromatic, purplish- or bluish-black granules (Plate VI, 12). They usually completely fill the cytoplasm. The nucleus stains even less deeply than that of eosinophils and may be partly hidden by the granules. The granules are peroxidase negative. They are also water-soluble. As a result they may be dissolved in the process of staining and washing and the cells may then appear to have a vacuolated and slightly acidophilic cytoplasm with only a few basophilic granules or none at all.

Basophils are quite as persistently active as neutrophils. The nucleus, however, is not usually subjected to the distortion common in neutrophils and often appears in the anterior end of the moving cell. With neutral red the granules take

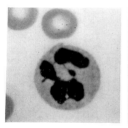 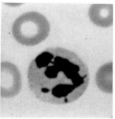 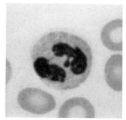 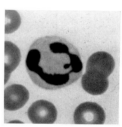

Fig. 4–5.—Granulocytes, to show the sex chromatin. The characteristic drumsticks found in the female are shown in the two cells on the left; the thin strand of chromatin joining the head to a nuclear lobe can be seen clearly. In the two cells on the right, "small clubs" are present such as may be seen in males. These should not be confused with drumsticks. (Wright's stain × 1300.)

a deep maroon color and do not appear very refractile. Similar but larger cells found in tissues are known as *mast cells*. The latter, however, show little motility and when stained, unlike the basophil leukocytes, are found to possess granules which are uniform in size and seldom overlie the small, round, eccentrically placed nucleus.[10a]

Macropolycytes.—"Macropolycyte" (Plate VI, *11*) is the name sometimes given to unusually large (16 to 25 μ) polymorphonuclear neutrophils possessing nuclei with 6 to 10 lobes.[24] Such cells are rarely seen in health and are found in the blood particularly in cases of pernicious anemia where they probably reflect the development in the marrow of a pathological series of cells (p. 480). They have been distinguished from *polycytes* and *propolycytes*, polymorphonuclear leukocytes with hypersegmented or complex nuclei but of the usual size which have been observed in cases of acute and chronic infection, usually when the polynuclear count was returning or about to return to its normal state.[36b] The abnormal dimensions of macropolycytes have been explained on the basis of plurinuclearity.[40a]

Determination of Genetic Sex.—A small mass, usually adjacent to the nuclear membrane, which stains deeply with hematoxylin, Feulgen reagent, and thionin and is approximately 0.7 by 1.2 μ in size, is known as the sex chromatin

body. This has been shown to be present in 80 to 90 per cent of the somatic cells of the normal female. A similar structure is present in approximately 1 per cent of the polymorphonuclear leukocytes of the female. There it takes the form of a "drumstick." This is a spherical body, about 1 μ in diameter, which is attached to the side of the lobulated nucleus by a thin stalk (Fig. 4–5). This must be distinguished from small sessile appendages attached to the body of the nucleus by a thick stalk, racquet-like bodies, or small lobes at the extremities of the nucleus, all of which may be seen in either sex.[1c] It has been claimed that a sex chromatin body can also be identified in lymphocytes, monocytes and non-segmented leukocytes as a planoconvex or elliptical mass of dark-staining chromatin closely applied to the inner aspect of the nuclear membrane.[35a]

Pelger-Huët Anomaly of the Granulocytes.—Rod-like, dumbbell, peanut-shaped and spectacle-like nuclei in granulocytes, instead of cells with the normal degree of segmentation, characterize this hereditary anomaly (Fig. 4–6). The chromatin of these nuclei, as well as that of the lymphocytes and monocytes appears unusually coarse.[38c] The anomaly may be mistaken for the increase in the number of unsegmented forms of granulocytes which occurs in association with infections. No difference in phagocytic activity of the cells, as compared with that of normal cells, has been observed

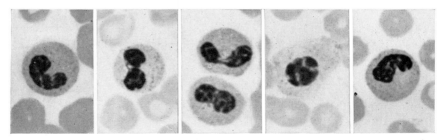

Fig. 4–6.—Pelger-Huët anomaly of the granulocytes. The various unusual forms of the nucleus are shown. (Wright's stain × 1220).

and the carriers manifest no lowered resistance to infection. Penetrance of this non-sex-linked, autosomal dominant anomaly seems to vary since full and partial carriers of the trait have been described.[44] A similar anomaly was discovered in rabbits and thus it became possible to produce the homozygous state experimentally.[19b] This was either lethal or was accompanied by skeletal and other anomalies, as well as round nuclei instead of the bilobed nuclei of the heterozygous state. The homozygous condition has also been described in the human in the offspring of consanguinous parents.[2b] In almost all the neutrophils the nucleus was round and eccentric, with a very coarse and fragmented chromatin structure. Observed mainly in Holland, Germany and Switzerland where an incidence of about 1 to 4000 was found,[12b] the condition has also been encountered in other parts of the world. The anomalous appearance of the cells, which may be the consequence of an arrest or dysplasia of nuclear chromatin synthesis, is demonstrable in the bone marrow as well as the blood. In a special type of the heterozygous condition, the "Stodmeister type," nearly all of the nuclei are found to be round, with a fine but exceedingly compact nuclear structure, and chromatin threads may radiate from the nucleus into the surrounding cytoplasm.[44] The nuclei have been compared to pomegranates. Cells resembling the typical hetero-

zygous and homozygous forms have been observed in patients with acute and chronic myelogenous leukemia, in Fanconi's anemia and following prolonged exposure to myelotoxic therapeutic agents.[11a]

Hereditary Hypersegmentation of Neutrophils.[44a]—This anomaly has been less extensively studied than its counterpart, the Pelger-Huët anomaly. There is a suggested association between the "drumstick" count and the lobe count in this condition.[28b] Another inherited anomaly is characterized by the presence of substantial numbers of *giant neutrophils* with multilobed nuclei (macropolycytes).[9a]

Alder's Constitutional Granulation Anomaly[1a]—This is characterized by heavy azurophilic granulation of the neutrophils, eosinophils and basophils, as well as in some monocytes and lymphocytes. Variations and "incomplete" forms have been described.[18d] It is likely that this is a manifestation of a metabolic disorder, perhaps hereditary in nature, in which there is a derangement of cellular metabolism of protein and polysaccharides.[28d] *Gargoylism* and Morquio's disease are thought to be caused by the same metabolic derangement.[17a,18e]

Chediak-Steinbrinck-Higashi Anomaly.[7a,21a]—Abnormalities in the granulation and nuclear structure of all types of leukocytes, with gigantic and monstrous malformation of peroxidase-positive granules, cytoplasmic inclusions and Döhle bodies (see below) characterize this serious disorder in which albinism and other skin changes, psychomotor underdevelopment, photophobia, roentgenologic changes of bones, lungs and heart, and hepatosplenomegaly, lymphadenopathy, anemia, thrombocytopenia and leukopenia occur in addition.[40] There is increased susceptibility to infections, which often result in death in childhood. The disorder may be recessively inherited but is not sex-linked.[44b]

Döhle Bodies.—These are discrete, round or oval bodies ranging in diameter from just visible size to 1 to 2 μ which stain sky blue to gray blue in color with Romanowsky stains. They have been observed in the cytoplasm of neutrophils in the blood of patients suffering from infections or burns.[65a] Their significance is unknown.

Lymphocytic Series

The **lymphocyte** is formed in lymphoid tissue in many parts of the body, especially the lymph glands, the spleen, and the subepithelial lymphoid tissues such as tonsils, adenoids, Peyer's patches and appendix.[29] Some consider thymus lymphocytes to differ from those derived from lymph nodes.[15b] Lymphocytes probably constitute 0.5 to 1.0 per cent of the body weight.[47]

The lymphocyte is generally small (10 μ) but larger forms (10 to 20 μ) are common (Plate VI, *17* to *21*). In the stained cell (Wright's stain) the nucleus stains deeply (purplish-blue) and is composed of dense aggregates of chromatin. The margin of the nucleus is sharply defined. The nucleus is usually round but may be slightly indented, and is eccentrically placed in a sky-blue cytoplasm. The latter may form only a fine rim about the nucleus or it may be quite abundant. Usually granules are absent from the cytoplasm but in some cells several bright reddish-violet (azurophil) granules are found. These differ from

the granules of the myeloid series of cells in that they fail to give the oxidase or peroxidase reaction.

The lymphocyte is actively motile[14] and moves in a characteristic manner. The nucleus is found at the anterior end and the pseudopodia are inconspicuous (Fig. 4–4). The cytoplasm may be seen to pass through "constriction rings" which appear to be "static;" that is, they retain their position in relation to objects external to the cell.[38] As in the stained cells, the nucleus may be round, slightly oval, or indented and even horseshoe-shaped, and there is a variable amount of cytoplasm. The cell outline is definite and clear-cut. The mitochondria, staining with Janus green, characteristically appear as short, thick rods which may clump at one side opposite or overlying the indentation of the nucleus, or they may encircle the nucleus in a single or double row. Neutral red bodies may or may not be present. If present they may be 4 to 10 in number, are usually small and deep red in color, and are generally scattered without pattern throughout the cytoplasm and may lie over the nucleus. Rarely the neutral red bodies are relatively large and numerous. Occasionally they may congregate in the region of the indentation of the nucleus, thus resembling monocytes.[26]

In contrast to the granulocytic series, there is no clearly defined maturation cycle for lymphocytes. Attempts to classify lymphocytes as "young," "mature" and "old,"[46] whether on the basis of supravital staining (Table 4–2, p, 232) or according to their appearance in Wright's stained preparations, are not well founded. It is a common assumption that large and medium-sized lymphocytes are less mature than small lymphocytes, but this is an uncertain foundation for classification. Differentiation according to the degree of basophilia of the cytoplasm, as well as the presence or absence of nucleoli is better founded.[43]

15

It has been suggested that the site of origin of lymphocytes may account for their form, large lymphocytes with kidney-shaped nuclei arising from the spleen while the small round ones come from lymph nodes.[22] Other views concerning the significance of morphologic differences in the lymphocytes will be discussed later (p. 261).

Lymphoblasts.—The cell from which the lymphocyte is thought to be derived is known as the *lymphoblast* (Plate VI, *16*, Fig. 4–1). The difficulty of distinguishing these cells from myeloblasts has been mentioned already (p. 217). The situation becomes even more difficult if one follows the neo-unitarians (Downey), for this school holds that there are two morphological lymphoblast types: (1) The normal form which is intermediate between the reticulum and the lymphocyte of the blood; and (2) the pathological form seen in leukemia which may be derived from Downey's myeloblast (Fig. 1–3, p. 37).

As seen in the circulating blood in cases of acute lymphoblastic leukemia, lymphoblasts are characterized by a large nucleus made up of a chromatin structure which is finer than that of the mature lymphocyte but is more coarse than that of the myeloblast (Plate XVI, p. 934). There is a well-defined, fairly dense, nuclear membrane and nucleoli, usually only one or two, are present. Their outlines are sharp and suggest the presence of a nucleolar membrane. The cytoplasm stains clear blue. In unstained films the cytoplasm is distinctly yellowish. In supravitally stained preparations many short, thick mitochondria may be seen scattered throughout the cytoplasm or, more often, in a characteristic position close to the nucleus. Neutral red bodies are absent. Although in flat slide-cover-slip preparations lymphoblasts appear to be non-motile, in hanging-drop preparations their movement is quite characteristic.[37] The

nucleus is at the anterior end while at the posterior end a narrow band of cytoplasm protrudes, giving the whole cell the appearance of a hand mirror (Fig. 4–4). The movement is stately and in one direction, as if purposeful. De-Bruyn[10] found, however, that myeloblasts give the same appearance when moving on a flat surface.

The peculiar lymphocytes seen in cases of infectious mononucleosis are described in the chapter dealing with that disease (p. 1112).

Plasma Cells.—The term plasma cell is usually applied to large, spherical or ellipsoidal cells possessing abundant, deep blue cytoplasm and an eccentrically placed round or oval nucleus containing large dense masses of chromatin arranged in a wheel-spoke fashion ("Radkern") (Plate XVIII, p. 1070). There is usually a well-defined clear zone beside the nucleus and the cytoplasm often contains vacuoles.[32] Cells such as these but containing granules and hyaline bodies with acidophilic staining qualities have been called **Russell body cells.**[28a] In supravitally prepared films, the cytoplasm of plasma cells is deep yellowish-gray in color and contains numerous mitochrondria which vary in size and shape but are usually smaller than those of lymphocytes.[33]

The plasma cell is held to be a derivative of lymphocytes or primitive connective tissue cells, although many other types of cells have been named as its precursor.[32] A maturation cycle has been described. The *plasmoblast* is defined as any cell of the plasmocytic series which possesses fine nuclear chromatin as well as nucleoli.[8a] The nucleus is usually greater than 12 μ in diameter. Such cells are usually seen only in multiple myeloma and in plasma cell leukemia. In the *"proplasmocyte,"*[8a] nucleoli are still present but the chromatin is more coarse. The nucleus is usually 7 to 12 μ in diameter. The fully mature form (plasmocyte, plasma cell) has been described above. It possesses only minute or no nucleoli and the nucleus is usually less than 7 μ in diameter. It is rarely seen in normal blood but is normally present in the interstitial tissue of various organs and glands and is a prominent constituent of chronic inflammatory tissue.

Intracytoplasmic inclusions and crystal-like bodies in the cytoplasm of plasma cells, which have been called "*grape cells*" and "*morular cells*," because of their appearance, may be manifestations of immune responses.[47a] The globules stain positively in the periodic acid Schiff reaction and probably contain mucopolysaccharide.

Monocytic Series

Originally called "transitional cells" by Ehrlich because of the view that they represent a transition stage between the lymphocyte and the neutrophilic leukocyte, the monocytes were first clearly differentiated by Schilling (1912) and were later studied by Sabin and her associates who, as already stated (Chapter 1) regard these cells as being derived from a specific stem cell, the **monoblast.** This cell is described as possessing basophilic or grayish cytoplasm, fine, stringy chromatin and one or two large nucleoli. It is 14 μ or greater in diameter and non-motile. In the unstained state the cytoplasm is slightly yellow and "muddy." Numerous fine, spherical or slender, rod-like mitochondria appear in supravitally stained cells, but neutral red vacuoles are either absent or only a very few fine bodies are found in the centrosphere. It is obvious that differentiation of this cell from the myeloblast is, to say the least, very difficult.

Monocytes.—The monocyte, on the other hand, is a well-defined cell which can be readily distinguished from other cells of the blood in well-stained preparations. It is usually larger than the other leukocytes, and possesses an abundant, opaque, grayish- or muddy-blue cytoplasm (Wright's stain) which is filled with myriads of very fine, lilac or reddish-blue granules (Plate VI, *22* to *25*). If the preparation is not overstained these granules resemble fine dust, but they may be confused with those of granulocytes if the stain is heavy. The granules can be demonstrated in films stained by the peroxidase method, but they are fewer and finer than in granulocytes.

There is no perinuclear clear zone as is so common in lymphocytes. The nucleus is large and is usually centrally placed. Even when it is eccentric in position a rim of cytoplasm can almost always be seen outside the peripheral portion of the nucleus. The latter may be round or oval but is usually reniform or horseshoe-shaped. Rarely it resembles a petaled flower. One of the most significant characteristics of this cell is the fine skein-like or lacy structure of the chromatin. This is so fine that the stained nucleus is lighter in color than that of the metamyelocyte or the lymphocyte, the two types of cells with which it is most often confused (Plate VII).

The motility of the monocyte is characteristic. The cell contour is much more delicate than in lymphocytes and is often irregular and wavy. There appears to be a delicate surface film which is in constant waving motion and the cell advances slowly by a sort of sliding movement. The protoplasm has a foamy, ground-glass appearance. In supravitally stained films, numerous (40 to 80) neutral red bodies varying in size from minute dust-like granules to large vacuoles, brick-red in color, are characteristically found. About a clear area (centrosphere) in the bay of the nucleus, two or more concentric rows of small neutral red vacuoles of uniform size may be seen. This "rosette" is much more common in the monocyte of the rabbit and guinea pig than in that of man and is not specific for the monocyte.[19] The mitochondria are very small and few in number and often they are found peripherally to the rosette. Their number varies with the age of the cell, being greater in the younger forms. The ground-glass appearance of the cytoplasm, the variability in the size of the neutral red vacuoles and their great number, the fine mitochondria and the characteristic motility of the monocyte distinguish this cell from the lymphocyte.

Monocytes normally are not found in bone marrow in large numbers but according to Sabin and her co-workers,[39] these cells may be stimulated to arise there in rabbits experimentally infected with bovine tuberculosis. In such experiments and in the peripheral lymph nodes of normal rabbits, transition forms between the monoblast and monocyte have been described.[16a]

Promonocytes. — The promonocyte or *young* monocyte (Plate XVII, p. 936) possesses fewer neutral red bodies than the monocyte; they are more uniform in size and in the earliest type there is but a single row of these red bodies about the centrosphere. The mitochondria are more numerous than in the mature cell. The nucleus is moderately indented and a nucleolus may be visible. The cell shows the characteristic contour and motility of monocytes.

Epithelioid Cell.—The epithelioid cell of tuberculosis is derived, according to the Sabin school, from the mature monocyte by condensation and proliferation of the rosette vacuoles so that a very large rosette of dust-like vacuoles is formed. There are few or no mitochondria. The cytoplasm is abundant and the whole cell is usually larger than the monocyte. The nucleus is indented or oval. The nuclear chromatin is heavy. In motility this cell resembles the monocyte. Its contour is varied and phagocytosis is often seen. The **Langhans' giant cell** is thought to be a multinucleated epithelioid cell formed by amitotic division of the nucleus of an epithelioid cell.[16,21]

Macrophage, Clasmatocyte or Histiocyte.—The tissue macrophage, clasmatocyte or histiocyte (Fig. 4–7) is also thought by these[21] and other[13] workers to be derived from the monocyte, although it is admitted that monocytes may not be the sole source of clasmatocytes. Some may originate from reticulum cells. They are large cells (15 to 80 μ), their contour is irregular, and their motility is similar to that of monocytes. Transient bleb-like and filiform pseudopodia may be seen. The cytoplasm is abundant and neutral red bodies of varied size and color are present in variable numbers and manifest no characteristic distribution.[9] Mitochondria are usually absent. The nucleus is elongated, indented or egg-shaped. Phagocytosis is a striking characteristic. When stained with Wright's stain the nuclear chromatin is seen to be "spongy" and the nuclear membrane is distinct (Fig. 4–7). The cytoplasm is sky-blue, often opaque and contains numerous, moderately coarse, azure granules as well as vacuoles. The granules are often grouped about the nucleus. Owing to the marked fragility of this cell it may appear broken up, or little but the nucleus may be found.

The **morphological characteristics of the various leukocytes** are summarized in Tables 4–1 and 4–2. Nucleated forms of the erythrocyte series can usually be readily distinguished from the leukocytes. In Romanowsky stained films, confusion arises only when the cytoplasm of the cells is basophilic. Even then a small area of the pink-staining cytoplasm of erythrocytes can usually be made out near the nucleus. The latter not infrequently is more pyknotic than is ever seen in leukocytes. When the chromatin is arranged in wheel-spoke fashion, the erythroblast may resemble a small plasma cell. In microblasts only a small amount of cytoplasm is usually present and at first glance the cell may resemble a small lymphocyte (Plate IV).

PLATE VII

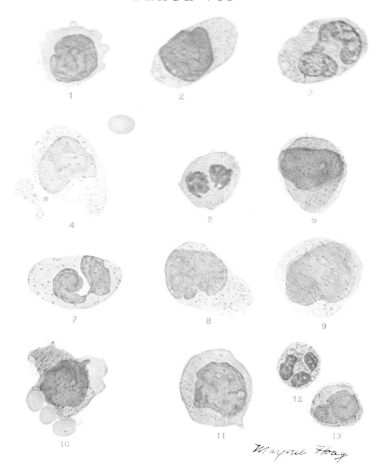

Monocytes from the blood of a patient who died of miliary tuberculosis.
Similar cells were seen in the tissues about the tuberculous nodules.

No. 11 is a typical monocyte, nos. 1, 2 and 6 have nuclei which are a little darker and are somewhat more stippled but are otherwise typical monocytes. No. 13 is a small monocyte. No. 9 most probably is a monocyte even though the nucleus is somewhat less distinct than in the other cells.

"Toxic" monocytes with altered nucleus and granules are illustrated by nos. 3 and 7. Nos. 4, 8 and 10 are monocytes with histiocytic characteristics.

No. 5 is in mitosis. The cytoplasm is basophilic. The cell may be lymphoid in origin.

No. 12 is a polymorphonuclear leukocyte showing "toxic" granulation.

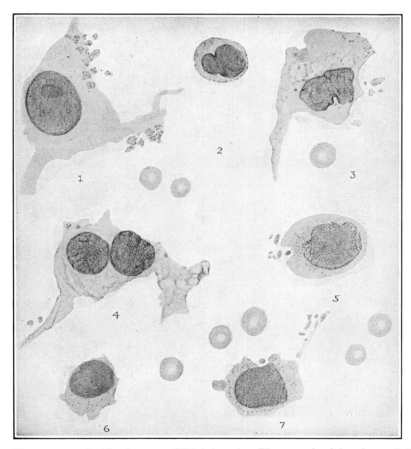

FIG. 4–7.—Clasmatocytes in blood smears, Wright's stain. Photograph of drawings. *1, 2,* and *3* are from a case of dementia paralytica in which frequent convulsions occurred; *5, 6* and *7,* from a case of monocytic (histiocytic) leukemia. *1* is an extremely large histiocyte. Several platelets seem to have become phagocytized; the nucleolus in the spongy nucleus is prominent. *2* is an ordinary monocyte. The fine granules in the grayish-blue cytoplasm and the fine chromatin network of the indented nucleus are to be noted. *3* is a histiocyte with a large amount of ingested debris. Vacuole formation is common in these cells. *4* is the possible beginning of a giant cell. This has occurred in a histiocyte that has probably undergone amitotic division of the nucleus. Note the phagocytized platelets and the vacuoles. *5* is the perfect histiocyte. Note the spongy character of the nuclear chromatin and the perinuclear arrangement of the granules. *6* is apparently a transition between the typical histiocyte of *5* and *7* and the typical monocyte of *2.* There is more pseudopod formation, a rounder nucleus and coarser granules than in the ordinary monocyte. *7* is another typical histiocyte seen in a more "active" stage than cell *5.* (Dameshek, courtesy of Arch. Int. Med.)

Microblasts, however, are much smaller (4 to 6 μ) than lymphocytes. Greatest difficulty arises in distinguishing polychromatophilic erythroblasts and still younger forms of the erythrocyte series from the "blast" cells of the leukocytic series. The appearance of erythroblasts when stained by the Romanowsky method has already been described in detail (Chapter 2, p. 86).

The nucleated cells of the red cell series are non-motile and in wet films are found to have a rounded, distinct border with homogeneous, non-granular cytoplasm in which a yellow tint of hemoglobin may be evident. The nu-

Table 4-1—Morphologic Characteristics of the Leukocytes (Wright's Stain)

Type of cell	Size	Nucleus						Cytoplasm			
		Position	Shape	Color	Chromatin	Nuclear membrane	Nucleoli	Relative amount	Color	Perinuclear clear zone	Granules
1. Granulocytes: (a) Myeloblast	10–18 μ	Eccentric or central	Round or oval	Light reddish purple	Very fine mesh-work	Very fine	2–5	Scanty	Blue	None	Only a few (azurophilic)
(b) Myelocyte	12–18 μ	Eccentric	Oval or slightly indented	Reddish purple	Fine but becomes gradually more coarse	Indistinct	Smaller, fewer	Moderate	Bluish pink	None	Red or blue-black, fine or coarse
(c) Metamyelocyte ("Juvenile" form)	10–18 μ	Central or eccentric	Horse-shoe or sausage	Light purplish blue	Basi- and oxy-chromatin clearly distinguished	Present	None	Plentiful	Pink	None	Neutrophilic, eosinophilic or basophilic
(d) Polymorphonuclear neutrophil	10–15 μ	Central or eccentric	2–5 or more lobes	Deep purplish blue	Rather coarse	Present	None	Plentiful	Faint pink	None	Fine pink or violet-pink

	Size	Position	Shape	Color	Chromatin		Nucleoli	Amount	Cytoplasm color		Granules
(e) Polymorphonuclear eosinophil	10–15 μ	Central or eccentric	2–3 lobes	Paler purplish blue	Coarse	Present	None	Plentiful	Bluish pink	None	Large, coarse, uniform in size, crimson-red, numerous
(f) Polymorphonuclear basophil	10–15 μ	Central	2–3 lobes	Pale purplish blue	Coarse, overlaid with granules	Present	None	Plentiful	Faint pink	None	Large, coarse, uniform, bluish-black
2. Lymphocytes (a) Lymphoblasts	10–18 μ	Eccentric or central	Round or oval	Light reddish purple	Moderately coarse particles, "stippled"	Fairly dense	1–2	Scanty	Clear blue	Present	None
(b) "Mature" lymphocyte	7–18 μ	Eccentric	Round or slightly indented	Deep purplish blue	Large masses of moderate or large size, or pyknotic	Dense	None	Scanty or plentiful	Sky-blue, deep blue or even very pale pink	Present if cytoplasm is dark	None or few azurophilic
3. Monocyte	12–20 μ	Eccentric or central	Round, oval, notched, or horseshoe	Pale bluish violet	Fine reticulated, skeinlike or lacy	Present	None	Abundant	Grayish or cloudy blue	None	Abundant, fine, lilac or reddish blue
Clasmatocyte	15–80 μ	Central	Elongated, indented or oval	Pale bluish violet	Spongy	Distinct	None	Usually abundant	Opaque sky blue	None	Numerous, moderately coarse azure granules and vacuoles

Table 4-2—Morphologic Characteristics of the Leukocytes (Supravital Stain)

Type of cell	Size, microns	Contour	Type of motility	Nucleus			Cytoplasm			Mitochondria		Physical state	Evidence of phagocytosis
				Shape	Chromatin	Nucleoli	Relative amount	Color	Neutral red vacuoles	Size	Distribution		
1. Myeloid series:													
(a) Myeloblast	14–20	Smooth and sharp	None	Round or oval	Loose meshwork	2–5	Scanty	Slightly yellow	None	Spherical	Numerous diffuse	Gel	None
(b) Myelocyte	16–24	Distinct, smooth	None	Round or oval	Gradually more dense	Gradually disappear	Moderate	Gray	Refractile, bright red A = 3–10 B = 30–100 C = full amt.	Spherical	Diffuse, few in C type	Gel, sol in C type	None
(c) Metamyelocyte	12–18	Irregular	Slightly ameboid	Reniform or horseshoe	Moderately dense	None	Plentiful	Gray	Beginning streaming	Spherical	Few	Sol	Slight to moderate For bacteria, débris, etc.
(d) Polymorphonuclear neutrophil	12–15	Irregular Repeated pseudopod formation	Actively ameboid	Lobulated Dragged behind except in basophil	Coarse	None	Plentiful Clear ecto- and endoplasm except in basophil	Homogeneous and clear	Yellowish pink tiny, refractile	Spherical	Rare	Sol	
(e) Eosinophil			Less Active						Bright yellow, large, oval, refractile				
(f) Basophil			Active						Deep maroon, non-refractile, all streaming				

2. Lymphoid series:													
(a) Lymphoblast	10–20	Sharp	None	Round or oval	Sparse	1–2	Scanty	Yellow	None	Short plump rods	Numerous esp. close to nucleus	Gel	None
(b) "Young" lymphocyte	9–18	Sharp	Nucleus at front, static constriction rings	Round or indented	Slight	0–1	More	Grayish yellow	None or many. Any distribution	Short plump rods	Numerous esp. at one side of N.	Sol	None
(c) "Mature" lymphocyte	7–18	Sharp	Nucleus at front, static constriction rings	Round or indented	Moderate	0	Usually plentiful	Gray	None or many. Any distribution	Short plump rods	10–20	Sol	None
(d) "Old" lymphocyte	7–15	Sharp	Nucleus at front, static constriction rings	Usually round	Coarse	0	Usually scanty	Colorless	None or many. Any distribution	Smaller	0–10	Sol	None
3. Monocytic series:													
(a) Monoblast	12–18	Sharp or slightly irregular	None	Round or oval	Very sparse	1–2	Scanty	Slightly yellow and "muddy"	None, or very fine in centrosphere	Fine spheres or slender rods	Numerous	Gel	None
(b) "Young" monocyte	12–18	Irregular and lacelike	Bleblike pseudopodia, surface film type	Indented	Slight	0–1	Moderate	Colorless and muddy	Numerous small, rosette arrangement	Fine, dust-like	Moderate number about rosette	Sol	Uncommon
(c) "Mature" monocyte	16–20	Irregular and lacelike	Bleblike pseudopodia, surface film type	Markedly indented	Moderate loose mesh	0	Abundant	Colorless and muddy	Very numerous, vary in size, occas. rosette	Fine dust-like	Few	Sol	Moderate
(d) Clasmatocyte	15–80	Irregular	Bleblike pseudopodia, surface film type	Elongated, indented or oval	Moderate	0–1	Usually abundant	Colorless	Often many but vary in number, size and color	Delicate filaments	Few or none	Sol	Usually for particles or whole cells

cleus is round or oval and is centrally placed, occupying most of the space. The chromatin gives the nucleus a vesicular appearance. One or two large nucleoli are present. If supravitally stained, no neutral red staining bodies will be found, but many coarse, rod-shaped coccoid mitochondria may be seen scattered without pattern in the cytoplasm.

The student will find it valuable when learning to identify the various cells of the blood, to systematically seek all the morphological criteria which have been enumerated here. By doing so he will acquire the habit of seeing all he is looking at, and in time he will learn to identify cells because of a number of characteristics which he unconsciously perceives. The actual identification of cells regarding which there may be some doubt can be made only by weighing the evidence for and against each type being considered. It must be kept in mind that practically no character of a cell is entirely specific. Thus, a perinuclear clear zone is sometimes seen in cells other than lymphocytes and a rosette of neutral red bodies has been observed in many types of blood and connective tissue cells other than the monocyte.[19]

CHEMICAL COMPOSITION AND METABOLISM OF LEUKOCYTES

With the development of appropriate technics of microchemistry and histochemistry[28c] and in consort with the growth of knowledge of metabolism, including enzymology, a picture of the chemical constitution and metabolic activities of the leukocytes is being formed. Investigation in this field has been stimulated by the hope of discovering differences in the metabolic activities of normal and leukemic leukocytes[2a] as well as by the desire to differentiate lymphoblastic from myeloblastic leukemias by histochemical reactions.[42]

In addition to a water content of 82 per cent, leukocytes contain nucleoproteins, phospholipids and measurable traces of sodium, potassium, zinc, magnesium, calcium, chloride, inorganic phosphorus and bicarbonate ion.[14e] Their content of glycogen, alkaline phosphatase and a large variety of enzymes as well as histamine and a number of miscellaneous substances has been found to differ in the various types of leukocytes and varies in different diseases.

Glycogen has been identified in the cytoplasm of neutrophilic leukocytes and metamyelocytes. The amount increases as the granulocyte matures.[36e] It is of interest that the glycogen within myeloid leukocytes, which presumably serves as a storehouse of reserve energy, remains relatively unchanged post-prandially when blood glucose rises and is unaltered in poorly controlled diabetics with marked elevations in blood sugar levels. In addition, leukocyte glycogen levels are changed very little by cortisone and ACTH therapy.[44e] In contrast, leukocyte glycogen has been observed to be substantially lower than normal in chronic myelocytic leukemia, high in polycythemia vera with leukemoid features, and above normal in the neutrophilic leukocytoses of infection. Lymphocytes and "blast" cells are either glycogen-free or extremely poor in glycogen content. Eosinophils possess glycogen[1d] and basophils may possibly contain it.[40d] Monocytes usually possess none.[1d]

Glycolytic metabolism in leukocytes is predominantly aerobic. Studies of the respiratory activity of leukocytes, originally undertaken to determine whether leukemic leukocytes resemble malignant cells in aerobic and anaerobic glycolysis, Pasteur effect and respiratory rate, have not yet been fully resolved. However, it does appear that oxygen consumption, glucose utilization and lactic acid production are significantly higher in normal than in leukemic homogenates, and that glucose utilization and lactic acid production are greater in cells from myelocytic than lymphocytic leukemia.[2a] There probably are qualitative as well as quantitative differences.[44c] The various phosphorylated intermediates of glycolysis have been demonstrated.[45] Deficiency of hexokinase, the enzyme responsible for the initial phosphorylation of glucose, is the most likely rate limiting factor responsible for the observed lower glycolytic activity in leukemia.[2a]

Leukocyte alkaline phosphatase is an enzyme capable of hydrolyzing phosphorus from a wide variety of phospho-monoesters. Activity of this enzyme has been shown both by histochemical (p. 418) and biochemical methods to be much lower than normal in the neutrophils of chronic leukemia[30a] and of paroxysmal nocturnal hemoglobinuria, whereas it is greatly increased in polycythemia vera, myelofibrosis, thrombocythemia, physiological leukocytosis and leukemoid reactions. Although increases have been observed following the administration of ACTH or adrenocorticosteroids, not all clinical "stressful" circumstances evoke the increased leukocyte-phosphatase response.[44d] When graded from 0 to 4 plus, as described elsewhere (p. 418), the sum of the grades for the alkaline phosphatase content of 100 neutrophilic "band" and segmented cells was 25 and under in 90 per cent of cases of chronic myelocytic leukemia. In contrast, the mean values were 76 ± 12.3 in normal persons, 146 in leukocytosis, 107 in polycythemia vera and 119 in myelofibrosis.[24a] The high levels of enzyme activity observed in polycythemia vera contrast with normal levels in other forms of polycythemia.[33a] Higher values were reported in acute lymphoblastic leukemia in contrast to zero values in acute myeloblastic leukemia.[20a] Values in Hodgkin's disease were high, in chronic lymphocytic leukemia and in lymphosarcoma and reticulum cell sarcoma within or just above or below the normal range.[20a] In pa-

tients with chronic myelocytic leukemia who developed prolonged remissions, return of the enzyme level to normal was noted.[33a] The significance of the observed differences in leukocyte alkaline phosphatase activity is obscure and exceptions to the usual activity patterns have been noted but the alkaline phosphatase test has found considerable usefulness in helping to differentiate chronic myelocytic leukemia from certain syndromes which superficially resemble it.

In addition to glycogen, nucleoproteins, as discussed in an earlier chapter (p. 42), and phospholipids are found in leukocytes. The specific granules of neutrophils appear to contain phospholipids, while in most eosinophils the granules consist of protein surrounded by phospholipid.[5] The eosinophilic granules may contain other lipid substances as well. In monocytes the region of the attraction sphere often contains numerous phospholipid-containing granules. In addition, mitochondria, found in all varieties of cells, appear to be rich in phospholipids. The lipid composition of the leukocytes in leukemia is normal.[5a]

Leukocytes possess a variety of enzymes in addition to those mentioned already: nuclease, several proteolytic enzymes,[33b] peptidase,[35b] lipase,[44c] esterase,[1] amylase, adenosinase, catalase,[41b] acid phosphatase, cathepsin,[2,17] arginase,[36d] glyoxalase,[29b] and a bactericidal agent (lysozyme).[15c] Myeloperoxidase is abundant in granulocytes and gives chloromatous tumor tissue (p. 937) its characteristic color. Eosinophils and, to a lesser extent, basophils, are particularly rich in arylsulfatase.[44c] Oxidase is present in the myeloid leukocytes and in many monocytes. Peroxidase is found in the neutrophilic granules.[20b] These granules may also contain a hyaluronic acid ester.[25] Nucleotidase, which is an acid phosphatase, measures ten times greater in granulocytes than in lymphocytes.[43a] It has been suggested that neutrophils contain growth-activating substances (trephones)[7] and may aid in the coagulation of blood.

β-glucuronidase has been found in substantial amounts in neutrophilic leukocytes and in eosinophils whereas lymphocytes contain little.[44c] Low levels of activity have been observed in chronic lymphocytic and in acute leukemias and normal or elevated values in chronic myelocytic leukemia. Glucuronic acid is also present in leukocytes in significant amounts. In chronic myelocytic leukemia low normal to low values have been found and consistently low values were observed in chronic lymphocytic leukemia and in nonleukemic lymphocytosis. The functions of these substances are obscure.

The sulfhydryl content of leukocytes is several times as great as that of erythrocytes.[18c,44c] In the cells of chronic lymphocytic and acute leukemias, as well as in infectious mononucleosis, less than the normal quantities have been found, whereas in chronic myelocytic leukemias normal or increased values have been reported.[18c] There is evidence that both *l*-cystine (or *l*-cysteine) and sulfate are of importance in the metabolism of leukocytes.[45c]

Half of the normal blood histamine is located in the basophils, about a third in eosinophils and probably most of the remaining sixth in neutrophils.[18b] Lymphocytes, monocytes, erythrocytes and platelets contain little or none. Consistent with this is the observation that the total blood histamine is greatly increased in chronic myelocytic leukemia and moderately increased in polycythemia vera, in contrast to normal or low values in leukocytoses of other etiology.[44c] It is possible that the various granulocytes carry different concentrations of histamine under different conditions.

In addition to the protein and phospholipid already mentioned, the granules of *eosinophils* have been reported to contain desoxyribonucleic acid, high concentrations of arginine[36] and, on the basis of less good evidence, iron,[6] phosphorus, tyrosine and glycogen.[44f] The granules of *basophilic* leukocytes, which are very soluble in water, like the mast cells of the tissues carry an acid substance identical with or closely related to ·heparin.[23b,25] This acid may be bound by the base, histamine.[18b]

FUNCTION AND BIOLOGIC PROPERTIES OF THE LEUKOCYTES

Heretofore our concepts of the functions of the leukocytes were based largely on inference and were founded to a great extent on the variations which have been observed to occur in the blood and in the tissues in pathological conditions. Greater interest and a more direct approach to the problem, the development of new cytological, cytochemical and optical technics,[36c] and the demonstration of the influence of hormones on the leukocytes, have added much to our knowledge concerning these cells.[38a,40b]

The leukocytes are concerned in various defensive and reparative functions of the body. They play important roles in the destruction of invading antigen and, probably, in the production, or at least transportation and distribution of antibody. The motility of the leukocytes has been described already. Those observed in the blood stream are chiefly cells *en route* to tissues where they will carry on their activities. The direction in which they move is thought to be governed by chemical substances emanating from foreign particles or products set free when tissues are injured.[31] Hence the term **chemotaxis.**[29a] This property has been observed chiefly in polymorphonuclear leukocytes but has been noted also in eosinophils. Considered at one time to be lacking in monocytes, it has been shown by the use of appropriate technics that monocytes are no less subject to chemotaxis than granulocytes.[19c] No means have been found so far, however, which reveal chemotaxis in lymphocytes.

Chemotaxis appears to be important chiefly as a reaction by means of which leukocytes are attracted to infecting organisms from a distance. Although emigration of leukocytes from blood vessels is widely regarded to be the result of chemotaxis, experimental studies have shown that emigration may occur without chemotaxis. This phenomenon is made possible by changes in the vascular endothelium.[29a]

Phagocytosis[3,34,38b] is another important property of the leukocytes. In the case of the neutrophils, phagocytosis is especially directed against bacteria and small particles; hence the neutrophils are called microphages. Such cells were shown to contain a bactericidal substance, "phagocytin."[21c] The monocytic series of cells characteristically engulfs not only bacteria but also protozoa, particulate matter and even red corpuscles. They are, therefore, called macrophages. It has been postulated that phagocytosis is the result of interplay of surface forces and is accompanied by a spontaneous decrease in the free energy of surfaces.[3] Wood observed that leukocytes can very promptly phagocytize virulent organisms in the absence of antibody after trapping them against surfaces of suitable physical properties by a process referred to as "surface phagocytosis."[46a] This important phenomenon makes it possible for untreated patients to resist infection until antibodies come to the rescue. The "L.E. cell" (p. 419) is a manifestation of phagocytosis which has been found to be extremely useful in the recognition of disseminated lupus erythematosus.

The neutrophilic leukocytes play a key role in **inflammation.** Viewed through the electron microscope,[36a] they were found to lose their specific granulation rapidly after arrival at the site of inflammation. At the same time the endoplasmic reticulum was modified and hyperactivity of the Golgi apparatus developed. Only after disappearance of the granulation did phagocytic activity take place. Other investigators showed that in the absence of neutrophils from the circulating blood, the early stages of the acute inflammatory cycle are inhibited.[35d] Thus, early lymphocytic infiltration and the development of hematogenous macrophages are delayed and local edema of the connective tissues fails to develop. The phagocytic activity of the polymorphonuclear leukocytes and intracellular destruction of bacteria were found, *in vitro*, to be favored by opsonic factors present in fresh serum and by the availability of glucose.[8] Antibacterial factors ("leukins") have been prepared from rabbit polymorphonuclear leukocytes.[40c]

Injury to polymorphonuclear leukocytes causes them to release endogenous pyrogen.[46a] Menkin[31] postulated that the injury of cells leads to the release of a number of different factors, which he named leukotaxine, exudin, necrosin and pyrexin, and he identified leukocytosis-promoting and leukopenia-producing substances. To the interplay of these factors he attributed the localization and the ultimate disposal of the irritant and the final repair of the injured area. The various systemic effects associated with inflammation he attributed to these products of cell injury. His findings must yet be confirmed. Others have described various other substances alleged to stimulate or inhibit production of leukocytes but the adequacy of the technical procedures employed is open to question.[19c]

The relation of leukocytes to **antibody formation** has been the subject of considerable study. Largely because the output of antibody may be depressed through blockage of the macrophages, antibody formation was at first attributed to the action of the reticulo-endothelial system. More recently lymphoid tissue has been credited with this activity. Noting that the conspicuous cells of acute splenic tumor are lymphoid, Rich, Lewis and Wintrobe[38] suggested that one function of the lymphocyte is concerned with the body's reaction to foreign protein. McMaster[30] had already offered evidence of agglutinin formation in the local lymph nodes draining the area of intradermal injection of antigen into mice, before detectable antibody appeared in the blood. Harris et al., in a series of studies,[20] showed that antibodies to typhoid antigen or to sheep erythrocytes injected in rabbits appeared in highest titer in the lymphocytes present in the efferent lymph draining the injected area. This was accompanied by a rise in the output of lymphocytes and by hyperplasia of lymphatic tissue. They also found that the concentration of ribonucleic acid in aqueous extracts of lymph nodes had risen to more than twice its normal value by the second to fifth day following the injection of antigens into the foot, after which it declined. The peak of this change occurred at or slightly before the appearance of the maximal concentration of antibodies in the same node. Non-antigenic materials, when injected into the foot, did not give rise to these changes. Thus, from their data it appeared that the antibody was produced in the lymphocytes rather than being absorbed from the surrounding lymph plasma.

Others found that the lymphocytes of normal rabbits contain a globulin identical with the normal serum gamma globulin of the rabbit.[11b] The observed effects of the adrenocorticosteroids on lymphatic tissue (p. 49) led to the suggestion that the rate of liberation of antibody from lymphoid tissue is under the control of the pituitary-adrenal cortical secretions.

Nevertheless, these observations do not necessarily indicate that the lymphocyte is the source of antibody or that antibody production is under the control of the adrenals. No increment of serum gamma globulin or augmented antibody response has been found to follow the administration of ACTH and, in rabbits at least, release of antibody can take place in adrenalectomized animals.[35]

On the other hand, there is considerable evidence that plasma cells are actively involved in antibody production.[15a] Thus, Bjornboe and Gormsen[4] found that hyperimmunization in rabbits caused marked proliferation of plasma cells in the spleen and other organs, and Fagraeus[15a] showed that antibody is formed in tissue cultures of spleens of rabbits previously injected with typhoid bacilli. He observed that the red pulp, which contains abundant plasma cells, formed larger amounts of antibody than the white pulp, which consists of lymph follicles. It has been shown that the cytoplasm of the plasma cell, rather than that of the mature lymphocyte, possesses high concentrations of ribonucleic acid, a substance which is involved in protein production.[14b] Again, the lymphoid cells of antibody-forming lymph nodes, which in vitro agglutinated on their surface the bacteria to which the animals had been immunized, were identified as plasma cells.[14b] Other experiments can be cited.[15a] In addition, there is the well recognized association in human subjects of hyperglobulinemia and an increase in plasma cells. Finally, the opportunity to study patients with agammaglobulinemia has furnished significant evidence in regard to the cell responsible for antibody production. The profound immunological handicap of such individuals has been shown to be associated with a deficiency of plasma cells and failure of plasma cell development from reticulum in response to antigenic stimuli.[5c] In the immunologically normal child born to a woman with acquired agammaglobulinemia, the capacity to synthesize gamma globulin and antibody developed concurrently with the capacity to produce plasma cells.

Some investigators regard it as possible that antibody production commences in young or undifferentiated cells[15a] and that, in some unexplained manner, both plasma cells and lymphocytes play a role.

There is, thus, considerable uncertainty concerning the function of the *lymphocyte*. Perhaps this is because the lymphocyte is not the kind of structure which the polymorphonuclear leukocyte or the red corpuscle are considered to be. Instead of being a cell with a differentiating life cycle which terminates in the small lymphocyte stage, it may be a totipotential structure which can migrate and hypertrophy, and may give rise to mononuclear cells, epithelioid cells and even giant cells, as many investigators have insisted.[5b,29] The small lymphocyte may be a resting cell rather than a senile one. It can hardly be denied that the lymphocyte must somehow play an important role in the defenses of the body. It is situated strategically in the lymph nodes throughout the body and responds whenever infection develops. It is the details that are obscure. The lymphocyte may be important in providing the structure from which other cells are formed and may furnish the means for walling off an area of inflammation. It may well be a depot of specific nucleic acids which can thus be readily transported and supplied[23c] and, through its content of appropriate enzymes, the lymphocyte may provide a means for the destruction of toxic products of protein metabolism.[14b] A role in the transference of fat from intestinal epithelium to the lacteals has been denied.[27]

As already indicated, the **monocytes** are scavengers for a wide variety of particulate materials as well as bacteria.[43b] The first leukocytes to appear on the field of inflammation are usually the neutrophils and the macrophages. The former predominate but after about three days macrophages preponderate, the granulocytes having disintegrated. Macrophages contain nucleases, proteinases and carbohydrases, as do microphages, but they differ from granulocytes in that they are rich in lipases.[2c] This presumably enables them to digest bacteria with a lipoid capsule and explains the well-recognized rôle of the monocyte in tuberculosis[39] and in leprosy. Clasmatocytes have been found, in animal experiments, to appear after the struggle between the body's defenses and the microörganism is complete. It may be mentioned here that the structure and functional activity of the macrophage cells, like those of the lymphocyte, appear to be regulated by the adrenal cortex.[18]

Because they are normally more abundant in tissue fluid than in blood and are found within the epithelial lining of the bowel, the respiratory tract and the skin, an important role in detoxification[44f] has been attributed to the **eosinophils.** These cells increase in number following the injection of foreign protein and during the decomposition of body protein. Consequently it is held that eosinophils are concerned in the disintegration and removal of protein. The Charcot-Leyden crystals, so regularly found wherever eosinophil leukocytes are being broken down, probably represent crystalline protein formed on a nidus derived from the inner substance of the eosinophilic granules.[45d] The constitution of these granules was mentioned earlier (p. 236). Histamine is claimed to have a chemotactic effect on eosinophils.[1b] Eosinophilia is characteristic of allergic reactions. The eosinophilic response, however, unlike the anaphylactic reaction, was not found to be abolished by antihistamine drugs[39a] and its meaning in relation to hypersensitivity is still obscure.[41] The relation of eosinophilic leukocytes to the pituitary and adrenal hormones has been discussed already

(p. 49). Repeated failure of adreno-corticotrophic hormone to produce eosinopenia strongly suggests non-functioning adrenals but eosinophil response tests with epinephrine cannot be so construed.[47e]

Basophilic leukocytes are very numerous in the blood of many of the amphibia and it has been suggested, therefore, that they may represent in man a functionless evolutionary rest. However, from the fact that these cells and the mast cells of the connective tissue[17b] appear in greater numbers only during the healing phase of inflammation or in chronic inflammation, and from the observation that their metachromatic granules contain heparin, it seems plausible that they function in inflammation by delivering anti-coagulants to facilitate absorption or to prevent clotting of blood and lymph in the obstructed tissue.[14b] The significance of their high content of histamine (p. 236) is obscure. Mast cells may produce hyaluronic acid, thus contributing to the ground substance, and they may produce and release 5-hydroxytryptamine.[17b]

LEUKOKINETICS. DYNAMICS OF LEUKOCYTE PRODUCTION AND CIRCULATION

In an earlier chapter (p. 41) the multiplication and maturation of cells in the bone marrow were discussed and current data concerning mitosis, turnover time and total cell population were presented. Additional quantitative data concerning the leukocytes can now be presented.

Granulocytes. — The granulocytes or, more specifically, the neutrophilic series of cells and the lymphocytes must be considered separately. The source and the functions of these two cell series are quite different and their fate likewise probably differs. The neutrophil is almost certainly an end product and, quite probably, once it has passed out of the intravascular compartment, it never returns. On the other hand, there are reasons to suspect that recirculation of lymphocytes occurs and some believe that this cell can be the progenitor of a number of different cell types. As to other types of cells, namely eosinophils, basophils and monocytes, little in the way of quantitative data is available.

The earliest attempts to study the dynamics of leukocyte production and circulation[60] involved the use of homologous transfusions and cross circulation procedures. Genetic and immunologic incompatibilities and the prompt removal of transfused leukocytes by the lungs,[3a] as well as by the liver and spleen[45a] greatly limited the value of such observations. A more physiological approach was provided by the injection of C^{14}-adenine or radioactive phosphorus, which became incorporated in the deoxyribonucleic acid of the leukocytes[35] or by the use of radioactive (S^{35}) l-cystine[45b] which labels the protein. A very useful technic has been developed in our laboratories by Athens, Cartwright and co-workers, who have employed diisopropylfluorophosphate, the phosphorus being radioactively tagged (DFP^{32}).[1e] This compound is a potent and irreversible inhibitor of cholinesterase and of other esterases and certain proteolytic enzymes. It rapidly forms an irreversible bond with the protein to which it becomes attached and the diisopropylphosphate which is released when the protein is degraded is not reutilized in the body. By appropriate technics DFP^{32} can be used as a label for granulocytes both *in vivo* and *in vitro*.

In addition to the limitations inherent in the technics employed in the early investigations, two important considerations were overlooked. These studies did not measure the life span of leukocytes. The term "life span" is a misnomer when applied to the granulocytes since their functions are carried out chiefly in the

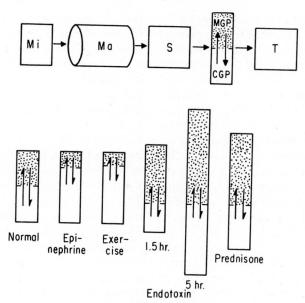

Fig. 4–8.—Kinetic model of granulocyte production and alterations in blood granulocyte pool under various circumstances. Mi refers to mitotic pool; Ma, maturation pool; S, storage pool; MGP (marginal granulocyte pool) and CGP (circulating granulocyte pool) make up the total blood granulocyte pool; T, refers to tissue pool.

tissues and no method has been found whereby their survival there might even be estimated. This is an important difference in the study of leukokinetics as compared with erythrokinetics. Furthermore in a number of the earlier studies, the existence of a large, intramedullary pool of granulocytes was ignored and the fact that cells in the marrow, as well as those in the blood, would be labeled by some of the *in vivo* procedures was not fully appreciated. It has been estimated that the ratio of marrow to blood granulocytes is about 25 to 30 to 1.[11]

A kinetic model for the granulocytes is presented in Figure 4–8. This is a simplified scheme and embodies a great many assumptions. Some of the difficulties and uncertainties which beset the student of leukokinetics were mentioned in an earlier chapter in the discussion of the multiplication and maturation of the cells of the bone marrow (p. 45). "Mi" represents the cells undergoing mitosis, namely myeloblasts, promyelo-

cytes and myelocytes, the "mitotic" or proliferating pool. It is not known how many divisions take place in each of these stages of the granulocyte but it may be significant that the average percentages of these cells, as normally found in the bone marrow, namely 2, 5 and 12 per cent (Table 1–2, p. 65), are roughly consistent with the unproven assumption that only one division takes place as each of these cells is transformed to the next stage. The percentage of metamyelocytes usually found in normal bone marrow, namely 22 per cent, is consistent with another assumption, namely that the myelocyte divides only once to produce the metamyelocyte. The latter cell is thought to be incapable of further division and is considered in the model to be in the "maturation" or differentiating pool (Ma). The "storage pool" (S) contains the mature polymorphonuclear neutrophils. In normal marrow the number of these cells is approximately equal to the number of metamyelocytes.

16

The development of granulocytes probably represents a continuous process involving cell division, growth and maturation. In the mitotic pool, division and maturation occur simultaneously and ultimately the cells pass into the maturation pool, where proliferation does not occur. Presumably, under normal conditions a specific period of time is required for the process of maturation, after which the cells proceed in an orderly manner into the storage pool, whence they leave in random fashion. The size of the mitotic pool has been estimated to be about 2.6×10^9 cells per Kg. body weight. That of the maturation pool may be of the order of 6.3×10^9/Kg. and the storage pool approximately 2.5×10^9/Kg.[11] Estimates of the time a cell spends in the intramedullary pool (Mi + Ma + S) have ranged from three to 11 days.[1e]

It has not been appreciated, as a rule, that a large proportion of granulocytes in the blood are not in the main stream of the circulation. As will be pointed out shortly (p. 243), it is well known that various physiologic influences, such as exercise, excitement and other factors, may be associated with a substantial increase in the leukocyte count. This was long attributed to release of leukocytes sequestered in the spleen. However, various observers have recorded the fact that such changes also occur in splenectomized persons. The DFP[32] technic,[1e] in particular, as well as some earlier studies, have shown that there are in essence two "pools" of granulocytes in the blood, a circulating granulocyte pool (CGP) and a marginated granulocyte pool (MGP). These are almost equal in size ($30.7 \pm 11.8 \times 10^7$ cells/Kg. body weight and $34.6 \pm 15.6 \times 10^7$, respectively) and are in dynamic equilibrium. Exercise or the administration of epinephrine increases the size of the circulating granulocyte pool by about 50 per cent but the total blood granulocyte pool is unchanged. The administration of endotoxin was found to have two effects.[1e] At the end of 90 minutes there was a modest increase in the total number of granulocytes in the blood but, in particular, many leukocytes entered the marginal pool, thus lowering the number in the active circulation. At the end of five hours there was a marked increase in the total granulocyte pool, presumably as the result of the outpouring of cells from the storage pool of the bone marrow. The administration of steroids also produced an increase in the size of the total blood pool, probably for the same reason.

Granulocytes have been labeled successfully in vitro with DFP[32] and the undamaged cells have been returned to their donor, thus making possible an estimate of their "blood transit time." Half of the labeled cells ($T\frac{1}{2}$) are removed, on the average, in 6.6 hours.[1e] From these and other studies it appears that the average time granulocytes spend in the circulation is nine hours.[1e,8b] It is likely that they leave the circulation in random fashion. From leukophoresis and other experiments[8b] it is probable that granulocytes which have crossed the endothelial barrier between blood and tissues do not re-enter the circulation, at least not in significant numbers. The number of granulocytes which pass through the blood each day (granulocyte turnover rate, GTR) has been calculated from these data to be 172×10^7 cells/Kg., or 7.2×10^7 per hour.

One more estimate can be made on the basis of current information. From the figures for pool sizes quoted earlier (p. 46) and from the value for granulocyte turnover rate given above, it would appear that the turnover time for the mitotic, maturation and storage pools of the bone marrow may be in the range of 159 to approximately 256 hours. Consequently, the "life span" of granulocytes up to the point of their entry into the tissues may be estimated as being of the order of 6½ to 11 days.

Needless to say, the above are approximations which can be expected to be modified by further observations. Furthermore, they refer to average values in a normal man. Some of the alterations which occur in response to physiologic requirements have been mentioned already. Studies based on the technic of leukophoresis have shown that the normal animal replenishes the circulating blood by calling upon stores of cells as well as by an increased production rate.[8b] Acceleration of production of granulocytes can be postulated as occurring in several ways. Thus (1) more stem cells may differentiate into myeloblasts, (2) more mitoses may take place, (3) mitosis may become more rapid and the intermitotic interval may be shortened. An increase in the quantity of cells in the circulation would occur if, in addition, granulocytes were released more rapidly from the bone marrow and the bone marrow stores were drained. Finally, granulocytes can be mobilized quickly from the marginal pool of the blood. On the other hand, the total number of cells in the blood can be influenced by the rate of passage of granulocytes into the tissues as well as by alterations in the number of cell deaths, in the circulation as well as in the marrow. Granulocytes can be found in the saliva, in the tracheobronchial tree and in the gastrointestinal tract. What proportion is lost by these routes and whether or not their presence there is accidental or serves a useful purpose, is unknown. It seems most likely that the majority are lost through disintegration and dissolution in various organs, particularly in the liver, spleen and lymph nodes.[47d]

It is obvious that application of the technics mentioned to the study of leukocytosis and leukopenia, as well as in the investigation of the various forms of leukemia, including the leukopenic forms, should be rewarding.

Lymphocytes.—In view of the uncertainties concerning the nature and functions of the lymphocyte (p. 239), it is not surprising that considerable confusion has revolved about the kinetics of lymphocyte production and distribution. DNA-labeling experiments indicated a very prolonged life span for the bulk of lymphocytes (100 to 200 days) but about 20 per cent of the cells seemed to have a mean age of three to four days.[35c] It is difficult to reconcile these findings with the evidence of rapid proliferation of lymphoid tissue and the observation that lymphocytes disappear rather quickly if production is terminated.[8b] Part of the paradox may be resolved by evidence which indicates that recirculation of lymphocytes occurs.[15b,18a] Another consideration is that large and medium lymphocytes may have a life history quite distinct from that of the small lymphocyte. Finally, fragments of the latter may be reutilized.[19a]

In chronic lymphocytic leukemia the life span of lymphocytes was found to approximate that of the longer-lived type of normal cells.[45b] The life span of the immature cells of acute leukemia may be very brief.

NORMAL VALUES FOR LEUKOCYTES

It is generally stated that the leukocyte count of the normal adult is 5000 to 10,000 cells per c.mm. with an average of 7000 (See p. 249). Values above 10,000 are usually considered as representing *leukocytosis* whereas those below 5000 indicate *leukopenia*.

Physiological Leukocytosis. — Actually, the situation is more complex than appears from this simple statement. In 11 per cent of apparently normal persons values above 10,000 per c.mm. are found.[50] Then again, it appears that in some individuals the leukocyte count is normally well below 10,000 and this figure

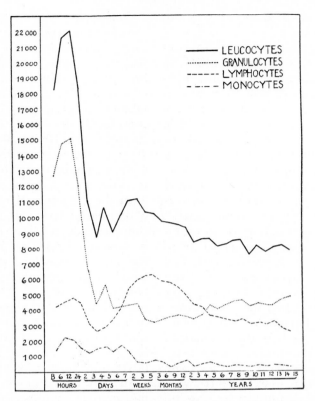

Fig. 4–9.—Average values for total leukocytes, granulocytes, lymphocytes and monocytes from birth to fifteen years of age. (Kato, courtesy of Jour. Pediatrics.)

in them is distinctly in the region indicating a pathological leukocytosis. The leukocyte count differs according to the state of physical and mental rest, and with reference to many other factors. A number of the factors producing a "*physiological*" leukocytosis may be considered.

In the **newborn infant,** values above 10,000 are the rule and counts as high as 45,000 have been recorded, although very low values, even 3600, are sometimes found.[50] The maximum leukocyte count is usually attained at the end of the first twenty-four hours. The cells are chiefly polymorphonuclear neutrophils, particularly single and bilobed forms. On the third or fourth day, the count usually drops quickly and then fluctuates[54] as shown in Figure 4–9. From the

third week on, the relative proportion of neutrophils and lymphocytes is reversed and this relative lymphocytosis continues until four years of age or even later. Adult proportions are probably reached at about puberty. During *infancy*, however, the leukocyte count may be very irregular. Until twenty-six weeks of life variations from 5000 to 24,000 may occur in the absence of demonstrable disease.[65] In the majority of normal infants the range of leukocyte counts is 8000 to 16,500.

In childhood, the range of variation tends to decrease and the general average becomes lower as adult age is approached. Thus, for the age groups four to seven, and eight to eighteen years the range is given as 6000 to 15,000, and 4500 to 13,500, respectively, with averages of

10,700 and 8300, respectively.[50] No significant difference, as compared with adults, has been observed in the **aged.**[61b]

Fluctuations occur *during a single day*, as well as *from day to day*. The suggestion that these follow a characteristic hourly rhythm has not been confirmed,[48a,56] nor has the occurrence of a "digestive" leukocytosis (that is, following meals) been established.[64d] Light influences the diurnal variation.[63d] Under conditions of complete physical and mental relaxation, a *basal level* of 5000 to 7000 cells isusual.[50] The random activity of ordinary routine may be associated with a moderate increase and a somewhat higher level is common in the afternoon. Under all these conditions, however, the leukocyte count tends to remain within the range of "normal." In protracted heavy manual work, neutrophilic leukocytosis, lymphopenia and eosinopenia have been observed.[53] With **strenuous exercise** the leukocyte count may rise as high as 35,000. The increment in cells is made up chiefly of polymorphonuclear neutrophils and is probably due to a redistribution of forms normally shunted out of active circulation. This type of leukocytosis may occur even in splenectomized animals.[50] As discussed earlier (p. 241), mobilization of cells from the marginal granulocyte pool probably accounts, in large measure at least, for the increased numbers of cells. The leukocytosis appears with remarkable rapidity (*e.g.*, 35,000 after a quarter-mile run completed in one minute) and recedes to normal within an hour. The magnitude of the leukocytosis associated with exercise appears to depend primarily on the intensity of the activity, rather than upon the duration.[49c] Fatigue approaching exhaustion is accompanied by neutrophilia, with neutrophils ranging from 80 to 90 per cent. **Convulsive seizures,** such as those of epilepsy, are followed by the same effects on the leukocyte count as violent exercise. Electrically induced convulsions are followed by a reduction in eosinophils and lymphocytes and a rise in neutrophils.[47c] **Epinephrine** causes a marked leukocytosis which manifests two phases.[49e,63c] In the first, which is maximal at about 17 minutes after the injection, the neutrophils, lymphocytes and eosinophilis are increased. During the second phase the neutrophils rise again but the lymphocytes and eosinophils are reduced in number.[63c] Epinephrine evokes leukocytosis even in the absence of the spleen.[59] During attacks of **paroxysmal tachycardia** leukocytosis of 13,000 to 22,000 has been observed.[58]

An important consideration from the viewpoint of differential diagnosis is the fact that **pain** without associated infection has been observed to cause leukocytosis and so also have nausea and vomiting. This cellular change is not due to new formation of cells but is caused by their mobilization from the lungs, liver, spleen and other organs, where they lie within or in close proximity to the smaller blood vessels. It can be distinguished from the leukocytosis of infection by the increase of young cells in the latter.

Leukocytosis is of frequent occurrence in patients with **emotional disorders** (fear and panic reactions, depression with anxiety [agitation], subacute and persistent anxiety states). The degree of leukocytosis has been noted to be related often to the intensity of the psychopathological emotion.[61]

Ether anesthesia produces leukocytosis but this does not occur following narcosis with barbital compounds. Emotional and reflex reactions as well as struggling during the stage of excitement probably account for the leukocytic increase.

During the ovulatory period, eosinopenia and a slight rise in the number of leukocytes as well as increased levels of 17-hydroxycorticosteroids have been reported.[62] Slight leukocytosis occurs during **pregnancy,** and neutrophilia increases as term approaches.[64a] The onset of labor is accompanied by neutrophilic leukocytosis, which is sometimes very pronounced (34,000), and this continues for a day after delivery, only receding to normal after four or five days. These changes are accompanied by a reduction in the number of circulating eosinophils.[49a]

Conclusive demonstration of the effects of **climate** or **season** on the leukocyte count is lacking. It was claimed that meterologically conditioned fluctuations occur.[63] Heat and intense solar radiation are said to cause leukocytosis.[55] Artificially induced heat causes lymphocytosis.[49d] Sunlight and ultraviolet radiation are reported as causing lymphocytosis. Acute anoxia, both anoxic and anemic, causes leukocytosis.[49] This is neutrophilic in type and does not develop in adreno-demedullated rats. In the first few days after arrival at high altitudes some leukocytosis, accompanied by lymphopenia and eosinopenia, has been observed. Slight lymphocytosis and eosinophilia soon develop, however.[64c]

Many of the physiologic variations in the leukocytes which have been described above can be explained as manifestations of stimulation of the adrenal cortex (p. 49). It is noteworthy in this connection that the administration of cortisone or hydrocortisone was found to be followed by increased blood levels of 17-hydrocorticosteroids which attained their maximal elevation in one hour.[61a] This was succeeded by eosinopenia and lymphopenia which became maximal in four to eight hours and bore a close relation to the quantity of hormone administered. Neutrophilia occurred less constantly and was not found to be well correlated in time or degree to the changes in eosinophils and lymphocytes.

The above observations have led to new interest in the *normal eosinophil count* and in its *physiologic variations*. Methods for making absolute eosinophil counts will be described later (p. 391). Although, on the basis of the differential count and the total leukocyte count, the normal eosinophil count is generally regarded as ranging from 50 to 250 cells per c.mm. (p. 249), absolute counts yield higher maximal values, up to about 550 per c.mm.[64b] There is a cyclic diurnal variation, some finding a decrease in number in the morning[64b] while others have stressed that there is no pattern common to all subjects and that significant, random day to day differences are found within the same subject.[47b] Emotional stress may be associated with a decrease in the total eosinophil count.[57] Cyclic changes during the different phases of the menstrual cycle have been reported, progressive eosinopenia occurring during the whole of the intermenstrual period.[61c]

SYSTEMS FOR DIFFERENTIAL COUNTING

Following the perfection of methods for enumerating the blood corpuscles and the introduction of the blood stains, the next technical advance in the study of the leukocytes was **Arneth's classification** (1904) of the leukocytes of the myeloid series according to the shape and number of lobes forming their nucleus (Fig. 4–10). He believed that the nucleus gradually becomes more indented as it develops, subsequently dividing into two, then three and more lobes. The formation of a segmented neutrophil from a metamyelocyte has been observed in tissue culture.[47f] Although Arneth's hypothesis is accepted, his classification is rarely followed. He divided the granulocytes into five classes and a number of subdivisions, making a total of 20 in all. Not only is such a classification too complex for ordinary use, but emphasis is laid on the separation of the older types of polymorphonuclear leukocyte, a task which experience has indicated is un-

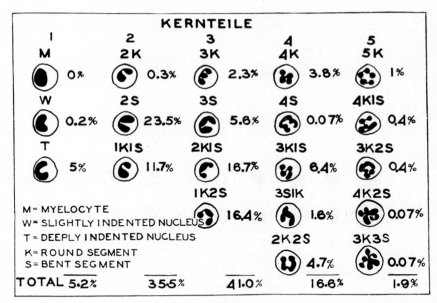

FIG. 4–10.—Arneth's classification of neutrophilic leukocytes. The number of each of the cell types which he considered normal is shown in per cent. (Wintrobe, courtesy of Bull. New York Acad. Med.)

necessary. Cooke and Ponder's classification, though much more simple, is also open to the last criticism.[52]

In classifying the granulocytes, Arneth tabulated them across a page with the first class (single-lobed nucleus) to the left and the last class at the right (Fig. 4–10). Thus the term *"shift to the left"* was introduced to describe an increase in the single and bilobed (and thus younger) forms, while *"shift to the right"* implies an increase in the older forms.

In **Schilling's classification** (1911)[52] the neutrophils are divided into four groups: (1) myelocytes; (2) juveniles, in which the nucleus is indented; (3) "stab-kernige" or staff cells with unsegmented but T-, V-, or U-shaped nuclei; and (4) segmented neutrophils. Schilling used the term *"regenerative shift"* in referring to the rapid outpouring of leukocytes from the marrow in response to an acute need, as indicated by the appearance of younger forms (juveniles and even myelocytes). He also introduced the concept of a *"degenerative"* shift to the

left. By this he meant a failure to mature as the result of the depression of marrow function. When the "shift" is of this type, an increased number of immature forms is found in the blood but the nuclei of many of these are narrow, deeply staining and little or no structural detail can be made out ("stab-kernige" or staff cells).[63b] Such cells, it is assumed, can mature no further.

The significance of **qualitative changes in the cytoplasm** has also been emphasized.[51a,52] In severe infections and other toxemias, deeply staining, basophilic granules are found in the neutrophils. These *"toxic granules"* may be large or small. If small, they are distributed among the normal, pinkish granules. If large, few or no normal granules are found in the affected cells and only the diffusely scattered, coarse, irregular, dark granules are found. Abnormality of the cytoplasmic structures of the neutrophils is also indicated by bluish staining or vacuolization of the cytoplasm[63a] and by the appearance of

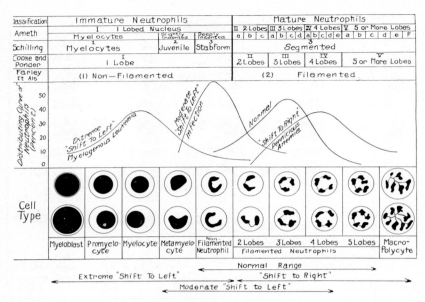

Fig. 4–11.—Diagram illustrating several classifications of the neutrophils. Note that all the classifications agree in a common dividing line between mature and immature cells. The Schilling classification further subdivides only the immature cells. The Cooke and Ponder and the Arneth classifications further subdivide only the more mature cells. (Haden, Principles of Hematology.)

the cells after staining by the peroxidase method. Normally, neutrophilic cells are full of peroxidase staining granules. When toxic basophilic staining is demonstrable by one of the Romanowsky staining methods, few peroxidase reacting granules are found in the cells. The cytoplasmic abnormalities may occur in segmented or in non-segmented neutrophils. It is thought that the "toxic" changes in these cells are manifestations of cell damage.[51a]

A great number of methods for differential counting, "hemograms," indexes and formulae, have been described (Fig. 4–11). It would serve no useful purpose to discuss them in any detail. They introduce no morphological criteria in addition to those described above but instead, in the writer's opinion, enshroud a relatively simple subject with an air of complexity and mysticism.

The interpretation of the neutrophil picture will be considered in subsequent pages where the significance of alterations in other types of leukocytes will also be discussed.

The Technic of the Differential Count.—A uniformly thin smear of blood on a cover-slip is the most satisfactory kind of preparation. Smears drawn or pulled on slides are less suitable because the larger leukocytes tend to accumulate at the margins while the smaller cells (lymphocytes) are distributed in the central portion of the films. Ideally, one should enumerate all the leukocytes on both cover-slips, thus identifying all the cells in a single drop of blood. This being usually impractical, as large an area as possible should be covered, 100 cells being considered a minimum. It is preferable to examine both cover-slip preparations even if this small number is counted. The oil-immersion magnification should be used. A mechanical stage is invaluable.

A matter of great importance in the interpretation of the leukocyte count, is an understanding of *the significance of a change in the percentage of cells*, let us say from 70 per cent polymorphonuclears to 80 per cent. As already stated, the error due to chance distribution is considerably lessened as more cells are enumerated. Goldner and Mann[51] published "confidence curves" from which one may estimate the probable error of a differential count when various numbers of cells are counted. According to these curves, if 200 cells are counted, one may, nineteen times out of twenty, expect the true proportion of polymorphonuclears to be somewhere between 63.6 and 76.4 per cent when the count is found to be 70 per cent. Accordingly, a count of 80 per cent on the same patient at another time could probably be considered as being significantly increased. However, if the count was made on only 100 leukocytes, the difference would be scarcely significant.

It is necessary to lay some emphasis on the subject of error in leukocyte counting because, in general, physicians are not sufficiently critical of this, just as they may too readily accept at face value many other laboratory procedures. Because the results are expressed numerically, many derive a false sense of accuracy from them. It is important to scrutinize the figures as carefully as one examines the patient. In fact, it is probably even more important to do so because the physician usually examines the patient himself, whereas the laboratory studies are often left to an assistant.

Good staining is, of course, a prerequisite for satisfactory work. It may be pointed out that "toxic" changes in neutrophils must be distinguished from the effects of poor staining. It is rare to find that all leukocytes in a smear show abnormal staining of the nuclei of the neutrophils and toxic granules in their cytoplasm. Such a finding should arouse suspicion of faulty technic and must be checked by the examination of a smear of normal blood stained at the same time.

Differences in interpretation naturally introduce great variations in the differential count. Even a well-trained observer may have difficulty in distinguishing some segmented forms from non-segmented neutrophils. The filament, non-filament count was introduced to make this distinction easier.[52] By "*filamented*" *cells* is meant those in which two or more lobes are united by a filament of chromatin. All other cells, even though they may appear segmented, are classed as non-filamented. This arbitrary method of classification, however, defeats the purpose of a differential count. The writer recommends the avoidance of formulas and rules and advises instead careful scrutiny of each cell, bearing in mind the fact that when one deals with living cells it may be expected that some will not fit exactly into a rigid classification.

Normal Values for Different Types of Leukocytes.—The values for the different types of leukocytes in the normal

Table 4–3—Relative and Absolute Values for Leukocyte Counts in Normal Adults per c.mm. Blood

Type of cell	Per cent	Absolute number		
		Average	Minimum	Maximum
Total leukocytes	...	7,000	5,000	10,000
Myelocytes	0	0	0	0
Juvenile neutrophils	3–5	300	150	400
Segmented neutrophils	54–62	4,000	3,000	5,800
Eosinophils	1–3	200	50	250
Basophils	0–0.75	25	15	50
Lymphocytes	25–33	2,100	1,500	3,000
Monocytes	3–7	375	285	500

adult are given in Table 4–3. In this table the juvenile neutrophils include Schilling's "stab" forms. He gave the normal values for the latter as 3 to 5 per cent and for juvenile, non-stab forms, 0 to 1 per cent.

As already stated, because of the element of chance in distribution of cells, a variation from the normal values for neutrophils can hardly be considered significant unless it differs by at least 10 per cent, and for cells found in smaller numbers the probable error is much greater.

Normally, myelocytes are not found in the blood. It was shown, however, that concentrates of leukocytes, as in the buffy coat, will yield metamyelocytes and even myelocytes, and atypical mononuclear cells as well as nuclear fragments of megakaryocytes.[49b]

Leukocyte Resistance.—Studies of osmotic and mechanical resistance of leukocytes have been carried out[64] but their importance for clinical medicine is obscure.

VARIATIONS OF LEUKOCYTES IN DISEASE

Alterations in the total number of leukocytes and in their relative proportions are of considerable significance as measures of the reaction of the body to noxious agents. In many instances the alterations in the total and relative numbers of the leukocytes are of such a character that the nature of the noxious agent may be suspected. The changes which occur may involve all three types of leukocytes and may be observed not only in acute infections but in many chronic ailments as well.[131]

Leukocytosis. Neutrophilia.—Leukocytosis refers to an increase in the total number of leukocytes above the normal; that is, an increase in the count above 10,000 or 11,000 per c.mm. Generally leukocytosis is due to an increase in the number of cells of the neutrophilic series and thus the term is often used synony-

Table 4–4—Causes of Neutrophilia*

1. Acute infections, especially coccal
     certain bacilli, fungi, spirochetes, viruses and parasites
     Localized infections
     Certain general infections, such as rheumatic fever, diphtheria, smallpox
     Development of complications in diseases usually not associated with neutrophilia

2. Intoxications
     (a) Metabolic; uremia, diabetic acidosis, eclampsia, gout, burns
     (b) Poisoning by chemicals and drugs; lead, mercury, digitalis, epinephrine, insect venoms;
          black widow spider
          foreign proteins, after a preliminary leukopenia

3. Acute hemorrhage

4. Postoperatively

5. Non-inflammatory conditions, such as coronary thrombosis

6. Malignant neoplasms when growing rapidly, especially in gastro-intestinal tract, liver, bone
     marrow

7. Sudden hemolysis of red corpuscles

8. Physiological in the newborn, during labor, after strenuous exercise, after repeated vomiting,
     convulsions, paroxysmal tachycardia.

9. Myelocytic leukemia and erythremia.

* Tables 4–4 to 4–13 from Wintrobe: Bull. New York Acad. Med., *15*, 223, 1939.

mously with the designation *neutrophilia*. Usually neutrophilia is "absolute;" that is, not only is the proportion of the neutrophilic leukocytes increased above the normal (62 per cent), but their total number per c.mm. is generally increased and, as a consequence, the total leukocyte count rises above normal.

In certain pathological conditions leukocyte counts of 15,000 to 25,000 are common and values as high as 40,000 are not unusual. Occasionally higher counts, even up to 100,000 per c.mm. may be found. (See Leukemoid Pictures.)

Causes of Neutrophilia.—Neutrophilia (Table 4–4) is found in:

1. Acute *infections* caused by *cocci* (staphylococcus, streptococcus, pneumococcus, gonococcus, meningococcus, micrococcus catarrhalis) and by *some bacilli* (E. coli, Ps. aeruginosa, C. diphtheriae, P. tularensis) as well as certain *fungi* (Actinomyces), *Spirochetes* (L. icterohemorrhagiae), *viruses* (rabies, poliomyelitis, herpes zoster), *rickettsia* (typhus) and *parasites* (liver fluke, coccidioidosis). Thus neutrophilia is found in the following *localized infections*: abscess, furunculosis, osteomyelitis, tonsillitis, otitis media, pyelitis, cholecystitis, salpingitis; as well as in the following *generalized infections*: acute rheumatic fever, scarlet fever, smallpox, chickenpox, diphtheria, erysipelas, endocarditis, septicemia, appendicitis, peritonitis, meningitis, gonorrhea, anthrax, cholera and plague.

In these conditions leukocyte counts of 15,000 to 25,000 are usually found. In pneumonia, higher counts (20,000 to 40,000) are characteristic. Immediately following the crisis a shower of myelocytes may appear in the peripheral blood.[123] In bronchopneumonia a moderate leukocytosis is common, although this depends on the cause of the infection. Of all the exanthems, leukocytosis is most marked in scarlet fever in which condition it may be as high as 40,000.

Usually leukocytosis is absent in typhoid fever, paratyphoid fever, tuberculosis, measles, glanders and epidemic mumps. In these conditions leukocytosis suggests complication or localization, *e.g.*, in tuberculous meningitis leukocytosis is common. It is also found in tuberculous peritonitis and, if blood has escaped into the pleural cavity, in tuberculous pleurisy.

2. *Intoxications.*—These may be: (*a*) Those associated with *metabolic* disorders such as uremia, diabetic acidosis, eclampsia and gout. In diabetic acidosis counts as high as 25,000 may be found. In azotemia the leukocytosis is especially marked if pericarditis occurs. The leukocytosis in gout occurs during acute attacks and may reach values as high as 30,000. Leukocyte counts as high as 80,000 have been found in cases of severe burns.

The neutrophilic increase in eclampsia is at least in part caused by the convulsions, and muscular activity probably accounts for the slight leukocytosis of delirium tremens. Leukocytosis is also found in intestinal obstruction and in strangulated hernia but many insist that this does not occur until peritonitis has set in. Leukocytosis is frequently found in association with burns. This is accompanied by neutrophilia, a "shift to the left" and the presence of "toxic" and "degenerative" forms.[127a]

(*b*) Leukocytosis has been described following *poisoning* by the following *chemicals and drugs*: lead, mercury, illuminating gas, potassium chlorate, digitalis, epinephrine, camphor, antipyrin, acetanilid, phenacetin, pyridine, pyrogallol, turpentine, benzene derivatives, arsphenamin; as well as in cases of *poisoning by insect venoms*, such as that of the black widow spider. It has been reported that leukocytosis can be induced by the intramuscular injection of methyl-acetamide, especially if it is combined with *p*-chloroxylenol.[134]

A number of the drugs mentioned have also been found to cause marked reduction in the leukocyte count, particularly in the neutrophils. This effect may depend on the degree of poisoning, leukocytosis occurring when the effect is temporary and less serious. Some of these drugs no doubt cause leukocytosis because vomiting or convulsions are induced.

In lead colic leukocyte counts as high as 20,000 may be found.

(c) Following the injection of *foreign protein* there is a preliminary leukopenia which is followed by leukocytosis. The latter is found also in serum disease and transiently during a Jarisch-Herxheimer reaction. The injection of vaccine is followed by leukocytosis.

3. Following *acute hemorrhage*. Leukocytosis will develop within an hour or two of the hemorrhage. The leukocytosis is greater when the hemorrhage has occurred into the peritoneum, the pleura, against the dura or into a joint cavity, than when it is external. In ruptured tubal pregnancy the count may be as high as 22,000. In cases of fractured skull in which bleeding against the dura has occurred or in spontaneous subarachnoid hemorrhage, even higher counts are sometimes found. A value as high as 31,000 has been observed following rupture of the spleen. Large external hemorrhages cause leukocytosis probably through stimulation of the bone marrow. In the case of internal bleeding, since even small hemorrhages may cause marked neutrophilia, absorption of some unusually stimulating substance probably plays a rôle.

4. *Postoperatively*, neutrophilia occurs for twelve to thirty-six hours, perhaps as the result of the extensive tissue injury and liberation of protein.

5. In *certain non-inflammatory conditions* such as coronary thrombosis. The leukocytosis of coronary thrombosis is valuable in distinguishing this disease from angina pectoris.

6. *Malignant neoplasms* may cause leukocytosis when the neoplasm is growing rapidly. When the liver, gastro-intestinal tract or bone marrow is involved, the count may be exceptionally high. In such cases the whole clinical picture may suggest leukemia.[95]

7. Following the *sudden hemolysis of red corpuscles* very marked leukocytosis may occur.

As already mentioned, leukocytosis of the neutrophilic type may occur, without associated infection or disease, in the newborn, during labor and after strenuous exercise, as well as following repeated vomiting or convulsions, in dehydration and in paroxysmal tachycardia.[58] Neutrophilia also occurs in chronic myelocytic leukemia and in erythremia. In leukemia there is usually a marked "shift to the left" and myelocytes predominate. A few cases of leukemia have been observed in which the predominating cells in the blood were polymorphonuclear leukocytes (See Chapter 19.)

Factors Affecting the Magnitude of Neutrophilia.—The magnitude of the increase in the total neutrophil count (Table 4–5) generally depends on:

1. *The cause of the neutrophilia.* Thus, pyogenic bacteria, particularly cocci, call forth a neutrophilic response when they invade the body tissue, whereas other bacteria, such as typhoid and tubercle bacilli have no such effect. Pneumococci generally cause a more marked neutro-

Table 4–5—Factors Influencing the Magnitude of Neutrophilia

1. The cause of the neutrophilia; pyogenic, especially coccal *vs.* typhoid or tubercle bacilli
2. Localization of the process; then even tubercle bacilli may cause neutrophilia
3. Virulence of the organism, reactivity of the patient
   Numerical increase = resistance of the individual
   Percentage increase ⎫
   Toxic changes ⎭ = effort of the response

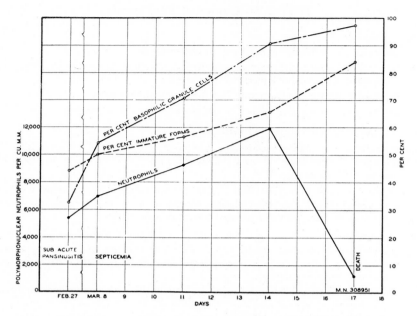

Fig. 4–9.—The neutrophilic leukocytes in a fatal case of acute pansinusitis and cavernous sinus thrombosis followed by septicemia. The leukocytic picture was unfavorable throughout. (Bethell, courtesy of J. Lab. & Clin. Med.)

philia than do other types of cocci. But it must be kept in mind that neutrophilia is not necessarily the result of an infection; thus, neutrophilia is common in uremia.

2. *The localization of the process.* A generalized infection, even when it is the result of an invasion of cocci, as in streptococcal septicemia, is often not associated with an increase in the total leukocyte count, whereas a more localized process tends to stimulate neutrophil formation. The latter may occur even when the invading organism is one which usually is associated with leukopenia; *e.g.*, neutrophilia is common in tuberculous meningitis.

3. *The virulence of the invading organism, the reaction of the patient,* and his general resistance are also concerned in determining the magnitude of the neutrophilic increase. Thus, neutrophilia will be absent when the infection is very mild. It is also lacking, however, when the infection is overwhelming or

the patient is too feeble and non-resistant. A good example of the effect of overwhelming infection is the leukopenia of acute fulminating appendicitis.

4. *In children* a given stimulus tends to produce a more marked increase in the total neutrophil count than in adults.

As a general rule, the total numerical increase of neutrophils may be regarded as indicating the resistance of the individual to an infection. The percentage increase of these cells and the qualitative changes, on the other hand, indicate the effort of the response and the severity of the infection. It is in these respects that a detailed differential count in which the number of young granulocytes is determined and the qualitative changes in their nuclei, cytoplasm and granules are noted, is important. Thus, in the presence of an overwhelming infection, even though the total leukocyte count may not be increased, there is a marked "shift to the left," the nuclei of many of the

Table 4–6—Causes of Leukopenia

1. Certain infections
   - (a) Bacterial; *e.g.*, typhoid, paratyphoid, undulant fever.
   - (b) Infections caused by viruses and rickettsia; *e.g.*, influenza, measles, rubella, infectious hepatitis, Colorado tick fever, sandfly fever.
   - (c) Protozoal infections; *e.g.*, malaria, relapsing fever, kala-azar.

2. All types of overwhelming infections; *e.g.*,miliary tuberculosis, septicemia.

3. Cachectic and debilitated states and inanition.

4. Certain conditions of unknown cause; *e.g.*, cirrhosis of the liver, Felty's syndrome, lupus erythematosus disseminatus, "primary splenic neutropenia," cyclic neutropenia, chronic hypoplastic neutropenia.

5. Hemopoietic disorders, especially those involving the spleen: Banti's disease, Gaucher's disease; also in pernicious anemia (relapse), chronic hypochromic anemia, aplastic anemia, myelophthisic anemia, "aleukemic" leukemia, agranulocytosis.

6. As the effect of:
   - (a) Chemical and physical agents which regularly produce marrow hypoplasia and aplasia if a sufficient dose is given (ionizing radiation, mustards, urethane, myleran, benzene, antimetabolites).
   - (b) Chemical agents which are occasionally associated with leukopenia (amidopyrine, antithyroid drugs, anticonvulsants, sulfonamides, antihistaminics, various anti-microbial agents, etc. See Table 21–1, p. 1098).

7. In anaphylactoid shock and in early stages of reaction to foreign protein.

juvenile neutrophils are pyknotic and toxic granulation is found in their cytoplasm. The juvenile neutrophils may outnumber the segmented forms and myelocytes may appear.

Successive, detailed blood examinations are thus of considerable value as an index of prognosis. Furthermore, "physiological" leukocytosis may be distinguished from the pathological type by the fact that the former is unaccompanied by qualitative changes in the cells. In general, the following principles may be accepted:

1. A slight neutrophilia with a slight increase in the juvenile neutrophils suggests a mild infection, very good resistance or favorable localization of the infective process.

2. A marked leukocytosis with moderate "shift to the left" (as much as 25 per cent juveniles) and only moderate toxic granulation (*e.g.*, 20 per cent) suggests a severe infection well handled.

3. A falling total leukocyte count with a relatively great increase in the immature granulocytes is an unfavorable sign, especially when accompanied by an increase of toxic granulation (Fig. 4–9). These qualitative changes are of less serious omen if they are accompanied by a high total leukocyte count.

Leukopenia.—Leukopenia is the term applied to a reduction in the leukocyte count below normal. Usually the reduction in cells is due to a marked decrease in the cells of the granulocytic series. When the leukopenia is marked, however, all types are affected.

Causes of Leukopenia.—The causes of leukopenia (Table 4–6) may be enumerated as follows:

1. As a *characteristic of certain infections.* These include:

(a) *Bacterial* infections: typhoid, paratyphoid and sometimes tularemia. In a series of 888 cases of brucellosis, leukopenia was present in one-third.[73d] When typhoid is ushered in by bronchitis, moderate leukocytosis may occur at first.

(*b*) Infections caused by *viruses* and *rickettsia*: influenza (except at the onset), measles,[68] rubella[97] and, until the fourth day, smallpox; infectious hepatitis, psittacosis, dengue, Colorado tick fever,[90g] tsutsugamushi fever (scrub typhus), pappataci fever (sand-fly fever). In influenza the leukocyte count may fall as low as 1500. If complications arise, leukocytosis may develop. In *infectious hepatitis*, leukopenia due to reduction both in granulocytes and lymphocytes begins in the first twenty-four to forty-eight hours of fever and is associated with the primary, preicteric phase of the disease.[88a] Subsequently, relative, and even absolute lymphocytosis follows and numerous atypical lymphocytes are common.

(*c*) *Protozoal* infections: malaria, kala-azar,[73b] oriental sore, relapsing fever. In malaria slight leukocytosis (11,000 cells per c.mm.) may develop for a short time during the paroxysm, but shortly after its onset leukopenia ensues. In relapsing fever the leukopenia is found between the periods of fever. While there is fever, leukocytosis as high as 15,000 cells per c.mm. may occur.

2. In *all types of overwhelming infection*; *e.g.*, miliary tuberculosis, septicemia. In fatal cases of pneumonia counts as low as 150 per c.mm. have been observed.

3. *Cachectic and debilitated states* and inanition. The possible role of nutritional factors will be discussed below.

4. In certain conditions of unknown cause. In *portal cirrhosis of the liver* there is a tendency to leukopenia and absolute monocytosis.[98] Leukopenia is found in 66 per cent of cases of *lupus erythematosus disseminatus*[74c] (p. 1029). In *Felty's syndrome*, a condition characterized by arthritis and splenomegaly (p. 1056), leukopenia of about 3000 cells per c.mm. and affecting all types of leukocytes, is the third of a characteristic triad. Leukopenia sometimes occurs in infectious mononucleosis (Chapter 21). "Primary splenic neutropenia" periodic or cyclic neutropenia and other chronic neutropenias of obscure etiology are described elsewhere (p.1103).

5. *Hemopoietic disorders*; Chronic anemias such as pernicious anemia and chronic hypochromic anemia; aplastic anemia, myelophthisic anemia; *disorders involving the spleen* such as "Banti's disease" (Chapter 20), Gaucher's disease, "aleukemic" leukemia; and in the condition agranulocytosis (Chapter 21).

6. As the effect of certain *chemical* and *physical* agents. The different chemical agents which may produce leukopenia are discussed in the chapter on agranulocytosis (p. 1096). The effects of irradiation are considered on page 557.

7. In *anaphylactoid shock* and in the early stage of the reaction to foreign protein parenterally introduced.

Leukopenic Index (Vaughan). — This refers to leukopenia which is said to occur in allergic individuals following the ingestion of food to which they are sensitive. The patient, previously fasting and at rest, is given the test food. Leukocyte counts are made before and at fifteen-minute intervals in the first hour and at thirty-minute intervals in the second hour following ingestion. A decrease in the leukocyte count of 1000 or more cells per c.mm. is interpreted as indicating incompatibility of the food.

This test has been the subject of considerable criticism on the ground that many factors, recognized as well as obscure and not easily controlled, are capable of affecting the number of leukocytes and that consequently the test is misleading. There is, furthermore, a large unavoidable error in leukocyte counting (p. 391) which must also be considered in evaluating the results.

Neutropenia Without Leukopenia. —In some instances there may be neutropenia (reduction in the number of neutrophils below normal) without leukopenia, the deficit being made up by an increase in the other cells. Thus, a leukocyte count of 7600 per c.mm. with 0.5 per cent neutrophils was reported in a case of typhoid fever.[67] Less marked modifications of the leukocytic picture are not uncommon.

Rarely, *leukopenia* may be *due to a reduction in the lymphocytes*. This has been described in miliary tuberculosis, following excessive exposure to irradiation and in systemic lupus erythematosus. The action of certain chemical agents is much more pronounced on lymphocytes than granulocytes (*e.g.*, nitrogen mustards, p. 1037). *Lymphopenia* is encountered in some lymphadenopathies, especially Hodgkin's disease, and has been noted in cardiac failure, uremia and cholemia.[122] It follows administration of adrenocorticotropic hormone or adrenal cortical hormone. Three cases have been described in children in which there was extreme atrophy of lymphoid tissue with virtual absence of lymphocytes from the blood.[80a]

Pathogenesis of Leukopenia.— Various mechanisms may be concerned in the production of leukopenia. In anaphylactoid shock the neutrophilic leukocytes collect in the internal organs.[72] Within an hour of the intravenous injection of killed bacteria or other foreign protein, the leukocyte count may fall to a quarter, or less, of its former level. It has been observed by means of a transparent chamber inserted in the ears of rabbits that, in response to intravenous injections of appropriate doses of glycogen, gum acacia and other substances, the leukocytes cease to move along the walls of the veins and adhere to the walls of the vessels and to each other.[82a] This effect is transient but is accompanied by marked leukopenia.

The pathogenesis of the leukopenia seen as a characteristic of certain infections or of that found in association with overwhelming infections is quite obscure. The leukocytic response to inflammation was discussed in an earlier section (p. 236).

The significance of alterations in the fragility of the phagocytizing neutrophil[83a] is uncertain. The leukopenia associated with splenic disorders has been attributed to "hypersplenism," a concept implying a hormonal or sequestrational effect which, though very plausible, remains to be demonstrated more conclusively (p. 1051). The leukopenia accompanying marrow metastases has been attributed to "crowding out" of the marrow by the new growths, a view generally accepted but by no means proved.

The rôle of leukocyte agglutinins and the mode of action of amidopyrine and certain other drugs in producing leukopenia is discussed in Chapter 21; individual sensitivity appears to be an important factor. Other chemical and physical agents produce leukopenia consistently if they are given in doses of sufficient size. Their action is due to destruction of leukocyte-forming tissue. Thus, it has been observed that lymphocytorrhexis and aplastic degeneration of the bone marrow follows the administration of the vesicant nitrogen and sulfur mustards such as bis-(β-chloroethyl) methylamine hydrochloride.[85a] Marrow protected from exposure to these agents continues to flourish. The mode of action of benzene and arsenicals is discussed in Chapter 11.

There is considerable evidence that nutritional deficiency may produce leukopenia. The role of nutritional factors in hemopoiesis was discussed earlier (p. 129). Here it may be pointed out that in the pig tryptophane deficiency was found to be associated with leukopenia[73c] and in experimental rats granulocytopenia and anemia have been produced by means of deficiencies of pantothenic acid,[66a] riboflavin[81b] or protein. The granulocytopenia developing in these rats and in rats receiving sulfasuxidine or thiourea plus thyroxin,[66a] could be corrected by the administration of folic acid. Leukopenia associated with protein deficiency can be relieved by increasing the quantity of protein in the diet.[86] The leukopenia observed in pernicious anemia is, no doubt, nutritional in origin for it is relieved by the administration of folic acid, or vitamin B_{12}. The cause of the leukopenia seen in chronic hypochromic anemia is not clear but may well also be nutritional in character. What rôle specific nutritional deficiencies play in the causation of the leukopenia accompanying various cachectic and debilitated states remains to be determined.

Eosinophilia.—Eosinophilia is the term applied to an increase in the number of eosinophilic leukocytes above the normal (250 per c.mm.). It is seen (Table 4–7) in the following conditions:

Table 4–7—Causes of Eosinophilia

1. Allergic disorders: bronchial asthma, urticaria, angioneurotic edema, hay fever.
2. Skin diseases: especially pemphigus and dermatitis herpetiformis.
3. Parasitic infestations: especially parasites which invade the tissues; e.g., trichinosis, echinococcus disease; less regularly in intestinal parasitism.
4. Loeffler's syndrome; "tropical eosinophilia."
5. Certain infections; e.g., scarlet fever, chorea, erythema multiforme.
6. Certain diseases of the hemopoietic system: chronic myelocytic leukemia, erythremia, Hodgkin's disease, after splenectomy, pernicious anemia.
7. Following irradiation.
8. Miscellaneous disorders: periarteritis nodosa; tumors of the ovary or those involving serous surfaces or bones; sarcoidosis; certain poisons.
9. As a familial anomaly.

1. In *allergic disorders*: bronchial asthma, urticaria, angioneurotic edema, hay fever. Usually the eosinophilia is moderate (4 to 11 per cent) but in some instances it may be much higher; e.g., bronchial asthma, leukocyte count 20,000, eosinophils 20 per cent; angioneurotic edema, leukocyte count as high as 44,000, eosinophils 27 to 85 per cent.[103] Eosinophils are usually abundant in nasal discharges,[75] sputum, and skin wheals[93] of allergic individuals. In a case of fatal bronchial asthma a large preponderance of eosinophils was found in the bone marrow and tremendous infiltrations of these cells were observed in the myocardium.[73e]

2. In *skin diseases*: The highest and most constant eosinophilia (10 to 60 per cent, sometimes with leukocytosis) has been observed in pemphigus and in dermatitis herpetiformis. Eosinophilia has been found in association with the following: exfoliative dermatitis, psoriasis, pruritus, prurigo, eczema, dermatitis venenata, ichthyosis, mycosis fungoides, pityriasis rubra, facial granulomas[74a] and scabies. The development of eosinophilia may possibly depend on the underlying nature of the skin disturbance; that is, whether it is allergic or infectious, due to nutritional deficiency or due to other causes. The degree of eosinophilia in many instances appears to vary with the extent of the skin involvement.

3. In *parasitic infestations*: Parasites which invade the *tissues* cause the most pronounced eosinophilia. The most striking example of this is the eosinophilia encountered in *trichiniasis*, described by T. R. Brown in 1897. The change in the blood appears about one week after ingestion of the infected food and often reaches its maximum at the end of the third week. It usually lasts for as long as six months and has been reported to persist in some instances for years. Values as high as 85 per cent with absolute eosinophil counts as high as 15,000 per c.mm. have been found. It is noteworthy, however, that eosinophilia may be absent throughout the infection and in severe fatal infections eosinophilia is generally absent.[115]

In *echinococcus* disease, eosinophilia is usually mild but occasionally it is pronounced. It is more likely to occur when slow leakage of cyst fluid into the surrounding tissue is occurring.[91a] When

17

suppuration develops, eosinophilia disappears and neutrophilia develops. In amebic abscess of the liver, eosinophilia is not found, neutrophilic leukocytosis being common.[95a] In the early stages of *cysticercosis*, moderate eosinophilia is found but this disappears when encystment occurs.[79] In *coccidioidal granuloma*, eosinophilia is sometimes found.[117] Eosinophilia has been observed in human *toxoplasmosis*.[125a] In *schistosomiasis* (S. mansoni) eosinophilia may be marked during the incubation period.[118] The *liver fluke*, Clonorchis sinensis, causes marked eosinophilia.[69] Eosinophilia was observed only in a third of a series of cases of *filariasis*[70b] but has not been found in trypanosomiasis or in kala-azar. From 50 to 85 per cent eosinophils may be found in the blood in gnathostomiasis[78] and 78 per cent was found in *Capillaria hepatica* infection.[74b]

In *malaria* the presence and degree of eosinophilia is variable. Thus, in a series of 100 patients convalescent from malarial attacks the range of eosinophils, in absolute numbers, was 0 to 1350 per c.mm. with an average of 250, as compared with 0 to 700, average 145, in a control group of non-infected subjects. Eosinophilia diminished as time progressed but lasted for at least eight weeks. A pronounced fall by some 50 per cent was observed twenty-four to thirty-six hours before the onset of malarial symptoms. After the febrile period, in cases in which treatment was given, the eosinophil count rose and regained its previous level in about ten days.[96b]

Intestinal parasitism is less regularly associated with eosinophilia than are some of the instances of tissue invasion mentioned above, and the eosinophilia is never as marked. However, eosinophilia of 10 to 30 and even 69 per cent[66b] may occur in infestation by *Uncinaria*[92] and *Strongyloides* during the early stage of active infection; in Ascaris infestation;[67b] and in Taenia infections during periods of diarrhea or abdominal pain. Infestations

with Enterobius vermicularis (Oxyuris), Trichocephalus trichiuris,[109] the amebae[91] and the flagellates are usually not associated with eosinophilia.

4. In *Loeffler's syndrome*, a peculiar type of transitory lung infiltration presumed to be due to a hyperimmune hypersenstivity reaction, eosinophilia is a characteristic finding[78d,81a] A clinical and blood picture identical with that described for Loeffler's syndrome has been observed in cases of cutaneous helminthiasis, a "creeping eruption" usually caused by *Ancylostome brasiliense*.[133] Transitory pulmonary infiltration with eosinophilia has been described also in clonorchiasis,[73a] Ascaris,[67b,113] Trichina, and amebic infestation, in tuberculosis, brucellosis, pollinosis[133] and in coccidioidomycosis.[130b] A disorder described in *young children* which is characterized by hepatomegaly, pulmonary infiltrations, asthmatic complaints, joint symptoms, urticaria, convulsions, eosinophilia and hyperglobulinemia may be due to invasion by nematode larvae ("*visceral larva migrans*" [117b]).

Under the title of "*tropical eosinophilia*," a condition of unknown etiology was described in India[128b] and in South-East Asia[77a] which begins gradually with malaise, weight loss, low grade fever, a paroxysmal dry hacking cough and physical findings similar to those of bronchial asthma. There is leukocytosis and high eosinophilia. The spleen may be palpable. Roentgenograms reveal diffuse bilateral mottling of the lung fields resembling the picture of acute miliary tuberculosis. After several weeks a chronic subfebrile state is reached in which paroxysms of coughing and wheezing may persist but weight loss usually ceases. Increased bronchial markings, like those seen in chronic bronchitis, are found in roentgenograms at this stage. Symptomsmay persist for a long time unless arsenotherapy or diethylcarbamazine,[78b] is given, to which the response is striking. Tropical eosinophilia, like Loeffler's syndrome, probably represents a hyperimmune reaction and is attributable to a variety of parasites, mainly microfilariae.[128a]

5. With *certain infections*, moderate eosinophilia may occur: most noteworthy is *scarlet fever*. In the early stage of this disease eosinophilia of 5 to 8 per cent and even as high as 17 per cent may be found, especially when constitutional symptoms are mild and the rash slight.[84] This may aid differentiation from diphtheria, in which condition leukocytosis occurs without eosinophilia. In *chorea*, eosinophilia is common and may reach values as high as 26 per cent.[69a] It is of interest that this occurs also in *erythema multiforme* but not in acute rheumatic fever.[125] It has been stated that moderate eosinophilia occurs in *gonorrhea* when the posterior urethra, epididymis or prostate is involved. Eosinophilia has been reported in *leprosy*.[92a]

During infections in which neutrophilia occurs, eosinophils are generally reduced in number or disappear entirely. This phenomenon has been called *"Simon's septic factor"* and now can be attributed to the action of the adrenal cortical hormone. Recovery in such cases is often marked by eosinophilia.

6. In *certain diseases of the hemopoietic system*: in *chronic myelocytic leukemia* an increase in all types of granulocytes usually occurs. In such a case, although the eosinophils may not be more than proportionately increased, their absolute number is usually high. In *erythremia*, eosinophilia is not unusual. In about 20 per cent of cases of *Hodgkins's disease* a slight or moderate eosinophilia occurs. In rare cases it has been as high as 90 per cent.[121] Following *splenectomy* for any cause, eosinophilia together with lymphocytosis often replaces the neutrophilia which first appears. This may persist for several months.

Several cases of marked eosinophilia, leukocytosis and splenomegaly have been described in which the clinical and post-mortem picture suggested leukemia.[88] (See *Eosinophilic Leukemia*, Chapter 19.)

In *pernicious anemia* eosinophilia of even 20 to 60 per cent may develop. This was particularly common following the use of uncooked liver but had often been noted even before liver therapy was introduced (see p. 480). In *sickle cell anemia* eosinophilia is found occasionally.

7. Following slight or moderate repeated *irradiation* by roentgen rays, one of the effects observed may be eosinophilia (7 to 23 per cent) (see p. 557).

8. Eosinophilia has also been noted in a *miscellaneous* group of disorders: *periarteritis nodosa* (in about 18 per cent of cases, with eosinophilia as high as 84 per cent in 1 case[106]); *tumors of the ovary*, various other neoplasms, especially those metastasizing[90e] or involving serous surfaces or bones or when necrosis of tumor tissue occurs; extensive caseous tuberculosis of the lymph nodes;[71] and following poisoning by copper sulphate, camphor, pilocarpine and phosphorus.

9. A number of instances of eosinophilia have been observed which occurred in the majority of the members of several families.[124] All of the conditions which might have caused this abnormality, with the possible exception of trichiniasis, were satisfactorily ruled out. It was therefore suggested that these represented a *familial anomaly*.

Basophilic Leukocytosis.—The introduction of methods for enumerating basophilic leukocytes directly (p. 392) has yielded normal values[48,70a] similar to those calculated from the total and differential count (p. 249). These cells are often *increased* in chronic myelocytic leukemia, polycythemia vera, myeloid metaplasia, following splenectomy, in chlorosis, in some chronic hemolytic anemias, as well as in Hodgkin's disease, chronic inflammations of the accessory sinuses, smallpox and chickenpox, following the injection of foreign protein,[6] in myxedema and in some cases of nephrosis.[52a,70a] In hyperthyroidism[52a,70a] they are *decreased*. A decrease also occurs following radiation or chemotherapy,[83c] in pregnancy, following treatment with glucocorticoids[70a] and during the acute stage of infections.[105a] Mast cells may be increased in the bone marrow in urticaria pigmentosa[113b] and in the exudate in non-specific ulcerative colitis[114] without noticeable basophilic leukocytosis appearing in the blood.

Lymphocytosis.—Lymphocytosis is the term applied to an increase above normal in the number of lymphocytes. It is important to distinguish a relative increase in these cells from an absolute one, for it is the latter which is of significance.

As already stated, the blood of *infants* contains a high proportion of lymphocytes as compared with that of adults. Their number gradually decreases as maturity is approached but conditions which interfere with growth, such as rickets and malnutrition, may inhibit this natural decrease or cause an increase in lymphocytes.

Lymphocytosis (Table 4–8) is characteristic of *lymphocytic leukemia* and of *infectious mononucleosis* (See Chapters 19 and 21). Minot's cases of lymphocytosis in *purpura hemorrhagica* may have been examples of infectious mononucleosis.[104] During the stage of *convalescence* from an acute infection, lymphocytosis is common.[116] It is rare during the active stage of acute infections except in *pertussis*, in which disease lymphocytosis is characteristic. This is sometimes of extreme degree (145,000 per c.mm.).[111] This change in the blood commences in the early catarrhal stage and persists until well into convalescence. Usually the total leukocyte count in this disease is about 20,000 and the lymphocytes constitute 60 per cent or more of this number.[130] High leukocyte counts have been observed

particularly in cases complicated by pneumonia.[66]

Under the title of **acute infectious lymphocytosis,** Smith[122a] described a benign condition characterized by pronounced lymphocytosis which seems to be distinct from infectious mononucleosis.

Table 4–8—Causes of Lymphocytosis

1. Certain acute infections: pertussis, infectious mononucleosis, acute infectious lymphocytosis.
2. Exanthems, after the initial stage especially in mumps and German measles.
3. Chronic infections; such as tuberculosis, secondary and congenital syphilis, undulant fever, infectious hepatitis.
4. During the stage of convalescence from an acute infection.
5. Thyrotoxicosis (usually only relative lymphocytosis).
6. Infants and young children, especially in the presence of rickets and malnutrition.
7. Lymphocytic leukemia.
8. Relative lymphocytosis, in most conditions associated with neutropenia.

The great majority of the reported cases have been in children.[67a,120] The onset is marked by varying degrees of constitutional reaction, there having been no symptoms whatever in most of the cases whereas in others vomiting, diarrhea, irritability, fever and abdominal signs and symptoms even sufficient to suggest an acute surgical condition have been observed. In other instances symptoms of an upper respiratory infection, or signs of involvement of the nervous system have been reported and even skin involvement (morbilliform, maculopapular) has been described.[120] Symptoms, when present, have been of only a few days' duration. The leukocytosis, on the other hand, has persisted for three to seven weeks. Leukocyte counts reaching 40,000 per c.mm. and even over 100,000 have been more common than lower ones. The great majority of the cells (60 to 92 per cent) have been "adult" small lymphocytes, not unlike those seen in chronic lymphocytic leukemia. Absolute eosinophilia, even of marked degree, has been observed in many cases.[67a] Lymph node enlargement and splenomegaly have been conspicuous by their absence. No anemia or thrombocytopenia has been observed. The sternal marrow has shown an increase in the percentage of lymphocytes (30 to 40 per cent) of normal type. In 2 cases biopsy of lymph nodes revealed degeneration of the lymph follicles and striking proliferation of the reticuloendothelium of the sinuses.[122a] In other instances degenerative changes have not been observed.[67a] The heterophil agglutination test has been uniformly negative. An increase in lymphocytes in the spinal fluid has been reported in occasional cases. The disease appears to be both infectious and contagious but all attempts to disclose the etiologic agent have failed. The incubation period may be twelve to twenty-one days. The outcome has been uniformly favorable. The condition has been confused most often with chronic lymphocytic leukemia and with infectious mononucleosis.

Lymphocytosis may occur in the *exanthems* after the initial stage, and has been observed particularly in mumps (44 to 68 per cent)[129] and in German measles.[89] In the latter condition the lymphocytes have been described as "atypical" (See below). Occasionally absolute lymphocytosis is found in *undulant fever.*[73d] It is associated with *tuberculous* infection where the resistance is good.[132] In the *secondary* stage of *syphilis* lymphocytosis may occur along with leukocytosis and in *congenital syphilis* counts as high as 60,000 due chiefly to lymphocytosis have been reported.[76]

In *thyrotoxicosis* Kocher (1908) described leukopenia due to a reduction mainly of granulocytes, relative and absolute lymphocytosis and moderate eosinophilia. While this is found in many cases, the changes are inconstant and may be slight in degree. They cannot be regarded as a reliable index of prognosis or of return to normal following treatment.[78e] It is of interest, however, that the lymphocytic infiltration of the thyroid gland is correlated with the degree of lymphocytosis, and hyperplasia of lymphoid organs such as the lymph nodes and spleen may be associated. It is likely that these manifestations are the expression of a relative deficiency of adrenal steroids.

Moderate exposure to dry heat, sunlight, the short ultraviolet rays[74] (less than 300 $\mu\mu$) and roentgen rays[106a] have been shown to cause in experimental animals, after an initial reduction in lymphocytes, a marked lymphocytosis which persists for several weeks.

Relative lymphocytosis will be found in all of the conditions associated with neutropenia.

From time to time attention has been called to **morphologic variations in lymphocytes in disease.** Wiseman's Y:M:O ratio of lymphocytes (p. 225) attracted little clinical application but, in other studies which were concerned with the relation of endocrine organs to lymphatic tissue, it was observed that, in response to stress, lymphocytes may appear which are characterized by nuclear and cytoplasmic distortion and a greater quantity of cytoplasm than is evident in lymphocytes found under normal conditions.[80b] The cytoplasm of these cells is less basophilic than is seen normally. It is claimed that stress stimuli not only cause a reduction in the number of normal lymphocytes, an effect mediated by adrenocortical secretions, but also produce a nonadrenocortically mediated response which is characterized by an increase in the number of "stress" lymphocytes. These correspond to the type II lymphocyte of Downey (p. 1113). Such cells are found not only in infectious mononucleosis but in a variety of other conditions, including infectious hepatitis,[88a] serum sickness and chronic infections.[80b] An increase in the size of lymphocytes in the blood has also been described in the presence of adrenal insufficiency and in hyperthyroidism.[88c] This disappears on appropriate therapy of the underlying condition.

Plasma Cells.—Plasma cells are rarely found in the circulating blood and their significance is quite obscure. In *rubella* as many as 19 per cent have been observed[90a] while in *scarlatina, measles* and *chickenpox*[90c] they are less numerous.[89] They may be increased in serum reactions, multiple myeloma, benign lymphocytic meningitis,[132a] skin diseases and, sometimes, in infectious mononucleosis. In plasma cell leukemia they are the predominating cells.

Monocytosis.—Monocytosis (Table 4–9) refers to an increase in the number of monocytes above the normal (500 per c.mm.). This is found:

Table 4–9—Causes of Monocytosis

1. Certain bacterial infections: tuberculosis, subacute bacterial endocarditis, brucellosis, rarely in typhoid.
2. During subsidence of acute infection and recovery phase of agranulocytosis.
3. Many protozoal and some rickettsial infections: malaria, Rocky Mountain spotted fever, typhus, kala azar, trypanosomiasis, Oriental sore.
4. Hodgkin's disease; also in diseases of disturbed lipoid metabolism, such as Gaucher's disease.
5. Monocytic leukemia.
6. Tetrachlorethane poisoning.

1. In *certain bacterial infections*, which include tuberculosis, subacute bacterial endocarditis and brucellosis. Monocytosis may occur in typhoid[80] and may develop in pneumonia as an accompaniment of the increased activity of the myeloid system. In rabbits monocytosis occurs in infection by B. monocytogenes[107] (see p. 1109).

During the subsidence of acute infections, monocytosis may develop temporarily. It has also been noted during the recovery phase of agranulocytosis (p. 1105).

The role of the *monocyte in tuberculosis* was the subject of intensive study.[80] It was shown that this cell is an important part of the cellular reaction to the tubercle bacillus. The lipoids of this organism are phagocytized by monocytes, are partially degraded within them and cause their transformation to epithelioid cells. Thus, it is the chief cell in new tubercle formation. This activity is reflected in the circulating blood and it is now generally accepted that monocytosis in a tuberculous patient is an unfavorable sign. In following the course of patients with tuberculosis, considerable attention is given to the *ratio of monocytes to lymphocytes*, for the latter vary inversely with the former in this disease and lymphocytosis occurs when a tuberculous lesion is healing. The normal average M:L ratio is 943:2805; that is, an "index" of 2.9.[100] A very unfavorable ratio would be 3469:2799 (index 0.8); a favorable one is 854:3047 (index 3.6).

In *endocarditis* caused by *Streptococcus viridans*, the total leukocyte count may be normal, subnormal or increased. The increase may be due to neutrophilia, particularly when infarction or thrombosis is occurring;[112] or it may be due to monocytosis and these cells may constitute even one-third of all the leukocytes. Monocytosis may occur in the absence of leukocytosis and its magnitude is subject to great fluctuations.[90f] Undifferentiated reticuloendothelial cells may be found in the blood as well as intermediate stages between such cells and monocytes. These cells may exhibit vacuoles in their cytoplasm and sometimes have been found to have engulfed red cells, neutrophils or lymphocytes. They are more abundant in blood obtained from the ear lobe than from the finger.[78a] In one study it was noted that the number of these circulating macrophages[90f] was greater in patients with sterile blood cultures than in positive cases.[90] *Phagocytic reticuloendothelial cells* have been found in 15 to 30 per cent of cases. Although a rare cell of this sort may be seen in a variety of other disorders,[9] except when there is reason to consider trypanosomiasis or malaria, their presence should bring bacterial endocarditis to mind.[90]

2. In many *protozoal* and some *rickettsial infections*: malaria, Rocky Mountain spotted fever, kala-azar (as high as 40 per cent monocytes),[6] Oriental sore, trypanosomiasis and in some cases of syphilis,[130a] especially dementia paralytica.[9]

3. In *Hodgkin's disease* monocytosis is common, and it may also be found in Gaucher's disease,[6] Niemann-Pick's disease and in Hand-Schüller-Christian's xanthomatosis.

4. In tetrachorethane poisoning.[105]

5. In *monocytic leukemia* (see Chapter 19).

INTERPRETATION AND PROGNOSTIC VALUE OF THE LEUKOCYTE PICTURE

The above outline of the conditions in which characteristic changes in the leukocytic picture occur indicates how study of the leukocytes may be of value as an aid in diagnosis. A painstaking differential count may be helpful in discovering cryptic infections of subacute and chronic type in which there is no increase in the total leukocyte count. The leukocyte picture may also be useful as a guide to prognosis (Table 4–10).

Generally, three phases can be observed in the leukocytic picture. During the progressive stage of an infection neutrophilia predominates and the severity of the infection as well as the reaction of the patient may be gauged by the magnitude of the leukocyte count, the degree of "shift to the left," and the presence of toxic cytoplasmic granulation. Thus, a slight neutrophilia with slight nuclear shift to the left suggests a mild infection, whereas a moderate leukocytosis, moderate shift to the left, together with disappearance of eosinophils and decrease

Table 4–10—Estimation of Prognosis From Leukocytic Count—Significant Factors

1. Magnitude of leukocyte count.
2. Proportion of immature cells.
3. Number of "toxic" forms of leukocytes.
4. Degree of reduction in number of eosinophils.
5. Degree of reduction in number of lymphocytes.
6. Degree of increase in monocytes (tuberculosis).

of lymphocytes, signifies a moderately severe infection. As already stated, still more marked leukocytosis or a fall in the leukocyte count, with an even greater "shift to the left" than before, are grave signals. Unfavorable signs in the leukocyte picture are listed in Table 4–11.

Table 4–11—Unfavorable Signs in the Leukocytic Picture

1. Extremely high total number of leukocytes with high percentage of neutrophils; or
2. Failure to develop leukocytosis.
3. High proportion of immature cells especially if they outnumber mature forms.
4. Absence of eosinophils.
5. Marked absolute reduction of lymphocytes.
6. Presence of numerous toxic, degenerative forms.

Except in certain diseases, such as tuberculosis, in which an increase in the number of monocytes is an unfavorable sign, the reappearance of these cells in the course of an acute infection usually indicates the beginning of the recovery stage. Their return is often followed by the reappearance of eosinophils. Finally, lymphocytosis develops during the period of convalescence. The changes in the blood picture during recovery are shown in Table 4–12.

Table 4–12—Changes in Blood Picture During Recovery

1. Falling total leukocyte count with diminishing proportion of neutrophils.
2. Decrease of immature forms.
3. Temporary increase of monocytes.
4. Reappearance or increase of eosinophils.
5. Increase in number of lymphocytes.
6. Absence or decrease of toxic forms.

In tuberculosis, as already mentioned, monocytosis occurs when the disease is progressive and the number of monocytes in relation to the number of lymphocytes is increased. Improvement is associated with a fall in the number of monocytes and an increase in the total number of lymphocytes. These changes may appear some time prior to other indications of a change in the status of the patient and are thus of great prognostic value. Medlar devised a leukocytic index based on four variables, namely, total leukocyte count and the proportions of neutrophils, lymphocytes and monocytes, which he found very useful in the evaluation of the clinical status of tuberculous patients.[101]

LEUKEMOID BLOOD PICTURES

Under the head of leukemoid pictures may be grouped a number of case reports of unusual reactions in association with a variety of infections, intoxications and malignant disorders. In some of these cases it was only the magnitude of the leukocytic reaction, or its unusual quality which suggested leukemia.[82c] In many, however, severe anemia accompanied the leukocytic change and nucleated red corpuscles of various types were found as well. In a number of instances, moreover, the clinical picture, because of fever, hemorrhage, splenomegaly or ade-

nopathy, suggested leukemia. The true diagnosis often was evident only on postmortem examination and it may well be emphasized that the differentiation of leukemoid reactions from true leukemia is often extremely difficult, if not impossible, to make during life. Differentiation has not always been possible even at autopsy. This topic will be considered further in a later section (p. 948). The value of splenic puncture in aiding the differentiation of leukemoid reactions from true leukemia has been discussed already (p. 71). The alkaline phosphatase reaction (p. 235) may prove to be useful since high levels have been observed in leukemoid reactions, in contrast to the low values found in myelocytic leukemia.[96a]

1. **Infections.**—Leukemoid reactions have been observed in association with bacterial, spirochetal, viral and protozoal infections.[90b] Exceptionally high leukocyte counts have been encountered in cases of pneumonia, rupture of encapsulated empyema into the pleural cavity (71,500),[127] pneumococcal endocarditis (76,800),[128] meningococcal meningitis (60,000), diphtheria (70,000), bubonic plague (100,000) and septicemia (112,000).[94] In these conditions the reaction was myeloid in type and a marked shift to the left was noted. Marked leukocytosis with lymphocytosis has also been described, as in whooping cough (199,000)[128c] chickenpox (81,200),[85] congenital syphilis (105,000),[76,128] infectious mononucleosis (63,000) infectious lymphocytosis (147,000)[120] and dermatitis herpetiformis.[82b]

It is in association with *tuberculosis* that leukemoid pictures have been described most frequently. The tuberculosis has usually been miliary or it involved the lymph nodes or spleen particularly. The leukocytic picture has resembled that of acute myeloblastic leukemia[90d,113a] in most instances and severe anemia, fever and splenomegaly have made this diagnosis seem very plausible.[77,96] Counts

Table 4–13—Leukemoid Blood Pictures

1. Infections presenting pictures resembling
   Myelocytic or myeloblastic leukemia: pneumonia, meningococcus meningitis, diphtheria, tuberculosis.
   Lymphocytic leukemia: whooping cough, chickenpox, infectious mononucleosis, infectious lymphocytosis, tuberculosis.
   Monocytic leukemia: tuberculosis.
2. Intoxications: eclampsia, severe burns, mercury poisoning.
3. Malignancy, especially with bone metastases; also multiple myeloma, myelosclerosis, Hodgkin's disease.
4. Severe hemorrhage; sudden hemolysis of blood.

as high as 156,000 and 115,200 have been reported with approximately 50 per cent myeloblasts. Lymphocytic,[84a] monocytic[84b] and neutrophilic[90b] leukemoid reactions have also been described. It is of interest that it has been possible to produce leukocytosis as great as 124,000 by the injection of tuberculin in sensitized rabbits.[83] This increase, however, was due chiefly to the presence of adult cells.

2. **Intoxications.**—Rare instances of marked leukocytosis in eclampsia (100,000) and following severe burns (80,000) have been described. In a case of mustard gas poisoning 91 per cent of the leukocytes were myelocytes although the total count was only 5400.[94] Poisoning following the use of 33 per cent mercury ointment produced a leukocyte count of 69,500 with 24 per cent myelocytes and a clinical picture very suggestive of subacute or chronic myelocytic leukemia.[81] The alleged production of leukemia by multiple bee stings[110] is not very convincing. It seems more probable that the cases described were instances of true leukemia and that the insect bites were incidental. A strangely varying leukemoid picture was described in a case of acute glomerulonephritis.[90b]

3. **Malignancy.**—A number of instances of leukemoid pictures in association with malignancy without bone metastasis have been described (carcinoma of colon with metastasis to the spleen,[81,102] carcinoma of the stomach with lymphoid reaction,[70] carcinoma of the lung,[82c] adrenal and renal carcinoma with widespread metastases showing necrosis[88b]). However, except when severe hemorrhage was associated,[94] the majority of the cases reported have been those in which extension to the bone marrow had taken place.[92b] The picture may suggest myelocytic[95] or lymphoid leukemia.[119]

In cases of *multiple myeloma*[94] and in *osteosclerosis*,[89a] leukemoid pictures have also been described. Very high leukocyte counts (250,000) have been reported in rare instances of *Hodgkin's disease*.[73]

The patient described by Fraser[83b] as one of *exfoliative dermatitis* with a leukemoid blood picture was found to be living and well fourteen years later.[116a]

4. Severe **hemorrhage** and the **sudden hemolysis** of blood may be followed by marked leukocytosis (106,000) of the myeloid type.[94] In *pernicious anemia*, such a reaction has also been observed (69,000 leukocytes, 18 per cent myelocytes) during remission following liver therapy[82] or in the presence of an infection (p. 454). This has also been described in pernicious anemia of pregnancy following folic acid therapy.[117a,120a]

BIBLIOGRAPHY

Morphology, Function and Biologic Properties of the Leukocytes

1. ACKERMAN, G. A.: Histochemical Demonstration of Indoxyl Acetate Esterase Activity in Normal Human Blood and Bone Marrow, Lab. Invest., *9*, 298, 1960.

1a.ALDER, A.: Über konstitutionell bedingte Granulationsveränderungen der Leukozyten, Deutsches Arch. f. klin. Med., *183*, 372, 1939; Schweiz. med. Wchnschr., *80*, 1095, 1950.

1b.ARCHER, R. K.: Eosinophil Leucocytes and their Reactions to Histamine and 5-Hydroxytryptamine, J. Path. & Bact., *78*, 95, 1959; Australasian J. Exper. Biol. & Med. Sc., *38*, 147, 1960.

1c.ASHLEY, D. J. B.: The Technic of Nuclear Sexing, Am. J. Clin. Path., *31*, 230, 1959.

1d.ASTALDI, G., BERNARDELLI, E. and RONDANELLI, E. G.: Richerche sul contenuto in glicogeno delle cellule del sangue e del midollo osseo, Haematologica, *36*, 749, 1952.

1e.ATHENS, J. W. *et al.* Leukokinetic Studies, Blood, *14*, 303, 1959; J. Clin. Invest., *39*, 1481, 1960; *in The Kinetics of Cellular Proliferation*, edited by F. Stohlman, Jr., New York, Grune & Stratton, 1959, p. 231; J. Clin. Invest., *40*, 159, 1961.

2. BARNES, J. M.: The Enzymes of Lymphocytes and Polymorphonuclear Leukocytes, Brit. J. Exper. Path., *21*, 264, 1940.

2a.BECK, W. S. and VALENTINE, W. N.: The Carbohydrate Metabolism of Leukocytes: A Review, Cancer Research, *13*, 309, 1953; J. Biol. Chem., *232*, 251, 1958; Ann. New York Acad. Sc., *75*, 4, 1958; J. Biol. Chem., *232*, 271, 1958.

2b.BEGEMANN, N. H. and CAMPAGNE, A. V. L.: Homozygous Form of Pelger-Huët's Nuclear Anomaly in Man, Acta haemat., *7*, 295, 1952.

2c.BERGEL, S.: Weiteres zur lipoidspaltenden Funktion der Lymphozyten, Beitr. z. path. Anat. u. z. allg. Path., *73*, 404, 1925.

2d.BERNARDELLI, E. and RONDANELLI, E. G.: Sullo svolgimento e sul significato della segmentazione nucleare del granulocito, Biol. Lat., *6*, 395, 1953.

3. BERRY, L. J. and SPIES, T. D.: Phagocytosis, Medicine, *28*, 239, 1949.

3a.BIERMAN, H. R.: The Hematologic Role of the Lung in Man, Am. J. Surg., *89*, 130, 1955; Am. New York Acad. Sci., *59*, 850, 1955.

4. BJØRNEBOE, M. and Gormsen, H.: Experimental Studies on Rôle of Plasma Cells as Antibody Producers, Acta path et microbiol. scandinav., *20*, 649, 1943.

5. BLOOM, M. L. and WISLOCKI, G. B.: The Localization of Lipids in Human Blood and Bone Marrow Cells, Blood, *5*, 79, 1950.

5a.BOYD, E. M.: The Lipid Composition of the White Blood Cells in Leukemia, Arch. Path., *21*, 739, 1936.

5b.BRAUNSTEINER, H., PAERTAN, J. and THUMB, N.: Studies on Lymphocytic Function, Blood, *13*, 417, 1958.

5c.BRIDGES, R. A., CONDIE, R. M., ZAK, S. J. and GOOD, R. A.: The Morphologic Basis of Antibody Formation Development during the Neonatal Period, J. Lab. & Clin. Med., *53*, 331, 1959.

6. BUNTING, C. H.: The Granular Leukocytes, *in* Cowdry, E. V., *Special Cytology*, New York, Paul B. Hoeber, Inc., *2*, 684, 1932.

7. CARREL, A.: Leukocytic Trephones, J.A.M.A., *82*, 255, 1924.

7a.CHEDIAK, M. M.: Nouvelle anomalie leucocytaire de caractère constitutionnel et familial, Rev. d'hémat., *7*, 362, 1952.

8. COHN, Z. A. and MORSE, S. I.: Functional and Metabolic Properties of Polymorphonuclear Leucocytes, J. Exper. Med., *111*, 667, 1960.

8a.Committee for Clarification of the Nomenclature of Cells and Diseases of the Blood and Blood-Forming Organs, Am. J. Clin. Path., *18*, 443, 1948; Third, Fourth and Fifth Reports, Am. J. Clin. Path., *20*, 562, 1950.

8b.CRADDOCK, C. G., JR., PERRY, S., VENTZKE, L. E. and LAWRENCE, J. S.: Evaluation of Marrow Granulocytic Reserves in Normal and Disease States, Blood, *15*, 840, 1960; Am. J. Med., *28*, 711, 1960; *in The Kinetics of Cellular Proliferation*, edited by F. Stohlman, Jr., New York, Grune & Stratton, 1959, p. 242; Blood, *14*, 50, 1959.

9. DAMESHEK, W.: The Appearance of Histiocytes in the Peripheral Blood, Arch. Int. Med., *47*, 968, 1931.

9a.DAVIDSON, W. M., MILNER, R. D. G. and LAWLER, SYLVIA D.: Giant Neutrophil Leucocytes: An Inherited Anomaly, Brit. J. Haemat., *6*, 339, 1960.

10. DEBRUYN, P. P. H.: Locomotion of Blood Cells in Tissue Cultures, Anat. Rec. *89*, 43, 1944; *ibid.*, *95*, 177, 1946.

10a.DOAN, C. A. and REINHART, H. L.: The Basophil Granulocyte, Basophilcytosis, and Myeloid Leukemia, Basophil and "Mixed Granule" Types, Am. J. Clin. Path., *11*, 1, 1941.

11. DONOHUE, D. M., GABRIO, BEVERLY W. and FINCH, C. A.: Quantitative Measurement of Hematopoietic Cells of the Marrow, J. Clin. Invest., *37*, 1564 and 1571, 1958.

11a.DORR, A. D. and MOLONEY, W. C.: Acquired Pseudo-Pelger Anomaly of Granulocytic Leukocytes, New England J. Med., *261*, 742, 1959.

11b.DOUGHERTY, T. F. and WHITE, A.: Influence of Hormones on Lymphoid Tissue Structure and Function, Endocrinology, *35*, 1, 1944; Am. J. Anat., *77*, 81, 1945; J. Immunol., *52*, 101, 1946; J. Lab. & Clin. Med., *32*, 584, 1947; Bull. New York Acad. Med., *24*, 26, 1948; Physiol. Rev., *32*, 379, 1952; *in The Kinetics of Cellular Proliferation*, edited by F. Stohlman, Jr., New York, Grune & Stratton, 1959, p. 264.

12. DOWNEY, H.: The Myeloblast, *in* Cowdry, E. V., *Special Cytology*, New York, Paul B. Hoeber, Inc., *2*, 653, 1932.

12a.DUSTIN, P., JR. and HARVEN, E. DE: La régulation hormonale de l'éosinophilie sanguine et son méchanisme, Rev. d'hémat., *9*, 307, 1954; Sang, *28*, 581, 1957.

12b.EBBING, H. C.: Beiträge zur Genetik der Pelger-Anomalie, Schweiz. med. Wchnschr., *89*, 1082, 1959.

13. EBERT, R. H. and FLOREY, H. W.: The Extravascular Development of the Monocyte Observed *in vivo*, Brit. J. Exper. Path., *20*, 342, 1939.

14. EBERT, R. H., SANDERS, A. G. and FLOREY, H. W.: Observations on Lymphocytes in Chambers in the Rabbit's Ear, Brit. J. Exper. Path., *21*, 212, 1940.

14b.EHRICH, W. E.: The Functional Significance of the Various Leukocytes in Inflammation, J. Mt. Sinai Hosp., *15*, 337, 1949; Proc. Soc. Exper. Biol. & Med., *74*, 732, 1950.

14c.ENDRES, G. and HERGET, L.: Mineralzusammensetzung der Blutplättchen und weissen Blutkörperchen, Ztschr. f. Biol., *88*, 451, 1929.

15. ESSELLIER, A. F., JEANNERET, R. L. and MORANDI, L.: The Mechanism of Glucocorticoid Eosinopenia, Blood, *9*, 531, 1954.

15a.FAGRAEUS, A.: Cellular Reaction in Antibody Formation, Acta haemat., *20*, 1, 1958.

15b.FICHTELIUS, K.-E.: A Difference between Lymph Nodal and Thymic Lymphocytes Shown by Transfusion of Labelled Cells, Acta anat., *32*, 114, 1958; Acta haemat., *19*, 187, 1958; *ibid.*, *22*, 322, 1959.

15c.FLANAGAN, P. and LIONETTI, F.: Lysozyme Distribution in Blood, Blood, *10*, 497, 1955.

16. FORKNER, C. E.: Origin and Fate of Two Types of Multinucleated Giant Cells in Circulating Blood, J. Exper. Med., *52*, 279, 1930.

16a.———— The Origin of Monocytes in Certain Lymph Nodes and Their Genetic Relation to Other Connective Tissue Cells, J. Exper. Med., *52*, 385, 1930.

17. FRAENKEL-CONRAT, J. and CHEW, W. B.: Catheptic Activity of Leukocytes in Normal and Leukemic Subjects. Blood, *16*, 1447, 1960

17a.FRICKER-ALDER, H.: Die Aldersche Granulationsanomalie, Schweiz. med. Wchnschr., *88*, 989, 1958.

17b.FULTON, G. P., MAYNARD, F. L., RILEY, J. F. and WEST, G. B.: Humoral Aspects of Tissue Mast Cells, Physiol. Rev., *37*, 221, 1957.

18. GORDON, A. S. and KATSH, G. F.: The Relation of the Adrenal Cortex to the Structure and Phagocytic Activity of the Macrophagic System, Ann. New York Acad. Sc., *52*, 1, 1949; *ibid.*, *59*, 907, 1955.

18a.GOWANS, J. L.: The Life-History of Lymphocytes, Brit. M. Bull., *15*, 50, 1959; J. Physiol., *146*, 54, 1959.

18b.GRAHAM, H. T., LOWRY, O. H., WHEELWRIGHT, F., LENZ, M. A. and PARISH, H. H., JR.: Distribution of Histamine among Leukocytes and Platelets, Blood, *10*, 467, 1955.

18c.GREEN, R. and MARTIN, S. P.: The Nonprotein Soluble Sulfhydryl Content of Human Leukocytes and Erythrocytes in Infection and Leukemia, J. Lab. & Clin. Med., *45*, 119, 1955.

18d.GRGIC, Z. and KALAFATIC, Z.: Drei Fälle von inkompletter Alder-Anomalie, Schweiz. med. Wchnschr., *88*, 994, 1958.

18e.GRIFFITHS, S. B. and FINDLAY, M.: Gargoylism: Clinical, Radiological and Haematological Features in Two Siblings, Arch. Dis. Childhood, *33*, 229, 1958.

19. HALL, B. E.: A Critical Review of the Hematological Literature Dealing With the Results of the Supravital Staining Method, Folia hæmatol., *43*, 206, 1930.

19a.HAMILTON, L. D.: Control and Functions of the Lymphocyte, Ann. New York Acad. Sc., *73*, 39, 1958.

19b.HARM, H.: Beiträge zur Morphologie und Genetik der Pelger-Anomalie bei Mensch und Kaninchen, Ztschr. menschl. Vererb., *30*, 501, 1952; Acta. haemat., *10*, 96, 1953.

19c.HARRIS, H.: Chemotaxis of Granulocytes, J. Path. & Bact., *66*, 135, 1953; Brit. J. Exper. Path., *34*, 276 and 599, 1953.

20. HARRIS, T. N., GRIMM, E., MERTENS, E. and EHRICH, W. E.: The Rôle of the Lymphocyte in Antibody Formation, J. Exper. Med., *81*, 73, 1945; *ibid.*, *83*, 373 and 84, 157, 1946; J. Biol. Chem., *179*, 369, 1949; J. Exper. Med., *90*, 169, 1949; *ibid.*, *100*, 269, 1954.

20a.HAYHOE, F. G. J. and QUAGLINO, D.: Cytochemical Demonstration and Measurement of Leucocyte Alkaline Phosphatase Activity in Normal and Pathological States by a Modified Azo-Dye Coupling Technique, Brit. J. Haemat., *4*, 375, 1958.

20b.Henning, N., Demling, L. and Härtlein, U.: Die Serumperoxydase, ein Gradmesser des pathologisch gesteigerten Granulocytenzerfalls, Deutsch. Arch. f. klin. Med., *196*, 233, 1949.

21. Hetherington, D. C. and Pierce, E. J.: The Transformation of Monocytes into Macrophages and Epithelioid Cells in Tissue Cultures of Buffy Coat (Demonstrated by Trypan Blue), Arch. f. exper. Zellforsch., *12*, 1, 1931.

21a.Higashi, O.: Congenital Gigantism of Peroxidase Granules, Tohoku, J. Exper. Med., *59*, 315, 1954.

21c.Hirsch, J. G.: Phagocytin: a Bactericidal Substance from Polymorphonuclear Leucocytes, J. Exper. Med., *103*, 589, and 613, 1956.

22. Isaacs, R.: Blood Cell Morphology in Constitutional Types and Heredity, Medical Papers Dedicated to Dr. Henry A. Christian, Baltimore, Waverly Press, Inc., 1936.

23a.Jordans, G. H. W.: Hereditary Granulation Anomaly of the Leucocytes (Alder), Acta med. scandinav *129*, 348, 1947.

23b.Jorpes, E., Odeblad, E. and Boström, H.: An Autoradiographic Study on the Uptake of S^{35}-labelled Sodium Sulphate in the Mast Cells, Acta haemat., *9*, 273, 1953.

23c.Kelsall, Margaret A. and Crabb, E. D.: Lymphocytes and Plasmacytes in Nucleoprotein Metabolism, Ann. New York Acad. Sc., *72*, 293, 1958.

24. Kennedy, W. P. and MacKay, I.: The Macropolycyte in Health and Disease in Iraq, J. Path. & Bacteriol., *44*, 701, 1937.

24a.Koler, R. D., Seaman, A. J., Osgood, E. E. and Vanbellinghen, P.: Diagnostic Value of the Leukocyte Alkaline Phosphatase Test, Am. J. Clin. Path., *30*, 295, 1958.

25. Laves, W. and Thoma, K.: Histoenzymatische Untersuchungen an den Granulationen der weissen Blutkörperchen, Virchow's Archiv., *318*, 74, 1950.

25a.Lawrence, J. S.: Physiology and Functions of the White Blood Cells, J. A. M. A., *157*, 1212, 1955.

26. Lawrence, J. S. and Todd, H.: Variations in the Characteristics of Lymphocytes in Supravital Preparations, Folia hæmatol., *44*, 318. 1931.

27. Leach, E. H.: The Role of Leukocytes in Fat Absorption, J. Physiol., *93*, 1, 1938.

28. Lewis, W. H.: On the Locomotion of the Polymorphonuclear Neutrophiles of the Rat in Autoplasma Cultures, Bull. Johns Hopkins Hosp., *55*, 273, 1934.

28a.Lisco, H.: Russell Bodies Occurring in the Lymph Follicles of the Intestinal Tract of Pigs, Anat. Rec., *82*, 59, 1942.

28b.Lüers, Th.: Das numerische Verhalten der geschlechtsspezifischen Kernanhänge bei der erblich-konstitutionellen Hochsegmentierung der Neutrophilenkerne Undritz, Schweiz. med. Wchnschr., *90*, 246, 1960.

28c.Marionone, G.: Problèmes de cytochimie quantitative des cellules des organes hémopoiétiques, Rev. d'hémat., *9*, 341, 1954.

28d.Mauri, C. and Soldati, Maria: Les caractéristiques cytochimiques des granulations cellulaires de Alder, J. Suisse de Méd., *88*, 992, 1958.

29. Maximow, A. A.: The Lymphocytes and Plasma Cells, *in* Cowdry, E. V, *Special Cytology* New York, Paul B. Hoeber, Inc., *2*, 603, 1932.

29a.McCutcheon, M.: Chemotaxis in Leukocytes, Physiol. Rev., *26*, 319, 1946.

29b.McKinney, G. R.: Glyoxalase Activity in Human Leukocytes, Arch. Biochem. & Biophys., *46*, 246, 1953.

30. McMaster, P. D. and Hudack, S. S.: The Formation of Agglutinins within Lymph Nodes, J. Exper. Med., *61*, 783, 1935; *ibid.*, *66*, 73, 1937.

30a.Meislin, A. G., Lee, S. L. and Wasserman, L. R.: Leukocyte Alkaline Phosphatase Activity in Hematopoietic Disorders, Cancer, *12*, 760, 1959.

31. Menkin, V.: Biology of Inflammation, Science, *123*, 527, 1956; Blood, *11*, 243, 1956. Proc. Soc. Exper. Biol. & Med., *104*, 312, 1960.

32. Michels, N. A.: The Plasma Cell, Arch. Path., *11*, 775, 1931.

33. Miller, F. R.: The Induced Development and Histogenesis of Plasma Cells, J. Exper. Med., *54*, 333, 1931.

33a.Mitus, W. J., Bergna, L. J., Mednicoff, I. B. and Dameshek, W.: Alkaline Phosphatase of Mature Neutrophils in Chronic Forms of the Myeloproliferative Syndrome, Am. J. Clin. Path., *30*, 285, 1958; New England J. Med., *260*, 1131, 1959.

33b.Mounter, L. A. and Atiyeh, W.: Proteases of Human Leukocytes, Blood, *15*, 52, 1960.

34. Mudd, S., McCutcheon, M. and Lucké, B.: Phagocytosis, Physiol. Rev., *14*, 210, 1934.

35. Murphy, J. B. and Sturm, E.: The Lymphoid Tissue and Antibody Formation, Proc. Soc. Exper. Biol. & Med., *66*, 303, 1947.

35a.Murthy, M. S. N. and von Haam, E.: The Occurrence of the Sex Chromatin in White Blood Cells of Young Adults, Am. J. Clin. Path., *30*, 216, 1958.

35b.Nour-Eldin, F. and Wilkinson, J. F.: The Estimation of Peptidase Activity in the White Blood Cells by Paper Chromatography, J. Clin. Path., *9*, 175, 1956.

35c. OTTESEN, J.: On the Age of Human White Cells in Peripheral Blood, Acta physiol. scandinav., 32, 75, 1954.

35d. PAGE, A. R. and GOOD, R. A.: A Clinical and Experimental Study of the Function of Neutrophils in the Inflammatory Response, Am. J. Path., 34, 645, 1958.

36. PERUGINI, S. and SOLDATI, M.: Ricerche citochimiche sulla componente proteica delle cellule ematiche, Riv. Istoch. norm. pat., 1, 217, 1954.

36a. POLICARD, A., COLLET, A. and PRÉGERMAIN, S.: Etude au microscope électronique des modifications infrastructurales présentées par les polynucléaires neutrophiles, Rev. hémat., 14, 97, 1959.

36b. PONDER, E.: The Polycyte, J. Lab. & Clin. Med., 27, 866, 1942.

36c. REBUCK, J. W. and CROWLEY, J. H.: A Method of Studying Leukocytic Functions in Vivo, Ann. New York. Acad. Sc., 59, 757, 1955.

36d. REYNOLDS, J., FOLLETTE, J. H. and VALENTINE, W. N.: The Arginase Activity of Erythrocytes and Leukocytes with Particular Reference to Pernicious Anemia and Thalassemia Major, J. Lab. & Clin. Med., 50, 78, 1957.

36e. RHEINGOLD, J. J. and WISLOCKI, G. B.: Histochemical Methods Applied to Hematology, Blood, 3, 641, 1948.

37. RICH, A. R., WINTROBE, M. M. and LEWIS, M. R.: The Differentiation of Myeloblasts From Lymphoblasts by Their Manner of Locomotion, Bull. Johns Hopkins Hosp., 65, 291, 1939.

38. RICH, A. R., LEWIS, M. R. and WINTROBE, M. M.: The Activity of the Lymphocyte in the Body's Reaction to Foreign Protein, as Established by the Identification of the Acute Splenic Tumor Cell, Bull. Johns Hopkins Hosp., 65, 311, 1939.

38a. RICHTER, K. M.: Studies on Leukocytic Secretory Activity, Ann. New York Acad. Sc., 59, 863, 1955.

38b. ROBINEAUX, R.: Mouvements cellulaires et fonction phagocytaire des granulocytes neutrophiles, Rev. d'hémat., 9, 364, 1954.

38c. ROSSE, W. F. and GURNEY, C. W.: The Pelger-Huët Anomaly in Three Families and Its Use in Determining the Disappearance of Transfused Neutrophils from the Peripheral Blood, Blood, 14, 170, 1959.

39. SABIN, F. R.: Studies of Living Human Blood Cells, Bull. Johns Hopkins Hosp., 34, 277, 1923.

39a. SAMTER, M.: The Response of Eosinophils in the Guinea Pig to Sensitization, Anaphy-laxis and Various Drugs, Blood, 4, 217, 1949; ibid., 8, 1078, 1953.

40. SARAIVA, L. G. et al.: Anomalous Panleukocytic Granulation, Blood, 14, 1112, 1959.

40a. SCHWARZ, E.: Cellular Gigantism and Pluripolar Mitosis in Human Hematopoiesis, Am. J. Anat., 79, 75, 1946.

40b. SIERACKI, J. C.: The Neutrophilic Leukocyte, Ann. New York Acad. Sc., 59, 690, 1955.

40c. SKARNES, R. C. and WATSON, D. W.: Characterization of Leukin, J. Exper. Med., 104, 829, 1956.

40d. SMITH, C.: Glycogen in Basophilic Leucocytes in Human Blood Smears, Proc. Soc. Exper. Biol. & Med., 72, 209, 1949.

41. SPEIRS, R. S.: Advances in the Knowledge of the Eosinophil in Relation to Antibody Formation, Ann. New York Acad. Sc., 73, 283, 1958.

41a. STEINBERG, B. and MARTIN, R. A.: Plasma Factor Increasing Circulatory Leukocytes, Am. J. Physiol., 161, 14, 1950; Fed. Proc., 9, 345, 1950.

41b. STERN, K. G.: Über die Katalase farbloser Blutzellen, Ztschr. f. Physiol. Chem., 204, 259, 1932.

42. STORTI, E. and PERUGINI, S.: Richerche di citochimica ematologica. Le reazioni dei polisaccaridi applicate alla diagnostica citologica delle leucosi acute, Il Progresso Medico, 8, 257, 1952.

42a. SUNDBERG, R. D. and DOWNEY, H.: Comparison of Lymphoid Cells of Bone Marrow and Lymph Nodes of Rabbits, Am. J. Anat., 70, 455, 1942.

43. SUNDBERG, R. D.: Lymphocytes and Plasma Cells, Ann. New York Acad. Sc., 59, 671, 1955.

43a. SWENDSEID, M. E., WRIGHT, P. D. and BETHELL, F. H.: Variations in Nucleotidase Activity of Leukocytes. Studies with Leukemic Patients, J. Lab. & Clin. Med., 40, 515, 1952.

43b. TOMPKINS, E. H.: The Monocytes, Ann. New York Acad. Sc., 59, 732, 1955.

44. UNDRITZ, E.: Les malformations héréditaires des éléments figurés du sang, Sang, 25, 296, 1954; Folia haemat., 1, 268, 1957.

44a. UNDRITZ, E.: Eine neue Sippe mit erblich-konstitutioneller Hochsegmentierung der Neutrophilenkerne, Schweiz. med. Wchnschr., 88, 1000, 1958.

44b. UNDRITZ, E.: Die Chediak-Steinbrinck-Anomalie oder erblich-konstitutionelle Riesengranulation (Granulaganten) der Leukocyten, Schweiz. med. Wchnschr., 88, 996, 1958.

44c. VALENTINE, W. N.: The Biochemistry and Enzymatic Activities of Leukocytes in

Health and Disease, *in Progress in Hematology*, New York, Grune & Stratton, 1956, p. 293; Am. J. Med., *28*, 699, 1960.

44*d*.VALENTINE, W. N., FOLLETTE, J. H., HARDIN, E. B., BECK, W. S. and LAWRENCE, J. S.: Studies on Leukocyte Alkaline Phosphatase Activity: Relation to "Stress" and Pituitary-Adrenal Activity, J. Lab. & Clin. Med., *44*, 219, 1954; *ibid.*, *49*, 723, 1957.

44*e*.VALENTINE, W. N., FOLLETTE, J. H. and LAWRENCE, J. S.: The Glycogen Content of Human Leukocytes in Health and in Various Disease States, J. Clin. Invest., *32*, 251, 1953.

44*f*.VAUGHN, J.: The Function of the Eosinophile Leukocyte, Blood, *8*, 1, 1953.

45. WAGNER, R.: Enzyme Studies on White Blood Cells. Arch. Biochem., *26*, 123, 1950; *ibid.*, *39*, 174, 1952; *ibid.*, *54*, 174, 1955; Arch. Biochem. & Biophys., *61*, 278, 1956; Ann. New York Acad. Sc., *75*, 16, 1958.

45*a*.WEISBERGER, A. S., HEINLE, R. W., STORA-ASLI, J. P. and HANNAH, R.: Transfusion of Leukocytes Labeled with Radioactive Phosphorus, J. Clin. Invest., *29*, 336, 1950.

45*b*.WEISBERGER, A. S. and LEVINE, B.: Incorporation of Radioactive L-Cystine by Normal and Leukemic Leukocytes *in Vivo*, Blood, *9*, 1082, 1954.

45*c*.WEISBERGER, A. S. and SUHRLAND, L. G.: Comparative Incorporation of S^{35} L-Cystine and S^{35} Sodium Sulfate by Normal and Leukemic Leukocytes, Blood, *10*, 458, 1955.

45*d*.WELSH, R. A.: The Genesis of the Charcot-Leyden Crystal in the Eosinophilic Leukocyte of Man, Am. J. Path., *35*, 1091, 1959.

46. WISEMAN, B. K.: Criteria of the Age of Lymphocytes in the Peripheral Blood, J. Exper. Med., *54*, 271, 1931.

46*a*.WOOD, W. B., JR. and Co-workers: Studies on the Mechanism of Recovery in Pneumococcal Pneumonia, J. Exper. Med., *84*, 365, 1946; *ibid.*, *90* 555, 1949; *ibid.*, *94*, 521, 1951; *ibid.*, *110*, 1005, 1959.

47. YOFFEY, J. M.: The Lymphocyte Problem, Nature, *183*, 76, 1959; Blood, *15*, 82, 1960.

47*a*.ZLOTNICK, A., GERICHTER, C. B. and NIR, I.: Experimental Production of "Grape Cells" and Their Relation to the Serum Gamma Globulin and Seromucoids, Blood, *14*, 564, 1959.

Normal Values, Physiologic Variations, and Systems for Differential Counting

47*b*.ACLAND, J. D. and GOULD, A. H.: Normal Variation in the Count of Circulating Eosinophils in Man, J. Physiol., *133*, 456, 1956.

47*c*.ALTSCHULE, M. D., ALTSCHULE, L. H. and TILLOTSON, K. J.: Changes in Leukocytes of the Blood in Man After Electrically Induced Convulsions, Arch. Neurol. & Psych., *62*, 624, 1949; J. Clin. Endocrinol., *9*, 440, 1949.

47*d*.AMBRUS, J. L. and AMBRUS, CLARA M.: Regulation of the Elimination of Leukocytes, *in* Homeostatic Mechanisms, Brookhaven Symposia in Biology: No. 10, Upton, N. Y., 1957, p. 84.

47*e*.BEST, W. R., KARK, R. M., MUEHRCKE, R. C. and SAMTER, M.: Clinical Value of Eosinophil Counts and Eosinophil Response Tests, J. A. M. A., *151*, 702, 1953.

47*f*.BOLL, I.: Ausreifung eines Myelocyten zum Segmentkernigen, Folia haemat., *3*, 78, 1958.

48. BOSEILA, A.-W. A.: The Normal Count of Basophil Leucocytes in Human Blood, Acta med. scandinav., *163*, 525, 1959.

48*a*.CASEY, A. E.: The Diurnal Levels of Blood Leukocytes in the Normal Rabbit, Proc. Soc. Exper. Biol. & Med., *45*, 863, 1940.

49. CRESS, C. H., CLARE, F. B. and GELLHORN. E.: The Effect of Anoxic and Anemic Anoxia on the Leucocyte Count, Am. J. Physiol., *140* 299, 1943.

49*a*.DAVIS, M. E. and HULT, B. E.: Changes in Circulating Eosinophils in Women During the Menstrual Cycle and Reproduction, J. Clin. Endocrinol., *9*, 714, 1949.

49*b*.EFRATI, P. and ROZENSZAJN, L.: The Morphology of Buffy Coat in Normal Human Adults, Blood, *16*, 1012, 1960.

49*c*.FARRIS, E. J.: The Blood Picture of Athletes as Affected by Intercollegiate Sports, Am. J. Anat., *72*, 223, 1943.

49*d*.FORWELL, G. D.: The Response of the Leukocyte Count in Man to Environmental Heat and to Exercise, J. Physiol., *124*, 66, 1954.

49*e*.GABRILOVE, J. L., VOLTERRA, M., JACOBS, M. D. and SOFFER, L. J.: The Effect of the Parenteral Injection of Epinephrin on Leukocyte Counts in Normal Subjects and in Patients with Addison's Disease, Blood, *4*, 646, 1949.

50. GARREY, W. E. and BRYAN, W. R.: Variations in White Blood Cell Counts, Physiol. Rev., *15*, 597, 1935.

51. GOLDNER, F. M. and MANN, W. N.: The Statistical Error of the Differential White Count, Guy's Hosp. Rep., *88*, 54, 1938.

51*a*.GORDIN, R.: Toxic Granulation in Leukocytes, Acta med. scandinav., Supp. 270, 1952.

52. HADEN, R. L.: Qualitative Changes in Neutrophilic Leukocytes, Am. J. Clin. Path., 5, 354, 1935.

52a.INAGAKI, S.: The Relationship between the Level of Circulating Basophil Leucocytes and Thyroid Function, Acta endocrinol., 26, 477, 1957.

53. KARVONEN, M. J. and KUNNAS, M.: Factor Analysis of Haematological Changes in Heavy Manual Work, Acta physiol. scandinav., 29, 220, 1953.

54. KATO, K.: Leucocytes in Infancy and Childhood, J. Pediat., 7, 7, 1935.

55. KENNEDY, W. P. and MACKAY, L.: The Normal Leucocyte Picture in a Hot Climate, J. Physiol., 87, 336, 1936.

56. KENNON, B., SHIPP, M. E. and HETHERINGTON, D. C.: A Study of the White Blood Cell Picture in Six Young Men, Am. J. Physiol., 118, 690, 1937.

57. KERR, A. C.: The Effect of Mental Stress on the Eosinophil Leucocyte Count in Man, Quart. J. Exper. Physiol., 41, 18, 1956.

58. LEVINE, S. A. and GOLDEN, R.: Some Observations on Paroxysmal Rapid Heart Action With Special Reference to Roentgen-ray Measurements of the Heart In and Out of Attacks, Arch. Int. Med., 29, 836, 1922.

59. LUCIA, S. P., LEONARD, M. E. and FALCONER, E. H.: The Effect of the Subcutaneous Injection of Adrenalin on the Leukocyte Count of Splenectomized Patients, Am. J. Med. Sc., 194, 35, 1937.

60. McCALL, M. S., SUTHERLAND, D. A., EISENTRAUT, A. M. and LANZ, H.: The Tagging of Leukemic Leukocytes with Radioactive Chromium and Measurement of the in Vivo Survival, J. Lab. & Clin. Med., 45, 717, 1955.

61. MILHORAT, A. T., SMALL, S. M. and DIETHELM, O.: Leukocytosis During Various Emotional States, Arch. Neurol. & Psychiat., 47, 779, 1942.

61a.NELSON, D. H., SANDBERG, A. A., PALMER, J. G. and TYLER, F. H.: Blood Levels of 17-Hydroxycorticosteroids following the Administration of Adrenal Steroids and Their Relation to Levels of Circulating Leukocytes, J. Clin. Invest., 31, 843, 1952.

61b.OLBRICH, O.: Blood Changes in the Aged, Edin. Med. J., 64, 306, 1947.

61c.PATHAK, C. L. and KAHALI, B. S.: Cyclic Variations in the Eosinophil Count during the Phases of the Menstrual Cycle, J. Clin. Endocrinol., 17, 862, 1957.

62. PEPPER, H. and LINDSAY, S.: Levels of Eosinophils, Platelets, Leukocytes and 17-Hydroxycorticosteroids during Norm Menstrual Cycle, Proc. Soc. Exper. Biol. & Med., 104, 145, 1960.

63. PETERSEN, W. F. and BERG, M.: Meteorological Influences on Leukocyte Curve, Proc. Soc. Exper. Biol. & Med., 30, 830, 1933.

63a.PONDER, E. and PONDER, R. V. O.: The Cytology of the Polymorphonuclear Leucocyte in Toxic Conditions, J. Lab. & Clin. Med., 28, 316, 1942.

63b.ROHR, K.: Zur Differenzierung der neutrophilen Leukocyten, Acta. hæmatol., 1, 98, 1948.

63c.SAMUELS, A. J.: Primary and Secondary Leucocyte Changes Following the Intramuscular Injection of Epinephrine Hydrochloride, J. Clin. Invest., 30, 941, 1951.

63d.SHARP, G. W. G.; The Effect of Light on Diurnal Leucocyte Variations, J. Endocrin., 21, 213, 1960.

64. STORTI, E. and PEDERZINI, A.: Clinical Significance of the Leukocytic Resistance, Acta med. scandinav., 154, 417, 1956; Rev. hémat., 14, 431, 1959.

64a.STURGIS, C. C. and BETHELL, F. H.: Quantitative and Qualitative Variations in Normal Leukocytes, Physiol. Rev., 23, 279, 1943.

64b.UHRBRAND, H.: The Number of Circulating Eosinophils, Acta med. scandinav., 160, 99, 1958.

64c.VERZÁR, F.: Die Zahl der Lymphocyten und eosinophilen Leukocyten in 1800 und 3450 m Höhe, Schweiz. med. Wchnschr., 82, 324, 1952.

64d.WACHHOLDER, L., BECKMANN, A. and WALTER, H.: Anderungen des Weissen Blutbildes nach Nahrungsaufnahme, Pflügers Archiv., 251, 459, 1949.

65. WASHBURN, A. H.: Blood Cells in Healthy Young Infants, Am. J. Dis. Child., 50, 395, 1935.

65a.WEINER, W. and TOPLEY, E.: Döhle Bodies in the Leucocytes of Patients with Burns, J. Clin. Path., 8, 324, 1955.

Variations of Leukocytes in Disease

66. ALBERT, J. and JONGCO, A. P.: Leukemoid Blood as Malignant Sign in Pertussis, Philippine M. A. J., 21, 63, 1941.

66a.ASHBURN, L. L., DAFT, F. S. and FAULKNER, R. R.: Hematopoiesis in Pantothenic Acid-Deficient Rats, Blood, 2, 451, 1947.

66b.ASHFORD, B. K., PAYNE, G. C. and PAYNE, F. K.: Acute Uncinariasis From Massive Infestation and Its Implications, J.A.M.A., 101, 843, 1933.

67. AUSTIN, J. H. and LEOPOLD, S. S.: An Extraordinary Polymorphonuclear Leukopenia in Typhoid Fever, J.A.M.A., 66, 1084, 1916.

67a.BARNES, G. R., JR., YANNET, H. and LIEBERMAN, R.: A Clinical Study of an Institutional Outbreak of Acute Infectious Lymphocytosis, Am. J. Med. Sc., *218*, 646, 1949.

67*b*.BEAVER, P. C. and DANARAJ, T. J.: Pulmonary Ascariasis Resembling Eosinophilic Lung, Am. J. Trop. Med., *7*, 100, 1958.

68. BENJAMIN, B. and WARD, S. M.: Leukocytic Response to Measles, Am. J. Dis. Child., *44*, 921, 1932.

69. BERCOVITZ, Z.: Clinical Studies on Human Infestations With the Liver Fluke (Clonorchis sinensis), Am. J. Trop. Med., *11*, 43, 1931.

69*a*.BERGER, H. C.: Eosinophilia Occurring in Chorea, Am. J Dis. Child., *21*, 477, 1921.

70. BICHEL, J.: Lymphatic Leukemia and Lymphatic Leukemoid States in Cancer of the Stomach, Blood, *4*, 759, 1949.

70*a*.BRAUNSTEINER, H. and THUMB, N.: Quantitative Veränderungen der Blutbasophilen und ihre klinische Bedeutung, Acta haemat., *20*, 339, 1958; Rev. hemat., *15*, 241, 1960.

70*b*.BROWN, T. McP., STIFLER, W. C., JR. and BETHEA, W. R., JR.: Early Filariasis, Bull. Johns Hopkins Hosp., *78*, 126, 1946.

71. BRUMLIK, J. and SIKL, H.: Eosinophil Leukemia With Lymph Node Tuberculosis or Leukemoid Reaction With Eosinophilia, Folia hæmatol., *43*, 1, 1930.

72. BULL, C. G.: The Fate of Typhoid Bacilli When Injected Intravenously Into Normal Rabbits, J. Exper. Med., *22*, 475, 1915.

73. BURHAM, C. F.: Hodgkin's Disease, J.A.M.A., *87*, 1445, 1927.

73*a*.CARTWRIGHT, G. E.: An Unusual Case of Clonorchiasis with Marked Eosinophilia and Pulmonary Infiltrations, Am. J. Med., *6*, 259, 1949.

73*b*.CARTWRIGHT, G. E., CHUNG, H. L. and CHANG, A.: Studies on the Pancytopenia of Kala-Azar, Blood, *3*, 249, 1948.

73*c*.CARTWRIGHT, G. E., WINTROBE, M. M., BUSCHKE, W. H., FOLLIS, R. H., JR., SUKSTA, A. and HUMPHREYS, S.: Anemia, Hypoproteinemia and Cataracts in Swine Fed Casein Hydrolysate or Zein, J. Clin. Invest., *24*, 268, 1945.

73*d*.CASTANEDA, M. R. and GUERRERO, G.: Studies on the Leucocytic Picture in Brucellosis, J. Infect. Dis., *78*, 43, 1946.

73*e*.CHAFEE, F. H., ROSS, J. R. and GUNN, E. M.: Eosinophilia in Fatal Asthma, Ann. Int. Med., *17*, 45, 1942.

74. CLARK, J. H.: The Action of Light on the Leucocyte Count, J. Am. Hyg., *1*, 39, 1921.

74*a*.COBANE, J. H., STRAITH, C. L. and PINKUS, H.: Facial Granulomas with Eosinophilia, Arch. Dermat. & Syphilol., *61*, 442, 1950.

74*b*.COCHRANE, J. C., SAGORIN, L. and WILCOCKS, M. G.: Capillaria Hepatica Infection in Man, South African M. J., *31*, 751, 1957.

74*c*.COPELAND, G. D., VON CAPELLER, D. and STERN, T. N.: Systemic Lupus Erythematosus, Am. J. M. Sc., *236*, 318, 1958.

75. COWIE, D. M. and JIMENEZ, B.: Cytologic Examination of Nasal Smears of Sensitized and Nonsensitized Persons With Nasal Symptoms, Arch. Int. Med., *57*, 85, 1936.

76. CUMMER, C. L.: Anemia and Other Blood Changes in Syphilis, J.A.M.A., *91*, 689, 1928.

77. CUSTER, R. P. and CROCKER, W. J.: The Myeloleukæmoid Blood Picture Associated With Tuberculosis, Folia hæmatol., *46*, 359, 1932.

77*a*.D'ABRERA, V. St. E.: The Aetiology of 'Tropical Eosinophilia' with a Preliminary Note on the Pathology of the Syndrome, Ceylon M. J., *4*, 195, 1958; Med. J. Australia, *1*, 517, 1959.

78. DAENGSVANG, S.: Human Gnathostomiasis in Siam with Reference to the Method of Prevention, J. Parasitol., *35*, 116, 1949.

78*a*.DALAND, GENEVA A., GOTTLIEB, L., WALLERSTEIN, O. and CASTLE, W. B.: Hematologic Observations in Bacterial Endocarditis, J. Lab. & Clin. Med., *48*, 827, 1956.

78*b*.DANARAJ, T. J.: The Treatment of Eosinophilic Lung (Tropical Eosinophilia) with Diethylcarbamazine, Quart. J. Med., *27*, 243, 1958.

78*c*.DAUGHADAY, W. H., WILLIAMS, R. H. and DALAND, G. A.: The Effect of Endocrinopathies on the Blood, Blood, *3*, 1342, 1948.

78*d*.DIAZ-RIVERA, R. S. *et al.*: Infiltrative Eosinophilia, Ann. Int. Med., *45*, 459, 1956.

79. DIXON, H. B. F. and SMITHERS, D. W.: Epilepsy in Cysticercosis (Tænia solium), Quart. J. Med., *3*, 603, 1934.

80. DOAN, A. and WISEMAN, B. K.: The Monocyte, Monocytosis and Monocytic Leukosis, Ann. Int. Med., *8*, 383, 1934.

80*a*.DONOHUE, W. L.: Alymphocytosis, Pediatrics, *11*, 129, 1953.

80*b*.DOUGHERTY, T. F. and FRANK, J. A.: The Quantitative and Qualitative Responses of Blood Lymphocytes to Stress Stimuli, J. Lab. & Clin. Med., *42*, 530 and 538, 1953; *ibid.*, *45*, 485, 1955.

81. DOWNEY, H., MAJOR, S. G. and NOBLE, J. F.: Leukemoid Blood Pictures of the Myeloid Type, Folia hæmatol., *41*, 493, 1930.

81*a*.ELDRIDGE, F.: Pulmonary Infiltration with Eosinophilia and the Alveolar-Capillary Block Syndrome, Am. J. Med., *25*, 796, 1958.

81b.ENDICOTT, K. M., KORNBERG, A. and OTT, M.: Hemopoiesis in Riboflavin-Deficient Rats, Blood, 2, 164, 1947.

82. ERCKLENTZ, B. W.: Leukämoide Reaktion bei Leberremission einer Anæmia Perniciosa, Folia hæmatol., 53, 382, 1935.

82a.ESSEX, H. E. and GRAÑA, A.: Behavior of the Leukocytes of the Rabbit During Periods of Transient Leukopenia Variously Induced, Am. J. Physiol., 158, 396, 1949; ibid., 172, 231, 1953.

82b.EVEN-PAZ, Z. and SAGHER, F.: High Leucocytosis (Leukaemoid Reactions?) in Dermatitis Herpetiformis, Brit. J. Dermat., 71, 325, 1959.

82c.FAHEY, R. J.: Unusual Leukocyte Responses in Primary Carcinoma of the Lung, Cancer, 4, 930, 1951.

83. FELDMAN, W. H. and STASNEY, J.: Leukemoid Response of Tuberculous Rabbits to Administration of Tuberculin, Am. J. Med. Sc., 193, 28, 1937.

83a.FLANAGAN, C. J.: Mechanical Fragility of Human Neutrophilic Erythrophagocytes, Proc. Soc. Exper. Biol. & Med., 90, 580, 1955.

83b.FRASER, J. F.: Exfoliative Dermatitis, Arch. Dermat. & Syphilol., 48, 42, 1943.

83c.FREDRICKS, R. E. and MOLONEY, W. C.: The Basophilic Granulocyte, Blood, 14, 571, 1959.

84. FRIEDMAN, S.: Eosinophilia in Scarlet Fever, Am. J. Dis. Child., 49, 933, 1935.

84a.GARDNER, F. H. and METTIER, S. R.: Lymphocytic Leukemoid Reaction of the Blood Associated with Miliary Tuberculosis, Blood, 4, 767, 1949.

84b.GIBSON, A.: Monocytic Leukæmoid Reaction Associated with Tuberculosis and a Mediastinal Teratoma, J. Path. & Bacteriol., 58, 469, 1946.

85. GOLDMAN, D.: Chickenpox With Blood Picture Simulating That in Leukemia, Am. J. Dis. Child., 40, 1282, 1930.

85a.GRAEF, I., KARNOFSKY, D. A., JAGER, B. V., KRICHESKY, B. and SMITH, H. W.: The Clinical and Pathologic Effects of the Nitrogen and Sulfur Mustards in Laboratory Animals, Am. J. Path., 24, 1, 1948.

86. GUGGENHEIM, K. and BUECHLER, E.: The Effect of Quantitative and Qualitative Protein Deficiency on Blood Regeneration. I. White Blood Cells, Blood, 4, 958, 1949.

88. HARRISON, F. F.: Eosinophilia With Splenomegaly, Am. J. Med. Sc., 179, 213, 1930.

88a.HAVENS, W. P., JR. and MARCK, R. E.: The Leukocyte Response of Patients with Experimentally Induced Infectious Hepatitis, Am. J. M. Sc., 212, 129, 1946.

88b.HENSLER, L.: Hohe Leukocytose durch Karzinom, Schweiz. med. Wchnschr., 83, 1032, 1953.

88c.HERNBERG, C. A.: Observations on the Size of Lymphocytes in the Blood in Addison's Disease; Panhypopituitarism, and Cushing's Syndrome during Treatment. Also Thyrotoxicosis, Acta med. scandinav., 144, 380, 1953; ibid., 149, 37, 1954.

89. HICKLING, R. A.: The Significance of Hæmic Plasma Cells in Various Infective Conditions, J. Hyg., 24, 120, 1925.

89a.HILL, J. M. and DUNCAN, C. N.: Leukemoid Reactions, Am. J. Med. Sc., 201, 847, 1941.

90. HILL, R. W. and BAYRD, E. D.: Phagocytic Reticuloendothelial Cells in Subacute Bacterial Endocarditis with Negative Cultures, Ann. Int. Med., 52, 310, 1960.

90a.HILLENBRAND, F. K. M.: The Blood Picture in Rubella, Lancet, 2, 66, 1956.

90b.HILTS, S. V. and SHAW, C. C.: Leukemoid Blood Reactions, New England J. Med., 249, 434, 1953.

90c.HOLBROOK, A. A.: The Blood Picture in Chickenpox, Arch. Int. Med., 68, 294, 1941.

90d.HUGHES, J. T., JOHNSTONE, R. M., SCOTT, A. C. and STEWART, P. D.: Leukaemoid Reactions in Disseminated Tuberculosis, J. Clin. Path., 12, 307, 1959.

90e.ISAACSON, N. H. and RAPOPORT, P.: Eosinophilia in Malignant Tumors, Ann. Int. Med., 25, 893, 1946.

90f.JAFFE, R. H.: Reticulo-Endothelial System, in Handbook of Hematology, Hal Downey, Ed. Paul B. Hoeber, N. Y., 1938, II, pp. 1061 and 1323.

90g.JOHNSON, E. S., NAPOLI, V. M. and WHITE, W. C.: Colorado Tick Fever As a Hematologic Problem, Am. J. Clin. Path., 34, 118, 1960.

91. KAMPMEIER, R. H. and HINEMAN, E. H.: Amebic Dysentery, J. Lab. & Clin. Med., 22, 985, 1937.

91a.KATZ, A. M. and PAN, C.-T.: Echinococcus Disease in the United States, Am. J. Med., 25, 759, 1958.

92. KELLER, A. E., GOOGE, J. T., COTTRELL, H. B., MILLER, D. G. and HARVERY, R. H.: Clinical Study Under Controlled Conditions of 1083 Children With Hookworm, J.A.M.A., 105, 1670, 1935.

92a.KIANG, S. and CHOA, G. H.: The Blood Picture in Leprosy, Am. J. Med. Sc., 217, 269, 1949.

92b.KNICK, B. and SCHILLING, F.: Leukämoide Reaktion und intermittierendes Charcotsches Fieber als klinisches Syndrom bei malignem Gallenwegverschluss und Meta-

18

stasenleber, Schweiz. med. Wchnschr., *90*, 464, 1960.

93. KNOTT, F. A. and PEARSON, R. S. B.: Eosinophilia in Allergic Conditions, Guy's Hosp. Rep., *84*, 230, 1934; *ibid.*, *85*, 94, 1935.

94. KRUMBHAR, E. B.: Leukemoid Blood Pictures in Various Clinical Conditions, Am. J. Med. Sc., *172*, 519, 1926.

95. KUGELMEIER, L. M.: Leukämoide Reaktionen bei Carcinom, Folia hæmatol., *53*, 370, 1935.

95a.LAMONT, N. McE. and POOLER, N. R.: Hepatic Amoebiasis, Quart. J. Med., *27*, 389, 1958.

96. LENHARTZ, H.: Zusammentreffen von akuter Miliartuberkulose und akuter Myeloblastenleukämie, Beitr. z. Klin. d. Tuberk., *79*, 501, 1932.

96a.LEONARD, B. J., ISRAËLS, M. C. G. and WILKINSON, J. F.: Alkaline Phosphatase in the White Cells in Leukaemia and Leukaemoid Reactions, Lancet, *1*, 289, 1958.

96b.LOWE, T. E.: Eosinophilia in Tropical Disease, Med. J. Australia, *1*, 453, 1944.

97. MACBRYDE, C. M. and CHARLES, C. M.: Differential Diagnosis of Rubella, Arch. Int. Med., *56*, 935, 1935.

98. MASINA, N.: Das Blutbild bei Leberzirrhose mit besonderer Berücksichtigung der Monozytengranulation, Folia hæmatol., *46*, 335, 1932.

100. MEDLAR, E. M.: Further Studies on the Pathological Significance of the Leucocytic Reaction in Tuberculosis, Am. Rev. Tuberc., *31*, 611, 1935.

101. MEDLAR, E. M., LOTKA, A. J. and SPIEGELMAN, M.: Leucocytic Counts in Tuberculosis, Am. Rev. Tuberc., *42*, 444, 1940; *cf.* Am. Rev. Tuberc., *44*, 58, 1941.

102. MEYER, L. M. and ROTTER, S. D.: Leukemoid Reaction in Malignancy, Am. J. Clin. Path., *12*, 218, 1942.

103. MILLER, T. G. and PEPPER, O. H. P.: Metabolic Studies of Angioneurotic Edema, Arch. Int. Med., *18*, 551, 1916.

104. MINOT, G. R.: Purpura Hemorrhagica With Lymphocytosis, Am. J. Med. Sc., *192*, 445, 1936.

105. MINOT, G. R. and SMITH, L. W.: The Blood in Tetrachlorethane Poisoning, Arch. Int. Med., *28*, 687, 1921.

105a.MITCHELL, R. G.: Basophilic Leucocytes in Children in Health and Disease, Arch. Dis. Childhood, *33*, 193, 1958.

106. MOWREY, F. H. and LUNDBERG, E. A.: The Clinical Manifestations of Essential Polyangiitis (Periarteritis Nodosa), with Emphasis on the Hepatic Manifestations, Ann. Int. Med., *40*, 1145, 1954.

106a.MURPHY, J. B. *et al.*: Effects of Dry Heat, Sunlight and X-rays on the Lymphocytes and the Relation of These Effects on resistance to Cancer, Tuberculosis and Poliomyelitis in Animals, J. Exper. Med., *29*, 1, 1919.

107. MURRAY, E. G. D., WEBB, R. A. and SWANN, M. B. R.: A Disease of Rabbits Characterized by a Large Mononuclear Leucocytosis, Caused by a Hitherto Undescribed Bacillus, *Bacterium Monocytogenes*, J. Path. & Bacteriol., *29*, 407, 1926.

109. OTTO, G. F.: Blood Studies on Trichuris-infested and Worm-free Children in Louisiana, Am. J. Trop. Med., *15*, 693, 1935.

110. PARRISIUS, W. and HEIMBERGER, H.: Akute Myelosen nach Bienenstichen und ihre Oxydasereaktion, Deutsch. Arch. f. klin. Med., *143*, 335, 1924.

111. PEARSON, W. J. and NEWNS, G. H.: Extreme Degree of Leukocytosis in Whooping Cough, Lancet, *2*, 254, 1937.

112. PEPPER, O. H. P.: Hematology of Subacute Streptococcus Viridans Endocarditis, J.A.M.A., *89*, 1377, 1927.

113. PERLINGIERO, J. G. and GYÖRGY, P.: Chronic Eosinophilia, Am. J. Dis. Child., *73*, 34, 1947.

113a.POLA, V.: Beitrag zum hämatologisch bunten Ablauf des myeloproliferativen Syndroms, Folia haemat., *77*, 26, 1960.

113b.POPPEL, M. H. *et al.*: The Roentgen Manifestations of Urticaria Pigmentosa (Mastocytosis), Am. J. Roentgenol., *82*, 239, 1959.

114. PRIEST, R. J., REBUCK, J. W. and HAVEY, G. T.: A New Qualitative Defect of Leukocyte Function in Ulcerative Colitis, Gastroenterology, *38*, 715, 1960.

115. REIFENSTEIN, E. C., ALLEN, G. E. and ALLEN, G. S.: Trichiniasis, Am. J. Med. Sc., *183*, 668, 1932.

116. REZNIKOFF, P.: White Blood Cell Counts in Convalescence From Infectious Diseases, Am. J. Med. Sc., *184*, 167, 1932.

116a.RICHTER, M. N.: (Personal communication.)

117. RIESMAN, D. and AHLFELDT, F. E.: Coccidioidal Granuloma, Am. J. Med. Sc., *174*, 151, 1927.

117a.RITCHIE, G. M.: Extensive Myeloid Response during Folic Acid Therapy in Megaloblastic Anaemia of Pregnancy, J. Clin. Path., *5*, 329, 1952.

117b.ROBERTS, M. H.: Extreme Eosinophilia in Childhood, South. M. J., *47*, 317, 1954.

118. RODRIGUEZ, M. R. and PONS, J. A.: Hematological Studies on Schistosomiasis Man-

soni in Puerto Rico, Puerto Rico J. Pub. Health & Trop. Med , *11*, 369, 1936.

119. SALA, A. M. and STEIN, R. J.: Carcinoma of the Breast With a Condition of the Blood Simulating Chronic Lymphatic Leukemia, Arch. Path., *23*, 531, 1937.

120. SCALETTAR, H. E., MAISEL, J. E. and BRAMSON, M.: Acute Infectious Lymphocytosis, Am. J. Dis. Child., *88*, 15, 1954.

120a.SCLARE, G. and CRAGG, J.: A Leukaemoid Blood Picture in Megaloblastic Anaemia of the Puerperium, J. Clin. Path., *11*, 45, 1958.

121. SEARS, W. G.: The Blood in Hodgkin's Disease, With Special Reference to Eosinophilia, Guy's Hosp. Rep., *82*, 40, 1932.

122. SHILLITOE, A. J.: The Common Causes of Lymphopenia, J. Clin. Path., *3*, 321, 1950.

122a.SMITH, C. H.: Infectious Lymphocytosis, Am. J. Dis. Child., *62*, 231, 1941; J.A.M.A., *125*, 342, 1944.

123. STEPHENS, D. J.: The Occurrence of Myelocytes in the Peripheral Blood in Lobar Pneumonia, Am. J. Med. Sc., *188*, 332, 1934.

124. STEWART, S. G.: Familial Eosinophilia, Am. J. Med. Sc., *185*, 21, 1933.

125. SWIFT, H. F., MILLER, C. P., JR., and BOOTS, R. H.: The Leucocyte Curve as an Index of the Infection in Rheumatic Fever, J. Clin. Invest., *1*, 197, 1924–25.

125a.SYVERTON, J. R. and SLAVIN, H. B.: Human Toxoplasmosis, J.A.M.A., *131*, 957, 1946.

127. THOMAS, H. M., JR.: Rupture of Encapsulated Empyema Into the Pleural Cavity, J.A.M.A., *72*, 29, 1919.

127a.VAN DUYN, 2D, J.: Degenerative White Blood Cell Picture as an Indication of Toxemia From Burns, Arch. Surg., *50*, 242, 1945.

128. WALLBACH, G.: Über die Grenzen zwischen Leukämie und Infekt, Folia hæmatol., *47*, 278, 1932.

128a.WEBB, J. K. G., JOB, C. K. and GAULT, E.

W.: Tropical Eosinophilia, Lancet, *1*, 835, 1960.

128b.WEINGARTEN, R. J.: Tropical Eosinophilia, Lancet, *1*, 103, 1943.

128c.WELSH, J. D., DENNY, W. F. and BIRD, R. M.: The Incidence and Significance of the Leukemoid Reaction in Patients Hospitalized with Pertussis, South. M. J., *52*, 643, 1959.

129. WIESE, O.: Beobachtungen bei Parotitis epidemica unter besonderer Berücksichtigung des Blutbefundes, Arch. f. Kinderh., *80*, 253, 1927.

130. WILDTGRUBE, F.: Whooping Cough: Leukocyte Picture, Ztschr. f. Kinderh., *50*, 152, 1930.

130a.WILE, U. J., ISAACS, R. and KNERLER, C. W.: The Blood Cells in Early Syphilis, Am. J. Syph., Gonor. & Ven. Dis., *25*, 133, 1941.

130b.WILLETT, F. M. and OPPENHEIM, E.: Pulmonary Infiltrations with Associated Eosinophilia, Am. J. Med. Sc., *212*, 608, 1946.

131. WINTROBE, M. M.: Diagnostic Significance of Changes in Leukocytes, Bull. New York Acad. Med., *15*, 223, 1939.

132. WISEMAN, B. K. and DOAN, C. A.: The Lymphatic Reaction in Tuberculosis, Am. Rev. Tuberc., *30*, 33, 1934.

132a.WOLF, P.: The Significance of Proplasmocytes and Atypical Plasma Cells in the Benign Lymphocytic Meningitis Syndrome, Blood, *9*, 971, 1954.

133. WRIGHT, D. O. and GOLD, E. M.: Loeffler's Syndrome Associated With Creeping Eruption, J.A.M.A., *128*, 1082, 1945.

134. ZONDEK, B. and BROMBERG, Y. M.: Leukocytosis Induced by Methyl-acetamide With p-Chloro-xylenol, Am. J. Med. Sc., *205*, 82, 1943.

135. ZUELZER, W. W. and APT, L.: Disseminated Visceral Lesions Associated with Extreme Eosinophilia, Am. J. Dis. Child., *78*, 153, 1949.

Chapter 5

Blood Platelets and Coagulation

THE BLOOD PLATELET

MANY investigators in the early part of the nineteenth century observed the blood platelets,[26a] but even Zimmermann (1860), Max Schultze (1865) and Osler (1874), who realized that these corpuscles were not artefacts, failed to recognize their true importance. Hayem (1878), like Zimmermann, thought that they developed into red blood cells. It remained for Bizzozero[4] (1882) to describe platelets as they appeared in the mesenteric vessels of rabbits and guinea pigs, to demonstrate their adhesive quality, their participation in thrombi, and their rôle in the coagulation of the blood. Wright's[29] important studies (1906) concerning the origin of the platelets will be discussed later.

Morphology. — Platelets are small, colorless, moderately refractile bodies, usually spherical, oval or rod-shaped. Under dark-field illumination they show a sharp contour, are translucent and may appear to possess a few immobile granules in the center. With the electron microscope[10b,13b] small mitochondria, dense granulations and clear areas, Golgi material and endoplasmic reticulum have been described. Contractile vacuoles and vacuoles of pinocytosis have been demonstrated by microcinematography of cells observed by phase contrast

(276)

microscopy. When stained by one of the Romanowsky methods, azure granules are seen in a hyaline, light blue cytoplasm. The granules may be so packed in the central portion of the platelets that they give the appearance of a nucleus. A nucleus, however, has never been satisfactorily demonstrated in the platelet, nor do the granules take the nuclear stains. Even the differentiation of a "hyalomere" and "granulomere," a smooth and a granular portion, may be purely artificial. Instantaneous fixation and staining with dyes like brilliant cresyl blue fails to show a sharp division into two portions. The platelet granules stain with neutral red, and a few mitochrondrial rods and granules stain with Janus green. Various factors affect platelet morphology, such as the nature of the contacting surface, the properties of the anticoagulant, its concentration and the thickness of the preparation.[5b]

Platelets generally vary from 2 to 4 μ in diameter and average 7 to 8 c.μ in volume.[22] Sometimes much larger platelets are found, particularly when blood regeneration is active. At such times platelets even 25 to 50 μ in length have been observed.[26] Bizarre forms appear under these circumstances: dumbbell, Indian club, comma, cigar and other unusual shapes.

If platelets are kept in moist preparations or in oxalated blood for some time, spine-like and filamentous processes may be formed. Stained preparations of such blood may show platelets which resemble flagellates, trypanosomes or piroplasma.

On the assumption that platelets undergo orderly "maturation" which is detectable by morphologic criteria, differential studies of platelets have been made. Platelets have been classified on the basis of size,[21] size and staining,[5] amount of granulation,[16] the shape, size and type of granulation,[1d] and the depth of coloring of the platelet hyaloplasm, the presence or absence of vacuoles, the size, number, position and intensity of staining of the granules, as well as the size and shape of the platelets as a whole.[14] On these grounds young and old forms, degeneration forms, normal and pathological "irritation" forms, and primitive types have been distinguished. Basophilic staining of the cytoplasm has been assumed to give evidence of youth, vacuolization of old age. Deep staining of the granules and eccentric position of the granules have been considered indications of full maturity. Small platelets have been said to have a higher agglutinative property than larger ones and to be, therefore, functionally more active.[21]

No one who has examined blood specimens from a variety of blood disorders can have failed to observe alterations, sometimes very striking ones, in the morphology of the platelets. Many of these changes are, no doubt, not artefacts. Their interpretation, however, is a matter of great difficulty in our present state of ignorance. The differential classification of platelets, therefore, although it is a subject of great interest and some promise, is at present one of mere speculation.

Physical and Chemical Properties. [16,26,28,30a]— Like red corpuscles, platelets were considered for a long time to have little intrinsic metabolic activity and now are known to be metabolically very active. Composed chiefly of protein (60 or more

per cent, dry weight), they also contain considerable lipid (15 per cent).[10] The total carbohydrate content is about 8.5 per cent. Calcium, Mg, Cu, Fe and Mn are present but Zn is absent.[30a] An important constitutent is a contractile actomyosin-like protein.[3b] There is disagreement concerning the ribonucleic acid content,[30a] some regarding this as the major nitrogenous constituent[12b] whereas others have not found this to be the case.[10a] There is no deoxyribonucleic acid.[30a] The lipids include phosphatidylethanolamine, phosphatidylserine, inositol phosphatide, lecithin and sphingomyelin.[16a] In addition to glycogen, a sulfated mucopolysaccharide is present[19] and a number of monosaccharides have been identified.[28b] Enzymes involved in glycolysis (both pentose-phosphate cycle and citric acid cycle), cellular respiration, phosphate splitting and transamination have been found.[28] Included among the more than 27 enzymes[30a] are nucleotidase,[23b] acid phosphatase,[27c] dehydrogenase,[14c] pyrophosphatase[7d] and acetylcholinesterase.[30] The vasoconstrictor substance, 5-hydroxytryptamine (serotonin) is transported in the blood by platelets, having been taken up, probably, from the gastrointestinal tract. During coagulation it is released into the serum by the action of thrombin.[12c] Platelets also can bind comparatively large quantities of histamine, epinephrine and norepinephrine[23c] but this is not thought to play any role under physiological conditions. Many of the components of the platelet can be demonstrated by histochemical methods.[12d]

Carbohydrate metabolism[6a] predominates, as judged by the respiratory quotient of 1.1.[28] The content of adenosine triphosphate (ATP) is 150 times that of red corpuscles. Similarities between the metabolism of skeletal muscle and platelets have been found. Like muscle, the platelet is capable of performing mechanical labor.

Most investigators distinguish megakaryocytes from polykaryocytes (osteoclasts?) which possess multiple separate nuclei[23a] (Plate II, p. 64). Megakaryocytes have

megakaryocyte is enveloped by a layer of viscous material outside the cell contour which disappears as the cell matures.[23f] In the preparation of smears this thin

Platelets manifest three important physical properties; namely, adhesiveness,
aggregation and agglutination.[5e] As soon
as a platelet comes in contact with a

cytoplasm of megakaryocytes. These
cells are so situated in the bone marrow
in relation to the blood vessels that small
projections or moderately long pseudo-

layer may be sheared off and pseudo-
thrombocytes formed.

A variety of technics have been devised for counting megakaryocytes.[22d]

**Site and Mode of Platelet Produc-
tion.**—It has been generally assumed
that the site of platelet production during
adult life is chiefly in the bone marrow.
Although megakaryocytes are normally
found in the lungs, it had been assumed
that these are effete cells. Howell and
Donahue[13] challenged this view on the
following grounds: (1) the platelet count
is generally higher in arterial as compared with venous blood; (2) fewer
platelets are found in the bone marrow
than in the spleen or lungs; (3) perfusion
of bone marrow yields few platelets
whereas perfusion of the lungs produces
many; (4) the megakaryocytes they observed in the lungs appeared to be
actively giving off platelets. They concluded that platelets are normally formed
in the lungs from megakaryocytes which
are not caught in the capillaries by
chance but are formed there in the same
manner as in the bone marrow. Others
have been unable to obtain satisfactory
evidence of platelet production in the
lungs.[12]

The manner of production of platelets
from megakaryocytes has been studied
by microcinematography of bone marrow
cultures.[3a,12h,14a] These photographs are
quite remarkable. As the nucleus becomes pyknotic, platelets appear to be
formed by the extension of numerous
long thin arms from the cytoplasm, much
in the manner of an octopus. These long
pseudopodia become thinner and thinner
until they become filiform. It has been
suggested that the filaments may become
caught in sinusoidal capillaries, segments
are broken off by the contractions of the
filaments and the platelets thus formed
are swept away by the blood current.

**Kinetics of Platelet Production,
Survival and Destruction.** — It has
been estimated that the maturation time

from a stem cell to a platelet-producing
megakaryocyte is about seven days and
that an average man may have 3.25 $\times$
10^8 megakaryocytes.[7a] The survival of
platelets in the circulation has been estimated in various ways, more recently by
tagging them *in vivo* with P^{32} and then
transfusing some of the tagged blood into
a compatible recipient;[1c] by tagging
platelets with Cr^{51} *in vitro* and observing
their survival after transfusion to normal
recipients; and by labelling platelets *in
vivo* with DFP^{32}. The use of the last agent
for labelling leukocytes was discussed in
the preceding chapter (p. 240). The
method[14d] has the advantage that damage
to platelets by their removal from the
body and handling is avoided. By the
last two methods survival times of nine
to eleven days[1] and eight to nine days[14d]
were obtained. These may be considered
to be the technics least open to criticism
and the results the best approximations
available at present.

The total number of circulating platelets in a normal average man may be of
the order of 1.05×10^{12}. On the assumption that the average platelet survival
time is ten days and assuming a platelet
volume of 4.2 c.μ, the total circulating
platelet mass would be 4.4×10^{12} c.μ.
Assuming that this is all derived from
megakaryocyte cytoplasm and on the
basis of estimates of the volume of megakaryocytes, it was calculated that the
turnover time of the megakaryocyte and
its younger forms is about 25 days.[7a]
This does not allow for platelet stores, but
it has been estimated that these are only
of the order of one or two times the
numbers in the circulation. Such reserves
may be present in the spleen and the
lungs. These may also be sites for their
removal when overcome by senescence,
providing they have not been destroyed
already in performing their functions.

Studies of the effects of platelet removal and reinjection of platelet-free
blood in dogs showed that the removal of

two to three blood volumes resulted in severe thrombocytopenia. Permanent recovery did not take place until two to three days after cessation of platelet removal.[7] Megakaryocyte hyperplasia was observed and ultimate recovery was preceded by a rise in platelet count to supranormal levels.

Such observations, as well as the remarkable constancy of the platelet count under normal conditions (p. 283), suggest that the production of platelets is well regulated. Nothing is known concerning the control mechanism. However, study of a patient with a congenital form of thrombocytopenic purpura provided evidence suggesting that a factor is present in normal plasma which stimulates megakaryocyte maturation.[23d]

Enumeration of Blood Platelets.— Scores of methods and modifications of methods for counting the platelets have been described, but no method is satisfactory in every respect. This is to be expected in dealing with structures whose property is ready agglutination and disintegration. Platelets are difficult to discern because of their small size; they become attached very readily to particles of débris on the glassware used or in the diluting fluid, and probably are not evenly distributed in the blood.[26] Yet, with care and experience, platelet counts can be performed which are sufficiently accurate to be useful.[5b]

Generally errors tend to give low platelet counts. However, this is not always the case, for fragmentation of platelets without complete dissolution, or the mistaking of particles of débris— crystals of some salts making up the diluting fluid, dye, bacteria, portions of hemolysed red corpuscles or broken leukocytes—may produce incorrectly high counts.

In general it may be emphasized that all glassware used must be scrupulously clean and diluting fluids should be fresh and frequently filtered. Diluting fluids should be sterilized, kept in glass-stoppered bottles, and stored at 2° to 4° C. when not in use. They should be filtered each time before use, and blank counts on the solution should be made at intervals in order to discover bacteria, molds or platelet-like bodies. Rees and Ecker solution (p. 282) which has stood for a time may cause hemolysis of red cells as the result of formic acid formation from oxidation of formaldehyde. Such solutions should be discarded. Some prefer to use 1 per cent ammonium oxalate as a diluent because this hemolyses red cells and leaves a clear background.[5b]

If blood is to be obtained by puncturing the skin, the hand should be washed thoroughly with soap and water and then cleansed with alcohol and ether or acetone.[20] It has also been recommended that the hand be first immersed in a warm bath and opened and closed for several minutes in order to produce active hyperemia. The finger is preferred to the lobe of the ear as a source of blood because hyperemia cannot be so readily produced in the latter and the fine hair there is said to favor adhesion of platelets. The skin puncture should be made with a sharp lancet.

Platelet counts are made either directly by enumerating them in a counting chamber, or indirectly by determining their proportion to the red corpuscles, a direct count being made of the latter. Usually whole blood, subsequently diluted, is used. In some rarely employed methods, the plasma alone is used.[26] In all cases it is wise to check the platelet count as obtained, by making a rough survey of the platelets as seen in a blood smear stained by one of the Romanowsky stains.

Indirect Methods.—The simplest procedure is to note the number of platelets as compared with the number of red corpuscles or leukocytes in a stained blood smear. *Fonio* placed a drop of 14 per cent aqueous solution of magnesium sulfate on the skin and punctured the finger through this in order to dilute the blood at once and to prevent disintegration of the platelets. *Olef's method*[20] is perhaps the best of the indirect procedures but is somewhat cumbersone. *Dameshek's method*[7b] is similar but more simple. The *diluting fluid* is made up by dissolving 8 Gm. of sucrose and 0.4 Gm. of sodium citrate in 100 ml. distilled water, to which is then added 0.15 Gm. brilliant cresyl blue. The resulting solution is mixed well and filtered. Three drops of a solution of formaldehyde (1:10) U.S.P., are added as a preservative. The first drop of blood obtained by puncturing a finger is discarded. A fairly large drop of the diluting fluid is placed over the puncture wound and the finger is gently squeezed so that a small amount of blood wells up into the drop of staining solution. The proportion of blood to stain should be about 1 to 5. The mixture of blood and stain is transferred to a cover-slip, which is then dropped on a slide. The preparation is examined under an oil immersion lens after fifteen to forty-five minutes. The ratio of platelets to red corpuscles is determined and their number calculated from the red cell count. Reticulocytes can be counted in the same preparation.

Platelet counts made by indirect methods tend to be higher than those obtained by direct methods of enumeration. This is attributable in part to the tendency of red cells to concentrate at the edge of the coverslip, thus giving a falsely high ratio of platelets to red cells in the central areas of the coverslip where the count is likely to be made.

Direct Methods.—These can be carried out on capillary or venous blood but platelet counts on finger blood are subject to greater errors than counts on venous blood.[5b] In collecting blood from a vein, a 20 gauge needle, with syringe attached, should be inserted into a cubital vein and such blood as is needed for

other purposes is collected in the syringe. The syringe is then removed, leaving the needle in place. One to 2 ml. blood is allowed to flow gently down the side of a tilted siliconized test tube (10 × 75 mm.). For platelet counts this is preferable to the collection of blood in the oxalate mixture used for other quantitative studies (p. 377). Whatever method is employed for collection or for dilution of blood, an important step which insures greater accuracy is the prompt dilution of the blood. This reduces the tendency of platelets to clump.[5b]

The *Rees and Ecker* diluting fluid consists of sodium citrate 3.8 Gm.; formaldehyde, neutral 38 per cent U.S.P., 0.22 ml.; brilliant cresyl blue 0.05 Gm.; distilled water to make 100 ml.

Blood is drawn in a red cell pipet to the 0.5 mark and the diluting fluid to 101, as for a red cell count. The diluted blood is thoroughly mixed for five minutes, preferably in a pipet rotor. The first four drops from the pipet are expelled and discarded and then *both* counting chambers of a hemocytometer are filled in the usual manner (p. 386). The hemocytometer is covered with one-half of a Petri dish containing a piece of wet filter-paper (to prevent drying out) and is set aside for fifteen minutes. The count is made under the high power of the microscope with the light partially cut down, using the whole of the finely ruled central ("red cell") area of each chamber. Thus a total of 50 groups of 16 small squares is counted. The result is multiplied by 2000 to give the number per c.mm.

In identifying the platelets, the observer should have the fingers of one hand on the fine adjustment of the microscope in order to obtain the critical focusing that reveals the characteristic highly refractile, silvery appearance of the platelets. They are lilac-colored, one-seventh to one-half the diameter of the red corpuscles, and usually oval, rod or comma-shaped. They may be seen singly or in groups. It is important to distinguish platelets from globules of oil, irregularly shaped débris floating on the upper layers of fluid, strings of cocci, and other particles which may be found moving about in the fluid as well as from tiny oily particles adhering to the counting chamber.

A serious handicap imposed by all direct methods for counting platelets is the difficulty in distinguishing platelets from other particles since the counting chamber does not permit the oil-immersion magnification to be used. This objection is met in part by the use of the *phase microscope*. In **Brecher's method**[5b] 1 per cent ammonium oxalate is used as the diluting fluid, a specially thin cover slip (No. 1 or 1½) is used on the counting chamber and appropriate adjustment of the phase microscope is made. Blood is collected in a siliconized test tube, as already described. Blood is drawn in a red cell pipette to the 1 mark with great accuracy and diluting fluid to the 101 mark. The pipette is shaken for approximately three minutes. Subsequent steps are similar to those described for the Rees and Ecker procedure but the count is made in five blocks of small squares in each counting chamber. The number of platelets in the total of ten squares is multiplied by 2500 to give the number per c.mm.

The *Brecher-Cronkite* method[5b] is the procedure we employ and prefer. It has the disadvantage of requiring special equipment (phase contrast microscope, a long working distance condenser with 43 × annulus, a 43 × phase objective (medium dark contrast), and 10 × oculars). Important advantages are the clearer background resulting from the hemolysis of the red cells produced by the diluting fluid and the greater ease of distinguishing platelets from extraneous particles.

Many other methods for platelet counting are in use, each with certain advantages and disadvantages.[4a,22c,25]

Volume Occupied by the Platelets. —The volume occupied by the platelets may be determined by means of a special "thrombocytocrit"[22,27] or, more simply, by observing the thickness of the platelet layer in a hematocrit which has been centrifuged after sedimentation has taken place (p. 381). If a hematocrit filled with blood is allowed to stand an hour or longer, the red cells settle to the bottom, the leukocytes settle more gradually and the platelets remain suspended in the plasma. If centrifugation is now carried out, slowly at first and then more rapidly, three layers of corpuscles may be made out; a creamy-white layer of platelets, a reddish-gray layer of leukocytes and a red layer of red corpuscles (Plate I and Fig. 8–3, p. 382). This method serves only as a rough guide because some of the platelets remain in the plasma in spite of centrifugation and others are mixed with the leukocytes.

Normal Values for Platelets.—Different values for normal have been recorded, depending chiefly on the method used. Employing the Rees and Ecker method, the mean platelet count in 80 healthy young adults was found to be 241,000 per c.mm.[23h] This is in agreement with the experience in the writer's laboratory. The standard deviation was 50,000, which would give a normal range of 140,000 to 340,000. In our hands the Brecher-Cronkite method gave an average value of 250,000 per c.mm., with 95 per cent of the counts ranging from 140,000 to 440,000.

Using his more refined procedure, Tocantins[26] found similar values. His figures were: cutaneous blood, 250,000; venous blood, 310,000; arterial blood, 350,000, with standard deviations of 58,500 to 128,000.

Indirect counting methods have, in general, yielded higher normal values. Thus, Olef,[20] using his own method, found an average count of 514,000 (437,000 to 586,000). By Dameshek's method,[7b] 500,000 to 900,000 platelets per c.mm. are normally found. As already stated, the highest counts recorded are not necessarily correct.

The volume of packed platelets in normal blood is about 0.3 ml. per 100 ml. blood[22] (about 0.3 mm. in the hematocrit).

Distribution of Platelets.—Platelets are found in the lumina of the blood vessels but, if one may judge by observation of the blood *in vivo* through "windows" in the ears of rabbits, their distribution is very irregular in the same vessels at different times.[3] They may be seen in the spleen, in the sinuses or between the cells of the pulp and they are present in great numbers in the capillaries of the liver and, particularly, of the lungs. Moderate numbers may be seen in the material obtained by puncture of the sternum. Platelets are not found in the lymph of the thoracic duct. It has been stated that fewer platelets enter the lungs than leave them.[13] These findings however, are not in agreement with other studies[12] and require confirmation. More platelets have been found in the arterial blood of the upper extremity than in venous or capillary blood[26] but, in these, as in the various studies already mentioned, the differences recorded are small when compared with the margin of error in platelet counting.

Physiological Variations in the Platelet Count.—The blood of *newborn infants* shows fewer platelets (150,000 to 250,000) than that of older infants, especially during the first forty-eight hours of life. At this time there may also be more variation in the size of platelets and in their staining reaction than is normal. The platelet count rises gradually to reach normal adult values at about three months of age.[17]

No differences between the sexes in platelet count have been demonstrated, but during the first day of *menstruation*

decreases of as much as 50 to 75 per cent have been recorded.[26] On the third or fourth day of menstruation the platelets increase again. Pohle[23] observed a slow progressive decrease during the fourteen days prior to menstruation and a rapid increase soon after the onset of the menses. During pregnancy there is no significant change but slight decreases have been described during the first stage of labor and on the first or second days postpartum.

Sudden changes in posture are said to cause a change in the platelet count and following violent *exercise* the number of platelets increases.[27b] A regular rhythm in relation to meals has been described but the evidence is not convincing. Lower counts have been reported in arterial blood during the spring months as compared with winter. A change to a high altitude may cause a more marked increase in platelets than in erythrocyte count.[26] The injection of *epinephrine* causes an increase in the platelet count within five minutes which lasts an hour and does not occur in splenectomized animals. Histamine has a similar effect. The intravenous injection of pyridine is also followed by thrombocytosis but, unlike the effect of epinephrine, this is accompanied by an increase in the stickiness of the platelets.[28c] Blood platelets do not appear to be influenced in any specific or significant way by adrenal cortical hormone but may be affected by the pituitary.[1b]

Variations in Platelets in Disease.—Numerous statements have been made regarding variations in platelet counts in disease but in so many instances the differences have been so small, or the technic of counting has been so questionable, that little credence can be given to these reports. Conditions in which thrombocytopenia is found are discussed fully in Chapter 17.

Trauma and asphyxiation may cause marked **increases in the platelet**

count. Fractures of bones, especially those of the neck of the femur, may be followed by thrombocytosis. An increase in the platelet count of 30 to more than 100 per cent may occur following *surgical operations.*[22a,28a] The maximal rise has been observed from the seventh to the twentieth postoperative day. Splenectomy is followed by a greater and more constant increase than other operations.[26]

Acute blood loss, obvious or occult, causes thrombocytosis but longstanding chronic hemorrhage may be associated with some thrombocytopenia. When there is massive gastro-intestinal bleeding the platelet count may be reduced during and for several days afterwards but this is followed by an increase during convalescence.[7e] An increase in platelets may occur also during the acute phase of rheumatic fever,[16] and in suppurative infections.

Thrombocythemia or **piastrinemia** are terms which have been applied to more persistently increased platelet levels, in contrast to the temporary instances of thrombocytosis described above. Thrombocythemia is commonly seen in myeloproliferative conditions such as chronic myelocytic leukemia and erythremia. It may occur also in Hodgkin's disease and is found in association with splenic atrophy,[12e] as well as after splenectomy.[12e] One or two instances of thrombocythemia have been observed also in association with carcinoma, Boeck's sarcoid, and splenic vein thrombosis.[23e] In addition, a few cases of thrombocythemia have been described in which no cause was apparent nor were there any apparent ill effects.[15a] A strange disorder marked by thrombocythemia and hemorrhage which may be a clinical entity will be discussed later (p. 850).

Variations in the Morphology of Platelets in Disease.—These variations have been mentioned already. Generally, more variation in size is found when the number of platelets is reduced than when it is normal. Unusually large platelets, sometimes with very coarse granules, have been observed frequently in purpura hemorrhagica. Basophilic platelets have been noted in thrombocytopenia and diminished platelet granulation has been reported. Particularly large or bizarre forms are found following splenectomy or whenever there is myeloid proliferation. In leuko-erythroblastosis exceptionally bizarre forms of platelets may be encountered.

Megakaryocytes in the Circulating Blood.—Megakaryocytes, or fragments of their nuclei or cytoplasm are sometimes found in the circulating blood. These nuclei stain deeply, are large, oval or irregular in shape, and may be surrounded by a small amount of cytoplasm. They have been seen a number of times in leuko-erythroblastosis (p. 587), myelocytic leukemia,[18] erythremia, Hodgkin's disease and in cases in which there was a leukocytic increase due to infection (*e.g.,* lobar pneumonia); isolated instances have also been reported in which these structures were observed in acute leukemia, aleukemic leukemia,[8a] purpura hemorrhagica during phases of platelet increase, pernicious anemia and plumbism. Megakaryocyte hyperplasia, sometimes associated with the presence of megakaryocytes in the blood, characterizes megakaryocytic leukemia (p. 940).

In various conditions calling forth abnormal or immature bone marrow elements, megakaryocytes have often been found packed in the lung capillaries.[18]

Functions of Platelets.—The platelets are concerned in hemostasis and thrombosis. By their agglutination they serve directly in sealing an injured blood vessel. They also play a part in the vasoconstrictive response observed when vessels are injured.[69] Whether any other purposes are served by their carrying various substances on their surface is unknown.

Platelets have been described as "packets of very active pharmacologic substances." Some of these compounds are adsorbed on the platelet surface. They include substances such as the vasoconstrictor, serotonin, (p. 277) and several coagulation factors. Roskam suggested that the latter maintain around the platelets the "plasma atmosphere."[74c] What substances are derived from the platelets themselves[78] and which ones have been adsorbed by them is disputed. Thus, the study of platelet extracts yielded "platelet factor 1," a term applied to an accelerator derived from platelets which catalyzes the conversion of prothrombin to thrombin.[86] Others, however, believe that this is simply adsorbed plasma coagulation factor V.[13a] Platelet factor 2 was described as a substance which accelerates the conversion of fibrinogen to fibrin under the influence of thrombin.[43] Platelet factor 3 has been defined as a lipoprotein which, in conjunction with a plasma substance ("cofactor I"), is capable of converting purified prothrombin to thrombin.[47] Platelet factor 4 has the property of neutralizing the action of heparin.[7f]

A number of experiments[72c] indicate, however, that certain clotting activities of platelets can be attenuated and then restored, as if adsorbed substances are removed and then replaced; for example by incubation in saline and then in plasma, the activity of platelets in the thromboplastin generation test can be attenuated and restored.[22b] Evidence has been presented for the presence of prothrombin and coagulation factors V, VII, VIII, IX and X in the "plasma atmosphere" of platelets.[5a] Antifibrinolytic activity[53a] and a fibrinogen-like substance which could be coagulated with thrombin[86] were also reported as platelet factors but may be only on their surface.

It seems clear, however, that certain constituents of platelets possess coagulant activity; for example, lipid constituents such as phosphatidylserine[84] (p. 277). It has been reported that the granulomere of platelets contains lipid phosphorus.[16b] For the contraction of the blood clot, viable platelets are required.[23j]

The physical properties of platelets and the changes they undergo in association with hemostasis and with coagulation have attracted considerable attention. An important property is platelet adhesiveness.[12g] When a small vessel is injured, platelets adhere to each other and to the edge of the injury, forming a platelet plug which covers the lesion.[74c] The formation of the platelet plug is the key event in normal hemostasis. At first the plug is permeable to the blood, but soon it becomes impermeable and the bleeding stops. The change in permeability is thought to be due to the phenomenon of *viscous metamorphosis*. This consists first in clumping of the platelets, then swelling of the mass and finally the release of granular material, possibly phospholipids, into the surrounding plasma. This reaction was found to precede the interaction of the coagulation factors which produce thromboplastin but was delayed in the absence of plasma thromboplastin antecedent (PTA) or Hageman factor.[23g]

There have been many suggestions concerning the factors which activate this process. It is thought that inactive precursors are transformed to an active principle. The activation product plays a trigger role in reactions leading to platelet clumping and viscous metamorphosis in native plasma. Thrombin has been found to induce viscous metamorphosis of platelets in the presence of calcium and a co-factor[58] but an intermediate product, formed early in blood coagulation, was also noted to release these platelet changes.[32,85] It has been suggested that viscous metamorphosis of platelets can develop in various ways and is released by different triggers.[85]

Coagulation is followed by *clot retraction*.[5a] Direct observation of coagulation has shown that soon after fibrin has been laid down, *intact* platelets in the interior of the mass converge toward the fibrin needles, adhere to them and form large knots at their intersections.[11] As the knots are being formed, the fibrin becomes bent, twisted and shortened. Retraction of the clot is more complete the higher the number of platelets and the greater the concentration of thrombin in relation to the quantity of fibrinogen.[72b] The number of platelets is important. When the platelet count is low the blood clot shows less adhesiveness, firmness, rigidity and contractility than is normal and, if blood has been collected in a vessel, it will not retain the shape of the vessel and will be heavier, softer and more jelly-like than the clot produced by normal blood.[24] It was found that clot retraction was absent when the platelet count was 70,000 or lower.[26] Glucose, phosphates, cysteine or glutathione and calcium are utilized in the process of clot retraction[5a] and glycolytic activity is increased with its onset.[3b] During clot retraction the ATP contained in platelets is partly consumed and more is produced by the glycolytic system. It appears that the major part of the ATP consumed during the retraction period is concerned in the contraction of the actomyosin-like protein of platelets.[3b]

When coagulation has taken place and fibrin has been formed, a thrombus is produced. Many factors influence *thrombosis*, among which are slowing of the circulation, changes in the vessel wall and agglutination of platelets. Platelet agglutination is favored by the presence of injured tissue or foreign particles in the circulation, such as staphylococci. The changes which occur in the platelets lead to the release of a potent diffusible vasoconstrictor which affects all the vessels of the surrounding area. Contraction of the clot leads to the expression of serum rich in nascent thrombin. At the same time new platelets adhere to the fibrin network of the clot, and in turn disintegrate. Release of more lipid follows and a cycle is thus established which causes enlargement of the thrombus. By successive formation and retraction of the new clots, the thrombus is propagated.

The concept that coagulation factors are adsorbed on the surface of platelets makes understandable the various views which have been expressed concerning the role of platelets in the coagulation of blood. These have ranged from claims for a position of prime importance to one of little significance.[61] It has been stated that platelets are essential for efficient clotting but that coagulation can occur in their absence.[39] It is generally acknowledged that agglutination of platelets may take place without coagulation; that coagulation may be initiated and proceed in the presence of few or even no platelets, as in lymph[61] or in glass tubes which present a relatively rough surface, in contrast to the great delay in coagulation in silicone treated tubes.[39] The distinction must be made between those activities which require the presence of viable, metabolically active platelets, such as viscous metamorphosis and clot retraction, and those functions in which platelets play a more passive role. For some activities, the viability of platelets is more important than their number.

HEMOSTASIS AND COAGULATION

Hemostasis.—The factors involved in the arrest of the flow of blood from a vessel (hemostasis) are of three types: (1) extravascular, as represented by subcutaneous tissue, muscle and skin, the usefulness of these tissues depending upon their mass, tonicity, tautness and resiliency; (2) vascular, comprising the blood vessels, these varying according to age, type, size, tone, location and nutritional state; and (3) intravascular, comprising all the factors concerned in the coagulation of blood.

When bleeding from a vessel occurs these forces normally function in a co-ordinated manner. Following injury, prompt vasoconstriction and retraction of the vessel occur. Normal tissue tone, together with the increased pressure on the vessel caused by egress of blood into the surrounding tissues tend to halt the escape of blood temporarily. Initial vasoconstriction is maintained for three to four minutes, during which time blood platelets agglutinate and adhere to the area of broken intima, as described above. The intravascular events which take place and the formation of the fibrin plug seals the gap in the broken vessel if it is not too large and tissue thromboplastin, as will be described below, causes clotting of the blood which has escaped into the tissues. Intravascular coagulation soon ceases because of intravascular forces which tend to keep the blood fluid (p. 295). Permanent hemostasis at the bleeding point occurs as the result of contraction and organization of the clot and, ultimately, healing of the wound.

It should be pointed out that, under normal conditions, an increase in the quantity of factors concerned in coagulation does not accelerate coagulation since they are already present in optimal amounts. Thus, stimulation of bone marrow activity with increased production of blood platelets, as occurs following hemorrhage, is of minor importance in accelerating coagulation for only a minimal number of platelets is needed for this process. The administration of vitamin K is of value when the quantity of prothrombin is reduced in amount and when liver function is adequate. The use of calcium is of no value since the levels encountered, even in conditions characterized by hypocalcemia, are still sufficient for clotting. However, conditions which render disintegration of platelets more likely, such as moist,

rough surfaces, and slowing of the blood stream, favor coagulation and the formation of thrombi.

Coagulation can be produced *in vivo* by the injection of tissue extracts or trypsin. The action of some snake venoms is directly on fibrinogen while others cause coagulation by converting prothrombin to thrombin.[44] Bacterial endotoxins are capable of stimulating coagulation.[59a] In animal experiments it was observed that arterial blood possesses hemostatic properties whereas venous blood does not.[41a] Evidence was obtained suggesting that the lung provides the blood with a cephalin-like hemostatic factor.

Local hemostasis is favored by two natural products, thrombin and fibrin. "Rabbit thrombin" and "thrombin topical," isolated from rabbit plasma and bovine plasma, respectively, are thrombic in nature and are useful hemostatics for small wounds.[80] Human thrombin preparations have been obtained by the conversion of human prothrombin with human thromboplastin of placental origin.[44a] Preformed fibrin, in the form of sheets or "foam," offers the advantage of serving as a dressing that is naturally absorbed during healing. Of artificial coagulants for local use, the venom of Russell's viper and that of the Australian tiger snake are effective.[58c]

Theories of Coagulation.[58c,59c] — The physical and chemical changes which result in the formation of a blood clot have been the subject of much investigation and speculation for centuries but they are still not fully understood. Malpighi (1666) was one of the first to consider the problem and, in the eighteenth century, Petit, Hewson, Chaptal and Hunter were concerned with it. In the next century, Buchanan, Lister, Denis and Hammarsten made contributions which set the stage for the concept proposed by Alexander Schmidt (1892);

namely, that the coagulation of blood is the consequence of a chain of reacting factors culminating in the conversion of fibrinogen into fibrin by a ferment called thrombin. It was recognized that thrombin is not present as such in the circulating blood and that an inactive precursor, prothrombin, is activated by another substance, probably lipoidal in nature. Recognition of the essential part played by calcium led to the development of the classical theory of the coagulation mechanism (Morawitz, 1905) in which four factors were regarded as necessary: thromboplastin, calcium, prothrombin and fibrinogen.

In the modern concept of coagulation, blood clotting is conceived as a dynamic process in which positive forces leading to coagulation are antagonized by negative contrary forces, the latter including natural anticoagulants and agents which remove the formed clot. The foundations for this concept were laid by Howell (1910).[49] It has also become clear that more than four factors are concerned, a

view first propounded by Nolf (1908)[61] and later supported by Bordet. It now appears that there are three distinct phases in the clotting of blood, namely, the formation of blood thromboplastin, the formation of thrombin and the production of fibrin.

Modern theories of coagulation will be more easily understood if the various factors and steps are first considered separately. Because there is less uncertainty concerning the nature of the end products of coagulation than there is concerning those which participate at earlier stages of the process, the various factors will be described more or less in reverse of the order of their formation.

Nomenclature.—The inherent complexity of the coagulation process has been compounded by the great number of terms which have been applied to the various factors involved. Fortunately, an international committee has agreed upon a uniform terminology.[89] This will be employed here. Synonyms will be found in Table 5–1.

Table 5–1—Synonyms for Various Coagulation Factors

International Nomenclature[89]	Synonyms
Factor I	Fibrinogen
Factor II	Prothrombin
Factor III	Thromboplastin
Factor IV	Calcium
Factor V	Proaccelerin,[63b] Labile Factor,[69] Accelerator Globulin (AcG),[87] Thrombogen[61]
(Factor VI	Accelerin)
Factor VII	Proconvertin ($\rightarrow$ convertin),[63b] Stable factor,[69] Serum prothrombin conversion accelerator (SPCA),[31a] Autoprothrombin I[75]
Factor VIII	Antihemophilic factor (AHF), Antihemophilic globulin (AHG), Thromboplastinogen,[69] Platelet cofactor I, Plasma thromboplastic factor A, Facteur antihémophilique A
Factor IX	Plasma thromboplastin component (PTC), Christmas factor, Platelet cofactor II, Autoprothrombin II,[75] Plasma thromboplastic factor B, Facteur antihémophilique B
Factor X	Stuart-Prower factor
PTA	Plasma thromboplastin antecedent
Hageman factor	

19

Fibrinogen (*Factor I*), **Thrombin and Fibrin.**—The end result of blood coagulation is the formation of a fine network of fibers that entangles the formed elements of the blood. This is the result of the conversion of fibrinogen to fibrin. Serum is therefore free of fibrinogen. Itself, one of the plasma proteins, fibrinogen is the least soluble of them all and is present in a concentration of about 0.3 Gm. per 100 ml. It is produced in the liver. It can be separated from plasma by salting out in the cold by half saturation with sodium chloride or quarter saturation with ammonium sulfate. Clinical methods have been devised for its measurement (p. 303). The plasma concentration is reduced in certain circumstances and, in one form of hemorrhagic disorder, fibrinogen is entirely absent (p. 883).

Fibrinogen is a protein of large molecular weight, about 341,000.[34] N-terminal amino acid analysis has indicated that it may be composed of six polypeptide chains. The fibrinogen of each of a number of species of mammals was found to have two tyrosyl residues but in other respects the species differed from one another; thus, perhaps, explaining the immunological species specificity of fibrinogen. In addition to the two tyrosyl residues, human fibrinogen was found to have two alanyl residues but two chains seemed to have no free N-terminal residues.

Thrombin is not normally present in the blood but is derived from prothrombin. Its activity is that of a proteolytic enzyme and it is comparable to the proteinase, papain, or to trypsin.[55c] Since its activity is inhibited by diisopropyl fluorophosphate, it may be an esterase.[59b] Preparations have been produced which are capable of clotting several hundred times their own weight of fibrinogen.[75b]

By electron microscopy it was observed that fibrinogen molecules are polymerized by the action of thrombin to form needle-shaped, crystal-like protofibrils which then become aligned into fiber strands by lateral association.[66] Chemically it appears that several steps take place. First fibrinogen is prepared for polymerization by enzymatic liberation of two soluble peptides.[46] Fibrin monomers are formed. These are readily soluble in urea and to this point the chemical reaction is readily reversible. The clot which ultimately develops, however, is insoluble in urea, a change which has been attributed to the intervention of a serum factor ("fibrin stabilizing factor") and calcium ions;[57] or thrombin may be responsible for the polymerization as well as the original proteolysis.[55d] N-terminal analysis of human fibrin showed the tyrosyl residues of fibrinogen still remaining but the other four chains all had glycyl end groups.[34] Both peptides liberated from fibrinogen contain arginine as the C-terminal amino acid.[55e]

Prothrombin. (*Factor II*).—In examining the literature on coagulation the reader must be prepared to distinguish between a hypothetical precursor of thrombin which was measured by tests now shown to depend on several variables, and "true" prothrombin, a substance which has been isolated from plasma in highly purified form and possesses well defined physical and chemical properties.[55b,75] These indicate that it is a glycoprotein of about 62,700 molecular weight and contains 18 amino acids, about 6.5 per cent carbohydrate as hexose and, in addition, glucosamine and neuraminic acid.[81] Prothrombin migrates with the α_2 globulins in electrophoretic analysis and behaves as a euglobulin. It is found in blood in a concentration of approximately 20 mg. per cent and is absent in serum. "Purified" prothrombin, however, is quite unstable.

The nature of the conversion of prothrombin to thrombin is uncertain.[78a] The amino acid composition of prothrombin and thrombin is similar[55b] and prothrombin can be converted to thrombin by sodium citrate without calcium ions or thromboplastin.[75a] These and other observations favor the suggestion that the conversion is an enzymatic process but other considerations support the view that autocatalysis is the fundamental process.[55d] Seegers and his associates have described a number of derivatives of prothrombin with different activities which can be produced under various conditions. These include biothrombin, citrate thrombin, thrombin-E (esterase) and thrombin-C (coagulating activity).[55d,75b] It has been suggested that the prothrombin molecule is broken into units by proteolysis and that at a certain point this is extensive enough to have esterase activity. If there is further activation, clotting activity appears. This, it is postulated, is due to the association of esterase molecules to form a dimer. The clotting activity does not persist, however, and this may be explained by dissociation of the molecule back to the esterase form.[55d] There is evidence that the molecular weight of thrombin is half of that of prothrombin, or even less. It appears that prothrombin loses a carbohydrate fragment in its conversion to thrombin.[35b]

Thromboplastin (*Factor III*).—The classical theory of blood coagulation attributed the initiation of clotting to a substance, thromboplastin which, in the presence of calcium ions, catalysed the conversion of prothrombin to thrombin. Modern views differentiate *tissue* thromboplastin and *blood* thromboplastin. The distinction is that, in the blood, thromboplastin activity arises during the process of coagulation whereas this activity is evident immediately in certain tissue extracts. Thromboplastin is widely distributed in the body as an intracellular substance and is found in highest concentration in the brain, lungs, placenta, thymus and testes. It can be demonstrated

whenever tissue cells are injured or ruptured. Human milk has high thromboplastic activity.[31c] Russell viper venom also has thromboplastic activity.[45b]

It now appears that even the term "tissue thromboplastin" is too broad and that more specific designation is necessary.[47] Thus, Chargaff[38] obtained from beef lung a very potent, homogeneous material with a molecular weight of about 170,000,000 which contained a variety of phosphatides, as well as protein, carbohydrate and ribonucleic acid. From brain an active lipid fraction has been derived which contains no protein.[47] The species from which thromboplastin is prepared is significant, as well as the tissue which is its source. Antigenic dissimilarity between tissue and blood thromboplastins has been demonstrated.[77]

Howell prepared from brain an ether soluble phospholipid factor, "cephalin," with thromboplastic activity.[49a] The nature of the phospholipid which contributes this activity is unsettled; that is, whether it is phosphatidyl ethanolamine, phosphatidyl serine, a mixture of these, or a mixture with lecithin.[16a,75d,79] Platelets, it will be recalled (p. 277) contain these substances. A phospholipid with thromboplastic activity has also been found in erythrocytes ("erythrocytin").[72a]

The nature of the thromboplastin activity has puzzled investigators for decades. Considered from time to time to be enzymatic, there is nevertheless increasing evidence opposing this view.[47]

Calcium (*Factor IV*).—Before the turn of the century calcium was recognized as playing a role in coagulation. The anticoagulant effect of oxalate is due to the precipitation of free calcium; that of citrate is through suppression of ionization, while ion-exchange resins and chelating agents remove it. Delayed coagulation *in vivo*, however, usually cannot be attributed to hypocalcemia since marked prolongation of coagulation time appears only at levels (2.5 mg. per cent) well below those which would produce clinical manifestations of hypocalcemia.[41] However, this may not hold true during massive exsanguino-transfusions.[76]

Calcium appears to be required in many phases of the clotting process. Details must await elucidation of the interactions which take place. The thrombin-fibrinogen reaction can take place without calcium but acceleration was observed in its presence.[74] Calcium was found to be required in the formation of urea-insoluble clots.[57] It may be utilized in the formation of a complex with factor IX[32] and may be concerned with the activity of factor VII.[56a]

Factor V.—The participation of still other factors in the coagulation process came to be recognized through the study of patients with coagulation defects. That hemophilia is not attributable to the absence of one of the four factors already discussed was disclosed when it was found that the addition of a fraction of normal plasma devoid of fibrinogen was capable of clotting hemophilic blood. Later, a disorder resembling hemophilia was discovered which was shown to be due to deficiency of still another substance. In the interval, the utilization of the "one-stage" and "two-stage" prothrombin tests in the study of bleeding disorders and investigation of the nature of the action of the anticoagulant, Dicumarol, led to the realization that what was originally considered to be a single compound, "prothrombin," was a mixture of active substances.[63b,70] These, and still other, newly discovered coagulation factors will be described, in turn.

Factor V is found in normal plasma but not in serum and is present in plasma treated with aluminum hydroxide. It is not adsorbed by barium sulfate. It is destroyed by heating to 56° C. for a half hour or by increasing the pH to 10.5, and deteriorates rapidly on standing at room temperature for 48 hours or on storage in the presence of oxalate or EDTA but not with citrate ions. It has the character of a globulin.[40a,63b]

Factor VI was so named because it was considered to be the active form of factor V.[63b]

Factor VII.[31]—Present in high concentration in serum, this material can be distinguished from Factor V by its stability both to heat and to storage and by the fact that it is adsorbed from serum with aluminum hydroxide and barium sulfate or most easily by means of an asbestos filter. Seegers considers this to be a derivative of prothrombin and consequently called it "autoprothrombin." Others deny this.[78a] Factor VII may be formed in the liver.[64] Its role in the coagulation process will be discussed shortly.

Factor VIII.—The antihemophilic factor is found in association with the euglobulins and fibrinogen of plasma, and is rather labile. It is not found in serum. It is adsorbed on Fuller's earth but not on barium sulfate, aluminum hydroxide or Seitz filter. Present in Cohn plasma fraction I, it can be separated from fibrinogen by solution and heating to 56° C. for two minutes. By a series of steps which include salt fractionation and ethanol precipitation, a purification factor of 200 has been attained but further purification has been difficult. Solubility properties of the concentrated material suggested that it is one of the cryoglobulins. Other properties of this factor will be discussed in a later chapter (p. 864).

Factor IX.—The factor linked with the disorder which parallels classical hemophilia, namely PTC (plasma thromboplastin component) deficiency (p. 875), like factor VII is present in normal serum and is adsorbed by aluminum hydroxide and barium sulfate. It is labile to heat but relatively stable on storage. It is not found in Cohn fraction I but is present in fractions III and IV₁. It is precipitated by 45 to 50 per cent ammonium sulfate and removed by a Seitz filter, whereas factor VIII is not. Other properties will be discussed later (p. 877).

Factor X.[89]—The Stuart factor, recognized through its deficiency in certain inherited and acquired disorders (p. 881), shows a striking resemblance to factor VII in a number of ways. It is present in plasma and in serum and is required for full coagulant activity of tissue and lipid thromboplastins. Electrophoretically it migrates with the albumin fraction of plasma by paper and curtain electrophoresis. It is stable at room temperature for a few days but is destroyed in serum in a few minutes at 56° C. It is adsorbed onto barium sulfate, aluminum hydroxide, tricalcium phosphate and Seitz filter.

Plasma Thromboplastin Antecedent (PTA).[89]—This is a stable factor present in plasma and in serum. It is maximally precipitated at 25 to 33 per cent ammonium sulfate saturation of normal plasma. It is present in Cohn fractions IV an III and is localized by electrophoresis in the β_2 globulin fraction. PTA deficiency has been observed in a numbe of cases with hemorrhagic manifestations (p. 877). A curious property of this factor is that PTA activity increases in PTA deficient plasma when it is stored in the refrigerator or frozen. In fact, the patient's own plasma will correct his clotting defect after storage. No international symbol has been assigned as yet to PTA factor.

Hageman Factor (HF).[89] — Also without a designated symbol is a factor lacking from the blood in a congenital coagulation abnormality known as the Hageman trait (p. 878). This is a remarkable condition in which the coagulation time of the blood is greatly prolonged but no hemorrhagic tendency results. It must be assumed that *in vivo*, as distinguished from the conditions in the test tube, a mechanism exists which does not require HF for coagulation to occur. The nature of HF is unknown but it can

be defined as a coagulation activity which is initiated by contact of blood with foreign surfaces[76b] of which glass is one of the most active. It appears that the same factor is involved in the release of plasma kinin, which contracts plain muscle and produces pain, and also is related to a substance which increases capillary permeability.[59] Hageman factor is present[53] in Cohn plasma fractions III, IV_1 and IV_4. Electrophoretically it migrates between the beta and gamma globulins and it is present in serum as well as plasma. It is non-dialyzable, poorly adsorbed by $BaSO_4$, resistant to heating at 60° C. for 15 minutes and is present in 25 to 33 per cent and 33 to 50 per cent $(NH_4)_2SO_4$ fractionated normal plasma precipitates. Since its activity can be inhibited by diisopropylfluorophosphate, it may be an esterase.[31d]

Interaction of the Various Components in the Process of Coagulation.—As stated earlier, the final phases of the coagulation mechanism are comparatively clear. The initial steps are still obscure. The scheme outlined in Figure 5–2 only lists the factors which are involved and separates tissue and blood thromboplastins since these seem to be slightly different from one another.

Factor VII does not appear to be necessary for thromboplastin generation in blood that is clotting or for prothrombin conversion by blood thromboplastin.[31] The only demonstrable clotting defect attributable to its lack is retarded or insignificant thrombin formation with tissue thromboplastin. Factors X and V are also concerned in the extravascular process of coagulation. As long as no tissue thromboplastin is present, no reactions take place. However, immediately after blood is brought into contact with tissue fluid, tissue thromboplastin, factor VII, calcium[48] and probably also factor X react with each other to form a product which, with the participation of factor V, causes prothrombin to be con-

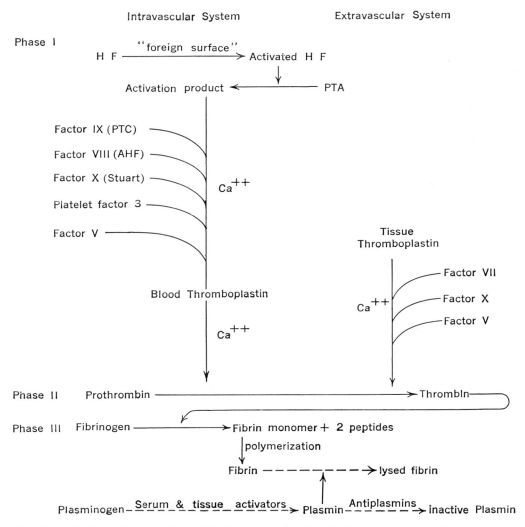

FIG. 5–2.—Outline of coagulation. The factors involved in the first phase of coagulation are shown more or less in the order in which they are thought to participate in the process. The counter forces are also indicated.

verted to thrombin. Names have been proposed for the intermediate products in these reactions but, until they can be more clearly identified than has been accomplished to date, there seems to be little reason to complicate matters by listing them.

The intravascular mechanism of coagulation has been difficult to elucidate because many factors seem to be involved. Furthermore, the trigger mechanism in this system has been poorly understood. It has long been recognized that contact with a foreign surface initiates the process of coagulation. Many explanations have been offered. Platelets were thought by Morawitz to play a part; then plasma factors,[39] Factor VIII (AHF),[69] Factor IX[73a] and Factor VII[73a] were believed to be involved. It was demonstrated subsequently that contact-activity may develop in plasma lacking all these clotting factors. Following this it appeared at first that both HF and PTA are concerned but it now seems most probable that HF is the only factor which is directly activated by surfaces.[76b] Both HF and PTA are inactive in their circulating, native forms. Contact activates HF which then reacts with PTA to produce an active prothromboplastic factor.[74a] The remaining reactions are obscure but it is clear that Factors IX, VIII and X are required and that a platelet substance, the lipoprotein factor 3, or simply certain lipid constitutents, is needed. As in the extravascular process of coagulation, Factor V is important in the ultimate development of the substance which promotes the conversion of prothrombin to thrombin.[43a]

Factors VIII and V disappear during the normal clotting process.[43a] This may mean that they serve as substrates. Factors IX, X and VII, HF and PTA are not consumed and consequently may be enzymatic.

In vivo, PTA must evidently be activated otherwise than by contact-activated HF, since the Hageman trait does not result in a bleeding tendency, while PTA deficiency does.

As indicated earlier, the exact role of calcium remains to be determined. In the diagram it is shown in those positions where its participation is thought to be important. There may be other steps in which it is needed, as well.

The role of platelets was discussed earlier (p. 285). Their high concentrations of adenosine triphosphate very probably plays an important role in the formation of thromboplastin.[35]

It would appear that the first phase of coagulation, the formation of thromboplastin, is a relatively slow process. The tissues have an advantage as compared with the blood, in that they are capable of supplying much more promptly a more or less complete thromboplastin. In the second phase active thrombo-plastin converts prothrombin into thrombin. Once a small amount of thrombin has been formed, according to Owren the activity of Factor V is greatly increased.[63b] Coagulation, in this view, is an auto-catalytic reaction which, once some thrombin has been formed, proceeds with ever increasing velocity. How the first traces of thrombin are formed, however, is not clearly understood.

Further investigation may shed more light on the paradoxes sometimes encountered clinically, such as prolonged bleeding time in the face of normal coagulation time, or vice versa, and alterations in capillary fragility with or without abnormalities in bleeding or coagulation times or of other tests of the coagulation process. Thus, in factor VII deficiency bleeding time may be prolonged whereas the coagulation time, prothrombin consumption and capillary fragility are usually normal. It has been suggested that this is indirect evidence of the importance of the tissue thromboplastin-prothrombin-converting mechanism in hemostasis, especially in stemming capillary bleeding,[31] since it is in relation to tissue thromboplastin that factor VII is needed. That HF is related to capillary permeability[59] was mentioned above. Since increased capillary permeability is observed in scurvy, it is interesting that in scorbutic guinea pigs a coagulation defect was demonstrated which closely resembled PTA and HF deficiencies in humans.[45a]

Natural Inhibitors of Coagulation. —Coagulation thus appears to be a dynamic process with positive forces leading to the solidification of the blood. The opposing forces which favor the fluid state are obscure. If it can be accepted that the speed of the clotting reaction depends on thrombin, this being the agent through which the autocatalytic reaction is mediated, some explanations can be offered.

An important safeguard is the relative

slowness of thrombin production. This is due in part to the absence of preformed thromboplastin and to the barriers which prevent the entrance of tissue thromboplastin, as well as the chemical stability of the various clotting factors. The unbroken continuity of the vascular endothelium is an important factor in preventing the formation of blood thromboplastin. Nevertheless, since trauma and disease may alter vascular endothelium and also permit entry of thromboplastic substances from the tissues, and since only local deposits of fibrin and platelets form when such injury occurs, negative or lytic factors must exist in the circulating blood. Several such inhibitors have been described: antithrombin, heparin and antithromboplastin.

Antithrombin. — After coagulation, thrombin disappears rapidly from the blood. Thrombin is promptly removed by virtue of its affinity for fibrin surface. This provides a ready means for preventing dangerous extension of a thrombus. These reactions can be observed if thrombin is injected intravenously: fibrin fibrils are formed and these in turn adsorb the thrombin. The fibrin fibrils are filtered off in the capillary network and are, presumably, destroyed.[71a] Thus fibrin can be regarded as a physiological antithrombin.

In addition to this mechanism, there appears to be a "natural" antithrombin in the blood. This has been separated by fractionating plasma with ammonium sulfate or by acidification and it can be concentrated with the α-globulin by electrophoretic separation.[58a] The reaction of this antithrombin with thrombin is thought to be stoichiometric.

From time to time various investigators have described a number of additional antithrombins.[76a] Those discussed above have been referred to as antithrombin I and antithrombin III, respectively. Still another antithrombin activity is that of heparin "co-factor" (see below) while a fourth is an antithrombin mechanism which has been observed after prothrombin activation.

Heparin[52] was first discovered in experiments designed to purify cephalin from tissues.[49] This highly active anticoagulant was extracted from liver but it is present in most of the tissues of the body and, as mentioned earlier (p. 236), is found in the granules of mast cells. The distribution of these cells among the smallest blood vessels and capillaries may signify that heparin is held strategically in locations where it may be used promptly to prevent local thrombosis. A normal constituent of blood, heparin is found in concentrations of 0.5 mg. per 100 ml.[44b]

Heparin is a sulfated mucopolysaccharide composed of glucosamine, glucuronic acid and sulfate ester groups.[44b] It is a polymer with a molecular weight of about 16,000 which is synthesized from glucose and inorganic sulfate.

The main effect of heparin has been thought to be antithrombic, through slowing of the rate of interaction of thrombin and fibrinogen and by augmenting the adsorption of thrombin on fibrin,[55] or by increasing the affinity of antithrombin for thrombin.[37] The plasma factor (heparin "co-factor") postulated as necessary for the antithrombic activity of heparin *in vitro* may be the same as normal antithrombin.[37] Heparin also markedly inhibits the formation of plasma thromboplastic activity. This, it has been suggested,[75c] is by way of its antithrombic effect which interferes with the formation of a thrombin-factor IX (PTC) complex necessary for factor IX activity.

Since it is nontoxic, heparin has been used widely in the treatment of thromboembolic disorders. Following injection heparin is rapidly cleared from the blood stream.[44b] The hypocoagulability of the blood of dogs in peptone or anaphylactic shock is probably attributable to heparin.[88]

On the other hand, the evidence that the anticoagulant described in the blood following heavy exposure to irradiation (atom bomb, roentgen rays) or nitrogen mustards[51] is heparin, is unconvincing.[52]

Protamine, a strongly basic protein, counteracts the effects of heparin, possibly by virtue of its electric charge, which neutralizes the negative charges of heparin, but it is also capable of interfering with factor IX activity and with thromboplastin generation, thus acting as an anticoagulant under certain circumstances.[75e]

A specific *antithromboplastin* is thought by some workers to explain the defect in hemophiliac blood (p. 864) and the rapid fall in thromboplastin titer observable in the thromboplastin generation test after a few minutes (p. 868).[32a] In fact, it has been claimed that there are two circulating antithromboplastins in plasma.[74d] Still other naturally occurring inhibitors of the first stage of coagulation have been described.[49b,74a]

In addition to these mechanisms for maintaining the fluidity of the blood, it has been suggested that clotting intermediates and thromboplastin are removed from the blood by reticuloendothelial cells.[77a]

The appearance of a circulating anticoagulant has been described as the cause of hemorrhagic disease in a number of instances (p. 884).

Clot Dissolution.—It has long been recognized that blood clots are not permanent structures and that nature has provided a mechanism for the dissolution of fibrin. This is achieved by proteolytic enzymes derived from the tissues and by the action of leukocytes but, in addition, *thrombolysis* is brought about by *plasmin*. This is a proteolytic enzyme derived from a precursor, plasminogen, which is carried in the globulin fraction of the plasma. Plasminogen activation occurs spontaneously or as a result of contact with activators of tissue, body fluid or

bacterial origin.[31b] The conversion of plasminogen to plasmin involves the loss of a peptide moiety. It appears that clot lysis takes place by a dual mechanism, of which the more important involves the diffusion or adsorption of plasminogen activators to the thrombus, activation of intrinsic clot plasminogen and autodigestion of the thrombus. A secondary mechanism involves digestion of the thrombus by extrinsic plasmin action. A plasminogen-like proenzyme has been demonstrated in organs rich in connective tissue, such as the aortic wall.[55a] Numerous attempts have been made to use plasmin or plasminogen activators to effect therapeutic thrombolysis.[31b]

Increases in thrombolytic activity have been demonstrated after exercise and in persons subjected to stressful stimuli, such as trauma or fear, epinephrine, nicotinic acid or pyrogens. This has also been observed in patients with liver disease and hematologic malignancies, and in some individuals with acute infections.[31b] The blood of victims of accidental death often is capable of liquefying fibrin.[32b] In Russia advantage was taken of the fluid nature of the blood of such corpses by collecting it without anticoagulants and using it for blood transfusion.

Abnormal bleeding due to fibrinolysis will be discussed in a later chapter (p. 884).

In some patients suffering from cancer and congestive heart failure there may be diminished thrombolytic activity.[31b] This is perhaps related to the frequent thromboembolic complications of these states.

The Development of "Deficiencies" of Clotting Components.—In a later chapter (p. 861) various disorders associated with the absence or insufficiency of different plasma coagulation factors will be discussed. It is generally assumed that these represent true deficiencies. It must be considered, however, that the lack of these clotting components may not be a lack in the strict sense. Just as in the case of hemoglobin a single alteration in the amino acid sequence of a polypeptide chain may lead to striking clinical manifestations, so also, perhaps, a gene responsible for the formation of one of the proteins essential in the process of coagulation may become defective and produce a compound which is unsuited for the specific reaction in which it is involved. Only a very small difference might suffice to prevent the normal reaction. Thereby, in effect, a "deficiency" may be produced. In reality, however, one deals in such cases with a genetic fault in construction of a protein rather than with total failure to produce the protein. Conceivably, also, such altered proteins might induce the formations of antibodies.

CLINICAL METHODS FOR THE MEASUREMENT OF DISTURBANCES OF HEMOSTATIC FUNCTION

Except for that which occurs during menstruation, the loss of blood is abnormal. Bleeding may arise from a great variety of causes and these may involve any of the systems of the body. The causes of hemorrhage and the various hemorrhagic conditions associated with disturbances in coagulation will be discussed in detail in Chapters 17 and 18. Methods for the study of disturbances in coagulation will, however, be described here. These vary in complexity. It is natural that, as more is learned about the intricate details of the coagulation mechanism, more and more procedures for the measurement of disturbances in coagulation are introduced. Some of the technics are impractical except in laboratories devoting special attention to the study of disorders in coagulation; others, though crude and simple to perform are valuable nevertheless, provided they are done carefully.

As a first step in the study of a suspected

hemorrhagic disorder, the coagulation time, clot retraction, platelet count, bleeding time and tourniquet test should be carried out (p. 301) A simple screening test for abnormal coagulation of the blood, based on the mixture of the suspected plasma and normal plasma, is an easy second step (p. 304). To this may be added the one-stage Quick "prothrombin time," (p. 302) now available in most laboratories. Requiring more experience but offering important information are other procedures, such as the prothrombin consumption test and the thromboplastin generation test.

Each laboratory engaged in the study of coagulation has its own favorites and tends to introduce modifications of the various procedures which have been described. These are intended to increase accuracy, reduce labor and provide the required information in the shortest possible periods of time. The methods described below are those used in our laboratory, under the direction of Dr. Paul Didisheim. References to other methods will also be given. Selection of the tests required in the study of a particular patient will depend on the nature of the problem.

Tests of Vascular Function. — 1. *Bleeding Time.*[82]—The original Duke method was based on measurement of bleeding following a moderately deep cut in the finger or ear lobe. Various modifications have been introduced,[30c] of which the *Ivy method*[50] is the one which is now most commonly employed. This is carried out in a less vascular area than the ear lobe and is performed under conditions in which an attempt is made to control variations caused by alterations in capillary tonus.

A blood pressure cuff is put on the arm above the elbow and inflated to 40 mm. Hg. An area of the forearm free of visible veins is cleaned with alcohol, and punctured by means of a Bard-Parker blade (No. 11) on which a small cork has been fixed to allow a wound 5 mm. deep. As a duplicate test, a similar wound is made 2 cm. above or below this site. With filter paper, all blood except that directly over the cut is blotted every 30 seconds. The clot must not be touched as it forms at the site of the cut since this may artificially prolong the bleeding time. Normally the bleeding time by this method is 1 to 9 minutes.

The wound should be dressed with "Bandaid," as bleeding may recur even in normal subjects.

2. Capillary Fragility Tests.—(Rumpel-Leede phenomenon, capillary resistance test, tourniquet test.) The simplest procedure is to apply a *blood pressure cuff* about the upper arm in the usual manner and keep it inflated for five minutes midway between systolic and diastolic pressure. The arm is first inspected for purpuric spots or pigmentation which might be mistaken for such spots. If the test is positive, a crop of purpuric spots will appear in the skin below the cuff within a few minutes after the cuff has been removed. Their number and size is roughly proportional to the bleeding tendency but may not coincide with the number of platelets. Rough quantitation may be achieved by recording, one minute after the pressure has been released, the number of petechiae in a circle 2 to 3 cm. in diameter which is (1) 4 cm. below the bend of the elbow; (2) on the extensor surface of the forearm midway between the elbow and the wrist; and (3) on the dorsal surface of the hand. Normally a few (0 to 20) tiny petechiae may appear (See Figure 17–2, p. 820).

The *suction cup* offers a simple and quick method of measuring capillary resistance. The Dalldorf modification[42] of the da Silva Mello instrument may be used.

It should be pointed out that the temperature of the room and of the patient's skin play an important part in the result. A week should be allowed to elapse before a capillary fragility test is repeated on the same arm.

Collection of Blood for Coagulation Tests.—Such tests are concerned with the clotting functions of the blood itself, as distinguished from blood which has come in contact with tissue factors. Consequently, a clean venepuncture made without traumatization is necessary. Suction should be avoided since air bubbles spoil the specimen. The needle must be new and sharp, 18- or 20-gauge, and tightly fitting; the disposable type (Monoject, Roehr Products Co., Inc.) is very good. The syringe must be clean and siliconized in order to minimize the activation of certain coagulation factors by contact with glass. (Siliclad, Clay Adams, Inc., diluted in water). The quantity of blood to be drawn should be calculated in advance and all necessary equipment must be ready in order to avoid undue delay.

In performing tests of coagulation, in order that comparison may be made with the normal and with previous measurements on the same individual, it is necessary that the same technic be followed each time, the same size glassware be used and temperature conditions be the same. Coagulation is more rapid the narrower the test tube and the nearer to physiological temperature (37°C.). Above and below this, coagulation is prolonged. Blood from a known normal person ("control") should be examined at the same time as that of the patient. The use of a stopwatch is most helpful in carrying out these tests and a waterbath at 37° C. is also important. In view of these requirements it is obvious that blood obtained by skin puncture is unsuitable for most of these tests. Admixture with tissue juice is impossible to prevent and the results can be wholly misleading.

The following will be found useful if a number of the tests listed below are to be carried out. If some are to be omitted or others added, appropriate modifications will naturally need to be made.

From the antecubital vein, 30 ml.

blood is withdrawn with a siliconized syringe and a sharp 18-gauge needle. Leaving the needle in the vein, one removes the syringe and a drop of blood is collected through the needle onto a siliconized glass slide. The needle is then withdrawn. This drop of blood is used for platelet counts (p. 282). The blood from the syringe is dispensed in the following manner, care being taken to let the blood run down the side of the test tubes without bubble formation. The stopwatch is started when blood is placed in the first tube:

2 ml. into each of 2 *new* 13 × 100 mm. Pyrex tubes (numbers 1 and 2).

2 ml. into each of 2 *siliconized* 13 × 100 mm. Pyrex tubes (numbers 3 and 4).

These four specimens are used for determination of coagulation time, clot retraction and clot lysis.

2 ml. into one *new* 13 × 100 mm. Pyrex tube (number 5). This is to be used for determination of prothrombin consumption (test number 13 below).

15 ml. into one *siliconized* 15 × 125 mm. Pyrex tube containing 0.15 ml. 38 per cent trisodium citrate (tube number 6). This provides plasma for use in the various tests and for the preparation of the platelet suspension used in the thromboplastin generation test (test 14, below).

2 ml. into a test tube containing 0.2 ml. double oxalate mixture (p. 378). This is used to measure volume of packed red cells and is needed for calculation of clot retraction (test 2, below).

2 ml. into one 13 × 100 mm. Pyrex tube which contains three glass beads (number 7) This is used for the preparation of the serum for the thromboplastin generation test (test number 14, below).

Tube no. 6 is stoppered immediately with Parafilm (Marathon Corp., Menasha, Wis.) inverted twice and stored at 2 to 5° C. until ready to centrifuge. Tubes 1 to 5, inclusive, and tube 7 are placed in a waterbath at 37° C. Tube 7

is tilted frequently until a good clot has formed.

If possible all *centrifugation* of blood for coagulation studies should be done at 2 to 5° C. Tube no. 6 is spun at 200 × G (*i.e.* 1000 r.p.m. in International PR–1 refrigerated centrifuge, flat head No. 269) for ten minutes. The platelet rich plasma (PRP) is pipetted off with a siliconized pipette into a siliconized 15 × 125 mm. tube, carefully avoiding erythrocytes. The volume is recorded. The tube from which the PRP was pipetted, as well as the tube containing PRP, is centrifuged at approximately 1700 G (3200 r.p.m., PR–1) for 45 minutes. The plasmas are then pooled in a single tube and stored at + 2° C., until used for prothrombin time and other tests on plasma. The platelet button remaining is saved for preparation of a platelet suspension.

The *concentration of citrate* in the plasma will naturally vary with the relative amounts of plasma and cells in the blood used. Since coagulation is inhibited by either excess citrate or excess calcium ion, a difference in citrate concentration may affect some of the tests for which the plasma is used. Such differences between control and patient specimens should be eliminated by measuring the volume of packed red cells and then adding the appropriate amount of citrate to the plasma with the lower citrate concentration.

A *buffer*[33a] is required for some of the following tests. This is composed of 5.878 Gm. sodium diethylbarbiturate, 7.335 Gm. sodium chloride and 215 ml. 0.1 N HCl. These are made up to one liter with distilled water. The pH should be 7.3 to 7.4.

Buffered saline is prepared by adding one part of the above buffer to nine parts 0.85 per cent NaCl.

Adsorbed plasma, required for some of these tests, is prepared by adding 0.2 ml. aluminum hydroxide gel ("Amphojel,"

Wyeth, unflavored) to 1 ml. plasma, inverting the tube several times and letting it stand at room temperature for five minutes. It is then centrifuged at 2000 r.p.m. for ten minutes and decanted. If many tests are to be performed, larger amounts (5 to 10 ml.) may be prepared in advance and stored frozen in small aliquots until needed.

1. **Coagulation Time**—This must be distinguished from "bleeding time" which has been described above. The test for "coagulation time" measures the clotting of whole blood in the absence of tissue factors. Although many different procedures have been proposed, the *method of Lee and White*, devised in 1913, remains the accepted technic. The principal modification has been the introduction of silicone, which permits measurement of coagulation time in siliconized test tubes, as well as in uncoated ones.

At five minutes after withdrawal of the blood in the manner described above, tube no. 1 is gently tilted 45° at one minute intervals until it can be inverted 180° without blood flowing. This time is recorded and the same procedure is repeated with tube no. 2. Handling favors coagulation and consequently the time for the second tube is taken as the true coagulation time since this was tilted less than no. 1.

At 15 minutes this procedure is repeated, at two minute intervals, with tube no. 3, then no. 4. Normal values in our laboratory are 6 to 17 minutes in glass; 19 to 60 minutes in siliconized tubes.

2. **Clot Retraction**[36a]—For a simple *qualitative* test the patient's and the control coagulation time tubes are allowed to remain in the water bath and are inspected one-half, one, two and four hours after the blood was drawn and then again at 24 hours after clotting. The extent of separation of the clot from the sides of the tube is noted. Normal blood begins to retract 30 minutes to an hour from the time it was drawn.

Quantitative Test (Didisheim).—One of the two siliconized coagulation time tubes is used, four hours after the blood was drawn. All the liquid (serum plus free red cells) is gently decanted from the clot and is placed in a siliconized conical graduated 15 ml. centrifuge tube. This is centrifuged at 3000 r.p.m. for five minutes. The serum volume is calculated by subtracting the volume of the cells at the bottom of the tube (C) from the total liquid volume (L). The clot is then submerged below the level of the serum in this tube and the total volume is read (T). The serum volume (L–C), times 100, is divided by the total volume (T) to determine the quantity of serum, in per cent, expressed from the retracted clot (S). The theoretical maximum amount of serum would be the same as the relative amount of plasma (P) in the blood (100 minus volume of packed red cells). This would indicate that all the plasma in the blood had become serum after clot retraction and that there was no serum left in the clot. S/P × 100 gives the value for serum as per cent of this theoretical maximum. The normal in our laboratory ranges from 55 to 95 per cent.

Other simple procedures have been described.[30b]

3. **Clot Lysis.**—A simple test only requires the inspection of the above coagulation time tubes by tilting them 90 degrees at 8, 24, 48 and 72 hours. If a clot was found initially and subsequently the blood has become completely fluid, lysis has taken place. This should not occur normally within 72 hours. Traces of clot may be looked for by pouring the contents of the tube onto a gauze square.

Various other technics have been described[54] which may be more sensitive. A satisfactory one is the *"euglobulin fibrinolysis time."* Four and two tenths ml. of distilled water and 0.3 ml. of plasma are added to a tube; 0.1 N HCl is then added drop by drop, with continuous mixing, until a pH of 5.2 to 5.4 is reached. The tube is then centrifuged at 600 G for three minutes. The clear supernate is discarded. The euglobulin precipitate is dissolved in 0.3 ml. of buffered saline and 0.1 ml. of a solution of thrombin (Bovine Topical; Parke, Davis, 2 N.I.H. units/ml.) is added to form a clot. The tube is incubated at 37° C. and observed at 15 minute intervals. Fibrinolysis time is the time at which a clot is no longer visible and only shreds of fibrin remain. Increased fibrinolysin is present if the patient's fibrinolysis time is significantly shorter than that of a series of control subjects.

4. **Prothrombin Time.**—The measurement of "prothrombin" led to a series of investigations which, in the last few decades, have shed considerable light on the process of coagulation. The procedure revolves about the capacity of the plasma to form thrombin, the visible clotting effect being due to the reaction of thrombin and fibrinogen. Of the two methods which originally were widely employed, the two-stage procedure of Warner, Brinkhous and Smith[45] is somewhat more specific but is considerably more time-consuming and, therefore, is less used now. By this method prothrombin is first converted completely to thrombin with an optimal amount of calcium and an excess of tissue thromboplastin. The amount of thrombin thus formed is measured by determining the highest dilution of the defibrinated plasma which will produce clotting of a standard fibrinogen solution in a specified period of time. For the test a tissue extract (thromboplastin) and a solution of fibrinogen, as well as other reagents are needed; the plasma being assayed must first be defibrinated with thrombin to rid it of the fibrin clot which would otherwise interfere with the measurement of thrombin; and serial dilutions of plasma are made before the prothrombin is converted to thrombin in the first step.

Simplicity and utility have favored the *one-stage, plasma prothrombin time of Quick*,[68] in spite of the recognized limitations of the method. A suspension of commercial tissue thromboplastin made from lyophilized, acetone-extracted rabbit brain (Difco Bacto-Thromboplastin) is prepared by suspending it in the diluent supplied. This is mixed occasionally for ten minutes while it is kept in the waterbath at 37° C. As soon as the sediment has settled the supernate is pipetted off into a tube which is kept in an ice bath. To a 12 × 75 mm. Pyrex tube in a 37° C. waterbath, 0.1 ml. plasma is added, followed by 0.1 ml. thromboplastin suspension. This suspension should be mixed thoroughly just before pipetting, to insure uniform distribution of thromboplastin particles. To this, 0.1 ml. 0.025 M $CaCl_2$ is added quickly with a blowout pipette, the stopwatch being started simultaneously. The tube is agitated immediately, for good mixing. Then, in bright direct illumination, the tube is tilted continually from vertical to almost horizontal position once per second until a gel appears. This is the endpoint. The test should be performed in duplicate. A control value of 11 to 16 seconds is satisfactory and this should be measured each time, together with the patient plasma. Results for patient and control should always be reported together. Reporting as per cent of normal on the basis of normal saline dilutions is of little value. Unused thromboplastin suspension can be kept in the frozen state for some weeks without appreciable loss of activity. The test can be made even more simple by the use of a commercial product (Simplastin, Warner-Chilcott) which contains thromboplastin and calcium already mixed.

Quick's method has been used successfully in the control of anticoagulant therapy even though it has certain limitations. It is non-specific, in that it not only detects deficiency of prothrombin but also of factors VII and X. This is an advantage, for these factors may decrease during anticoagulant therapy of the bishydroxycoumarin (Dicumarol) or phenylindandione type. However, there are a number of limitations. Quick's test is not sensitive to reduction in factor IX, which may also develop during such therapy. Furthermore, the Quick prothrombin time will be prolonged if there happen to be decreased levels of fibrinogen or factor V, which are uninfluenced by this type of therapy. Excesses of antithrombin or heparin will also prolong Quick's prothrombin time. Variations due to deterioration of thromboplastin can be met by running a simultaneous control. Finally, the test requires experience and skill, since the clotting times are short, particularly in the 50 to 100 per cent range. For these reasons, various modifications have been introduced. Of these, Owren's "P and P" test[62] (prothrombin and proconvertin), by providing a constant surplus of factor V and a constant level of fibrinogen and of oxalate concentration, offers many advantages, such as greater sensitivity in the near normal range, less random variability because irrelevant factors are supplied, and the combined effects of prothrombin and factors VII and X are measured. Still better, however, is Owren's "thrombotest"[63] which is sensitive to changes in both the extravascular and intravascular clotting systems, including depression of factor IX, to which the earlier procedures were not sensitive. The technic, furthermore, is very simple.

5. **Factor V Assay.**[77b]—"Aged plasma," deficient in factor V, is prepared by incubating normal oxalated plasma (9 volumes blood, 1 volume 0.1 M sodium oxalate) at 37° C. for 24 to 36 hours, then storing at −20° C. until needed. The prothrombin time of this plasma should be over a minute. To 0.1 ml. of this plasma, in a 12 × 75 mm. tube at 37° C., is added 0.1 ml. of a 1:10 dilution,

in buffer, of control (or patient) plasma. Then 0.1 ml. thromboplastin suspension and 0.1 ml. 0.025 M CaCl$_2$ are added and the stopwatch is started. The next steps are the same as in the test for prothrombin time. Duplicate determinations should be made. The results are expressed on the basis of a dilution curve. The normal is 60 to 140 per cent.

A newer method[34a] employs an artificial substrate which is prepared by incubation of a mixture of Russell's viper venom, cephalin and normal plasma, as the result of which factor V is specifically destroyed.

6. **Plasma Thrombin Time.**[56]—A solution of thrombin (Bovine Topical, Parke, Davis), in buffer is made up of such a strength that 0.1 ml. of the solution clots 0.1 ml. fresh normal plasma in 15 to 20 seconds. The test is then carried out on the patient's plasma. Prolongation of the plasma thrombin time is seen when there is afibrinogenemia, a marked increase in fibrinogen, increased heparin or antithrombin, or a deficiency of an albumin-like substance in plasma which aids the conversion of fibrinogen to fibrin.[52a]

7. **Fibrinogen.**—Control plasma, 0.5 ml., is placed in a 12 × 75 mm. Pyrex tube. Into another similar tube is placed an equal volume of patient plasma. For five minutes both tubes are kept in a water-bath which is carefully maintained at 55 to 58° C. The tubes are removed and the turbidities are compared. Significantly less turbidity in the patient's plasma suggests hypofibrinogenemia. Complete lack of turbidity indicates afibrinogenemia.

Quick[71] gives details of a satisfactory quantitative procedure.

8. **Presumptive test to distinguish between factor VIII (AHG), factor IX (PTC) and PTA deficiencies.**—Fresh patient plasma, 0.1 ml., is added to each of eight tubes. To tubes 1 and 2, 0.1 ml. of a 1:10 dilution in buffer of

fresh normal plasma is added; to tubes 3 and 4, 0.1 ml. of a 1:10 dilution of fresh normal adsorbed plasma; to tubes 5 and 6, 0.1 ml. of a 1:10 dilution of normal serum which has been adsorbed in the same way as used in the preparation of adsorbed plasma; to tubes 7 and 8, add only 0.1 ml. buffer. The tubes are placed in a waterbath at 37° C. and 0.1 ml. 0.025 M $CaCl_2$ is added to each tube. The clotting times are recorded.

In classical hemophilia (factor VIII deficiency) the plasma recalcification time, as measured in this way, will be markedly shortened in tubes 1 to 4, which all contain factor VIII. In PTC (factor IX) deficiency the plasma recalcification time will be shortened only in tubes 1 and 2, which contain factor IX, but not in tubes 3 to 6, where factor IX has been removed by adsorption. In PTA deficiency and in Hageman trait the recalcification time will be shortened in tubes 1 to 6, since these factors are present

adsorbed plasma defect and no serum defect in the thromboplastin generation test (TGT) (test 14, below). Such plasma should be stored in small aliquots in lusteroid tubes at −20° C. until needed. An electric chronometer which records in seconds up to 10,000 seconds (Labline) is very useful for this test.

A series of unscratched 12 × 75 mm. Pyrex tubes is placed in a 37° waterbath. First 0.1 ml. of the appropriate dilution of plasma is added to a tube, immediately followed by 0.1 ml. factor VIII-deficient plasma. Then 0.1 ml. 0.025 M $CaCl_2$ is added, 25 seconds after the addition of the diluted plasma. All tubes are gently tilted 45° every 50 seconds and the coagulation time is recorded. After all tubes are clotted, the results can be plotted on semilogarithmic paper. The patient's factor VIII level is expressed as per cent of normal plasma.

The table below indicates the plasma dilutions contained in each tube:

Tube number	1	2	3	4	5	6	7
0.1 ml. normal plasma, %	10	1	0.1	0.01	0.001	–	–
0.1 ml. patient plasma, %	–	–	–	–	–	10	1

in both plasma and serum and are not removed by adsorption. The differentiation of the last two disorders can be made on clinical grounds (p. 878).

9. **Quantitative Assay for Factor VIII.**—This is a modification of the test described by Lewis and Didisheim.[56] The test involves measurement of the recalcification clotting time of known factor VIII-deficient plasma to which varying dilutions, in buffer, of normal or patient plasma are added. These dilutions are prepared in siliconized tubes immediately before use.

The factor VIII deficient plasma for use in this test is obtained from a patient with known hemophilia who has a coagulation time in glass tubes exceeding an hour, a normal prothrombin time, an

Other satisfactory procedures have been described[35a,64]

10. **Quantitative Assay for Factor IX.**—This is identical to the factor VIII assay except that 0.1 ml. plasma from a patient with known severe factor IX deficiency is used instead (clotting time in glass, over 60 minutes; normal prothrombin time; serum defect and no adsorbed plasma defect in TGT).

The *partial thromboplastin time (PTT) test*[74b] has been found to be very useful in detecting mild deficiencies of factors VIII and IX.

11. **Simple Screening Test for Abnormal Coagulation of Blood.**—To a centrifuge tube containing 1.5 ml. of 0.2 molar sodium citrate, 13.5 ml. of the patient's blood is added carefully and

thoroughly mixed; the same is done with the "control" blood, using another centrifuge tube. Plasma is obtained by centrifugation of the citrated bloods at 2000 r.p.m. for five minutes. Both tubes should be spun at the same time under identical conditions. The plasmas are then mixed in a series of seven dry tubes to a final volume of 1 ml., as follows:

The tubes are placed in a waterbath at 37° C. To each tube 0.03 ml. 0.2 M $CaCl_2$ is added and mixed, starting the stopwatch at the same time. After 15 minutes, the tubes are tilted every minute and the clotting time is recorded. A circulating anticoagulant is considered to be present if the clotting time of the mixture of 1 part patient plasma and

			Tube Number				
	1	2	3	4	5	6	7
Source of Plasma			Volume of Plasma in Tube (ml.)				
Patient	1.0	0.8	0.6	0.4	0.2	0.1	0.0
Normal	0.0	0.2	0.4	0.6	0.8	0.9	1.0

The tubes are kept in a water bath at 37° C.

To each tube, 0.1 ml. of 0.2 molar calcium chloride solution is added and the contents of each tube are mixed. Each tube is tilted at 30 second intervals and the time when coagulation occurs is recorded. The tubes should be agitated as little as possible and must be kept in the waterbath. The end point is complete coagulation of the plasma.

This test will disclose defects in coagulation due to (1) deficiency of one or more of the plasma components necessary for coagulation since the coagulation time will be abnormal in tube 1 and will have been brought to normal by the addition of normal plasma in the remaining tubes; (2) the presence of a circulating anticoagulant, since in that case the coagulation time will diminish progressively in tubes 2, 3, 4, 5 and 6. If a plasma defect is suggested by the test, differentiation between the various hemorrhagic disorders may be made by means of the presumptive test to distinguish factor VIII and IX deficiencies (test 8, above).

12. **Test for Circulating Anticoagulants.**[83]—To a series of 12 × 75 mm. siliconized tubes the following are added with siliconized pipettes:

3 parts normal plasma is at least twice that of normal plasma alone.

Other good tests have been described.[40]

13. **Prothrombin Consumption Test.**—This test[72] is based on the principle that, by determining the prothrombin before and after coagulation is complete, a measure of the blood thromboplastin that converts prothrombin to thrombin is obtained. The same reagents are required as in Quick's method for determining prothrombin time.

Tube number 5 of the blood collected for coagulation studies (p. 299) is left undisturbed in the waterbath at 37° C. until two hours have elapsed, at which time the clot is rimmed with an applicator stick and the serum is decanted and centrifuged at 2000 r.p.m. for ten minutes in a refrigerated centrifuge. It is decanted again.

Adsorbed normal plasma (p. 300), 0.1 ml., thromboplastin suspension (see Prothrombin Time) 0.1 ml., and 0.025 M $CaCl_2$, 0.1 ml., are placed in a 12 × 75 mm. Pyrex tube in the waterbath at 37° C. Then 0.1 ml. of the above prepared serum is added and the stopwatch

Tube No.	1–2	3–4	5–6	7–8	9–10	11–12	13–14
Normal Plasma, ml.	0.30	0.27	0.24	0.20	0.15	0.10	0.00
Patient Plasma, ml.	0.00	0.03	0.06	0.10	0.15	0.20	0.30

20

started. The succeeding steps are the same as those for prothrombin time.

The validity of computing prothrombin consumption from one-stage prothrombin determinations has been questioned[43] on the ground that sera in the one-stage system frequently show more prothrombic activity than the parent plasma. This is attributed to the increased factor VII activity of serum. A practical two-stage method has been described.[43] In this the serum accelerator is inert and thus the total yield of thrombin is measured rather than the velocity of its evolution.

14. Thromboplastin Generation Test (TGT).[33]—This is a most useful method for differentiating abnormalities in coagulation in which there is impaired formation of blood thromboplastin, such as hemophilia (factor VIII) or PTC (factor IX) deficiency and conditions in which there is abnormal platelet function. It is based on the fact that normal plasma treated with $Al(OH)_3$ (which contains factors V, VIII, PTA and Hageman factor), platelets, and normal serum (which supplies factors IX and X, as well as Hageman factor and PTA) react to form blood thromboplastin in the presence of $CaCl_2$. A lack of any one of these seven factors will cause deficient thromboplastin formation and will be revealed by the test. If thromboplastin generation is deficient when the patient's adsorbed plasma, serum, platelet suspension and $CaCl_2$ are incubated together, then the defect can be narrowed down by one of several maneuvers. If thromboplastin generation is still deficient when the patient's adsorbed plasma, normal serum and normal platelets are incubated, then factor V or VIII deficiency exists. These two possibilities can easily be differentiated by the prothrombin time (see above), which is prolonged in factor V deficiency but not in factor VIII deficiency. Similarly, if the deficiency persists when normal adsorbed plasma,

patient's serum and normal platelets are incubated, then it must be due to factor IX or factor X deficiency. These likewise can be differentiated by the prothrombin time, which is normal in the former and prolonged in the latter case. If the defect is present in neither of the above circumstances but only when patient's adsorbed plasma, patient's serum and patient's or normal platelets are incubated, then the cause of the defective thromboplastin generation must be either Hageman trait or PTA deficiency. These can be differentiated on clinical grounds (p. 878). Finally, if the defect is present when normal adsorbed plasma, normal serum and the patient's platelets are incubated, then the patient has either thrombocytopenia or thrombocytopathia (p. 848). A normal platelet count would indicate that thrombocytopathia is the underlying fault.

A *platelet suspension* is prepared by resuspending the "platelet button" (see centrifugation of blood, p. 300) with 0.2 ml. buffer. As a stirring rod, a siliconized glass rod or a wooden applicator stick covered with silicone lubricant is used. About 10 ml. more buffer is added and the tube is centrifuged at 2000 G for five minutes. The supernate is discarded and the above procedure is repeated four times more. After discarding the fifth supernate, the washed platelet button is resuspended with a volume of buffer equal to one-third the original platelet-rich plasma volume. A uniform white suspension without large sedimenting particles should be attained. The *serum* for this test is prepared from tube number 7 of the blood collected for coagulation studies (p. 300). Four hours after the blood was drawn, the clot is rimmed, the serum decanted and then centrifuged at 2000 r.p.m. for ten minutes. This is decanted again. Glass beads and frequent tilting were used in the preparation of this serum to insure rapid and optimal conversion of prothrombin to thrombin with subsequent inactivation of thrombin by antithrombin. Significant amounts of prothrombin or thrombin in the serum can be a source of difficulty in the interpretation of this test.

Adsorbed plasma, prepared as already described, is needed, as well as 1 ml. of fresh control plasma and 1 ml. of the fresh patient plasma. The *substrate* required for the test is normal citrated plasma stored at −20° C. for not over three months. The absorbed plasma, serum, platelet suspension and substrate are all kept in an icebath during the test.

In carrying out the test 12 × 75 mm. Pyrex tubes are used throughout. Four tubes are prepared, each containing 0.1 ml. substrate. These are placed in a waterbath at 37° C. Adsorbed plasma is diluted 1:5 with buffer. Serum is diluted 1:10 with buffer. To a tube at 37° C. exactly 0.2 ml. diluted control serum, 0.2 ml. diluted control adsorbed plasma and 0.2 ml. control platelet suspension are added. To this 0.2 ml. 0.025 M CaCl₂ is added and a stopwatch is started. At 3, 5, 7 and 9 minutes, or until times no longer become shorter, 0.1 ml. 0.025 M CaCl₂ and 0.1 ml. of the above incubation mixture are added in that order to a tube at 37° containing 0.1 ml. substrate; a second stopwatch is started at the time of the addition of the incubation mixture. This tube is tilted as for prothrombin time. The second stopwatch is stopped when a gel or fibrin flecks appear. When all control reagents are incubated together (adsorbed plasma, serum and platelet suspension), the fastest of the four determinations should fall in the 8–15 second range. If, when all patient reagents are incubated together, the fastest of the four determinations is significantly longer (5 or more seconds) than when all control reagents are incubated together, then the following incubation mixtures should be similarly tested:

(1) patient's adsorbed plasma and normal serum and normal platelets;

(2) patient's serum and normal adsorbed plasma and normal platelets;

(3) patient's platelets and normal adsorbed plasma and normal serum;

(4) patient's adsorbed plasma and patient's serum and normal platelets

A reagent (TGTR) is available commercially (Warner-Chilcott) which supplies the necessary components for the TGT in dried form.

Thrombelastography.[46a] — This rather expensive instrument for the graphic demonstration of changes which occur during the clotting, retraction and lysis of blood has been used extensively by some investigators.[60] Different types of "coagulograms" are obtained in various hemorrhagic conditions but these do not appear to be sufficiently distinctive to be of much assistance in differential diagnosis.

Significance of Abnormalities in Coagulation and Capillary Fragility Tests.—The various causes of alterations from the normal in some of the tests which have been described are listed in Table 5–2. These will be discussed in detail in later chapters (pp. 816 and 861). Coagulation time will obviously be abnormal under a larger variety of circumstances. However, since the factors required for coagulation are normally present in excess, the coagulation time may be found to be normal even when a deficiency of one of these factors exists. Consequently more specific tests must be made if such a defect is suspected. Thus prothrombin time may be prolonged when coagulation time is normal. It is noteworthy that, if the blood ultimately clots, fibrinogen must be present.

It should be emphasized that *capillary resistance* is lowered under a large variety of circumstances in which there is no defect in blood coagulation. These include infectious diseases, particularly scarlet fever, measles and influenza, as well as chronic renal disease, hyperten-

Table 5-2—Causes of Alterations in Most Common Measures of Coagulation

Laboratory Finding	Condition	Mechanism
I. *Coagulation time* prolonged	A. Hemophilia	Deficiency of Factor VIII (AHF)
	B. Factor IX deficiency	Deficiency of Factor IX (PTC)
	C. PTA deficiency	Deficiency of PTA
	D. Hageman trait	Deficiency of Hageman factor
	E. "Hypoprothrombinemia"	When prothrombin time is greatly prolonged. Deficiency of prothrombin or of factors V, VII or X
	F. Afibrinogenemia or hypofibrinogenemia	Deficiency, rapid utilization or destruction of fibrinogen
	G. Hyperheparinemia	Excess heparin or heparinoid substances (heparin therapy, anaphylactic and peptone shock)
	H. Circulating anticoagulants	Anti-VIII, Anti-IX, Anti-V, etc.
II. *Prothrombin time* (one-stage) prolonged	A. Excess Dicumarol or related therapeutic agent or anticoagulant	Deficiency of prothrombin, factors VII and X
	B. "Parahemophilia"	Factor V deficiency
	C. "SPCA" deficiency	Factor VII deficiency
	D. Vitamin K deficiency	In newborn (hemorrhagic disease of newborn) and whenever absorption of vitamin K is impaired
	E. Liver disease	Reduction in prothrombin, factors V, VII, X and fibrinogen
	F. Circulating anticoagulants	Anti-prothrombin, antithromboplastin
III. *Prothrombin consumption* or *Thromboplastin generation* reduced	A. Thrombocytopenia	Impaired thromboplastin formation
	B. Thrombocytopathia	Diminished platelet factor 3
	C. Hemophilias	Deficiency of factors VIII, IX, or PTA
	D. Other deficiencies	Deficiency of factors V, X or Hageman factor
	E. Circulating antithromboplastin	Anti-VIII, anti-IX, anti-V, etc.
IV. *Bleeding time* prolonged	A. Thrombocytopenic purpura	Lack of platelets
	B. Any of the causes under I or II if sufficiently severe	Extreme deficiency of blood coagulation factors
	C. Vascular hemophilia (Angiohemophilia, von Willebrand's disease)	Deficiency of plasma factor necessary for normal bleeding time
	D. Thrombocytopathia	Diminished platelet factor 3
V. *Tourniquet test* positive	A. Nonthrombocytopenic purpuras	Damage to capillary endothelium
	B. Thrombocytopenic purpuras	Platelets too few to support capillaries under pressure
	C. Scurvy	Deficiency of intercellular cement substance
	D. Thrombocytopathia	Diminished platelet factor 3
VI. *Thrombocytopenia*	Thrombocytopenic purpuras, primary and secondary	Platelet antibodies, megakaryocyte damage, etc.
VII. *Clot retraction* poor	A. Thrombocytopenias of various types	Insufficient platelets to induce fibrin contraction
	B. Thrombasthenia	Impaired platelet aggregation

sion and diabetes with co-existent vascular disease. Increased capillary fragility may be observed also before the commencement of the menstrual period and even in a certain proportion of normal individuals in the absence of any associated abnormality.

The **paradox of prolonged bleeding time and normal coagulation time,** so characteristic of thrombocytopenic purpura, has not been fully explained. The prolonged bleeding in this condition which follows a minute sharp stab wound in the subcutaneous tissue, may be due to some obscure change in the capillary endothelium; or it may be attributable to the fact that the clot in this condition does not retract to squeeze out serum and thus assume a certain firmness, as it normally does, but remains a soft, non-retractile gel which is of little value as a mechanical plug. There is evidence,[58b] however, which indicates that the chief cause is defective capillary contractility. This may in turn be due to a reduction in the amount of vasconstrictor substance (serotonin) released, as the consequence of the diminished number of platelets. The normality of the test for coagulation time is explained by the fact that few platelets are needed to initiate the process of coagulation, if they are essential at all. Their deficiency is manifested, however, by the failure of the clot to contract.

In hemophilia, on the other hand, there is no abnormality of capillary endothelium and enough tissue factor and platelets are present to permit satisfactory closure of the small wound produced in the test for bleeding time. In larger wounds, however, clotting may occur on the surface of the bruised tissue thus closing the oozing capillaries, but coagulation is inadequate to stop bleeding from larger vessels and bleeding therefore continues. The nature of the coagulation defect in hemophilia will be discussed in a later chapter (Chapter 18, p. 863).

BIBLIOGRAPHY

Blood Platelets

1. Aas, K. A. and Gardner, F. H.: Survival of Blood Platelets Labeled with Chromium, J. Clin. Invest., 37, 1257, 1958.

1a. Ackerman, G. A. and Knouff, R. A.: Histochemical Differentiation of the Megakaryocytes in the Embryonic Liver, Blood, 15, 267, 1960.

1b. Adams, E.: Observations on the Influence of the Hypophysis and the Adrenal Cortex on Blood Platelet Levels, Blood, 4, 936, 1949.

1c. Adelson, E., Rheingold, J. J. and Crosby, W. H.: Studies of Platelet Survival by Tagging in vivo with P³², J. Lab. & Clin. Med., 50, 570, 1957.

1d. Arneth, J.: Über das qualitative Thrombozytenblutbild u.s.w., Klin. Wchnschr., 15, 964, 1936; Deutsch. Archiv. f. klin. Med., 179, 51, 1936; Folia hæmat., 55, 1, 1936; 56, 49, 1936; 57, 166, 1937.

3. Beecher, H. K.: Distribution of Platelets in Peripheral Blood, Acta med. scandinav., 87, 311, 1935.

3a. Bessis, M. and Burstein, M.: Études sur les thrombocytes, Rév. hémat., 3, 48, 1948; Compt. rend. Soc. de biol., 142, 647, 1948; Rev. hémat., 10, 753, 1955; ibid., 11, 162, 1956.

3b. Bettex-Galland, M. and Lüscher, E. F.: Studies on the Metabolism of Human Blood Platelets in Relation to Clot Retraction, Thromb. Diath. haemorrh., 4, 178, 1960.

4. Bizzozero, J.: Ueber einen neuen Formbestandtheil des Blutes und die Rolle bei der Thrombose und der Blutgerinnung, Virchows Arch. f. path. Anat., 90, 261, 1882.

4a. Björkman, S. E.: A New Method for Enumeration of Platelets, Acta haemat., 22, 377, 1959.

5. Blacher, L.: Recherches expérimentales sur les methodes d'exploration et sur la morphologie des thrombocytes ainsi que sur leur importance clinique, Sang, 9, 147, 1935.

5a. Bounameaux, Y.: Dosage des facteurs de coagulation contenus dans l'atmosphère plasmatique des plaquettes humaines, Rev. franç. étud. clin. et biol., 2, 52, 1957; Rev. hémat., 12, 16, 1957.

5b. Brecher, G. and Cronkite, E. P.: Morphology and Enumeration of Human Blood Platelets, J. App. Physiol., 3, 365, 1950; Proc. Soc. Exper. Biol. & Med., 78, 796, 1951; Am. J. Clin. Path., 23, 15, 1953.

5c. Braunsteiner, H., Fellinger, K. and Pakesch, F.: Structural Changes in the

Platelets As Observed by Electron Microscopy, Blood, *9*, 595, 1954.

6. BUNTING, C. H.: Blood Platelet and Megalokaryocytes, J. Exper. Med., *11*, 541, 1909; Bull. Johns Hopkins Hosp., *22*, 114, 1911; *Ibid.*, *31*, 439, 1920.

6a. CAMPBELL, E. W. *et al.*: Metabolic Activity of Human Blood Platelets, J. Lab. & Clin. Med., *47*, 835, 1956; Proc. Soc. Exper. Biol. & Med., *94*, 505, 1957.

7. CRADDOCK, C. G., JR., ADAMS, W. S., PERRY, S. and LAWRENCE, J. S.: The Dynamics of Platelet Production as Studied by a Depletion Technique in Normal and Irradiated Dogs, J. Lab. & Clin. Med., *45*, 906, 1955.

7a. CRONKITE, E. P.: Regulation of Platelet Production, *in Homeostatic Mechanisms*, Brookhaven Symposia in Biology: No. 10, Upton, N. Y., 1957, p. 96.

7b. DAMESHEK, W.: A Method for the Simultaneous Enumeration of Blood Platelets and Reticulocytes, Arch. Int. Med., *50*, 579, 1932.

7c. DANIELL, H. W.: Studies of Megakaryocyte Glycogen, Blood, *14*, 60, 1959.

7d. DATTA, N. and ZAJICEK, J.: Presence of Pyrophosphatase in Platelets, Acta haemat., *12*, 81, 1954; *ibid.*, *14*, 176, 1955.

7e. DESFORGES, J. F., BIGELOW, F. S. and CHALMERS, T. C.: The Effects of Massive Gastrointestinal Hemorrhage on Hemostasis, J. Lab. & Clin. Med., *43*, 501, 1954.

7f. DEUTSCH, E., JOHNSON, S. A. and SEEGERS, W. H.: Differentiation of Certain Factors Related to Blood Coagulation, Circulation Res., *3*, 110, 1955.

8. DOWNEY, H.: The Origin of Blood Platelets, Folia hæmat., *15*, 25, 1913.

8a. DOWNEY, H., PALMER, M., and POWELL, L.: The Origin of the Megakaryocytes in the Spleen and Liver in a Case of Atypical Myelosis, Folia hæmat., *41*, 55, 1930.

9. EAGLE, H.: Studies on Blood Coagulation, J. Gen. Physiol., *18*, 531, 1935.

10. ERICKSON, B. N., WILLIAMS, H. H., AVRIN, I. and LEE, P.: The Lipid Distribution of Human Platelets in Health and Disease, J. Clin. Invest., *18*, 81, 1939.

10a. FANTL, P. and WARD, H. A.: Nucleotides of Human Blood Platelets, Biochem. J., *64*, 747, 1956.

10b. FEISSLY, R., GAUTIER, A. and MARCOVICI, I.: L'ultrastructure des thrombocytes du sang humain normal, *in Proc. Fourth International Conference on Electron Microscopy*, Berlin, Springer-Verlag, 1960, p. 261.

11. FERGUSON, J. H.: Observations on the Alterations of Blood Platelets as a Factor in Coagulation of the Blood, Am. J. Physiol., *108*, 670, 1934.

12. FIDLAR, E. and WATERS, E. T.: The Origin of Platelets, Their Behavior in the Heart-Lung Preparation, J. Exper. Med., *73*, 299, 1941.

12a. FONIO, A.: Ueber die Wirkung des Hyalomers der Thrombocyten auf den Retraktionsvorgang, Acta haemat., *8*, 363, 1952.

12b. GREENE, R. W.: Effect of pH on Platelets and Identification of Ribonucleoprotein from Platelets, Proc. Soc. Exper. Biol. & Med., *87*, 412, 1954.

12c. GRETTE, K.: The Release of 5-hydroxytryptamine (Serotonin) from Blood Platelets during Coagulation, Scandinav. J. Clin. & Lab. Invest., *11*, 50, 1959.

12d. GUDE, W. D., UPTON, A. C. and ODELL, T. T. JR.: Blood Platelets of Human and Rat, Lab. Invest., *5*, 348, 1956.

12e. HARDISTY, R. M. and WOLFF, H. H.: Haemorrhagic Thrombocythaemia, Brit. J. Haemat., *1*, 390, 1955.

12f. HECKNER, F.: Polysacchariddarstellung in den Megakaryozyten, Acta haemat., *17*, 16, 1957.

12g. HELLEM, A. J.: The Adhesiveness of Human Blood Platelets *in Vitro*, Scandinav. J. Clin. & Lab. Invest. (Suppl.), *12*, 6, 1960.

12h. HIRAKI, K. and OFUJI, T.: Microcinematographic Observations on the Blood Cells and Their Clinical Applications, particularly by Means of Bone Marrow Culture, Acta haemat. japonica, *19*, 406, 1956.

13. HOWELL, W. H. and DONAHUE, D. D.: The Production of Blood Platelets in the Lungs, J. Exper. Med., *65*, 177, 1937.

13a. HJORT, P., RAPAPORT, S. I., and OWREN, P.A.: Evidence that Platelet Accelerator (Platelet Factor I) Is Adsorbed Plasma Proaccelerin, Blood, *10*, 1139, 1955.

13b. HUTTER, R. V. P.: Electron Microscopic Observations on Platelets from Human Blood, Am. J. Clin. Path., *28*, 447, 1957.

13c. JAPA, J.: A Study of the Morphology and Development of the Megakaryocytes, Brit. J. Exper. Path., *24*, 73, 1943.

14. JÜRGENS, R. and GRAUPNER, H.: Darstellung eines Entwicklungssystems der Thrombozyten: Zugleich ein Beitrag über das "Blutplättchenbild" der Blutkrankheiten, Folia hæmat., *57*, 263, 1937.

14a. KINOSITA, R., OHNO, S. and BIERMAN, H. R., Motion picture "Thrombopoiesis," City of Hope Medical Center, Duarte, California.

14b. KISSMEYER-NIELSEN, F.: Thrombopoiesis, Universitetsforlaget I Aarhus, 1954.

14c. KOPPEL, J. L. and OLWIN, J. H.: Dehydrogenase Activities of Human Platelets, Proc. Soc. Exper. Biol. & Med., *86*, 641, 1954.

14d. LEEKSMA, C. H. W. and COHEN, J. A.: Determination of the Life Span of Human

Blood Platelets Using Labelled Diisopropyl-
fluorophosphonate, J. Clin. Invest., *35*,
964, 1956.

15. LeSourd, L. and Pagniez, P.: Studies of
Platelets and Megakaryocytes, Compt. rend.
Soc. de biol., *58*, 109 and 562, 1906; *63*,
561, 1907; *65*, 400, 1908; *69*, 460, 1910;
71, 308 and 551, 1911; *74*, 580, 788 and
1259, 1913; *75*, 214, 1913; *76*, 587, 1914.

15a. Levinson, B., Jones, R. S., Wintrobe, M. M.
and Cartwright, G. E.: Thrombocythemia
and Pulmonary Intra-Alveolar Coagulum
in a Young Woman, Blood, *13*, 959, 1958.

16. MacKay, W.: The Blood Platelet: Its Clinical
Significance, Quart. J. Med., *24*, 285, 1931.

16a. Marcus, A. J. and Spaet, T. H.: Platelet
Phosphatides, J. Clin. Invest., *37*, 1836,
1958; J. Lipid Res., *1*, 179, 1960.

16b. Maupin, B.: Recherches sur les granules pla-
quettaires, Sang, *30*, 114, 1959.

17. Merritt, K. K. and Davidson, L. T.: The
Blood During the First Year of Life, Am.
J. Dis. Child., *46*, 990, 1933.

18. Minot, G. R.: Megacaryocytes in the Peripheral Circulation, J. Exper. Med., *36*, 1,
1921.

19. Odell, T. T., Jr. and Anderson, Bonnie:
Isolation of a Sulfated Mucopolysaccharide
from Blood Platelets of Rats, Proc. Soc.
Exper. Biol. & Med., *94*, 151, 1957; *ibid.*,
99, 765, 1958.

20. Olef, I.: The Enumeration of Blood Platelets,
J. Lab. & Clin. Med., *20*, 416, 1935.

21. ———— The Differential Platelet Count,
Arch. Int. Med., *57*, 1163, 1936.

22. ———— The Determination of Platelet
Volume, J. Lab. & Clin. Med., *23*, 166, 1937.

22a. Pepper, H. and Lindsay, S.: Responses of
Platelets, Eosinophils, and Total Leucocytes during and following Surgical Procedures, Surg. Gynec. & Obst., *110*, 319,
1960.

22b. Perry, S. and Craddock, C. G., Jr.: Platelet
Adsorptive Properties and Platelet Extracts
in Thromboplastin Generation, Blood, *8*,
177, 1958.

22c. Piette, M. and Piette, C.: Numération des
plaquettes sanguines utilisant un liquide
hypotonique a base de chlorhydrate de procaine, Sang, *30*, 144, 1959.

22d. Pizzolato, P.: Sternal Marrow Megakaryocytes in Health and Disease, Am. J. Clin.
Path., *18*, 891, 1948.

23. Pohle, F. J.: The Blood Platelet Count in
Relation to the Menstrual Cycle in Normal
Women, Am. J. Med. Sc., *197*, 40, 1939.

23a. Rebuck, J. W.: The Structure of the Giant
Cells in the Blood-Forming Organs, J. Lab.
& Clin. Med., *32*, 660, 1947.

23b. Salvidio, E.: Biochemical Aspects of Blood
Platelets, Acta haemat., *11*, 301, 1954.

23c. Sano, I., Kakimoto, Y., Taniguchi, K. and
Takesada, M.: Active Transport of Epi-
nephrine into Blood Platelets, Am. J.
Physiol., *197*, 81, 1959.

23d. Schulman, I., Pierce, Mila, Lukens, Abby
and Currimbhoy, Zinet: A Factor in
Normal Human Plasma Required for Platelet Production; Chronic Thrombocytopenia
Due to its Deficiency, Blood, *16*, 943, 1960.

23e. Schüpbach, A. and Herrmann, E.: Throm-
bosekrankheit bei essentieller (?) Thrombocythämie, Schweiz. med. Wchnschr., *84*,
95, 1954.

23f. Schwarz, E.: The Megakaryocyte, Arch.
Path., *47*, 545, 1949.

23g. Sharp, A. A.: Viscous Metamorphosis of Blood
Platelets, Brit. J. Haemat., *4*, 28 and 177,
1958.

23h. Sloan, A. W.: The Normal Platelet Count in
Man, J. Clin. Path., *4*, 37, 1951.

23i. Storti, E., Perugini, S. and Soldati, M.:
Cytochemical Investigations of Normal
Megakaryocytes and Platelets, Acta hae-
mat., *10*, 144, 1953.

23j. Szeinberg, A. and Moscowici-Gaffni, Dora:
Clot Retraction Activity of Platelets, Acta
haemat., *21*, 250, 1959.

24. Tocantins, L. M.: Platelets and the Structure
and Physical Properties of Blood Clots, Am.
J. Physiol., *114*, 709, 1936.

25. ———— Technical Methods for the Study of
Blood Platelets, Arch. Path., *23*, 850, 1937.

26. ———— The Mammalian Blood Platelet in
Health and Disease, Medicine, *17*, 175,
1938 (Bibliography).

26a. ———— Historical Notes on Blood Platelets,
Blood, *3*, 1073, 1948.

27. Van Allen, C. M.: The Volume Measurement of Blood Platelets, J. Lab. & Clin.
Med., *12*, 282, 1926–27.

27a. Vazquez, J. J. and Lewis, Jessica H.: The
Demonstration of a Common Antigen in
Human Platelets and Megakaryocytes,
Blood, *16*, 968, 1960.

27b. Wachholder, K., Parchwitz, Erika, Egli,
H. and Kesseler, K.: Der Einfluss körper-
licher Arbeit auf die Zahl der Thrombocyten und auf deren Haftneigung, Acta
haemat., *18*, 59, 1957.

27c. Wagner, R. and Yourke, A.: Alkaline and
Acid Phosphatases in White Blood Cells
and Blood Platelets, Arch. Biochem., *54*,
174, 1955.

28. Waller, H. D., Löhr, G. W., Frignani, F.
and Gross, R.: Uber den Energiestoff-
wechsel normaler menschlicher Thrombo-

zyten, Thromb. Diath. haemorrh., *3*, 520, 1959.

28a. WILLIAMS, J. H. and WARREN, R.: Endocrine Factors in the Alterations of the Blood Coagulation Mechanism following Surgery, J. Lab. & Clin. Med., *50*, 372, 1957.

28b. WOODSIDE, E. E. and KOCHOLATY, W.: Carbohydrates of Human and Bovine Platelets, Blood, *16*, 1173, 1960.

28c. WRIGHT, H. P.: The Sources of Blood Platelets and Their Adhesiveness in Experimental Thrombocytosis, J. Path. & Bacteriol., *56*, 151, 1944.

29. WRIGHT, J. H.: The Histogenesis of the Blood Platelets, J. Morphol., *21*, 263, 1910.

30. ZAJICEK, J. and DATTA, N.: Acetylcholine Esterase in Thrombocytes of Rat Blood, Acta haemat., *7*, 39, 1952; *ibid.*, *12*, 238, 1954; Acta physiol. scandinav. (Supp. 138), *40*, 1, 1957.

30a. ZUCKER, MARJORIE B. and BORRELLI, JENNIE: A Survey of Some Platelet Enzymes and Functions, Ann. New York Acad. Sc., *75*, 203, 1958; J. Clin. Invest., *38*, 148, 1959.

Coagulation

30b. ACKROYD, J. F.: A Simple Method of Estimating Clot Retraction with a Survey of Normal Values and the Changes That Occur with Menstruation, Clin. Sci., *7*, 231, 1949.

30c. ADELSON, E. and CROSBY, W. H.: A New Method to Measure Bleeding Time. The "Immersion" Method, Acta haemat., *18*, 281, 1957.

31. ALEXANDER, B.: Clotting Factor VII (Proconvertin): Synonymy, Properties, Clinical and Clinicolaboratory Aspects, New England J. Med., *260*, 1218, 1959.

31a. ALEXANDER, B., GOLDSTEIN, R. and LANDWEHR, G.: The Prothrombin Conversion Accelerator of Serum (SPCA), J. Clin. Invest., *29*, 881, 1950; *Ibid.*, *30*, 252, 1951.

31b. ALKJAERSIG, NORMA, FLETCHER, A. P. and SHERRY, S.: The Mechanism of Clot Dissolution by Plasmin, J. Clin. Invest., *38*, 1086, 1959; *ibid.*, *39*, 426, 1960.

31c. BACCHETTA, V. and SERAFINI, U. M.: Caratterizzazione biologica delle proprietà coagulanti del latte umano, Haematologica, *42*, 1583, 1957.

31d. BECKER, E. L.: Inactivation of Hageman Factor by Diisopropylfluorophosphate (DFP), J. Lab. & Clin. Med., *56*, 136, 1960.

32. BERGSAGEL, D. E.: The Role of Calcium in the Activation of the Christmas Factor, British J. Haemat., *1*, 199, 1955; *ibid.*, *2*, 113, 1956.

32a. BERRY, C. G.: Antithromboplastin: the Degeneration of Intrinsic Thromboplastin in Normal Serum, J. Clin. Path., *11*, 39, 1958.

32b. BIDWELL, E.: Fibrinolysins of Human Plasma, Biochem. J., *55*, 497, 1953.

33. BIGGS, R. and DOUGLAS, A. S.: The Thromboplastin Generation Test, J. Clin. Path., *6*, 23, 1953.

33a. BIGGS, ROSEMARY and MACFARLANE, R. G.: *Human Blood Coagulation and Its Disorders*, Ed. 2, Springfield, C. C Thomas, 1957.

34. BLOMBÄCK, B.: Studies on Fibrinogen: its Purification and Conversion into Fibrin, Acta physiol. scandinav. (Suppl. 148), *43*, 7, 1958.

34a. BORCHGREVINK, C. F., POOL, JUDITH G. and STORMORKEN, HELGE: A New Assay for Factor V (Proaccelerin-Accelerin) Using Russell's Viper Venom, J. Lab. & Clin. Med., *55*, 625, 1960.

35. BORN, G. V. R.: Changes in the Distribution of Phosphorus in Platelet-Rich Plasma during Clotting, Biochem. J., *68*, 695, 1958; Nature, *183*, 478, 1959.

35a. BOUNAMEAUX, Y.: Dosage du Facteur VIII en un temps, Acta haemat., *17*, 355, 1957.

35b. BOYLES, P. W., ASHLEY, CATHERINE C. and DUNAWAY, R. P.: Electrophoretic Studies of Purified Prothrombin and Thrombin, Am. J. Clin. Path., *34*, 214, 1960.

36. BUCKWALTER, J. A., BLYTHE, W. B. and BRINKHOUS, K. M.: Effect of Blood Platelets on Prothrombin Utilization of Dog and Human Plasmas, Am. J. Physiol., *159*, 316, 1949.

36a. BUDTZ-OLSEN, O. E.: *Clot Retraction*, Oxford, Blackwell Scientific Publications, 1951.

37. BURSTEIN, M. and LOEB, J.: Inhibition de la thrombinoformation par l'héparine, Rev. franç. étud. clin. et biol., *1*, 752, 1956.

38. CHARGAFF, E., BENDICH, A. and COHEN, S. S.: The Thromboplastic Protein, J. Biol. Chem., *156*, 161, 1944; *ibid.*, *161*, 389, 1945; *ibid.*, *173*, 253, 1948.

39. CONLEY, C. L., HARTMANN, R. C. and MORSE, W. I., II: The Clotting Behavior of Human "Platelet-Free" Plasma: Evidence for the Existence of a "Plasma Thromboplastin," J. Clin. Invest., *28*, 340, 1949; Bull. Johns Hopkins Hosp., *85*, 231, 1949; J. Clin. Invest., *29*, 1182, 1950; Bull Johns Hopkins Hosp., *88*, 321, 1951; J. Clin. Invest., *31*, 685, 1952; *ibid.*, *33*, 1423, 1954.

40. ———— Circulating Anticoagulants: A Technique for Their Detection and Clinical Studies, Bull. Johns Hopkins Hosp., *84*, 255, 1949.

40a. COX, F. M., LANCHANTIN, G. F. and WARE, A. G.: Chromatographic Purification of Human Serum Accelerator Globulin, J. Clin. Invest., *35*, 106, 1956.

41. CRANE, M. M. and SANFORD, H. N.: The Effect of Variations in Total Calcium Concentration Upon the Coagulation Time of Blood, Am. J. Physiol., *118*, 703, 1937.

41a. CRUZ, W. O., OLIVEIRA, A. C. and MAGALHAEAS, J. R.: Marked Differences in Behaviour of Arterial and Venous Blood in Haemostasis, J. Physiol., *142*, 242, 1958; Brit. J. Haemat., *5*, 141, 1959; Arch. Biochem. & Biophys., *85*, 550, 1959.

42 DALLDORF, G.: A Sensitive Test for Subclinical Scurvy in Man, Am. J. Dis. Child., *46*, 794, 1933.

43. DE VRIES, A., HERZ, N. and HEIMAN-HOLLANDER, E.: Observations on Prothrombin Consumption During Clotting of Normal Blood in Glass, Acta med. scandinav. *138*, 211 and 219, 1950.

43a. DOUGLAS, A. S. and BIGGS, R.: The Consumption of Some Components Involved in Physiological Blood Coagulation, Glasgow M. J., *34*, 329, 1953; J. Physiol., *122*, 538, 1953; Brit. J. Haemat., *2*, 153, 1956.

44. EAGLE, H.: Recent Advances in the Blood Coagulation Problem, Medicine, *16*, 95, 1937 (Bibliography).

44a. EDSALL, J. T., FERRY, R. M. and ARMSTRONG, S. H., JR.: The Proteins Concerned in the Blood Coagulation Mechanism, J. Clin. Invest., *23*, 557, 1944.

44b. EIBER, H. B. and DANISHEFSKY, I.: Synthesis and Metabolism of Radioactive Heparin, A. M. A. Arch. Int. Med., *102*, 189, 1958; Proc. Soc. Exper. Biol. & Med., *98*, 672, 1958.

45. FERGUSON, J. H., LEWIS, JESSICA H. and FRESH, J. W.: The Two-Stage "Prothrombin" Assay in Study of Bleeding and Clotting Disorders, Yale J. Biol. & Med., *28*, 253, 1955/6.

45a. FLUTE, P. T. and HOWARD, A. N.: Blood Coagulation in Scorbutic Guinea-Pigs: a Defect in Activation by Glass Contact, Brit. J. Haemat., *5*, 421, 1959.

45b. GEORGATSOS, J. G., HUSSEY, CLARA V. and QUICK, A. J.: Synergistic Action of Russell Viper Venom and Tissue Thromboplastin Extracts, Proc. Soc. Exper. Biol. & Med., *97*, 674, 1958.

46. GLADNER, J. A., FOLK, J. E., LAKI, K. and CARROLL, W. R.: Thrombin-Induced Formation of Co-Fibrin, J. Biol. Chem., *234*, 62 and 67, 1959.

46a. HARTERT, H.: Die Thromboelastographie. Eine Methode zur physikalischen Analyse des Blutgerinnungsvorganges, Ztschr. f. d. ges. exper. Med., *117*, 189, 1951.

47. HECHT, E. R., CHO, M. H. and SEEGERS, W. H.: Thromboplastin: Nomenclature and Preparation of Protein-Free Material Differ-

ent from Platelet Factor 3 or Lipid Activator, Am. J. Physiol., *193*, 584, 1958.

48. HJORT, P. F.: Intermediate Reactions in the Coagulation of Blood with Tissue Thromboplastin, Scandinav. J. Clin. & Lab. Invest. (Suppl. 27), *9*, 7, 1957.

49. HOWELL, W. H.: Theories of Blood Coagulation, Physiol. Rev., *15*, 435, 1935.

49a. ———— The Isolation of Thromboplastin From Lung Tissue, Bull. Johns Hopkins Hosp., *76*, 295, 1945.

49b. ISRAELS, L. G., FOERSTER, J. and ZIPURSKY, A.: A Naturally Occurring Inhibitor of the First Stage of Blood Coagulation, Brit. J. Haemat., *6*, 275, 1960.

50. IVY, A. C., SHAPIRO, P. F. and MELNICK, P.: The Bleeding Tendency in Jaundice, Surg., Gynec. and Obst., *60*, 781, 1935.

51. JACOBSON, L. O., MARKS, E. K., GASTON, E., ALLEN, J. G. and BLOCK, M. H.: The Effect of Nitrogen Mustard and X Irradiation on Blood Coagulation, J. Lab. & Clin. Med., *33*, 1566, 1948.

52. JAQUES, L. B.: Blood Clotting and Hemostasis, Ann. Rev. Physiol., *16*, 175, 1954.

52a. JIM, R. T. S.: A Study of the Plasma Thrombin Time, J. Lab. & Clin. Med., *50*, 45, 1957.

53. JIM, R. T. S. and GOLDFEIN, S.: Hageman Trait (Hageman Factor Deficiency), Am. J. Med., *23*, 824, 1957.

53a. JOHNSON, S. A. and SCHNEIDER, C. L.: The Existence of Antifibrinolysin Activity in Platelets, Science, *117*, 229, 1953.

54. VON KAULLA, K. N. and SCHULTZ, R. L.: Methods for the Evaluation of Human Fibrinolysis, Am. J. Clin. Path., *29*, 104, 1958.

55. KLEIN, P. D. and SEEGERS, W. H.: The Nature of Plasma Antithrombin Activity, Blood, *5*, 742, 1950.

55a. KOWALSKI, E. et al.: On the Occurrence of a Plasminogen-like Substance in Human Tissues, Blood, *8*, 436, 1958.

55b. LAKI, K., KOMINZ, D. R., SYMONDS, P., LORAND, L. and SEEGERS, W. H.: The Amino Acid Composition of Bovine Prothrombin, Arch. Biochem., *49*, 276, 1954; Physiol. Rev., *34*, 730, 1954.

55c. LAKI, K., GLADNER, J. A., FOLK, J. E. and KOMINZ, D. R.: The Mode of Action of Thrombin, Thromb. Diath. haemorrh., *2*, 205, 1958.

55d. LANDABURU, R. H. and SEEGERS, W. H.: Activation of Prothrombin, Am. J. Physiol., *193*, 169, 1958; *ibid.*, *197*, 1178, 1959; *ibid.*, *198*, 173, 1960.

56. LEWIS, JESSICA H. and DIDISHEIM, P.: Differential Diagnosis and Treatment in Hemorrhagic Disease, A. M. A. Arch. Int. Med., *100*, 157, 1957.

56a. LEWIS, M. L. and WARE, A. G.: The Mechanism of Action of Human Accelerator Globulin and Its Relation to Other Clotting Factors, Blood, 9, 520, 1954.

57. LORAND, L.: Interaction of Thrombin and Fibrinogen, Physiol. Rev., 34, 742, 1954.

58. LÜSCHER, E. F.: Viscous Metamorphosis of Blood Platelets and Clot Retraction, Vox sanguinis, 1, 133, 1956.

58a. LYTTLETON, J. W.: The Antithrombin Activity of Heparin, Biochem. J., 58, 8 and 15, 1954.

58b. MACFARLANE, R. G.: The Mechanism of Haemostasis, Quart. J. Med., 10, 1, 1941.

58c. MACFARLANE, R. G.: Normal and Abnormal Blood Coagulation: A Review, J. Clin. Path., 1, 113, 1948 (Bibliography); Blood Coagulation, Physiol. Rev., 36, 479, 1956.

59. MARGOLIS, J.: Hageman Factor and Capillary Permeability, Australian J. Exper. Biol. & M. Sc., 37, 239, 1959; J. Physiol., 151, 238, 1960.

59a. MCKAY, D. C. and SHAPIRO, S. S.: Alterations in the Blood Coagulation System Induced by Bacterial Endotoxin, J. Exper. Med., 107, 353 and 369, 1958.

59b. MILLER, K. D. and VAN VUNAKIS, HELEN: The Effect of Diisopropyl Fluorophosphate on the Proteinase and Esterase Activities of Thrombin and on Prothrombin and Its Activators, J. Biol. Chem., 223, 227, 1956.

59c. MILSTONE, J. H.: On the Evolution of Blood Clotting Theory, Medicine, 31, 411, 1952.

60. DE NICOLA, P.: Thrombelastography, Springfield, C. C Thomas, 1957.

61. NOLF, P.: The Coagulation of the Blood, Medicine, 17, 381, 1938; Sang, 29, 321, 1948.

61a. OWEN, C. A., JR., MANN, F. D., HURN, M. M. and STICKNEY, J. M.: Evaluation of Disorders of Blood Coagulation in the Clinical Laboratory, Am. J. Clin. Path., 25, 1417, 1955.

62. OWREN, P. A.: A Quantitative One-Stage Method for the Assay of Prothrombin, Scandinav. Jour. Clin. & Lab. Invest., 1, 81, 1949; ibid., 3, 201, 1951.

63. OWREN, P. A.: Thrombotest, Lancet, 2, 754, 1959.

63a. OWREN, P. A.: Prothrombin and Accessory Factors, Am. J. Med., 14, 201, 1953.

64. POOL, JUDITH G. and ROBINSON, JEAN: In vitro Synthesis of Coagulation Factors by Rat Liver Slices, Am. J. Physiol., 196, 423, 1959; ibid., 199, 139, 1960.

65. POOLE, J. C. F.: The Significance of Chylomicra in Blood Coagulation, Brit. J. Haemat., 1, 229, 1955; Quart. J. Exper. Physiol., 41, 31 and 36, 1956; ibid., 42, 285, 1957.

66. PORTER, K. R. and HAWN, C. V. Z.: Sequences in the Formation of Clots from Purified Bovine Fibrinogen and Thrombin: A Study with the Electron Microscope, J. Exper. Med., 90, 225, 1949.

68. QUICK, A. J.: Determination of Prothrombin, Am. J. Med. Sc., 190, 501, 1935; Proc. Soc. Exper. Biol. & Med., 42, 788, 1939; Am. J. Clin. Path., 15, 560, 1945.

69. ——— The Physiology and Pathology of Hemostasis, Philadelphia, Lea & Febiger, 1951.

70. ——— On the Constitution of Prothrombin, Am. J. Physiol., 140, 212, 1943; J. Lab. & Clin. Med., 34, 1203, 1949; Am. J. Physiol., 160, 572, 1950.

71. QUICK, A. J.: Hemorrhagic Diseases, Philadelphia, Lea and Febiger, 1957.

71a. QUICK, A. J. and FAVRE-GILLY, J. E.: Fibrin, a Factor Influencing the Consumption of Prothrombin in Coagulation, Am. J. Physiol., 158, 387, 1949; Angiology, 10, 386, 1959; Am. J. Physiol., 197, 791, 1959.

72. ——— The Prothrombin Consumption Test, Blood, 4, 1281, 1949.

72a. QUICK, A. J.: Influence of Erythrocytes on the Coagulation of Blood, Am. J. M. Sc., 239, 51, 1960.

72b. QUICK, A. J., SHANBERGE, J. N. and STEFANINI, M.: The Role of Platelets in the Coagulation of the Blood, Am. J. Med. Sc., 217, 198, 1949; Science, 112, 558, 1950; Am. J. Med. Sc., 220, 538, 1950.

72c. RACCUGLIA, G.: Factor VIII (Antihemophilic Factor) and Factor V (Proaccelerin) Activity of Platelets, Proc. Soc. Exper. Biol. & Med., 104, 309, 1960.

73. RAMOT, B., ANGELOPOULOS, B. and SINGER, K.: Plasma Thromboplastin Antecedent Deficiency, Arch. Int. Med., 95, 705, 1955; J. Lab. & Clin. Med., 46, 80, 1955.

73a. RAPAPORT, S. I.: The Effect of Glass upon the Activity of the Various Plasma Clotting Factors, J. Clin. Invest. 34, 9, 1955.

74. RATNOFF, O. D. and POTTS, A. M.: The Accelerating Effect of Calcium and Other Cations on the Conversion of Fibrinogen to Fibrin, J. Clin. Invest. 33, 206, 1954.

74a. RATNOFF, O. D. and ROSENBLUM, J. M.: Role of Hageman Factor in the Initiation of Clotting by Glass, Am. J. Med., 25, 160, 1958; J. Clin. Invest., 40, 803, 1961.

74b. RODMAN, N. F., JR., BARROW, EMILY M. and GRAHAM, J. B.: Diagnosis and Control of the Hemophilioid States with the Partial Thromboplastin Time (PTT) Test, Am. J. Clin. Path., 29, 525, 1958.

74c. ROSKAM, J.: Faits et hypothèses dans les domaines de l'hémostase spontanée, de la thrombose et de la coagulation, Schweiz. med. Wchnschr., *90*, 947, 1960; Bull. Acad. roy. med. Belgique, *25*, 160, 1960.

74*d*. Scott, T. G., Symons, C. and Markham, R. L.: Antithromboplastin in Human Serum and Plasma, Nature, *186*, 248, 1960.

75. Seegers, W. H. and Alkjaersig, N.: Comparative Properties of Purified Human and Bovine Prothrombin, Am. J. Physiol., *172*, 731, 1953; Am. J. Clin. Path., *25*, 983, 1955; Am. J. Physiol., *182*, 443, 1955; *ibid.*, *183*, 111, 1955; *ibid.*, *184*, 259, 1956.

75*a*. Seegers, W. H., McClaughry, R. I. and Fahey, J. L.: Some Properties of Purified Prothrombin and Its Activation with Sodium Citrate, Blood, *5*, 421, 1950.

75*b*. Seegers, W. H. and McGinty, D. A.: Further Purification of Thrombin, J. Biol. Chem., *146*, 511, 1942; Canadian J. Biochem. & Physiol., *37*, 775, 1959; Nature *185*, 930, 1960.

75*c*. Shanberge, J. N., Barlas, Angela and Regan, Ellen E.: The Effect of Protamine on Thromboplastin Generation, J. Lab. & Clin. Med., *52*, 744, 1958; *ibid.*, *54*, 501, 1959

75*d*. Slotta, K. H.: Thromboplastin. I. Phospholipid Moiety of Thromboplastin, Proc. Soc. Exper. Biol. & Med., *103*, 53, 1960.

76. Soulier, J.-P.: Les modifications du Ca^{++} dans les transfusions massives et la circulation extracorporéale utilisant du sang citraté, Rev. hémat., *13*, 437, 1958.

76*a*. Soulier, J.-P.: Les inhibiteurs naturels de la coagulation, Sang, *30*, 262, 1959.

76*b*. Soulier, J.-P. and Prou-Wartelle, O.: New Data on Hageman Factor and Plasma Thromboplastin Antecedent, Brit. J. Haemat., *6*, 88, 1960.

77. Spaet, T. H. and Cintron, J. R.: Induction in Rabbits of Activity against Human Blood Thromboplastin, Blood, *15*, 772, 1960.

77*a*. Spaet, T. H. and Kropatkin, Mona: Effect of Intravenous Blood Thromboplastin Intermediates on Clotting in Rats, Am. J. Physiol., *195*, 77, 1958; Proc. Soc. Exper. Biol. & Med., *104*, 498, 1960.

77*b*. Stefanini, M.: New One-Stage Procedures for the Quantitative Determination of Pro-

thrombin and Labile Factor, Am. J. Clin. Path., *20*, 233, 1950.

78. ———— Basic Mechanisms of Hemostasis, Bull. New York Acad. Med., *30*, 239, 1954.

78*a*. Streuli, F.: On the Purification and Conversion of Human Prothrombin, Thromb. Diath. haemorrh., *3*, 194, 1959.

79. Therriault, D., Nichols, T. and Jensen, H.: Purification and Identification of Brain Phospholipides Associated with Thromboplastic Activity, J. Biol. Chem., *233*, 1061, 1958.

80. Tidrick, R. T., Seegers, W. H. and Warner, E. D.: Clinical Experience With Thrombin as an Hemostatic Agent, Surgery, *14*, 191, 1943.

81. Tishkoff, G. H., Pechet, L. and Alexander, B.: Some Biochemical and Electrophoretic Studies on Purified Prothrombin, Factor VII (Proconvertin) and Factor X (Stuart), Blood, *15*, 778, 1960.

82. Tocantins, L. M.: The Bleeding Time, Am. J. Clin. Path., *6*, 160, 1936.

83. ———— The Coagulation of Blood, Methods of Study, New York, Grune & Stratton, 1955.

84. Troup, S. B., Reed, C. F., Marinetti, G. V. and Swisher, S. N.: Thromboplastic Factors in Platelets and Red Blood Cells, J. Clin. Invest., *39*, 342, 1960.

85. Waaler, B. A.: Contact Activation in the Intrinsic Blood Clotting System, Scandinav. J. Clin. & Lab. Invest. (Suppl.), *11*, 1, 1959.

86. Ware, A. G., Fahey, J. L. and Seegers, W. H.: Platelet Extracts, Fibrin Formation and Interaction of Purified Prothrombin and Thromboplastin, Am. J. Physiol., *154*, 140, 1948; Am. J. Physiol., *190*, 1, 1957.

87. Ware, A. G. and Seegers, W. H.: Serum Ac-Globulin, Am. J. Physiol., *152*, 567, 1948; Blood, *5*, 303, 1950.

88. Waters, E. T., Markowitz, J. and Jaques, L. B.: Anaphylaxis in the Liverless Dog, and Observations on the Anticoagulant of Anaphylactic Shock, Science, *87*, 582, 1938; J. Physiol., *99*, 454, 1941.

89. Wright, I. S., Koller, F. and Streuli, F.: New Blood Clotting Factors, Thromb. Diath. haemorrh. (Suppl.), *4*, 1, 1960.

The Blood as a Whole

THE TOTAL QUANTITY OF BLOOD

In clinical practice one is accustomed to think of the constituents of the blood in terms of a given unit of volume and little attention is usually paid to their total quantity. Under certain circumstances and in various diseases, alterations occur in the total quantity of corpuscles or of plasma, or both.

Methods for Determination.—The direct method of blood volume estimation was employed in 1854 by Welcker who bled animals to death, washed out the vessels with water, and extracted the hemoglobin still remaining in the tissues by mincing the organs and placing them in water for several days, after the bile, intestinal contents and urine had been removed.[22] He concluded that the blood volume of mammals constitutes 7.7 per cent of the body weight. This value was confirmed in man by Bischoff whose subjects were two condemned criminals.[22]

Other methods are less exhaustive but also less accurate. They depend upon the introduction of some foreign substance into the blood and estimation of the dilution this substance has undergone after a given interval of time. To such a procedure certain obvious objections come to mind. For one, it may be pointed out that the circulation is not equally active in all parts of the body at the same time and an injected substance may not reach one of the so-called "blood depots." Such inadequate mix-

ing is a serious source of error. Then again, absorption of the foreign substance into the tissues and its rapid excretion or destruction is another cause for error. Furthermore, the injected substance is one which is either diluted in the plasma or becomes a constituent of the corpuscular component of the blood. Consequently only the volume of the plasma or the size of the red cell mass is calculated from the dilution of the introduced substance, and the total blood volume must be estimated from the relative quantities of plasma and red cells as measured in the hematocrit. In addition to these, two basic technical problems were the need to develop accurate methods for the determination of the test substance in the blood and questions related to the interpretation of the time concentration curves obtained.

It has been shown that the *"venous" hematocrit* overestimates the proportion of red cells in the circulating blood as a whole. The volume of packed red cells in the capillary bed is substantially lower than in venous blood so that the *"body" hematocrit*, the average value for the body as a whole, is approximately 91 per cent of the volume of packed red cells in venous blood.[2b] Under most conditions the ratio of "venous" to "body" hematocrit is a constant one,[15,15b] so that a correction factor of 0.91 could be used. However, in anemic, splenomegalic patients the abnormal concentration of red corpuscles in the spleen makes up for the relatively low concentration in vessels of the body smaller than the jugular or ante-cubital veins, with the result that the ratio of body to venous hematocrit is closer to 1.0 than to 0.91.[28] The ratio may similarly depart from the usual one in conditions of prolonged oligemic shock where capillary blood flow is altered radically, as well as in patients with congestive cardiac failure.[2b]

Another source of error in the estimation of total blood volume on the basis of the ratio of plasma to the volume of packed red cells is the fact that some plasma is "trapped" in the column of packed red cells as measured in the hematocrit. However, a correction for this can be made, as is discussed elsewhere (p. 407).

Over the years many different procedures were devised in attempts to measure the total quantity of blood in man and in various animals. These included the injection of isotonic sodium chloride solutions,[3] or of tetanus anti-toxin,[1c] acacia[19,19a] or homologous precipitating antiserum.[5] The use of carbon monoxide as a label for hemoglobin, introduced in 1882 and improved in recent years,[21c] was shown to give significantly higher (16 per cent) values than are obtained by other methods,[21] due to the fact that hemoglobin in bone marrow, muscles and elsewhere, and other extravascular pigments, are tagged, in addition to the hemoglobin in the circulation. Subsequently, the introduction of the dye dilution method[17] provided a simple and attractive technic which could be applied widely and thus many investigators became interested. Finally, the introduction of radioactive elements in physiological studies led to a geometric acceleration of investigations in this field. The first result was an accumulation of discordant values. Now, however, many of the problems involved in the measurement of blood volume are understood, even if not completely solved, and one can define precautions that must be taken and the values which can be obtained under a variety of circumstances.[14]

Plasma Volume Methods.—The introduction of the non-toxic, slowly diffusing blue dye, T–1824 ("Evans blue"), solved some of the problems presented by the original "brilliant vital red." The use of T-1824 involves the injection of a known quantity of dye and the subsequent withdrawal of samples of blood at appropriate intervals for determination of dye dilution. The fact that this dye is firmly bound to the plasma albumin prevents its rapid elimination from the blood stream.[13] Special precautions must be taken to determine the exact amount of dye injected and that present in the samples.[14] Methods have been devised for extraction of the dye, thus permitting greater accuracy in measurement.[2] Graphic analysis of the time-concentration curve on a semi-log plot and back extrapolation of the disappearance curve provides the accepted means of arriving at the value for the initial concentration of dye needed for calculating the plasma volume.

Serum albumin tagged with radioactive iodine ("RISA"),[4,14,15a,26] gives results comparable with the T-1824 method[24] and, because the half-life ($T\frac{1}{2}$) of I^{131} is only eight days, determinations can be repeated more frequently. It is subject to errors similar to those of the dye method, but the method also has certain advantages.[29a]

Red Cell Volume.—The Ashby technic of differential agglutination of red cells (p. 163) has been used for the estimation of red cell volume and can be performed with considerable accuracy and without special equipment but the technic is tedious and scrupulous care is required.[1a] For these reasons it is rarely used and isotopic methods are preferred.[14] These include the use of Fe^{59}, P^{32} and Cr^{51}.

The *radioactive iron* method involves the administration of Fe^{59} to a donor to allow incorporation of the iron into his red corpuscles and the subsequent transfusion of such blood into the subject.[12,15] The dilution of the transfused blood is then determined by measuring the radioactivity of the recipient's blood. This method is now rarely used.

A simpler technic consists in the introduction of *radioactive phosphorus* (P^{32}) into erythrocytes *in vitro* and their subsequent return to the circulation where their dilution is measured.[2a] Thus, no problem of securing a donor and no concern regarding blood types arises. Many improvements on the original technic have been introduced.[19b] The $T\frac{1}{2}$ of P^{32} is 14.3 days.

Radioactive chromium (Cr^{51}), already discussed as providing a simple means for measuring the life span of red cells (p. 164), has come to be widely used for measurement of red cell volume as well.[12a,21b] This isotope is held more avidly by red cells than is radioactive phosphorus.[21b] The amount commonly used is well below the safe radiation dosage for humans. Since there is no significant loss of Cr^{51} to the plasma for 24 hours or more, only one or two samples need be taken at whatever postinjection time is considered necessary for complete mixing in the circulation.

Method.—A modification of the method of Read[21b] is as follows: Approximately 5 to 10 ml. of ACD solution (p. 356) is withdrawn from a sterile, siliconized 100 ml. glass blood collection bottle by means of a sterile 50 ml. syringe and a number 20 spinal needle (at least $2\frac{1}{2}''$ long). The syringe and needle are then used to draw approximately 40 ml. blood from the subject. The contents are injected into the blood bottle and thoroughly mixed. About 100 μc. (microcuries) of radioactive sodium chromate is added. This should be of high enough specific activity that no more than 25 μg. (micrograms) of chromium metal will be present per 1 ml. red blood cells. After mixing, the blood is incubated at 37° C. for 45 to 60 minutes, with occasional

remixing. Ascorbic acid (at least 50 mg.) is added. This reducing agent prevents further uptake of Cr^{51} by red cells. After 10 minutes the labelled red cells are washed three times with saline: the bottle containing the labelled blood is placed in a large centrifuge cup (250 ml.), balanced with another cup containing an empty ACD blood bottle and centrifuged for 10 minutes at 1000 r.p.m. The supernatant solution is removed by means of a sterile 50 ml. syringe and needle. This should be disposed of as provided for radioactive materials. Sterile isotonic saline is added to the ACD bottle in excess, the contents are mixed and the procedure is repeated two more times. After the last washing, the contents of the bottle are reconstituted to the original volume with saline.

The labelled red cells are then drawn into a sterile 50 ml. syringe. This, together with the needle, is weighed and about 2 ml. is then injected into a 100 ml. flask and the syringe is weighed again. The ejected red cells are diluted with saline to 100 ml. and constitute the "standard." The labelled red cells remaining in the syringe are injected into the subject and the syringe and needle are weighed once more.

Five ml. aliquots of venous blood are collected from the subject in oxalate (p. 378) 15, 30 and 45 minutes after the injection of blood. Hematocrit determinations are carried out on each. Two ml. blood is pipetted accurately into the counting container of a well type scintillation counter. After centrifuging, duplicate counts are made after the counting containers have been placed in a well type counter. On the basis of the measured volume of packed red cells in each of these samples and the known volume of blood used (2 ml.), the number of counts per ml. red cells can be calculated.

If the counts in the "standard" have also been determined, the number of counts injected (c.p.m.) can be calculated from the ratio of the weight of blood injected to the weight of blood in the standard; thus,

$$\frac{\text{weight of blood injected}}{\text{weight of blood used for standard}} \times \text{counts in standard} \times 100 = \text{c.p.m. injected}$$

The counts in each of the three post-infusion aliquots are averaged or are fitted by the best possible line and extrapolated to the ordinate of a graph in which counts are plotted against time. The red cell volume can then be calculated, as follows,

$$\frac{\text{c.p.m. injected}}{\text{c.p.m./ml. red cells from extrapolate}} = \text{red cell volume, ml.}$$

Methods are available whereby simultaneous measurements can be made of plasma volume by means of I^{131} or Cr^{51} Cl_3, red cell volume with Cr^{51} and even extracellular fluid volume, using S^{35}-tagged sulfate.[7a,25]

Normal Values.—Attempts to compile tables of normal values for man and other species have met serious difficulties for many reasons, including, in particular the fact that procedures have varied in detail, making comparisons difficult, and also because there has been no agreement concerning a suitable and uniform basis of comparison. Body surface area, height and weight have all been used. It is known that there is an increase in blood volume with increases in these parameters.[15c] It was claimed that the correlation between surface area and blood volume is greater than with weight,[22] but this, if true, applies only to persons exhibiting no marked disturbance in weight to height relationship.[9] Red cell mass was found to be related to lean body mass rather than to total body weight.[20a] In the lower animals blood volume has been found to be proportional to body weight.[3a]

In comparison to average values, the total blood volume per unit of surface area was said to be high in muscular and obese persons, and low in thin individuals. In terms of units of body weight, the blood volume was high in muscular and thin individuals and low in obese persons.[9]

The mean circulating *red cell volume* in normal male medical students in Boston was found to be 2208 ml. as measured by the radioiron method[12] and 2351 ml. (standard deviation 290 ml.) by the radioactive chromium technic.[12a] The respective mean red cell volumes per Kg. body weight were 29.7 and 31.8 ml. (standard deviation 3.5) and the mean red cell volumes per square meter of surface area were 1.15 and 1.21 liters (standard deviation 0.12). In a series of 25 normal males,[1f] mean red cell mass, measured with radioactive phosphorus, was 30.1 ml. (standard deviation 5.74) per Kg. body weight. Thus, in relation to weight an average figure for young normal males at sea level is 30.5 ml./Kg. For the female the corresponding figure would be 23.4 ml./Kg.[14]

Plasma volume in a series of 25 normal adult males[1f] was 43.6 ± 5.79 and 45.5 ± 5.43 ml. per Kg. body weight as measured by the iodinated albumin and Evans' blue methods, respectively. The corresponding figure for the female is 43.1 ml./Kg.[14]

Total blood volume in terms of body weight is greater in *males* than in *females*, due chiefly to the higher red cell volume of the male. Average values for the

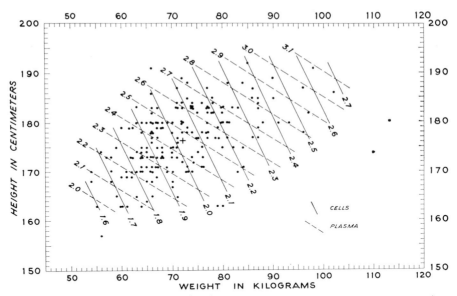

FIG. 6–1.—Red cell (Vrbc) and plasma (Vpl) volumes in relation to height and weight (Wennesland *et al.*, courtesy of J. Clin. Invest.)[29]

Each solid circle represents one subject, plotted according to his height and weight. The average of the heights and weights is shown by +. The solid and dashed contour lines give the mean predicted Vrbc and Vpl, respectively, to the nearest 0.1 L. The mean predicted volumes of a man 175 cm. tall and weighing 70 Kg. are: Vrbc = 1.98 L., Vpl = 2.40 L., and Vwb (volume whole blood) = 4.38 L. Values are uncorrected for trapped plasma and for differences between body hematocrit and venous hematocrit. Vrbc includes leukocytes and platelets.

The contour lines were constructed by introducing the successive mean values for Vrbc and Vpl in their respective regression equations and computing the height for a given weight or vice versa.

two sexes, respectively, are 75.5 and 66.5 ml./Kg.[14] Thus the blood of the young healthy adult makes up 7 to 8 per cent of the body weight.

A chart derived from a study of 201 men[29] carefully screened for health and classified as to age, habits of physical activity and somatotype is shown in Figure 6–1. The red cell volumes were measured with Cr^{51} tagged cells; the plasma and whole blood volumes were derived indirectly from venous hematocrits. Correction factors for plasma trapping and for body: venous hematocrit ratio (p. 407) were not made because, as already discussed, those applying to data on healthy subjects do not necessarily apply to subjects with disease. The volume of packed cells as measured in the hematocrit was read to the top of the buffy coat and thus includes packed leukocytes and platelets, as well as red

cells. Regression equations were derived from the data. The subjects ranged in age from 19 to 52 years. In this sample, age, somatotype and habits of physical activity were found to influence the variance of the data only slightly, after effects of height and weight were accounted for. Muscularity was found to have a slight positive effect while both linearity and obesity had negative effects on the residuals about the height × weight regression planes. Increasing grades of habitual physical activity also had a slight positive effect. This is consistent with the concept that the red cell mass tends to rise with increasing muscle mass but the claim that large differences exist in athletically trained men and women, as compared with inactive persons[17a] requires further study since the conclusions were based on measurements by the CO method.

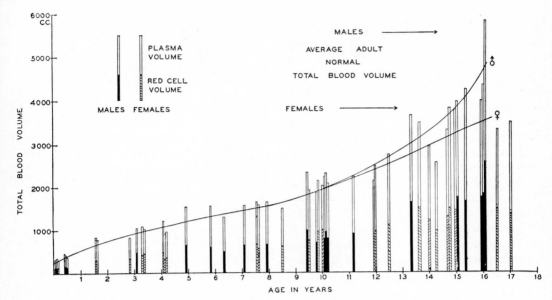

Fig. 6–2.—The plasma, red cell and total blood volume in 50 normal infants and children. The solid lines represent the averages for total blood volume for the entire group. (Brines, Gibson and Kunkel, J. Pediatrics.)

It was reported that there is a tendency for plasma and total blood volumes per unit size to decrease in the sixth decade of life[9] but there is no agreement on this point.[2c,24a,25c]

At *birth* the total blood volume is about 300 ml.[20] (87.9 ml./Kg.[25a]). When measurements were made with the dye, T-1824, a significant increase in circulating plasma, erythrocyte and total blood volumes, approximately 23 per cent, was observed during the first few hours of life.[25a] An average increase in total blood volume, without relation to body weight of 62 ml. was noted. Its source was obscure. In the first 12 weeks of life a reduction in red cell mass occurred and neonatal values were only restored at about 16 weeks. Average values were not considered reliable in the first 11 months of life owing to the wide range of values which were observed. In another study,[20] when P[32] and T-1824 were both used, values for plasma volume of 41.3 ml./Kg. and total blood volume of 84.7 ml./Kg. were obtained in infants. After infancy (Fig. 6–2), blood volume

increases gradually until puberty, when the volume increases more rapidly in males than in females.[19] Both plasma and total blood volumes have been found to be more closely related to physical size than to age.[23,25b]

Physiological Variations. — The total blood volume tends to remain relatively constant and quick adjustments take place[16] in spite of the administration of fluids intravenously as well as by mouth. Even blood transfusions cause only temporary increases in total blood volume in the normal individual, the fluid portions of the blood being rapidly removed by the kidneys and tissues. *Bed rest* is associated with a reduction in blood volume, due almost entirely to a contraction of the plasma volume.[27]

In *pregnancy*, both plasma and total blood volume increase.[8,17c] The greatest increase in plasma volume per unit of body weight occurs during the first trimester, when weight gain is the least, but the greatest absolute increase in blood volume occurs during the last half of pregnancy.[17c] At term the increase in plasma

21

volume may amount to 40 per cent and the increment in total blood volume may be 32 per cent or greater, but individual variations are very great.[18a] This explains why losses of blood are borne so well by the parturient woman. Postpartum, the blood volume returns to normal within a week. The relation of changes in blood volume to the "physiological" anemia of pregnancy will be discussed later (p. 575).

Variations in Disease.—The immediate effect of hemorrhage is a reduction in total blood volume but the plasma, in particular, is restored very quickly by the passage of fluid from the tissues. Even the corpuscular constituents of the blood can be restored to some extent by the liberation of cells from the storage depots of the body. However, if the reduction in circulating blood volume is excessive, shock supervenes.

The changes in blood volume which occur in various diseases cannot be considered in detail here and the interested reader is referred to the various reviews [1d,7,14,22] and the rather voluminous modern literature on shock, hemoconcentration and related subjects. In polycythemia vera, as will be shown later, a markedly increased cell and total blood volume is characteristic of the disease.[11] Contrary to earlier reports,[12,22] the blood volume in secondary polycythemia is also increased.[1d]

In anemia, the reported results have been conflicting but in general it appears that the total blood volume is little reduced, an increase in plasma volume making up for the reduced corpuscular volume.[11] In chronic leukemia increases in total blood volume due to an increase in plasma as well as cells have been recorded[1d] (p. 948). This is true also of other conditions in which splenomegaly occurs, such as cirrhosis of the liver, hemolytic jaundice and Banti's disease.

Data for various *animals* have been published (dog,[3a,15b,17b,19,19a,21a,22] cat,[19a] rabbit,[1,3a,5,19a] rat,[1e] goat,[3a] horse[3a]).

THE SPECIFIC GRAVITY OF BLOOD

The specific gravity of blood, that is, the ratio of the weight of the blood to the weight of the same volume of water at a temperature of 4° C., may be determined directly by weighing a given volume of blood. Schmaltz[36] described a capillary pycnometer for this purpose. Such a method, however, is very time consuming. Hammerschlag[31] devised an indirect method which depends upon the use of two miscible liquids of different specific gravities, in which a drop of blood is suspended by delivering it cautiously from a pipet bent at right angles near its tip. He used a mixture of chloroform and benzol. By altering the quantity of each, a mixture can be obtained in which the blood neither rises nor falls, indicating that its specific gravity is the same as that of the mixture. This is then determined by means of a pycnometer or areometer. The procedure must be carried out very quickly and is not entirely satisfactory. Consequently, numerous modifications have been devised.

In the falling drop method of Barbour and Hamilton,[30] a 10 c.mm. drop of the fluid to be measured is timed as it falls over a distance of 30 cm. through a mixture of xylene and bromobenzene in a tube of 7.5 mm. bore. Its falling time is compared with that of a 10 c.mm. drop of standard potassium sulfate solution of known density. By the use of an alignment chart correcting for room temperature, the unknown density is calculated. The method has been modified and improved by Kagan.[32]

Reznikoff's method[35] is suitable for the determination of the specific gravity of the red blood corpuscles because neither of the liquids he used, benzyl benzoate and cottonseed oil, dissolves any of the constituents of the erythrocyte or enters into a chemical or physical reaction with the corpuscles. A series of mixtures varying from 5 parts of each fluid to 10 parts of benzyl benzoate alone, gives a range in specific gravity of 1.017 to 1.115. A set of small Wassermann tubes containing 2 ml. of each mixture is prepared. By varying the quantity of either fluid 0.02 ml., the specific gravity is altered by 0.002. The red cells are prepared by centrifuging defibrinated blood and carefully removing the supernatant plasma. A drop of the packed red cells is placed in each tube and the tube in which the drop neither rises nor falls indicates the specific gravity of the cells. Reznikoff[35] found this relatively simple method to agree by 0.1 per cent with results obtained by the time consuming pycnometer method.

The normal specific gravity of blood as determined by the pycnometric method is given as 1.048 to 1.066 with reported averages of 1.052 to 1.063. It is slightly higher in men (1.057) than in women (1.053). There is a normal diurnal variation of about 0.003, the specific gravity being generally lower in the afternoon and after meals and higher after exercise and during the night.[34] The specific gravity of the blood serum is 1.026 to 1.031 while that of the erythrocytes is 1.092 to 1.095.[33]

The specific gravity of the blood depends on a number of factors, particularly the quantity and hemoglobin content of the red corpuscles and the protein content of the plasma. Since these are usually measured independently, few have been interested in studying the specific gravity of blood in various disease conditions.[34,37,38] The requirements of war, however, and the need for a quick and ready means for measuring the hemoglobin content, volume of packed cells and plasma protein concentration of blood, led to the development of a specific gravity method for this purpose.[33a]

The **copper sulfate method** for measuring specific gravity has a number of advantages as compared with the methods previously used. No precision instruments are required. The temperature coefficient of expansion of copper sulfate is like that of blood (consequently accurate temperature regulation is unnecessary), the substance used is not toxic and it does not give rise to explosive vapors. The dispersion of blood in copper sulfate is sufficiently slow to permit accurate observations to be made. The procedure consists in letting drops of plasma or whole blood fall into a graded series of solutions of copper sulfate of known specific gravity and noting whether the drops rise or fall in the solutions. Each drop on entering the solution becomes encased in a sack of copper proteinate and remains as a discrete drop without change of gravity for fifteen or twenty seconds, during which its rise or fall reveals its gravity relative to that of the solution. The method is capable of measuring gravities to ± 0.00005, the degree of accuracy depending on the number of standard copper sulfate solutions used. Even when only 16 solutions are used, with intervals of 0.004, gravities are accurate to ± 0.001. A practical feature is the fact that the copper sulfate solution automatically cleans itself. Within a minute or two after the test is completed the material of the drop settles to the bottom. Thus, solutions can be used a number of times.

A saturated copper sulfate solution is prepared by pouring 4 pounds of "fine crystals" of $CuSO_4.5H_2O$ into a 4-liter bottle; to this about 2500 ml. of distilled water is added and the bottle is stoppered and shaken vigorously for a total of five minutes. The temperature of this solution is taken and then the solution is immediately decanted off the crystals and is filtered through cotton or dry filter paper into a clean, dry 4-liter bottle to remove fine suspended crystals. This solution must be used at once to make up a stock solution of gravity 1.100. Depending on the temperature of the saturated solution a certain volume is diluted with a specific quantity of distilled water as indicated in a table supplied in the original publication. Next, from the stock copper sulfate solution of gravity 1.100, standard solutions of lower specific gravity ranging from 1.075 to 1.008, or any lesser number, in accordance with the purpose for which the method is to be used, are prepared.

Whole blood delivered directly from a syringe and needle after withdrawal from a vein, blood collected in an anticoagulant, plasma or serum is used in the test. For very precise determinations tables must be consulted which give the correction to be made for the effect on specific gravity of the quantity of anticoagulant employed and for serum when this has been used instead of plasma. If the ammonium-potassium oxalate mixture (p. 378) is used as anticoagulant in the concentration of 1 mg. per ml. of blood, no correction is needed. The drop of plasma, serum or whole blood is delivered from a height of about 1 cm. above the solution from a medicine dropper or from a syringe needle. The size of the drops does not have to be constant, hence no special pipet is needed for delivering them. The delivered drop breaks through the surface film of the solution and penetrates 2 or 3 cm. below the surface. Within five seconds the momentum of the fall is lost and the drop then either begins to rise or continues to fall. The gravity of the drop relative to the solution does not change appreciably until the drop has been immersed in the solution for another ten or fifteen seconds. Thus, there is ample time to note its behavior during this interval. If the drop is lighter than the test solution it will rise perhaps only a few millimeters and may begin to sink immediately afterwards. If the drop is of the same specific gravity as the standard test solution it will become stationary for this interval and then fall. If the drop is heavier it will continue to fall during the interval.

The method is very useful. A 4-ounce bottle of standard serves for about 100 tests.* It has been calculated that the gravity method indicates the plasma protein content of blood within ±0.3 Gm. per 100 ml. The estimation of cell volume and hemoglobin concentration is based on the assumption that the gravity and hemoglobin concentrations of the red cells are constant. In normal blood the mean deviation of hemoglobins estimated from specific gravity as compared with those determined by oxygen capacity was ±0.65 per cent. The maximum deviation was 2 per cent. The mean deviations of volume of packed red cells determined by centrifuge as compared with those calculated from gravities was ±1.9 per cent of the mean normal. The extreme deviations were from +7.3 to −3.7 per cent, equivalent to +3.4 to −1.7 ml. of cells per 100 ml. blood. In blood with cells of abnormal hemoglobin concentration the calculation of hemoglobin and of volume of packed red cells from gravity values is, of course, not as accurate as in blood with cells of normal composition.

A simple two bottle kit for large scale use in mass casualties has been devised.[33b]

THE BLOOD VISCOSITY

The simplest and most satisfactory method[40] for the measurement of the blood viscosity, is by means of the viscosimeter of Hess.[41] The instrument is based on Poiseuille's law; namely, that the flow rate of fluids in capillaries of equal caliber, under the same pressure and at the same temperature, depends upon the inner friction (viscosity). In the viscosi-

---

* Portable kits may be obtained from E. Machlett & Son, 230 E. 23rd St., New York 10, N. Y.

meter, blood and, in another tube, distilled water, are drawn under equal pressure through capillary tubes of equal caliber and length into graduated tubes. The blood is forced to reach a certain point. The volume of distilled water which has been drawn up under this pressure is indicated by the graduated tube containing the water. Since volume is inversely proportional to viscosity, the reading on the water tube indicates the viscosity of the blood in relation to that of distilled water. The test requires only 1 drop of blood and may be carried out in thirty seconds. Detailed instructions are given by Bircher.[39]

The *relative viscosity of the blood of healthy adults* ranges from 3.5 to 5.4 (average 4.5). According to Hess,[41] the viscosity of the blood of men is greater by 0.5 than that of women, and in children it is less than in adults.

Blood viscosity is dependent upon a number of factors, most important of which is the quantity of erythrocytes. According to Hess, the relationship of the volume of packed red cells to viscosity is hyperbolic but Nygaard and his associates[44] concluded that within a range of 15 to 50 ml. of packed cells, the correlation is linear. In cases of polycythemia, however, the viscosity was actually higher than values calculated from their formula. It has been shown that the influence of various factors which determine the blood viscosity is rapidly intensified by increases in concentration.

The quantity of leukocytes is of significance only when they are greatly increased in number. This is true particularly in cases of myelocytic leukemia because the myeloid leukocytes are larger than lymphocytes. The increased blood viscosity in leukemia is probably responsible for some of the symptoms of this disease, such as dizziness, roaring sensation in the ears and perhaps even priapism. Stephens[45] observed blood viscosities greater than 9 in cases of chronic myelocytic leukemia and demonstrated that blood circulation time was greatly delayed.

The influence of blood platelets on viscosity is not clear.[40] An increase of carbon dioxide in the blood is said to increase viscosity through changes in osmotic relationships. Venous blood has been found to possess a higher viscosity than arterial blood. Colloidal constituents of the plasma also affect viscosity. The viscosity of the blood serum itself is 1.6 to 2.2, that of the plasma about 20 per cent higher.

Naegeli[43] considered viscosimetry to be an important adjunct in routine blood examinations in the sense that a change in many factors is at once reflected by alterations in blood viscosity. In Naegeli's clinic, charts were devised whereby, from the viscosity of the plasma and whole blood, the protein content of the plasma and the volume of packed red cells could be calculated. Viscosimetry received considerable attention in European clinics[42] but has been little used in the United States.

SUSPENSION STABILITY OF THE BLOOD— THE SEDIMENTATION TEST

The blood is essentially a suspension of corpuscles in plasma. In 1918 Fahraeus,[54] while seeking an early test for pregnancy, discovered that the suspension stability of the blood is altered in pregnancy but he found that the speed of sedimentation is also accelerated in many diseases. A test was thus discovered which, because of its simplicity and its wide applicability, soon became very popular.

Variations in the suspension stability of the blood probably led to the development of the theory of the four humors of the ancient Greeks. When blood is withdrawn from a healthy person, it clots quickly and two portions, the clot and the serum, are formed. In the presence of disease, sedimentation of the red corpuscles may be so accelerated that some of the corpuscles quickly settle to the bottom of the vessel in which the blood has been collected and, since they are deprived of oxygen, appear very dark. Above this, the corpuscles still containing oxyhemoglobin, and therefore appearing red, will be found. The rapid sedimentation of the erythrocytes permits some separation of the leukocytes and these, especially when there is leukocytosis, form, together with fibrin, a well-defined grayish-white layer in the uppermost portions of the clot. These three portions of the blood were named respectively, "melancholia" or "black bile," "sanguis" or true blood and "phlegma" or "mucus." The blood serum itself formed the fourth humor, "cholera" or "yellow bile." Ill health was attributed to the failure of the four humors to mix. Not until the time of Paracelsus, it seems, was it considered possible that this separation into several layers might be the result rather than the cause of disease. The grayish-white layer of fibrin and leukocytes continued for centuries to occupy the attention of physicians, being referred to as "crusta inflammatoria," "buffy coat" or "size." Venesection was practiced in order to rid the body of this noxious substance.

The Nature of the Sedimentation Phenomenon.—Much remains to be learned about the true nature of this phenomenon. More than two hundred and fifty years ago, Hewson[59] recognized that the determining factor is contained in the plasma for, when the corpuscles of "sizy" blood were transferred to normal plasma, sedimentation was no longer accelerated. He also observed that the sinking speed of corpuscles is greater in plasma than in serum. Nasse[59] later demonstrated that changes in the specific gravity of the plasma could not be the determining factor, for the dilution of

blood with a weak solution of sodium chloride actually delayed sedimentation. On the other hand, the addition of gum acacia accelerated the sinking velocity. These findings, together with the demonstration that the addition of fibrinogen leads to a greatly increased sedimentation rate,[57] and the fact that the plasma fibrinogen is usually increased when the sedimentation rate is accelerated, led to the assumption that increased sedimentation velocity is the result of an increase in the quantity of fibrinogen in the plasma.[56, 61]

The addition of other protein fractions to blood also leads to an acceleration of sedimentation,[54] but the effect is less marked than that produced by the addition of fibrinogen. Close correlation between plasma globulin and sedimentation rate has been observed,[47, 57] particularly in cases of liver disease in which the plasma fibrinogen was low. Electrophoretic studies have shown as good correlation of sedimentation rate and alpha globulin levels as with fibrinogen levels.[65b] A fraction of plasma containing alpha and beta globulins was found to be about one-third as effective in accelerating sedimentation of red corpuscles as fibrinogen.[56b] Gamma globulin proved least effective; pure albumin inhibited sedimentation. It appears that sedimentation rate is not controlled by the absolute concentration of the total plasma proteins or of the protein fractions, but depends on the relation of the various fractions to one another. In artificial systems a linear relation to the concentration of macromolecules has been observed.[57a] It has been shown that the action of "faster" fractions such as fibrinogen and euglobulin can be inhibited by nucleoprotein and globoglycoid.[56a] It has also been reported that acceleration of erythrocyte sedimentation is caused by the presence of specific plasma proteins, "agglomerins."[64a]

No relationship has been found be-

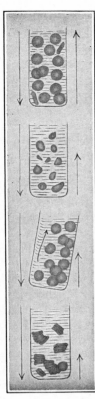

Normal blood. *RF* almost = *DF*.

Anemia. *RF* < *DF*.
  Less retardation from displacement of plasma by red corpuscles.

Inclined tube. *RF* < *DF*. Plasma streams along upper side of tube under the glass, exerting no retarding effect.

Increased rouleau formation. *RF* < *DF* because *RF* depends on relative surface. The larger the volume, the smaller the relative surface.

Fig. 6–3.—The effect of certain factors on sedimentation rate. Arrows pointing downwards represent the downard force of the red corpuscles (*DF*). Arrows pointing upwards represent the retarding effect (*RF*) of the medium and the limitation produced by the end of the tube.

tween sedimentation rate and blood sugar, aëration of the blood or loss of carbon dioxide, or blood calcium or phosphorus. [59,69] It has been reported that the addition of lecithin to blood delays sedimentation while cholesterol has an accelerating effect.[63] The type III pneumococcus polysaccharide produces accelerated sedimentation, and so also does hyaluronic acid. It has been suggested that all highly asymmetrical molecules of large size cause an increase of red cell sedimentation.[61c] Sodium salicylate has been observed to cause a marked reduction of sedimentation rate but this appears to be correlated with the plasma fibrinogen level which, in turn, seems to be related to the total quantity of salicy-

late received by the patient rather than to the quantity of salicylate in the plasma. It has been suggested that the change in fibrinogen may represent an effect of salicylate on the liver.[62f]

In Figure 6–3 are represented some of the physical forces concerned. Settling occurs because the density of the red corpuscles is greater than the density of the medium. The fall of the red corpuscles causes an upward displacement of the medium, thus producing an upward current and a retarding force. In blood drawn from normal persons the concentration of the red corpuscles is relatively great, and a relatively large volume of plasma must be displaced upward if much sedimentation is to occur.

Actually the downward and upward forces in normal blood are nearly equal and consequently little settling occurs.

When the number of red corpuscles is less than normal, there is less retardation of sedimentation by the red corpuscles themselves. No matter how high the column of blood may be, its length is not infinite and retardation is produced by the cells striking the bottom and piling up on one another. Obviously, the fewer the cells the less this effect will be. Methods have been described for "correcting" for the effect of anemia.[64,70] These are discussed more fully below.

The statements which have been made refer to a column of blood which stands in the vertical position. Any deviation from the vertical causes an acceleration in the rate of sedimentation. This is due to the fact that the plasma streams along the upper side of the tube from which the red corpuscles have already settled out and the latter therefore encounter less hindrance from displacement of the medium. This physical principle has been adopted in the development of the angle centrifuge.

The factor which is of chief importance in affecting the sedimentation rate in disease is the size of the sedimenting particle. The larger the volume of the particle, the smaller is the relative surface. The upward or retarding force is a function of the surface area exposed to the medium. The downward force depends on the weight of the particle. While increases above normal in the volume of the individual red corpuscles tend to accelerate their rate of sedimentation, such differences as may be encountered have a comparatively slight effect on sedimentation rate. In the presence of certain conditions, however, the *aggregation* of the red corpuscles is greatly affected, probably because of an alteration in their surface charges. Rouleau formation is greatly increased and this results in the production of corpuscular aggregates of large volume but relatively small surface area. An acceleration in sedimentation rate is the result. This is the chief cause of the acceleration encountered in the presence of disease and in pregnancy. The reason for the increased aggregation is quite obscure. One can only say that variations in sedimentation rate result from changes in the surface charge of the red corpuscles which cause them to aggregate and that these changes are related to alterations in the plasma, particularly in the physical state of the plasma colloids. Changes on the surface of red cells have been observed by electron microscopy.[60a] An attempt has been made to explain rouleau formation as a flocculation reaction between plasma proteins and the lecithoprotein surface of the erythrocyte.[57b]

By capillary microscopy and the observation of the blood in the retinal vessels, variations in the degree of aggregation of the corpuscles *in vivo*, similar to those seen in the test tube, have been described. Fahraeus[54] suggested that aggregation of corpuscles in the central stream of blood vessels permits rapid movement and allows the leukocytes to occupy the peripheral current whence they may readily pass into the tissues. There is disagreement as to whether rouleaux, aggregation and stasis within the capillaries account for the phenomenon of "sludging" of blood.[53,60a]

Methods.—Blood is collected and mixed with an anticoagulant. It is then placed in a tube which is fixed in a vertical position. The *time* required for the upper level of sedimenting corpuscles to fall a specified distance is measured (Linzenmeier method); or, as generally preferred, the *distance* the corpuscles have fallen in an arbitrary period of time is noted (Westergren method). Cutler[51] advocated readings at five-minute intervals for an hour and others make readings one and two hours after the tube has been filled. When frequent readings are

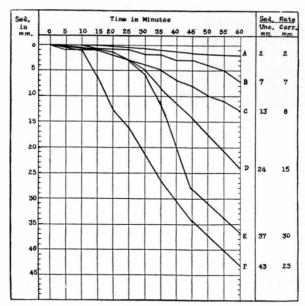

Fig. 6–4.—Sedimentation curves in the normal and in various disorders. *A*, normal; *B*, mild tonsillitis; *C*, mitral insufficiency with active rheumatic infection; *D*, chronic bilateral salpingitis and endocervicitis; *E*, bronchitis and bronchiectasis; *F*, acute pharyngitis, laryngitis and bronchitis. Both the "corrected" and "uncorrected" sedimentation rates are recorded in the last column. (Wintrobe, Med. Clin. North America, courtesy of W. B. Saunders Company.)

made, the results may be plotted graphically (Fig. 6–4). By this means every variation from an almost horizontal line to one which falls quickly in a vertical direction may be encountered. Cutler[51] demonstrated by means of such curves that the process of sedimentation consists of three phases; namely, (1) a preliminary period during which aggregation of the red corpuscles takes place, (2) a period of rapid fall and (3) the phase of packing when the corpuscular masses, in accumulating at the bottom of the tube, slow up the rate of sedimentation. Photographic apparatus has been devised for recording these curves.[62b]

If a record is made of the erythrocyte sedimentation at frequent intervals, it is possible to measure the phase of rapid sedimentation which is, of course, the significant phase. When readings are made only at the end of one hour, the figure obtained is influenced by packing of the corpuscles. In the Rourke-Ernstene method[64] the rate of sedimentation per minute is calculated. It was found that there is a closer correlation between the corrected sedimentation index of Rourke and Ernstene and the plasma fibrinogen concentration than between the quantity of fibrinogen and sedimentation rate as measured by any other method.[57] The chief drawback of the method is that it is somewhat time consuming for routine work. A nomogram for use in conjunction with this method has been devised.[62c]

The method we employ[70] is as follows:

1. Five ml. of venous blood are collected by means of a dry syringe and needle and mixed in a small bottle containing 4 mg. solid potassium oxalate and 6 mg. solid ammonium oxalate. This concentration of oxalate does not alter the sedimentation rate as compared with that of blood collected in heparin. Sequestrene may be used instead.[61b] Less

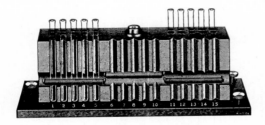

Fig. 6–5.—Support for holding hematocrits during sedimentation test. The stand can be adjusted to a perfectly horizontal position by turning the thumb screws at the base and noting the position of the bubble in the spirit level attached to the top of the block. Hematocrits placed in the V-shaped indentations at the front of the block will then be in a strictly vertical position. (Courtesy of Arthur H. Thomas Company.)

than 1 ml. of blood is needed for the sedimentation test. The remainder can be used for other blood examinations.

2. The blood so collected should be used for the determination of sedimentation rate within two hours of its time of collection. Further delay may be associated with increased suspension stability of the blood.

3. The hematocrit is filled with blood to the 10 cm. mark. The upper level of sedimenting corpuscles may be read at frequent intervals or, more simply, a single reading may be made at the end of one hour.

4. Since sedimentation rate increases with temperature,[61a] the sedimentation test should be carried out at a temperature not less than 22° C. nor greater than 27° C. Within this range variations resulting from differences in temperature are small. If the blood used has previously been kept in a refrigerator it should be permitted to attain the above temperature before being used.

5. The hematocrit should be kept in an exact vertical position during the sedimentation of the blood corpuscles for, when the instrument stands at an angle of even 3 degrees from the vertical, significant acceleration of sedimentation takes place. (A stand which can be

easily adjusted to a perfectly horizontal position is shown in Fig. 6–5).

6. After sedimentation rate has been determined, the hematocrit containing the blood should be centrifuged and the volume of packed red cells determined. In the same tube the volume of packed leukocytes and platelets, and the icterus index can also be measured (see p. 177).

It should be stressed that the hematocrit *must* be fixed in a vertical position. In a shorter and wider bored tube than that of the writer (Fig. 8–2, p. 379) this is less important. The quantity of anticoagulant used is also important, for an excess of oxalate will slow sedimentation. In regard to the influence of temperature, it has been suggested that the sedimentation tube be kept in an incubator at 37.5° C. during the test, with the object of securing comparable results and because the blood is in a more natural environment. While this is true, it is doubtful whether enough is to be gained to offset the added trouble. Graphs for correcting the effect of temperature have been devised.[61a, 68]

Because the relative quantities of plasma and red corpuscles influence sedimentation rate,[52, 70] various methods for "correction" for anemia have been devised.[47a, 58, 70] These have been criticized on the ground that aggregation of the red corpuscles and the size of the particles thus produced is a far more important factor leading to rapid or slow sedimentation of red corpuscles than the degree of anemia and that consequently correction for anemia may give misleading results.[65] Furthermore, differences in the size[62d] and hemoglobin content[62g] of the red corpuscles also affect the sedimentation rate and these have even been claimed to be as important as plasma factors.[62e] Anisocytosis may interfere with rouleau formation and poikilocytosis such as that encountered in sickle cell anemia actually prevents the formation of rouleaux. In sicklemia sedimentation is very slow even when there is marked anemia.[48] The most serious objection to correction for anemia is the fact that all methods of correction are crude and artificial. Furthermore, many who use such corrections do not recognize their artificiality and tend to make more of this ultra-refinement than it merits. It seems best, therefore, to abandon correction of sedimentation rate for anemia. It is our practice, however, to simultaneously record the volume of packed red cells, giving thus an indication of the presence or absence of anemia and its degree.

A number of technical variations have been introduced,[54a] including "micro-methods,"[52,60b,67] sedimentation at an angle of 45° C. in order to accelerate the process,[48a,68a] and improvements in the Westergren method.[52a] It has also been pointed out that the Wintrobe method gives more misleading results than the Westergren technic, chiefly because of the narrower bore of the Wintrobe tube.[65a] The question is whether this disadvantage outweighs the gain from the simultaneous determination of volume of packed red cells, leukocytes and platelets, as well as icterus index, which the smaller tube affords.

Normal Values and Physiological Variations.—The sedimentation rate depends on the type of tube in which it is carried out. When the technic we have described[70] was employed, the sedimentation rate ranged from 0 to 6.5 mm. at the end of one hour in 86 per cent of 137 healthy young adult males and from 0 to 15 mm. in 88 per cent of 100 healthy young women. The average in men was 3.7 mm. and in women 9.6 mm. The difference between the normal sedimentation rate in men and women is largely accounted for by the difference in the quantity of sedimenting red corpuscles. When these sedimentation rates were "corrected" to a volume of packed red cells of 47 ml. per 100 ml. of blood, the sedimentation rate in 72 per cent of the men and women ranged between 0 and 6 mm. and, in an additional 16 per cent, it was 7 to 10 mm.

In boys twelve to twenty years of age, using our method, Gallagher[55] found the "uncorrected" sedimentation rate to range from 1 to 20 mm. at the end of one hour. The average was 4.7 mm. and in 93 per cent the rate was 10 mm. or less. Others[57c] found the sedimentation rate in normal children four to fifteen years of age, regardless of sex, to range from 0 to 20 mm. but in 5 to 10 per cent the rate was higher than 20 mm. Smith[67] found the average rate of settling in infants and children twelve days to fourteen years of age to range, by his method, from 3 to 13 mm. at the end of one hour, with an average of 9 mm. In the blood of the newborn infant with its high volume of packed red cells, sedimentation rates of 0 to 2 mm. are usually found.

The rate of sedimentation under normal conditions is relatively constant. It varies more in women than in men and the causes of this are not fully understood. Some of the fluctuation is related to menstruation but these changes are so small that they are of no clinical significance. In association with *pregnancy*, on the other hand, there is a definite acceleration which begins at about the tenth or twelfth week. The rate gradually increases and does not return to normal until the third or fourth week postpartum.[59,69] In *old age* the erythrocyte sedimentation rate increases.[46,62a]

Variations in Disease.—The sedimentation test is a nonspecific reaction which may be compared with the body temperature, the pulse rate and the leukocyte count, in that it gives information of a general character. It is a measure of the presence and intensity of morbid processes within the body. The test is a useful supplement to these clinical methods because it may be accelerated when the temperature, pulse and even the leukocyte count are normal, particularly in chronic disorders and in localized inflammatory diseases.

In general, sedimentation rate is increased in all acute general infections while, in localized acute inflammatory conditions, variations in sedimentation rate depend on the nature and severity of the morbid process. Thus, in acute catarrhal inflammation the rate tends to be normal, whereas in localized acute suppurations, such as pelvic inflammatory disease, there may be a pronounced acceleration even when the pulse and temperature are normal. Again, in chronic localized infections the rate varies with the extent and nature of the infection. Uncomplicated new growths are not necessarily associated with rapid sedimentation even when malignant. In the case of the latter, sedimentation tends to be accelerated when the tumor is very vascular, when there is a tendency to break down and when there is much reaction about the tumor.[59]

One of the most important uses of the sedimentation test is in calling attention to the presence of more or less occult diseases and for this reason it is as valuable a routine procedure in examination as is urinalysis or the estimation of blood pressure. Not infrequently the sedimentation rate may be found accelerated when clinical and other laboratory studies are negative. If technical error can be ruled out, such a finding should be considered a challenge to the acumen of the physician and diligent search must be made for its cause. Although in our present state of ignorance regarding the exact nature of this phenomenon one cannot insist that an accelerated sedimentation rate always indicates the presence of disease or pregnancy,[46] in clinical practice it may well be regarded as such until the physician is thoroughly satisfied that the patient is perfectly well. On the other hand, it must be pointed out that a normal sedimentation rate does not necessarily mean that all is well and, occasionally,

especially in cachexia, the rate will be found normal in the presence of serious disease.[69] Normal rates have also been found in neoplastic conditions of the liver, cirrhosis[47] and chronic passive congestion.

As an aid in differential diagnosis, the sedimentation test is very useful. Other things being equal, an accelerated rate suggests organic disease rather than a functional disorder, an inflammatory condition rather than a tumor and malignancy instead of benign tumor. The test has been found helpful in differentiating coronary thrombosis from angina pectoris,[66, 71] carcinoma of the stomach from benign ulcer, rheumatoid, tuberculous, gouty[56b] or gonococcal arthritis from osteoarthritis, pelvic inflammatory disease from uncomplicated ovarian cyst or catarrhal appendicitis.[69] However, there are many complications involved in the use of the sedimentation test as an aid to differential diagnosis. Thus, whereas in early ectopic pregnancy the rate is little affected, an accelerated rate is found if the gestation is of ten or twelve weeks' duration, or when hemorrhage or infection has developed. Again, an accelerated rate in abortion may be due to the pregnancy, simple retention of uninfected products of gestation or infection, although in the last instance the sedimentation rate would be very rapid.

It is as a guide to the progress of an infection which has already been recognized that the sedimentation test has proved its chief usefulness. This is particularly true in regard to pulmonary tuberculosis, in which disease the test has received extensive study and wide application. It has been repeatedly shown that the sedimentation rate reflects the intensity of the tuberculous infection more accurately than many of the guides heretofore used.[51] At the Trudeau Sanatorium it was found that in some instances an increase in rate gave warning of relapses before new shadows were found in the roentgenogram.[60] In patients not under constant observation whose temperature could not be regularly recorded, and in those receiving pneumothorax therapy, the test was of great value.[51] Again, in rheumatic carditis the sedimentation rate has often been a useful guide to the state of repair, remaining accelerated when the temperature, leukocyte count and even pulse were normal, and presaging a relapse when other signs were quite negative.[49,56] To cite one more example, in infections such as scarlet fever, failure of the accelerated rate to return to normal has often been the first clue to the development of some complication.[50] But it must be remembered that the method is not infallible.[62] In one series of more than 5000 cases of tuberculosis, a normal sedimentation rate was found in as many as 2.1 per cent of cases in which the sputum was positive for tubercle bacilli and in some of which even cavities were present.[46a]

BIBLIOGRAPHY

Blood Volume

1. ARMIN, J., GRANT, R. T., PELS, H. and REEVE, E. B.: The Plasma, Cell and Blood Volumes of Albino Rabbits as Estimated by the Dye (T 1824) and ^{32}P Marked Cell Methods, J. Physiol., 116, 59, 1952.
1a. BARNES, D. W. H., LOUTIT, J. F. and REEVE, E. B.: A Comparison of Estimates of Circulating Red Blood Cell Volume Given by the Ashby Marked Red Cell Method and the T1824-Hæmatocrit Method in Man, Clin. Sci., 7, 135 and 155, 1948.
1c. VON BEHRING: Die Antitoxinmethode zur Blutmengebestimung, München. med. Wchnschr., 58, 655, 1911.
1d. BERLIN, N. I., HYDE, G. M., PARSONS, R. J. and LAWRENCE, J. H.: The Blood Volume in Various Medical and Surgical Conditions, New England J. Med., 247, 675, 1952.
1e. BERLIN, N. I., HUFF, R. L., VAN DYKE, D. C. and HENNESSY, T. G.: The Blood Volume of the Adult Rat, as Determined by Fe^{59} and P^{32} Labelled Red Cells, Proc. Soc. Exper. Biol. & Med., 71, 176, 1949.
1f. BRADY, L. W., COOPER, D. Y., COLODZIN, M., McCLENATHAN, J. E., KING, E. R., and

WILLIAMS, R.: Blood Volume Studies in Normal Humans, Surg., Gynec. & Obst., 97, 25, 1953.
1g. BRINES, J. K., GIBSON, J. G., 2D, and KUNKEL, P.: The Blood Volume in Normal Infants and Children, J. Pediatrics, 18, 447, 1941.
2. CAMPBELL, T. J., FROHMAN, B. and REEVE, E. B.: A Simple, Rapid and Accurate Method of Extracting T-1824 from Plasma, Adapted to the Routine Measurement of Blood Volume, J. Lab. & Clin. Med., 52, 768, 1958.
2a. CHAPLIN, H., JR.: Precision of Red Cell Volume Measurement Using ^{32}P-Labelled Cells, J. Physiol., 123, 22, 1954.
2b. CHAPLIN, H., JR., MOLLISON, P. L. and VETTER, H.: The Body-venous Hematocrit Ratio, J. Clin. Invest., 32, 1309, 1953.
2c. COHN, J. E. and SHOCK, N. W.: Blood Volume Studies in Middle-Aged and Elderly Males, Am. J. Med. Sc., 217, 388, 1949.
3. COHNSTEIN, J. and ZUNTZ, N.: Untersuchungen über den Flüssigkeits-Austausch zwischen Blut und Geweben unter verschiedenen physiologischen und pathologishen Bedingungen, Arch. f. d. ges. Physiol., 42, 303, 1888.
3a. COURTICE, F. C.: The Blood Volume of Normal Animals, J. Physiol., 102, 290, 1943.
4. CRISPELL, K. R., PORTER, B. and NIESET, R. T.: Studies of Plasma Volume Using Human Serum Albumin Tagged with Radioactive Iodine,^{131} J. Clin. Invest., 29, 513, 1950.
5. CULBERTSON, J. T.: The Determination of the Plasma Volume and the Blood Volume of the Rabbit by the Injection of Homologous Anti-crystallized-Egg-Albumin-Serum, Am. J. Physiol., 107, 120, 1934.
7. ERLANGER, J.: Blood Volume and Its Regulation, Physiol. Rev., 1, 177, 1921.
7a. FUDENBERG, H., BALDINI, M., MAHONEY, J. P. and DAMESHEK, W.: The Body Hematocrit/ Venous Hematocrit Ratio and the Splenic "Reservoir," Blood, 17, 71, 1961.
8. GEMZELL, C. A., ROBBE, H., and SJÖSTRAND, T.: Blood Volume and Total Amount of Haemoglobin in Normal Pregnancy and the Puerperium, Acta obst. et gynec. scandinav., 33, 289, 1954.
9. GIBSON, J. G. and EVANS, W. A.: The Relation of Plasma and Total Blood Volume to Venous Pressure, Blood Velocity Rate, Physical Measurements, Age and Sex in Ninety Normal Humans, J. Clin. Invest., 16, 317, 1937.
11. GIBSON, J. G., HARRIS, A. W. and SWIGERT, V. W.: Macrocytic and Hypochromic Anemias Due to Chronic Blood Loss, Hemolysis and Miscellaneous Causes, and Poly-

cythemia Vera, J. Clin. Invest., *18*, 621, 1939.

12. GIBSON, J. G., WEISS, S., EVANS, R. D., PEACOCK, W. C., IRVINE, J. W., JR., GOOD, W. M. and KIP, A. F.: The Measurement of the Circulating Red Cell Volume by Means of Two Radioactive Isotopes of Iron, J. Clin. Invest., *25*, 616, 838, and 848, 1946.

12a. GRAY, S. J. and STERLING, K.: The Tagging of Red Cells and Plasma Proteins with Radioactive Chromium, J. Clin. Invest., *29*, 1604, 1950; *ibid.*, *32*, 991, 1953.

13. GREGERSEN, M. I., GIBSON, J. G. and STEAD, E. A.: Plasma Volume Determinations With Dyes; Errors in Colorimetry; Use of the Blue Dye T–1824, Am. J. Physiol. (Proc.), *113*, 54, 1935; *see also* Am. J. Physiol., *120*, 494, 1937; J. Lab. & Clin. Med., *23*, 423, 1938; Am. J. Physiol., *125*, 142, 1939; *Ibid.*, *138*, 698, 1943; *Ibid.*, *163*, 517, 1950.

14. GREGERSEN, M. I. and RAWSON, RUTH A.: Blood Volume, Physiol. Rev., *39*, 307, 1959.

15. HAHN, P. F., ROSS, J. F., BALE, W. F., BALFOUR, W. M., and WHIPPLE, G. H.: Red Cell and Plasma Volumes (Circulating and Total) as Determined by Radio Iron and by Dye, J. Exper. Med., *75*, 221, 1942; Am. J. Physiol., *136*, 314, 1942; *Ibid.*, *141*, 363, 1944.

15a. HLAD, C. J., JR. and TANZ, ROSE: An Analysis of Technical Errors in Radioalbumin Blood Volume Methods and Presentation of a Modified Method, J. Lab. & Clin. Med., *52*, 289, 1958.

15b. HOPPER, J., JR., TABOR, H. and WINKLER, A. W.: Simultaneous Measurements of the Blood Volume in Man and Dog by Means of Evans' Blue Dye, T–1824, and by Means of Carbon Monoxide, J. Clin. Invest., *23*, 628, 636, 1944.

15c. INKLEY, S. R., BROOKS, L. and KRIEGER, H.: A Study of Methods for the Prediction of Plasma Volume, J. Lab. & Clin. Med., *45*, 841, 1955.

16. KALTREIDER, N. L. and MENEELY, G. R.: The Effect of Exercise on the Volume of the Blood, J. Clin. Invest., *19*, 627, 1940.

17. KEITH, N. M., ROWNTREE, L. G. and GERAGHTY, J. T.: A Method for the Determination of Plasma and Blood Volume, Arch. Int. Med., *16*, 547, 1915.

17a. KJELLBERG, S. R., RUDHE, U. and SJÖSTRAND, T.: Increase of the Amount of Hemoglobin and Blood Volume in Connection with Physical Training, Acta physiol. scandinav., *19*, 146, 1949.

17b. KRIEGER, H., STORAASLI, J. P., FRIEDELL, H. L. and HOLDEN, W. D.: A Comparative Study of Blood Volume in Dogs, Proc. Soc. Exper. Biol. & Med., *68*, 511, 1948.

17c. LUND, C. J. and SISSON, T. R. C.: Blood Volume and Anemia of Mother and Baby, Am. J. Obst. & Gynec., *76*, 1013, 1958.

18a. McLENNAN, C. E. and THOUIN, L. G.: Blood Volume in Pregnancy, Am. J. Obst. & Gynec., *55*, 189, 1948.

19. McQUARRIE, I. and DAVIS, N. C.: Blood Volume as Determined by the Change in Refractivity of the Serum Non-protein Fraction After Injection of Certain Colloids Into the Circulation, Am. J. Physiol., *51*, 257, 1920.

19a. MEEK, W. J. and GASSER, H. S.: Blood Volume, Am. J. Physiol., *47*, 302, 1918–19.

19b. MOLLISON, P. L., ROBINSON, MARGARET A. and HUNTER, DENISE A.: Improved Method of Labelling Red Cells with Radioactive Phosphorus, Lancet, *1*, 766, 1958.

20. MOLLISON, P. L., VEALL, N. and CUTBUSH, M.: Red Cell and Plasma Volume in Newborn Infants, Arch. Dis. Child., *25*, 242, 1950.

20a. MOLDOWNEY, F. P.: The Relationship of Total Red Cell Mass to Lean Body Mass in Man, Clin. Sci., *16*, 163, 1957.

21. NOMOF, N., HOPPER, J., JR., BROWN, E., SCOTT, K. and WENNESLAND, R.: Simultaneous Determinations of the Total Volume of Red Blood Cells by Use of Carbon Monoxide and Chromium[51] in Healthy and Diseased Human Subjects, J. Clin. Invest. *33*, 1382, 1954.

21a. PRICE, P. B. and LONGMIRE, W. P.: The Use of T-1824 in Plasma Volume Determinations, Bull. Johns Hopkins Hosp., *71*, 51, 1942; *69*, 327, 1941; *75*, 14, 1944.

21b. READ, R. C.: Studies of Red-Cell Volume and Turnover Using Radiochromium, New England J. Med., *250*, 1021, 1954; A. M. A. Arch. Int. Med., *100*, 259, 1957.

21c. ROOT, W. S., ROUGHTON, F. J. W. and GREGERSEN, M. I.: Simultaneous Determinations of Blood Volume by CO and Dye (T-1824) under Various Conditions, Am. J. Physiol., *146*, 739, 1946.

22. ROWNTREE, L. G., BROWN, G. E., and ROTH, G. M.: *The Volume of Blood and Plasma in Health and Disease*, Philadelphia and London, W. B. Saunders Company, 1929.

23. RUSSELL, S. J. M.: Blood Volume Studies in Healthy Children, Arch. Dis. Childhood, *24*, 88, 1949.

24. SCHULTZ, A. L., HAMMARSTEN, J. F., HELLER, B. I. and EBERT, R. V.: A Critical Comparison of the T-1824 Dye and Iodinated Albumin Methods for Plasma Volume Measurement, J. Clin. Invest., *32*, 107, 1953.

24a. SCHMIDT, L. A., III *et al.*: Blood Volume Changes in the Aged, Surgery, *40*, 938, 1956.

25. SHIRES, T., WILLIAMS, J. and BROWN, F.: Simultaneous Measurement of Plasma Volume, Extracellular Fluid Volume, and Red Blood Cell Mass in Man Utilizing I[131], S[3·]O₄, and Cr[51], J. Lab. & Clin. Med., *55*, 776, 1960.

25a. SISSON, T. R. C., LUND, C. J., WHALEN, LORRAINE E. and TELEK, AMALIA: The Blood Volume of Infants, J. Pediat., *55*, 163, 1959; *ibid.*, *56*, 43, 1960.

25b. SJÖSTRAND, T.: A Method for the Determination of Carboxy-Hæmoglobin Concentrations by Analysis of the Alveolar Air, Acta physiol. scandinav., *16*, 201 and 211, 1948; *ibid.*, *18*, 324, 1949; Physiol. Rev., *33*, 202, 1953.

25c. SKLAROFF, D. M.: Isotopic Determination of Blood Volume in the Normal Aged, Am. J. Roentgenol., *75*, 1082, 1956.

26. STORAASLI, J. P., KRIEGER, H., FRIEDELL, H. L. and HOLDEN, W. D.: The Use of Radioactive Iodinated Plasma Protein in the Study of Blood Volumes, Surg., Gynec. & Obst., *91*, 458, 1950.

27. TAYLOR, H. L., ERICKSON, L., HENSCHEL, A. and KEYS, A.: The Effect of Bed Rest on the Blood Volume of Normal Young Men, Am. J. Physiol., *144*, 227, 1945.

28. VEREL, D.: Observations on the Distribution of Plasma and Red Cells in Disease, Clin. Sci., *13*, 51, 1954.

28a. VEREL, D., BURY, J. D. and HOPE, A.: Blood Volume Changes in Pregnancy and the Puerperium, Clin. Sci., *15*, 1, 1956.

29. WENNESLAND, R. *et al.*: Red Cell, Plasma and Blood Volume in Healthy Men Measured by Radiochromium (Cr[51]) Cell Tagging and Hematocrit, J. Clin. Invest., *38*, 1065, 1959.

29a. ZIPF, R. E., WEBBER, J. M. and GROVE, G. R.: A Gravimetric Technique for the Determination of Plasma Volumes with Radio-iodinated Human and Serum Albumin, J. Lab. & Clin. Med., *45*, 648 and 800, 1955.

Specific Gravity

30. BARBOUR, H. G. and HAMILTON, W. F.: The Falling Drop Method for Determining Specific Gravity, J. Biol. Chem., *69*, 625, 1926.

31. HAMMERSCHLAG, A.: Eine neue Methode zur Bestimmung des spezifischen Gewichts des Blutes, Ztschr. f. klin. Med., *20*, 444, 1892.

32. KAGAN, B. M.: A Falling Drop Method for the Determination of Specific Gravity, J. Clin. Invest., *17*, 369, 1938; J. Lab. & Clin. Med., *26*, 1681, 1941.

33. LEAKE, C. D., KOHL, M. and STEBBINS, G.: Diurnal Variations in the Blood Specific Gravity and Erythrocyte Count in Healthy Human Adults, Am. J. Physiol., *81*, 493, 1927.

33a. PHILLIPS, R. A., VAN SLYKE, D. D., HAMILTON, P. B., DOLE, V. P., EMERSON, K., JR., and ARCHIBALD, R. M.: Measurement of Specific Gravities of Whole Blood and Plasma by Standard Copper Sulfate Solutions, J. Biol. Chem., *183*, 305, 1950.

33b. POLLER, L.: An Evaluation of the Copper Sulphate Blood Specific Gravity Method with Reference to the Control of Fluid Therapy in Mass Casualties, Acta haemat., *21*, 242, 1959.

34. POLOWE, D.: The Specific Gravity of the Blood: Its Clinical Significance, J. Lab. & Clin. Med., *14*, 811, 1929.

35. REZNIKOFF, P.: A Method for the Determination of the Specific Gravity of Red Blood Cells, J. Exper. Med., *38*, 441, 1923.

36. SCHMALTZ, R.: Untersuchung des spezifischen Gewichtes der menschlichen Blutes, Deutsch. Arch. f. klin. Med., *47*, 145, 1891.

37. STRASSER, U.: Die Pyknometrie des Blutserums in Dienste der Klinik, Wien. Arch. f. inn. Med. *19*, 451, 1930.

38. TERRY, R. J. and SEIB, G. A.: On the Specific Gravity of the Blood, Anat. Rec., *36*, 279, 1927.

Blood Viscosity

39. BIRCHER, M. E.: Clinical Diagnosis by the Aid of Viscosimetry of the Blood and the Serum With Special Reference to the Viscosimeter of W. R. Hess, J. Lab. & Clin. Med., 7, 134, 1921 (Bibliography); II. The Value of the Refracto-viscosimetric Properties of the Blood Serum in Cancer, *Ibid.*, 7, 660; III. The Value of the Refracto-viscosimetric Properties of the Blood Serum in Tuberculosis, *Ibid.*, 7, 733.

40. HEILMEYER, L.: *in* Hirschfeld, H., and Hittmair, A., *Handbuch der allgemeinen Hämatologie*, Berlin, Urban & Schwarzenberg, 2, Part 1, 373 (Bibliography), 1933.

41. HESS, W. R.: Viscosität des Blutes und Herzarbeit, Vierteljahrs-schr. d. Naturf.-Gesellsch, Zürich, 1906.

42. LAWRENCE, J. S.: The Plasma Viscosity, J. Clin. Path., *3*, 332, 1950.

43. NAEGELI, O.: *Blutkrankheiten und Blutdiagnostik*, Berlin, Julius Springer, p. 38, 1931.

44. NYGAARD, K. K., WILDER, R. M., and BERKSON, J.: The Relation Between Viscosity of the Blood and the Relative Volume of Erythrocytes (Hematocrit Value), Am. J. Physiol., *114*, 128, 1935.

45. STEPHENS, D. J.: Relation of Viscosity of Blood to Leukocyte Count, With Particular Refer-

ence to Chronic Myelogenous Leukemia, Proc. Soc. Exper. Biol. & Med., *35*, 251, 1936.

Suspension Stability of the Blood

46. ANSELL, BARBARA and BYWATERS, E. G. L.: The "Unexplained" High Erythrocyte Sedimentation Rate, Brit. M. J., *1*, 372, 1958.

46a.BANYAI, A. L., and CALDWELL, E.: Normal Sedimentation Rate in Open Pulmonary Tuberculosis, Am. Rev. Tuberc., *38*, 491, 1938; Arch. Int. Med., *72*, 245, 1943.

47. BENDIEN, W. M. and SNAPPER, I.: Zusammenhang zwischen der Senkungsgeschwindigkeit der roten Blutkörperchen und dem Eiweissspektrum, Biochem. Ztschr., *235*, 14, 1931.

47a.BEST, W. R.: A Slide Rule to Correct the Sedimentation Rate for Anemia, Am. J. Clin. Path., *20*, 87, 1950.

48. BUNTING, H.: Sedimentation Rates of Sickled and Non-sickled Cells From Patients With Sickle Cell Anemia, Am. J. Med. Sc., *198*, 191, 1939.

48a.CANTARELLI, G., DI MASSIMO-SIMONETTI, S. and NARDI, E.: La velocità di sedimentazione delle emazie, Policlinico (sez. med.), *66*, 1, 1959.

49. COBURN, A. F. and KAPP, E. M.: Observations on the Development of the High Blood Sedimentation Rate in Rheumatic Carditis, J. Clin. Invest., *15*, 715, 1936.

50. COOKSON, J. S.: Erythrocyte Sedimentation Rate in Scarlet Fever and Its Complications, Brit. J. Dis. Child., *33*, 251, 1936.

51. CUTLER, J. W.: The Practical Application of the Blood Sedimentation Test in General Medicine, Am. J. Med. Sc., *183*, 643, 1932.

52. ———— A Standardized Technique for Sedimentation Rate, J. Lab. & Clin. Med., *26*, 542, 1940

52a.DAWSON, J. B.: The E. S. R. in a New Dress, Brit. M. J., *1*, 1697, 1960.

53. DITZEL, J.: Relationship of Blood Protein Composition to Intravascular Erythrocyte Aggregation (Sludged Blood), Acta med. scandinav. (Suppl. 343), *164*, 11, 1959.

54. FAHRAEUS, R.: The Suspension Stability of the Blood, Acta med. scandinav., *55*, 1, 1921 (Bibliography); Acta med. scandinav., *161*, 151, 1958.

54a.FRIMBERGER, F.: Differential-Blutsenkung, Folia haemat., *2*, 280, 1958; *ibid.*, *3*, 3, 1958.

55. GALLAGHER, J. R.: The Value of the Blood Sedimentation Test in the Routine Medical Examination of Adolescents and in Certain of Their Diseases, Am. J. Med. Sc., *188*, 450, 1934.

56. GILLIGAN, D. R. and ERNSTENE, A. C.: The Relationship Between the Erythrocyte Sedimentation Rate and the Fibrinogen Content of Plasma, Am. J. Med. Sc., *187*, 552, 1934.

56a.GORDON, C. M., and WARDLEY, J. R.: The Effect of the Plasma Proteins Upon the Sedimentation Rate of Human Blood, Biochem. J., *37*, 393, 1943.

56b.HADEN, R. L. and KINELL, J.: The Sedimentation Rate in Gout, J. Lab. & Clin. Med., *27*, 725, 1942.

57. HAM, T. H. and CURTIS, F. C.: Sedimentation Rate of Erythrocytes, Medicine, *17*, 447, 1938 (Bibliography).

57a.HARDWICKE, J., and SQUIRE, J. R.: The Basis of the Erythrocyte Sedimentation Rate, Clin. Sci., *11*, 333, 1952.

57b.HIRSCHBOECK, J. S.: Lecithin and the Erythrocyte Factor in the Blood Sedimentation Phenomenon, Blood, *2*, 578, 1947.

57c.HOLLINGER, N. F., and ROBINSON, S. J.: A Study of the Erythrocyte Sedimentation Rate for Well Children, J. Pediat., *42*, 304, 1953.

58. HYNES, M. and WHITBY, L. E. H.: Correction of Sedimentation Rate for Anemia, Lancet, *2*, 249, 1938.

59. KATZ, G. and LEFFKOWITZ, M.: Die Blutkörperchensenkung, Ergebn. d. inn. Med. u. Kinderh., *33*, 266, 1928 (Bibliography).

60. KELLEY, W. O.: The Erythrocyte Sedimentation Rate in Estimating Activity in Pulmonary Tuberculosis, Am. Rev. Tuberc., *34*, 489, 1936.

60a.KNISELY, M. H., BLOCH, E. H., BROOKS, F., and WARNER, L.: Microscopic Observations of the Circulating Blood of Nine Healthy Normal Horses, All of Which had Unagglutinated Circulating Blood Cells and High *in Vitro* Erythrocyte Sedimentation Rates, Am. J. Med. Sc., *219*, 249, 1950; Science, *115*, 46, 1952.

60b.LANDAU, A.: Microsedimentation, Am. J. Dis. Child., *45*, 692, 1933.

61. LUCIA, S. P., BLUMBERG, T., BROWN, J. W., and GOSPE, S. M.: The Relation Between the Suspension Stability of Erythrocytes and Various Constituents of Pathologic Human Blood, Am. J. Med. Sc., *192*, 179, 1936.

61a.MANLEY, R. W.: The Effect of Room Temperature on Erythrocyte Sedimentation Rate and Its Correction, J. Clin. Path., *10*, 354, 1957.

61b.MELVILLE, I. D. and RIFKIND, B. M.: The Use of a Sequestrene-citrate Mixture in the Estimation of the Blood Sedimentation Rate, J. Clin. Path., *12*, 258, 1959; Brit. M. J., *1*, 107, 1960.

61c. MEYER, K., HAHNEL, E. and FEINER, R. R.: Experiments on Erythrocyte Sedimentation Rate, Proc. Soc. Exper. Biol. & Med., *58*, 36, 1945.

62. NOEHREN, T. H.: Normal Sedimentation Rates in Active Pulmonary Tuberculosis, J. Lab. & Clin. Med., *32*, 526, 1947.

62a. OLBRICH, O.: Blood Changes in the Aged, Edinburgh Med. J., *55*, 100, 1948.

62b. OLMSTED, F. and HAINLINE, A., JR.: Automatic Photographic Recording of Sedimentation Rates, Am. J. Clin. Path., *24*, 1030, 1954.

62c. ORDWAY, N. K. and SINGER, R. B.: A Simplified Sedimentation Rate Technique with Combined Chart and Correction Nomogram, J. Lab. & Clin. Med., *33*, 511, 1948.

62d. PHEAR, D.: The Influence of Erythrocyte Factors on Their Sedimentation Rate, J. Clin. Path., *10*, 357, 1957.

62e. POOLE, J. C. F. and SUMMERS, G. A. C.: Correction of E. S. R. in Anemia, Brit. Med. J., *1*, 353, 1952.

62f. RAPOPORT, S. and GUEST, G. M.: Effect of Salicylate on Plasma Fibrinogen and Sedimentation Rate in Rheumatic and Non-Rheumatic Patients, Proc. Soc. Exper. Biol. & Med., *61*, 43, 1946.

62g. ROGERS, K. B.: Effect of Hypochromasia on the Specific Gravity and Sedimentation Rate of Red Cells, Brit. Med. J., *1*, 1109, 1952.

63. ROPES, M. W., ROSSMEISL, E. and BAUER, W.: The Relationship Between the Erythrocyte Sedimentation Rate and the Plasma Proteins, J. Clin. Invest., *18*, 791, 1939.

64. ROURKE, M. D. and ERNSTENE, A. C.: A Method for Correcting the Erythrocyte Sedimentation Rate for Variations in the Cell Volume Percentage of Blood, J. Clin. Invest., *8*, 545, 1930.

64a. RUHENSTROTH-BAUER, C., BRITTINGER, G., GRANZER. E. and NASS, G.: The Mechanism and the Significance of the Sedimentation Rate of Red Blood Cells, Deutsches med. Wchnschr., *85*, 808, 1960.

65. SCHUSTER, N. H.: Sedimentation Rate in Relation to the Red Cell Count: The Problem of Correction, Tubercle, *19*, 529, 1938.

65a. SHANNON, F. T. and BYWATER, E. G. L.: Cause of Anomalous Results in the Erythrocyte Sedimentation Rate Using Wintrobe's Method, Brit. M. J., *2*, 1405, 1957.

65b. SHEDLOVSKY, T. and SCUDDER, J.: A Comparison of Erythrocyte Sedimentation Rates and Electrophoretic Patterns of Normal and Pathological Human Bloods, J. Exper. Med., *75*, 119, 1942.

66. SHOOKHOFF, C., DOUGLAS, A. H. and RABINOWITZ, A.: Sedimentation Time in Acute Cardiac Infarction. Ann. Int. Med., *9*, 1101, 1936.

67. SMITH, C. H.: A Method for Determining the Sedimentation Rate and Red Cell Volume in Infants and Children With the Use of Capillary Blood, Am. J. Med. Sc., *192*, 73, 1936.

68. WARTMAN, W. B.: Effect of Room Temperature on Sedimentation Rate of Red Blood Cells of Man, Am. J. Med. Sc., *212*, 207, 1946.

68a. WASHBURN, A. H. and MEYERS, ALDULA, J.: The Sedimentation of Erythrocytes at an Angle of 45 Degrees, J. Lab. & Clin. Med., *49*, 318, 1957.

69. WINTROBE, M. M.: The Erythrocyte Sedimentation Test, Internat. Clin., 46th ser., *2*, 34, 1936 (Bibliography).

70. WINTROBE, M. M., and LANDSBERG, J. W.: A Standardized Technique for the Blood Sedimentation Test, Am. J. Med. Sc., *189*, 102, 1935.

71. WOOD, P.: The Erythrocyte Sedimentation Rate in Diseases of the Heart, Quart. J. Med., *5*, 1, 1936.

Chapter 7

Blood Groups and Blood Transfusion

THE advances which have been made in our knowledge of the blood groups have been so great that the geneticist, the anthropologist and the jurist each in his own field, have found this information useful. Furthermore, as an example of the impact, one on the other, of scientific discovery and political and economic affairs, the development of this field of knowledge is significant since it was the recognition of the value and need for blood and blood fractions in war that gave the great impetus to the study of blood preservation, stock-piling and blood banking which made blood transfusion so readily available.

It has become evident that blood transfusion is a most effective therapeutic tool when judiciously applied. However, the use of blood and blood products has become so commonplace that the dangers as well as the advantages of these valuable therapeutic agents have been multiplied manifold. It is not sufficiently realized that the indiscriminate use of blood is a waste of funds and efforts, and a source of danger to the patient.

Before considering the indications for blood transfusions, the choice of methods and the effects, both good and bad, of the administration of blood and blood products, it will be advantageous to describe the different blood groups and to discuss certain matters relating to technic.

THE BLOOD GROUPS

The ABO System.—In 1901 Landsteiner demonstrated that, according to whether the red cells contain one (A) or another (B), agglutinogen, or both (AB) or neither (O), human beings could be classified into four groups. He also showed that there are antibodies (agglutinins) to A and B, named α and β, and that a person's serum does not contain the antibody for the antigen present in his own red cells but carries antibodies against the agglutinogens he does not possess. Landsteiner's nomenclature for the four blood groups is now in general use but for a time it was rivaled by those of Moss and Jansky, group I of Moss corresponding to Landsteiner's AB, group II corresponding to A, group III to B and group IV to O.

Subgroups of A were described in 1911 when it was demonstrated that nearly all anti-A sera are composed of qualitatively different fractions; namely, anti-A proper (α) which reacts with agglutinogens A_1 and A_2 and anti-A_1 (α_1) which reacts only with agglutinogen A_1. The anti-A agglutinins are present in all B and O sera but the quantities of α and α_1 vary. These subgroups of A increase the number of groups in the ABO system from four to six, A_1, A_2, B, A_1B, A_2B, and O.

The significance of the subgroups of A in blood grouping will be considered later. It may be added here, however, that rare sera from A_1 and A_1B individuals (1 out of 250) contain agglutinins reacting with A_2 blood, that is, α_2. These agglutinins, however, are not specific for A_2 cells for they react with all group O cells more intensely than with A_2 cells. For this reason they are also known as anti-O agglutinins. This observation has led to the suggestion that O has a positive character rather than the negative one implied by Landsteiner.

It is becoming evident that the ABO blood group system is not as simple as was once assumed. Thus, an agglutinogen, A_3, has been described which seems to be a weaker form belonging to the A_1A_2 series.[76a] Again, there appear to be genes which modify the expression of the A_1A_2BO genes, such as the "Bombay" phenotype, in which the very rare gene x in double dose prohibits the B and O genes from putting antigen into red cells and into saliva.[45] Another very rare gene, y, in double dose modifies the development of the A antigen. The phenotypes A_x and A_m may be due to the yy genes.[92] The phenotype A_x may be the same as what has been reported as A_4, A_5, A_z, A_0 and C. The suggestion that group O serum may contain another antibody, besides α and β, anti-C, the so-called "cross-reacting antibody," has not found support.[39a]

Failure of a strong A antigen to agglutinate with anti-A serum led to the discovery of another blood group, A_g.[87]

Although, so far, no clear division of B into subgroups has been made, some observations in this direction have been reported.[26a] It appears possible, furthermore, that a B-like antigen may be acquired in association with illness.[9a,30b]

It was observed that anti-O sera could be divided into two kinds; namely, those inhibited by the addition of saliva of secretors (p. 347) of any group (called "anti-H") and those not inhibited ("anti-O").[56a] The H antigen seems to be present in almost all human red cells but varies in quantity according to the ABO group. The reactivity of the various groups with anti-H serum is greatest with group O and least with group A_1B in the following order: $O > A_2 > A_2B > B > A_1 > A_1B$. Some have postulated that the H substance may represent the "positive" character of O referred to above.

"Immune" anti-A and anti-B, as opposed to "natural" antisera, have been described.[101a] The fact that these antibodies are associated with the more serious forms of ABO hemolytic disease of the newborn (p. 764) may be related to the smaller size of these antibody molecules and their easier passage through the placental barrier, as compared with "natural" antibodies. Antigens with at least some of the serological properties of A and B are to be found in the red cells and tissues of a very wide range of animals.[62a] Plants have been discovered to have agglutinins for human blood group antigens, a finding which may offer biochemists a new approach to the study of the antigens. The chemistry of these antigens is being elucidated by Kabat[2a] and others.

The blood group substances are widely distributed in human tissues.[82b] A and B antigens occur in platelets (p. 840) and perhaps in leukocytes.

It is clear that much more remains to be learned about the ABO blood group system. The possibility exists that the ABO system is the result of gene interaction between expressor and suppressor groups. A detailed discussion will be found in the monograph of Race and Sanger.[70]

The MNSs and Related Blood Groups.—The agglutinogens M and N were discovered by Landsteiner and Levine in 1927 by means of immunization experiments in which human blood was injected into rabbits. Three blood groups were identified, M, N and MN. Twenty years later the antibody anti-S was discovered and, in 1951, anti-s. These were shown to be closely associated with M and N, probably existing as closely linked loci on a single chromosome.[77] The antibody "anti-U." discovered as the result of a fatal transfusion reaction in a Negro woman,[101] probably is the result of a third allele at the Ss locus, S^u, or is anti-Ss.[70]

Not to be outdone by other blood group-systems, the MN system is developing more complexities. There appear to be three alleles, M_1, M_2 and N.[77] Another allele,[1a] probably, is the rare antigen M^g. On the same chromosome [33a,55a] but not allelic are Hu, He, Mi^a, Vw (Gr) and Vr.

From a clinical standpoint these antigens are important if antibodies arise as immune responses in man. Anti-M, anti-N, anti-Hu and anti-He seldom are found under such circumstances[70] although isosensitization to the M agglutinogen may occasionally cause a transfusion reaction or erythroblastosis fetalis[14a] and in several instances anti-N was regarded as the cause of a hemolytic reaction.[89] On the other hand, anti-S, anti-s, anti Ss (anti-U), anti-Mi^a and anti-Vw have been encountered a number of times as immune responses to transfusion or in pregnancy[70] (p. 764).

The P Blood Groups.—Landsteiner and Levine demonstrated still another system, P+ and P— by immunization experiments in rabbits. Subsequently the antigen Tj^a was found and later was shown to be part of the P system. Contrary to earlier views, this now emerges as a strong system with regularly occurring antibody, like anti-A and anti-B in the ABO system but more violent than these in hemolytic power.[70] It is now thought that there are three alleles at the P locus, P_1, P_2 (previously called p) and p (previously called Tj^b), and a fourth (P^k) has been described.[52] The antibodies are anti-P_1 (previously anti-P) and anti-$P+P_1$ (previously anti-Tj^a). With suitable technic anti-P_1 is found in the serum of P_2 persons[35] and on rare occasions this antibody can be stimulated by transfusion. Anti-$P+P_1$ occurs regularly in the serum of all people lacking the antigen P.

The Rh System.—Rh refers to a factor present in human red cells which was discovered in 1940 by Landsteiner and Wiener[41] through the use of sera prepared by the injection of the red corpuscles of Rhesus monkeys in rabbits, guinea pigs and other animals. It was found that the red cells of about 85 per cent of white persons were agglutinated by the anti-Rhesus (anti-Rh) serum, whereas the remainder failed to react in this way. The former were referred to as Rh positive, the latter Rh negative.

The importance of this observation became apparent when it was shown that anti-Rh could be a cause of hemolytic transfusion reactions[98] and that Rh incompatibility between mother and child is the most frequent cause of erythroblastosis fetalis[43] (p. 756).

Complexity in the field began to develop when it was discovered that, whereas the animal anti-rhesus agglutinins are all of the same specificity, the anti-Rh agglutinins of human sera have several different specificities. These were found to correspond to three Rh factors. It was also observed that, whereas human serum usually contains only one sort of Rh agglutinin, there are some which possess two Rh agglutinins.

Table 7-1—Frequency of Some Rh Types Among Caucasoids in New York City[100a] Together with Corresponding Wiener and Fisher Nomenclature

Genetic and Antigenic Constitution				Reactions with Antisera					
Fisher's Nomenclature	Wiener's Designation			Anti-Rho (D)	Anti-rh' (C)	Anti-rh" (E)	Anti-hr' (c)	Anti-hr" (e)	Frequency %
	Genes	Agglutino-gens	Blood Factors Present						
Rh positive									
CDe/CDe	R^1	Rh_1	$Rh_0rh'rh_1hr''Rh^AHr_0$	+	+	−	−	+	43.0
cDE/cDE	R^2	Rh_2	$Rh_0rh''hr'Rh^AHr_0$	+	−	+	+	−	15.0
cDe/cde	R^0	Rh_0	$Rh_0hr'hr''hrRh^AHr_0$	+	−	−	+	+	2.7*
CDE/CDE	R^z	Rh_z	$Rh_0rh'rh''Hr_0$	+	+	+	−	−	0.2
Rh negative									
cde/cde	r	rh	$hr'hr''hrHr_0$	−	−	−	+	+	38.0
Cde/Cde	r'	rh'	$rh'rh_1hr''Hr_0$	−	+	−	−	+	0.6
cdE/cdE	r''	rh''	$rh''hr'Hr_0$	−	−	+	+	−	0.5
CdE/CdE	r_y	rh_y	$rh'rh''Hr_0$	−	+	+	−	−	0.01

* Frequency 42.5% among Negroids in New York City[18]

Adding still further complexity was the discovery in the serum of the Rh-positive mother of an erythroblastotic infant, of an agglutinin which acted upon all Rh-negative bloods as well as on certain Rh-positive bloods.[42] This not only explained certain instances of intra-group sensitization in Rh-positive individuals,[9] but also indicated that Rh-negative blood, while lacking the agglutinogen characterizing "positive" bloods, itself carries some factor (Hr). Ultimately, by the use of the three Rh antisera (anti-Rh$_o$ [D], anti-rh' [C] and anti-rh" [E] and two anti-hr sera (anti-hr' [c] and anti-hr" [e]) it was possible to separate eighteen Rh blood types. The most common of these, with their approximate frequencies in New York City, are shown in Table 7–1.

Wiener postulated that the genes responsible for the various antigens occupy a single locus on a chromosome, there being a series of multiple alleles. Fisher, on the basis of the work of Race and his associates,[71] suggested that three genes are responsible for the Rh antigens rather than one and that each of these genes is responsible for at least two alternate forms, C or c, D or d, E or e. Each chromosome carries three genes, which may be CDE, CDe, cDE, or other combinations. Since every person carries a chromosome from each parent, various combinations (genotypes) of these would be found, such as CDe/cde, CDe/CDe, cde/cde, cDE/cde and CDe/cDE, to mention the most common. On the basis of this theory, it was predicted that additional antisera must exist even though they are rare. The discovery of anti-e[71] partially fulfilled these predictions but the reported anti-d is in doubt.[70]

A number of alleles of these Rh antigens have been discovered.[70] These include the fairly common C^w, C^{x68} and C^u. The last may have many varieties. Only one allele of D has been reported, D^u, but there are different grades of D^u and other inherited varieties of D prob-

ably exist. D^u is common in Negroes. It can stimulate anti-D in a dd person and some D^u people have made anti-D. E^w is a very rare allele of E but E^u is much less uncommon. Examples have also been described of Rh chromosomal deletion (-D-).[8c]

Another antigen, f, was indicated by discovery of the antibody anti-f.[75a] This antibody may not be of any great practical importance in routine Rh blood group work but it implies the existence of another pair of Rh antigens, f and F. The newest of the Rh antibodies is anti-V.[24] This gene, which is common in Negroes but rare in white persons may represent another pair, Vv, it may be an allele of f, or perhaps is the product of interaction between c and e.[76b] The appearance of many irregular Rh antibodies probably depends on the phenotypic effect of closely linked loci; that is, on whether they exist on the same or on opposite chromosomes (so-called "cis" and "trans" positions.)[69a, 70a, 74a]

Still another "factor," G, has been discovered in Cde cells.[38] This caused sensitization of the Rh negative mother.

Race and Sanger now visualize at least four sites on the Rh chromosome that can be occupied by alleles, arranged in the order D, C, E and f[70] (Fig. 7–1). In their view, the existence of at least three sites where Mendelian substitution can go on is unassailable and the chief point of difference with Wiener's hypothesis is whether the several sites are to be placed within or without the boundary of one gene, a question which, they point out, would be difficult to settle in view of present ignorance concerning the boundaries of a gene.

Wiener makes a distinction between an *agglutinogen*, a substance present on the surface of red blood cells that is identified by certain agglutination reactions with diagnostic reagents, and *blood factors*. The latter are those attributes of the agglutinogen molecule (electric charges, arrangement of polar groups and other configurational details on the surface of the molecule) that enable it to combine with antibodies. In general each agglutinogen is characterized by multiple blood factors.[100a] Thus, "standard" Rh-positive blood is thought to have, besides factor Rh_o, all the factors Rh^A, Rh^B, Rh^C and Rh^D. However, rare Rh-positive individuals have been found by Wiener and his associates[86a] with blood lacking one or more of the associated factors who can be sensitized to the missing blood factor. The resulting antibody resembles anti-Rh_o in specificity except for its failure to clump the patient's own cells and the cells of certain other rare Rh-positive individuals.

For practical purposes there is no difference between Wiener's series of alleles and the closely or completely linked loci postulated by the British. The British notation, however, is much simpler. It is unfortunate that to the inherent complexities of the subject there have been added the difficulties which arise from disagreement concerning nomenclature and different interpretations of recorded observations.[10] Some geneticists point out that neither of the rival hypotheses is established and the suggestion has been made that there is but a single Rh gene with several mutable sites, a view which would include both of the apparently exclusive claims.[9b]

In Table 7–1 both the terminologies of Fisher and of Wiener are used but, in other discussions in this volume, that of Fisher will be employed.

The commonly used terms "Rh positive" and "Rh negative" were first used when the complexity of the Rh system was not appreciated. It happened, however, that the antiserum which paralleled the anti-rhesus serums and gave positive reactions in 85 per cent of white persons was anti-Rh_o (anti-D). This is still employed as the standard anti-Rh serum and consequently the terms "Rh positive"

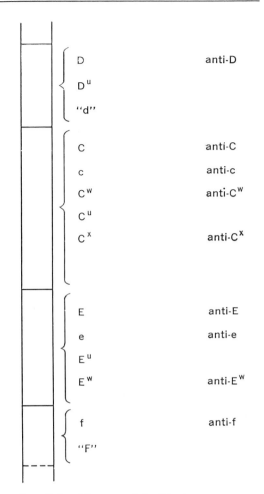

Fig. 7–1.—Diagram of the Rh chromosome, together with antibodies specific for the gene products. "d" and "F" are hypothetical. (Modified from Race and Sanger[70]).

tive" and "Rh negative" refer to the presence of the D antigen.

Kell, Lewis, Lutheran, Duffy, Kidd and Other Blood Groups.—The Kell, Lewis and Lutheran blood groups were all discovered in 1946 and were named after the person in whose blood they were discovered. Anti-K (*Kell*) antibody was found in the serum of the mother of a child with probable erythroblastosis.[70] By means of the antibody found in serum of the mother (Mrs. Cellano) of another child suffering from this disorder,[46] another agglutinogen was found which is very common (99.8 per cent) and is allelic with K. This was therefore designated k. These agglutinogens were found to be independent of known blood groups and it is assumed that there are three genotypes, KK, Kk and kk. The Kell antibody is not usually detected by routine cross-matching technics but can be demonstrated by means of the indirect Coombs test.[33]

Unlike Kell, the Lewis and Lutheran blood groups were not discovered because of the trouble produced by antibodies for these groups. They seem to be comparatively innocent inherited characteristics. The mode of inheritance of the *Lewis* genes (Le^a, Le^b) is by no means clear.[58] Very few instances of hemolytic reaction caused by anti-Le^a have been reported.[53a] The Lewis system may be primarily an antigen system of the saliva and serum and only secondarily an antigen system of the red cells. It has been found that all persons whose red cells were Le(a+) were also salivary nonsecretors of A, B or H substance.[70]

The antigen of *Lutheran* is determined by the presence of a gene *Lu^a* whose frequency is low (3.9 per cent in English people[58]). The allele of this gene, *Lu^b*, was found in the blood of a woman who had had a mild hemolytic transfusion reaction.[32a] Anti-Lu^a has not been found to cause sensitivity reactions although Lu^a is moderately antigenic in man. In contrast to anti-Kell, its reactions are stronger at lower temperatures than at 37° C.

The *Duffy* system[15] is determined by a pair of allelic genes, Fy^a and Fy^b, each of which gives rise to a detectable antigen. Anti-Fy^a occurs in humans as a result of isoimmunization[11d] but very few examples of pure anti-Fy^b are known.[70]

The *Kidd* system has been considered as depending on two allelic genes, *Jk^a* and *Jk^b*, but a third gene, *Jk*, has been reported.[79] Although Jk^a is a rather

weak antigen, several instances of isoimmunization have been reported.[75] There are only three examples[70] of anti-Jk^b.

It shall be seen whether or not the above blood group systems will remain comparatively simple. The Kell system is already expanding. Related alleles Kp^a, Kp^b, and K$_o$ have been described.[2,11a]

There is increasing evidence that the antigen Di^a (*Diego*) defines another locus controlling antigens of the red cells and saliva.[41b] This antigen is not found, except as an extreme rarity, in the blood of Europeans and West Africans but it is found in the blood of South American Indians, Japanese and Chinese and is generally presumed to be a Mongolian character. Like other blood group antigens, it is inherited as a dominant character.

Still another blood group system (*Sutter*)[29a] is defined by the blood group antigen, Js^a and its postulated allele, Js^b. The antigen was found in 20 per cent of Negroes.

In addition to the above nine blood group systems which are well established and the two newest ones, Diego and Sutter, other systems have been described. A number of these have been referred to as "*private*" (Be^a, By, Rm, Wr^a, Levay and others); that is, they are of such infrequent occurrence that they appear to be almost the private property of particular families. It has been pointed out, however, that what may seem to be a "private" antigen in one race may be common in another. What is more, further investigation sometimes has revealed that some of the antigens were related to known blood group systems.[70]

"*Public*" antigens are those which are possessed by the vast majority of people. These include the antigens Vel,[8] Yt^a[27] and I.[70]

Human *sera*, like red cells, can be grouped. One group system, the haptoglobins (Hp), was discussed earlier (p.

168). Another is the Gm group.[41a] While the former are referable to that part of the α_2 globulins that is capable of binding hemoglobin, the Gm groups appear to be due to differences in the γ-globulins.

Blood Chimeras.—This refers to an occurrence, apparently quite rare in humans, in which examination of blood groups in non-identical twins shows that each twin possesses red cells only some of whose ancestors were directly inherited, the rest having been acquired as grafts *in utero* of immigrant embryonic cells from the opposite twin. Grafting of leukocytes, as well as red cell precursors, probably does take place.[3b]

Ethnological Distribution of Blood Groups.—The reader interested in the details of distribution of the blood groups throughout the world should consult the excellent monographs of Mourant[58] and Boyd.[7] Only very limited consideration can be given here to the great mass of interesting data which have been accumulated.

Group O is in most parts of the world the most common group of the ABO system and attains a peak among North, Central and South American Indians[64] (Table 7–2). The proportion falls with the Australian aborigines and the predominance of group O is superseded by that of group B among the Chinese and Asiatic Indians and by that of group A among the Eskimos.[66] Among the white population of the United States, group A is almost equally common.[36] In Negroes, A is less frequent than O.[100] The frequencies of M and N are about equal in many parts of the world but M has been found to be more common than N among North American Indians, Eskimos[66] and Asiatic Indians whereas N predominates among the Australian aborigines. P is much more common in the blood of American Negroes than in that of American whites.

In regard to the Rh system, it is of interest that most people not of European origin are Rh positive. In Asia, the Pacific area and among the American Indians, the closely linked chromosomic combinations CDe and cDE are the principal ones found. African Negroes are principally cDe. On the other hand, Europeans such as the Dutch and, particularly, the Basques have been found to be Rh negative in exceptionally high proportions.

Relation to Genetics and to Anthropology. — Bernstein, in 1924,[58] worked out the genetics of the ABO system and showed that it depends on the presence of three allelic genes, A, B and O (sometimes called p, q and r). Gene A determines the presence of the A substance or antigen on the red cells, whether A be present on both chromosomes or only on one. The same holds for gene B. When A is on one chromosome and B on the other, the red cells carry AB. The O gene does not give rise to either of these antigens. Thus the genotype for group A blood may be AA or AO; for group B, BB or BO; for group O it is OO. The same principle. apply in regard to the subgroups of As

The inheritance of all the other blood groups has been investigated extensively. An exhaustive discussion together with frequency data will be found in the excellent monograph of Race and Sanger.[70]

The blood groups are highly valuable for studies of genetics and anthropology since they are sharply distinguishable "all or none" characteristics which do not shade into each other. They owe nothing to environment in their inheritance nor are they subject to variations because of natural selection, as is the case, for example, with skin color. Hence the blood groups are especially fitted to throw light on moderately remote as well as the recent origins of mankind. For these purposes, MNSs, the Rh system, $A_1 A_2 BO$ and the Kidd system have been found to be especially useful.

Table 7-2—Distribution of ABO, MN, and Rh Blood Groups[7,58,70,94]

	ABO				MN			Rh-Hr						
	O	A	B	AB	M	MN	N	cde	CDe	cDE	CDe-cDE	cDe	Cde	cdE
American Indians (Utah)	97.4	2.6	0	0	58.7	34.6	6.7	0	33.7	28.8	37.5	0	0	0
Australian aborigines	48.1	51.9	0	0	2.4	30.4	67.2	0	58.2	8.5	30.4	1.3	1.7	0
Basques	57.2	41.7	1.1	0	23.1	51.6	25.3	28.8	55.1	7.8	6.0	0.6	1.8	—
English	47.9	42.4	8.3	1.4	28.7	47.4	23.9	15.3	54.8	14.7	11.6	2.3	0.6	0.7
Negroes (U. S. A.)	51.5	29.5	15.5	3.5	23.0	51.5	25.5	8.1	20.2	22.4	5.4	41.2	2.7	0.5
White (U. S. A.)	42.2	39.2	13.5	5.1	29.9	50.2	19.9	13.5	33.5	13.0	13.8	2.5	0.5	0.5
Chinese	30.7	25.1	34.2	10.0	33.2	48.6	18.2	1.5	60.6	3.0	34.1	0.9	0	0
Asiatic Indians	32.5	20.0	39.4	8.1	—	—	—	7.1	70.5	5.1	12.8	1.9	2.6	0

Based on gene frequencies, various interesting tentative racial classifications have been made. Defining "race" as a population which differs significantly from other human populations in regard to the frequency of one or more of the genes it possesses, Boyd[7] at first distinguished six groups, later 13, as follows:

A. *Europeans.* These could be subdivided among (1) Early Europeans; (2) Lapps, with the highest N frequencies in Europe, a high value of Fy^a, very low B frequency, A_2 frequencies three times those found anywhere else in the world, relatively infrequent Rh negative (r) gene and high R^2; (3) Northwest, (4) Eastern and Central and (5) Mediterranean Europeans, with variations from those of the Lapps and shifting to a very high frequency of the Rh negative gene in the Basques. The preponderance of Rh negative and extremely low frequency of Group B were considered characteristics of the Early Europeans;

B. (6) *Africans* (south of the Sahara), with a tremendously high incidence of Rh positive and a rather high incidence of B;

C. in *Asia* (7) the Asian race and (8) the Indo-Dravidian;

D. the *American Indians* (9) with probably no B or Rh negative and low N;

E. the *Pacific group* consisting of (10) Indonesian, (11) Melanesian and (12) Polynesian; and

F. (13) the *Australian aborigines*, with high incidence of N and no Rh negative.

These and other related topics were thoughtfully discussed by Mourant.[58]

It seems reasonable to suppose that these are but the crude beginnings as far as the newer knowledge of the migration of races, genetic drift and selection and related topics is concerned. With the discovery of still more blood groups, and especially with such markers as the Diego factor, and with the contributions which the great variety of abnormal hemoglobins are making to this field, it may be expected that a most interesting picture will be unfolded.

Medicolegal Applications.[18,37,56]— With the ABO system and the two subgroups of A, the MNSs groups, P, the Rh system, Lutheran, Lewis and Kell, the total number of possible different combinations or serologically recognizable phenotypes is 23,616 and the number of genotypes is 972,000.[51] Because of technical and other difficulties, the P, Lewis, Kell, Duffy and Kidd systems have not been recommended for use in problems of parentage or identity.[63] Nevertheless, even if only the ABO, MN and Rh blood groups of the mother, child and alleged father are known, it is possible to exonerate 51 per cent of all men wrongfully accused of paternity.[82] Blood group investigation has been relied upon extensively in the Scandinavian countries and to an increasing degree in the United States in courts of law. Blood groups are also of practical importance in helping to decide whether twins are monozygotic or dizygotic.[70]

Secretors and Nonsecretors.—The antigens A, B and H are present in saliva. The ability to secrete them is inherited as a Mendelian dominant character (*Se*) which is not linked to the ABO genes. It was mentioned earlier that persons whose red cells are Le^a positive are salivary nonsecretors of A, B or H substance whereas those who are Le^b are secretors. The secretor gene, which is independent of the Lewis gene, thus tends to interact with it.

It appears that there are two distinct forms of the ABH antigens: (1) a water-soluble form not present in the red cells or serum but present in most of the body fluids and organs of a secretor; and (2) an alcohol soluble form, not influenced by the secretor gene, which is present in all tissues (except the brain) and in the red cells, but not present in the secretions.[70] As a consequence it is possible to apply blood grouping to the examination of dried stains of saliva, seminal stains and muscle extracts.

Blood Groups and Human Disease.—It may well be that blood groups are examples of balanced polymorphism and, if this is true, different combinations of genotypes may have different survival values. This topic has attracted much attention in recent years.

The rôle of blood group sensitization in the pathogenesis of erythroblastosis fetalis will be discussed later (p. 756). Another example of the rôle of blood groups in the development of disease is found in the demonstration of an identifiable "warm" antibody, such as anti-e, in a patient with acquired hemolytic anemia whose own red cells were of a genotype containing the corresponding antigen (p. 616). In addition, there are two other areas where, in particular, there may be reasons to consider the association of the blood groups and disease; namely, fertility, and certain disorders of the upper part of the gastrointestinal tract.

Concerning the association between ABO blood groups and fertility, published data are conflicting and difficult to interpret.[70,71b] It is also hard to evaluate the significance of reports concerning the relationship of these blood groups and prematurity and stillbirth,[69] or blood group "conflicts" and aberrant salivary secretion in spontaneous abortion.[53] However, in relation to the association between blood group A and gastric cancer,[1,3a] and with pernicious anemia, the evidence is very much more substantial and that indicating a very high incidence of duodenal ulcer in people of group O[11b] is considered by some to be "overwhelming."[70] The interesting observation has also been made that duodenal ulceration was commoner in nonsecretors than in secretors.[11b]

Similar studies have been carried out with reference to many other diseases, but less strong evidence has been uncovered concerning the association of blood groups and these diseases.[70] The studies are of great interest and importance. Investigations of this kind, however, must be interpreted with great caution as the sources of error and chances for misinterpretation are very great.[50]

METHODS OF BLOOD TYPING

In the charming style in which their fascinating monograph[70] has been written, Race and Sanger point out, "Blood group tests need some delicacy of hand and a great deal of concentration of mind. The importance of placing the right serum and the right cells in the right tube and of correctly recording the results is almost too obvious to mention. Yet to achieve accuracy a long apprenticeship in error seems necessary. A friendly but silent atmosphere is essential. Given silence, there is still danger of the mind wandering; this it must not be allowed to do, however routine the tests may be, however primrose the alternative paths." One wonders how often failure to attend to this admonition has resulted in the untimely death of the recipient of a blood transfusion.

Blood typing and matching require red corpuscles, serum or plasma and testing sera of high titer. The suspension of red corpuscles may be obtained by placing one drop of blood from the finger into 3 ml. of physiological solution of sodium chloride or by making such a dilution in a white cell counting pipet; or better still, venous blood is obtained, 0.5 ml. of blood is expelled into a test tube containing about 10 ml. of physiological sodium chloride solution, the tube is gently shaken to wash the cells, the supernatant fluid is poured off after centrifugation and fresh saline solution is added to make a 1 or 2 per cent suspension.

Red cell concentrations greater than 1 or 2 per cent should be avoided; otherwise the cells may absorb all the agglutinins present in weak or diluted sera and fail to agglutinate with such sera. If agglutination does occur it may be weaker or may develop more slowly than usual. Until the test is carried out, however, the red cells should be kept in concentrated form since they retain their sensitivity better in this way.

Unless the testing sera are of high titer, the reaction may be so slight as to be overlooked. The red cells of infants are of especially low sensitivity and require sera of high titer to avoid incorrect grouping. With inadequate testing sera it is not very unusual to mistake A_2B blood for group B or A_2 for group O. This is due to the fact that a serum may contain much α_1 (anti-A_1) agglutinin and little α (anti-A); the latter is necessary for the demonstration of the A_2 agglutinogen. The importance of this is evident when it is realized that a fifth of all group A persons are A_2 and a third of group AB are in actuality A_2B. It is essential, therefore, that all group B sera used for typing purposes be titrated against known A_2 cells as well as A_1 cells. Typing sera are usually obtained from donors deliberately immunized against blood group factors.[102]

Testing sera should be inactivated or stored in a refrigerator for a week before use; when they are fresh, complement is present and hemolysis may occur. Then the red corpuscles may disappear before agglutination has been observed. It is also noteworthy that testing sera deteriorate and it is necessary, therefore, to test the contents of each new vial against known cell suspensions.

The **technic of blood typing** is as follows:

One drop of anti-B serum is placed on the left side of a glass slide and one drop of anti-A serum on the right side. One drop of unknown cell suspension is mixed with each of these sera and the slide is then tilted back and forth for three to five minutes. The drops may then be covered with cover-slips to facilitate examination under the microscope. Clumping which is visible with the naked eye (Fig. 7–2) occurs in accordance with the types of agglutinogens in the tested blood (see below).

The above technic is that commonly used but a more satisfactory procedure is carried out in *small test tubes* (inside diameter 7 mm.). One drop each of unknown cell suspension, saline and testing serum are mixed in such a tube. Blood suspensions of known groups should be put up at the same time to serve as controls. The tubes are centrifuged at about 2000 r.p.m. for about one minute. They are then replaced in a rack, which is shaken. When agglutination has not occurred the sediment of packed red cells at the bottom of the tube can be shaken up into an even suspension. Positive reactions are indicated by the persistence of clumps of red cells the size of which depends on the intensity of the reaction (Fig. 7–3). If desired, the contents of each tube can be examined microscopically.

If clumping occurs only in the anti-B serum which contains β agglutinins, the red corpuscles must contain B agglutinogens; if clumping occurs only in the anti-A serum, which contains α agglutinins, the red corpuscles must have A agglutinogens; if clumping occurs in both sera, containing α and β agglutinins, the red corpuscles must have A and B agglutinogens; and if no clumping whatever occurs, there must be no agglutinogens (group O).

Accordingly, blood from donors can be given to members of their own blood group, or to those of group AB, who have no agglutinins; and, theoretically, blood from group O can be given to members of all groups (the so-called "universal donor"), the agglutinins found in group O blood plasma being rapidly diluted and made ineffectual. Actually, how-

Serum A (anti-B)   *Serum B (anti-A)*

Blood Group O

A

B

AB

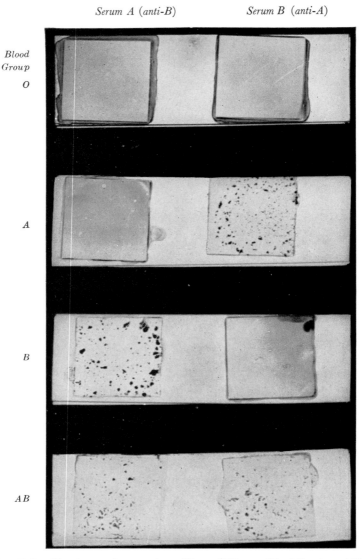

Fig. 7–2.—Blood grouping on glass slides. (Wiener, *Blood Groups and Transfusion,* courtesy of Charles C Thomas.)

ever, unless certain precautions are taken, it is unwise to employ universal donors (see p. 363).

Errors in Blood Typing and Their Prevention.—With the discovery of a number of new blood groups and with the increasing likelihood of isoimmunization as the result of the liberal use of blood transfusion, the problem of ade-

quate blood typing and the need for the employment of technics which will reveal "intra-group" iso-agglutinins has become more important than ever. Whenever practical the blood of the patient should be typed as completely as possible and this should be done in advance since it is a time-consuming process. This is especially important in patients with

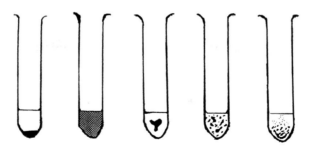

Fig. 7–3.—Blood grouping by the centrifuge method. (Wiener, Blood Groups and Transfusion, courtesy of Charles C Thomas.) *Test Tube 1:* The mixture of cell suspension and serum is centrifuged, and as a result the blood cells are packed at the bottom of the tube. *Test Tube 2:* After shaking, the sedimented cells break up into an even suspension—negative reaction. *Test Tube 3:* Shaking fails to separate the packed cells which float about in one clump—strong positive reaction. *Test Tube 4:* Positive reaction of moderate strength. *Test Tube 5:* Same as 4, after standing a short time.

hemolytic disorders who often receive many transfusions. Agglutination tests should be carried out not only in saline to detect ABO incompatibility but by other methods as well, as will be discussed shortly. In addition to tests of the patient's red cells, it is well also to check the patient's plasma or serum against known group A and group B cells. By thus determining the iso-agglutinin content of the serum, the results of the tests on the red cells are checked and technical and recording errors are discovered.[83,93]

In *all* instances prior to the use of blood for transfusion, *cross-matching* must be carried out. For this test the red corpuscles of the donor are mixed with the serum of the recipient and *vice versa*. This is best done by the test tube method described above. If time permits, the mixtures of cells and serum should be allowed to stand one hour at 37° C. before centrifuging. If no agglutination is seen in either mixture, even when examined under the low power of the microscope, the donor may be used for the transfusion.

It is often assumed that simple direct matching is sufficient to rule out incompatibilities when blood which is homologous both as to ABO group and Rh is administered. This, unfortunately, does not always suffice in those who have had repeated transfusions or pregnancies and may thus have become sensitized to other blood factors (see p. 763).

Confusion in typing and matching may occur as the result of *pseudoagglutination* or *autoagglutination*. The former term refers to rouleau formation and clumping which occur when the sedimentation rate of the blood is accelerated. This is more likely to cause confusion when the slide method of typing is employed and disappears when pressure is exerted on the cover-slip or when saline is added. Since the patient's serum, and particularly his plasma, contains the factors causing rapid sedimentation of red corpuscles, pseudo-agglutination may cause difficulty when the patient's serum is cross-matched against the blood of prospective donors. Dilution of the serum one or two times abolishes pseudo-agglutination.

Autoagglutination refers to the agglutination of the red cells of the individual by his own serum or plasma. Its most troublesome form is cold hemagglutination (p. 169). Although this phenomenon, like group specific isoagglutination, persists in spite of considerable dilution, it occurs usually at low temperatures whereas specific isoagglutination is little affected by changes of temperature from 0° to

37° C. Consequently, if the test is performed at 37° C., particularly with red cells washed with normal saline solution at this temperature, auto-agglutination can be avoided.

If in blood grouping an "AB reaction" is obtained, a control test of the patient's cells in his own serum should be set up. If the reaction has been caused by autoagglutinins, agglutination will take place under these circumstances as well.

Autoagglutinins may cause confusion when the patient's serum is cross-matched against the blood of prospective donors. They can be removed from the serum by separating the serum from the cells at 0° to 5° C. since the red corpuscles absorb them at this temperature.

Erythrocytes from old blood samples may sometimes be agglutinated by sera irrespective of their blood groups. This phenomenon of *panagglutination* may, therefore, be a cause of error in blood typing. It has been shown that this "Huebener-Thomsen-Friedenreich phenomenon" is due to the fact that filtrates of certain bacteria contain an enzyme which acts on human red cells, changing a latent antigen to an active one ("T-antigen"). A similar phenomenon has been described as occurring transiently *in vivo*.[72]

Irregular and atypical isoagglutinins which occur naturally, such as subgroups of A and the agglutinogens P and M, generally give much weaker reactions than typical iso-agglutinins and only exceptionally[4] act at 37° C. Since they are observed usually only in the cold they have been confused with cold hemagglutinins. Other irregular isoagglutinins resulting from isoimmunizations, especially the Rh-Hr antibodies, generally react at body temperature and may be quite potent, giving rise to dangerous hemolytic transfusion reactions. Special procedures are required to detect some of these.

Special Procedures for the Detection of Isoagglutinins.—Experience with Rh sensitization led to the discovery of "*Rh blocking iso-antibodies*," so named because they combine specifically with Rh-positive erythrocytes without producing any visible reaction except that the erythrocytes lose their capacity of being agglutinated even by potent anti-Rh sera. As a result, violent hemolytic reactions may occur without isoagglutinins being detected by the saline technic. These can be demonstrated, however, if the cells are suspended in compatible plasma or in human or bovine albumin.

The theoretical implications of these observations need not be discussed here but it may be stated that they have led to the recognition of at least two, and possibly three or even four forms of agglutinins.[70] "*Saline agglutinins*" are those demonstrable in saline dilutions of red corpuscles and they are visualized as being bivalent and therefore being capable of uniting with the antigen of two red corpuscles, thereby producing agglutination. "*Albumin agglutinins*," on the other hand, are those which are demonstrable only when suspended in 20 per cent albumin or a similar medium. They are visualized as being univalent ("*incomplete*") and capable of uniting with the antigen of only one red corpuscle. When this union has taken place they are no longer capable of agglutinating (thus the term, "blocking antibody") and require a serum factor to bring them together. This serum factor is adsorbed onto only such specifically sensitized corpuscles. Apparently this serum factor is readily dissociated on dilution with saline and consequently an agglutination test as ordinarily carried out in a saline suspension of red corpuscles is negative.[94]

A great variety of technics have been described for Rh testing.[70] Deserving special mention is a capillary tube method which has been found very satisfactory for routine Rh testing.[11] In a very simple slide test,[26] approximately 0.2 ml. of whole group O, Rh-positive blood is mixed with an equal amount of the serum to be tested on a glass slide. After gentle warming over a 25-watt bulb and gentle tilting of the slide, readily discernible agglutinates appear within a few seconds to three minutes, if the test is positive. A control test with Rh-negative blood is run at the same time. This test serves to demonstrate antibodies of either of the above mentioned types and has been found positive in 99.8 per cent of cases of Rh sensitization. Errors in interpretation arise as the result of rouleau formation; the rouleaux, however, can be dispelled by adding a drop of saline. A standard tube procedure has also been described.[26]

Other media, besides albumin or serum, have been found to encourage incomplete antibody to agglutinate red cells, especially *polyvinylpyrrolidone* (P.V.P.), which is probably superior to albumin.[38a] To 0.5 ml. of a 5 per cent buffered solution of P.V.P. 0.1 ml. whole blood or packed red cells is added, mixed and allowed to stand at room temperature until settling is evident (about 15 minutes). Then 15 ml. physiologic saline is added and the tube is inverted two or three times. The intensity of agglutination or rouleau formation can be read microscopically within a few minutes after the saline dilution has been made. The presence of short chains of 2 to 4 red cells is scored as 1 +, longer chains and occasional clumps as 2 +, many aggregated rouleaux and numerous clumps as 3 +, and coarse macroscopic clumps as 4 +.

Even more sensitive are tests based on the discovery that some *proteolytic enzymes*, such as papain and ficin, modify the red cell envelope and render treated red cells agglutinable to saline dilutions of albumin-active antisera. Simplified tests have been described.[70,79b]

The *Coombs* or *antiglobulin test*[12] is the most useful and sensitive, even though it is a more laborious procedure for the detection of incomplete antibodies. It depends on the use of an anti-human globulin serum prepared by injection of human globulin into rabbits. This will agglutinate red corpuscles which have been sensitized and thus have antibody globulin absorbed on some points on their surface, but normal erythrocytes are not agglutinated by this serum. The *"direct"* test is carried out with thrice washed (saline) patient's red corpuscles and serves to detect incomplete antibody on the cells. The *"indirect"* test is used to detect incomplete antibodies in the patient's serum and is therefore useful in the study of intra-group hemolytic reactions. Serum suspected of containing, for example, incomplete anti-D antibody is incubated with a sample of normal D (Rh-positive) and dd (Rh-negative) cells which are also homologous to the ABO group. The cells are then washed free of serum and rabbit anti-human globulin serum is added. If the suspected serum contains anti-D, this antibody will have become attached to the D red corpuscles and they will be agglutinated by the antiglobulin serum.

In addition to its usefulness in the study of Rh antibodies, the Coombs test serves to demonstrate the Kell, Kidd and Duffy systems of blood groups and is important in the study of the hemolytic anemias (p. 622). As indicated in Table 7–5, the various other technics which have been mentioned each has its usefulness.

A *fluorescent antibody method* for the identification of blood group antigens in erythrocytes and the demonstration of minor cell populations[11c] gives promise as a procedure for the exploration of many problems in immunohematology.

BLOOD TRANSFUSION

The transfusion of blood from one dog to another was achieved successfully in the 17th century[55b] but the transfusion of blood from man to man, with rare excep-

23

tions, was not accomplished until the mysteries of serological incompatibility were disclosed and subsequently classified, as discussed above. In the earlier attempts, blood was collected in paraffin-lined containers or "direct" transfusions were given, in which communications were made between the vessels of the donor and the recipient. Sodium citrate was introduced as an anticoagulant for blood in 1914 and two decades later it was shown that cadaver blood, because of the fibrinolysis which takes place after death, can be used for transfusion without mixing it with anticoagulants. Since a cadaver yields from two to four liters of blood, this technic has been exploited in Russia.[67] It was not, however, until the concept of "blood banks" was introduced and the exigencies of the second World War stimulated the investigation of methods for blood preservation[65] that blood became readily available and blood transfusion became very popular. This, however, has not been an unmixed blessing for familiarity has bred thoughtlessness and now, in civilian practice at least, blood transfusion is carried out all too frequently when it is not required and without due consideration of the risks involved.

Indications.—By far the most important uses of whole blood transfusion are to restore blood volume after hemorrhage, trauma or burns and to maintain the concentration of circulating hemoglobin at an adequate level in those types of anemia which cannot be relieved by specific measures such as iron or vitamin B_{12} therapy.

As an emergency measure to restore the blood volume following *acute hemorrhage*, whole blood transfusion has no equal. Blood plasma and the "plasma expanders" are but second and third best, respectively, although they are useful until the typing and matching have been done. The extent to which blood may be lost when acute hemorrhage has

occurred and the quantities of blood needed following trauma or burns are often underestimated. In anemia from acute blood loss, transfusion is indicated if symptoms of oxygen want are developing but it is unnecessary to wait for the classical signs of restlessness, pallor, dyspnea, a rising pulse rate and a falling blood pressure. It is noteworthy that the blood volume deficit may be as great as 20 per cent without hypotension developing as long as the subject remains in the horizontal position.

In cases of *acute hemolytic anemia*, blood transfusion must be approached with caution since the transfused cells may be destroyed as readily as those of the recipient in cases of the acquired type.[9] Consequently, it is wise to defer transfusion in the hope that the patient may reach a balance between destruction and formation of cells spontaneously and to reserve the blood for use only when the anemia is developing rapidly for, in such cases, the danger of death or of serious ill effects from shock is greater than the potential hazards of the administration of blood. In the more chronic forms of hemolytic anemia, where the hemolytic process has reached a state of equilibrium, blood transfusion as a rule offers little for the patient. In hemolytic disease of the newborn, blood transfusion can be curative and here exchange transfusion has an important place (p. 761).

On the other hand, in *anemias of gradual onset* the indications for blood transfusion are much more limited. A *deplorable practice* is the rule which some physicians follow of transfusing if the hemoglobin value is below an arbitrarily set figure. The insistence of some surgeons that the hemoglobin concentration be "normal" prior to surgery is a form of superstition. The concept of "chronic shock" has no foundation in fact. Blood transfusion is not a tonic, nor is it a placebo. In cases of chronic anemia it should be realized that the anemia has developed so gradually that the patient has become accustomed to the new hemoglobin level. Such symptoms as may be present are due to the underlying disease of which the anemia is itself a symptom. As a rule in such cases a new equilibrium between red cell production and destruction has been reached and blood transfusions only serve to alter this balance temporarily. At the same time they subject the patient to unnecessary risks.

It is true, of course, that a certain level of hemoglobin is needed, below which the physiologic adjustments to anemia (p. 436) begin to fail and such symptoms as excessive weakness, orthopnea and even angina and restlessness will develop. Such complaints can be avoided by blood transfusion but, as a rule, they do not appear in adults until the volume of packed red cells has dropped below 25 ml. per cent and the hemoglobin is under 8 Gm. Children tolerate well even lower levels. It may be added that, even when the anemia is severe, a decision for or against transfusion depends on the nature of the anemia. Thus, before the discovery of liver therapy, transfusion was the most useful method of treatment in pernicious anemia. Now it is almost never required. It is extremely rare, indeed, that the patient's condition is so critical that he cannot wait two or three days for vitamin B_{12} to take effect. When one considers the danger of transfusion reactions and the fact that they are more serious the more anemic the patient, it is evident that transfusion should be avoided even when the hemoglobin is as low as 7 Gm. Recovery can be brought about by vitamin B_{12} therapy without any risk, provided the diagnosis is correct. Again, in iron deficiency anemia, the administration of iron, by mouth, is the most effective as well as the least expensive method of treatment and is entirely devoid of risk. Even when surgical measures are necessary in such cases,

unless an emergency exists, it is far better to restore the patient's health by physiological means, such as a good diet and the administration of the specific antianemic substance which is lacking than to "prime" the patient artificially.

In chronic anemias not due to lack of specific antianemic substances such as iron or vitamin B_{12}, a decision concerning the need for blood transfusion should be made according to the severity of the anemia, within the limitations discussed above, and also in accord with the possibilities of successful treatment of the underlying disease. Thus, in acute lymphoblastic leukemia, corticosteroid therapy is likely to produce a remission and blood transfusion may be withheld unless the anemia is very severe. On the other hand, in the acute myeloblastic and monocytic forms, the prospect of even temporarily successful treatment with metabolic antagonists is not as great and blood transfusion will be needed. Again, in chronic myelocytic leukemia, the chance of successful therapy with busulfan is good and blood transfusions are usually not necessary. In many instances of acquired hemolytic anemia corticosteroid therapy is effective and the risks of transfusion can be avoided. In the hereditary varieties of hemolytic anemia, blood transfusion has no place at all, unless the anemia is very severe and, even then, is helpful only temporarily. On the other hand, in aplastic anemia, blood transfusion is all that is available to support life and to keep the patient in a relatively comfortable state. Furthermore, in some cases, spontaneous recovery ultimately occurs.

There is no sound basis for the use of transfusion in the management of the great majority of infections. Although blood transfusions have been employed effectively for the transfer of specific immune antibodies from convalescent donors to susceptible contacts where measles, mumps, and yellow fever have been present in epidemic form, and immune transfusions have been considered of value in treating certain infections, notably herpes ophthalmia and scarlet fever, other and more convenient measures are available for most of these conditions.

For the relief of the anemia of nephritis, blood transfusion is all that is available. Hypertension and uremic symptoms are not contraindications to transfusion and instances of nephritis and anemia have been described in which transfusion was followed by distinct improvement in the function of the kidneys.[57] Such benefit, however, is uncommon. In other cases of chronic anemia, blood transfusion is justifiable if the anemia is severe and surgical measures are indicated at once; when the diagnosis is obscure, the patient's condition critical, and diagnositic procedures are necessary to clarify the clinical picture; or when there is extensive edema due to a marked lowering of the plasma proteins.

In addition to raising the hemoglobin level and restoration of depleted blood volume, blood or plasma transfusion may furnish *substances which are specifically lacking*. Plasma protein was mentioned above. Fresh normal plasma is capable of restoring all clotting factors and is necessary for supplying factor V and antihemophilic globulin. The quantity of factor V decreases rapidly on storage and the quantity of antihemophilic globulin also falls, the amount depending on the conditions of storage.[79a] Transfusion of fresh blood or plasma is the most rapid means of raising the prothrombin content of the plasma. Even stored blood will supply factor IX (PTC), as well as PTA (p. 293), factor VII and fibrinogen.

It often has been observed that distressing oozing of blood in acute leukemia or in aplastic anemia may cease following blood transfusion. To what extent this is attributable to the administration of blood platelets is uncertain.

Platelets isolated from fresh, human blood and preserved for long periods of time were found to be effective in decreasing bleeding time, reversing capillary fragility and raising the platelet count modestly for 12 hours or longer.[85a] Sometimes prothrombin consumption improved as well. As a temporary source of viable platelets, fresh blood collected in silicone-coated or plastic equipment (p. 357) may have real value. Further progress in this field can be expected. As a method of treating conditions where leukocytes are needed, blood transfusion is of no value.

Collection and Preservation of Blood.—The procedure which is now universally used is the collection of venous blood from healthy donors in suitable containers under appropriate conditions of sterility and with measures to prevent coagulation. Such blood may be stored for as long as 21 days and is easily transported. When this is stored in "banks," donors receive credit and are entitled to blood of an appropriate blood group for themselves, their family or their community when it is needed.

Glass *containers* for the blood so collected have been used most generally but plastic containers are receiving increasing attention. Obvious advantages are their lightness in weight, the fact that they are not breakable and that they permit a closed gravity technic for collection and rapid administration by external pressure. Methods have been developed whereby they can be used to facilitate the separation of plasma and red corpuscles.[30] Since they present non-wettable surfaces they offer conditions for optimal platelet survival.[81a] They have not been found superior, however, to conventional glass bottles insofar as the preservation of erythrocytes is concerned. Materials which may have toxic effects may be leached from either type of container.[81a]

Acid-citrate-dextrose (ACD) *solution* is

now generally used as the anticoagulant for blood. The addition of dextrose to the sodium citrate employed previously was found to slow the decrease in diphosphoglycerate and adenosine-triphosphate (ATP) which takes place in stored blood. The formula now commonly employed (National Institutes of Health, formula B) consists of trisodium citrate (dihydrous) 1.32 Gm.; citric acid (monohydrous) 0.48 Gm.; dextrose (monohydrous) 1.47 Gm.; distilled water, to make up 100 ml. Blood collection bottles contain 120 ml. of this solution, to which 480 ml. blood are added.

The preservation of red corpuscles is improved by taking precautions that air be completely displaced by the blood mixture, thereby reducing hemolysis,[23] as well as by rapid cooling after collection, and storage at 4° C.

The use of ion exchange resins and chelating compounds has not been found to offer advantages over ACD solution.[81a] However, a *citrate-phosphate-dextrose solution*[30a] may offer an advantage as compared with ACD solution in avoiding the hypokaliemia and hypocalcemia associated with the administration of hyperphosphatemic blood when multiple transfusions must be given. Efforts to improve the viability of red cells in the circulation have not been very successful but it has been possible to devise means for the storage of blood for long periods of time. Thus, in glycerol solution red cells have been maintained at −80 and −120° C. for 19 months without any more injury than is demonstrable in blood kept for 21 days at 4° C.[85b]

Effects of Blood Preservation on Corpuscular and Other Components of Blood.—When freshly collected ACD blood is transfused, an average of 5 per cent of the cells is lost during the first 48 hours post-transfusion. Approximately 90 per cent of the *red corpuscles* survive in usable form at the end of 14 days' storage but only 70 per cent remain after 24 days.

After 21 days' storage all the transfused red cells disappear within a period of 100 days rather than in 115 days, as occurs when fresh blood is given.[81a] Most blood banks consider blood unsuitable for transfusion after 21 days. The deterioration which occurs in stored cells is manifested by increased fragility and decreased utilization of glucose. The organic phosphates gradually disappear whereas inorganic phosphate accumulates.[3] As discussed in an earlier chapter, the preservation of red cells *in vitro* can be enhanced by the addition of purine ribosides (p. 126). These permit generation of ATP and temporary healing of the "storage lesion."

Leukocytes are not well preserved in stored blood. The polymorphonuclear forms, in particular, show nuclear changes within a few hours and are reduced to 50 per cent of their number in 48 hours. The phagocytic and bactericidal activity of blood is modified in three to 14 days and complement disappears but natural and immune antibodies are quite stable when stored *in vitro*.

Platelet preservation during storage of blood is improved if platelet loss during collection is minimized by the use of silicone-coated and plastic surfaces during blood collection.[60] Plastic (Fenwall) bags have been used with some success to protect platelets against destruction and, when several have been placed in series, they have been used to separate platelet-rich plasma for transfusion in cases of serious bleeding due to thrombocytopenia. It has been found that loss of *factor V* activity during blood collection and storage is directly related to the degree of platelet loss and to the number of platelets present in the blood at the time of collection.[60] Likewise *antihemophilic globulin activity* was most stable in stored blood when platelet loss was minimal. Factor VII activity, on the other hand, was least in blood which had minimal platelet loss.

Other preservatives for platelets are being explored.[2c] Further exploitation of biomechanical equipment which permits separation of the various constituents of the blood immediately after phlebotomy offers promise.[85a] Lyophilization of platelets has yielded disappointing results.[37b]

Administration of Red Cells Alone. —Certain advantages are to be derived from the administration of concentrated suspensions of red corpuscles instead of whole blood.[30] In patients with reduced cardiac reserve who do not require the constituents of the plasma and in subjects needing red cells mainly and receiving repeated transfusions, removal of the plasma reduces the volume which must be introduced and avoids the introduction of sodium and potassium. It has been calculated that ACD-preserved blood contains 16.8 mEq. of sodium, up to 20 mEq. of potassium, has a pH ranging from 7.0 to 6.5 and introduces a volume of 575 ml. instead of 300 ml., since the anticoagulant solution augments the volume of the 500 ml. of blood. In exchange transfusions and, it is claimed, in cases of hepatic disease, a functional hypocalcemia is produced because the citrate ion in ACD solution is present in excess of the amount needed to complex calcium.

The simplest procedure is to pack the red corpuscles by centrifugation of freshly drawn ACD blood, draw off the plasma and transfuse the remaining cell suspension; or simpler still, the plasma is removed from the sedimented cells of stored blood. Some resuspend the corpuscles in saline or in dextrose and saline. For those who are sensitive to plasma (p. 360), washed red cells must be given. These simple procedures unfortunately carry the risk of bacterial contamination of the blood. It must therefore be administered within a few hours of preparation.

Since some patients may become immunized to the leukocytes and possibly also to platelets in transfused blood, technics have been devised for the preparation of buffy-coat poor blood.[10a]

Route of Administration.—The usual site for transfusion is one of the antecubital veins of the forearm but the superficial veins of the neck and legs may be used and, in infants with open fontanelles, the superior sagittal sinus has been utilized. The amount of blood given varies, according to requirements, from 500 to 1000 ml., or more, in adults. Excluding replacement in hemorrhage, in children no more than 5 ml. per pound body weight (11 ml. per Kg.) should be given, usually at the rate of 15 to 20 drops per minute.

When for various reasons (peripheral circulatory failure, extensive skin burns, *etc.*) veins are not accessible for transfusions, blood and other suitable fluids may be given *via the bone marrow*. In *adults* the sternum is the site of election. Sternal puncture is done as described elsewhere (p. 54) and a few drops of marrow are withdrawn, thus making sure that the needle is in the proper location. A syringe containing the material to be administered is then inserted into the needle and the material is injected as fast as the resistance offered to it will allow. Special apparatus[84] has been devised (p. 55). It is convenient, if more than 50 ml. of fluid is to be injected, to attach tubing to the sternal puncture needle and to connect this with a manually operated two-way stopcock. This in turn is connected with the syringe on the one hand and the container holding the fluid to be injected, on the other. Thus it is unnecessary to disconnect the syringe each time it must be filled. If still more rapid injection is needed than is possible through one needle, a second one can be placed in the sternum. In such a case one needle should be placed in the body of the sternum, the other in the manubrium.

In children, especially in those under four years of age, the cavity of the sternum is not large enough to permit its use for infusion. The marrow cavity of the proximal end of the tibia is the site of choice.[84] The technic in general is similar to that for sternal puncture.

If continuous infusion is attempted *via* the bone marrow, dropping of pressure in the tubing should be avoided for, in such a case, marrow may enter the lumen of the needle and clot.

The administration of fluids *via* the marrow is not without danger and should not be attempted when veins are accessible. The procedure is contraindicated in case of severe systemic infections. Even in their absence secondary infection may occur. In children, if the sternum is used there is the danger of passing through the whole of the sternum, thus penetrating the mediastinum. The possibility of fat embolism seems to be small but small amounts of air are less well tolerated in the bone marrow than by vein. Varying degrees of pain are experienced by many patients during the administration.

For extreme emergencies, as in the treatment of shock resulting from a rapid decrease in blood volume where conventional methods of therapy have failed, a technic for *intra-arterial* transfusion has been developed.[74] The procedure is based on the principle that, under a pressure greater than that of the mean arterial blood pressure, an infusion will enter the arterial system and flow will be conducted through the entire system, as far proximally as the aortic valves. The result is an immediate increase in arterial pressure and blood volume. Transfusions into peripheral arteries, however, are subject to difficulties due to spasm and to dangers from subsequent ligation or thrombosis and there is no unanimity of opinion concerning the need for them. Transfusion into the abdominal aorta at the level of the third lumbar vertebra has been proposed as a means of avoiding some of these dangers.[34] *Intraperitoneal* transfusion was found to be a simple procedure which can be accomplished quickly and easily.[91]

Beneficial Effects.—The beneficial effects of transfusion are noticeable more or less in direct proportion to the need for blood. When the blood volume is greatly reduced or the hemoglobin concentration has fallen rapidly to a critical level, following transfusion, restlessness and sweating disappear, respiration becomes more quiet, the color improves and the pulse rate and blood pressure approach normal. If there has been bleeding, oozing may cease within a few minutes. A transfusion of 500 ml. in an adult will elevate the red blood cell count and hemoglobin about 10 per cent within twenty-four hours. To increase the red cell count by 1,000,000 cells per c.mm. 15 ml. of blood per Kg. body weight are required.[93] Transfused platelets may remain in the circulation three or four days. Transfused leukocytes, on the other hand, are almost immediately removed from the circulating blood.[55] In addition to these effects, there may be diuresis and a visible diminution of edema if the patient has been edematous; an elevated temperature if due to the anemia may subside within a few hours; and the basal metabolic rate, if elevated, becomes lower within a few days.[85]

The delayed effects of transfusions are not so obvious. It is well known that temporary remission sometimes followed repeated transfusions in pernicious anemia. This may have been due to the administration of anti-anemic substance by this means. The cessation of bleeding in hemorrhagic disorders even for some time after the platelets introduced had probably been destroyed and the rare onset of temporary remission in acute leukemia following blood transfusion are unexplained. The effects of blood transfusion in suppressing erythropoiesis, first suggested by the experiments of Boycott and Oakley,[6] were discussed in an earlier chapter (p. 47).

Potential Unfavorable Effects of Blood Transfusion.—These may be classified in several categories: (1) simple febrile and allergic reactions, including plasma and leukocyte sensitivity; (2) those caused by overloading of the circulation; (3) reactions due to incompatibility; (4) those related, in particular, to massive transfusions; and (5) miscellaneous ill effects, such as the transmission of infections, especially serum hepatitis, thrombophlebitis, air and fat embolism and transfusion siderosis.

(1) *Simple febrile reactions* have been observed, according to various reports,[71a] in 0.65 to 19.8 per cent of cases. A more recent figure is 3.55 per cent.[71a] A chill and subsequent fever may follow within an hour after the transfusion, or it may be delayed for 24 hours. Headache, nausea and vomiting may occur. The reaction may be mild and, if there is only fever, the patient may not be aware of it; or it may be more alarming. It usually lasts only a few hours. Improperly prepared diluting fluids with excessive acid or alkali, soluble toxic substances in new rubber tubing or improperly cleaned tubing, insufficiently sterilized and improperly distilled water and sodium chloride solutions which may contain small amounts of bacterial protein[47] are among the causes of such febrile reactions. There have been fewer reactions since plastic tubing, which is used only once and then is discarded, has become available. The age of the blood was found not to be a factor if it was administered within 14 days of collection.[71a] The reaction rate increases with the number of previous transfusions. Such patients sometimes develop cold antibodies and may react with a chill if the blood is given without warming.

Allergic reactions, characterized simply by urticaria or occasionally by swelling of lymph nodes and sore throat, eosinophilia, joint pains and fever occur in at least 1 per cent of cases.[93] They may develop some days after the transfusion. Angioneurotic edema and asthma have been observed. These reactions are sometimes due to transfer of reagins in the donor's plasma to which the patient is sensitive. Such a transfer is less likely to occur if blood is drawn from donors who have fasted for several hours.

Plasma sensitivity has been observed most frequently in patients with hemopoietic disorders who have received multiple transfusions.[14] Chills, fever, backache, pain in the legs and intestinal peristalsis may occur. Although serological tests reveal no incompatibility, the incrimination of the plasma rather than other factors can be demonstrated by injecting, intravenously in the patient, 20 to 30 ml. of plasma, preferably but not necessarily from the donor whose blood is suspected. If plasma sensitivity is present, a reaction will occur within 30 minutes. Plasma sensitivity is especially common in paroxysmal nocturnal hemoglobinuria (p. 642). The offending plasma factor is heat-labile and can be removed by washing the red corpuscles free of plasma.

In patients who have received a large number of blood transfusions, *antibodies against the administered leukocytes*[16] (p. 1100), have been demonstrated.[8b, 65a] The reactions bore a striking resemblance to those caused by bacterial pyrogens and were sometimes severe and even life threatening. They could be prevented by removal of the buffy coat prior to transfusion.

(2) The administration of excessively large quantities of blood, or even smaller amounts if given rapidly ("speed reaction"), especially when there is myocardial weakness, can cause *circulatory failure*. This is often signalized by the onset of a series of short, sharp coughs, precordial and back pain, dyspnea,

Table 7–3—Transfusion Reactions

Type	Cause	Frequency Per Cent
Pyrogenic	Bacterial pyrogens, etc.	1.0–5.0
Urticarial	Sensitivity to (?)	0.8–1.1
Hemolytic	Mismatched blood	0.1–0.5
Isosensitization	Sensitization through repeated transfusions and in pregnancy	Not rare
Circulatory overload	Injudicious augmentation of blood volume	Not rare
"Cold reaction"	Cold agglutinins (?)	Not rare
Transmission of disease	Homologous serum jaundice	0.45–1.0
	Syphilis, malaria, etc.	Rare
Febrile	Leukoagglutinins	After 10–20 transfusions
Serum sickness	Unknown	Rare
Plasma sensitivity	Heat-labile plasma factor	Esp. in PNH
Infectious	Grossly contaminated blood	Rare
Air embolism	Entry of air into veins	Rare
Fat embolism	Transfusion via bone marrow	Rare
Hypocalcemia	Exchange transfusions	Not rare
Hemorrhagic diathesis	Massive transfusions, etc.	Rare (?)

cyanosis and finally a productive cough.[20] These symptoms may develop at any time from one to twenty-four hours after transfusion, and death may result from pulmonary edema. Overloading of the cardiovascular system can be prevented by transfusing blood from which most of the plasma has been removed, and by giving the blood slowly by the gravity-drip method, with the patient in a propped up position if there is any question of cardiac failure. The rate of administration should not exceed 1 ml. per pound of body weight per hour and often may well be slower than this. Only when there has been acute and severe hemorrhage does blood need to be given quickly.

(3) The administration of *incompatible blood* is usually associated with the onset of symptoms before much blood has been introduced and, if the transfusion is stopped, no serious harm may result. The symptoms observed include restlessness, anxiety, flushing of the face, precordial oppression and pain, an increase in pulse and respiratory rate, generalized tingling sensations and pain in the back and thighs. Nausea and vomiting may fol-

low and cyanosis, shock with cold, clammy skin, coma and a failing pulse may develop. A chill, followed by a rise of temperature to 105° F. or higher, and possibly delirium may ensue. Not infrequently a hemorrhagic tendency develops immediately after the transfusion and blood may ooze from the site of the transfusion or from mucous membranes.[52a] Thrombocytopenia, hypoprothrombinemia and hypofibrinogenemia may be associated.[39e] Leukopenia is followed by leukocytosis. Hemoglobinemia can be detected by examining the blood plasma. Hemoglobinuria and jaundice, as well as oliguria or even anuria may follow, but hemoglobin may be present only in the first urine specimen passed after the transfusion and hemoglobinuria and jaundice may not be observed.[20,31] The symptoms may develop rapidly and subside in large measure after twenty-four hours, only to be followed by a progressing state of uremia; or they may seem to be insignificant at first and yet are followed by the signs of severe renal impairment. The latter may be succeeded after several days by diuresis and recovery may then occur, if proper care is given

(p. 369) or uremia may persist and death ensue. Death has occurred as late as the seventh to nineteenth day following transfusion, while diuresis and recovery have appeared as late as the sixteenth day.[31]

The mechanism involved in the production of the *renal failure* which has followed the administration of incompatible blood has been clarified by clinical and experimental studies. The primary factor is a disruption of the renal tubule due to focal cortical ischemia.[62b] This occurs at random among nephrons and in any part of a nephron. Contrary to earlier views, hemoglobinemia *per se* is not the primary cause of the disorder. Injections of hemoglobin into normal animals have not produced hemoglobinuric nephrosis. Considerable evidence has been presented[40] which shows that the precipitation of hemoglobin in renal tubules depends upon functional abnormality of the nephrons. This is the consequence, probably, of the circulatory failure associated with transfusion reactions. Multiple variables probably then operate: the degree of peripheral vascular failure, the amount of reduction in urine volume, and the influence of the hydrogen ion concentration of the urine in favoring precipitation of hemoglobin in the renal tubules, thereby producing mechanical blockage. Only as governed by these various factors does the extent of hemoglobinemia affect the quantity of hemoglobin precipitated in the kidney.

The administration of incompatible blood may sometimes be carried out without the immediate development of symptoms or at least of alarming complaints. This is of course more likely if the patient is already in shock or is receiving anesthesia, but fatal reactions have been reported in patients whose condition at first was good. This has been observed particularly where the transfusion reaction was due to anti-Rh sensitization from previous transfusions.[21]

Such sensitization, however, is not always slow in producing symptoms for in an Rh-negative woman who has had an infant with erythroblastosis, blood transfusion may promptly cause a serious if not fatal reaction.[25]

Laboratory tests which should be carried out in the investigation of a suspected case of hemolytic transfusion reaction[19] include examination of the blood and urine of the patient for hemoglobinemia, bilirubinemia and urinary pigments as well as for the agglutinogen and agglutinin content of the blood; examination of a pre-transfusion sample of the patient's blood and the pilot tube of the blood that was cross-matched for the recipient, as well as of the blood which was actually given. Furthermore, the administered blood should be examined for bacteria. This should include a search for anaerobic organisms and for cold saprophytes as well as for routine organisms. Saline, serum and antiglobulin typing and matching tests should be carried out on the collected blood specimens and the blood and urine of the recipient should be re-examined repeatedly for the late appearance of signs of increased blood destruction, if these are not found at first, and for the appearance of antibodies which may not be detectable at first. The blood and urine should be watched closely to detect developing azotemia.

Statistics differ as to the frequency of various types of incompatibility in the causation of transfusion reactions but many will agree that human error resulting in the administration of ABO incompatible blood is the chief cause.[21] In this system, as mentioned earlier, the presence of weak A_2 or A_2B agglutinogens in the donor's blood has caused errors in typing. Again, the "universal" group O donor has sometimes been the source of a higher titer of anti-A and anti-B agglutinins than is usual and serious reactions have occurred. The weak sub-group of A known as A$_x$ (p. 339) was associated with a non-fatal hemolytic transfusion reaction in one case.[78]

Pooled plasma may be a cause of hemolysis as the result of the presence of high titers of anti-A.[76] Thus prolonged administration of untitered pooled plasma to recipients of group A, and probably B, is potentially dangerous.

The Dangerous Universal Donor.—In emergency situations, large transfusions of group O blood have been given successfully to patients of group A, B and AB when the titer of iso-agglutinins was low.[13] The titer of agglutinins was tested by diluting the serum of the donor 1:200 and then mixing it with a suspension of appropriate red cells. When agglutination did not occur under these conditions, the blood was regarded as safe. Additional qualifications which should be demanded of "safe universal" group O blood would be that it be truly group O and not A$_2$ or A$_2$B mistaken for O, Rh-negative and lacking anti-O, anti-M and anti-P agglutinins. With the isolation of the group-specific A and B substances, it is possible to reduce the titer of the agglutinins α and β in group O blood by adding these substances to the blood.[102]

Nevertheless, the use of "universal" group O blood in ordinary practice cannot be recommended. Cases have been observed in which severe hemolytic reactions occurred when neutralization by soluble A and B substance was incomplete[28] and even when the anti-A agglutinin titer of the donor's blood was not unusually high.[80] The dangerous anti-A antibodies in such cases have shown characteristics of an "immune" type of antibody in that they agglutinated more readily at 37° C. than at lower temperatures and in serum or albumin rather than in saline, fixed complement and acted as hemolysins and were relatively impervious to the addition of soluble A and B substance. Such agglutinins have been encountered particularly in persons who

have been immunized with horse serum or other similar agents which might have stimulated the production of such "immune" antibodies[80] as well as in group O mothers immunized by type A or B infants.

Rh-Hr System.—The discovery of the Rh system of blood groups and the recognition of still other groups clarified many instances of hemolytic transfusion reaction which would be incomprehensible otherwise since ABO incompatibility could be excluded. Of the causes of such "intra-group" hemolytic reactions Rh sensitivity (D) is by far the most common.[25] Fortunately anti-Rh agglutinins do not develop in significant titer in all Rh-negative men or non-gravid women to whom Rh cells are given;[25] otherwise transfusion reactions would occur more often than they do. It has been estimated that about 50 per cent develop some degree of sensitization following a single transfusion, while a small proportion fail to show any sensitization even after repeated transfusion.[56] The size of the transfusion is not important but the spacing is significant, long intervals favoring sensitization more than short ones.

Of the various components of the Rh-Hr system, anti-D (anti-Rh$_o$) is by far the most common antibody causing reactions and anti-D plus anti-C (anti-Rh$_1$) is another frequent cause. Anti-c (anti-hr'), anti-E (anti-rh'') and anti-D plus anti-E (anti-Rh$_2$) are not rare but other antibodies involving this system are found in less than 1 per cent of cases.

In an earlier section certain Rh allelomorphs were mentioned for which specific antisera have not been found, the antibodies for these antigens seeming to be inseparable from certain anti-D, anti-C, anti-c and Anti-E sera.[70] Of these, D^u appears to be quite important because it is sufficiently antigenic to provoke an immune response, with transfusion reactions or erythroblastosis fetalis resulting

Table 7–4—Approximate Frequency of Occurrence of Rh Antibodies

Fisher Terminology	Wiener Terminology	Approximate Percentage Frequency[56,58,70]
Anti-D	Anti-Rh$_0$	40–70
Anti-D + anti-C	Anti-Rh$_1$	8–30
Anti-c	Anti-hr'	1–2
Anti-E	Anti-rh″	1–10
Anti-D + anti-E	Anti-Rh$_2$	2–4
Anti-C	Anti-rh'	<1
Anti-C^w	Anti-rh^w	<1
Anti-e	Anti-hr″	*
Anti-d	Anti-Hr$_0$	?

< Indicates "less than"
* Some examples reported

and yet, since it gives weaker reactions than other "Rh-positive" bloods, a D^u carrier may be mistaken for Rh-negative (dd).[39] Routine use of the Coombs technic in typing for Rh antigens can prevent this error. Among the other Rh allelomorphs, anti-C^w and anti-E^w have been known to cause erythroblastosis fetalis.[32]

Table 7–4 indicates that antibodies to "Rh-negative" blood are not so rare and this should emphasize the fact that the *transfusion of Rh-positive patients with Rh-negative blood is potentially dangerous.* In a number of cases transfusion reactions due to this cause have been observed.[95] These have usually been so mild in degree as to be passed off as pyrogenic reactions but death due to this cause has been reported.

In Table 7–5 the clinical importance of the various blood groups in causing sensitization and transfusion reactions or hemolytic disease of the newborn, is indicated. It is noteworthy how important the Kell factor is from the standpoint of sensitization. Fatal transfusion reactions have been observed.[66a] It may be added that a number of the "private" blood group antigens (p. 344) have been associated with hemolytic disease.[70]

Hemolytic Transfusion Reactions in the Absence of Demonstrable Incompatibility.— Several cases have been described in which transfused red cells were rapidly destroyed even though no antibody was demonstrable at the time of transfusion. In a number of instances antibody was discovered some days after transfusion or was known to have been present some time before.[29] In one instance, however, exhaustive studies failed to reveal an antibody.[81] It may well be that gradually increasing transfusion requirements in patients receiving very many transfusions are due to undetected sensitization. It would be of interest to study such cases by a double labelling technic[55b] in which the suspected incompatible cells are labelled with Cr^{51} and, as a control, the recipient's own cells are labelled with P^{32}.

(4) *Reactions Associated with Massive Blood Transfusions.*—With the advent of modern surgical technic and the very liberal use of whole blood transfusions, two types of problems have been introduced; namely, metabolic effects resulting from the use of large amounts of "bank blood" and hemorrhagic manifestations.

The sudden infusion of large volumes of ACD solution may cause hyperkaliemia[54] and potassium intoxication may occur.[41c] In addition hypocalcemia may develop temporarily and striking electrocardiographic changes may ensue (prolongation of QT interval, depression of T wave and of P wave voltage).[61] Time

Table 7–5—Blood Groups: Clinical Importance and Sensitivity to Agglutination

System	Isoantibodies		Components Important in Sensitivity Reactions			Sensitivity to Agglutination by Various Technics			
	Natural	Isoimmune	Frequently	Rarely	Unknown	Saline	Albumin	Trypsin	Antiglobulin
ABO	Regularly present[1]	Common	A, B	—	A_1, B_1, O	++	+	+	++
Rh-Hr	Rarely, if ever	Common	D, c, E	C, C^w, D^u, E^w, e	d (?), f	±	+	++	++
Kell	None	Occasional	K[2]	k	—	±	±	±	++
Kidd	None	Rarely	—	Jk^a	Jk^b	±	—	—	++
{M-N	Rare	Rare	—	M, N	—	++	+	—	+
{S-s	Rare	Rare	—	S, s, U, Mi^a, V_w	—	±	±	+	+
Duffy	None	Rarely	—	Fy^a	—	±	—	—	++
Lewis	Infrequent	V. rarely	—	Le^a	Le^b	++	++	++	+
Lutheran	None	1 case	—	—	Lu^a	++	++	++	±
P	Regularly	—	—	Anti-P_1	—	++	+	+	±

The blood group systems have been listed in the order of their clinical importance. The order of genetic importance is MNSs, Rh-Hr, ABO and Kidd. Those most readily useful in medicolegal work are ABO, MN and Rh-Hr; because anti-sera are scarce or for other reasons, other blood factors are rarely or never used.

[1] Except during neonatal period.
[2] By no means comparable in frequency with ABO or Rh-Hr system.
Queries indicate single or at least exceedingly rare exceptions.
Key to sensitivity: ++ indicates preferred technic; + means almost always positive; ± may be positive or negative; — almost always negative.

here appears to be an important factor because at slower rates there is opportunity for calcium to be mobilized from body stores and other adjustments can take place.

Blood drawn in ACD solution has a pH of 7.0 and, in time, may attain a pH of 6.6 on storage as the result of continued glycolysis.[30a] If massive transfusions are given, an immediate post-transfusion acidosis may occur.[48] In several hours this is followed by the gradual development of metabolic alkalosis, due to the metabolic breakdown of sodium citrate. The metabolic alkalosis is most marked on about the third post-transfusion day.[48] For these reasons, fresh blood is preferred in exchange transfusions and in operations involving cardiac shunts.

When massive whole blood transfusions are administered rapidly an abnormal bleeding tendency may occur. This was found to be associated with thrombocytopenia and was attributed to replacement of the recipient's blood by blood containing nonviable platelets.[39b] Others have noted fibrinolysis and decrease in factor V activity and have attributed the bleeding to the effect of a multiplicity of factors.[104]

(5) *Miscellaneous Ill Effects.*—Syphilis,[73] malaria,[2d] hepatitis[62] and even brucellosis[103] have been transmitted by blood transfusion. Screening of blood by serological tests for syphilis is not entirely adequate since in the most infectious phase of the disease (late primary, early secondary) such tests are negative. *Treponema pallidum* is destroyed, however, if blood is kept at a refrigerator temperature for ninety-six hours.[86] *Plasmodia* may survive refrigeration and storage. Cinchonization of the donor is sometimes practiced in malarial countries. A more serious hazard, however, is transmission of the virus of *hepatitis*, which is very hardy and is dangerous even when greatly diluted. As little as 2 ml. of blood can infect the recipient. This is

why pooled plasma proved to be so dangerous, since virus in one bottle was thereby widely distributed. Fibrinogen, anti-hemophilic globulin and human thrombin have also been found to carry the virus.[90] No satisfactory method has yet been discovered for detection or destruction of the virus. Tests of hepatic function in the donor have revealed abnormality in some, but not all, asymptomatic carriers.[2b, 62] The administration of blood and of certain blood products, therefore, must be regarded as carrying a calculated risk. In spite of all precautions the minimal incidence of viral hepatitis is between 0.26 and 1 per cent following the use of whole blood and ranges from 1 to 20 per cent following the use of pooled plasma.[62] Storage of pooled plasma in a liquid state for six months at room temperature appears to be suitable for eradicating the virus.[2]

Another serious, although fortunately uncommon hazard, is from the administration of *contaminated blood*. This is due to the accidental introduction of saprophytic bacteria into the bottle of blood. Gram-positive saprophytes, such as diphtheroids, generally produce only fever. However, gram-negative chromogens have been responsible for the production of profound shock that is almost always fatal.[80a] The gram-negative bacteria appear to be capable of utilizing citrate as the sole source of carbon and can multiply in the refrigerator at 4 to 8° C. One group (*Pseudomonas achromobacter*) is clearly saprophytic. The second group is of the coli-aerogenes variety and exhibits good growth in the incubator and at room temperature but not always in the refrigerator. After a latent period of 30 minutes or more, fever, hypotension and pain in the abdomen and extremities develop and death from shock may take place within six hours. Severe vomiting and diarrhea occur and, if the patient survives for 24 hours, signs of renal failure develop. A hemorrhagic diathesis may ensue.[39b] Differentiation from a reaction due to the administration of incompatible blood can be made by microscopic examination of a Gram stain of blood remaining in the bottle and by the absence of evidences of a hemolytic reaction. Treatment[8a] depends mainly on the continuous intravenous administration of pressor drugs such as levarterenol. Antibiotics are of lesser importance but the addition of 20 mg. tetracycline to each liter of blood has been advocated as a prophylactic measure.[8a]

Thrombophlebitis is not rare when transfusions are given repeatedly and especially if small needles are used or small veins are punctured, particularly in the lower extremities.

Hemosiderosis closely resembling hemochromatosis may result from the administration of large numbers of transfusions.[37a]

Fat embolism may occur if positive pressure is used when blood is being given via the bone marrow or in those who have bony injuries. Secondary osteomyelitis or mediastinitis and cardiac tamponade may follow such transfusions. *Air embolism*, resulting from the accidental introduction of air as, for example, through ill-fitting tubing or when blood is introduced under pressure, is usually well-tolerated but may be dangerous in a gravely ill patient.

Prevention of Transfusion Reactions.—It is the general experience that reactions following transfusions are reduced in number when scrupulous care is taken in preparing the apparatus. If rubber tubing is used it should be cleansed with sodium hydroxide solution, then thoroughly rinsed with sterile distilled water and promptly dried and sterilized. Needles should be cleaned with hydrogen peroxide, rinsed thoroughly with distilled water and alcohol and ether run through them. Cleanliness of tubing is more easily checked by the use of transparent rubber. The solutions used must be prepared with sterile, triple distilled water and must be free of bacterial protein.[47] "Cold reactions" can be avoided if some of the transfusion tubing is allowed to rest in a water bath maintained at body temperature, thus allowing the blood to be warmed before it enters the patient's vein.

The donor should be in good health, preferably young, and should have fasted for the preceding six hours. He must be questioned regarding symptoms of allergy, syphilis, jaundice and malaria particularly. A sensitive flocculation test for syphilis can be carried out with little delay but in addition the donor should be examined for evidence of early syphilis or other disease if the blood is to be used at once. As stated earlier, the danger of transmitting syphilis is greatly reduced if the blood is stored.

The possible sources of error in blood typing, and methods for their avoidance have been discussed already (p. 350). It is clear that one cannot rely solely on the saline cross-matching procedure. This not only fails to elicit many potent antibodies of the Rh system, but may also fail to detect numerous other immune antibodies with the potential capacity to cause serious transfusion reactions. The likelihood of various agglutinins being detected by the different technics is indicated in Table 7–5. The indirect antiglobulin (Coombs) test is a most valuable procedure; but, it should be noted that, whereas this is very helpful in detecting anti-Rh, anti-Kell, anti-Duffy and anti-Kidd antibodies, it may fail to demonstrate a number of agglutinins detectable by the serum or albumin technics (anti-A_1, anti-A_2, anti-Le^a, anti-P_1).

New test samples of the patient's blood for cross matching should be obtained prior to *each* spaced transfusion even though the interval between transfusions may be only a few days. It must be borne in mind also that in patients suffering from acquired hemolytic anemias the autoagglutinins commonly associated with such anemias may not only interfere with the usual transfusion compatibility tests, but may also obscure the true identity of the patient's blood group. In such patients, in particular, saline, serum and albumin (or P.V.P.) technics must be employed and tests may need to be carried out at different temperatures, such as 37 and 18° C.

Since multiple isoantibodies may occur in pregnancy, it is imperative that the serum of the mother be used to match directly the donor blood for exchange transfusions in hemolytic disease of the newborn.[90]

It is good practice, when possible, to avoid transfusing a woman with the blood of her husband (or his blood relatives) since she presumably has had, or will have, babies who have inherited his blood factors and she may become sensitized to them.

Except in emergency and particularly when repeated transfusions are being given, the first 50 or 100 ml. of blood should be given slowly in order to determine whether a reaction will occur. If a chill or other untoward symptoms appear, the infusion should be interrupted. Fatal reactions have been observed only when large quantities of blood (over 300 ml.) have been given.[98] The "*biological test*" of Wiener[93] consists in the comparison of the icterus index of the blood plasma or serum of the patient before and one hour after the injection of 50 ml. of blood. This is recommended for use where all other methods of testing for compatibility have failed to reveal incompatibility and yet the possible occurrence of a hemolytic reaction is suspected owing to the fact that the patient has already received several transfusions or is postpartum. The test is not without considerable danger, however, for highly sensitized patients showing no positive *in vitro* reaction may nevertheless have a moderate reaction to as little as 5 or 10 ml. of incompatible blood. Furthermore, the injected red cells are potentially antigenic. Mollison's double tagging procedure (p. 364), if practicable, is much safer.

Another source of danger is in overlooking the fact that immediately following the transfusion of incompatible blood and for two or three days thereafter, there is a negative phase in which the isoantibody titer is low on account of the absorption of the isoagglutinins by the incompatible blood cells. Examination of the blood in this phase may lead to an erroneous result and transfusion seven to ten days following the sensitizing injection at a time when the isoagglutinin titer has risen to its peak, may lead to a fatal reaction. Furthermore, it should be kept in mind that if the blood of an Rh-negative person is tested within a few hours or even a day or two of an Rh-positive transfusion, there may be an appreciable number of Rh-positive erythrocytes present, even when the patient has shown clinical signs of hemolysis. Therefore the patient may appear to be Rh-positive and additional errors may be committed. After a large transfusion of group O blood has been given, group specific blood should not be administered for at least two weeks.[13]

It has been pointed out[17] that patients with chronic leukemia of any type have very weak isoagglutinins. In such patients cross-matching tests may not indicate incompatibility and yet a reaction *in vivo* may occur.

With the prevalent use of "bank blood" it is important to bear in mind that hemoglobinuria, occasionally associated with oliguria or anuria has followed the transfusion of blood hemolyzed as a result of exposure to excessive freezing or heat or due to prolonged storage.[93] The administration of grossly contaminated blood can be avoided by examining a stained smear of the blood for bacteria immediately preceding its administration.[8a] The ill effects of contamination of blood from which plasma has been withdrawn to provide concentrates of red corpuscles can be prevented by not permitting such blood to stand more than an hour before it is given.

Treatment of Reactions. — The most common reaction after transfusions is the pyrogenic effect which almost inevitably occurs in a small proportion of transfusions. The chill and rise in temperature can be prevented or greatly modified by the administration of acetyl-salicylic acid (0.65 Gm.) prior to transfusion. This drug will not mask a serious reaction. If a chill occurs the patient will be more comfortable if covered with warm blankets. These should be removed as soon as the chill is over. Calcium gluconate (10 ml. of a 10 per cent solution) injected intravenously will stop a chill if given early, particularly if morphine sulfate (0.016 Gm.) is given hypodermically at the same time. It is generally unwise to administer acetyl-salicylic acid once fever has developed.

For allergic reactions the anti-histaminics are valuable and phenolated (0.5 per cent) calamine lotion may allay the itching of urticaria.

The development of pulmonary edema should be anticipated in patients with poor cardiac reserve. Blood should be given slowly, the patients should be in the sitting position if possible, and the lungs should be examined frequently for the appearance of rales. If pulmonary edema develops it is treated by the injection of morphine sulfate (0.016 to 0.032 Gm.), the application of tourniquets to the extremities ("bloodless phlebotomy"), and the inhalation of oxygen by a suitable method. The transfusion should be interrupted and, if necessary, blood should be withdrawn. If the patient has not been digitalized previously, digitalization should be accomplished at once by the intravenous injection of a rapidly acting preparation.

The mortality from transfusion of blood incompatible with respect to the major blood groups has been stated to be as high as 50 per cent, but this figure probably ignores the milder reactions of this type from which patients have recovered. The recipient's chances of survival probably depend not only on the amount of incompatible blood injected but also on the isoagglutinin titer, the prior condition of the patient and whether or not the reaction developed under anesthesia and was therefore overlooked for a time. The occurrence of a reaction to incompatible blood during a surgical procedure may not be detected unless close attention is paid to the development of jaundice, oliguria and hemoglobinuria.

The management of reactions following the administration of incompatible blood has been greatly improved as the effects of such an unfortunate eventuality have become better understood. Since shock may be an important factor in the development of renal shutdown, during the *first phase*[59] of the hemolytic transfusion reaction, adequate compatible blood should be given to combat anemia and hypovolemia. However, if there is any question as to blood compatibility, blood transfusions are better not given and plasma or other fluids should be used instead for, as pointed out already (p. 367), erroneous conclusions may be reached when blood is examined for agglutinins immediately after a transfusion reaction has occurred. Pressor substances such as levarterenol may be helpful. On the basis of animal experiments it was concluded that the precipitation of heme pigments in the kidneys is favored by an acid reaction and alkalinization of the urine therefore was recommended (4 to 5 grams of sodium bicarbonate or lactate orally or parenterally) to prevent this. However, the value of this procedure once the kidneys have been injured may be questioned since renal ischemia rather than the precipitation

24

of heme pigments in the tubules is probably the etiologic factor in the acute renal failure which may follow the transfusion of incompatible blood (p. 362). Furthermore, the administration of excess sodium salts to patients who are developing severe oliguria presents the double hazard of alkalosis and tetany, in addition to subsequent congestive heart failure and pulmonary edema.

During the *second phase*, that of renal insufficiency, which begins approximately twenty-four hours after the incompatible blood has been given and may last for many days, it is important (1) not to attempt to force damaged kidneys into action; (2) to limit the fluid intake during this oliguric period to the insensible water loss plus other fluid output. Usually 400 to 500 ml. per day plus a volume equal to the urinary output will suffice. However, in the presence of fever, diarrhea, vomiting, wound drainage or other losses, these also must be replaced; and (3) to maintain adequate nutrition and electrolyte balance. These aims may be accomplished by (1) keeping an accurate record of fluid output and intake and maintaining fluid balance; (2) providing adequate calories by mouth or, if nausea or vomiting supervene, by giving 50 per cent dextrose or invert sugar in water continuously through a plastic catheter in the cephalic or brachial vein of the arm; (3) replacing of electrolytes which are lost. The intake should be potassium free. Repeated measurements of the carbon dioxide combining power of the plasma and the serum Na, K and Cl should be made. Daily electrocardiograms will help in recognizing the development of hyperkaliemia. Mild sedation may be required during this period but should be avoided if possible. In critical situations, dialysis with the artificial kidney may be lifesaving.

In the *final phase*, during the period of tubular recovery and regeneration, there is copious diuresis and loss of salt and water. These must be replaced. This may necessitate parenteral administration but as recovery takes place oral administration may suffice. The sodium chloride and water needs may be very large in an occasional patient but usually 4 to 4.5 grams sodium chloride and 2500 ml. water daily will be adequate.[82a]

BIBLIOGRAPHY

1. AIRD, I., BENTALL, H. H., MEHIGAN, J. A., FRASER ROBERTS, J. A.: The Blood Groups in Relation to Peptic Ulceration and Carcinoma of Colon, Rectum, Breast, and Bronchus, Brit. M. J., 2, 4883, 1954; *ibid.*, 1, 1163, 1960.

1a. ALLEN, F. H., CORCORAN, PATRICIA A., KENTON, H. B. and BREARE, NANCY: M^g, a New Blood Group Antigen in the MNS System, Vox sanguinis, 3, 81, 1958.

2. ALLEN, F. H., JR., LEWIS, SHEILA J. and FUDENBERG, H.: Studies of Anti-Kp^b, a New Antibody in the Kell Blood Group System, Vox sanguinis, 3, 1, 1958.

2a. ALLEN, P. Z. and KABAT, E. A.: Immunochemical Studies on Blood Groups, J. Immunol., 82, 340, 1959.

2b. ALSEVER, J. B.: The Blood Bank and Homologous Serum Jaundice, New England J. Med., 261, 383, 1959.

2c. BALDINI, M., EBBE, SHIRLEY and DAMESHEK, W.: The Use of a Special Preservation Medium for the Maintenance of Platelet Viability at 4 C, Blood, 15, 909, 1960.

2d. ANTSCHELEWITSCH, W. D.: Transfusion von konserviertem Malarikerblut, Folia haemat., 57, 406, 1937.

3. BARTLETT, G. R. and BARNET, H. N.: Changes in the Phosphate Compounds of the Human Red Blood Cell during Blood Bank Storage, J. Clin. Invest., 39, 56, 1960.

3a. BEASLEY, W. H.: Blood Groups of Gastric Ulcer and Carcinoma, Brit. M. J., 1, 1167, 1960.

3b. BOOTH, P. B. *et al.*: Blood Chimerism in a Pair of Twins, Brit. M. J., 1, 1456, 1957.

4. BOORMAN, K. E., DODD, B. E., LOUTIT, J. F. and MOLLISON, P. L.: Some Results of Transfusion of Blood to Recipients with "Cold" Agglutinins, Brit. M. J., 1, 751, 1946.

6. BOYCOTT, A. E. and OAKLEY, C. L.: Regulation of Marrow Activity; Experiments on Blood Transfusions and on Influence of Atmospheres Rich in Oxygen, J. Path. & Bact., 36, 205, 1933.

7. BOYD, W. C.: *Genetics and the Races of Man*, Boston; Little, Brown & Co., 1950; Boston, Boston University Press, 1958.

8. BRADISH, ELIZABETH B. and SHIELDS, WILMA F.: Another Example of Anti-Vel, Am. J. Clin. Path., *31*, 104, 1959.

8a. BRAUDE, A. I.: Transfusion Reactions from Contaminated Blood, New England J. Med., *258*, 1289, 1958.

8b. BRITTINGHAM, T. E. and CHAPLIN, H., JR.: Febrile Transfusion Reactions Caused by Sensitivity to Donor Leukocytes and Platelets, J. A. M. A., *165*, 819, 1957.

8c. BUCHANAN, D. I.: Blood Genotypes —D—/—D— and CDe/—D—, Am. J. Clin. Path., *26*, 21, 1956.

9. CALLENDER, S. T. and PAYKOC, Z. V.: Irregular Haemagglutinins after Transfusion, Brit. M. J., *1*, 119, 1946.

9a. CAMERON, C. *et al.*: Acquisition of a B-Like Antigen by Red Blood Cells, Brit. M. J., *2*, 29, 1959.

9b. CARLSON, E. A.: The Bearing of a Complex-Locus in Drosophila on the Interpretation of the Rh Series, Am. J. Human Genet., *10*, 465, 1958.

10. CASTLE, W. B., WINTROBE, M. M. and SNYDER, L. H.: On the Nomenclature of the Anti-Rh Typing Serums: Report of the Advisory Review Board, Science, *107*, 27, 1948.

10a. CHAPLIN, H., JR., BRITTINGHAM, T. E. and CASSELL, MONA: Methods for Preparation of Suspensions of Buffy Coat-Poor Red Blood Cells for Transfusion, Am. J. Clin. Path., *31*, 373, 1959.

11. CHOWN, B., LEWIS, M. and BRYCE, A.: On the Detection, Differentiation and Titration of Anti-Rh Antibodies, Canad. M. A. J., *59*, 379, 1948; J. Clin. Path., *1*, 73, 1948. *See also* J. Clin. Path., *4*, 55 and 464, 1951.

11a. CHOWN, B., LEWIS, MARION and KAITA, KIROKO: A "New" Kell Blood-Group Phenotype, Nature, *180*, 711, 1957; *ibid.*, *183*, 1586, 1959.

11b. CLARKE, C. A., EVANS, D. A. P., McCONNELL, R. B. and SHEPPARD, P. M.: Secretion of Blood Group Antigens and Peptic Ulcer, Brit. M. J., *1*, 603, 1959.

11c. COHEN, FLOSSIE, ZUELZER, W. W. and EVANS, MARGARET M.: Identification of Blood Group Antigens and Minor Cell Populations by the Fluorescent Antibody Method, Blood, *15*, 884, 1960.

11d. COMPTON, A. and HABER, JANE M.: The Duffy Blood Group System in Transfusion Reactions, Blood, *15*, 186, 1960.

12. COOMBS, R. R. A., MOURANT, A. E. and RACE, R. R.: A New Test for the Detection of Weak and "Incomplete" Rh Agglutinins, Brit. J. Exper. Path., *36*, 225, 1945; J. Path. & Bact., *59*, 105, 1947.

13. CROSBY, W. H. and AKEROYD, J. H.: Some Immunohematologic Results of Large Transfusions of Group O Blood in Recipients of Other Blood Groups, Blood, *9*, 103, 1954.

14. CROSBY, W. H. and STEFANINI, M.: Pathogenesis of the Plasma Transfusion Reaction with Especial Reference to the Blood Coagulation System, J. Lab. & Clin. Med., *40*, 374, 1952.

14a. CROWLEY, L. V., RICE, J. D., JR. and BREEN, MARY: High Titered Anti-M Isoagglutinins in Human Blood, Am. J. Clin. Path., *28*, 481, 1957.

15. CUTBUSH, M., MOLLISON, P. L. and PARKIN, D. M.: A New Human Blood Group, Nature, *165*, 188, 1950.

16. DAUSSET, J.: Iso-leuco-anticorps, Acta haemat., *20*, 156, 1958.

17. DAVIDSOHN, I.: A Method for Recognition of Blood Subgroups A_1 and A_2, J. A. M. A., *112*, 713, 1939.

18. DAVIDSOHN, I., LEVINE, P. and WIENER, A. S.: Medicolegal Application of Blood Grouping Tests, J. A. M. A., *149*, 699, 1952.

19. DAVIDSOHN, I. and STERN, K.: Diagnosis of Hemolytic Transfusion Reactions, Am. J. Clin. Path., *25*, 381, 1955.

20. DEGOWIN, E. L.: Grave Sequelæ of Blood Transfusions, Ann. Int. Med., *11*, 1777, 1938.

21. ——— Isoimmunity to the Rh Factor as a Cause of Blood Transfusion Reactions, J. Lab. & Clin. Med., *30*, 99, 1945.

23. DEGOWIN, E. L., HARRIS, J. E., PLASS, E. D., HARDIN, R. C. and SWANSON, L. W.: Studies on Preserved Human Blood, J. A. M. A., *114*, 850, 855, 858, 859, 1940; *ibid.*, *115*, 895, 1940.

24. DENATALE, A., CAHAN, A., JACK, J. A., RACE, R. R. and SANGER, R.: V, a "New" Rh Antigen, Common in Negroes, Rare in White People, J. A. M. A., *159*, 247, 1955.

25. DIAMOND, L. K.: The Clinical Importance of the Rh Blood Type, New England J. Med., *232*, 447 and 475, 1945.

26. DIAMOND, L. K. and ABELSON, N. M.: The Demonstration of Anti-Rh Agglutinins, J. Lab. & Clin. Med., *30*, 204, 668 and 821, 1945.

26a. DUNSFORD, I., STACEY, S. M. and YOKOYAMA, M.: A Rare Variety of the Human Blood Group B, Nature, *178*, 1167, 1956.

27. EATON, B. R., MORTON, J. A., PICKLES, M. M. and WHITE, K. E.: A New Antibody,

Anti-YT^a, Characterizing a Blood-Group Antigen of High Incidence, Brit. J. Haemat., 2, 333, 1956.

28. ERVIN, D. M. and YOUNG, L. E.: Dangerous Universal Donors, Blood, 5, 61 and 553, 1950.

29. FUDENBERG, H. and ALLEN, F. H., JR.: Transfusion Reactions in the Absence of Demonstrable Incompatibility, New England J. Med., 256, 1180, 1957.

29a.GIBLETT, ELOISE R. and CHASE, JEANNE: Js^a, a 'New' Red-Cell Antigen Found in Negroes; Evidence for an Eleventh Blood Group System, Brit. J. Haemat., 5, 319, 1959.

30. GIBSON, J. G., II: Use of Separated Human Red Cells, New England J. Med., 250, 976, 1954.

30a.GIBSON, J. G., II, MURPHY, W. P., JR., SCHEITLIN, W. A. and REES, S. B.: The Influence of Extracellular Factors Involved in the Collection of Blood in ACD on Maintenance of Red Cell Viability during Refrigerated Storage, Am. J. Clin. Path., 26, 855, 1956; ibid., 28, 569, 1957; New England J. Med., 262, 595, 1960.

30b.GILES, CAROLYN M. et al.: A Weak B Antigen, probably Acquired, Brit. M. J., 2, 32, 1959.

31. GOLDRING, W. and GRAFE, I.: Nephrosis with Uremia Following Transfusion with Incompatible Blood, Arch. Int. Med., 58, 825, 1936.

32. GREENWALT, T. J. and SANGER, R.: The Rh Antigen E^w, Brit. J. Haemat., 1, 52, 1955.

32a.GREENWALT, T. J. and SASAKI, T.: The Lutheran Blood Groups: a Second Example of Anti-Lu^b and Three Further Examples of Anti-Lu^a, Blood, 12, 998, 1957.

33. GROVE-RASMUSSEN, M., DREISLER, N. and SHAW, R. S.: A Serologic Study of 8 Samples of Anti-Kell Serum, Am. J. Clin. Path., 24, 1211, 1954.

33a.VAN DER HART, Mia et al.: Vr, an Antigen Belonging to the MNSs Blood Group System, Vox sanguinis, 3, 261, 1958.

34. HAXTON, H. A.: Intra-Aortic Blood-Transfusion, Lancet, 1, 622, 1953.

35. HENNINGSEN, K.: Investigations of the Blood Factor P, Acta path., 26, 640 and 769, 1949; Rev. d'hémat., 5, 276, 1950.

36. HERVEY, G. W., DIAMOND, L. K. and WATSON, V.: Geographic Blood Group Variability in the United States, J. A. M. A., 145, 80, 1951.

37. HIRSZFELD, L. and MILGROM, F.: Sur L'Application des Examens de Groupes Sanguins dans les Recherches de Paternité, Rev. d'hemat., 4, 6, 1949.

37a.HUGHES, J. T. and TRUELOVE, L. H.: Transfusional Haemosiderosis Simulating Haemochromatosis, J. Clin. Path., 11, 128, 1958.

37b.JACKSON, D. P. et al.: Effectiveness of Transfusions of Fresh and Lyophilized Platelets in Controlling Bleeding Due to Thrombocytopenia, J. Clin. Invest., 38, 1689, 1959.

38. JAKOBOWICZ, RACHEL and SIMMONS, R. T.: Iso-Immunization in a Mother Which Demonstrates the "New" Rh Blood Antigen G (rh^G) and Anti-G (rh^G), Med. J. Australia, 2, 357, 1959.

38a.JANDL, J. A. and CASTLE, W. B.: Agglutination of Sensitized Red Cells by Large Anisometric Molecules, J. Lab. & Clin. Med., 47, 669, 1956.

39. JONES, A. R., DIAMOND, L. K. and ALLEN, F. H.: A Decade of Progress in the Rh Blood-Group System, New England J. Med., 250, 283 and 324, 1954.

39a.JONES, A. R. and KANEB, LORRAINE: Some Properties of Cross Reacting Antibody of the ABO Blood Group System, Blood, 15, 395, 1960.

39b.KREVANS, J. R. and JACKSON, D. P.: Hemorrhagic Disorder Following Massive Whole Blood Transfusions, J. A. M. A., 159, 171, 1955; Tr. A. Am. Physicians, 69, 155, 1956.

39c.KREVANS, J. R., JACKSON, D. P., CONLEY, C. L. and HARTMANN, R. C.: The Nature of the Hemorrhagic Disorder Accompanying Hemolytic Transfusion Reactions in Man, Blood, 12, 834, 1957.

40. LALICH, J. J. and SCHWARTZ, S. I.: The Role of Aciduria in the Development of Hemoglobinuric Nephrosis in Dehydrated Rabbits, J. Exper. Med., 92, 11, 1950; Am. J. Path., 31, 153, 1955.

41. LANDSTEINER, K. and WIENER, A. S.: Studies on an Agglutinogen (Rh) in Human Blood Reacting with Anti-rhesus Sera and with Human Isoantibodies, J. Exper. Med., 74, 309, 1941.

41a.LAURELL, A. B. and GRUBB, R.: The Hp and Gm Groups and Secretor Characters of 46 Blood Donors, Vox sanguinis, 2, 312, 1957.

41b.LAYRISSE, M., SANGER, RUTH and RACE, R. R.: The Inheritance of the Antigen Di^a: Evidence for Its Independence of Other Blood Group Systems, Am. J. Human Genet., 11, 17, 1959; Caracas, La Fundación Creole y la Fundación Eugenio Mendoza, 1960.

41c.LEVEEN, H. H. et al.: Hemorrhage and Transfusion as the Major Cause of Cardiac Arrest, J. A. M. A., 173, 770, 1960.

42. LEVINE, P.: On the Hr Factor and the Rh Genetic Theory, Science, *102*, 2636, 1945; *cf.* WIENER, A. S., *ibid.*, *102*, 479, 1945.

43. LEVINE, P., KATZIN, E. M. and BURNHAM, L.: Isoimmunization in Pregnancy: Its Possible Bearing on Etiology of Erythroblastosis Fetalis, J. A. M. A., *116*, 825, 1941.

45. LEVINE, P. *et al.:* Gene Interaction Resulting in Suppression of Blood Group Substance B, Blood, *10*, 1100, 1955.

46. LEVINE, P., WIGOD, M., BACKER, A. M. and PONDER, R.: The Kell-Cellano (K-k) Genetic System of Human Blood Factors, Blood, *4*, 869, 1949; Science, *109*, 464, 1949.

47. LEWISOHN, R. and ROSENTHAL, N.: Prevention of Chills Following Transfusion of Citrated Blood, J. A. M. A., *100*, 466, 1933.

48. LITWIN, M. S., SMITH, L. L. and MOORE, F. D.: Metabolic Alkalosis following Massive Transfusion, Surgery, *45*, 805, 1959.

50. MANULLA, A.: Blood Groups and Disease-Hard Facts and Delusions, J. A. M. A., 167, 2047, 1958.

51. MATHER, K.: Human Blood-Groups, Advanc. Sci., *5*, 305, 1949.

52. MATSON, G. A. *et al.:* A "New" Antigen and Antibody Belonging to the P Blood Group System, Am. J. Human Genet., *11*, 26, 1959.

52a.McKAY, O. G., HARDAWAY, R. M., III, WAHLE, G. H., JR., EDELSTEIN, R. and TARTOCK, D. E.: Alterations in Blood Coagulation Mechanism after Incompatible Blood Transfusion, Am. J. Surg., *89*, 583, 1955.

53. McNEIL, C., WARENSKI, L. C., FULLMER, C. D. and TRENTELMAN, E. F.: A Study of Blood Groups in Habitual Abortion, Am. J. Clin. Path., *24*, 767, 1954; *ibid.*, *28*, 469, 1957.

53a.MERRILD-HANSEN, B. and MUNK-ANDERSEN, G.: Haemolytic Transfusion Reaction Caused by Anti-Le^a, Vox sanguinis, *2*, 109, 1957.

54. MILLER, G., McCOORD, A. B., JOOS, H. A. and CLAUSEN, S. W.: Studies of Serum Electrolyte Changes During Exchange Transfusion, Pediatrics, *13*, 412, 1954.

55. MINOT, G. R. and ISAACS, R.: Transfusion of Lymphocytes: Their Rapid Disappearance from the Peripheral Circulation in Man, J. A. M. A., *84*, 1713, 1925.

55a.MOHN, J. F. *et al.:* On the Relationships of the Blood Group Antigens Mi^a and Vw to the MNSs System, Am. J. Human Genet., *10*, 276, 1958.

55b.MOLLISON, P. L.: Blood-Group Antibodies and Red-Cell Destruction, Brit. M. J., *2*, 1035 and 1123, 1959.

56. MOLLISON, P. L., MOURANT, A. E. and RACE R. R.: The Rh Blood Groups and Their Clinical Effects, Medical Research Council Memorandum 19, His Majesty's Stationery Office, London, 1948.

56a.MORGAN, W. T. J. and WATKINS, W. M.: The Detection of the Blood Group O Gene and the Relationship of the So-Called O Substance to the Agglutinogens A and B, Brit. J. Exper. Path., *29*, 159, 1948.

57. MOSENTHAL, H. O. and ASHE, B.: Transfusion of Blood in Bright's Disease, Am. J. M. Sc., *180*, 476, 1930.

58. MOURANT, A. E.: *The Distribution of the Human Blood Groups,* Springfield, Ill., Charles C Thomas, 1954.

59. MUIRHEAD, E. E., HALEY, A. E., HABERMAN, S. and HILL, J. M.: Acute Renal Insufficiency Due to Incompatible Transfusion and Other Causes, with Particular Emphasis on Management, Blood, *3*, Supp. No. 2, 101, 1948.

60. MUSTARD, J. F.: Platelets in Stored Blood, Brit. J. Haemat., *2*, 17, 1956; *ibid.*, *3*, 50 and 202, 1957.

61. NAKASONE, N., WATKINS, E., JR., JANEWAY, C. A. and GROSS, R. E.: Experimental Studies on Circulatory Derangement Following the Massive Transfusion of Citrated Blood, J. Lab. & Clin. Med., *43*, 184, 1954.

62. NEEFE, J. R., NORRIS, R. F., REINHOLD, J. G., MITCHELL, C. B. and HOWELL, D. S.: Carriers of Hepatitis Virus in the Blood and Viral Hepatitis in Whole Blood Recipients, J. A. M. A., *154*, 1066, 1954; Am. J. Clin. Path., *25*, 158, 1955.

62a.NEIMANN-SØRENSEN, A.: Blood Groups of Animals in Relation to Human Blood Groups, Acta haemat., *20*, 225, 1958.

62b.OLIVER, J., MacDOWELL, M. and TRACY, A.: The Pathogenesis of Acute Renal Failure Associated with Traumatic and Toxic Injury, Renal Ischemia, Nephrotoxic Damage and the Ischemuric Episode, J. Clin. Invest., *30*, 1307, 1951.

63. OWEN, R. D., STORMONT, C., WEXLER, I. B. and WIENER, A. S.: Medicolegal Applications of Blood Grouping Tests, J. A. M. A., *164*, 2036, 1957.

64. OTTENSOOSER, F. and PASQUALIN, R.: Blood Types of Brazilian Indians (Matto Grosso), Am. J. Human Genet., *1*, 141, 1949.

65. PARPART, A. K., GREGG, J. R., LORENZ, P. B., PARPART, E. R. and CHASE, A. M.: Whole Blood Preservation, J. Clin. Invest., *26*, 641, 1947.

65a.PAYNE, ROSE and ROLFS, MARY R.: Further Observations on Leukoagglutinin Transfusion Reactions, Am. J. Med., *29*, 449, 1960.

66. PAULS, F. P., VICTORS, B. B. and DODSON, M. W.: Distribution of Blood Groups among the Eskimos, Indians, and Whites of Western Alaska, Am. J. Human Genet., 5, 252, 1953.

66a. PESCHEL, E. et al.: Acute Tubular Necrosis after Transfusion Reaction Due to Anti-Kell Antibodies, J. A. M. A., 167, 1736, 1958.

67. PETROV, B. A.: Transfusion of Cadaver Blood, Surgery, 46, 651, 1959.

68. PLAUT, GERTRUDE, BOOTH, P. B., GILES, CAROLYN M. and MOURANT, A. E.: A New Example of the Rh Antibody, Anti-C^x, Brit. M. J., 1, 1215, 1958.

69. PLOTKIN, S. A.: The A-B-O Blood Groups in Relation to Prematurity and Stillbirth, J. Pediat., 52, 42, 1958.

69a. RACE, R. R.: Blood Groups and Human Genetics, J.A.M.A., 174, 1181, 1960.

70. RACE, R. R. and SANGER, R.: *Blood Groups in Man*, Springfield, Ill., Ed. 3, Charles C Thomas, 1958.

70a. RACE, R. R., SANGER, RUTH and LAWLER, SYLVIA D.: The Rh Antigen Called cl: a Revocation, Vox Sanguinis, 5, 334, 1960.

71. RACE, R. R., TAYLOR, G. L. and Associates: Recognition of Rh Genotypes in Man, Nature, 152, 300 and 563, 1943; *ibid.*, 153, 52, 560 and 771, 1944; *ibid.*, 155, 112 and 542, 1945.

71a. RAMGREN, O., SKÖLD, E. and TENGBERG, J-E.: Immediate, Non-Haemolytic Reactions to Blood Transfusion, Acta med. scandinav., 162, 211, 1958.

71b. REED, T. E. and AHRONHEIM, J. H.: An Association between ABO Blood Groups and Fertility in a Normal American Population, Nature, 184, 611, 1959.

72. REEPMAKER, J.: Relation between Polyagglutinability of Erythrocytes *in Vivo* and the Hübener-Thomsen-Friedenreich Phenomenon, J. Clin. Path., 5, 266, 1952.

73. REIN, C. R., WISE, F. and CUCKERBAUM, A. R.: The Control and Prevention of Transfusion Syphilis, J. A. M. A., 110, 13, 1938.

74. ROBERTSON, R. L., TRINCHER, I. H. and DENNIS, E. W.: Intra-Arterial Transfusion, Surg., Gynec. & Obst., 87, 695, 1948.

74a. ROSENFELD, R. E. and HABER, GLADYS V.: An Rh Blood Factor, rhi (Ce) and its Relationship to hr (ce), Am. J. Human Genet., 10, 474, 1958.

75. ROSENFIELD, R. E., VOGEL, P., GIBBEL, N., OHNO, G. and HABER, G.: Anti-Jk^a: Three New Examples of the Isoantibody, Am. J. Clin. Path., 23, 1222, 1953.

75a. ROSENFIELD, R. E., VOGEL, P., GIBBEL, N., SANGER, R. and RACE, R. R.: A "New"

76. RUTZKY, J., COHEN, FLOSSIE and ZUELZER, W. W.: Anti-A Agglutinins in Pooled Plasma as a Cause of Hemolytic Anemia, Blood, 11, 403, 1956.

76a. SALMON, C., SCHWARTZENBERG, L. and ANDRÉ, R.: Observations serologiques et genetiques sur le groupe sanguin A$_3$, Sang, 30, 227, 1959.

76b. SANGER, RUTH et al.: An Rh Antibody Specific for V and R'^{s}, Nature, 186, 171, 1960.

77. SANGER, R., RACE, R. R., WALSH, R. J. and MONTGOMERY, C.: An Antibody Which Subdivides the Human MN Blood Groups, Heredity, 2, 131, 1948; Am. J. Human Genet., 3, 332, 1951; Nature, 186, 642, 1960.

78. SCHMIDT, P. J., NANCARROW, J. F., MORRISON, ELEANOR G. and CHASE, C.: A Hemolytic Reaction Due to the Transfusion of A$_x$ Blood, J. Lab. & Clin. Med., 54, 38, 1959.

79. SILVER, R. T., HABER, JANE M. and KELLNER, A.: Evidence for a New Allele in the Kidd Blood Group System in Indians of Northern Mato Grosso, Brazil, Nature, 186, 481, 1960.

79a. SPAET, T. H. and GARNER, E. S.: Studies on the Storage Lability of Human Antihemophilic Factor, J. Lab. & Clin. Med., 46, 111, 1955.

79b. STAPLETON, R. R. and MOORE, B. P. L.: A Tube Test for Rh Typing Using Papain and Incomplete Anti-D, J. Lab. & Clin. Med., 54, 640, 1959.

80. STEVENS, A. R. and FINCH, C. A.: A Dangerous Universal Donor, Am. J. Clin. Path., 24, 612, 1954.

80a. STEVENS, A. R., JR., LEGG, J. S., HENRY, B. S., DILLE, J. M., KIRBY, W. M. M. and FINCH, C. A.: Fatal Transfusion Reactions from Contamination of Stored Blood by Cold Growing Bacteria, Ann. Int. Med., 39, 1228, 1953.

81. STEWART, J. W. and MOLLISON, P. L.: Rapid Destruction of Apparently Compatible Red Cells, Brit. M. J., 1, 1274, 1959.

81a. STRUMIA, M. M.: The Preservation of Blood for Transfusion, Blood, 9, 1105, 1954; J. Lab. & Clin. Med., 53, 106, 1959.

82. SUSSMAN, L. N.: Pitfalls of Paternity Blood Grouping Tests, Am. J. Clin. Path., 33, 406, 1960.

82a. SWANN, R. C. and MERRILL, J. P.: The Clinical Course of Acute Renal Failure, Medicine, 32, 215, 1953.

82b. SZULMAN, A. E.: The Histological Distribution of Blood Group Substances A and B in Man, J. Exper. Med., 111, 785, 1960.

Rh Antibody, Anti-f, Brit. M. J., 1, 975, 1953.

83. TAYLOR, G. L., RACE, R. R., PRIOR, A. M. and IKIN, E. W.: A Reliable Technique for the Diagnosis of the ABO Blood Groups, J. Path. & Bact., *54*, 81, 1942.

84. TOCANTINS, L. M., O'NEILL, J. F. and JONES. H. W.: Infusions of Blood and Othei Fluids *via* the Bone Marrow, J. A. M. A., *117*, 1229, 1941; Ann. Surg., *114*, 1085, 1941.

85. TOMPKINS, E. H., BRITTINGHAM, H. H. and DRINKER, C. K.: The Basal Metabolism in Anemia with Especial Reference to the Effect of Blood Transfusion, Arch. Int. Med., *23*, 441, 1919.

85*a*.TULLIS, J. L., SURGENOR, D. M. and BAUDANZA, PHILIPPA: Preserved Platelets: Their Preparation, Storage and Clinical Use, Blood, *14*, 456, 1959.

85*b*.TULLIS, J. L. *et al.:* Studies on the *In Vivo* Survival of Glycerolized and Frozen Human Red Blood Cells, J. A. M. A., *168*, 399, 1958.

86. TURNER, T. B. and DISEKER, T. H.: Duration of Infectivity of Treponema Pallidum in Citrated Blood Stored under Conditions Obtaining in Blood Banks, Bull. Johns Hopkins Hosp., *68*, 269, 1941.

86*a*.UNGER, L. J., WIENER, A. S. and KATZ, L.: Studies on Blood Factors Rh^A, Rh^B and Rh^C, J. Exper. Med., *110*, 495, 1959; J. Lab. & Clin. Med., *54*, 835, 1959.

87. VAN LOGHEM, J. J., JR., DORFMEIER, H. and VAN DER HART, MIA: Two A Antigens with Abnormal Serologic Properties, Vox sanguinis, 2, 16, 1957.

89. VAN LOGHEM, J. J., JR., KLOMP-MAGNÉW and VAN DER HART, M.: De aanwezigheid van het koude agglutinine anti-N in twee menselijke sera, Bull. Centraal Lab. v. d. Bloedtransfusiedienst, 2, 3, 1952.

90. VOGEL, P.: Current Problems in Blood Transfusion, Bull. New York Acad. Med., *30*, 657, 1954.

91. WAITE, M. E., COLUCCI, D. D. and GLASER, J.: Blood Transfusion by the Intraperitoneal Route, A. M. A. J. Dis. Child., *91*, 561, 1956.

92. WEINER, W. *et al.:* A Gene, y, Modifying the Blood Group Antigen A, Vox sanguinis, *2*, 25, 1957.

93. WIENER, A. S.: *Blood Groups and Transfusion,* 3rd ed., Springfield, Ill., Charles C Thomas, 1943 (Bibliography).

94. ———Rh Factors in Clinical Medicine, J. Lab. & Clin. Med., *30*, 957, 1945 (Review).

95. ———Intragroup Incompatibility with Respect to the Hr Blood Factors as a Cause of Minor Hemolytic Transfusion Reactions, J. Lab. & Clin. Med., *33*, 985, 1948.

98. WIENER, A. S. and PETERS, H. R.: Hemolytic Reactions following Transfusion of Blood of the Homologous Group, Ann. Int. Med., *13*, 2306, 1940; Arch. Path., *32*, 227, 1941.

100. WIENER, A. S., SONN, E. B. and BELKIN, R. B.: Distribution and Heredity of the Human Blood Properties, A, B, M, N, P and Rh, J. Immunol., *50*, 341, 1945.

100*a*.WIENER, A. S. and UNGER, L. J.: Rh Factors Related to the Rh$_0$ Factor As a Source of Clinical Problems, J. A. M. A., *169*, 696, 1959; Blood, *14*, 522, 1959; J. A. M. A., *172*, 1158, 1960.

101. WIENER, A. S., UNGER, L. J. and GORDON, E. B.: Fatal Hemolytic Transfusion Reaction Caused by Sensitization to a New Blood Factor U, J. A. M. A., *153*, 1444, 1953.

101*a*.WINSTANLEY, D. P., KONUGRES, ANGELYN and COOMBS, R. R. A.: Studies on Human Anti-A Sera with Special Reference to So-called "Immune" Anti-A, Brit. J. Haemat., *3*, 341, 1957; *ibid.*, *4*, 261, 1958.

102. WITEBSKY, E., KLENDSHOJ, N. C. and SWANSON, P.: Preparation and Transfusion of Safe Universal Blood, J. A. M. A., *116*, 2654, 1941; *ibid.*, *128*, 1091, 1945; Blood, *5*, 123, 1950; Am. J. Clin. Path., *24*, 321, 1954.

103. WOOD, E. E.: Brucellosis as a Hazard of Blood Transfusion, Brit. M. J., *1*, 27, 1955.

104. ZUCKER, M. B. *et al.:* Generalized Excessive Oozing in Patients Undergoing Major Surgery and Receiving Multiple Blood Transfusions, J. Lab. & Clin. Med., *50*, 849, 1957.

Chapter 8

The Principles and Technic of Blood Examination

In connection with some of the subjects discussed in the preceding pages, the details of certain technical procedures were given. In this chapter the principles and technic of the remaining methods will be discussed.

OBTAINING THE SPECIMEN

Small Samples.—For small quantities of blood, puncture of the finger or, in the case of infants, the plantar surface of the heel is adequate. These are the sources of choice for samples used for qualitative blood examinations (blood smears) even when blood has been drawn from a vein for quantitative studies. Blood smears made from venous blood may be unsatisfactory for several reasons. If the blood in the needle is used, endothelial cells from the lining of the vein may mix with the blood and cause confusion[48a] (Fig. 8–1 and Plate II, E, p. 64). They are especially likely to be found if the needle is slightly barbed. If the smears are made from blood in the bottle after mixture with anticoagulant, crystals of the latter may be engulfed by the leukocytes. Other contaminants may also be encountered which will cause confusion, such as fungus spores or bacteria. Furthermore, if the leukocytes are not fixed as soon as they are withdrawn from the body, their nuclei may assume bizarre forms.

(376)

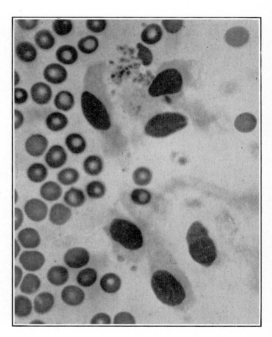

Fig. 8–1.—Endothelial cells from the lining of a vein in a blood smear. Platelets have been caught up by the syncytium of cells. Wright's stain, × 900.

Blood from the ear lobe has been found to contain significantly more hemoglobin than venous or finger-tip blood[5d] and is also not very reliable for leukocyte counts.[35c]

The part to be punctured must not be cyanotic or edematous. If it is cyanotic or cold it should be immersed in water at

38° to 40° C. for three to five minutes. If the finger is used, the side will be found less sensitive than the ball of the finger. In the ear the edge of the lobule is used. The skin is cleansed with alcohol and then rubbed dry for, if it is moist, a rounded drop will not form. The application of a thin film of sterile petroleum jelly to the site chosen for puncture facilitates the formation of well-rounded drops of blood and helps to prevent clotting. This step is recommended in infants if it is desired to avoid venipuncture and yet to collect 0.5 ml. or more of blood for hematocrit studies.

It has been found that instruments such as needles, blades or lancets which are used repeatedly may transmit infectious hepatitis from one patient to another since the hepatitis virus is not destroyed by alcohol. Consequently, a disposable stylet should be used for puncture of the skin.

The puncture is made by a quick stroke which should be sufficiently deep to produce a spontaneous flow of blood. The first drop or two should be discarded. Slight pressure may be made along the sides of the finger some distance from the wound. Undue pressure in securing drops of blood should be avoided as this will cause dilution of the blood with tissue fluid or, if exerted close to the wound, will stop the flow of blood altogether.

Collection of Blood from Veins.— When several blood examinations of a quantitative character are to be carried out, it will be found more satisfactory to collect blood from a vein rather than to make a number of dilutions in several pipets at the bedside. Blood will thus be available for repetition of unsatisfactory counts and for additional tests which may be found desirable after the patient is no longer near by. The blood counts, moreover, may be made at any time that is convenient, although it is best to carry them out within about three hours after the blood has been drawn. Platelet counts are best done within an hour.

It has been shown repeatedly that there is no difference in counts made on venous blood as compared with capillary blood, if proper precautions to secure a freely flowing sample are observed in each instance.[53] In fact, in samples of venous blood there is less chance of error due to cold, edema or other local factors which may interfere with accuracy when blood is obtained from the finger. Venous blood may be used for erythrocyte, reticulocyte, platelet, and white cell counts, hemoglobin, sedimentation rate, volume of packed cells, icterus index, and fragility tests. At the same time blood may be taken for coagulation time, clot retraction time, van den Bergh, Wassermann and other hematological, serological or chemical examinations.

The venipuncture is best made in one of the antecubital veins, but when this fails one of the small veins of the hand, wrist or ankle can sometimes be entered (No. 23 needle). In infants, the superior longitudinal sinus or the external jugular vein is used, but this should be attempted only by one who has had considerable experience.

A suitable vein having been found, the area to be punctured is cleansed with 70 per cent alcohol and a tourniquet applied about 2 inches above the bend of the elbow. The tourniquet should be so adjusted that a slight pull will release it. If the veins are not readily seen, the patient should be instructed to open and close his fist a few times or the site may be gently slapped. In obese patients the veins may be more readily felt than seen. The tourniquet should not be applied so tightly that the arterial flow is cut off; nor should it be applied for longer than two minutes since the blood may then be altered in concentration.

The syringe and needle used must be clean and *dry*, as otherwise hemolysis will occur. A 20- or 18-gauge, sterile hypodermic needle with a short bevel should be employed. Needles with long bevels are unsatisfactory because, if the vein is superficial, the point of the needle may be within the vein while the proximal end of the bevel is still outside the skin. The forearm of the patient is held firmly with one hand and the skin over the vein is drawn tense by means of the thumb, while the needle is inserted beneath the skin with the other. The syringe is so held that the bevel of the needle is turned up. The skin should be punctured first, a little away from the vein, it being better not to puncture both the skin and vein at the same point.

The needle should not be withdrawn until the tourniquet has been released, to prevent formation of a hematoma. The flow of blood from the puncture wound is stopped by pressing directly upon it a piece of sterile gauze. The blood collected is expelled into a small glass vial or bottle fitted with a cork and containing an anticoagulant. This bottle should be made of thick glass so that it will not be easily broken; it should be of such dimensions that it will hold about 5 ml. of blood and will allow a pipet to be readily passed to the bottom. (Smaller vials should be used if smaller quantities

* Holobaugh[26] has described a simple method for opening syringes clogged with blood. "Two pieces of soft rubber tubing, each 30 to 40 cm. in length (such as are used for tourniquets), are the only equipment required. The first is wrapped tightly around the barrel of the syringe in a counterclockwise direction so as to cover the whole barrel with one or more spirals of flattened tubing. This is then held tightly with the left hand while the second tube is wrapped tightly around the handle of the plunger in a clockwise direction, piling up to several thicknesses which can readily be grasped in the right hand. Force is then applied with the two hands to produce a clockwise rotation of the plunger within the barrel. Usually very little force is required but, if necessary, a powerful, steady torsion can be applied because of the improved grip and increased leverage. Careful and complete winding of both tubes will prevent injury to the operator if breaking of the glass should occur."

are to be obtained by heel puncture in an infant.) Before emptying the syringe* into the bottle, the needle should be removed, as hemolysis may result from forcing the blood through the needle. The bottle should be kept tightly corked even when a sample is to be removed within a few minutes. The blood must be thoroughly mixed before each sample is withdrawn. If these precautions are not taken, evaporation of plasma may take place, thus concentrating the mixture; or sedimentation of the corpuscles may occur with the result that varying counts will be obtained, depending on whether the sample is taken from the upper, middle or lower portions of the blood. When the blood is not in use, it should be kept in a refrigerator.

Anticoagulants.—We have found a mixture of dry ammonium and potassium oxalate[25] to be very satisfactory. The former salt causes the red corpuscles to swell and the latter leads to shrinkage. When 6 mg. of ammonium oxalate and 4 mg. of potassium oxalate are used for 5 ml. of blood, no shrinkage in the volume of packed red cells takes place and the other corpuscular constituents are also unchanged. Such a mixture is most easily prepared by dissolving 1.2 Gm. ammonium oxalate and 0.8 Gm. potassium oxalate in 100 ml. neutral distilled water (to prevent deterioration 1 ml. of 40 per cent formalin is added). From a buret 0.5 ml. of this solution is measured into each of a series of bottles and this is then allowed to dry.

The effects of various anticoagulants have been studied.[35] Divergences in results can probably be explained in part by the fact that the salts used were not dried before they were weighed. When this precaution was taken, it was found that a 1.6 per cent solution of potassium oxalate is isotonic with human blood. The use of anticoagulant solutions instead of the dried salts is undesirable, however, in routine hematological work for, if quantitative studies are to be made, a correction for the dilution of the blood is necessary.

Heparin is sometimes used but it is expensive and, since it may not mix readily with blood, tiny clots form unless great care is taken.* However, by comparison with hemophiliac blood to which no anticoagulant need be added, it has been found that heparin does not alter the size of the corpuscular constituents of the blood. For this reason, heparinized blood is generally used as the standard for comparison of the effects of various inorganic anticoagulants.

Ethylenediamine tetra-acetate (dipotassium) ("Sequestrene," "Versene," "EDTA") has an advantage over the double oxalate mixture described above in that platelets are better preserved. The appropriate concentration to achieve anticoagulation and avoid alteration in cell volume is 1 mg. per 1 ml. blood. A solution containing 1.0 Gm. of the anticoagulant in 100 ml. distilled water is prepared and 0.5 ml. is measured by means of a buret into a series of blood bottles and allowed to dry overnight at room temperature. This will provide sufficient anticoagulant for 5 ml. blood.

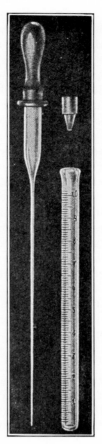

Fig. 8–2.—Author's hematocrit, pipet and bulb used for filling it, and cap for hematocrit. Two-thirds actual size. (Tice's *Practice of Medicine;* courtesy of W. F. Prior Company, Inc.)

MACROSCOPIC EXAMINATION OF THE BLOOD

The study of venous blood with the aid of the hematocrit (Fig. 8–2) is a procedure of great value in diagnosis and should be employed in the routine examination of every patient. By a series of steps in which the same sample of blood and the same instrument is used, information is gained regarding the presence and intensity of morbid processes within the body (sedimentation rate); the presence of anemia, polycythemia, leukopenia, leukocytosis or alterations in the quantity of blood platelets; and the appearance (color, opacity) of the blood plasma.[55]

Technic.—After the blood, collected as already described, has been thoroughly mixed, it is drawn into a capillary pipet (Fig. 8–2) and by means of this it is expelled into the hematocrit. This is done by passing the pipet to the bottom

* We have found the following to be the most satisfactory method for preparing heparin. It is dissolved in water in such a concentration that there will be 7.5 mg. per 1 ml. of water. This amount is placed in a blood bottle and allowed to dry at room temperature. A thin film of heparin (which mixes with blood quite readily) will be formed along the sides and bottom of the bottle. This amount of heparin will prevent the coagulation of 5 ml. of blood.

of the hematocrit and, as pressure is applied to the bulb and the blood slowly forced out, the pipet is withdrawn. This must be done at such a rate that bubbles of air will not form in the hematocrit tube. The hematocrit is filled exactly to the 0 mark at the left side of the scale. With a little practice this can be done quickly and accurately.

The hematocrit is then allowed to stand vertically for one hour and the sedimentation rate is determined (Fig. 6–5). The significance and technical details of this procedure have been outlined fully in Chapter 6 (p. 325). After the sedimentation rate has been measured, the hematocrit is centrifuged.

Before centrifugation the hematocrit may be sealed with the rubber cork supplied, but if it has been filled to the 0 mark this is unnecessary since evaporation will only affect the plasma, the upper level of which has already been read.

The object of centrifugation is to secure such complete packing of the corpuscles that no plasma remains between them and yet distortion or expulsion of some of their contents does not occur. When the cells are densely packed and there is little or no intervening plasma, the column of red corpuscles in the hematocrit is translucent (*Koeppe's criterion*). This is probably attributable to the fact that when the cells are in intimate contact there is so little change of refractive index that the scattering of light is reduced and the suspension appears translucent.

To secure optimal packing of the cells we use a force of 2260 × gravity (G). This force (relative centrifugal force [R.C.F.], expressed in number times gravity) depends upon the distance of the particle from the center of revolution (radius, r) as well as upon the number of revolutions of centrifugation per minute (r.p.m.). This relationship is expressed by the formula:

$$R.C.F. = 0.000,011,18 \times r \times r.p.m.^2$$

We define the radius (r) as the distance from the center of the drive shaft of the centrifuge to the bottom of the hematocrit as it is held horizontally in the centrifuge cup. (Reasons for this definition of radius are given on page 407). With the appropriate head, this radius in a No. 2 International centrifuge is 22.5 cm. which, at 3000 r.p.m., will produce 2264 × G. Centrifugation at this speed is carried out for thirty minutes in order to secure complete packing.

Completeness of packing under any given set of conditions is indicated by failure to secure further packing on repeated centrifugation for succeeding intervals of time. However, failure to attain further packing does not indicate that optimal packing as described above has been attained. This depends on the production of the necessary R.C.F. Since centrifuges with quite different radial distances may be used, it is necessary to determine the speed which must be attained to produce the desired R.C.F. with one's own centrifuge. Substituting in the formula given above an R.C.F. of 2260 × G, the equation may be written:

$$r.p.m. = \sqrt{\frac{202,146,700}{r}}$$

Thus, by measuring the radius of a particular centrifuge (or for the particular centrifuge head if more than one type is used), one may calculate the speed of centrifugation required to achieve the necessary R.C.F. The revolutions per minute should be determined by means of a tachometer since the attainable speed indicated on the face of the centrifuge is not necessarily correct. Furthermore, this should be checked from time to time since the efficiency of a centrifuge may decrease in time.

It should be emphasized that prolongation of the time of centrifugation does not make up for deficiencies in R.C.F.

Unless the centrifuge is capable of producing the number of revolutions per minute required by its radius to attain the necessary R.C.F., centrifugation even for several hours will not produce complete packing.

If a tachometer is not available, a simple way in which the necessary working conditions of a centrifuge can be worked out is to fill hematocrits in pairs with blood samples representing normal, anemic and polycythemic values and to determine the volume of packed red cells of one of each pair of tubes in an instrument of known R.C.F. The speed, or rheostat setting, of the instrument in question at which the hematocrits must be centrifuged to attain the levels found in the machine used as the standard, can be taken as the required speed of centrifugation. Trial by this method will indicate that certain small, inexpensive, table model angle centrifuges provide the necessary R.C.F. to achieve complete packing. They have the small disadvantage that the cells in the hematocrit are packed at an angle and the true value must therefore be estimated.

It has been observed that the addition of fibrinogen to blood accelerates the rate of settling of the red corpuscles and shortens the time required for centrifugation.[16a]

Volume of Packed Red Cells.—The volume of packed red cells may be read directly from the numbers on the right side of the scale. This scale is divided into centimeters and millimeters and, since the inside bore of the hematocrit is uniform and meets the bottom at right angles, the accuracy of the scale can be easily measured by comparison with a good millimeter rule. If the hematocrit has been filled to "10" (which is to the right of the scale and is opposite the 0 mark at the left of the scale), the level at which the packed red corpuscles are found, if multiplied by 10, will give the volume per 100 ml. of blood.

At the uppermost level of the packed red cells, immediately adjacent to the reddish-gray layer of packed white corpuscles, a narrow black band will be seen. The writer had always assumed that this represents a layer of erythrocytes in which the oxyhemoglobin has been reduced by the metabolic activity of the leukocytes. Baumberger[16] proved this to be the case. The reading of "volume of packed red cells" is made at the uppermost level of the black line.

The volume of packed red corpuscles affords the same kind of information as does the red cell count or hemoglobin. However, this information is obtained very easily and with great accuracy (0.59 $\pm$ 0.092 per cent).[56] This procedure is therefore the most useful single criterion of the degree of anemia or polycythemia at present available. In the routine examination of a patient, if the volume of packed red cells is normal nothing further need be done unless clinical examination makes additional studies seem necessary. If it is abnormal, blood is available for red cell counts and hemoglobin determinations and the mean size and hemoglobin content of the corpuscles can be calculated (p. 402).

Reddish-gray Layer of Packed Leukocytes and Platelets.—Above the deep red layer of packed red corpuscles, a reddish-gray layer of packed leukocytes and platelets is found (Fig. 8–3). In normal blood this varies from 0.5 to 1 mm. in thickness, each 0.1 mm. corresponding approximately to 1000 leukocytes per c.mm. When the platelet count is approximately normal, the thickness of this reddish-gray layer may be used as a rough index of the leukocyte count. When the leukocyte count is greater than 12,000 per c.mm. the correlation between the thickness of the leukocyte layer and the white cell count is less accurate than when the count is below this value; but even for counts as high as 30,000 per c.mm. the thickness of

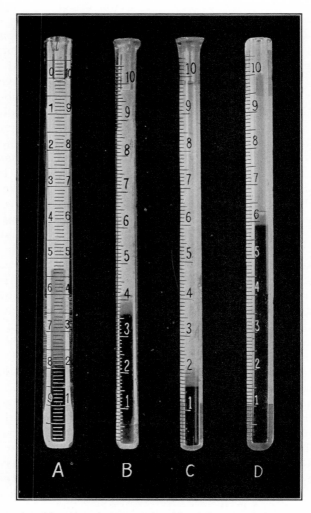

Fig. 8–3.—Photographs of hematocrits containing blood from cases of leukemia and polycythemia. *A*, Chronic lymphocytic leukemia: vol. packed W.B.C. and platelets, 26.5 ml. per 100 ml. blood; vol. packed R.B.C., 20.5 ml. The leukocyte count was 900,000 per c.mm., platelets numbered 180,000, erythrocytes, 2,330,000. *B*, *C*, Chronic myelocytic leukemia. The respective erythrocyte counts were 4 and 2.3 millions per c.mm., but the leukocyte and platelet counts were approximately the same (W.B.C., 42,000 and 35,000, respectively; platelets, 360,000 and 325,000). *D*, Erythremia, showing an increase in all the corpuscles of the blood. R.B.C. 6,700,000, W.B.C. 24,400, platelets 430,000. The successive layers of packed platelets, leukocytes and red corpuscles are particularly clear in *B*, *C* and D.

the reddish-gray layer is a remarkably useful guide. When leukocytosis is marked, relatively more packing of leukocytes tends to occur than in normal blood and 0.1 mm. corresponds more nearly to 2000 leukocytes per c.mm. than to 1000.

The thickness of the layer above the packed red corpuscles depends on a number of factors; namely, the number of leukocytes, the kind of leukocytes, and the quantity of platelets. Since lymphocytes are smaller than the cells of the myeloid series, when there is relative lymphocytosis

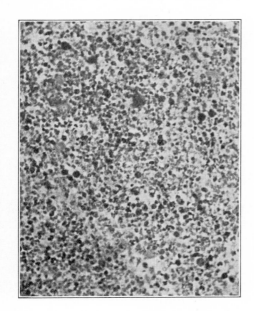

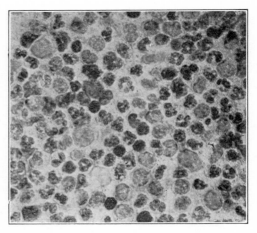

FIG. 8–5.—The reddish-gray layer below the cream-colored layer in the hematocrit shown in figure 8–3, *B* and *D*. It is composed almost entirely of leukocytes. (× 700.)

FIG. 8–4.—Microscopic view of the topmost, cream-colored layer in the hematocrit shown in figure 8–3, *C*. It is composed almost entirely of platelets. (× 700).

the layer will be narrower for a given quantity of corpuscles than when myeloid leukocytes predominate. Again, if the platelets are reduced in number the layer is correspondingly narrower. In cases of leukopenia, and particularly when this is accompanied by thrombocytopenia, the layer of corpuscles above the red cells is barely perceptible. On the other hand, when the platelets are more numerous than usual, and sometimes even when they are present in normal numbers, it is possible to distinguish two portions in the layer above the red corpuscles (Fig. 8–3 *B*, *C*, *D*). Uppermost will be found a cream-colored layer which on aspiration, smear, and microscopic examination (Fig. 8–4) is found to consist practically entirely of platelets. The reddish-gray layer below this consists almost exclusively of leukocytes (Fig. 8–5). In cases of chronic myelocytic leukemia and in erythremia, in which both the number of leukocytes

and the quantity of platelets are increased-the three well-defined layers of corpuscle, present a very striking picture. Separartion of the corpuscles into layers is aided by a period of sedimentation preceding centrifugation.

Measurement of the corpuscular layer above the layer of packed red cells is not recommended as an alternative to leukocyte or platelet counts. It is evident, however, that this can serve as a useful rough guide and is important in routine studies in calling attention to alterations in the numbers of these corpuscles.

Color and Opacity of Blood Plasma.—The procedure described also permits observation of the color and opacity of the blood plasma (Plate I, frontispiece). It is not at all unusual in medical practice to encounter degrees of jaundice which are not sufficiently marked to be perceived by physical examination ("latent" jaundice). The icterus index of the plasma is easily measured in the hematocrit by comparison with standards in tubes of the same size. (See Chapter 3, p. 177.) Lipemia is also easily detected, the plasma appearing quite opaque in

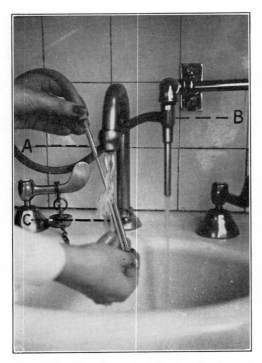

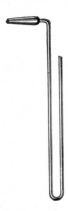

Fig. 8–7.—Tube for cleaning hematocrit by suction. (Courtesy of Will Corporation, Rochester, N. Y.)

Fig. 8–6.—Simple method for cleaning hematocrit. *A* is the type of capillary pipet used in filling hematocrits. It is attached by rubber tubing to a Chapman suction pump (*B*). The capillary pipet is passed to the bottom of the hematocrit (*C*); the water and the suction are turned on. By holding the hematocrit under running water, water is drawn in as the blood is withdrawn.

such instances. Other abnormalities may also be discovered occasionally, as we did in a case of multiple myeloma.[57] In this case cloudy plasma and a yellowish-gray layer 10 mm. in thickness were found above the packed corpuscles. The unusual color and the fact that the leukocyte and platelet counts were already known to be below normal, led to further study. It was noted that the cloudiness of the plasma increased when the tube was kept in a refrigerator and disappeared at room temperature. Further investigation revealed multiple myeloma, a diagnosis which had not been suspected until these observations in the hematocrit had been made.

Cleaning the Hematocrit.—The simplest method of cleaning the hematocrit is with the aid of a Chapman suction pump (Fig. 8–6). A capillary pipet (*A*) is attached by a piece of rubber tubing to the suction pump (*B*) and, with the pipet passed to the bottom of the hematocrit (*C*), the faucet is turned on. The hematocrit with the capillary pipet inside is held under the running water as shown in Figure 8–6. The suction not only withdraws the blood from the hematocrit but draws water into the instrument. When it has been thoroughly cleaned, the hematocrit is removed from the current of water and the water within it is withdrawn by suction. If it is allowed to stand in an inverted position, drying will be completed. When it is necessary to use the instrument immediately, rinsing with alcohol or ether will hasten drying. From time to time the hematocrit may need to be filled with strong acid in order to remove a thin film of coagulated protein which may accumulate on the glass.

A device which makes cleaning still easier consists of a U-shaped, chromium plated metal tube to the longer portion of which is attached, at right angles, a short, beveled arm (Fig. 8–7). The latter is attached to rubber tubing connected with a suction pump. The hematocrit, inverted on the metal tube, is placed into a beaker containing water. When the suction is turned on, the blood will be withdrawn from the hematocrit and water will follow. A device based on this principle whereby several hematocrits can be cleaned at one time is also obtainable.

OTHER METHODS FOR DETERMINING VOLUME OF PACKED RED CELLS

The hematocrit was introduced in the latter part of the last century (Hedin, Blix, 1890; Daland, 1891). **Daland's hematocrit**[9] consisted of two graduated capillary tubes and a small hand centrifuge. The tubes were filled with blood and, before coagulation could take place, were centrifuged by hand for three minutes as rapidly as possible (about 8000 to 10,000 r.p.m.). The method was not very accurate and the procedure was consequently neglected.

The Van Allen hematocrit, which enjoyed a brief popularity, has the serious drawback that it is difficult to prevent leakage of blood during centrifugation, since the instrument is open at both ends. It was this which led the writer in 1929 to devise a hematocrit (Fig. 8–2) in which leakage is impossible. Only 1 ml. blood is required to fill it and, if less than this amount is available, the tube can be filled only partly, an appropriate calculation being made to determine the volume of packed red cells per 100 ml. blood.

Nevertheless, in certain types of work, especially if small animals are being used, even 0.5 ml. is difficult to obtain readily. This fact has led to the introduction of a number of *micro-hematocrits*. Some of these are sealed at one end[36,36f,46b,50a,51a] and others are open at both ends.[17,23,30,36c,37,48c] Of these, the high-speed, closed-end capillary tube of Strumia,[51a] the open-end method of Guest,[36b] and the

very simple open-end tube of McInroy[36c] seem to be the best. For these as little as 0.05 ml. blood is required.

The refractometer and the viscosimeter have been used for cell volume determinations and accurate conductivity[50] and colorimetric methods have been described,[44] but they are not applicable to clinical work. Shohl's method[49] depends on the impedance of light produced by a suspension of red corpuscles. A photoelectric colorimeter is required but a single drop of blood will suffice.

The accuracy of the hematocrit method as a means of measuring the size of red corpuscles is discussed elsewhere (p. 407).

THE ENUMERATION OF RED CORPUSCLES

The **principle** consists in the accurate dilution of a measured quantity of blood with a fluid which is isotonic with the blood and which will prevent its coagulation. A dilution of 1 to 200 is usually necessary because normal blood is so concentrated that the individual corpuscles in undiluted blood can scarcely be distinguished in a counting chamber. The diluted blood is placed in a counting chamber and the number of cells in a circumscribed volume is enumerated.

Apparatus. — The Thoma diluting *pipet*, a modification of that of Potain and Malassez, is now generally employed. It consists of a capillary tube graduated in tenths, which opens into a bulb containing a glass bead. The bulb, when filled to the mark above it (101), will hold 100 times the quantity of fluid contained in the 10 divisions of the capillary tube.

Trenner devised an "automatic" pipet consisting of a capillary tube ending abruptly in a bulb, the sides of which meet the capillary portion at right angles. The bulb contains exactly 200 times the volume held in the capillary.

Hayem's solution (sodium sulfate, 2.5

25

Gm.; sodium chloride, 0.5 Gm.; mercuric chloride, 0.25 Gm.; distilled water, 100 ml.), and *Toison's fluid* (sodium chloride, 1 Gm.; sodium sulfate, 8 Gm.; methyl violet [5 B], 0.025 Gm.; neutral glycerin, 30 ml.; and distilled water, 180 ml.) are generally used as diluting fluids but 0.9 per cent saline or Ringer-Locke's solution are also quite satisfactory.

The specific gravity of Toison's fluid is higher than that of the other solutions mentioned and therefore the red corpuscles do not settle out in it as readily. Besides, the white corpuscles are stained blue and therefore can be distinguished and enumerated in the same preparation as the red cells. However, the dilution used for enumerating red cells is too great to afford very accurate leukocyte counts. A further disadvantage is that fungi grow in it rather readily, a fact which necessitates frequent filtering.

Hayem's solution, for best results, should not be more than two or three weeks old. When this fluid is used, coarse particles may be observed occasionally which are produced by *clumping of the red corpuscles.* Such clumping may be due to cold hemagglutinins (p. 169), in which case it can be prevented by warming the Hayem's solution before use. It may also be produced by precipitation of globulins by the heavy metal in the diluting fluid. In multiple myeloma and in kala-azar clumping is usually due to the latter cause. In cirrhosis of the liver and atypical pneumonia, cold hemagglutinins may be found. Such pseudo-agglutination is avoided if Gower's solution* is used[8] or, better still, if 0.01 Gm. gelatin is added to 100 ml. of the Hayem's solution.[51c]

The *counting chamber* now used is the product of modifications suggested by workers in many countries. Invented by Cramer in 1855, the counting chamber

* Gowers' solution: Sodium sulfate, 12.5 Gm.; acetic acid, 33.3 Gm.; distilled water, 100 ml.

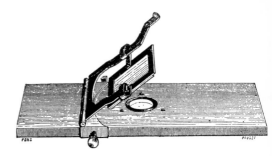

Fig. 8–8.—Early type of counting chamber and cover-glass.

was modified by Alferow (1884) who utilized the principle of the loose cover-glass suggested by Hayem and Natchet (1875). Gowers (1877) suggested that the rulings be made in the counting chamber rather than in the eyepiece of the microscope as the original technic called for. Further modifications were introduced by Bürker (1911) and Neubauer, whose ruling is still employed[43] (Fig. 8–9).

The counting chamber is a heavy glass slide in the center of which are two ruled platforms. These are separated from each other by one moat and from elevated bars on each side by transverse moats. These lateral bars are so ground that a cover-slip resting on them lies exactly 0.1 mm. above the ruled platforms. On each platform is engraved a ruled area 3 mm. on each side (9 mm. square). This area is divided into 9 large squares which are again subdivided, the 8 outside squares being divided into 16 smaller squares and the central square being subdivided into 400 small squares. Each of the largest squares is 1 mm. on the side, or 1 sq. mm. in area. Each of the medium squares is 0.25 mm. on the side, while each of the small squares is 0.05 mm. on the side or 0.0025 sq. mm. in area. In the original Neubauer ruling the 400 smallest squares in the central square millimeter are arranged into 16 groups of 25 small squares each by means of an extra line in the

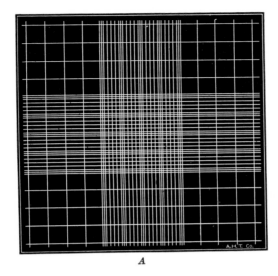

A

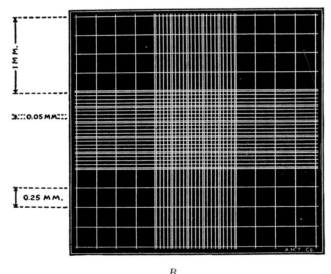

B

FIG. 8–9.—*A*, Original Neubauer ruling (1907) with triple lines used in Spencer "bright-line" chamber. *B*, "Improved" Neubauer ruling (1924) with double line surroundng each group of sixteen small squares used in all-glass chambers to produce the optical phenomenon of a single translucent boundary line.

middle of every fifth square (Fig. 8–9 *A*). In the improved ruling (Fig. 8–9 *B*), the 400 smallest squares in the central square millimeter are arranged into 25 groups of 16 squares, separated by "split" boundary lines.

Method.—In making a red blood cell count, blood is drawn by suction into a Thoma red cell pipet to the 0.5 mark or if there is marked anemia, to the 1 mark. This must be done meticulously since any error is magnified 200 times by the subsequent dilution. If there is a slight excess of blood above the 0.5 mark it may be drawn down by touching the point of the pipet lightly with a blotter or cloth.

(A great excess of blood should not be drawn into the pipet since, even though it is withdrawn, enough blood will adhere to the sides of the pipet to vitiate the results. It is better to clean the pipet and start again.) The blood adhering to the outside of the pipet is next wiped off and the diluent is drawn in until it fills the bulb and reaches the mark 101. If blood is being obtained from the finger, the steps up to this point must be carried out without delay. Otherwise coagulation is likely to begin before the blood is mixed with the diluting fluid and the cells will be clumped in the preparation; or coagulation may take place in the capillary of the pipet.

In the Trenner pipet the required amount of blood can be measured more easily than in the Thoma pipet. Blood is drawn into the pipet until it is three-fourths full. Suction is then discontinued and, if the pipet is being held in a nearly horizontal position, blood will continue to rise until it reaches the extremity of the capillary where it automatically stops. The diluent is then drawn up as with the Thoma pipet.

While drawing in the diluent, the pipet is revolved between the finger and the thumb in order to mix the blood thoroughly with the diluent. After the desired quantity of solution has been drawn into the pipet, it is held horizontally and shaken for about one-half minute in order to secure thorough mixing. For this purpose the pipet may be held loosely in one hand while the attached rubber tubing is revolved between the thumb and forefinger of the other hand. Shaking constantly in any one direction should be avoided. The mixing should be repeated each time before expelling a drop for examination. A number of mechanical devices for shaking blood cell counting pipets have been described.[7,40,41a]

The cover-glass is next placed on the counting chamber. If the apparatus is clean, concentric color rings ("Newton's rings") will be visible when the surface of the applied cover-slip is held toward the light at, or slightly below, the level of the eyes.*

Several large drops of fluid are expelled from the pipet and discarded. This is done in order to remove the fluid in the capillary portion of the pipet which has not come in contact with the blood. A small quantity of diluted blood is then placed between the cover-glass and the ruled platform of the counting chamber. The fluid will run under the cover-glass by capillary attraction. The platform should be completely covered with fluid and none should run over the sides.

After a few minutes have been allowed for the blood to settle, the slide is examined to ensure even distribution of the cells in the chamber. If distribution is satisfactory, the cells are counted. The high-power objective of the microscope should be used. In the Neubauer ruling the small squares in the central square millimeter are employed in the enumeration of red cells. In the improved Neubauer chamber the number of cells in the four corner groups of 16 squares and in one central group is recorded.

Some cells will be found lying outside the specified area, touching the lines of division. Those cells which lie on the dividing lines to the left or above the section being counted are included, whereas those lying outside the specified area but touching dividing lines to the right or below are omitted.

If the dilution has been 1 to 200 (blood drawn to the 0.5 mark), then the total number of cells found in five groups of 16 squares is multiplied by 10,000 in order to give the number of cells per c.mm. of blood. If the dilution has been 1 to 100, the total number of cells is multiplied by 5000.

* If the chamber is made of opaque glass, Newton's rings cannot be seen.

The smallest squares have an area of 0.0025 sq. mm. and are 0.1 mm. deep, being thus 0.00025 c.mm. in volume. Since 80 such squares are counted, a volume of 0.00025×80 or 0.02 c.mm. has been covered. In order to give the value per 1 c.mm. the number of cells counted must be multiplied by 1/0.02, or 50. However, since the dilution was 1 to 200, the multiplication factor is 50×200 or 10,000.

A necessary prerequisite for accurate counts is apparatus free from dust or grease. The counting chamber is washed with lukewarm water or it may be wiped with alcohol. Pipets should be thoroughly washed[5] with water, alcohol and ether, these being added in amounts equal to at least three fillings of the pipet with each liquid. In expelling these fluids it will be found convenient to place the rubber tubing over the long arm of the pipet and force the fluid through the short arm. Finally the pipet must be thoroughly dried. If many counts are being done, much time in cleaning pipets will be saved if a suction apparatus is set up. This is easily done by fixing a Chapman pump to a water faucet. From time to time pipets, cover-slips and counting chambers (if cut from one piece of glass) should be washed with pure nitric acid or sulphuric acid to remove any traces of blood protein that may have accumulated. Acid should be carefully washed away before the instruments are used again. A horsehair—never a wire—should be used in removing blood which has clotted in the pipets. It is extremely important to avoid making even the slightest crack in the bore of the pipet.

Pipets may be calibrated by gravimetric or colorimetric methods.[11,14] A simpler procedure, if apparatus of highest accuracy is desired, is to purchase pipets, counting chambers and cover-glasses certified by the U.S. Bureau of Standards; if this is too expensive, one such set in the laboratory can be used as a basis of comparison.

Critique of Method.—In addition to the errors which may be introduced through the use of faulty apparatus, it is necessary to guard against errors from imperfect dilution, from failure to mix the blood and diluting fluid thoroughly, and from imperfect filling of the chamber. An important source of error in red cell counting is in the filling of the counting chamber. The speed of filling the chamber and differences in the bore of the pipets produce significant differences in hemocytometer counts.[36a] Hemolysis in the counting chamber may also contribute to the error. Proper sampling is important and is attained by securing a free flow of blood if it is obtained from the finger or ear lobe, or by thoroughly mixing the blood each time before a sample is withdrawn if it has been collected from a vein and placed in a bottle.

It has been shown that persons not specially trained tend to count fewer cells than are actually present in the several fields of the counting chamber.[3] This must be avoided. It is best to make at least two complete dilutions and counts in every case. Much more is gained from the standpoint of accuracy by doing this than by filling both sides of the counting chamber from the same pipet and enumerating the cells in 10 groups of squares rather than 5. Statistical analyses indicate that the probable minimum error of red cell counts is 7.8 per cent,[3c] even in the hands of trained technicians. There is no doubt that the error frequently is much greater than this (10 to 15 per cent or more). Statistical studies of various practices designed to improve the accuracy of erythrocyte counts, such as the rejection of counts in which the distribution of cells appears to be unduly irregular, have shown that such rejection— or the unconscious equalization which the establishment of arbitrary standards tends to induce—not only fails to improve accuracy but increases work.[33a,46c] The best practice consists in the performance of counts with as much care as to equipment, sampling and technic as is possible; data should be rejected only when technic has been imperfect and never on statistical grounds. The mean of two or more separate, carefully performed dilutions and counts should be the recorded count.

Electronic Apparatus.—The photoelectric procedures which were first devised for the counting of blood cells[5a,5b] depended on principles of turbidity and, as such, failed to compensate for the influence of differences in the size of cells. Two types of apparatus are now available which have overcome some of the objections to the earlier procedures.

(1) *"Flow-through" System* ("Coulter counter").[5c,36a] This instrument is based on the principle that cells are poor electrical conductors as compared with a saline solution. A dilute suspension of red corpuscles in 0.9 per cent solution of sodium chloride (to which 0.2 ml. of a 2.5 per cent solution of albumin has been added to make the suspension stable) is drawn through a minute aperture conducting an electric current between platinum electrodes. Each cell passing through the aperture displaces an equal volume of the solution of electrolyte and thereby modulates the electric current. The resulting pulses are amplified and automatically counted and they are simultaneously displaced on the screen of an oscilloscope. All of the cells contained in 0.5 ml. of the suspension are counted, except when two or more cells enter the aperture together. These coincidences increase with greater concentrations of cells. The dilution customarily used (1:50,000) was found to be optimal. The instrument has a threshold-control dial that can be set for the minimal size of the cells to be counted.

A number of sources of error, such as bubbles inside the aperture tube or in the suspension of red cells, cotton fibers or dirt, or inadequate rinsing of the aperture tube, can be readily recognized and avoided. Since the counter will register white as well as red blood cells, very high leukocyte counts will introduce significant errors if the results are not corrected by simultaneous white blood cell counts. Microcytosis or macrocytosis has not been found to induce errors. The accuracy and reproducibility of results with this apparatus was found to be of the order of 2 per cent. Thus it permits a significant increase in accuracy, as well as an increase in speed and reduction in the fatigue of the operator.

(2) *Double-scan Principle.*[35f]—A chamber of known depth is filled with diluted blood and enlarged images of the red cells are projected on to a scanning slit, of known width, and are placed in front of a photomultiplier tube. The chamber is moved to and fro by a cam and between each excursion is moved sideways by an intermittent drive. In effect, the aperture sweeps over an area of the chamber determined by the number and length of its excursions, the width of the slit and the optical magnification. Other machines of this type have been described.[8c]

Sources of error include spurious counts from small artifacts, extra counts from cell images overlapping the slit edges, counts missed by the coincident arrival of two images in the slit and extra counts produced by the summation of fractional images. Replicate counts on the same samples of normal blood were found to have coefficients of variation ranging from 2 to 2.5 per cent. However, when microcytosis or macrocytosis was present this increased to a range of 3 to 6.4 per cent.

ENUMERATION OF WHITE CORPUSCLES

The *enumeration* of the leukocytes is carried out according to the same principles as the erythrocyte count with the following differences: (1) because they are less numerous, the dilution of the blood need not be as great. A special pipet which allows a dilution of 1 to 20 is used; (2) the diluent is usually one which destroys the red corpuscles, such as 3 per cent acetic acid. This may be colored with gentian violet (Türk's solution*) thus making the leukocytes more visible; (3) the count is made in five large (1 sq. mm.) squares of the Neubauer counting chamber (Fig. 8–9). Satisfactory distribution of the cells in the counting chamber is indicated by variations between the 5 squares of not more than 8 cells when the total count is about normal. The number of cells found in the 5 squares is multipled by 40 to find the number per c.mm. ($\times$ 20 for the dilution, $\times \dfrac{1}{1 \times 1 \times 0.1 \times 5}$ for the volume counted). When the leukocyte count is exceptionally high, as in cases of leukemia, the dilution should be made in an erythrocyte pipet and an appropriate allowance made for the greater dilution.

Precautions like those mentioned for erythrocyte counting must be observed in order to ensure accuracy. Thorough mixing of the sample in the pipet is very important. It is a common fault to shake the pipet in one direction only. Furthermore, it should be kept in mind that the error is less, the larger the area counted. Whenever possible the count should be made in two chambers; it is still better to make two separate dilutions.

Inherent Errors in Leukocyte Counting.—It is generally agreed by those who have investigated the subject, that the apparatus of responsible manufacturers in the hands of *experienced* workers, introduces almost negligible

* Türk's Diluting Fluid: glacial acetic acid, 3 ml.; Gentian violet, 1 ml.; distilled water to make 100 ml.

variations as the result of filling the sampling pipet, dilution of the sample, variations in the calibration of the appliances, and the personal factor of counting. Bryan et al.[6] found the chief errors to occur in the mixing of the cells and diluting fluid, filling the counting chamber by capillarity and settling of the cells by chance on the ruled field of the counting chamber. The mean error due to these causes, they found, may amount to as much as 600 cells when the leukocyte count is normal (7000) and an area of only 4 sq. mm. (one chamber) is counted, or about 425 cells if the count is made in two chambers. When the leukocyte count is, say 16,000, the probable error is about 900 if the count is made in one chamber only. Others have found the error to be as high as $\pm$ 20 per cent when only one chamber is used and $\pm$ 15 per cent when two chambers are employed. The error is reduced if the cover-slip is so placed on the counting chamber that the ruled areas lie midway between an edge of the cover-slip and the nearer edge of the central trough.[28] An extensive study of the error in blood cell counts has been made by Berg.[2a]

The Coulter counter (p. 390) can be employed for leukocyte as well as for red cell counts.[1] The standard error of the apparatus is in the range of 1 or 2 per cent and, for the entire procedure, was found to be 7.56 per cent.[46]

A difference between "capillary" and venous blood may appear more readily in leukocyte counts than in red cell counts, the capillary count sometimes being 1000 or 1500 cells higher. The difference is probably due to local stasis of leukocytes.

Eosinophil and Basophil Counts. —Interest in the *enumeration of eosinophils* has led to the development of methods for direct counting of these cells since the irregular distribution of eosinophils in a blood smear makes inaccurate calculation of their absolute number from the proportion in the smear and the total leukocyte count. Several types of diluting fluids have been used, these depending on acetone, propylene glycol or urea as the diluent.[50b] To these, dyes have been added to stain the cells and other agents have sometimes been included to cause rupture of cells other than eosinophils. *Pilot's solution* combines the advantages of the different procedures.[35d] Propylene glycol is used as the vehicle. This renders the red corpuscles relatively non-refractile and invisible, acts as a vehicle for stains and, being viscous, does not evaporate quickly. By the use of a small amount of sodium carbonate all leukocytes other than the base-resistant eosinophils are lysed. Phloxine stains these cells red.

The diluting fluid consists of propylene glycol, 50 ml.; distilled water, 40 ml.; phloxine (1 per cent aqueous stock solu-solution) 10 ml.; sodium carbonate (10 per cent aqueous stock solution) 1 ml.; heparin sodium 100 units. The sodium carbonate must be measured especially carefully. The addition of heparin to this fluid in a concentration of one unit per ml. prevents clumping of the leukocytes on standing.[35d] The mixture is filtered and kept in a well-stoppered bottle. It is usable for at least one month.

Blood is drawn in each of two white cell pipets to the 1.0 mark and the diluting fluid to the 11 mark. After shaking the pipets for two minutes, the first four drops from each pipet are expelled and one chamber of the Neubauer counting chamber is filled from each. All the precautions for filling pipets and counting chambers which have been described already should be taken. The filled counting chamber is allowed to stand for fifteen minutes under an inverted Petri dish containing wet filter paper. This allows lysis and staining of cells without evaporation. The number of eosinophils in all 9 large squares in each of the two filled chambers

is now counted under low power magnification. The number of eosinophils per c.mm. is the number counted multiplied by 10 (for the dilution) and divided by 1.8. The count should be done within three hours of the collection of the blood and preferably sooner.

Another diluting fluid which has been devised consists of Bromcresol blue (Eastman No. 745) 25 mg. in 50 ml. distilled water.[36e] A leukocyte dilution pipet is used and the count is made in the counting chamber. The eosinophil granules are stained dark purple and stand out in contrast against other leukocytes, which are colored pale yellow. Very small purple granules in the neutrophils are easily distinguished from the large granules of the eosinophils.

Because of the small number of cells counted, the *error in eosinophil counts* is greater than that involved in total leukocyte counts. When two pipets and two chambers are used, as described above, the inherent error of the count, expressed as two coefficients of variation, is approximately 35 per cent when the number of eosinophils is 175 per c.mm. Special counting chambers have been devised to permit the counting of larger numbers of cells, thus reducing the error approximately in half. The Fuchs-Rosenthal and Speirs-Levy[50b] counting chambers are both satisfactory.

Basophilic leukocytes can be counted by the use of a method which depends on toluidine blue to stain the cells.[38] A proposed modification is the use of lead acetate solution to fix the basophil leukocytes.[28a]

HEMOGLOBINOMETRY

In spite of the fact that it is one of the most useful procedures in clinical medicine, the measurement of hemoglobin has been one of the least satisfactory. This has been due to the fact that an unfortunate proposal introduced at the turn of the century became a habit and also because instruments for the accurate measurement of hemoglobin for a long time were not readily available.

Hayem's proposal that hemoglobin be expressed in per cent resulted in confusion both because no standards were then available to correspond to 100 per cent and also because the normal hemoglobin value differs in males and females and in children of different ages, as pointed out elsewhere (p. 104). As a result, even though normal data have now been gathered in different parts of the world, it is impossible to designate a single value which truly represents 100 per cent. Unfortunately, manufacturers of hemoglobinometers, confronted by the lack of a scientific basis, arbitrarily chose a wide range of values as the equivalent of 100 per cent, from 13.8 Gm. to 17.2 Gm. (and even 21 Gm.!) per 100 ml. blood. Consequently, the same sample of blood could be read as 101 per cent on one instrument and 81 per cent (and even 67 per cent) on another.

The fallacy of expressing hemoglobin in per cent is gradually becoming generally recognized. However, the errors involved in instrumentation are still very great and are not fully appreciated. This is attributable in part to the grossly inaccurate hemoglobinometers which have been in use, in part to the lack of good, inexpensive instruments and in part because of the need for a satisfactory method of calibration and standardization. These defects, fortunately, can all now be corrected.

Types of Instruments. — These range from the grossly inaccurate and inexcusable Tallqvist scale to highly expensive electrophotometers. The Tallqvist, designed in 1900, is a series of lithographed colors supposedly representing hemoglobin values in grades of 10 to 100 per cent. The undiluted blood, collected on a piece of absorbent paper, is compared with these. The margin of error is somewhere between 20 and 50 per cent. Remarkable is the fact that this worthless procedure is still used by some physicians.

Other hemoglobinometers[48] include the relatively inexpensive Sahli in which blood collected in a pipet is diluted with hydrochloric acid and the resulting mixture is compared with a color standard; somewhat more expensive but more easily operated instruments with a fixed light source which do not require dilution of the blood; and the electrophotometers. The latter are mainly of two types; namely, filter photometers and spectrophotometers. In the filter photometer white light is passed through filters in order to obtain light of a wave length range which will correspond to the region of the spectrum absorbed most effectively by the colored solution. This filtered light passes through a fixed thickness of solution and the percentage of the selected range of light transmitted by the solution is detected by a photoelectric cell and recorded by a galvanometer. The intensity of the light is made constant by adjusting the galvanometer to an arbitrary value, such as a reading of 100 per cent transmission, with a tube of the same thickness as that containing the colored solutions but holding instead only a blank solution. The concentration of the colored substance is proportional to the optical density.

In the spectrophotometer a narrow band of light of a particular wave length is passed through the unknown solution and the light absorption in this wave length range is measured.

All instruments naturally require calibration and need to be checked from time to time for various sources of error. Before these are discussed the various methods of handling blood for hemoglobin examination will be considered briefly.

Procedures for Hemoglobin Measurement.—These can be classified in four categories.

A. **Colorimetric Procedures.** — By visual means or by photoelectric methods hemoglobin is measured as oxyhemoglobin or it is first converted to acid hematin, alkaline hematin, cyan-methemoglobin, cyan-hematin, or pyridine-hemochromogen. (a) *Oxyhemoglobin*. In Dare's instrument (1900), in which blood is drawn by capillary attraction between two glass plates, one transparent and the other translucent and white, the color of the blood was matched with a rotating circular disk of tinted glass of varying thickness and depth of red color. Though much more expensive than the Tallqvist, the Dare gave reading which were as much as 20 to 30 per cent in error. In other instruments (Gowers' [1878], Fleischl-Miescher, Burker) blood was diluted with water and matched by eye with various standards such as picrocarmine solution or a wedge of glass.

One of the great disadvantages of the oxyhemoglobin method is the difficulty of matching shades of red by eye. This objection is met in the adaptation of the procedure to photometry, as in the method of Evelyn and Malloy.[12] Still better is dilution of the blood with dilute ammonia for, in the latter, oxyhemoglobin is very stable. The ammonia water is made up by adding 0.48 ml. concentrated NH_4OH to 1000 ml. distilled water. The water must be glass distilled for it has been shown that the presence of minute amounts of copper in distilled water or other diluents employed in photometric oxyhemoglobin determinations may cause the oxyhemoglobin to be converted rather rapidly to methemoglobin and low values will result.[11a] Of the ammonia water, 10 ml. is placed in a test tube and to this is added 0.02 ml. (20 c.mm.) or 0.05 ml. of blood, depending on the type of photometer being used, this being measured in a suitable, calibrated pipet. Care must be taken to wash all the blood out of the pipet. The

hemoglobin reading can be made at any time within a period of 12 or more hours. Readings in the photoelectric colorimeter are made with a 540mμ filter. A tube containing only ammonia water is used for the blank or center setting. The hemoglobin concentration is read directly from a chart or graph which relates optical density to Gm. per 100 ml. blood.

The Spencer hemoglobinometer is portable but somewhat expensive. It depends on the matching of a thin layer of undiluted, hemolysed blood through a green filter against a standardized glass wedge with transmission in the green. A fixed light source is used. This permits matching at the point of greatest sensitivity of the eye.

(b) *Acid Hematin Methods.*[39] — *Sahli* (1895) suggested that blood be diluted with 0.1 N hydrochloric acid, the hemoglobin of the blood being thus converted to acid hematin which is brown in color. Into an empty graduated tube hydrochloric acid is placed to the level of the 10 mark. Blood, drawn into a measuring pipet, is added and thoroughly mixed with the acid, care being taken not to form bubbles of air. The resulting dark brown fluid is then diluted with water until a match with the brown glass standard is attained, when the hemoglobin value is read from the scale by noting the height of the column of the diluted acid hematin.

A practical objection to the Sahli method is the necessity of adding water until a match is attained. This is not only tedious and time consuming but, if the match point is passed, the whole procedure must be repeated. Nevertheless, the acid hematin method is in common use for clinical hemoglobinometry because the brown color match is more easily made than the red of the "direct" methods. Several disadvantages must be recognized, however.

1. The color of an acid hematin preparation gradually increases in in-

tensity. It has been shown that the rate of formation of the color of acid hematin follows a rectangular, hyperbolic curve ending at infinity. However, the changes after forty minutes are so slight that, for practical purposes, the maximum color is reached at the end of one hour. Nevertheless, this delay in making hemoglobin readings is often impractical. Attainment of maximum color may be hastened by heating at 55° to 60° C. for seven minutes, but this may cause the solution to become cloudy and in any case it is often inconvenient to heat the acid hematin. In practice it is the custom, therefore, to make readings at a specified interval following mixture of the blood and acid, generally after ten minutes, because 95 per cent of the final color is attained in this time. It is obviously necessary that the same time interval be observed on each occasion the instrument is used, and it should be standardized under these conditions.

2. A truly satisfactory standard for comparison has not been devised. Brown glass, although it is the simplest standard, never allows a perfect match. One must learn to make the best possible match and to make a comparison of intensity as much as of shade.

3. As in all colorimetric work, the source of light and the personal equation introduce errors. Matching by daylight is generally easier than by artificial light, but the intensity of daylight is variable. In making comparisons, several rapid readings must be made and the average of these taken; otherwise the eye will become fatigued and erroneous readings accepted.

(*c*) *Alkali-hematin Method.*—The color of blood diluted with acid is affected by non-hemoglobin substances (protein, lipoid) in both plasma and cell stroma, owing to the fact that the acid hematin is in colloidal suspension rather than a true solution. This, incidentally, makes the acid-hematin method unsatisfactory for photometry. The addition of excess alkali as, for example, 10 per cent by volume of 10 per cent sodium hydroxide solution, produces a true solution of hematin and a much better solution of plasma proteins and fat.[59]

It has been observed, furthermore, that from 2 to 12 per cent of the total hemoglobin of the blood circulates in an inactive form, chiefly as carboxyhemoglobin, methemoglobin and sulfhemoglobin.[1a] In alkaline solutions of pH 10, these abnormal forms of hemoglobin are converted to hematin whereas this cannot be accomplished with acid. However, the fact that the blood of the newborn and young infant carries a small amount of fetal hemoglobin, which is alkali-resistant (p. 34), introduces an error which, in the newborn, may be significant.

In the method of Wu,[59] 0.05 ml. of blood is treated with 4 ml. of N/10 HCl, left at room temperature for forty minutes, and then diluted to 5 ml. with N/1 NaOH. Clegg and King[8a] dilute 0.05 ml. of blood to 5 ml. with N/10 NaOH. This is heated in a boiling-water bath for four to five minutes, cooled, and read against an appropriate standard.

(*d*) *Cyan-methemoglobin Method.*[8b]—Ferricyanide converts hemoglobin iron from the ferrous to the ferric state to form methemoglobin, which then combines with potassium cyanide to produce the stable pigment, cyanmethemoglobin. These two reactions are rapid and stoichiometric. Drabkin's diluent solution consists of $NaHCO_3$ 1.0 Gm., potassium cyanide (KCN) 50 mg., potassium ferricyanide ($K_3Fe[CN]_6$) 200 mg. and distilled water to 1 liter. This is a clear solution, pale yellow in color. If it develops turbidity it should be discarded. It should be kept in a brown bottle and a fresh solution should be made up once a month. The concentration of cyanide in the reagent is so low that as much as four liters would be required to produce a lethal effect in man.

An accurately measured volume of blood (0.02 ml.) is diluted in an accurately measured volume of the diluent. In most photometers 5 ml. of diluent are used, a 251-fold dilution. The optical density of this solution is then compared with that of the standard. The optical density is taken to be directly proportional to the concentration of the pigment. The color intensity is measured in a photometer set at the 540 mμ band.

(e) *Cyan-hematin Method*.[31]—This method has a high degree of accuracy. Two hundredths of a milliliter of blood are mixed with 1.98 ml. 0.1 N hydrochloric acid and left for ten minutes to complete the transformation to acid hematin. Then 2 ml. of 2 per cent sodium cyanide are added and the solution is mixed. The standard solution consists of pure crystalline hemin (8.57 per cent iron), 28.8 mg., which are weighed into a one liter volumetric flask. To this 200 ml. of 5 per cent sodium cyanide are added, and then water, until the flask is nearly full. The mixture is left at room temperature and occasionally shaken until all the hemin has been dissolved. It is then made up to the mark and mixed. The color intensity is measured in any colorimeter or photometer, visual or photoelectric, with a light filter with maximum transmission between 530 and 550 mμ and transmitting a fairly broad band in the green part of the spectrum (480 to 600 mμ). In the hematin standard the hemin is used in the theoretical proportion of 4 molecules of hemin to one of hemoglobin.

(f) In the method of Rimington[46a] all heme pigments present in the sample, whether they be derived from oxy-, met-, or sulfhemoglobin, are converted into *pyridine-hemochromogen* and the intensity of absorption of the latter is measured after calibration against crystalline hemin. The smell of pyridine is very unpleasant and the technic is very exacting.

B. **Gasometric Methods.**—*The oxy-*gen capacity of the blood* may be determined by the method introduced by Haldane and Smith (1897). As improved by Van Slyke (1924), an accuracy of 0.5 per cent may be attained in experienced hands. The method is somewhat time consuming, however, and the apparatus expensive, and the procedure therefore has limited application. Hemoglobin is calculated on the assumption that 1 gram of hemoglobin combines with 1.34 ml. of oxygen.

By this method only "active" hemoglobin, namely, that which potentially may carry hemoglobin, is measured. Hemoglobin values measured by oxygen-capacity have been found to be 2 per cent lower than those determined by iron methods.[31a]

Hoppe-Seyler introduced the *carbon monoxide method* in 1892. This was adapted for use with the Gowers hemoglobinometer by *Haldane* in 1900. Blood was diluted with water and then saturated with coal gas. The standard consisted of a 1 per cent solution of animal blood having an oxygen capacity of 18.5 volumes per cent (13.8 Gm. hemoglobin per 100 ml.) which had been saturated with carbon monoxide and hermetically sealed. Palmer[48] modified the technic for use with the Duboscq colorimeter. Robscheit applied Palmer's procedure to Sahli's principle with satisfactory results.[48] Jenkins[29] attained an accuracy of 1 per cent by applying the principle of the flicker-photometer to the method, thus eliminating errors introduced by variations in the observer's sense of color. The need for coal gas is an obvious objection to the carbon monoxide method.

C. **Specific Gravity of Blood**—The copper sulfate method described in the preceding chapter (p. 322) can be used for calculation of hemoglobin on the assumption that the corpuscular hemoglobin concentration is constant.[51d] Although this assumption is admittedly incorrect, the technic is useful for mass surveys.

D. **Chemical Methods.**—The *iron of the hemoglobin molecule* can be detached by the action of sulfuric acid and, after the proteins have been precipitated, the quantity of iron can be measured by comparison with the color of a standard solution of known iron content.[58] Various methods are available for the iron analysis, of which the titanous chloride method is probably the best.[31a] It is assumed that only insignificant quantities of iron are found in the plasma; the plasma iron actually represents less than 0.4 per cent of all the iron in normal blood. Depending on the degree and type of anemia, the plasma iron would scarcely ever form more than 1.4 per cent.

One factor which has not been resolved is the iron content of the hemoglobin molecule. The figure which is generally quoted (0.334 per cent) appears to be a misquotation of the data of Hüfner who actually cited the figure 0.336 per cent.[44a] This was based on five determinations, which ranged from 0.328 to 0.342 per cent. Other reports give figures ranging from 0.335 to 0.340 per cent.[3a] The difficulty in establishing this value arises from the fact that crystalline hemoglobin has not been prepared in an absolutely pure and dry state.

The *benzidine* test for blood has been modified for use as a hemoglobin method and is quite accurate even for minute amounts of blood.[4] A spectrophotometric method based on this procedure has also been described for quantitating hemoglobin in plasma or serum.[27a]

Choice of Methods and Instruments.—The authoritative study under the auspices of the British Medical Research Council[35e] showed that the dilution methods of hemoglobinometry (Haldane, Gowers, Sahli) are, on the whole, less reliable than other methods. Even with a single "average" observer, significance could not be attached to differences less than 10 per cent. The methods using whole blood were, on the whole, slightly better than the dilution procedures. These investigators found acid hematin procedures less reliable than the alkali-hematin methods, for reasons already cited. They concluded that oxyhemoglobin is the derivative of choice for hemoglobin estimation and recommended the gray-wedge photometer[31b] as a simple hemoglobinometer for general use. This is an instrument designed to measure the optical density of colored liquid which can be used in daylight or, with a specially designed lamp, by artificial light.

In the United States, the acid-hematin method with the Sahli type of instrument is in common use because it is relatively inexpensive. Better but more expensive is the type of instrument with a fixed light source in which oxyhemoglobin is matched through a filter and no dilution of blood is required. The cyanmethemoglobin method, however, is receiving wide acceptance as a practical and dependable technic, especially since this is the recommended procedure for calibration of instruments (see below). It offers certain advantages; namely, (1) the absorption band of cyanmethemoglobin in the region of 540 mμ is broad rather than sharp, so that its solutions are suitable for use in filter type photometers as well as in narrow band spectrophotometers; and (2) all forms of hemoglobin likely to be found in blood, with the exception of sulfhemoglobin, are quantitatively converted to cyanmethemoglobin upon the addition of a simple reagent.[10b]

Calibration of Instruments.—Instruments as obtained on the open market are not all well or uniformly standardized. The error may be as great as 20 per cent or more. This criticism applies to the very expensive as well as the cheaper instruments. It is not generally appreciated that the photoelectric principle does not guarantee the accuracy of a hemoglobinometer. It is necessary to calibrate the instrument under the conditions of its operation and to recheck the calibration from time to time. Furthermore, the blood diluting pipets must be calibrated[51b] and the cuvettes must be matched. The physician using a simple type of hemoglobinometer which is not of the photoelectric type should at least compare the results he obtains with his instrument with those of a properly calibrated photoelectric apparatus.

The photometer itself first requires calibration.[10c] The method varies with the type and make of the instrument. If it is a spectrophotometer the wave length setting should be checked, and adjusted if necessary. Some instruments are provided with factory calibrated standard filters for this purpose. For those not so provided a solution of known absorption maximum should be used. The accuracy of the meter reading should also be checked.

A variety of excellent methods are available for standardization of instruments. The iron method, for example, is very good but unfortunately it is technically difficult and requires considerable skill.[51b] Oxygen capacity is likewise a good procedure but this too requires the skill of a person trained in this procedure. Furthermore, as already stated, this measures only "active" hemoglobin. Crystalline hemin has been proposed as a standard[8a] and the method has been modified[1c,26a] from time to time but the procedure presents difficulties from the standpoint of purity.

A panel of the United States National Research Council concluded that, in respect to simplicity and adaptability, the cyanmethemoglobin method is the method of choice for calibration of instruments.[7a] Solutions of the pigment can be prepared simply and inexpensively from crystalline hemoglobin and are stable for years when preserved at refrigerator temperatures. Furthermore, they can be accurately standardized and, as stated earlier, cyanmethemoglobin because of its broad absorption band in the region of 540 mμ is adaptable to a variety of photometric instruments and cuvettes. The standard of reference is crystalline human hemoglobin prepared by the method of Drabkin.[10b] This is characterized spectrophotometrically on the basis that the extinction coefficient of one milligram atom of iron (c = 1 mg. atom of iron per liter, d = 1 cm.), in the form of cyanmethemoglobin at a wave length of 540 mμ, is 11.5. The iron content of hemoglobin is assumed to be 0.338 per cent (w/w), which corresponds to a molecular weight for hemoglobin of 16,520 per gram atom of iron. A factor of 1,65$\overline{2}$ should therefore be used in calculating hemoglobin in mg. per 100 ml. from millimoles per liter.

Standards which carry the certification label of the College of American Pathologists are available from several commerical sources. The Panel recommended that the standard be distributed as a single concentration of not less than 55 mg. of cyanmethemoglobin per 100 ml., in brown glass containers and in sterile condition. They are known to be stable for nine months. Full details concerning recommended standardization procedures have been published.[7b]

Error of Methods.—It is essential that the physician be aware of the error in the method of hemoglobinometry on which he is relying. Lack of such information will obviously lead to misleading conclusions. Thus a patient may be regarded as anemic, who is not—a rather common error; or anemia, a valuable sign of disease, may be overlooked when it is present. When the error of the method is known, even a relatively cheap and simple hemoglobinometer is useful for certain purposes. The error of a method, furthermore, must not only be known but it should be weighed against the practicality of the procedure. It is of little help in routine work that the gasometric method of Van Slyke can be carried out to an error of only 0.5 per cent by a skilled technician. This is important only from the standpoint of the use of the procedure for calibration purposes. It is very valuable to know, on the other hand, that the cyanmethemoglobin method in a correctly calibrated and maintained electrophotometer can carry an error as low as ± 2 per cent. It is also important to bear in mind that hemoglobin pipets purchased on the open market may carry an error as great as 5 per cent.[34b]

Measurement of Heme Pigments Other Than Hemoglobin.—When abnormal pigments are present in sufficient concentration they can be detected readily and their nature suspected from the color of the blood, as discussed in an earlier chapter (p. 193). More exact identification requires the use of a spectroscope or other equipment. The hand spectroscope suffices if their concentration is relatively high. If it is less than 10 per cent, as well as for quantitative measurements, it is necessary to resort to spectrophotometric,[24b] colorimetric[12a] and gasometric[51e] procedures.[51b]

The *collection of the blood* specimens must be carried out with special care and should be prompt since, with the exception of sulfhemoglobin, the abnormal pigments disappear rapidly on removal of the causative agent or on institution of therapy. In obtaining the specimen every precaution must be taken to prevent hemolysis. If hemoglobinemia is suspected, part of the blood should be allowed to clot. After allowing this to stand for an hour in the refrigerator, the blood is centrifuged without dislodging the clot. If carbon monoxide exposure is suspected, the blood should be collected in small tubes which are tightly stoppered, using dry sodium citrate as an anticoagulant. For most other purposes, dry oxalate is preferable to heparin as an anticoagulant but the latter is preferable if methemoglobin is suspected since oxalate increases the pH of the blood and favors the conversion of neutral methemoglobin to alkaline methemoglobin.[51b]

Centrifugation of the blood will reveal plasma which, if it contains oxyhemoglobin will be pink or red and if methemoglobin or methemalbumin is present it will be brown. Spectroscopic examination will reveal a band at 576 mμ if oxyhemoglobin is present. A band in the region of 620 to 630 mμ indicates that either methemalbumin or methemoglobin is present. These can be distinguished by adding (with a dropper, not a pipet) two drops of a 5 per cent solution of potassium cyanide to 2 ml. plasma. If methemalbumin is present the band will remain fixed; if the pigment is methemoglobin, it will disappear and the specimen will change in color from brown (or black) to dark red. The differentiation of bilirubin and carotene, pigments producing a yellow color, has been discussed already (p. 177).

The presence of an abnormal pigment in the plasma does not absolve the red cells. The plasma must therefore be decanted off and the red corpuscles washed with physiological saline so that they may be examined separately.

In examining for *methemoglobin* and *sulfhemoglobin*, whole blood or washed red corpuscles are added to distilled water in a ratio of 1:10 or 1:100, depending upon the concentration of the abnormal pigment. A few ml. of the hemolysed blood is placed in each of two test tubes. The first tube is then examined with the hand spectroscope. Methemoglobin produces a dark band at 630 millimicrons in the red region of the spectrum (Plate VII). To the second tube two or three drops of 5 per cent solution of potassium cyanide are added. If the pigment is methemoglobin, the band will disappear. Sulfhemoglobin produces a dark band at 618 mμ which is difficult to distinguish from that of methemoglobin in the hand spectroscope but it can be recognized by the fact that it is not removed by the addition of cyanide. Hydrogen peroxide (3 per cent) causes both of these bands to disappear.

The bands of *carboxyhemoglobin* are difficult to distinguish from those of oxyhemoglobin since they are very similar, being only a little nearer to the violet end of the spectrum. However, simple clinical procedures can be used.[7b] Thus, in dilute solutions oxyhemoglobin appears yellowish-red, whereas carboxyhemoglobin is pinkish or bluish-red. To demonstrate this requires only the addition of a drop of blood to 5 ml. of water and the serial dilution of the hemolysed blood. The suspected blood is compared with normal blood treated in the same way. An alkali test is also useful. Two drops of normal blood and two drops of the suspected blood are placed side by side on a spot plate. Two drops of 25 per cent sodium hydroxide are added to each. Normal blood turns a brownish color whereas carboxyhemoglobin does not change color.

Spectrophotometry offers more precise as well as quantitative information. The essential principle[10c] consists in the determination of the optical densities at various wave lengths of a dilute solution of hemolysed normal blood and repetition of the same procedure on the suspected sample. Details are given in an excellent monograph by Heilmeyer.[24b]

THE MEASUREMENT OF THE SIZE AND HEMOGLOBIN CONTENT OF RED CORPUSCLES

One wonders whether Leeuwenhoek, in sleepless and imaginative moments, visualized the extent of the studies of which his own observation was probably the first. If he did, he probably did not suspect that it would be more than two centuries after he compared the diameter of red corpuscles with that of a grain of sand, that further attempts, not very much more refined, would be made to study the size of these cells. Although Thomas Young in 1813 showed the value of the principle of diffraction for the measurement of small objects, including red cells, it was more than a century afterwards that Pijper rediscovered the value of diffraction for this purpose (1919). It was not until the latter half of the nineteenth century, moreover, that the diameter of red corpuscles in various diseases was measured and the significance of variations in the size and hemoglobin content of erythrocytes began to be appreciated. In 1864, Welcker demonstrated that the diameter of the red cells in chlorosis is less than normal and Sorensen pointed out that an increase in the size of the cells is one of the most characteristic features of the blood in pernicious anemia (1876). During the last quarter of the nineteenth century, the blood was the object of study by many investigators. Hayem introduced the color index (1878). Malassez described the normal variation in the diameters of red corpuscles, and also calculated the "titre hémoglobique" in micromicrograms. Following the introduction of the hematocrit, Capps introduced the volume index (1903) and made important observations in the anemias. Price-Jones' painstaking measurements of the diameters of red cells, which are responsible for the attention which ultimately came to be paid to cell size, were commenced in 1910. The relationship of hemoglobin to volume of cells attracted Malassez' interest and similar studies were made by Hart (1881), Herz and Bönninger (1919). Haden introduced the term "saturation index" (1923). The terms "mean corpuscular volume," "mean corpuscular hemoglobin" and "mean corpuscular hemoglobin concentration" and methods for their calcula-

PLATE VIII

SPECTRUMS OF HEMOGLOBIN

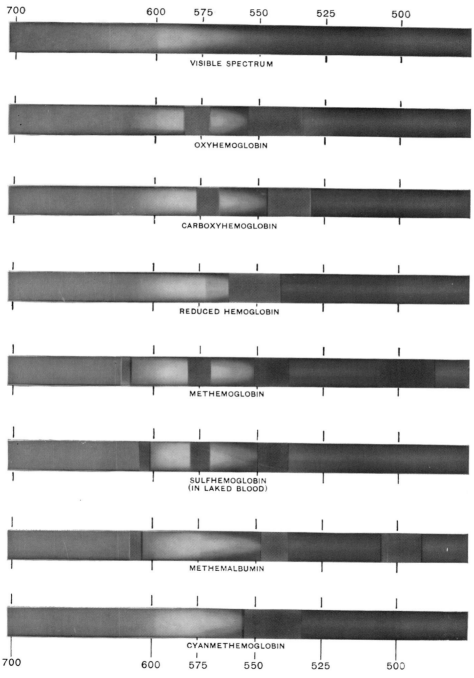

(Prepared by Captain V. E. Martens, MC, USN, U. S. Naval Medical School, Bethesda, Maryland.)

(From Clinical Laboratory Diagnosis, Levinson and MacFate, 1956)

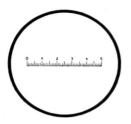

Fig. 8–10.—Micrometer disk.
(Courtesy of Carl Zeiss, Inc.)

A simpler but less accurate method consists in the measurement of the cells as seen in the microscope. A disk on which a scale has been etched (*micrometer disk*, Fig. 8–10) is placed in the eyepiece of any microscope. A thin portion of a film of blood is brought into view and the diameter of all cells which appear beneath the scale, is measured. The film of blood is slowly moved and measure-

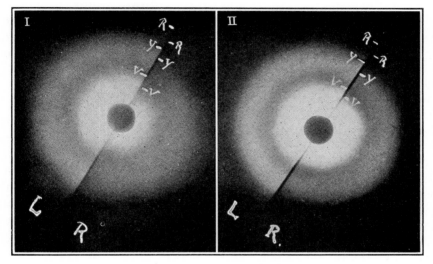

Fig. 8–11.—*I*, Diffraction patterns of "normal" blood (left) and blood from a case of pernicious anemia (right). *V*, inner edge of violet circle; *R*, outer edge of red circle; *Y*, yellow circle. *II*, Normal blood (left); blood from a case of subacute combined degeneration of the cord (right). (Pijper, courtesy of Lancet.)

tion were introduced in 1929 by Wintrobe.[52]

The Determination of the Size of the Red Corpuscles.—(*a*) **The measurement of cell diameter** can be accomplished by measuring the individual cells, or by measuring their diffraction patterns.

1. The method used by *Price-Jones*[45] in his pioneer studies is relatively accurate but laborious. It consisted in the projection of a stained blood film on paper, outlining the cells in pencil, and measurement of the maximum and minimum diameters of each of 500 or 1000 cells. Less time consuming modifications have been devised.[26b]

ments of cells crossing the scale are continued until 500 or more cells have been measured. The micrometer disk must be calibrated for the particular tube length and lenses employed by means of a micrometer slide or with the aid of a hemocytometer, the smallest squares of which are 50 μ to the side. This is done by noting how many of the divisions on the disk correspond, as seen through the microscope, to a given number of divisions on the micrometer slide. Since the distance between the latter is known, the value of each division on the disk is readily calculated.

It is important that a uniform technic be followed and that measurements be made of the cells of a few normal individuals before the procedure is applied to clinical or experimental work. Variations in methods of collecting, fixing, staining and mounting may cause apparent or actual alterations in the diameters of erythrocytes. Because red corpuscles on drying shrink from 0.7 to 1.0 μ[44] and since wet films of blood require less manipulation than stained films, the measurement of cells in wet preparations is recommended.

The diameters of the erythrocytes may be recorded graphically to show the number of cells of various sizes. This has come to be known as the "Price-Jones curve" (Figs. 9–4, 10–6 and 10–8 pp. 455, 479 and 488).

2. The mean diameter of the red cells may be measured very easily by making use of the fact that a beam of white light passing through a film containing numerous small particles is diffracted by the edges of these particles to produce a set of circular concentric spectra. All the individual spectra can be made to coincide on a screen by means of a positive lens between the light and the blood film and, from the radius of the yellow circle, the mean diameter can be calculated.[42] It has been pointed out that some idea of the degree of variation in the diameter of the cells can be gained

instruments all based on the same principle, have been described (halometer, eriometer, erythrocytometer).[20,21]

(b) **The Measurement of the Volume of the Red Corpuscles.**—The mean volume of the corpuscles may be calculated when the erythrocyte count and the volume of packed red cells are known. The result may be expressed in absolute terms or in the form of an index, the **"volume index."** The latter expresses the mean volume of the cells in proportion to the mean volume of cells in normal blood and is calculated from the formula,

$$\text{Volume Index} = \frac{\text{vol. packed red cells, ml. per 100 ml.} \times 2.3}{\text{red cell count, millions per c.mm.} \times 20}$$

As the normal red cell count, 5,000,000 cells has been chosen (therefore the count multiplied by 20 gives per cent), while for normal mean volume of packed red cells 43.2 ml. per 100 ml. of blood should be used (therefore the volume found, multiplied by 2.3 $\left(\dfrac{100}{43.2}\right)$ gives the volume in relation to the normal).

The mean volume of the cells in absolute terms, may be calculated from the formula,

$$\frac{\text{Mean corpuscular volume}}{\text{(M.C.V.)}} = \frac{\text{vol. packed red cells, ml. per 1000 ml.}}{\text{red cell count, millions per c.mm.}}$$

by measuring the violet and the red circles of the diffraction pattern (Fig. 8–11).

This method was introduced by Pijper (1919).[42] Since that time numerous

This formula was designed in order that the result may be expressed in cubic microns (c.μ).

Example: R.B.C., 3,600,000; vol. packed R.B.C., 39.2 ml. per 100 ml. of blood.

$$\text{Then, mean corpuscular volume} = \frac{392}{3.6} = 109 \text{ c.}\mu,$$

$$\text{and volume index is } \frac{39.2 \times 2.3}{3.6 \times 20} = 1.25.$$

The electronic cell counter (p. 390) can be employed to record red blood cell frequency distribution curves.[16] This is done by increasing the threshold systematically and recording the differences in counts at various cell sizes. To secure absolute values, the relation of the threshold scale to cell volume must be known.

(c) **The Measurement of Mean Corpuscular Thickness.**—The thickness of red corpuscles, like their diameter, can be measured microscopically as they lie on edge in wet films. The mean thickness may also be estimated from the mean corpuscular volume and the mean diameter, by regarding the cells as short cylinders. Thus,

$$\text{Mean corpuscular thickness (M.C.T.)}$$

$$= \frac{\text{mean corpuscular volume}}{\pi \left(\dfrac{\text{mean diameter}}{2} \right)^2}$$

The Estimation of the Hemoglobin Content of the Red Corpuscles.—Such measurements are necessarily indirect and are derived from the hemoglobin content of the blood, the red cell count and the volume of packed red cells.

(a) The ratio of hemoglobin to red cell count, which indicates the weight of hemoglobin in the average corpuscle, may be expressed in relation to the normal or in absolute terms. The former, **"color index,"** is derived thus,

$$\text{Color index} =$$

$$\frac{\text{hemoglobin, per cent (Gm. per 100 ml. } \times \text{ 6.9)}}{\text{red cell count, millions per c.mm. } \times \text{ 20}}$$

As for volume index, 5,000,000 red corpuscles has been chosen as "normal," while for the equivalent of 100 per cent hemoglobin 14.5 gm. may be considered "normal." The reasons for this choice have been discussed elsewhere (p. 104).

The same function, measured in absolute terms, is derived as follows:

$$\textbf{Mean corpuscular hemoglobin} \\ \textbf{(M.C.H.)}$$

$$= \frac{\text{hemoglobin, Gm. per 1000 ml.}}{\text{red cell count, millions per c.mm.}}$$

The formula has been calculated so that the result may be given in micromicrograms ($\gamma\gamma$) (millionth of a millionth of a gram or Gm. $\times$ 10^{-12}).
Example: R.B.C., 3,600,000; hemoglobin, 13.6 Gm.
Then, mean corpuscular hemoglobin is

$$\frac{136}{3.6} = 38\gamma\gamma.$$

and color index is $\dfrac{13.6 \times 6.9}{3.6 \times 20} = 1.3$.

(b) An even more important ratio, as will be shown in the chapters on the anemias is that of hemoglobin to volume of packed red cells. This measures the concentration of hemoglobin in the average red corpuscle, as if the erythrocyte carried hemoglobin in solution.

In relative terms, the **"saturation index"** is derived, as follows:

$$\text{Saturation index} =$$

$$\frac{\text{hemoglobin, per cent (Gm. 100 ml. } \times \text{ 6.9)}}{\text{vol. packed red cells, per cent (ml. per 100 ml. } \times \text{ 2.3)}}$$

In absolute terms,

Mean corpuscular hemoglobin concentration (M.C.H.C.)

$$= \frac{\text{hemoglobin, Gm. per 100 ml.} \times 100}{\text{vol. packed red cells, ml. per 100 ml.}}$$

The result is expressed in per cent.
Example: Hemoglobin, 13.6 Gm.; vol. packed red cells, 39.2 ml. per 100 ml. of blood.
Then mean corpuscular hemoglobin concentration $= \frac{13.6}{39.2} \times 100 = 35\%$ and saturation index is $\frac{13.6 \times 6.9}{39.2 \times 2.3} = 1.0$.

With the aid of the chart shown in Figure 8–12 or by the use of a slide rule,[3b, 39a] the corpuscular constants can be easily calculated.

The **difference between mean corpuscular hemoglobin** (M.C.H.) **and mean corpuscular hemoglobin concentration** (M.C.H.C.) should be clearly understood. The former measures the *weight* of hemoglobin in the average red corpuscle and expresses the result in parts of a gram (micromicrograms). The latter (M.C.H.C.) indicates the *concentration* of hemoglobin in the average red corpuscle, the ratio of weight of hemoglobin to the volume in which it is contained, and the result is expressed in per cent. The distinction is an important one. In most types of anemia increases or decreases in the average size of the red corpuscles (M.C.V.) are associated with corresponding increases or decreases in the weight of hemoglobin (M.C.H.) carried in the corpuscles. The ratio of these to one another is indicated by the mean corpuscular hemoglobin concentration (M.C.H.C.), which remains normal in the types of anemia just mentioned. There is an important group of anemias, however, in which the reduction in the weight of hemoglobin in the average corpuscle is even greater than the decrease in the average cell size. This is indicated by a reduction below normal in M.C.H.C. The latter, therefore, serves to identify this type of anemia. M.C.H.C. is, in fact, a much more valuable measurement than M.C.H. for, whenever the latter is not altered proportionately with mean corpuscular volume, the lack of correlation is indicated by a change from the normal in M.C.H.C.

It is noteworthy that, except in hereditary spherocytosis (p. 648), an increase above normal in M.C.H.C. does not occur. It appears that there is a maximal concentration of hemoglobin in red corpuscles and that this maximal concentration is maintained in the normal individual and in many cases of anemia. Only *reductions* below normal in M.C.H.C. have been observed.

A misunderstanding as to the meaning of color index has led to a mistaken impression regarding the hemoglobin content of the red corpuscles in pernicious anemia. Because the color index is increased in this disease it has been assumed that the red corpuscles in this condition are "hyperchromic" or supersaturated with hemoglobin. This is not true. The weight of hemoglobin in the average cell, as measured by M.C.H. or by color index, is increased but this increase is only proportional to the increase in the average size of the cells. M.C.H.C. is not increased. The darker appearance of these corpuscles when examined under the microscope, and the lack of the normal central pallor, is due to their increased thickness.

Relative Value of Indexes and Corpuscular Constants.—The advantage offered by the calculation of volume index, color index and saturation index is that the volume and hemoglobin content of the red corpuscles are expressed in relation to the normal in such a way that the index for normal blood is 1.0,

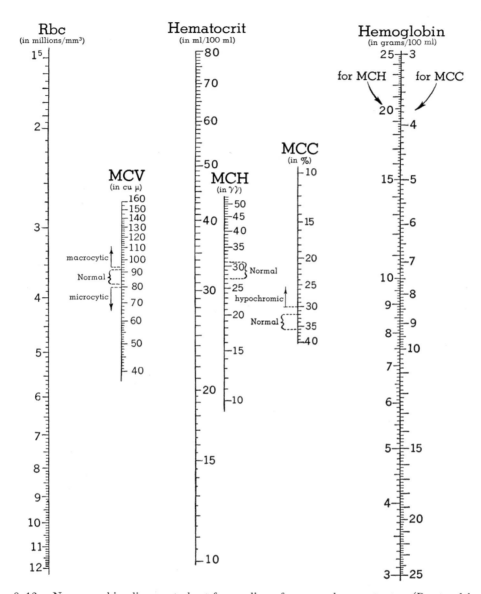

Fig. 8–12.—Nomographic alignment chart for reading of corpuscular constants. (Prepared by Dr. Robert E. Mason.) For mean corpuscular volume (M.C.V.) join the value for red cell count and volume of packed cells ("hematocrit") by means of a ruler, preferably a transparent one. (A very satisfactory one is prepared by scratching a straight line on a strip of clear x-ray film and filling it in with ink.) The reading is made where the line intersects M.C.V. Similarly where a line joining R.B.C. and Hemoglobin intersects M.C.H. the reading for mean corpuscular hemoglobin is made; where a line joining Hemoglobin and Hematocrit intersects M.C.C. the reading for mean corpuscular hemoglobin concentration is made. Note that the left side of the Hemoglobin scale is used for M.C.H., the right side for M.C.C. (See page 1137.)

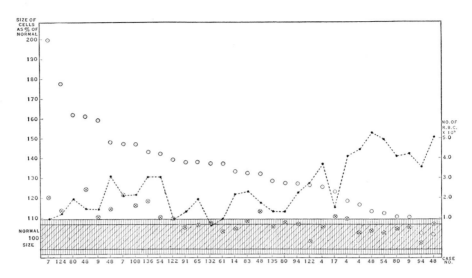

FIG. 8–13.—The comparative value of mean corpuscular volume (M.C.V.) determinations and mean cell diameter values in the diagnosis of macrocytosis. Thirty-two determinations in 14 cases of pernicious anemia and 5 cases of sprue in all stages of severity. The values for mean corpuscular volume and mean cell diameter are expressed as per cent of normal, 87 c.μ being taken as the mean normal corpuscular volume and 7.9 μ the mean normal diameter. The values for M.C.V. have been arranged in order of magnitude and the corresponding cell diameter and red cell count have been placed in the corresponding vertical position. ⊕ is the M.C.V., ⊗ the cell diameter, and ● the red cell count for each patient. The larger vertically shaded portion denotes the normal range of variation in M.C.V. and the smaller diagonally shaded area the normal range of cell diameter as indicated by the coefficients of variation for these values, 9 per cent and 6.3 per cent, respectively.

a value easily remembered. Unfortunately, however, it is impossible to set any single value for red cell count, hemoglobin or volume of packed red cells which truly represents normal. The method therefore gives only approximate results since it is based on an assumption which is not strictly correct. As generally carried out, the results have often been actually misleading. The indexes possess the additional disadvantage that they indicate less clearly what it is that they measure than do the absolute measurements, mean corpuscular volume, mean corpuscular hemoglobin, and mean corpuscular hemoglobin concentration, as the misunderstanding regarding the significance of the increased color index in pernicious anemia illustrates. The value of the corpuscular constants as an aid in the classification and treatment of anemia

is discussed more fully in the next chapter (p. 428).

Relative Value of Volume and Diameter Measurements. — As between measurement of mean corpuscular volume or mean diameter, it will generally be found of more advantage to determine the former. In the anemias, alterations in the size of corpuscles occur in all dimensions. Consequently, changes in the size of cells which may be too slight to be perceived by mean diameter measurements are so magnified when changes in all the dimensions of the cells are determined, as is done in volume calculations, that they can be readily appreciated (Fig. 8–13). Since red cell counts are regularly done and hematocrit determinations are carried out very easily, the calculation of mean corpuscular volume is no more troublesome than the measurement of cell diameter by one of the diffraction methods. The chief merit of diameter studies lies in the demonstration of the degree of variation, information which can be roughly but usually adequately obtained by examination of the blood film. Only occasionally is it necessary to study the diameter of the cells more exactly than can be done by simple inspection of the blood smear, and then it is preferable to use the microscopic-method rather than the diffraction technic since the latter gives only average values.

Accuracy of Hematocrit Method.— The hematocrit method as a means of determining the size of corpuscles has been criticized by Ponder.[44] His criticism that "constant volume" is not a perfectly accurate criterion for the necessary time for centrifugation of the hematocrit, is justified; and his dislike of "Koeppe's criterion," the translucent, "laked" appearance of cells following prolonged centrifugation, also has merit. The failure of the height of the column of cells in the hematocrit to change further, as well as the translucent appearance, depends on the speed of centrifugation. When the hematocrit is spun at 1800 r.p.m. there will occur no further packing after a certain time no matter how much longer centrifugation is continued, whereas centrifugation at 3000 r.p.m. will produce a change in a short time. Centrifugation at still greater speeds will cause still further packing. Ponder admits, however, that there may be an ideal centrifugal force for packing. That this probably is in the neighborhood of 2260 × G (p. 380), is suggested by the fact that the mean corpuscular volume for normal blood as determined by the author's method is exactly the same as that derived by Ponder by his colorimetric method, namely 87 c.μ.

It is clear, however, that under the conditions employed in clinical work, some plasma is trapped in the red cell column. This has been measured in various ways (dye or iodinated albumin dilution, radioactive iron) but also, unfortunately, under different conditions so that estimates of the quantity of trapped plasma have ranged from 2 to 5 and even 8.5 per cent. A careful study of the factors concerned has revealed that the two major ones are the mean effective radius of centrifugation (MERC) and the time of centrifugation.[7c] It has been shown, for example, that more plasma is trapped in the upper third of the packed cell column of normal blood than in the lower two-thirds.[34a] If the MERC is calculated as the distance from the middle of the packed cell column to the center of the centrifuge, it is obvious that the relative centrifugal force (RCF, p. 380) will be significantly different when the height of the red cell column is 20 mm. or 65 mm. It is for this reason, incidentally, that in defining desirable RCF we have chosen to define radius as the distance from the center of the centrifuge shaft to the *bottom* of the hematocrit; in clinical work one deals with columns of packed red cells ranging from less than 10 mm. to more than 70 mm.

Another important factor is the time of centrifugation. It has been pointed out that in a blood of low packed cell volume, the column will settle to a state of high volume concentration within the first two minutes of centrifugation and will be subjected to the maximum force determining tight packing during the succeeding twenty-eight minutes if the time of centrifugation is thirty minutes. On the other hand, blood of high packed cell volume settles to a state of high volume concentration less rapidly and may be subjected to tight packing only for the last fifteen to twenty minutes. It has been found that these differences become less important as the duration of centrifugation is increased from thirty to thirty-five minutes.[7c] In blood samples with hematocrit readings 33 per cent or higher, there is a direct correlation between the amount of plasma trapped and the height of the red cell column.[10d] Below this level, no plasma trapping has been demonstrated. Other factors which influence trapping, such as plasma specific gravity, the degree of oxygenation of the red cells and variations in sedimentation rate, have a negligible effect under conditions of centrifugation which are adequate insofar as RCF is concerned. More plasma is trapped if the red cells are spherocytic than when they are normal.[14a] Calibration curves, whereby corrections for trapped plasma can be made have been provided.[7c]

These considerations emphasize the importance of adequate and standard conditions for centrifugation of the hematocrit. Allowances for trapped plasma can be made when total blood volume is measured (p. 317). The use of a correction factor for routine clinical measurements of volume of packed red cells would serve no useful purpose, however, since in routine hematological procedures only comparative values for volume of packed red cells are needed and, furthermore, the standards which are in general use today were established without correction for trapped plasma.

Accuracy of Corpuscular Constants.—The corpuscular constants can, in trained hands, be measured with a high degree of accuracy. In the author's laboratory the coefficients of variation when five determinations were made on the same sample of blood were, in four experiments, for mean corpuscular volume 0.04 to 1.63 per cent; for mean corpuscular hemoglobin 0.13 to 2.08 per cent, and for mean corpuscular hemoglobin concentration 0.72 to 1.46 per cent. As judged by ± three average standard deviations, mean corpuscular volume if carefully performed should be correct to ±2.7 c.μ, mean corpuscular hemoglobin to ±1.0$\gamma\gamma$, mean corpuscular hemoglobin concentration to ±0.8 per cent.[54,56]

On the other hand, there is no doubt that, because red cell counting is so open to error, gross inaccuracies may occur in the determination of mean corpuscular volume. Biggs and Macmillan[3c] concluded that the probable minimum error is 7 to 9 per cent, this difference in estimate of error as compared with that of the writer being due to their higher estimate of the probable minimum error of red cell counting. One can go even further and say that in some hands the calculation of mean corpuscular volume is worthless and can be misleading. Undoubtedly, in all instances, whether the technic is beyond criticism or where it is only mediocre, the examination of the blood smear by the physician himself is extremely important. In this way gross errors are not likely to pass unnoticed and a visual picture of the blood morphology can be obtained; in addition, sometimes important information may have been overlooked by persons less directly interested in the patient. The English workers found that mean cell diameter, as measured by a modification of the Price-Jones method,[26b] can be carried out with considerable precision.[3c] However, the time required to perform the measurements is a cause for serious objection.

Because hemoglobin can, with proper instrumentation, be measured with a relatively much higher degree of accuracy (2 to 3 per cent[3c]) than red cell count and since hematocrit determinations are quite precise (0.5 per cent probable minimum error[3c]), mean corpuscular hemoglobin concentration is a relatively accurate measurement (2 to 3 per cent error[3c]). The same criticism applies to mean corpuscular hemoglobin and color index as to mean corpuscular volume since these depend upon the accuracy of the red cell counts.

The **volume-thickness index**[18] (the ratio of the actual mean corpuscular volume to the mean corpuscular volume calculated from the measured mean corpuscular diameter) offers nothing which cannot be derived much more readily and more clearly from a consideration of the mean volume, diameter and thickness of the cells in any sample of blood and comparison with the normal values for these measurements.

CARE AND PREPARATION OF SLIDES AND COVER-GLASSES

A good grade of glassware should be used. The glassware must be flat since blood will not spread on concave or convex surfaces. Square cover-glasses, 22 mm. to the side are better than round ones for blood work. Those of No. 2 thickness (0.17 to 0.25 mm.) are more easily handled than thinner ones (No. 1, 0.13 to 0.17 mm.) but the focal distance of some microscopes may be too short for their use.

1. **Gross Cleaning.**—Either of the following methods is satisfactory:

(*a*) Wash with soap and water, then with abundant clean hot water (never allow the water to cool before all the soap has been removed), followed by distilled water. Finally put into 95 per cent alcohol.

(*b*) Soak in acid (concentrated nitric acid or a mixture of sulfuric acid, 250 ml.; potassium bichromate, 100 Gm.; and water, 750 ml.) for four to six hours. Wash thoroughly in clean water, then distilled water. Finally run through two thorough washings with 95 per cent alcohol. Keep in alcohol in a closed container.

2. **Fine Cleaning.**—(*a*) Keep in alcohol, then when needed polish with a clean cloth absolutely free from grease and dust (old linen preferable); or (*b*) take from alcohol and polish. Keep glassware in a clean, dry, well-closed receptacle until used. Pick up glassware with clean forceps. Dust off with clean camel hair brush before using.

EXAMINATION OF THE WET FILM OF BLOOD

A simple and useful, and yet a very much neglected method of blood examination is one in which a drop of blood from the finger or ear lobe is placed on a cover-glass. The latter is inverted on a glass slide and the preparation is rimmed with petroleum jelly or paraffin. The drop of blood should be only slightly larger than a pinhead. If the glassware is clean and the cover-glass is deposited gently on the slide, the blood will spread out evenly under the weight of the cover-glass. Pressure should not be applied. The specimen is first examined with the low power of the microscope in order to determine whether it is satisfactory, and then the oil-immersion lens is used.

Wet preparations yield a great deal of information and permit a rapid survey which will indicate whether or not a more detailed examination will be necessary. If the drop of blood is of the correct size, the red corpuscles will lie slightly separated from one another and their size, shape and color may be noted. This technic is necessary for the demonstration of sickling of the red corpuscles. It is valuable also for the demonstration of parasites in blood, some organisms being more easily detected by their pigment (malaria) or by the currents and disturbance they produce in wet films (spirochetes, trypanosomes) than after they have been stained. Rouleau formation may be observed, and, after the specimen has stood for ten or fifteen minutes, increase or decrease of fibrin may be roughly gauged. In these preparations the motility of the leukocytes is preserved and their activity and phagocytic power may be studied. Supravital staining is a modification of this technic, dye being added for the purpose of staining the mitochondria and vacuoles (see below).

Dark-field Illumination. — Dark-field illumination facilitates the examination of the wet blood film[24] (see Fig 4–2, p. 217). The leukocytes are exceptionally well seen by this method, for their granules are refractile and set off the nucleus in sharp contrast. Erythrocytes are readily made out because the pericellular membrane is highly refractile. Normoblasts may be distinguished by a faintly perceptible perinuclear membrane. Unstained reticulocytes cannot be distinguished but, after staining with brilliant cresyl blue, the reticulum stands out strikingly. Blood platelets are easily seen because of their refractility and, in addition, numerous small round or dumbbell-shaped particles ("blood dust," hemokonia of Müller) which manifest active Brownian movements are found. Fibrin crystals appear as fine, slightly refractile needles. Malaria plasmodia stand out with clarity, the pigment being highly refractile. Since the parasites remain viable for ten to sixteen hours in these preparations, their growth and development may be observed.

Supravital Staining. — Supravital staining, introduced by Cowdry,[10] was developed and popularized by Simpson and, particularly, by Sabin and her students. The *technic* is as follows:[13]

Solution 1: 125 mg. vital neutral red (National Aniline or Grübler) dissolved in 50 ml. neutral absolute ethyl alcohol.

Solution 2: 125 mg. vital Janus green (National Aniline or Grübler) dissolved in 62.5 ml. neutral absolute ethyl alcohol.

Solution 3: 1.1 ml. of Solution 1 dissolved in 10 ml. neutral absolute ethyl alcohol.

Solution 4: 2 drops of Solution 2 added to 3 ml. of Solution 3.

Slides are prepared as follows: (*a*) by means of a pipet, flood with Solution 4 the surface of a chemically clean slide; (*b*) the slide is held sideways with one corner in the mouth of the bottle so as to permit the excess of dye to drain back into bottle; (*c*) the excess of dye on the dependent edge of the slide is quickly wiped away; (*d*) the remaining alcohol on the slide is evaporated by immediately holding it over a piece of wire gauze under which a gas flame is burning. In this way a thin even film of dye is left on the slide. The stained side of the slide is marked.

The subsequent steps are the same as the examination of the wet film of blood. A drop of blood is obtained on a clean cover-slip and allowed to fall gently on the prepared slide. The preparation is rimmed with petroleum jelly. The blood may be examined within fifteen to thirty minutes or, if delay is necessary, the preparation may be stored in the icebox at a temperature of about 4° C. for as long as twenty-four hours. A warm chamber in which the microscope can be placed facilitates supravital study of blood, but it is not essential.

Schwind[48a] recommended pinacyanol in preference to Janus green.

For successful supravital staining it is necessary (1) to have clean glassware, (2) to avoid the use of so great a concentration of dye that the cells are killed. The quantity of dye recommended for Solution 4 will usually be found suitable for normal blood, but the amount used for abnormal bloods should be adjusted according to the number of leukocytes. Death of a cell is indicated by staining of the nucleus. In a good preparation the Janus green stains the mitochondria a brilliant blue green, while the neutral red stains the specific granules and vacuoles of the leukocytes in varying shades depending on their pH: basophilic granules are brick red, neutrophilic granules faint pink and eosinophilic granules bright yellow. (For detailed descriptions of leukocytes stained "supravitally," see Chapter 4 and Table 4–2, p. 232).

For the study of bone marrow, lymph nodes, or other tissues where there is an abund-

ance of colorless cells to be stained, the following solutions are required:

Solution 5: 150 drops of Solution 1 dissolved in 10 ml. of neutral absolute ethyl alcohol.

Solution 6: 8 drops of Solution 2 are added to 3 ml. of Solution 5.

Slides are prepared with Solution 6 in the same manner as with Solution 4. Solutions 4 and 6, being mixtures of neutral red and Janus green, deteriorate after about twenty-four to forty-eight hours and must be freshly prepared each time they are needed. The remaining solutions, if kept in glass-stoppered, alkali free bottles in a cool, dark place, are quite stable. Excess of alkali causes the neutral red solution to become muddy yellow in color.

For the study of cells from organs or dense tissues, if a thin film of intact tissue cannot be obtained, the cut surface is scraped with a sharp scalpel and the tissue accumulating on the knife blade is placed on a slide prepared with Solution 6. If the tissue is very dry, a drop of normal salt solution may be added. A cover-slip is then applied and is rimmed with petroleum jelly.

Phase-Contrast and Electron Microscopy. — Differences of optical path are translated by phase-contrast microscopy into light and shade. Particles which differ in refractive index from the medium in which they are immersed consequently appear brighter or darker than their surroundings. This technic, therefore, offers a means for the study of the finer structure of living cells which has not been readily available heretofore. Thus chromatin, mitochondria, the centrosome and the specific granules of the cells can be seen clearly, often more distinctly than in stained preparations.[2c,37a] Howell-Jolly bodies can be recognized as bright "shining balls" inside the erythrocyte, Heinz-Ehrlich bodies as distinct, dark bodies. The various forms of granulocytes can be differentiated by the

different appearance of their granulation. The cells of infectious mononucleosis manifest a black and coarse granulation in their cytoplasm which differentiates them from monocytes and ordinary lymphocytes. In certain types of reticulum cells and especially in myeloma cells dark, drop-shaped formations have been observed adjacent to the nuclear membrane which have not been found in other cells. Distinguishing features have also been described in leukemic and lymphosarcoma cells, lymphoblasts and myeloblasts,[37a] as well as in other types of tumor cells. Auer bodies and nucleoli are particularly well seen.[2c]

When microcinematography is combined with phase microscopy cellular activities can be seen which have passed unobserved by ordinary technics. Uses of microcinematography are illustrated in Figures 4–3 and 4–4 (pp. 218 and 220).

Although it requires special conditions of fixation, dehydration, embedding and sectioning, *electron* microscopy, by making possible the study of cellular detail at magnifications of more than 100,000, has provided extremely valuable information concerning the structure of the cells of the blood[14b] as well as their function[2c] (See Chapters 3 and 4).

PREPARATION OF BLOOD SMEARS

Cover-glass Technic.—Although it is somewhat more difficult to learn, the preparation of blood films on coverglasses is preferable to the use of slides because thinner preparations and a more even distribution of the leukocytes can be obtained. Scrupulously clean glassware is essential. The cover-glasses may be handled with forceps but this is unnecessary except for removing them from the container in which they are kept. When they are to be used immediately they may be placed cornerwise into slits made in a cardboard box, in the manner

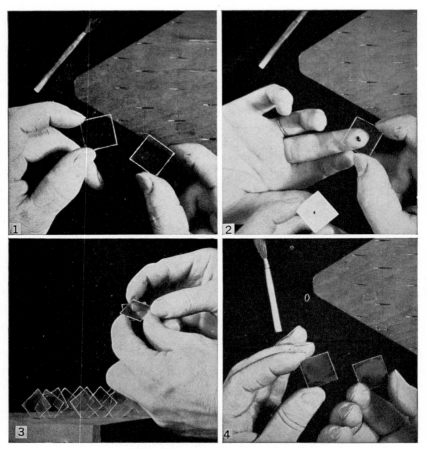

Fig. 8–14.—The preparation of blood films by the cover-glass method. (Haden, Clinical Laboratory Methods, courtesy of C. V. Mosby Company.)

shown in Figure 8–14, *3*, or on a holder made by folding a small piece of paper crosswise. For making the smear, the cover-glasses are held, one in each hand, in such a way that only the edges are touched (Fig. 8–14, *1*). The cover-glass in the right hand is held *just over* a freshly drawn drop of blood (Fig. 8–14, *2*). The blood will reach the glass by capillary attraction. The drop should be about 2 to 3 mm. in diameter. Touching the skin with the cover-glass must be carefully avoided. This cover-glass is then gently placed on the cover-glass held in the left hand in the crosswise fashion shown in Figure 8–14, *3*. If the glass-ware is clean, the blood will spread quickly and evenly between the two surfaces. A moment is allowed for this to occur and, *just before* spreading is complete, the two cover-glasses are separated by a sliding (not lifting) movement. This is done by holding one corner of each cover-glass in each hand and separating the hands by a horizontal motion. If one waits too long before the cover-glasses are separated, clotting will commence and it will be found difficult to pull them apart. If the cover-glasses are not drawn in a strictly horizontal direction, holes in the preparation will result. If the operation has

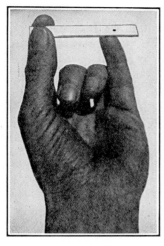

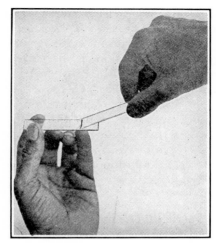

A   *B*

Fig. 8–15.—The preparation of blood films by the slide method (Bass and Johns, courtesy of the Williams & Wilkins Company). *A*, Slide with drop of blood on it held in the proper position for spreading. *B*, Slides held in proper position preparatory to spreading the blood by pushing the upper slide to the left.

been carried out successfully, the blood will be spread evenly and the red corpuscles will neither be overlapping nor in rouleaux.

Slide Technic.—A drop of blood larger than that used for the cover-glass method, is placed on the surface of a slide near one end. The slide is then held between two fingers and steadied with the little finger of the left hand, as shown in Figure 8–15 *A*, with the drop of blood on the upper surface and towards the right. The blood may be spread by means of another glass slide or with the aid of a small glass rod to which another glass rod has been fused in such a way that the two form a T. The cross-beam of the T is the spreader. The width of the spreader is preferably slightly less than that of the slide on which the smear is to be made. If a slide is used as the spreader it may be made slightly narrower by breaking off the corner. This is not essential, however.

The spreader is held just to the left of the drop of blood and then it is pulled back to the edge of the drop (Fig. 8–15,*B*). The latter will then spread out behind the spreader, which is next pushed to the left. The movement must be a rather quick but steady one. The smear will be thin or thick, according as the movement is slow or rapid, and depending on the angle at which the spreader slide is held. This angle should be about 30 degrees.

A good smear should be smooth, homogeneous and without serrations, have even edges and should occupy approximately the middle third of the slide. Smears on slides are excellent when only the red corpuscles are to be examined or a search is to be made for parasites, because more fields may be examined. For differential counts, however, they are less satisfactory than smears on cover-glasses, for the large leukocytes (polymorphonuclears and monocytes) are pushed to the edges and the lymphocytes remain scattered throughout the smear.

Fixation of Smears.—The blood is allowed to dry on the glass in the open air. *With most stains fixation is brought about in the first minute when the undiluted stain, which contains alcohol, is applied to the smear.* If the stain is an aqueous one and preliminary fixation is necessary, this may be accomplished by heating the slides at 120° to 125° C. for a few minutes; or by passing them through a small flame three or four times; by immersion for five minutes in absolute alcohol; or by immersion for one minute in a 1 per cent solution of formalin in 50 per cent alcohol.

THE STAINING OF BLOOD SMEARS

The foundations for the morphological study of the blood were laid by Ehrlich's investigations of the anilin dyes, commenced in 1877 while he was still a student.[33] Originally, simple dyes were used in the clinical laboratory and tissues were stained successively if more than one color was desired. The majority of the anilin dyes are in the form of salts of acids or bases. During the process of staining, compounds are probably formed between the basic dyes and the acid nuclear substances of cells, and between the acid dyes and the basic protoplasm. Ehrlich combined acid and basic dyes (so-called "neutral" dyes) and showed that in this way the staining principles of the original components were preserved and, in addition, new staining properties dependent upon the union of the component dyes were developed. These were therefore termed polychrome dyes. For many years **Ehrlich's triacid stain** was used routinely. It is now of historical interest only, because it is relatively difficult to use and the results are imperfect.

Jenner (1889) introduced an important simplification of technic when, instead of using two separate aqueous solutions to be mixed freshly each time, he collected the precipitate formed when eosin and methylene blue are mixed and redissolved it in methyl alcohol to obtain a single solution which was both fixative and stain. **Jenner's stain** or the **May-Gruenwald stain*** as an essentially similar stain is called in the German literature, is very simple to apply. However, the stain fails to demonstrate nuclear detail in leukocytes or granules in platelets, and the nucleus of malarial parasites is invisible.

The next discovery of importance in staining technic was that of Romanowsky (1890), who observed that, by mixing old, mold-covered solutions of methylene blue with eosin, a stain was produced which brought out details which the Jenner or May-Gruenwald stains failed to show. A purplish-red stain, methylene azure, which is an oxidation product of methylene blue, is produced when moldy methylene blue is mixed with eosin. Malachowski (1891) subsequently demonstrated that this new metachromatic stain can be obtained consistently by alkalinization of methylene blue and the subsequent addition of eosin, thus making it unnecessary to wait for mold formation to occur.

The numerous **modifications of the Romanowsky method,** which followed these discoveries, differ chiefly in the manner by which methylene blue is "polychromed." These include the stains of Reuter (1901), Leishman (1901), Wright (1902), Hastings (1905), and Wilson (1907). The appearance of the blood corpuscles after staining with these different solutions is practically the same. Since Wright's stain is the one in common

---

* *May-Gruenwald stain:* 100 ml. absolute methyl alcohol are warmed to 50° C. To this is added, in minute portions, 0.3 Gm. of May-Gruenwald dye powder. After each addition of the dye the solution is shaken vigorously. When solution is complete, it is allowed to stand twenty-four hours. It is then filtered into a dark bottle and stored in a cool place. For staining, the stock solution is diluted with an equal quantity of buffer solution, pH 6.8. The stain solution must be made up fresh daily.

use, it will be described in detail. The factors influencing the Romanowsky staining of blood films have been discussed in detail by Lillie.[35b]

Wright's stain is made by heating methylene blue with sodium bicarbonate, after which the mixture is combined with eosin. The dye may be purchased as a powder which is then dissolved in in methyl alcohol or, more simply, a ready-made solution may be obtained.

Technic.—Fresh smears are preferable. The air-dried blood film is placed with the smeared side upwards on a support (*e.g.*, a cork) from which it can be readily picked up. For slides various types of staining trays may be purchased, or one is made by fixing two glass rods on a tray at a distance from one another which is somewhat less than the length of a glass slide.

The blood smear is completely covered with stain which is allowed to remain for one minute, this procedure serving to fix the smear. The stain is then diluted with distilled water. This is added drop by drop, using approximately the same number of drops of water as had been used of dye. A greenish metallic scum should appear and the margins should show a reddish tint. In adding the water, care should be taken that the solution does not run over the edges of the cover-glass or slide.

After three or four minutes, the stain is washed off with water until the film is yellowish or pink. It is important to commence washing while the cover-glass is still horizontal and the stain is still on it, as otherwise a scum which is difficult to remove by subsequent washing tends to settle on the smear. The stain should be "floated" off the slide by adding water, first very slowly and then more briskly while the slide is still in a horizontal position. If the cover-glass is held with forceps, fluid should not be allowed to collect at the tip of the forceps and then run over the preparation, for streaking

will occur. This may be avoided by letting excess of water run towards the forceps. After the preparation has been thoroughly washed, it is stood on edge to dry, or it may be dried between filter papers. When it is thoroughly dry, the preparation, if it is a cover-glass, is mounted in neutral Canada balsam.

In a good stain, the film will appear pink to the naked eye; microscopically the erythrocytes will be pink, the nuclei of the leukocytes purplish-blue, neutrophil granules violet-pink or lilac, eosinophil granules red, and the basi- and oxychromatin of the nuclei will be clearly differentiated. The areas between the cells will be clear with no film or precipitated stain visible.

It is soon learned by those who use Wright's or similar stains that perfect results are sometimes not obtained even when the technic described is rigorously followed. Each supply of stain may require some modification in the time of staining or in the degree of dilution of the stain. Again, unless the distilled water is neutral, variations in the results of staining will occur. Furthermore, after the stain has stood for some time, it may become too alkaline and may need to be neutralized.

If the whole smear is too blue, this may be due to insufficient washing, too prolonged staining or the use of too alkaline a preparation.

In alkaline preparations, nuclear chromatin is deeply stained, and erythrocytes stain blue or green. The cytoplasm of lymphocytes becomes gray or lavender and the granules of the neutrophils become intensely overstained and appear larger than normal. Eosinophil granules become deep gray or blue.

To improve the color, less stain or more diluent may be used, or the time of staining may be decreased and the time of washing increased. To counteract the effects of an excess of alkali in the stain, several drops of Haden's acid buffer* may be added to the diluted stain or, if the stain is very alkaline, buffer may be used as a diluent in the place of distilled water. More simply, a drop of weak acetic acid solution may be added to the stain if it is too alkaline, or a drop or two of weak ammonia water is employed when it is too acid. Sometimes the stain is improved by diluting it with an equal part of absolute methyl alcohol.

Acidity of the staining solution is indicated by pale blue-staining of the nuclei of the leukocytes and of other structures which should be stained a more vivid blue, by bright red or orange coloring of the erythrocytes and brilliant staining of the eosinophils. Excessive washing or understaining will produce pale nuclei just as occurs when the stain is acid, but the erythrocytes will also be pale and the eosinophil granules will appear blurred.

A poorly stained smear may sometimes be saved by washing very rapidly with a dash of 95 per cent alcohol and then washing immediately with water. It is then re-stained.

The *reaction of the distilled water* used may be tested with the aid of hematoxylin.[15] A few crystals, picked up with a pair of forceps, are placed in a test tube which has been previously rinsed with the water to be tested. Approximately 5 ml. of water are poured into the test tube. If the water is neutral it will become a pale lavender-pink within two minutes. If it is acid it becomes yellow and remains so longer than five minutes. If it is alkaline it becomes reddish-purple immediately, or before one minute. On standing, water usually becomes acid in

reaction, in which case 1 per cent potassium carbonate is used; if it is alkaline, 1 per cent hydrochloric or acetic acid is used. The neutralizing agent is added a drop at a time to the stock bottle of water and the reaction tested each time until the water turns pink without a trace of yellow in two minutes.

An important reason for difficulty with the use of Wright's and similar polychromed stains is the fact that they are alkaline solutions in which the concentrations of the dye are continually changing due to the progressive oxidizing action of the alkali.[33] Two additional variables are alterations in the concentration of solvent (methyl alcohol) as the result of evaporation, and variations in the degree of dilution of the stain when water is added during staining.

Giemsa's stain (1902) represents an attempt to correct the first of these variables by using purified dyes. However, although with Giemsa's method the azurophilic property of the polychrome dyes is preserved, erythrocytes are poorly stained and neutrophil granules are pale. **Pappenheim,** by his **panoptic method** successfully remedied this by fixing and staining smears with May-Gruenwald solution and then restaining with diluted Giemsa's stain. Strumia[51] further improved this technic by combining the May-Gruenwald and the Giemsa stains in one solution. Lillie has described the preparation of a Giemsa stain of quite constant composition and performance.[35a] A stable modification of the Pappenheim stain has also been devised.[27] The J.S.B. stain[35g] is claimed to be superior to Wright's stain, especially in hot climates.

Kingsley[32] devised a **stain** which is claimed to be an improvement over all the technics heretofore proposed. Purified dyes are used which offer all the staining properties of methylene blue, methylene azure and eosin. Variations in the results of staining caused by the necessity of adding water to the stain, as with Wright's stain, are eliminated,

* Haden's phosphate buffer solution: Recrystallized primary (monobasic) potassium phosphate 6.63 Gm., recrystallized secondary sodium phosphate (exposed to air for two weeks to lose its water of crystallization) 3.20 Gm. (or anhydrous secondary (dibasic) sodium phosphate (Merck) 2.56 Gm.), distilled water to make 1000 ml. The solution should have a pH of 6.4.

and the procedure is more rapid than that for Giemsa's stain as usually employed. Only one variable factor remains, namely, the time of staining. An additional advantage of this stain, according to Kingsley, is the fact that it may be used to demonstrate megakaryocyte and platelet granules in tissues and to stain frozen sections rapidly. For the latter purposes appropriate treatment before and after staining is, of course, necessary.

Peroxidase Staining.—The differentiation of leukocytes is sometimes facilitated by taking advantage of the presence of an oxidizing ferment in myeloid leukocytes. The *oxidase reaction* involves the transference of oxygen from the air while the *peroxidase* staining methods depend on the use of hydrogen peroxide as the source of oxygen. The latter are more commonly used. The oxidizing ferment in myeloid cells causes the oxidation and deposition of benzidine by hydrogen peroxide.

Many methods have been recommended. **Goodpasture's technic** has been most generally used.[2] The blood film, made in the usual manner, is covered with the stain* for one minute. An equal amount of a freshly made 1 to 200 dilution of hydrogen peroxide is then added to the stain and the preparation allowed to stand three or four minutes. The film is next washed and allowed to dry. The peroxide solution is prepared by adding 2 drops of fresh hydrogen peroxide to 15 ml. of distilled water.

By this method nuclei appear clear red, cytoplasm pink and red cells a smooth buff color. Neutrophilic granules of myelocytes or polymorphonuclear leukocytes are stained deep blue and are

* *Goodpasture's peroxidase stain*, as modified by Beacom,[2] consists of the following: Alcohol 100 ml., sodium nitroprusside 0.05 Gm., benzidine C.P. (Harmer) 0.05 Gm., basic fuchsin 0.05 Gm. The nitroprusside is dissolved in 1 to 2 ml. of water, mixed with alcohol and then the other ingredients are added. This stain will keep for eight months.

well defined. Eosinophilic granules are dark blue but basophilic granules are not shown. No granules are seen in the lymphocytes. Granules which are fewer in number and less well defined than in the myeloid series of cells are seen in most monocytes.

The following method (Washburn, modification of Osgood and Ashworth[41]) has been satisfactory:

Solution 1.—Benzidine base, 0.3 Gm. is dissolved in 99 ml. of ethyl alcohol and to this is added 1 ml. of a saturated aqueous solution of sodium nitroprusside. This staining solution will remain active for eight to ten months.

Solution 2.—A dilute solution of hydrogen peroxide is made just before use by adding 0.3 ml. of fresh 3 per cent hydrogen peroxide to 25 ml. of distilled water. Films of blood, dried in air, are stained, preferably within three to four hours or at least within twelve hours of the time of collection of the blood. Ten drops of solution 1 are placed on the slide and allowed to remain for one to one and a half minutes; 5 drops of solution 2 are added directly and allowed to stand three to four minutes. The slide is then washed thoroughly in tap water for three to four minutes and counterstained with Wright's stain.

The **copper peroxidase method of Sato and Sekiya** in our hands has been the most consistently successful method. Solution A† is applied to a fresh dry blood smear for thirty to sixty seconds.

† *Sato and Sekiya peroxidase stain*, Solution A: Copper sulphate solution 0.5 per cent. Solution B: Rub 0.2 Gm. of benzidine (benzidin. puriss. Merck or benzidin base, Merck) with a few drops of water in a mortar. To this are added 200 ml. of water at room temperature and a *saturated* solution of benzidine is thus prepared. The preparation is filtered and 4 drops of hydrogen peroxide (3 per cent) are added. If this preparation is kept in the dark when not in use, it will last a year. It may be tested by mixing Solutions A and B in a test tube. If this mixture does not become blue, the reagents are at fault. Most often difficulties arise because the benzidin solution (Solution B) is not saturated.

This is then poured off, or gently washed off and Solution B is applied for two minutes. This is poured off and the counterstain applied for two minutes. The smear is then washed thoroughly and dried. As counterstain, safranin (1 per cent aqueous solution) or carbol fuchsin (1 part in 5) may be used. By this method the cytoplasm of the myeloid leukocytes is stained blue and the peroxidase-positive granules bluish-green with the eosinophil and basophil granules intensely blue; monocytes are faintly stained and their granules appear small though distinctly blue. Lymphoid elements show no trace of blue or green but appear red. Red cells and platelets remain unstained either by peroxidase or by counterstain except when carbol fuchsin is used. (See Plate XIV, p. 924.)

For successful staining, it is important that fresh blood be used for the oxidizing ferment in the leukocytes disappears rapidly.

Leukocyte Alkaline Phosphatase.[29a] —Dry, unstained blood smears are immersed for 30 seconds at 0° C. in a fixative solution consisting of formalin (36 to 39 per cent formaldehyde) 10 ml., in absolute methyl alcohol 90 ml. They are then washed in running water for 10 seconds and incubated in a substrate mixture for 10 minutes at room temperature. The substrate mixture consists of sodium alpha napthyl acid phosphate 35 mg., Fast Blue RR 35 mg., and propanediol buffer (0.05 M) 35 ml., and has a pH of 9.5. The smears are washed in running water again for 10 seconds and then are counterstained with Mayer's aqueous hematoxylin.[7b] Following this the smears are washed again in running water for 10 seconds and are air dried. They are then mounted in balsam.

Neutrophilic leukocytes are the only cells which take up the stains. The granules stain from a pale brown color to deep black. In normal subjects, most of the neutrophils are unstained. In

blood from cases of infection, ploycythemia vera, myelofibrosis and other types of myeloid reactions, alkaline phosphatase staining is increased whereas in acute and chronic myeloid leukemia the reaction is decreased. The amount of staining can be graded as follows: 0, colorless; 1 +, diffuse pale brown cytoplasm, no granules; 2 +, brown cytoplasm with or without occasional clumps of brownish-black precipitate; 3 +, brownish-black, unevenly distributed granular precipitate; 4 +, uniform deep black granular precipitate.

The test is of some value in distinguishing a nonleukemic myeloid reaction from chronic myelocytic leukemia (See p. 235).

Various other stains have been described for various special purposes: (1) a dithizone stain which brings out the *granules of myeloid cells*, thus complementing the peroxidase stain;[36d] (2) a modification of the Feulgen stain for *deoxyribonucleoprotein* which is useful in demonstrating nucleoli in nuclei, since the latter will take the stain and the nucleoli will appear as unstained spaces;[16b] (3) a methyl-green-pyronin stain which affords some measure of the *ribonucleoprotein* content of leukocytes;[41b] (4) smears previously stained by the Romanowsky method can be stained by the *periodic-acid-Schiff* (*PAS*) *reaction* to facilitate cell identification.[22a]

Choice of Methods for Microscopic Study of Leukocytes.—For a quick survey of the appearance and activity of the leukocytes, the examination of the unstained wet film of blood is a valuable procedure. Dark-ground illumination facilitates this but phase-contrast microscopy is even better. The addition of dyes in the so-called supravital technic, by staining the mitochondria and granules facilitates differentiation and yet complicates the technic very little. Since the nuclei of the cells are not stained, the important nuclear detail which dry, stained preparations offer is lacking, but on the other hand it is possible to observe their motility, mitochondria and vacuolar apparatus. Due to lack of nuclear staining, lymphocytes and nucleated red corpuscles are easily missed. Polychromatophilia and stippling cannot be demonstrated in supravital preparations, but on the other hand reticulocytes can only be demonstrated by staining while wet. The proponents of the supravital method claim that the staining reaction for each cell type is specific and that cells can be differentiated more accurately than by the use of the Romanowsky stains. Such specificity has been denied by other observers.[22,34] It has been the custom for the advocates of each of these methods to work almost exclusively with one technic or the other. This has resulted in increased efficiency with the method favored and ignorance of the other. This is unfortunate for the methods are essentially complementary and both should be used when differentiation is difficult. For routine work, the permanence of the preparations and the ease with which they can be transported and examined, make the staining of fixed, dry preparations the method of choice.

Demonstration of L. E. Phenomenon.[24a]—Since a variety of hematological abnormalities are encountered in cases of systemic lupus erythematosus, the "L. E. test" becomes an important procedure in the study of disorders of the blood. This test depends on the presence in the blood serum of a factor, a component of the serum gamma globulin, which dissolves nuclei by depolymerization of deoxyribonucleic acid. The nuclei are usually derived from polymorphonuclear leukocytes and lymphocytes. The chromatin of the cell nuclei loses its structural pattern and becomes a relatively homogeneous, swollen mass which ruptures the nuclear membrane. Such lysed nuclear material attracts phagocytic cells, usually neutrophilic polymorphonuclear leukocytes, which tend to cluster about it and form a "rosette." Ultimately the material is engulfed by one or more of the phagocytes, thus producing the "L. E. cell." In addition, "tart cells" have been described which consist of monocytes containing an engulfed nucleus with well preserved nuclear structure. Nucleophagocytosis or "tart cells" can be distinguished from L. E. cells by the fact that in nucleophagocytosis the phagocytized nucleus usually maintains an intact chromatin pattern, and the chromatin is more dense and tends to become vacuolated. The circumference of the phagocytized nucleus may even appear to be "condensed," giving the impression of a thick rim and may resemble a tart.

The L. E. cell is claimed by many investigators to be specific for lupus erythematosus. A phenomenon showing some resemblance to this has been described in the blood and bone marrow of patients with symptoms of drug allergy and serum disease. This differs from the L. E. phenomenon in that the inclusion bodies are not homogeneous and still possess a clear chromatin structure. Furthermore, in such cases phagocytosis of lymphocytes, platelets and red corpuscles may be observed as well.

The test requires (1) a source of the L. E. cell factor, (2) nucleoprotein with which this factor reacts, and (3) phagocytic cells to engulf the lysed nuclear material produced by the interaction of the L. E. cell factor and the nucleoprotein. The L. E. cell factor has been demonstrated in the gamma globulin fraction of the plasma and is relatively stable, maintaining its potency for long periods if kept frozen. Boiling destroys its activity. The L. E. cell reaction, being a biochemical one, requires time and the proper temperature to permit optimal reaction. Many methods have been devised for the test.[24a,50c,60] A popular one involves the removal of approximately 10 ml. blood by venipuncture from the individual suspected of having the disease. This is placed in a sterile, dry, chemically clean centrifuge tube of sufficient size and allowed to clot and remain at room temperature for about two hours. The serum is then decanted and discarded and the remaining clot is forced through a screen of fine mesh to defibrinate it. The resulting fluid portion of the clot is collected in a chemically clean, sterile Petri dish and is then transferred to one or two hematocrits for centrifugation. The latter is carried out at 1,500 to 1,800 r.p.m. for about five minutes. The serum is then discarded and the buffy cellular layer is collected with a pipet and is transferred to a small, paraffined receptacle, where it is remixed. Drops of suitable size are then transferred to chemically clean, glass slides or coverslips and smears are made in the usual fashion. These are stained in the same way as blood smears.

In certain cases a positive test is not obtained by one method and yet occurs with another. An essential requirement is the production of sufficient leukocyte trauma to permit the reaction to occur. Equal to, or perhaps even better than the above sieved clot technic is the *"rotary method."*[60] Five ml. of freshly drawn blood are placed in a dry test tube containing no more than 0.75 mg. of heparin. The use of excessive amounts of heparin depresses the L. E. phenomenon.[10] Within two hours 3 ml. of this blood are transferred to a test tube ($\frac{1}{2}'' \times 4''$) containing five glass beads, 5 mm. in diameter. The tube is placed in a rotor[7] and is rotated for 30 minutes at room temperature. Following this 1 ml. blood is transferred to a hematocrit and centrifuged at 1000 r.p.m. for ten minutes. The buffy coat is then pipetted off, smeared on cover-slips and stained with Wright's stain.

The preparation is first examined under low power in order to find areas where suspicious material is present in greater abundance. Under oil immersion magnification the L. E. cell is recognized by the presence of a relatively smooth, homogeneous, nuclear mass which stains a pale blue color and is less prominent than the host nucleus. The latter is compressed to the periphery of the cell by the cytoplasmic inclusion. The phagocytic cell is usually a polymorphonuclear neutrophil, less often an eosinophil. (See also Plate XV, p. 926).

The following technical procedures have been discussed in the preceding chapters:

CHAPTER 1.
    Bone marrow:
        Technic of marrow puncture and trephining.
        Methods of preparation of bone marrow for examination, including dry imprints and smears.
        Sections of bone marrow.
        Method of staining.
    Spleen and lymph node examination.

CHAPTER 2.
    Erythrocytes:
        Identification and classification of different types of nucleated red cells and abnormal forms.
    Enumeration of reticulocytes.
    Demonstration of siderocytes.

CHAPTER 3.
    Erythrocyte fragility tests.
    Study of pigment metabolism:
        Demonstration of hemosiderin.
        Icterus index and van den Bergh tests.
        Measurement of urobilinogen and urobilin in urine and stools.
        Test for porphobilinogen.

PLATE IX

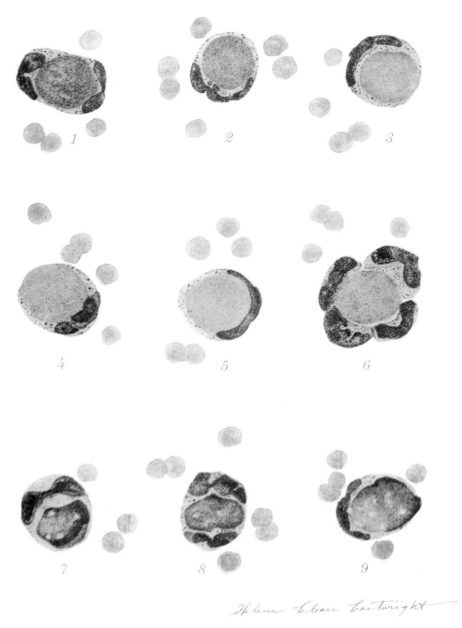

Helene Clare Cartwright

"L.E." Cells and "Tart" Cells (Nucleophagocytosis). Cells 1 to 6 are from the blood of a patient with disseminated lupus erythematosus. Cells 1, 2 and 3 show the characteristic progressive loss of nuclear detail and staining quality which take place in affected nuclei. Cell 1 by itself could not be identified as an L.E. cell. Cells 3, 4 and 5, however, are typical, fully developed L.E. cells and show the complete loss of nuclear detail. No. 6 is a small "rosette". As yet the nuclear mass has not been engulfed by any one of the phagocytes.

Nucleophagocytosis (cells 7, 8 and 9) must be distinguished from the L.E. phenomenon. Note that the engulfed material in 7, 8 and 9 retains some of its original chromatin pattern. The nuclear chromatin stains more darkly than in fully developed L.E. cells and is condensed about the edges. Vacuolization is also present.

Principles of technics for the study of abnormal hemoglobins.
Life span of red corpuscles.
Study of erythrokinetics, including ferrokinetics.

CHAPTER 4.
Leukocytes:
Identification and methods of classification of different types.
Study of leukokinetics.

CHAPTER 5.
Blood platelets and coagulation:
Enumeration of blood platelets.
Clinical methods for measurement of disturbances of coagulation, including coagulation time, retraction time of blood clot, clot lysis, bleeding time, capillary fragility tests, simple screening test for abnormal coagulation of the blood, quantative determination of "prothrombin," plasma thrombin time, prothrombin consumption test, thromboplastin generation test, assays for factors VIII and IX, test for circulating anticoagulant and fibrinogen content of plasma.

CHAPTER 6.
Measurement of total plasma volume and total red cell volume.
Measurement of specific gravity and of viscosity of blood.
Sedimentation test.

CHAPTER 7.
Methods of blood typing.
Blood transfusion.

Other technical procedures will be described in the following pages, as they bear on the topics discussed. These include:

CHAPTER 10.
Use of radioactive vitamin B_{12} in diagnosis.

CHAPTER 12.
Tests for inclusion bodies, Heinz bodies, GSH instability.

CHAPTER 13.
Tests for sickle cells, quantitation of alkali-resistant hemoglobin.
Hemoglobin electrophoresis, quantitation of hemoglobin A_2.

BIBLIOGRAPHY

Principles and Technic of Blood Examination

1. AKEROYD, J. H., GIBBS, MARY B., VIVANO, S. and ROBINETTE, R. W.: On Counting Leukocytes by Electronic Means, Am. J. Clin. Path., *31*, 188, 1959.

1a.AMMUNDSEN, E. and TRIER, M.: On the Blood Content of Inactive Hemoglobin. With Special Consideration of Hemoglobin Standardization, Acta med. scandinav., *101*, 451, 1939; J. Biol. Chem., *138*, 563, 1941.

1b.BAUMBERGER, J. P.: A Note on the "Black Line" in Hematocrit Determinations, J. Lab. & Clin. Med., *27*, 1084, 1942.

1c. BAVISOTTO, V. S., PRITHAM, G. H. and CHILCOTE, M. E.: Improvement of a Hemin Standard by Recrystallization, Proc. Soc. Exper. Biol. & Med., *81*, 280, 1952.

2. BEACOM, D. N.: A Modification of Goodpasture's Technic for the Peroxidase Reaction in Blood Smears, J. Lab. & Clin. Med., *11*, 1092, 1926.

2a.BERG, W. N.: Blood Cell Counts, Their Statistical Interpretation, Am. Rev. Tuberc., *52*, 179, 1945.

2c. BESSIS, M.: Phase Contrast Microscopy and Electron Microscopy Applied to the Blood Cells, Blood, *10*, 272, 1955; Rev. hémat., *12*, 43, 1957.

3. BERKSON, J., MAGATH, T. B. and BURN, M.: The Error of Estimate of the Blood Cell Count as Made With the Hemocytometer, Am. J. Physiol., *128*, 309, 1940.

3a.BERNHART, F. W. and STEGGS, L.: The Iron Content of Crystalline Human Hemoglobin, J. Biol. Chem., *147*, 19, 1943.

3b.BEST, W. R.: A Hematologic Slide Rule for

Calculating the Corpuscular Constants, J. Lab. Clin. Med., *34*, 434, 1949.

3c. BIGGS, ROSEMARY and MACMILLAN, R. L.: The Errors of Some Hæmatological Methods as They are Used in a Routine Laboratory, J. Clin. & Path., *1*, 269, 1948.

4. BING, F. C. and BAKER, R. W.: The Determination of Hemoglobin in Minute Amounts of Blood by Wu's Method, J. Biol. Chem., *92*, 589, 1931; *Ibid.*, *95*, 387, 1932.

5. BLOCH, O., JR.: A Simple Blood Pipette Cleaner, J. Lab. & Clin. Med., *24*, 749, 1939.

5a. BLUM, L. L.: The Photoelectric Determination of Erythrocyte Count, Am. J. Clin. Path., *15*, 85, 1945; *Ibid.*, *16*, 53, 1946.

5b. BRACKETT, F. S., MATTERN, C. F. T. and OLSON, B. J.: Appraisal of Instrument for Counting Erythrocytes by Scatter Photometry, Am. J. Clin. Path., *23*, 731, 1953.

5c. BRECHER, G., SCHNEIDERMAN, M. and WILLIAMS, G. Z.: Evaluation of Electronic Red Blood Cell Counter, Am. J. Clin. Path., *26*, 1439, 1956.

5d. BRÜCKMANN, G.: Blood From the Ear Lobe, J. Lab. & Clin. Med., *27*, 487, 1942.

6. BRYAN, W. R., CHASTIAN, L. L. and GARREY, W. E.: Errors of Routine Analysis in the Counting of Leukocytes, Am. J. Physiol., *113*, 416, 1935.

7. BRYAN, W. R. and GARREY, W. E.: A Mechanical Device That Produces Uniform Dispersion of Blood Cells in the Diluting Pipet, J.A.M.A., *103*, 1059, 1934.

7a. CANNAN, R. K.: Proposal for a Certified Standard for Use in Hemoglobinometry, Blood, *13*, 1101, 1958.

7b. CARTWRIGHT, G. E.: *Diagnostic Laboratory Hematology*, New York, Grune & Stratton, Ed. 2, 1956.

7c. CHAPLIN, H., JR. and MOLLISON, P. L.: Correction for Plasma Trapped in the Red Cell Column of the Hematocrit, Blood, 7, 1227, 1952.

8. CH'U, Y. and FORKNER, C. E.: Errors in Erythrocyte Counts Due to Hayem's Solution Avoided With Gowers' Solution, J. Lab. & Clin. Med., *23*, 1282, 1938.

8a. CLEGG, J. W. and KING, E. T.: Estimation of Hemoglobin by Alkaline Hematin Method, Brit. Med. J., *2*, 329, 1942.

8b. CROSBY, W. H., MUNN, J. I. and FURTH, F. W.: Standardizing a Method for Clinical Hemoglobinometry, U. S. Armed Forces Med. J., *5*, 693, 1954.

8c. CROSLAND-TAYLOR, P., STEWART, J. W. and HAGGIS, G.: An Electronic Blood-Cell-Counting Machine, Blood, *13*, 398, 1958.

9. DALAND, J.: Ueber das Volumen der rothen und weissen Blutkörperchen im Blute des gesunden und kranken Menschen, Fortschr. d. Med., Berlin, *9*, 867, 1891.

10. DUBOIS, E. L. and FREEMAN, VIVIAN: A Comparative Evaluation of the Sensitivity of the L. E. Cell Test Performed Simultaneously by Different Methods, Blood, *12*, 657, 1957.

10a. DRABKIN, D.: Crystallographic and Optical Properties of Human Hemoglobin, Am. J. Med. Sc., *209*, 268, 1945.

10b. ————The Standardization of Hemoglobin Measurement, Am. J. Med. Sc., *217*, 710, 1949.

10c. DRABKIN, D. L.: Spectroscopy, Photometry and Spectrophotometry. *In* Glasser, O. (editor): *Medical Physics*. The Year Book Publishers, Inc., Chicago, Ill., 1950. Vol. 2, pp. 1039–1089.

10d. EBAUGH, F. G., JR., LEVINE, P. and EMERSON, C. P.: The Amount of Trapped Plasma in the Red Cell Mass of the Hematocrit Tube, J. Lab. & Clin. Med., *46*, 409, 1955.

11. ELLERBROOK, L. D.: A Simple Colorimetric Method for Calibration of Pipets, Am. J. Clin. Path., *24*, 868, 1954.

11a. ELLERBROOK, L. D. and DAVIS, J. H.: Effect of Traces of Copper on Hemoglobin Determination, Am. J. Clin. Path., *24*, 607, 1954.

12. EVELYN, K. A.: A Stabilized Photoelectric Colorimeter With Light Filters, J. Biol. Chem., *115*, 63, 1936; *Ibid.*, *117*, 365, 1937; *Ibid.*, *126*, 655, 1938.

12a. EVELYN, K. A. and MALLOY, H. T.: Microdetermination of Oxyhemoglobin, Methemoglobin and Sulfhemoglobin in a Single Sample of Blood, J. Biol. Chem., *126*, 655, 1938.

13. FORKNER, C. E.: Origin and Fate of Two Types of Multinucleated Giant Cells in Circulating Blood, J. Exper. Med., *52*, 279, 1930.

14. FRANCIS, D.: Calibration of Micropipettes and Tubes Simplied, J. Lab. & Clin. Med., *22*, 718, 1937.

14a. FURTH, F. W.: Effect of Spherocytosis on Volume of Trapped Plasma in Red Cell Column of Capillary and Wintrobe Hematocrits, J. Lab. & Clin. Med., *48*, 421, 1956.

14b. GOODMAN, J. R., REILLY, E. B. and MOORE, R. E.: Electron Microscopy of Formed Elements of Normal Human Blood, Blood, *12*, 428, 1957.

15. GRADWOHL, R. B. H.: Reaction of Water on the Staining of Blood Smears, J. Missouri M. A., *33*, 14, 1936.

16. GRANT, J. L., BRITTON, M. C., JR. and KURTZ, T. E.: Measurement of Red Blood Cell Volume with the Electronic Cell Counter, Am. J. Clin. Path., *33*, 138, 1960.

16a. GRAY, S.: The Use of Fibrinogen in a Rapid Method of Determining Cell Volume, Am. J. Med. Sc., *207*, 29, 1944.

16b. GREIG, H. B. W: A Substitute for the Feulgen Staining Technique, J. Clin. Path., *12*, 93, 1959.

17. GUEST, G. M.: Modified Van Allen Hematocrit Tube Providing for Automatic Volume Adjustment of the Blood Sample, J. Lab. & Clin. Med., *24*, 75, 1938.

18. HADEN, R. L.: The Volume Thickness Index of the Erythrocyte of Man, J. Lab. & Clin. Med., *20*, 567, 1935

20. ———Diffraction Methods for Measuring the Diameter of the Red Blood Cell, J. Lab. & Clin. Med., *23*, 508, 1938.

21. ———A New Instrument for the Diffractometric Measurement of the Diameter of Red Blood Cells, J. Lab. & Clin. Med., *25*, 399, 1940.

22. HALL, B. E.: A Critical Review of the Hematological Literature Dealing With the Results of the Supravital Staining Method, Folia hæmatol., *43*, 206, 1930.

22a. HAYHOE, F. G. J., QUAGLINO, D. and FLEMANS, R. J.: Consecutive Use of Romanowsky and Periodic-Acid-Schiff Techniques in the Study of Blood and Bone-Marrow Cells, Brit. J. Hæmat., *6*, 23, 1960.

23. HAMRE, C. J.: The Capillary Hematocrit Method of Determining Blood Cell Volume, J. Lab. & Clin. Med., *25*, 547, 1940.

24. HANSEN-PRUSS, O. C.: The Circulating Blood Cells as Seen by Dark-ground Illumination, Am. J. Clin. Path., *6*, 423, 1936.

24a. HARGRAVES, M. M.: The L. E. Cell Phenomenon. *In Advances in Internal Medicine*, VI, p. 133, W. Dock and I. Snapper, Ed., Chicago, Year Book Publishers, Inc., 1954.

24b. HEILMEYER, L.: *Spectrophotometry in Medicine*, 1932, Trans. by A. Jordan, London, Eng., 1943, Adam Hilger, Ltd.

25. HELLER, V. G. and PAUL, H.: Changes in Cell Volume Produced by Varying Concentrations of Different Anticoagulants, J. Lab. & Clin. Med., *19*, 777, 1934.

26. HOLOBAUGH, G.: A Simple and Rapid Method for Opening Syringes Clotted With Blood, J. Lab. & Clin. Med., *22*, 208, 1936.

26a. HORECKER, B. L.: A Primary Standard for the Colorimetric Determination of Hemoglobin, J. Lab. & Clin. Med., *31*, 589, 1946; *Ibid.*, *33*, 783, 1948.

26b. HUMBLE, J. G. and BELYAVIN, G.: A Simplified Price-Jones Technique, J. Clin .Path., *1*, 77, 1948.

27. HUNT, G. A.: A Study of the Pappenheim Stain, J. Lab. & Clin. Med., *29*, 207, 1944.

27a. HUNTER, F. T., GROVE-RASMUSSEN, M. and SOUTTER, L.: A Spectrophotometric Method for Quantitating Hemoglobin in Plasma or Serum, Am. J. Clin. Path., *20*, 429, 1950.

28. HYNES, M.: The Distribution of Leucocytes on the Counting Chamber, J. Clin. Path., *1*, 25, 1947.

28a. INAGAKI, S.: Studies on the Fixing, Staining and Counting Methods for Basophil Leukocytes, Acta haemat. japonica, *18*, 635, 1955.

29. JENKINS, C. E.: A Flicker Hæmoglobinometer, Brit. J. Exper. Path., *11*, 261, 1930; *ibid.*, *12*, 212, 1931.

29a. KAPLOW, L. S.: A Histochemical Method for Localizing and Evaluating Leukocyte Alkaline Phosphatase Activity in Smears of Blood and Marrow, Blood, *10*, 1023, 1955.

30. KATO, K.: Use of Combination Microhemopipet, Am. J. Dis. Child., *59*, 310, 1940.

31. KING, E. J. and GILCHRIST, M.: Determination of Hæmoglobin by a Cyan-Hæmatin Method, Lancet, *2*, 201, 1947.

31a. KING, E. J., GILCHRIST, M., WOOTON, I. D. P., O'BRIEN, J. R. P., JOPE, H. M., QUELCH, P. E., PETERSON, J. M., STRANGEWAYS, D. H. and RAMSAY, W. N. M.: Determination of Hæmoglobin, A Comparison of Methods for Determining Iron Content and Oxygen Capacity of Blood, Lancet, *1*, 478, 1948.

31b. KING, E. J., WOOTTON, I. D. P., DONALDSON, R., SISSON, R. B. and MACFARLANE, R. G.: Determination of Hæmoglobin, Test of the M.R.C. Gray-Wedge Photometer, Lancet, *2*, 282, 478, 563, 971, 1948; *ibid.*, *1*, 1044, 1951.

32. KINGSLEY, D. M.: A New Hematological Stain, Stain Technol., *10*, 127, 1935.

33. ———Polychromed Methylene Blue as a Constituen of Romanowsky Stains, J. Lab. & Clin. Med., *22*, 736, 1937 (Bibliography).

33a. LANCASTER, H. O.: Accuracy of Blood Cell Counting, Australian J. Exper. Biol. & M. Sc., *31*, 603, 1953.

34. LAWRENCE, J. S. and TODD, H.: Variations in the Characteristics of Lymphocytes in Supravital Preparations, Folia hæmatol., *44*, 318, 1931.

34a. LEESON, D. and REEVE, E. B.: The Plasma in the Packed Cell Column of the Haematocrit, J. Physiol., *115*, 129, 1951.

34b. LOCHHEAD, H. B. and PURCELL, M. K.: Accuracy of Sahli Hemoglobin Pipets, Am. J. Clin. Path., *22*, 296, 1952.

35. LEICHSENRING, J. M., DONELSON, E. G., WALL, L. M. and OHLSON, M. A.: Evaluation of Oxalate Solutions for the Determination of Packed Cell Volume in Human Blood, J. Lab. & Clin. Med., *25*, 35, 1939.

35a.LILLIE, R. D.: A Giemsa Stain of Quite Constant Composition and Performance, Pub. Health Rep., 58, 449, 1943.

35b.————Factors Influencing the Romanowsky Staining of Blood Films and the Role of Methylene Violet, J. Lab. & Clin. Med., 29, 1181, 1944.

35c. LUCEY, H. C.: Fortuitious Factors Affecting the Leucocyte Count in Blood from the Ear, J. Clin. Path., 3, 146, 1950.

35d.MACFARLANE, J. C. W. and CECIL, G. W.: Eosinophil Counting: A Modification of Pilot's Method, Brit. M. J., 2, 1187, 1951.

35e.MACFARLANE, R. G., KING, E. J., WOOTTON, I. D. P. and GILCHRIST, M.: Determination of Hæmoglobin, Lancet, 1, 282, 1948; Ibid., 2, 563, 1948.

35f.MACFARLANE, R. G. et al.: An Automatic Apparatus for Counting Red Blood Cells, Brit. J. Haemat., 5, 1, 1959.

35g.MANWELL, R. D.: The J. S. B. Stain for Blood Parasites, J. Lab. & Clin. Med., 30, 1078, 1945.

36. MASON, S. J.: A New Method for the Determination of the Blood Cell Volume, J. Lab. & Clin. Med., 20, 318, 1934.

36a.MATTERN, C. F. T., BRACKETT, F. S. and OLSON, B. J.: Determination of Number and Size of Particles by Electronic Gating. I. Blood Cells, J. Appl. Physiol., 10, 56, 1957.

36b.McGOVERN, J. J., JONES, A. R. and STEINBERG, A. G.: The Hematocrit of Capillary Blood, New England J. Med., 253, 308, 1955.

36c.McINROY, R. A.: A Micro-Haematocrit for Determining the Packed Cell Volume and Hæmoglobin Concentration on Capillary Blood, J. Clin. Path., 7, 32, 1954.

36d.McNARY, W. F., JR.: Dithizone Staining of Myeloid Granules, Blood, 12, 644, 1957.

36e.McNARY, W. F., JR.: A New Diluting Fluid for Eosinophils, Using Bromcresol Purple, Am. J. Clin. Path., 30, 373, 1958.

36f.MEYERSTEIN, W.: Simple Sealed Hematocrit Tube, J. Physiol., 101, 5P, 1942; Ibid., 108, 32P, 1948.

37. MILLER, A. T., JR.: A Simple and Accurate Hematocrit Tube, J. Lab. & Clin. Med., 24, 547, 1939.

37a.MOESCHLIN, S.: Phase-Contrast Microscopy of Leukocytes, in The Leukemias: Etiology, Pathophysiology and Treatment, New York, Academic Press, Inc., 1957, p. 37.

38. MOORE, J. E., III and JAMES, G. W., III: A Simple Direct Method for Absolute Basophil Leukocyte Count, Proc. Soc. Exper. Biol. & Med., 82, 601, 1953.

39. NEWCOMER, H. S.: Absorption Spectra of Acid Hematin, Oxyhemoglobin and Carbon Monoxide Hemoglobin: A New Hemoglobinometer, J. Biol. Chem., 37, 465, 1919; Ibid., 55, 569, 1923.

39a.NICHOLAS, J. W.: A Slide Rule for Haematological Calculations, J. Clin. Path., 10, 208, 1957.

40. OLSEN, C.: A Simple Mechanical Device for Shaking Blood Cell Counting Pipettes, J. Lab. & Clin. Med., 22, 724, 1937.

41. OSGOOD, E. E. and ASHWORTH, C. M.: Atlas of Hematology, J. W. Stacey, San Francisco, 1937.

41a.PARRY, K. C. and SIMMONDS, G. E.: Blood Pipette Shaking Machine, J. Clin. Path., 3, 164, 1950.

41b.PERRY, S. and REYNOLDS, J.: Methyl-Green-Pyronin as a Differential Nucleic Acid Stain for Peripheral Blood Smears, Blood, 11, 1132, 1956.

42. PIJPER, A.: The Diffraction Method of Measuring Red Blood Cells, J. Lab. & Clin. Med., 32, 857, 1947.

43. PLUM, P.: Accuracy of Hæmatological Counting Method, Acta med. scandinav., 90, 342, 1936.

44. PONDER, E.: The Mammalian Red Cell and the Properties of Hæmolytic Systems, Protoplasma, Berlin, Gebrüder Borntraeger, 1934; Hemolysis and Related Phenomena, New York, Grune and Stratton, 1948.

44a.POOLE, J. C. F.: Hæmoglobin Standard, Lancet, 2, 116, 1954.

45. PRICE-JONES, C.: Red Blood Cell Diameters, London, Oxford Medical Publications, 1933.

46. RICHAR, W. J. and BREAKELL, E. S.: Evaluation of an Electronic Particle Counter for the Counting of White Blood Cells, Am. J. Clin. Path., 31, 384, 1959.

46a.RIMINGTON, C.: Hæmoglobinometry, Brit. Med. J., 1, 176, 1942.

46b.SABINE, J. C. and NICKOLAI, D. J.: A Microhematocrit Method and Its Use with Citrated Blood, Blood, 7, 1128, 1952.

46c.SCHNEIDERMAN, M., MANTEL, N. and BRECHER, G.: The Effect of Rejection Procedures on the Accuracy of Blood Counts, Am. J. Clin. Path., 21, 973, 1951.

48. SCHWENTKER, F. F.: The Estimation of Hemoglobin: A New Hemoglobinometer, J. Lab. & Clin. Med., 15, 247, 1929 (Bibliography).

48a.SCHWIND, J. L.: The Supravital Method in the Study of the Cytology of Blood and Marrow Cells, Blood, 5, 597, 1950.

48b.SHANBERGE, J. N.: Accidental Occurrence of Endothelial Cells in Peripheral Blood Smears, Am. J. Clin. Path., 25, 460, 1955.

48c.SHILS, M. E., SASS, M. and GOLDWATER, L. J.:

A Microhematocrit Method and Its Evaluation, Am. J. Clin. Path., 22, 155, 1952.

49. SHOHL, A. T., BLACKFAN, K. D. and DIAMOND, L. K.: Cell Opacity Method for Determination of Cell Volume on a Single Drop of Rat Blood, Proc. Soc. Exper. Biol. & Med., 45, 383, 1940.

50. SLAWINSKI, A.: A New Conductivity Method for the Determination of the Cell Volume of Blood, Biochem. J., 27, 356, 1933.

50a.SMITH, S. E.: A New Hematocrit Tube, J. Lab. & Clin. Med., 29, 301, 1944.

50b.SPEIRS, R. S.: The Principles of Eosinophil Diluents, Blood, 7, 550, 1952; J. Lab. & Clin. Med., 39, 963, 1952.

50c.SNAPPER, I. and NATHAN, D. J.: The Mechanics of the "L.E." Cell Phenomenon, Studied with a Simplified Test, Blood, 10, 718, 1955.

51. STRUMIA, M.: A Rapid Universal Blood Stain —May-Gruenwald-Giemsa in One Solution, J. Lab. & Clin. Med., 21, 930, 1936.

51a.STRUMIA, M. M., SAMPLE, A. B. and HART, E. D.: An Improved Micro Hematocrit Method, Am. J. Clin. Path., 24, 1016, 1954.

51b.SUNDERMAN, F. W., MACFATE, R. P., MAC-FADYEN, D. A., STEVENSON, G. F. and COPELAND, B. E.: Clinical Hemoglobinometry, Am. J. Clin. Path., 23, 519, 1953; ibid., 25, 695, 1955.

51c.TOMPKINS, E.: Methods to Increase Accuracy in the Use of Hayem's Solution for Red Blood Counts, J. Lab. & Clin. Med., 33, 1180, 1948.

51d.VAN SLYKE, D. D., PHILLIPS, R. A., DOLE, V. P., HAMILTON, P. B., ARCHIBALD, R. M. and PLAZIN, J.: Calculation of Hemoglobin from Blood Specific Gravities, J. Biol. Chem., 183, 349, 1950.

51e.VAN SLYKE, D. D., HILLER, A., WEISIGER, J. R. and CRUZ, W. O.: Determination of Carbon Monoxide in Blood and of Total and Active Hemoglobin by Carbon Monoxide Capacity. Inactive Hemoglobin and Methemoglobin Contents of Normal Human Blood, J. Biol. Chem., 166, 121, 1946.

52. WINTROBE, M. M.: Erythrocyte in Man, Medicine, 9, 195, 1930.

53. ———— Blood of Normal Young Women Residing in a Sub-tropical Climate, Arch. Int. Med., 45, 289, 1931.

54. ———— The Size and Hemoglobin Content of the Erythrocyte: Methods of Determination and Clinical Application, J. Lab. & Clin. Med., 17, 899, 1932.

55. ———— Macroscopic Examination of the Blood, Am. J. Med. Sc., 185, 58, 1933.

56. ———— Anemia, Arch. Int. Med., 54, 256, 1934.

57. WINTROBE, M. M. and BUELL, M. V.: Hyperproteinemia Associated With Multiple Myeloma, Bull. Johns Hopkins Hosp., 52, 156, 1933.

58. WONG, S. Y.: Colorimetric Determination of Iron and Hemoglobin in Blood, J. Biol. Chem., 77, 409, 1928. Modified by Ponder, Ibid., 144, 333, 1942

59. WU, H.: Studies on Hemoglobin, J. Biochem. (Japan), 2, 173 and 189, 1922.

60. ZINKHAM, W. H. and CONLEY, C. L.: Some Factors Influencing the Formation of L.E. Cells, Bull. Johns Hopkins Hosp., 98, 102, 1956.

Chapter 9

Anemia: General Considerations and Treatment

Definition of Anemia.—The term anemia, as it is generally used in clinical medicine, refers to a reduction below normal in the number of red corpuscles per c.mm., the quantity of hemoglobin, and the volume of packed red cells per 100 ml. of blood. Anemia, which thus refers to the concentration of oxygen-carrying substance in a certain volume of blood, is to be distinguished from **oligemia,** which signifies a reduction of the total amount of blood in the body; from **oligocythemia,** which refers to a deficiency in the total quantity of red corpuscles; and from **oligochromemia,** which signifies a reduction in the total quantity of hemoglobin.

The last mentioned terms are rarely used, because total blood volume is not measured frequently and clinical experience is based on measurements of the concentration of the red cells, hemoglobin or volume of packed red corpuscles in a unit of volume. In a sense the latter are, indeed, the more important measurements because they indicate how much oxygen can be carried to the tissues by a certain quantity of blood. This is, in the last analysis, the best measure of its functional efficiency. Furthermore, when anemia develops, although there may be an immediate oligemia if the anemia is due to actual loss of blood, the tendency is to make up for this loss immediately by an increase in

the fluid portion of the blood, thus bringing the total volume to normal once more. In anemias of gradual onset there is the same tendency to maintain a constant total volume of blood. Therefore, volume being relatively constant, measurements of the quantity of cells or hemoglobin in a unit volume of blood serve as a rough index of their total quantity. In certain conditions, however, as will be mentioned later, exceptions to this general rule occur.

Concept of the "Erythron."—The "erythron"[3] refers to the circulating red corpuscles as well as the organ from which they arise, namely, the bone marrow. It is a useful term because it emphasizes the functional unity of the red corpuscles and their precursors. The erythron has been compared[35] to the skin which, with its various layers, from the stratum germinativum to the stratum corneum, represents a widespread organ, consisting of several layers evolving eventually to a layer of essentially inert but functionally important cells, those of the corneum. In the same way one may think of the erythron with its primitive erythroblasts giving rise eventually, after a series of changes, to the non-nucleated, highly specialized red corpuscles. The interstitial tissue of the erythron is represented by the plasma and by the fat and reticulum of the bone marrow. When considered as a whole, the erythron is an

Table 9–1—Etiologic Classification of Anemia

I. Loss of Blood
   A. Acute posthemorrhagic anemia
   B. Chronic posthemorrhagic anemia

II. Excessive destruction of red corpuscles, resulting from
   A. Extracorpuscular causes
   B. Intracorpuscular defects, congenital (see IV, A below) and acquired

III. Impaired blood production resulting from deficiency of substances essential for erythropoiesis
   A. Iron deficiency
     Experimentally, also copper and cobalt deficiencies
   B. Deficiency of various B vitamins
     Clinically, B_{12} and folic acid deficiencies (pernicious anemia and related macr cytic, megalo-
     blastic anemias). Pyridoxine-responsive anemia.
     Experimentally, pyridoxine, folic acid, B_{12} and niacin deficiencies; possibly also riboflavin,
     pantothenic acid and thiamin deficiencies
   C. Protein deficiency
   D. Possibly ascorbic acid deficiency

IV. Faulty construction of red corpuscles
   A. Congenital or hereditary
     1. Sickle cell anemia and related disorders (hemoglobin C disease, etc.)
     2. Thalassemia
     3. Congenital hemolytic diseases
   B. Acquired
     1. Anemia associated with infection
     2. Anemia associated with various chronic diseases (renal ,etc.)
     3. Anemia in plumbism; following irradiation; in drug sensitivity (aplastic anemia)
     4. "Myelophthisic" anemias (leukemia, Hodgkin's disease, myelofibrosis, malignancy with
       metastases, etc.)
     5. Anemia in myxedema and in other endocrine deficiencies
     6. Anemia associated with splenic disorders: "hypersplenism"
   C. Unknown
     Miscellaneous hypersideremic anemias

organ much larger than the liver. Certain quantitative aspects of the erythron were discussed in an earlier chapter (p. 180).

Viewed from the standpoint of an organ, pathological changes in the erythron may be considered in the same way as disorders of other organs. The erythron may atrophy or hypertrophy, it may be damaged by infections and toxemia, it may be partially removed and it may be the seat of congenital disorders. It differs from other organs in that it is quite easy to obtain samples by which one can judge the state of destruction or repair and it has been possible to gather information regarding some of the specific substances necessary for its reconstruction. Perhaps because it is so accessible, it has been learned that the erythron is affected in a great variety of disorders.

Anemia may be classified in many different ways, none of which is wholly satisfactory. Thus, on etiologic grounds it may be attributed to (1) loss of blood, (2) excessive blood destruction, (3) impaired blood production as the result of deficiency of substances essential for erythropoiesis and (4) faulty construction of red corpuscles because of hereditary or congenital defects or as the consequence of some acquired disorder. Such a classification is presented in Table 9–1. This classification can be criticized, however, because it is, in part, based on assumptions which may be found to be incorrect, such as the implication that the anemia associated with infection is primarily the result of faulty construction of red corpuscles. Again, a certain amount of overlapping will be observed. Congenital hemolytic disease falls into two categories and pernicious anemia and certain other anemias, although true nutritional deficiencies, are in certain respects hemolytic anemias.

The time-worn division of anemia as primary (*i.e.*, resulting from fundamental disease of the hemopoietic system) and secondary, is no longer adequate. Anemia is now recognized as a symptom and in this sense is always "secondary." Even the classical form of "primary" anemia, pernicious anemia, has been shown to be the consequence of a defect in the gastrointestinal tract.

Morphological Classification.—Because the study of blood disorders naturally begins in the laboratory, a classification of anemia based on morphology[31] is useful. In the various types of anemia which have been mentioned, characteristic changes in the size and hemoglobin content of the red corpuscles occur and for this reason classification on morphological grounds is valuable in differentiating them. Treatment can be guided to some extent by the morphological type of anemia, as will be shown below. The classification is, therefore, of practical, clinical value.

When anemia develops, there may be a proportionate decrease in the number of corpuscles, the quantity of hemoglobin, and the volume of packed red cells. In such a case the cells have not, on the average, been changed in size or hemoglobin content and the anemia is called **normocytic.** Certain etiological factors, however, cause a greater decrease in number of cells than in hemoglobin or volume of packed cells. This is due to the fact that the majority of the red corpuscles which are produced are larger than normal; thus the term, **macrocytic**

anemia. On the other hand, the reverse of these changes may take place; namely, there may be a greater decrease in the quantity of hemoglobin and in volume of packed cells than in red cell count. In such cases the majority of corpuscles are smaller than normal, and the anemia is called **microcytic.**

It may be noted that in all the types of anemia mentioned so far, the change in hemoglobin and in volume of packed red cells has been proportionate. There may occur, however, a greater decrease in hemoglobin than in volume of packed cells as the result of a reduction in the quantity of hemoglobin in the majority of the cells in proportion to their size; thus the term hypochromic. Because in this type of anemia the corpuscles are usually also reduced in size, it is called **hypochromic microcytic** anemia. These four types of anemia are described further in Table 9–2.

The various clinical types of anemia, differentiated according to their fundamental cause, fit in a logical manner into the above four morphological groups. **Macrocytic anemias** (Table 9–3) fall into two main categories. The more consistent and usually the most striking instances of macrocytic anemia are those arising from lack of vitamin B_{12} or folic acid. Of these the most common example is pernicious anemia, the result of impaired absorption of vitamin B_{12} due to lack of the gastric "intrinsic factor." In other macrocytic anemias there may, for other reasons, be impaired absorption from the gastrointestinal tract of vitamin B_{12} or, more often, folic acid (sprue, idiopathic steatorrhea and certain other intestinal disorders); or there may be dietary deficiency of folic acid (nontropical nutritional macrocytic anemia, tropical macrocytic anemia), relative deficiency of vitamin B_{12} or folic acid (anti-epileptic drugs, antimetabolites), or other mechanisms may be involved. These will be discussed fully in the next

Table 9-2—Morphologic Classification of Anemias

Class and severity	No. of red corpuscles	Mean corpuscular volume Vol./R.B.C.	Mean corpuscular hemoglobin Hb./R.B.C.	Mean corpuscular hemoglobin concentration Hb./Vol.	Description
Macrocytic:					Red cells increased in volume; mean corpuscular hemoglobin proportionally increased; increase in size and hemoglobin content of red cells roughly inversely proportional to number of cells; mean corpuscular hemoglobin concentration remains normal throughout or may be slightly reduced.
Slight	—	+	+	0	
Moderate	——	++	++	0—	
Severe	———	+++	+++	0—	
Normocytic:					Reduction in the number of red cells without any, or at most only a slight increase in mean corpuscular volume and mean corpuscular hemoglobin; mean corpuscular hemoglobin concentration normal throughout.
Slight	—	0	0	0	
Moderate	——	+0	+0	0	
Severe	———	+0	+0	0	
Simple microcytic:					Reduction in volume and hemoglobin content characteristically less marked than reduction in number of red cells; mean corpuscular hemoglobin concentration normal or only slightly reduced.
Slight	—	0	0	0	
Moderate	——	—	—	0—	
Severe	———	——	——	0—	
Hypochromic microcytic:					Reduction in volume and hemoglobin content characteristically more marked than reduction in number of red cells; *mean corpuscular hemoglobin concentration characteristically reduced.*
Slight	0	—	—	—	
Moderate	—	——	———	——	
Severe	——	———	————	———	

Hb. indicates the quantity of hemoglobin in grams per 1000 ml. of blood; Vol. = volume of packed red cells in cubic centimeters per 1000 ml. of blood; R.B.C., the number of red cells in millions per cubic millimeter.

+ increase; — decrease; 0 no change from the normal; 0— no, or only slight decrease; +0 slight or no increase. The amount of increase or decrease is indicated by the number of plus or minus signs, respectively.

Table 9–3—Morphologic, Etiologic and Clinical Classification of Anemia

Type of anemia	Mean corpuscular volume (cμ)	Mean corpuscular hemoglobin concentration (%)	Cause	Clinical syndrome	Treatment
I. Macrocytic	>94*	>30	A. Deficiency of vitamin B$_{12}$ or folic acid (Megaloblastic, macrocytic anemias)	(1) Pernicious anemia (2) Sprue Idiopathic steatorrhea Some cases of intestinal stricture or resection, gastrocolic fistula, celiac disease (3) "Tropical" nutritional macrocytic anemia Less frequently, dietary deficiency in temperate zones. "Refractory megaloblastic" and "achrestic" anemia (4) Rare cases of carcinoma of the stomach Following total gastrectomy (5) Macrocytic anemia of pregancy (6) Megaloblastic anemia of infancy (7) Diphyllobothrium latum infestation (8) Antimetabolites and increased demands for hemopoietic factors	Vitamin B$_{12}$ Vitamin B$_{12}$ or folic acid
			B. Intense activity of bone marrow (?) (Non-megaloblastic macrocytic anemias)	Conditions usually associated with normocytic anemia (Type II), especially: (1) Sickle cell anemia (2) Macrocytic hemolytic anemias of obscure etiology (3) Chronic and extensive liver disease (4) Macrocytic anemia of hypothyroidism (5) "Internal radiation" (dial workers)	Transfusions and treatment of cause
II. Normocytic	80 to 94	>30	A. Sudden loss of blood	Acute posthemorrhagic anemia, including (1) Scurvy (2) Hemophilia (3) Purpura	1. Treatment of cause 2. Transfusions (N.B. precautions) 3. Cortisone and related compounds 4. Splenectomy in special circumstances
			B. Destruction of blood (for details see Table 12–1, p. 600) I. Extracorpuscular causes	Hemolytic anemia due to (1) Infectious, chemical, physical, vegetable and animal agents (2) Immune body reactions, isoagglutinins, cold, warm and blocking antibodies Paroxysmal "cold" hemoglobinuria (3) Underlying disease ("symptomatic") (4) Idiopathic	
			II. Intracorpuscular causes	(1) Hereditary spherocytosis (2) Sickle cell anemia and other hereditary hemoglobinopathies (3) Paroxysmal nocturnal hemoglobinuria	1. Transfusions (N.B. precautions) 2. Splenectomy in (1)

	MCV	Mechanism	Causes / Examples	Treatment
		C. Lack of blood formation (for details see Tables 11–1 and 11–2, pages 550 and 552)	(1) Primary refractory anemias, due to	
			1. Agents which regularly produce marrow hypoplasia (ionizing radiation, mustards etc.)	
			2. Agents occasionally associated with hypoplasia (anti-microbials, anticonvulsants, etc., etc.)	Removal of cause
			3. Unknown causes	Transfusions
				Good diet
			(2) Simple chronic anemia, associated with various inflammatory and non-inflammatory diseases, especially renal disease, malignancy and chronic infections	Treatment of caues
				Transfusions
				Good diet
			(3) "Myelophthisic" anemia, due to metastatic carcinoma in bone marrow, Hodgkin's disease, leukemia, multiple myeloma, myelosclerosis, marble bone disease	Same
		D. Hydremia(?) "Imperfect" formation of blood	"Physiologic" anemia of pregnancy	None
			Subacute and chronic inflammatory diseases and chronic non-inflammatory conditions	Transfusions and treatment of cause
III. Simple microcytic	<80†			
	>30			
IV. Hypochromic microcytic	<30	A. Deficiency of iron through	Diet deficient in foods containing iron, especially in infants	Iron in large doses, correction of cause
	<30	(a) Deficient diet	In association with achlorhydria	
		(b) Defective absorption	Following gastrectomy (total or partial)	
			Sprue, idiopathic steatorrhea, celiac disease, chronic diarrhea	
		(c) Continued loss of blood	Chronic alimentary or genito-urinary tract bleeding	
			Multiple hereditary telangiectasia	
		(d) Excessive demands† or iron	Requirements for growth	
			Repeated pregnancies	
			Chlorosis	
		(e) Above causes in various degrees and combinations	Chronic hypochromic anemia of women	
		(f) Deficient antenatal storage or postnatal supply	Hypochromic anemia of infants	
		B. Pyridoxine requirement	Pyridoxine-responsive anemia	Pyridoxine
		C. Deficiency of copper	Hypocupremic syndrome of infants	Copper and iron
		D. Genetic anomaly	Thalassemia major	
			Combination of thalassemia and abnormal hemoglobinopathies	
		E. Unknown	Miscellaneous hypersideremic anemias	Refractory to therapy

* The sign > indicates "greater than"

†The sign < indicates "less than."

chapter (p. 467). A finding common to these macrocytic anemias which is absent in the next group is the character of the bone marrow. It is *megaloblastic*.

Macrocytic anemia can also be encountered when there is no deficiency of vitamin B_{12} or folic acid. This is observed chiefly in conditions in which normocytic anemia is more often found. The macrocytosis is attributable in most instances to the intense bone marrow activity which accompanies them. The bone marrow in these cases is often hyperplastic but it is not megaloblastic. This topic will be considered again after the normocytic anemias have been discussed.

As one might imagine on purely theoretical grounds, anemia characterized by no change in the average size or hemoglobin content of the red corpuscles **(normocytic anemia)** may result from sudden loss of blood, destruction of blood, lack of blood formation, or dilution of the blood. Under all of these circumstances, other things being equal, the remaining red corpuscles are as normal in size or hemoglobin content as they were before blood loss, destruction or dilution had occurred.

Normocytic anemia is found in the various types of hemolytic anemia, in acute posthemorrhagic anemia and in many refractory ("aplastic") anemias. In leukemia, in cases of anemia associated with bone marrow metastases, in myelofibrosis and in other so-called "myelophthisic" anemias, the anemia is usually normocytic in type. In the so-called "physiological" anemia of pregnancy, it is thought that the anemia is often more apparent than real, there being a considerable increase in the total plasma volume.

In some of the types of anemia discussed, namely, in acute posthemorrhagic anemia, in the hemolytic anemias, and sometimes even in "aplastic" anemia, blood regeneration of varying degree occurs. When the stimulus to new blood formation is great and the capacity for hematopoiesis is good, a large number of immature cells may pass into the circulation. Immature cells, as stated in an earlier chapter (p. 90 and Fig. 2–2), are usually larger than their fellow mature corpuscles. Consequently, if the flow of new cells into the circulation is great enough, the average size of the cells in the blood stream may be increased to such an extent that the mean corpuscular volume is increased above normal; thus macrocytic anemia develops. Following acute blood loss, the macrocytosis, if it occurs at all, is short in duration and usually of small magnitude. In the hemolytic anemias, especially in the acute hemolytic anemias, macrocytosis may be marked and, in the chronic forms, it may be long continued. It is noteworthy that even in "aplastic" anemia (this term is used in the clinical sense as applying to states of inadequate blood formation in which there may be some remaining hematopoietic tissue, as well as to those in which there is total aplasia) the anemia may sometimes be moderately macrocytic rather than normocytic.

Microcytic anemia which is associated with little or no decrease in the hemoglobin content of the red corpuscles **(simple microcytic),** includes a rather ill-defined group of anemias associated with a great variety of subacute and chronic inflammatory diseases and non-inflammatory conditions, such as nephritis and various infections. In the same disorders the anemia may also be normocytic. The mechanism of this type of anemia is poorly understood, the morphological characteristics are not clear-cut, and in all probability several factors are concerned in the production of the anemia.

The fourth type of anemia, **hypochromic microcytic anemia,** is almost always the result of a deficiency of iron. This may be due to the long continued use of a diet poor in iron, it may be the result of defective absorption of iron, or it may be due to continued loss of blood or excessive demands for iron for other reasons, such as the requirements of the fetus. Frequently all these factors play a role. A variety of clinical syndromes fall in this category (Table 9–3). Also attributable to deficiency of iron is the hypochromic anemia of infants, which is probably due to defective antenatal storage as well as inadequate postnatal supply.

Anemia similar morphologically to that mentioned above, is found in thalassemia but it is not due to iron deficiency and iron therapy, unlike its effect in the common type of hypochromic microcytic anemia, is of no avail. This type of anemia has also been described in certain cases of refractory anemia associated with hypersideremia (p. 562) as well as in pyridoxine-responsive anemia (p. 136) and in cases of hypocupremia in infants (p. 141). Such causes of hypochromic microcytic anemia are extremely rare, however.

Morphological differentiation of anemias is useful not only as an aid in the recognition of various blood disorders, but it is valuable as a guide in treatment. In hypochromic microcytic anemia, thalassemia and the rare disorders above mentioned excepted, iron therapy is strikingly effective. In macrocytic anemia resulting from deficiency of vitamin B_{12} or folic acid, the administration of these substances is followed by a dramatic response. These forms of treatment are specific for the respective types of anemia and they are of no value in other anemias. It is obviously important to separate those forms of anemia which can be readily relieved from those which are more resistant to treatment.

GENERAL SYMPTOMATOLOGY OF ANEMIA

The development of symptoms in cases of anemia depends chiefly on three factors: the causative disorder, the degree of change in total blood volume, and the reduction in the oxygen-carrying power of blood with its consequent disturbance of cell nutrition and function. The red cell count itself is not necessarily an indication of the symptoms that may be expected.

If the anemia has been insidious in onset, adjustment to the reduced oxygen carrying power of the blood may be so good that the red cell count may be as low as 2,000,000 cells per c.mm. or the hemoglobin as low as 6 grams per 100 ml., without sufficient functional embarrassment occurring for the patient to appreciate his true condition. In children with severe anemia particularly, the absence of apparent restriction of their ability to take exercise has been often noted.[21] The physiological adjustment which takes place involves chiefly the cardiovascular system and will be discussed shortly.

The most prominent symptoms following the *sudden loss* of blood are those resulting from the reduction in the total blood volume and they are relieved in large measure when the loss of blood is replaced by absorption of fluid from the tissues or by artificial introduction of fluid. Symptoms of oxygen deprivation develop when about 50 per cent of the blood has been lost. When there is *rapid destruction* of blood the chief manifestations are connected with the disposal of the products of blood destruction; namely, jaundice and hemoglobinuria. The fever as well as the abdominal pain which are commonly encountered in such cases are probably in large measure effects produced by the excessive amount of breakdown products.

Integumentary System.—The most striking outward symptom of anemia usually is *pallor*. Although this is often manifest in the skin, it can be observed more constantly in the buccal and pharyngeal mucous membranes, the con-

28

junctivae, the lips, the lobes of the ears, the palms of the hands and the nailbeds. The bed of the fingernail, if it is not artificially colored, is more dependable as an index of pallor than is the skin. In the hands the skin of the palms first becomes pale. The skin creases, the "lines" which are the palmist's delight, lose their usual pink coloring only when the anemia is severe (hemoglobin less than 7 gm. per 100 ml.). In examining the hands it is important that they be normally warm, and that they be held at about the level of the heart. Cyanosis or abnormal constriction of the blood vessels should not cause one to be misled. The palms of the hands are often more helpful in estimating the degree of pallor than the skin elsewhere and they may be more helpful than the mucous membranes, which may be pigmented, or the conjunctivae, which may be inflamed.

In cases of profound acute blood loss there is seen a waxy, dead whiteness of the skin. In chronic intermittent loss of blood there is a distinctly sallow color. In the chronic anemia of women associated with blood loss, faulty diet and achlorhydria, the pallor is profound but the peculiar greenish sallowness, once considered pathognomonic of chlorosis, is often lacking. In pernicious anemia, a lemon-yellow pallor was described in the early accounts of the disease but it must be noted that this is observed only when the condition is well advanced. In leukemia, pallor is often marked and may be associated with a grayish tint of the skin.

In various systemic diseases, the pallor may be characteristic. In acute glomerulonephritis with general edema there is a curious pasty white skin even when little or no anemia is present. Sometimes the peculiar dead white skin of the legs may be traversed and overlaid by venules in such a manner as to justify the old-fashioned term, "marble-like" edema. In chronic nephritis without edema, on the other hand, even when a considerable degree of anemia is present, there may be little pallor.

In malignant disease, especially in cases of carcinoma of the stomach, the pallor may resemble that of pernicious anemia; it may have a peculiar, earthy, muddy hue; or it may be slight and insignificant. In mitral regurgitation, and especially in mitral stenosis, an existing anemia may be masked by the misleading redness of the patient's cheeks and lips. In advanced cases of aortic regurgitation, on the other hand, there may be an appearance of pallor without the existence of anemia.

It is important to bear in mind that the appearance of the skin is affected by the state of constriction or dilatation of the peripheral vessels, by the degree and nature of its pigmentation and by the nature and fluid content of the subcutaneous tissues. In syncope, pallor without anemia results from constriction of peripheral vessels. In nephritis with edema, as already mentioned, and in myxedema there may be pallor without anemia. Certain persons habitually have a pale skin and pallor is common in indoor workers. The generally pallid appearance of persons residing in tropical and subtropical climates was shown to be misleading.[34] If there is dilatation of peripheral vessels, on the other hand, there may be anemia without pallor ("chlorosis rubra"). Furthermore, jaundice, cyanosis, and skin pigmentation may mask anemia.

It is evident that the skin may be pale, yet not anemic; ruddy yet profoundly anemic; but, it is noteworthy, a person is never anemic with normal color in the visible mucous membranes.

Besides pallor, loss of normal *skin elasticity* and tone resulting in dry skin shrivelled in appearance; thinning, loss of luster and early graying of the *hair*; and *purpura* and *ecchymoses* may be found in the skin and mucous membranes.

The *nails*, especially in chronic hypochromic anemia, lose their luster, become brittle and break easily and may actually become concave instead of convex (Fig. 14–2). When nutritional deficiency is present symmetrical dermatitis may develop, there may be erythematous lesions on the hands, face, neck or elbows, fissures may be present at the angles of the mouth or glossitis may be found. *Chronic leg ulcers* may occur,[22] especially in hemolytic anemias (p. 602).

Respiratory and Circulatory Systems.—Respiratory symptoms in patients suffering from anemia are often noticeable only following exertion or excitement although, when the anemia is profound, there may be dyspnea and shallow breathing even at rest in bed. The occurrence of symptoms depends on the rapidity of the production of anemia, its severity, the age of the patient and the capacity of the cardiovascular system for adjustment.[32] The rapid development of anemia is accompanied by shortness of breath, tachycardia and pallor; if very severe, shock may develop. In chronic anemia moderate dyspnea and palpitation may be the only symptoms referable to the cardiovascular system but cases have been observed in which the clinical picture of congestive heart failure[1] or angina pectoris, or symptoms of intermittent claudication[24] were the presenting manifestations. Experimental studies have shown that up to a certain degree, increasing anemia is accompanied by a greater coronary flow per unit of left ventricular work; ultimately, however, when the hemoglobin level was reduced below approximately 50 per cent of normal, depression of ventricular function was observed, presumably because the coronary vessels had approached maximal dilatation.[8]

Clinical evidences of an adjusting circulation in cases of anemia are to be found in a rapid heart rate, increased arterial pulsation, increased pulse pressure and even capillary pulsation in the finger tips. The heart may be dilated and the pulse of low tension. The **physiologic adjustments to anemia** which take place in the cardiovascular system are schematically outlined in Figure 9–1. Cardiac output (liters/min/M^2) is generally increased on the basis of a narrowed arteriovenous oxygen difference.[7,27] Central venous and intracardiac pressures are not altered although at times right atrial pressures may be elevated. The velocity of blood flow is increased, hence circulation time is shortened. Since these adjustments are not accompanied by changes in either systemic or pulmonary artery pressures, peripheral vascular resistance is lowered. The total circulating blood volume may decrease,[2] although this is not always the case.[28] The oxygen dissociation curve is displaced to the right; that is, there is a reduction in the affinity of hemoglobin for oxygen.[23] Extraction of oxygen by the tissues is therefore facilitated and by this means tissue oxygen utilization can be maintained in spite of the narrowed arteriovenous oxygen difference and the rapid circulation time.

These changes may not take place in an orderly and uniform manner. Thus, little change in cardiac output has been demonstrated until moderate anemia has developed, at which stage the cardiac output may be altered greatly in association with comparatively small differences in the degree of anemia.[7] Similarly, alterations in total plasma volume may take place in step-wise shifts rather than at a gradual and continuous rate as indicated in the diagram. Again, the state of the small blood vessels is not uniform everywhere; thus, the blood flow in the hands and kidneys[6] may be greatly reduced. This may be a homeostatic device for the diversion of blood to tissues more sensitive to oxygen lack. In any event, the low renal blood flow

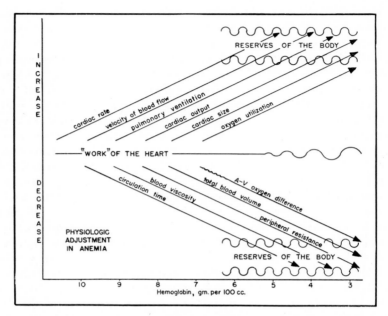

Fig. 9–1.—Diagrammatic presentation of physiologic adjustments in anemia.

is conceivably a cause of salt and water retention in anemia.[30]

Studies of the mechanical properties of the lungs in patients with anemia and during mild exercise revealed no abnormalities.[20] However, coincidentally with the cardiovascular changes, the rate and depth of respiration often are increased and the vital capacity, together with the reserve and complemental air volumes, are lowered.[2] The residual air is somewhat increased. Minute ventilation is increased.

With the decreased availability of hemoglobin as a buffer in carbon dioxide transport and with the reduced carbonic anhydrase activity, there is decreased ability to absorb carbon dioxide from the tissues for release via the lungs. The arterial oxygen tension is lower and the alveolar-oxygen tension gradient is higher than in normal subjects.[26] Nevertheless, at rest, anemic individuals are able to compensate satisfactorily in the delivery of oxygen and the transport of carbon dioxide. However, during strenuous exercise, the various hemodynamic adjustments do not suffice to prevent a marked depression of both oxygen intake and CO_2 production in comparison with those found in normal individuals exercising at comparable levels.[28]

When compensatory adjustments become imperfect or fail, the clinical picture of cardiac failure ensues. Cardiac enlargement accompanied by basilar systolic ejection murmurs, systolic, and occasionally diastolic apical murmurs may develop together with rales in the dependent portion of the lungs, enlargement of the liver, and dependent edema. The last may be the consequence of lowered renal blood flow, as mentioned above, but also is favored by such factors as hypoproteinemia and diminished tissue oxygen tension, which leads to increased capillary permeability.[12] The osmotic pressure of the plasma is not changed.

The commonest cardiac abnormality in anemia is the presence of murmurs. These are usually systolic in time and are most often heard at the apex, with the pulmonary area a close second.[14] A murmur at the aortic area is less common. Frequently murmurs are present at more than one site. They may be faint in character but often they are moderate in intensity and at times may be rough and arouse strong suspicion of organic valvular disease. Rarely a late diastolic or presystolic murmur is heard at the apex. Very occasionally an early blowing diastolic murmur may be heard in the third left interspace near the sternum. The murmurs are, as a rule, not widely transmitted and usually are easily distinguished from those of organic heart disease. In some cases, however, and particularly in sickle cell anemia, as will be discussed later, the cardiac murmurs may closely simulate and even be indistinguishable from those of organic disease of the heart.

In addition to murmurs there may be a curious humming sound over the vessels of the neck, the "bruit de diable." The greatly increased rapidity of the blood stream, the reduction in specific gravity and viscosity as well as loss of tone in the myocardium are factors in the production of the abnormalities in heart sounds.

In many cases of severe anemia, electrocardiographic changes have been noted. The most common change is depression of the RT (ST) junction with a U-shaped deformation of the ST segment and flat or inverted T waves, but without a corresponding change in the QRS complex. The changes often resemble those produced by digitalis. Changes in the duration of the electrical systole (QT interval) and disturbances in A–V conduction have been noted occasionally.

Neuromuscular System. — Headache, vertigo, faintness, increased sensitivity to cold, tinnitus or roaring in the ears, black spots before the eyes, muscular weakness and easy fatigability, irritability, lack of power of concentration, restlessness or drowsiness are common symptoms of anemia. It was common at one time for women, especially, to go through a large part of their life with a deficit of 30 to 40 per cent of hemoglobin. In consequence they suffered from a substandard physical state which resulted in chronic irritability of disposition and character that was indirectly a fertile source of mental ill-health. Thus anemia may lead to "neurotic" or psychasthenic disorders.[25] Headache due to anemia may be so severe as to simulate meningitis. Delirium is seldom seen except in pernicious anemia and in the terminal stage of leukemia. The development of many of these symptoms is not necessarily correlated with the degree of anemia.

Retinal hemorrhages occur frequently in pernicious anemia and in aplastic anemia and are common in leukemia. They may be flame-shaped, splinter, punctate, purpuric, preretinal and subhyaloid. Flame-shaped and punctate hemorrhages with white centers may be seen in severe anemia as well as in leukemia.[19] A peculiar tortuosity of the blood vessels is seen in sickle cell anemia (p. 677).

Paresthesias are common in pernicious anemia. They may be accompanied by signs and symptoms of extensive peripheral nerve and spinal cord disease. They may also be encountered in chronic hypochromic anemia but, in the latter, spinal cord degeneration is very rare. In leukemia, involvement of cranial and peripheral somatic nerves occurs but it is then almost always due to pressure or infiltration.

Alimentary System.—Symptoms referable to disturbed digestion, gastric or intestinal, are extremely frequent in anemia. They may lead to, be a part of, or aggravate the anemic condition. In pernicious anemia and less often in chronic hypochromic anemia, glossitis and atrophy of the tongue papillae are common. In aplastic anemia, as in granulocytopenia and acute leukemia, necrotic lesions in the mouth and pharynx may occur. Anorexia, nausea, flatulence, abdominal discomfort, constipation, diarrhea, vomiting, or abnormal appetite are common manifestations. Dysphagia may be encountered in chronic hypochromic anemia and occasionally in pernicious anemia.

Genito-urinary System.—Menstrual disturbances, most often amenorrhea, in the female and loss of libido in the male are frequently a manifestation of anemia. In the chronic hypochromic anemia of women the menstrual symptoms may be so pronounced as to bring these patients first to the gynecologist. Menorrhagia is not uncommon and may contribute largely to the persistence of the anemia; or amenorrhea may be succeeded by menorrhagia as the anemia is relieved.

It is not unusual to discover slight albuminuria and even evidence of distinct renal functional impairment in anemia.

Metabolism.—The state of nutrition, as far as quantity of superficial fat is concerned, may be moderately or well preserved. This was frequently noted in chlorosis, it is not unusual in chronic hypochromic anemia, and in pernicious anemia as Addison himself wrote: "The bulkiness of the general frame and the obesity often present a most striking contrast to the failure and exhaustion observable in every other respect." This does not deny, however, that in many cases of anemia, including pernicious anemia, there is weight loss and general undernutrition.

In severe anemia the basal metabolic rate may be increased. In leukemia such an increase is common and may be pronounced.

Fever of mild degree is common when anemia is severe. A well-marked febrile reaction is characteristically found when there is rapid blood destruction.

Other Systems.—Enlargement of the liver, spleen and lymph nodes occurs in various disorders of the blood and will be discussed later. **Splenomegaly** of varying degree occurs frequently, particularly in pernicious anemia, chronic hypochromic anemia, and the various hemolytic anemias. In some forms of anemia, such as the Banti syndrome, enlargement of the spleen is an essential characteristic. In acute anemia, except when the spleen is specifically involved, as in leukemia, splenic enlargement is unusual although, in acute hemolytic anemia, it may be found. A more detailed consideration of splenomegaly will be given in the description of the various specific types of blood disorders.

Localized *tenderness of bone*, especially the sternum, is found very frequently in leukemia and sometimes in multiple myeloma, but only rarely under other circumstances; for example, when bone marrow metastases are present or when there is exceptionally marked hyperplasia, such as may occur in hemolytic anemias.

TREATMENT OF ANEMIA

General Considerations.—In recent years there has been a vast improvement in the treatment of anemia. The measures which are available are presented in Table 9–4. From a period when nonspecific measures represented all that was available for the treatment of anemia we have passed to a period in which several types of anemia can be treated specifically and dramatic recoveries can be expected. Yet it is by no means unusual even today to encounter cases of anemia which have been treated inefficiently, inadequately, and incorrectly. Occasionally one even finds that patients have been treated for anemia whose blood is normal and who probably have not been anemic.

Several reasons can be offered to explain these inadequacies. The first is a failure to understand the *importance of*

Table 9–4—Therapeutic Measures for the Anemias

A. Agents which meet a deficiency
   (a) vitamin B_{12}—in pernicious anemia and related disorders
   (b) folic acid—in certain rare megaloblastic, macrocytic anemias
   (c) iron—in iron deficiencies
 and, perhaps less directly,
   (d) desiccated thyroid—in anemia of hypothyroidism
   (e) ascorbic acid—anemia of scurvy
   (f) steroids in Addison's disease

B. Agents which relieve or modify the underlying disorder
   (a) antibiotics and other measures for the treatment of various infections
   (b) chemotherapeutic agents and irradiation in leukemia, Hodgkin's disease and related disorders
   (c) other measures directed at the underlying disorder

C. Agents or measures which decrease the extent of blood destruction
   (a) adrenocorticosteroids in many instances of acquired hemolytic anemia
   (b) splenectomy in hereditary spherocytosis; less often in acquired hemolytic anemias

D. Measures which restore blood volume and temporarily relieve anemia
   (a) whole blood transfusion
   (b) administration of washed red corpuscles

E. Measures intended to stimulate erythropoiesis but of doubtful value
   (a) cobalt
   (b) adrenocorticosteroids
   (c) androgenic hormone

accurate diagnosis. It has been mentioned already in this chapter and will be considered more fully later that in the great majority of the macrocytic and of the hypochromic microcytic anemias, brilliantly successful treatment is possible. To achieve success, however, a thorough study of the patient and the blood picture is an essential prerequisite. The diagnosis should and almost always can be made before the use of therapeutic agents has obscured the whole clinical picture.

A deplorable factor is the promotion of "shotgun" remedies, even by pharmaceutical houses of good repute. These therapeutic agents are partly based on the results of experiments in animals which have not been shown to apply to man. They are also prepared with the attitude that some of the constituents of the mixture may be beneficial while the remainder will certainly do no harm. Thus, mixtures with attractive or impressive names and containing iron, copper, manganese, and other metals as well as various fractions of liver, gastric substances, and all the vitamins known and hypothetical, are recommended by "detail men" with imposing lists of references. Such mixtures are used sometimes even in the absence of a thorough blood examination, in the hope that something in the remedy will meet a therapeutic need. This practice is unwise because, even if one of the constituents of the remedy is needed, the amount of this substance in the mixture is usually too small to be as effective as it would be if it were given in optimal doses. The result is great waste of money and time for the patient and discredit to the physician (Table 9–5). "Shotgun" therapy cannot be condemned too strongly.

It is not generally realized that substances which have been shown in animal experiments to be required for blood formation are not necessarily useful therapeutically in patients with anemia. The reasons for this are several. First, the *requirements* for certain substances may

Table 9–5—Pros and Cons of "Shotgun" Antianemic Therapy

Advantages	Disadvantages
1. No diagnosis required	1. Underlying factor in pathogenesis of anemia may be overlooked and opportunity for early definitive therapy (*e.g.*, for carcinoma) may be missed.
2. Neurasthenics may inprove temporarily	2. No confirmation of diagnosis by response to a single, specific therapeutic agent.
3. A puzzling patient may seek a better physician	3. In recommended dosage often does not supply enough of the substance which may be required.
	4. Wasteful.
	(a) contains many substances not needed for treatment of patients.
	(b) cost of therapeutic agent multiplied 10– or 20-fold.

be so low that, even under the extraordinary circumstances under which man sometimes finds himself, anemia attributable to lack of such substances is unlikely to occur or may never develop. Those who assume that such substances must be used therapeutically in man fail to appreciate the fact that the experimental conditions under which certain deficiencies were produced were extremely artificial.

Storage is another safety factor. The body contains large metabolic pools which can be drawn upon. This explains in part why severe anemia does not develop when there is protein deficiency. It would explain the lack of iron deficiency anemia in a male adult if his diet excluded iron even for ten years.

It appears likely that *bacterial synthesis* provides us with still another protective factor. Thus, in order to produce folic acid deficiency in swine, we found it necessary not only to give a diet lacking this vitamin but to feed the animals succinylsulfathiazol in order to cut down the growth of bacteria in the bowel. In fact, to produce a consistent and severe anemia a folic acid antagonist had to be given as well.

Finally, for the development of certain types of anemia, certain *special conditions* must exist. These have been called "*conditioned deficiencies*" (p. 522). The best example of this is the role which lack of "intrinsic factor" plays in the development of vitamin B_{12} deficiency in pernicious anemia. Although the diet contains vitamin B_{12}, the victim of pernicious anemia is unable to absorb this essential substance because the necessary mechanism for its absorption is absent. Again, in pregnancy the need to supply the fetus, and in childhood and in adolescence the great needs for growth provide the "conditions" which lead to the development of iron deficiency.

In the **study of the patient from the standpoint of anemia,** it is important to ask certain questions in addition to the routine ones. One should inquire about the *family* history with especial reference to anemia, spells of jaundice, and bleeding disorders. The patient's *occupation* and his hobbies must be known in seeking out possible poisonous agents. It may be recalled that even women who do nothing more injurious than housewifery may use cleaning fluids and paints which may be harmful; or they may use hair dyes and depilatories that are injurious. The patient should be questioned about early graying of the hair, burning of the tongue, sores about the angles of the mouth, and discomfort and brittleness of the fingernails, for these are symptoms of the deficiency anemias which can be treated successfully. When there is achlorhydria it is very common for the patient to have a stool in the morning, immediately on arising, and one or two later in the day. Bouts of diarrhea are not uncommonly disguised as "intestinal flu." Inquiry about such bowel movements should be made. The possibility of blood loss must be kept in mind. In men there may be occult loss from the gastrointestinal tract. In women it is necessary to inquire about the actual amount of blood lost during menstruation and the number and frequency of pregnancies and abortions. In the case of a child or adolescent, the rate of growth may be significant. The dietary history is most important but is difficult to obtain accurately. It is obviously not sufficient to learn that the patient eats certain foods. It is important to know how much or how little of these foods is consumed. The patient must be questioned regarding the diet meal by meal, and quantitative information should be obtained as far as possible. Occasionally a statement regarding dietary idiosyncrasies is very helpful. Pains in the limbs, paresthesias, difficulty in walking, fever, abnormal color of the urine, bruises, ecchymoses, and purple spots on the skin are important points in the history. In all instances, the presence or absence of symptoms suggesting an underlying disease such as chronic renal disease, chronic infection or malignancy, must be looked into.

The *physical examination* should include the fundi and the nervous system. A neglected but useful procedure in the physical examination is careful palpation of the sternum for tenderness. It is uncommon in leukemia to find tenderness of the bones of the extremities, but rather frequently one will find a small, acutely tender area near the lower end of the sternum of which the patient may have been quite unaware and which can be easily overlooked unless it is particularly sought out. A systematic check for evidence of glandular enlargement must be made and an icteric tint in the sclerae

should not be overlooked. The heart cannot be ignored, for it may yield the first evidence of subacute bacterial endocarditis. Not only must one attempt to palpate the liver and spleen but the kidneys should be given attention, since hypernephroma may be the cause of obscure anemia. Neither the pelvic nor the rectal examination can be neglected, for these may reveal the first indication of the nature and cause of the anemia.

The physical examination may need to be supplemented by *roentgenography*. A roentgenographic film of the chest may reveal unsuspected mediastinal enlargement, while roentgenograms of the bones may lead to the discovery of tumors, myelosclerosis or periosteal elevations suggesting leukemia.

Examination of the blood microscopically, the stained blood smear or an unstained wet film of blood, should be done by the physician himself. Too much reliance is placed in clinical practice on technicians for blood examinations. While the quantitative determinations may be too time consuming to be done in person, examination of the smear can be done in a very short time with great profit and serves as a check on the work of the technician. It is necessary that an accurate hemoglobinometer be used. The use of such grossly inaccurate methods as is represented by the Tallqvist scale is inexcusable. They have led too often to the treatment of nonexistent anemia or to failure to recognize disease which is readily amenable to treatment. The value of the hematocrit as a simple, quick and accurate aid to the physician has been discussed (p. 379).

The fact should not be overlooked that the hemopoietic system functions as a physiologic unit. Consequently, when red cell formation is stimulated, it is found as a rule that there is, in addition, increased leukopoiesis and an increase in the quantity of platelets. Thus, following acute blood loss, there may be not only reticulocytosis but also moderate or even marked leukocytosis accompanied by an increase in the younger forms of leukocytes not ordinarily seen in such numbers in the blood ("shift to the left"). The quantity of platelets is also likely to be increased.

When erythropoiesis is impaired, owing to iron or to vitamin B_{12} or folic acid deficiency, one finds evidence of disturbed leukocyte and platelet formation as well. Thus, in pernicious anemia, leukopenia is a common accompaniment of the anemia and is usually associated with relative lymphocytosis and the presence of multi-segmented polymorphonuclear leukocytes. Thrombocytopenia often is also found.

Evidence of increased red cell destruction must also be sought out. The clue to this is generally given by the appearance of the plasma, which, in cases of increased blood destruction, is distinctly icteric. The van den Bergh reaction reveals this to be of the "indirect" type, and examination of the urine in such cases reveals an increased quantity of urobilinogen. It is useful, where the facilities exist, to measure the quantity of urobilinogen excreted in the stool as well. In relation to increased blood destruction, it is again important to look upon the hemopoietic system as a physiologic unit. Increased blood destruction, except in certain types of chronic hemolytic anemia, is accompanied not only by the chemical evidence just mentioned but also by reticulocytosis, leukocytosis, and thrombocytosis.

The anemia associated with chronic infection or with chronic renal disease, like aplastic anemia due to the action of a poison, is differentiated from the anemias due to nutritional deficiency and the anemias due to exaggerated blood destruction by the lack of evidence of hemopoietic activity. Thus, the anemia is usually normocytic and is accompanied by relatively little poikilocytosis or anisocytosis; reticulocytes are normal in number and nucleated red cells are not found in the blood smear; the leukocytes are not altered in number from the normal except in so far as they may represent a reaction to the underlying disorder.

Knowledge of the chemical processes concerned in erythropoiesis has not yet reached the point where chemical examination is of great practical value in the recognition and differentiation of the various types of anemia. Ultimately, this may become as important as the morphologic study of the blood. Thus, the plasma iron content is reduced below the normal in cases of iron deficiency, in association with the anemia of chronic infection, and in various types of anemia in which blood regeneration is active. It is increased in pernicious anemia in relapse and in hemolytic anemias. The plasma iron decreases to values below normal when blood regeneration occurs as the result of vitamin B_{12} therapy in pernicious anemia. In certain circumstances, particularly in the anemia of chronic infection, the content of free protoporphyrin in the erythrocytes is increased. In this type of anemia the serum copper is also in excess of the normal.

When the patient has been studied thoroughly in the manner indicated above, the number of instances in which examination of the bone marrow will be required is small. The indications for marrow puncture and biopsy were considered fully in an earlier chapter (65).

It is customary to think of the blood in relation to a unit of volume. It is not unusual to forget that the sample examined is only a portion of the whole mass of blood. Fortunately, the unit obtained by venipuncture or from the finger is reasonably representative, and it is rarely necessary to measure the blood volume; nor is it often practicable to perform the latter determination. It is necessary, nevertheless, to bear in mind the concept of total blood volume and to recall that an increase in the fluid portion of the blood—that is, an increase in the total plasma volume—may give a false impression of anemia, the total red cell mass having been reduced little or not at all. Of even greater importance is the fact that extracellular fluid deficit (dehydration) may mask an underlying anemia.

For diagnosis in the great majority of cases of anemia, the use of isotopic methods for the study of erythrokinetics (p. 185) is unnecessary. In general it may be said that these and other procedures which involve special laboratory equipment and technics such as are available only in certain centers are not required in the study of the great majority of cases, notwithstanding their importance in helping to elucidate the pathogenesis of many forms of anemia.

General Measures.—It is unnecessary to dwell on general measures in the treatment of anemia for they are similar to those employed in the treatment of all acute and chronic diseases. Physical rest, mental serenity, fresh air, sunshine and massage are valuable and important. As the patient improves in strength and well-being, exercise should be started gradually and persisted in systematically. Physical exertion to the point of actual fatigue should be avoided. It must be kept in mind that in anemia of long standing and high degree, the cardiovascular system is involved and, in elderly patients particularly, the cardiac reserve may be easily overtaxed.

Gastrointestinal disturbances must be treated as they arise. Constipation is common in anemic patients. Drastic purgation should be avoided. Contrary to the effect of small doses of iron, the larger amounts which are now employed may cause diarrhea. The latter can be prevented by commencing iron therapy with about half the ultimate dose and gradually increasing the amount. If this is done, an anemic patient, formerly constipated, may regain normal bowel movements. In achlorhydric patients, diarrhea may be troublesome or nausea may occur. These symptoms are sometimes relieved by the administration of dilute hydrochloric acid, 2 to 4 ml. in water or fruit juices, three times daily with meals. Glossitis can be relieved by appropriate therapy, depending on the nature of the deficiency, but this may have to be given parenterally to be effective (*e.g.*, vitamin B$_{12}$).

Respiratory and circulatory symptoms will be alleviated as the anemia is effectively relieved. Sometimes the development of anemia is sufficient to precipitate failure in a diseased cardiovascular system able to function adequately when the oxygen supply is normal. Digitalis therapy may be necessary. Anginal symptoms will often vanish as the blood count rises.

From the viewpoint of the nervous system, management is the same as in the treatment of nervous conditions unrelated to anemia. As indications arise, it is permissible to use sedatives such as the barbituric acid preparations. Those mixtures containing amidopyrine and other drugs of potentially toxic effect (p. 1097) should be scrupulously avoided. For treatment of the disturbances of gait and coördination which occur in pernicious anemia, physiotherapy is important and very valuable.

DIET IN ANEMIA

In an earlier chapter the substances needed for red cell production were discussed (p. 129). When any one of these is specifically lacking it should, if possible, be given. Normally these blood-building materials are obtained in food and thus a diet rich in these remains the most important adjunct in the treatment of anemia.

The classical experiments of Whipple and his co-workers[159] furnished the groundwork of our knowledge of the effect of various foods in hemoglobin production and were the studies which led to the discovery of the value of liver therapy in pernicious anemia. They may be regarded as having initiated the development of modern hematology, so profound was their influence in stimulating the shift in this field to physiological investigation as distinguished from morphological. This is true in spite of the fact that it is now recognized that the standard salmon-bread ration which these investigators fed dogs, made anemic by bleeding, was deficient in a number of respects and therefore the hemopoietic effect they observed can now be attributed to a variety of factors.

Animal organs, such as liver, kidney and chicken gizzard were found to be the most efficient of all the foods in favoring hemoglobin regeneration, whereas dairy products were the least valuable. Pig liver was found to be 40 per cent more effective than beef liver, and oysters were excelled only by liver. Fruits such as apricots, peaches, and prunes and even raisins, fresh grapes, and apples were found to be of greater value than the chlorophyll-containing vegetables, such as spinach and beet greens.

The results of these experiments can be used as a guide in the dietary management of anemia. To the anemic patient a well-balanced diet favoring the foods mentioned above should be given. They will furnish important proteins and minerals as well as vitamins. The concentrated carbohydrate foods, such as cakes, pastry, puddings and the like, should be avoided since their ingestion necessarily lessens the appetite for more valuable foods. For similar reasons, fats should not be given in excess.

The consistency of the diet and the number of feedings must be adjusted to the state of health of the patient. All food should be tastefully served and seasoned while cooking, and monotony in meals must be avoided.

Liver.—Liver is a complex mixture which contains various proteins, carbohydrates and fats, and their breakdown products, and it is very rich in vitamins, including vitamin B_{12}.

In the treatment of pernicious anemia, a liver diet is useful but not necessary now that vitamin B_{12} is available. This has greatly simplified the treatment and management of this disease. In related forms of macrocytic anemia, the value of liver may be just as great as in pernicious anemia but its influence in other types of anemia is not as striking. In hypochromic microcytic anemia, the foods mentioned are effective to some extent but their influence is small in comparison to the effect of iron.

AGENTS WHICH RELIEVE OR MODIFY THE UNDERLYING DISORDER

As implied several times already, the treatment of anemia involves primarily the eradication of the cause of the anemia, if that is possible, or at least modification of the underlying disorder. The general measures which have just been described are purely accessory to this objective. When the anemia is due to deficiency of a substance essential for erythropoiesis, such as vitamin B_{12}, folic acid or iron, administration of the agent which is lacking will be followed by a very gratifying therapeutic response. The uses of these anti-anemic substances will be discussed shortly. In the majority of cases of anemia, however, vitamin B_{12}, folic acid, liver extract and even iron have no value, since the anemia is not due to deficiency. In such cases less specific measures must be employed.

Blood transfusion is a valuable temporary measure for the treatment of

Table 9–6—Case Illustrating the Significance of the Type of Anemia

Male, 45 years of age, complaining of anemia.

P.I.: (1) weakness and dizziness began 8 months before. Crampy abdominal pain from time to time, stools occasionally mixed with blood. Physician found anemia and achlorhydria. Treatment: vitamin B_{12} and liver.

(2) weakness persisted, 20 lb. weight loss.

Physical Exam.: pallor, koilonychia, systolic apical and basal cardiac murmurs, indistinct oval mass. 3×4 cm., right side abdomen.

Blood: Severe hypochromic microcytic anemia (vol. pkd. RBC 22 ml., MCV 49, MCC 23); WBC 9,000; platelets 229,000.

Barium enema: midportion ascending colon narrowed 8 cm.

Conclusion: carcinoma of colon presented itself under guise of anemia. The clue was overlooked for 8 months.

anemia if employed judiciously. The indications for blood transfusion were discussed in an earlier chapter (p. 354) and the risks involved were also considered. Needless to say, if there is acute or chronic blood loss, the bleeding should be arrested. It does require emphasis that the presence of hypochromic microcytic anemia represents a challenge to the physician for it signifies in most cases that blood loss has been occurring for a long time and its source must be discovered. The finding of such anemia is often the first signal of the existence of an occult ulcerative lesion. This, in the male, is almost always in the gastrointestinal tract and should direct a search for peptic ulcer or for malignancy (Table 9–6). Although in the female menorrhagia or frequently repeated pregnancies may offer a ready explanation for the development of iron deficiency, this answer should not be accepted without sufficient evidence. In the adult, dietary iron deficiency alone is rarely if ever the cause of hypochromic microcytic anemia.

Infections, if of long standing, may produce anemia but this is usually one of the less prominent symptoms. Infections naturally deserve treatment in their own right, whether that be surgical or by means of *antibiotics*. It should not be forgotten that malarial infection produces anemia which is hemolytic in nature and can be severe.

Not to be overlooked in the treatment of anemia is the possibility of **removal from exposure to an offending agent.** In cases of acquired hemolytic anema and aplastic anemia this may be the most important action which can be taken (Table 9–7).

Irradiation, by means of roentgen therapy or radioactive phosphorus, and **chemotherapy** relieve anemia in leukemia, Hodgkin's disease and related conditions when these measures influence the disorder causing the anemia. Thus the administration of busulfan in chronic myelocytic anemia, steroid hormones and metabolic antagonists in acute leukemias, and nitrogen mustard in Hodgkin's disease, is associated often with disappearance of anemia as well as relief of other manifestations. In other conditions, such as the anemia associated with metastatic malignant tumors of the bone marrow, these measures are less effective. Details of the treatment of these and other related disorders will be discussed separately in later chapters.

Splenectomy is the only means by which the anemia of hereditary spherocytosis can be relieved permanently. This operation also has an important place in the treatment of purpura hemorrhagica. In acute hemolytic anemia of

Table 9–7—Case Illustrating Importance of Discovering Cause of Anemia

Male, 37 years of age, complaining of weakness and bleeding tendency.

P.I.: (1) Anemia discovered 7 months before. Treatment: liver capsules.
　　(2) Increasing anemia, cold, shaking chills, fever. More procrastination: liver shots, iron, six transfusions, pentnucleotide.
　　(3) G.I. series negative; stools negative for blood. More transfusions and injections.

Consultation: (1) physical examination revealed pallor, petechiae and ecchymoses of skin, mucous membranes and fundi; no splenomegaly, adenopathy or sternal tenderness.
　　(2) blood showed normocytic anemia (vol. pkd. RBC 19 ml., MCV 86, MCC 36), neutropenia (WBC 1650, neutrophils 11 per cent) and thrombocytopenia (platelets 60,000, bleeding time 35 min., clot retraction poor, tourniquet test positive).

Impression: Aplastic anemia

Additional History: Patient has epilepsy; Mesantoin therapy 2 years.

Summary: The hematologic findings led to further questioning which revealed a possible cause for the anemia. Cessation of Mesantoin therapy followed by recovery.

obscure etiology, splenectomy is of less definite value and the mortality is high (p. 629). The operation has been successful in certain instances of chronic hemolytic anemia of the "acquired" type, especially when spherocytosis has been a prominent feature and leukopenia as well as thrombocytopenia have been present also ("panhematopenia") (p. 1052). In general, however, unless there is some evidence to support the possibility that the condition is actually hereditary spherocytosis, splenectomy should be considered only after all other measures have failed. Complete relief of symptoms by splenectomy is reported in "primary splenic neutropenia" (p. 1103). In Felty's syndrome, a rare condition marked by anemia, leukopenia, arthritis and splenomegaly, splenectomy does not appear to be of lasting benefit. Splenectomy has been proven useless in sickle cell anemia, pernicious anemia and polycythemia vera and only rarely has it been found helpful in thalassemia (p. 712).

There is considerable difference of opinion regarding the place of splenectomy in the treatment of "splenic anemia" or the Banti syndrome. Frequently cases regarded as Banti's disease turn out to be examples of chronic hypochromic anemia, leukemia, or Hodgkin's disease. In these diseases splenectomy is not indicated. When they have been ruled out and tuberculosis and tumors and infections of the spleen have been successfully excluded, the presence of the Banti syndrome should be considered. The value in this condition of splenectomy combined with "shunt" operations is discussed fully in a subsequent chapter (p. 1063).

Adrenocorticotropic hormone (ACTH), and the *steroid hormones*, cortisone and related compounds, have turned out to be very useful agents for the control of many instances of acquired hemolytic anemia (p. 628) and are valuable for a time in the management of acute lymphoblastic leukemia, relieving the anemia of that condition as well as other manifestations (p. 983). They have been less convincingly effective in stimulating erythropoiesis even though it is clear that reticulocytosis follows their administration, even in pernicious anemia, and that erythroid hyperplasia may develop in the bone marrow and nucleated red cells may appear in the circulation.[33] The changes in the leukocytes which follow their administration were discussed in an earlier chapter (p. 49). The importance of myxedema as a cause of anemia and the value of *desiccated thyroid* in its relief are discussed elsewhere (p. 519).

Not only are the hormones of little value in *stimulating erythropoiesis*, but there is little else that is useful for this purpose. *Arsenic* in the form of Fowler's solution (Fig. 2–11, p. 114) or sodium cacodylate was used to stimulate blood regeneration in pernicious anemia before the discovery of liver therapy. A striking but irregular reticulocyte response was observed, as well as severe toxic and destructive changes in the megaloblasts, with inconstant increases in red cell count.[148] The effects of *cobalt*, which were discussed fully in an earlier chapter (p. 141), are in some respects similar to those of arsenic and appear to be nonspecific as well as unrewarding. Androgenic hormone has been used in the treatment of congenital hypoplastic anemia in children (p. 765) and in other anemias (p. 567) but its value has yet to be clearly demonstrated.

The rôle of *copper* and of *other minerals* and accessory substances in hemopoiesis was also discussed earlier (p. 139). They cannot be regarded as having a place in rational antianemic therapy. What minerals, in addition to iron, are required for erythropoiesis are needed in such minute amounts that these quantities are easily available in vegetables and other foods, and even as contaminants in therapeutic iron preparations.

With the exception of vitamin B_{12} and folic acid, the *vitamins* can also be dismissed from consideration in antianemic therapy unless a specific nutritional deficiency disorder is present. Thus, the administration of ascorbic acid when scurvy is present is associated with improvement but, as described earlier (p. 138), ascorbic acid does not appear to serve a specific function in hemopoiesis except in relation to the metabolism of folic acid. Again, even though experimental pyridoxine deficiency in animals is associated with the development of a striking anemia, naturally occurring pyridoxine deficiency anemia in man is unknown. The curious "pyridoxine-responsive" anemia which has been encountered in a few cases was discussed earlier (p. 136). An appropriate diet furnishes the vitamins which play a rôle in blood formation, particularly if it contains liver, and also supplies the necessary amino acids and other substances. Brewer's yeast, in doses of 12 Gm. daily, has been used as a dietary supplement, given with fruit juices, milk or soft drinks, as a paste on bread or crackers or as a dressing on vegetables. Although it is a good source of the B vitamins, as are the vitamin B tablets and capsules which are available in such abundance, multi-vitamin therapy is rarely necessary.

ADMINISTRATION OF SUBSTANCES SPECIFICALLY LACKING

Vitamin B_{12}, Folic Acid and Related Substances.—General Considerations.—In the discussion of the classification of anemia, it was pointed out that, of the two main categories of macrocytic anemia, the type characterized by megaloblastic bone marrow results from a lack of vitamin B_{12} or folic acid. There, also, the various clinical syndromes associated with these deficiencies were listed. In an earlier chapter, the development of our knowedge concerning the role of these B vitamins in hemopoiesis was described (p. 130) and in the next chapter the clinical manifestations of the macrocytic, megaloblastic anemias will be considered. Here it will be convenient to discuss the treatment of these conditions.

In 1926 Minot and Murphy[94] demonstrated the value of liver therapy in pernicious anemia. The induction of a remission in this disease required the consumption of half a pound of liver a day and tried the patience of the original investigators, not to speak of their subjects. Desiccated whole hogs' stomach, [117,121] as well as mammalian kidney and brain and brewers' yeast,[135] all of which were shown to be effective remedies in this disease, are now only of historical interest since completely satisfactory therapeutic results can be achieved by the administration of vitamin B_{12} or, in certain other megaloblastic macrocytic anemias, folic acid. Even the highly effective, concentrated liver extracts which were developed in the 1930's now find little use.[63]

The objectives of treatment in pernicious anemia and related macrocytic anemias are restitution of the blood count, reduction in the size of the red cells to normal, relief of all symptoms and rehabilitation of the patient. It is desirable, also, to administer anti-anemic substances in excess of basic requirements in order that a normal condition be maintained and a reserve supply be stored in the body. The amount of effective substance required to produce these results varies considerably in different patients. This is especially true if oral therapy is used, but has been observed also in patients treated parenterally. Other things being equal, more anti-anemic substance will be required if the patient is old, if he has liver disease, arteriosclerosis or other disorders, or suffers from an infection.[54] Infection of the genitourinary tract is a common and particularly troublesome source of difficulty. In a few, an *associated iron deficiency* will prevent the development of a complete remission until iron has been furnished. In a series of cases reported in England[70a] it was found that associated *ascorbic acid* deficiency inhibited the response to liver therapy. In one patient, choline was required for the treatment of a case of pernicious anemia.[99] In patients with changes in the nervous system, complete relief of symptoms may never occur but treatment with large doses of vitamin B_{12} must be continued for a long time for, with patience and persistence, some improvement will take place in most cases.

The *dietary management* of anemia has been discussed already (p. 443). The patient with megaloblastic, macrocytic anemia should be encouraged to take a normal diet if his condition permits and this, preferably, should include liver, meat, green vegetables and fruits.

The reticulocyte response is a useful, objective measure of the effectiveness of treatment. It is therefore very helpful in a given case to establish the diagnosis by appropriate means, as discussed in the next chapter, and then to make daily reticulocyte counts and other blood examinations at appropriate intervals with the view to confirming the diagnosis by the demonstration of a clear-cut therapeutic response. In pernicious anemia, in particular, where treatment should be continued for the remainder of the patient's life, good practice demands that the diagnosis be established on unequivocal grounds. One cannot condemn too strongly the all too prevalent practice of administering vitamin B_{12}, folic acid and other agents in "shotgun" form and seeking medical advice after this has been done or only when this has failed. Such "shotguns" will be useless if the anemia is not due to a deficiency and will rarely be completely effective if there is one. They usually serve only to confuse the clinical picture and make the establishment of a clear-cut diagnosis more difficult than it might have been otherwise.

Vitamin B_{12} and Liver Extracts, Oral and Parenteral.—Now that vitamin B_{12} is available, there is no apparent reason for the use of liver extract in the treatment of pernicious anemia.[63] The vitamin is cheaper, there is less discomfort at the site of injection and sensitivity reactions are most unusual. In other types of megaloblastic anemia, folic acid may be more effective than B_{12} (see below). Rarely a case is reported in which it appeared that crude liver extract had an effect which neither of these two vitamins afforded.[73,85,103] Such experiences have led to speculation concerning the existence of a third antianemic factor in liver and yeast ("Wills' factor,"[132] p. 509).

It is well established that gastrointestinal absorption of vitamin B_{12} is severely impaired in pernicious anemia. This is the consequence of deficiency of intrinsic factor. This substance in some manner binds the relatively small quantities of B_{12} in the normal diet and facilitates their absorption. However, when massive doses of B_{12} are given by mouth, gastrointestinal absorption can take place even in cases of pernicious anemia. Thus, complete clinical and hematologic remissions were observed in the greater proportion of patients given 100 to 150 μg. B_{12} daily, by mouth, without intrinsic factor[60,62] although on this dose, serum cobalamin levels remain low.[89a] Vitamin B_{12} (10 to 30 μg. daily) has even been shown to be effective when given by nasal instillation in isotonic sodium chloride solution and lactose powder.[97a] These doses contrast with a minimal effective daily intramuscular dose of 1 μg.

When intrinsic factor is given orally, with vitamin B_{12}, absorption is greatly enhanced. This can be demonstrated, for example, by the Schilling test (p. 490). However, attempts to develop commercial preparations of vitamin B_{12} with added hog duodenal mucosa for oral administration of the vitamin in pernicious anemia have met with a curious difficulty. In spite of good initial responses and even successful maintenance therapy for variable periods of time, a state of refractoriness has ultimately developed in the majority of cases.[59,125] Some preparations have led to the development of refractoriness more often than others. The decreased response to the enhancing effect of intrinsic factor on B_{12} absorption appears to depend on the development of an immune reaction to heterologous tissues.

Parenteral rather than oral therapy with vitamin B_{12} is therefore the treatment of choice for pernicious anemia. For a patient in relapse, between 1000 and 5000 μg.[97] should be given since the substance is needed not only to produce a remission but to replenish the greatly depleted body stores. It is best to give this amount in divided doses in the course of the first two weeks or more of therapy since otherwise much of the vitamin will be excreted before it can be used or stored. An injection of 100 μg. is a satisfactory amount to be given at one time.

The above amounts undoubtedly represent an excess of vitamin B_{12}. Thus a single parenteral dose of 1 mg. of vitamin B_{12} was observed to produce remissions and maintain patients in a normal state for periods of time ranging from 128 to 358 days.[129a] The writer has observed a remission lasting a year following a single injection of 15 μg. It is true that, as larger doses are given, a greater proportion of B_{12} is excreted.[97] Nevertheless, larger amounts, up to about 80 to 100 μg. daily, produce greater effects, the mean response being roughly proportional to the logarithm of the dose.[126] Furthermore, storage of vitamin B_{12} is relatively efficient.[74] The recommended dosage therefore represents a reasonable compromise between the objectives of maximal response and minimum waste of therapeutic agent.

Although patients with pernicious anemia can be maintained in an entirely satisfactory state of health on injections of 30 μg. once a month[86] or even 100 μg. every three months, it is probably safer to calculate maintenance therapy with vitamin B_{12} on the basis of at least 2 μg. per day; that is, injections of 60 to 100

29

μg. once a month or twice these amounts every two months.

Parenteral vitamin B_{12} therapy has been found to be effective in pernicious anemia, in the doses cited, even when neurologic manifestations were present,[127,130] including those which have developed under folic acid therapy.[55] An advantage of parenteral therapy is that the intake of the required dose is assured and the trouble and psychological effect of having to take medication daily are avoided. Parenteral therapy is also cheaper and is more likely to assure regular medical attention. Oral therapy, on the other hand, is undependable. Before the discovery of vitamin B_{12}, whole liver, proteolyzed liver[68a] (an enzymic digest of raw liver), autolysed liver,[61] fish liver,[66] desiccated hogs' stomach,[117] various aqueous concentrates of liver[105] and a variety of liver extracts were used when parenteral therapy was refused or contraindicated. Now that B_{12} is available, if parenteral therapy cannot be employed, daily oral dosage with vitamin B_{12} in amounts of 1000 μg. a day[89a] is probably preferable to the use of B_{12}-intrinsic factor mixtures. Such patients may, however, require closer supervision than those treated parenterally. Because the continued effectiveness of oral therapy in pernicious anemia is unpredictable, the U. S. Pharmacopeia standard of therapeutic potency, the U. S. P. unit, has been abandoned.[57]

In *tropical sprue* parenteral vitamin B_{12} therapy has also been found effective[122] although, in some cases, relapse developed after a temporary beneficial effect.[85] A good response to vitamin B_{12} therapy has been observed in cases of *nutritional macrocytic anemia*,[85,104] *megaloblastic anemia of pregnancy* and in the *megaloblastic anemia of infancy*[90,120] although in most instances of pregnancy anemia[58] and anemia in infancy[88,120,136] partial or complete failure of vitamin B_{12} therapy has been reported. In most cases of megaloblastic, macrocytic anemia other than pernicious anemia, folic acid deficiency is the cause and folic acid is therefore the therapeutic agent of choice.

The hematopoietic effects of certain analogs of vitamin B_{12}, such as vitamin B_{12b}, are similar to those of vitamin B_{12}.[60,63]

Folic Acid.—This vitamin, in doses of 5 to 20 mg. daily, by mouth, is capable of producing a hemopoietic response in many cases of pernicious anemia. However, in contrast to vitamin B_{12}, the effects are more variable. Thus reticulocyte responses and erythrocyte regeneration may be suboptimal,[63] macrocytosis may persist and, during maintenance therapy, the blood values may even decline.[80,96,131a] The lingual manifestations of pernicious anemia may respond well or poorly[116,129] but, what is more important, the compound *fails to protect patients against the development of changes in the nervous system.*[114,128,129] The explosiveness with which neurological changes have made their appearance in some patients with pernicious anemia receiving folic acid[114] led to the suggestion that the administration of this agent further depletes the body of vitamin B_{12}, a substance which is apparently essential for the integrity of the nervous system. It was observed that the administration of folic acid caused a lowering of the serum vitamin B_{12} levels of patients with pernicious anemia.[86]

The interrelationship between vitamin B_{12} and folic acid, already discussed elsewhere (p. 133), is therefore of practical importance. It seems likely that the normal daily requirement for folic acid is less than 0.5 mg.[89] The larger doses which are used to produce a hematologic remission in pernicious anemia may work by a mass action effect. It has been observed that, when hematologic relapse followed, this was associated with a hypocellular, non-megaloblastic bone marrow and the response to vitamin B_{12}

was a slow one unassociated with a marked reticulocyte response.[101] The reverse has also been reported; namely, the administration of vitamin B_{12} in one case of pernicious anemia and in one with nutritional megaloblastic anemia was followed by the development of glossitis and cheilosis which could be relieved by folic acid.[75] Thus, the administration of folic acid in unphysiologic amounts to patients with pernicious anemia may seriously disturb the balance between folic acid and vitamin B_{12} in an individual who is incapable of meeting increased demands because of a fault in the intrinsic factor mechanism for the absorption of vitamin B_{12}. Very occasionally, the reverse may also take place. For these reasons it is generally accepted that vitamin B_{12} and not folic acid is the agent of choice for the treatment of pernicious anemia.

For the treatment of other disorders characterized by megaloblastic bone marrow hyperplasia and macrocytic anemia, however, folic acid has been found of value and even superior to vitamin B_{12}. In sprue prompt and dramatic clinical and hematologic effects have been observed.[65,123] To achieve this, 10 to 30 mg. have been given orally per day, together with an adequate sprue diet, but as little as 2.5 to 5 mg. daily has been sufficient for maintenance therapy in many cases.[123] Cessation of diarrhea, relief of glossitis, flatulence, anorexia and nausea, hematologic improvement and some improvement in absorption of glucose, vitamins A and E and fats have been described.[65] The roentgenographic appearance of the bowel becomes normal. The best results have been seen in tropical sprue and in cases of relatively short duration. In non-tropical sprue less satisfactory or even poor results have been obtained with folic acid therapy.[67] In a number of cases the blood level has not been restored entirely to normal and macrocytosis has persisted.[67]

Good therapeutic responses have been obtained with folic acid in *nutritional macrocytic anemia*,[64,107,128] celiac disease,[125] megaloblastic anemia following gastrectomy[100] and ileosigmoidostomy,[128] macrocytic anemia of pregnancy,[67,98] and megaloblastic anemia of infancy,[88,136] in a number of instances when liver extract or vitamin B_{12} were ineffective. In cases of "refractory megaloblastic" and "achrestic" anemia, the administration of folic acid was effective where liver extract was of no value.[67]

Even in these disorders, however, folic acid has been of value only when the anemia was macrocytic, with megaloblastic bone marrow hyperplasia. When the anemia was of another type, no hemopoietic response or clinical benefit was observed.[78] It may also be mentioned that only those instances of leukopenia which accompanied a megaloblastic marrow reaction have been relieved by folic acid therapy, such treatment being entirely ineffective in other types of leukopenia.[52,67] It is also noteworthy that no changes in the nervous system have been observed to develop in normal subjects or in those with anemia other than pernicious anemia when folic acid was given.[76,129c]

Conjugates of folic acid, such as the diglutamic, triglutamic and heptaglutamic forms, have been shown to produce a hemopoietic response in pernicious anemia[131] but this is of no practical importance and carries the same risk as folic acid therapy. The therapeutic effectiveness of brewers' yeast in pernicious anemia[135] is probably attributable to its content of a folic acid conjugate.

Citrovorum Factor.—The effects of citrovorum factor or *folinic acid*, a compound closely related to folic acid (p. 132), are similar to those of folic acid and the contraindications as well as indications for its use appear to be the same.[129b] As with folic acid, citrovorum factor has been found effective in cases

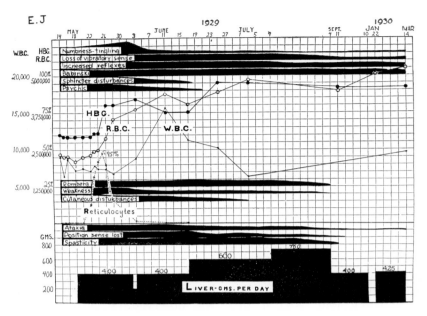

FIG. 9–2.—Changes in the symptoms and signs referable to disease of the nervous ystem as well as in the blood count, during prolonged treatment by liver in a case of pernicious anemia with combined degeneration. (Baker, Bordley and Longcope, Am. J. Med. Sc.)

of nutritional megaloblastic anemia when vitamin B_{12} therapy has failed.[129b] It has been administered orally in doses of 10 or more mg. daily and intramuscularly in doses of 2 to 6 mg. daily. In sprue it was not found to offer any advantages over folic acid.[123a]

Effects of Treatment. — Symptoms.—When treatment is effective, the results are clear-cut and can be dramatic. Symptomatic improvement may often be recognized before any change in the blood is noticeable. The patient becomes more alert, more coöperative, and appetite improves. If large doses are given parenterally, these signs may be noted in forty-eight hours; with oral therapy they appear within three to seven days. In the second week of treatment the pads of the fingers and palms, the chin, cheeks, and tip of the nose become flushed. The temperature and pulse become normal and gastrointestinal symptoms usually clear up in one or two weeks. In place of the characteristic

fiery red, sore tongue, a normal color returns and new papillae appear on the pink, smooth surface. The appetite may become ravenous. These changes may not be as striking with oral therapy as with parenteral treatment.

Dyspnea and weakness are relieved more slowly. Peripheral edema may even become more marked or become evident for the first time when the patient sits up. The creases in the palms of the hands do not take on their red color until the red cell count approaches 3,000,000 and the hemoglobin reaches about 7 Gm.

Paresthesias as well as other symptoms of nervous system involvement are slow to disappear unless they have been of short duration or of peripheral origin. A degree of fatigability, mental and physical, may persist for a very long time. This is to be expected for it is recognized that central nervous system regeneration does not take place.[69] It should not

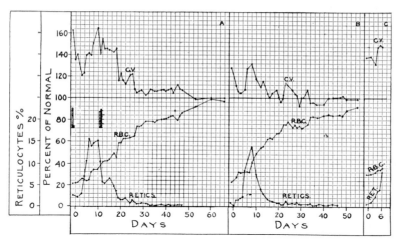

Fig. 9–3.—Variations in mean volume of red corpuscles compared with reticulocyte count in 3 cases of pernicious anemia. The mean corpuscular volume (*C.V.*) and the red cell count (*R.B.C.*) are represented as per cent of their respective average normal values. By this method the red cell count and mean corpuscular volume of a hypothetical normal individual would fall on the line at 100 per cent. Reticulocytes are recorded directly. The abscissa records days following the commencement of liver therapy. The columns represent absolute numbers of red corpuscles 6μ or less in diameter (hatched columns) and absolute numbers of reticulocytes (solid columns). Each division represents 50,000 cells per c.mm. (Wintrobe, courtesy of J. Clin. Invest.)

discourage the physician, and the patient should be prepared to expect only gradual improvement in the neurological symptoms. The patient can be told that persistent and long-continued treatment will bring some degree of symptomatic improvement of the neurological complaints in as many as 90 per cent of cases[127] and that arrest of the disease may be expected in all patients. The greatest part of the improvement takes place in the first six months of treatment. Sphincter control improves, ataxia decreases, and paresthesias may diminish or disappear (Fig. 9–2). Vibratory sensation, cutaneous and joint sensibility, and absent reflexes may return; a plantar extensor response has even been observed to become flexor. The upper limbs improve more than the lower. Factors contributing to improvement include training, gain in strength, recovery of lesions in the peripheral nerves, reversal of early lesions in the central nervous

system and arrest of others, as well as greater use of unaffected pathways.

Other signs of neural involvement may change very little. Those referable to involvement of the lateral columns such as spasticity are particularly resistant to treatment. Their appearance in a patient who previously showed chiefly posterior column changes may even give a false sense of improvement by the development of hyperreflexia.

Blood.—An increase in the percentage of **reticulocytes** is the earliest noteworthy effect on the blood. Their enumeration affords a simple and valuable method of determining the effectiveness of therapy. The *total number* of reticulocytes which are released from the bone marrow following treatment appears to be related directly to the degree of bone marrow involvement.[56] The *speed* with which they are released depends on the amount of effective anti-anemic substance administered and the rapidity with which it reaches the marrow. Thus, when an average therapeutic dose is given daily, the reticulocytes will usually begin to increase in number about three to five days following the commencement of treatment and a maximum percentage will be reached on the eighth to twelfth day. If a massive dose is given, the reticulocyte response may commence in forty-eight hours and reach a maximum in one hundred and four to one hundred and forty hours.[112] The *height* of the reticulocyte curve depends on the degree of anemia, varying inversely with the number of red corpuscles and the speed of the response.

A curve recording the changes in percentage of reticulocytes associated with effective treatment of pernicious anemia[93] and the related macrocytic anemias, has a characteristic shape (Fig. 9–3). Following the rapid rise, above described, there is a more gradual fall which, especially if treatment is somewhat irregular, may be broken by a second rise. The reticulocytes which appear early possess a great deal of reticulum, whereas cells which are found later contain less and less reticular substance. As the percentage of reticulocytes falls, the total number of red corpuscles increases and by the end of two weeks of treatment[113] the red cell count and, particularly, the volume of packed red cells will have increased substantially. If no complications develop in the course of four to eight weeks normal values should be attained.[82]

Formulas were devised whereby the expected maximum reticulocyte increase for any given red cell count could be predicted. The average expected maximum reticulocyte percentage following the daily *intramuscular* injection of 1 unit of liver extract was calculated from the formula,[83] in which R equals the maximum reticulocyte per cent reached during the course of the reticulocyte response and Eo the initial red blood cell count, in millions per c.mm., on the day therapy was started.

$$R = \frac{82 - 22\ Eo}{1 + 0.5\ Eo}$$

A corresponding increase can be expected following the administration of an average dose of vitamin B_{12}.

For calculating the expected increase in red cell count during the first two weeks of effective parenteral liver therapy in cases of pernicious anemia, Della Vida[69a] proposed the formula,

$$I = 0.93 - 0.214\ Eo$$

I represents the average weekly increase in red cells during the first two weeks of treatment and Eo is the red cell count before treatment.

Nucleated red corpuscles and other immature forms may appear in increased numbers when the reticulocyte response occurs. The *white cells* increase in number, chiefly as the result of the appearance of more polymorphonuclear neutrophils and, later, eosinophils.[118] Myelocytes and even myeloblasts may be found. In rare instances, such a marked leukocytosis with "shift to the left" develops as to simulate the blood picture of myelocytic leukemia.[71] Eosinophilia was frequently observed when raw liver therapy was used,[92] but it occurred also following other forms of liver treatment.[53] Platelets become more numerous.[102] The marked anisocytosis decreases and the numerous bizarre-shaped red corpuscles disappear. Mean corpuscular volume, after a preliminary increase[134] gradually decreases (Fig. 9–2) and the range found in good health returns, usually when the red cell count has reached normal.[133] Hemoglobin may not increase as rapidly as the number of cells and the values for mean corpuscular hemoglobin concentration may be subnormal for a time. The average diameter of the red cells may return to the values found in health (Fig.9–4) in a short time but completely normal mean diameter and normal variability in size may be very

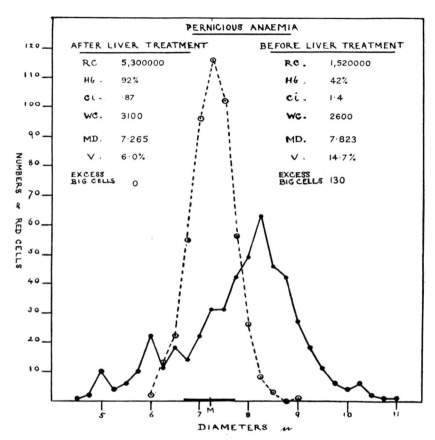

FIG. 9–4.—Complete recovery of average size and variability of the diameters of red corpuscles in pernicious anemia following treatment. In some instances there is recovery of average size but not of variability, and *vice versa*. (Price-Jones, courtesy of J. Path. & Bact.)

difficult to attain.[106] Restitution of the morphology of the blood as well as its quantitative characteristics should be a goal in treatment.

Bone Marrow.—Following effective therapy the marrow picture is altered with extraordinary rapidity. Within six to ten hours after the initial injection of liver extract the typical megaloblasts were found to be greatly reduced in number.[68] The same is true following vitamin B_{12} therapy. In many cases twenty-four hours following the injection the total number of nucleated cells may be substantially reduced.[119] In the succeeding twenty-four to forty-eight hours the number of nucleated cells fluctuates but in general a marked rise in their total number may be observed preceding by perhaps forty-eight hours the maximal increase in reticulocytes in the blood; following this the number of nucleated marrow cells falls slowly to reach normal levels. The cells taking part in the cellular increase prior to the reticulocyte peak are not megaloblasts. These cells disappear rapidly within twenty-four to forty-eight hours following the injection.[119] In their place are found smaller cells with comparatively irregular, lumpy and dark staining chromatin (normoblasts).[68] Basophilic and polychromatic normoblasts are succeeded by still more mature (orthochromatic) forms.

The remarkable rapidity with which the megaloblastic marrow picture is altered to a normoblastic one has been used as evidence that these two cell types belong to one developmental cell series[68] (see p. 94). Other explanations have been offered, however, such as the suggestion that multipolar mitosis takes place[87] and that normoblasts reappear by heteroplastic development from the reticulum and the myeloblasts and by homoplastic development from quiescent remnants of the normoblastic series present in the marrow during relapse.

Metabolism. — Pronounced metabolic changes are observed following effective therapy in pernicious anemia. The high plasma iron characteristic of pernicious anemia in relapse drops precipitously, even to subnormal values.[77] The protoporphyrin in the erythrocytes, normal or somewhat low in relapse, may tend to rise.[158] The excretion of coproporphyrin I, generally regarded as an index of hematopoietic activity and found elevated during relapse, is restored to normal by specific therapy, sometimes after a preliminary increase.[70] Megaloblastic bone marrow has been reported to contain no protoporphyrin.[119] Concomitant with the reappearance of normoblasts following therapy, protoporphyrin was found in the bone marrow and its quantity increased until just prior to the maximal rise in reticulocytes; following this a lower level was attained. Simultaneously with the reduction in the number of normoblasts in the marrow and in association with the increase of reticulocytes in the peripheral blood, the uric acid content of the blood and urine increases.[111,119] All of these changes are attributable to the increased hematopoiesis taking place immediately following therapy and the return to normal hematopoiesis which succeeds this stage.

Evidence of increased blood destruction disappears promptly with effective therapy. The plasma bilirubin falls at about the end of the first week and will usually be found within normal limits at the end of three or four weeks. Urobilinogen in the urine begins to decrease in amount at the end of the reticulocyte response[72,79] and falls to within normal limits in a few days. When remission is incomplete and slight anemia persists, slight plasma bilirubinemia and increase of urobilinogen excretion continue.

Other interesting metabolic changes which have been observed following therapy will be described later (see p. 485).

Untoward Effects.—Before the introduction of vitamin B₁₂ therapy in pernicious anemia, reactions to liver extract presented at times a difficult problem in management. These reactions were usually of the secondary type; that is, they did not follow the first injection of liver extract[115] but occurred after repeated injections had been given. Reactions were reported in 6.6 per cent[91] to almost 20 per cent of cases. The commonest reactions consisted of flushing, tachycardia, localized itching of the skin, sometimes accompanied by nausea, weakness and faintness. Occasionally more serious effects were observed[72a] and even death was recorded.[91] Methods for desensitization were described.[91]

Vitamin B₁₂ is essentially devoid of ill effects.[63] Hypersensitivity to folic acid is rare.[95]

Maintenance Therapy.—Details of dosage have been discussed already (p. 449). It must be emphasized that it is necessary to explain to the patient that treatment of pernicious anemia must be continued for life. Otherwise relapse will occur, possibly necessitating hospitalization and always with the risk of progression of neurological changes or their development if they have not been present before. During relapse, furthermore, resistance is lowered and infections may develop which, if they do not cause death, may become chronic and impair the response to vitamin B_{12} therapy.[93] The patient should be warned that relapse usually does not become noticeable to him immediately but may require several months to develop to the point where he himself becomes alarmed. Otherwise accidental failure to receive treatment for a short time without any obvious harmful results may cause the patient to doubt the importance of regular treatment. He should also be cautioned that the development of new symptoms is not usually to be attributed to the treatment (as the patient is wont to assume) but is probably the result of some complication or new illness, and calls for more therapy rather than less. The majority of patients will heed if the situation is carefully explained. A few, unfortunately, only learn by experience.

The patient should be re-examined at regular intervals. In addition to the physical examination, the blood should be checked at least once in two months. For this purpose the volume of packed red cells and survey of a stained blood film suffice, a more detailed study being made if these reveal any change from the normal.

In many cases of megaloblastic macrocytic anemia other than pernicious anemia, maintenance therapy may not be required. This is usually true of the megaloblastic anemia of pregnancy and that seen in infancy and is often the case in nutritional macrocytic anemia, provided a good diet containing adequate amounts of animal protein and vitamins is consumed.

IRON

Iron salts have been used by physicians since the time of Hippocrates. It has been stated that iron therapy takes its origin in sympathetic magic, the weakly sufferer having hoped to assume something of the strength of steel by drinking the water in which a sword had rusted.

Three centuries ago Syndenham introduced iron into clinical medicine for the treatment of the "chlorosis of hysteria" for which he found iron or steel filings, steeped in cold Rhenish wine, of great value. A rational basis for the use of iron was provided almost one hundred years later when iron was demonstrated in the ash of the blood and it was shown that the iron of the blood could be increased by feeding iron-containing foods.[143]

In 1832 Pierre Blaud emphasized the specific action of iron in the treatment of chlorosis and described the use of his deservedly famous pills (0.3 Gm. ferrous sulfate plus potassium carbonate, or approximately 0.1 Gm. ferrous carbonate per pill). He gave gradually increasing doses, from 2 pills on the first day to 12 on the sixteenth day. Many excellent observers, including Niemeyer and Osler, confirmed his findings. Yet, in the period 1890 to 1920 iron therapy became discredited, thanks to dogmatic statements by Bunge that inorganic iron is valueless in therapy and that only organic preparations should be used, as well as the result of von Noorden's teaching that no more than 0.1 Gm. of metallic iron is necessary. Furthermore, physicians failed to distinguish between iron-deficiency anemias and anemia due to other causes. It was not until chronic hypochromic anemia resulting from iron deficiency became a clearly defined syndrome and methods for its recognition came into general use that the value of large doses of inorganic iron, resurrected by Lichtenstein and by Meulengracht, once again received general recognition.[143]

The rôle of iron in hematopoiesis was discussed in an earlier chapter (p. 143). Here only iron therapy will be considered.

Relative Value of Various Forms of Iron.—Clinical experince is consistent regarding the effectiveness of inorganic iron salts, given by mouth, in the treatment of iron deficiency anemias and the greater efficiency of bivalent salts as compared with trivalent forms. However, what is true for man is not the case in all other species. Thus, in studies with radioactive iron it was observed that human subjects absorbed $1\frac{1}{2}$ to 15 times more ferrous than ferric iron, whereas dogs either absorbed both valence forms to a comparable degree or showed only preferential assimilation of ferrous salts.[151] This explains the disagreement between certain experimental observations in dogs and clinical experience in man.

It would appear that differences in the activity of ferric and ferrous compounds upon oral administration in man are largely due to differences in their adsorbability from the intestinal tract; thus it was observed that the parenteral injection of ferric iron produces more or less quantitative increases in circulating hemoglobin.[142,153]

A great variety of compounds for use in oral iron therapy have been promoted from time to time, with claims of greater effectiveness, greater tolerance and less toxicity.[157] No convincing evidence has been provided that any one of the compounds proposed is better in any way than *ferrous sulfate*, which is also the cheapest compound available. There is also no evidence that supplementation of ferrous sulfate with other substances, whether they be metals, such as copper or cobalt, or vitamins, such as vitamin B_{12}, folic acid or ascorbic acid, is of any value in accelerating the response to therapy with iron in cases of iron deficiency anemia. These mixtures only add to the cost.

Thus, in a well controlled study, ferrous gluconate, ferrous succinate and ferrous calcium citrate were not found to possess any advantage over ferrous sulfate.[147] The alleged advantage of ferrous gluconate over ferrous sulfate[152a] insofar as gastrointestinal tolerance is concerned is attributable to the larger size of the molecule and the consequent lower concentration of iron (12 per cent as compared with 20 per cent.)

Oral Administration of Iron.—The effective daily dose of ferrous sulfate is 0.6 to 0.8 Gm. per day, given in the form of tablets of 0.2 Gm. size. To avoid gastric irritation ferrous sulfate should be taken with or immediately after a meal. The daily dose should be divided roughly in accordance with the size of the meal. Two tablets may be readily tolerated after a large meal whereas one may cause discomfort if the stomach is empty.

Tolerance for iron salts is usually achieved by *giving a small dose at first* and increasing the amount in the course of three or four days to the full dose of three or four tablets. Without such a gradual increase in dosage not only gastric irritation but diarrhea may develop as well.

Tablets, pills or capsules containing iron salts are preferable to solutions of iron for the latter may oxidize, generally stain the teeth and are distasteful. Tablets of ferrous sulfate are usually specially coated to prevent oxidation to the ferric form.

Ferrous salts of iron cannot be given in a simple aqueous solution because oxidation will produce the ferric form; an elixir is commonly used. For young children, concentrates of ferrous sulfate which provide 60 mg. elemental iron per 2.4 ml. are available commercially. This can be added to orange juice or milk. If preferred, the following prescription is suitable *for a child*:

R—Dilute hypophosphorous acid   0.6 ml.
    Ferrous sulfate .   .   .   .   3.0 Gm.
    Dextrose .   .   .   .   .   30.0 Gm.
    Chloroform water to .   . 120.0 ml.
Sig.—4 ml. three times daily, p.c.

This dose, which furnishes 0.3 Gm. (4.5 gr.) ferrous sulfate daily, is suitable for infants and up to one or two years of age. Half as much again may be given children between two and six years of age and for those who are still older the dose may be doubled.

Another liquid form of iron consists of 0.2 Gm. iron ammonium citrate in water sweetened with glycerine. This dose, three times a day, is recommended for a child of three to six months. For children six to eighteen months of age, two or three times this amount may be given.

Ill effects from the oral administration of ferrous sulfate, when properly taken, are uncommon. When other compounds were used, serious ill effects were observed occasionally. Thus "iron encephalopathy" following the administration of 11 Gm. iron and ammonium citrate daily has been reported,[145] as well as a case in which ileus occurred from retention of iron in the cecum.[156]

The accidental ingestion of very large amounts of ferrous sulfate by children who have mistaken the tablets for candy has produced *serious ill effects*.[154] At one time 50 per cent of the reported cases had ended in death. In these instances 3 to 10 or more grams had been swallowed. The symptoms consist of two phases: (1) an earlier phase developing after ingestion which is marked by pallor, restlessness, nausea and often diarrhea and vomiting. This is followed by drowsiness and ultimately semiconsciousness or coma and finally by signs of peripheral circulatory collapse. If this does not prove to be fatal, (2) a period of rapid improvement for 12 to 24 hours may be followed by sudden death 24 to 48 hours after the ingestion of iron.

The ill effects of these excessive amounts of iron are attributable to the rapid absorption of the metal in amounts far above the iron-binding capacity of the plasma. Serum iron values as high as 3000 μg per cent have been observed. The iron also has a local escharotic action on the gastrointestinal mucosa and, in the liver, hemorrhagic necrosis of the peripheral or periportal portions of the lobules has been described.[149] Treatment consists of measures to combat shock and acidosis and to reduce further tissue damage by removing any iron tablets remaining in the stomach. The use of edathamil calcium-disodium by vein and disodium orthophosphate by mouth has been advocated.[138,155]

Parenteral Iron Therapy.[140]—Parenteral iron therapy should not be used if oral administration is possible. There are few legitimate *indications* for parenteral therapy. These are: (1) patients with iron deficiency anemia who are unable to tolerate iron by mouth; as, for example, in some cases of ulcerative colitis, persistent vomiting (as in pregnancy), disordered gastrointestinal function after gastrectomy and carcinoma of the stomach. In such patients iron by mouth may seriously aggravate symptoms. However, most patients with these and similar gastrointestinal disorders can take iron orally if proper instructions are given (p. 458). (2) Inability to absorb adequate amounts of iron taken by mouth. Such cases are rare.[137] In most of those who have been well studied, steatorrhea was present. However, in many cases of steatorrhea and even in sprue and after gastrectomy, iron is usually absorbed satisfactorily from the gastrointestinal tract. (3) Need for rapid restoration of normal hemoglobin level as, for example, when anemia is first discovered in the third trimester of pregnancy or when blood transfusion is contraindiated or unavoidable. It is rare that the need is this urgent.

The majority of preparations for parenteral therapy which have been available in the past contained so little iron that they had little or no value or the reactions to their use were so severe that their use had to be abandoned. Two compounds have, more recently, been more effective. One, however, iron-dextran[146] was found to be markedly sarcogenic in the rat[144] and its use was temporarily abandoned. Also available is the *saccharated oxide of iron*,[140,152] which must be given intravenously. This is an iron-sucrose complex containing 2 per cent ferric or ferrous iron, colloidally suspended.

If parenteral iron therapy is indicated, the total quantity given should not be greater than the amount needed to restore the hemoglobin to normal. A formula for calculation of the required amount has been devised on the basis of a hypothetical blood volume of 5000 ml. which allows 50 per cent extra iron to replace the depleted iron stores.[139] This is,

normal hb.—patient's hb., in Gm. per 100 ml. $\times$ 0.255 = Gm. Fe.

Because of possible toxic effects, only 50 mg. iron should be given at the time of the initial injection. Subsequent daily doses of 100 mg. are given until the calculated dose has been administered. It is important that a clean venepuncture be made and blood should be allowed to flow into the syringe and mix with the iron oxide solution. The latter is strongly alkaline and hypertonic and local induration, thrombophlebitis, transient venospasm and other local reactions may be produced. Other ill effects which may occur include headache, pain in the chest, back or extremities, symptoms suggestive of sympathetic stimulation (tachycardia, pallor, faintness), or of parasympathetic response (sweating, feeling of intense burning, lacrimation, nausea, bronchospasm, dyspnea), and, more rarely, symptoms of circulatory collapse. A variety of late reactions may occur as well.[140] Toxic reactions occur in at least 10 per cent of cases.

Effects of Iron Therapy.—If severe iron deficiency anemia is present, a vigorous response can be expected. The speed and magnitude of this effect depend on the route of administration and the amount of iron absorbed. With paren-

teral therapy there may be a subjective response in 24 to 72 hours but this may be masked by the toxic effects and, in any event, does not justify the risks of parenteral therapy. With oral therapy the response is somewhat slower. No benefit from iron therapy can be expected if iron deficiency is not present. However, its administration is justified prophylactically in pregnancy and during lactation, and in other circumstances in which the development of iron deficiency is likely.

An increase in the percentage of **reticulocytes** follows the institution of iron therapy. The increase is generally slower to appear and not as marked as may be observed following vitamin B_{12} therapy in pernicious anemia and, instead of being more or less inversely proportional to the number of red cells, the magnitude of the reticulocyte response is related to the quantity of hemoglobin.[150] The increase of reticulocytes is maximal usually on the fifth to the tenth day after the institution of iron therapy. Reticulocyte responses higher than would be expected on maximal oral therapy can be induced by iron given parenterally.[139,142]

Following the reticulocyte rise, the hemoglobin, volume of packed cells, and red cell count increase, and the size and hemoglobin content of the red cells gradually return to normal. The increased production of red cells may be so great for a time the erythrocyte count may be well above normal whereas the hemoglobin and the size of the cells are still below normal (Fig. 9–5). Therefore the red cell count is not a safe guide in estimating the need for further treatment. It is the hemoglobin and the size and hemoglobin content of the red corpuscles which must be followed.

The hemoglobin increase takes place in a characteristic manner. There is at first a lag of several days until the peak of the reticulocyte increase has been reached. Following this the hemoglobin

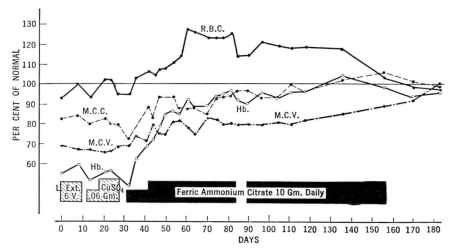

Fig. 9–5.—Blood changes in a case of chronic hypochromic anemia. All values are shown in proportion to the normal for the individual. Note the rapid increase in hemoglobin (Hb) following commencement of iron therapy and then the more gradual rise; the increase in the erythrocyte count (R.B.C.) to values above normal; and the eventual restoration of all values to normal, including those for mean corpuscular hemoglobin concentration (M.C.C.). (Wintrobe and Beebe, Medicine, courtesy of Williams & Wilkins Company.)

value rises at an average rate of 0.17 Gm. per 100 ml. per day. In many instances we have observed hemoglobin regeneration at the rate of 0.25 Gm. per 100 ml. per day, for two to four weeks. Only as normal values are approached does the rate of regeneration slow up. Parenterally administered massive doses of iron have been found to cause hemoglobin regeneration at a rate as high as 0.26 Gm. per day.[139]

The continuation of blood loss, if that is the cause of the iron deficiency, may reduce or nullify the effects of therapy, depending on the extent of the bleeding. *When some inhibiting factor is present*, blood regeneration will be slower than usual and may even fail to take place. The presence of infection or of nitrogen retention impairs the capacity of the bone marrow to regenerate hemoglobin, and a deficiency of thyroid secretion or failure to correct associated nutritional deficiencies may have the same effect. In the presence of severe damage to vital organs, as in cases of malignancy, moder-

ately satisfactory regeneration of hemoglobin may nevertheless occur if the anemia is due to lack of iron.

Symptomatic improvement occurs rapidly along with blood regeneration. The color improves, the skin becomes less dry and wrinkled and more elastic. Appetite is better and the patient's strength is regained. The tongue papillae become more normal in appearance and may be completely restored and, if koilonychia has been present, the brittle concave nails are eventually replaced by convex, smooth, and shiny ones (see Chapter 14). The enlarged spleen recedes and, although it is quite rare, we have even observed secretion of free hydrochloric acid to be restored. The "hemic" cardiac murmurs are slow to disappear.

BIBLIOGRAPHY

Anemia—General Considerations

1. Bartels, E. C.: Anemia as the Cause of Severe Congestive Heart Failure, Ann. Int. Med., *11*, 400, 1937.

2. BLUMGART, H. L. and ALTSCHULE, M. D.: Clinical Significance of Cardiac and Respiratory Adjustments in Chronic Anemia, Blood, *3*, 329, 1948.

3. BOYCOTT, A. E.: The Blood as a Tissue: Hypertrophy and Atrophy of the Red Corpuscles. Proc. Roy. Soc. Med., *23*, 15, 1929.

6. BRADLEY, S. E. and BRADLEY, G. P.: Renal Function During Chronic Anemia in Man, Blood, *2*, 192, 1947.

7. BRANNON, E. S., MERRILL, A. J., WARREN, J. V. and STEAD, E. A., JR.: The Cardiac Output in Patients With Chronic Anemia as Measured by the Technique of Right Atrial Catheterization, J. Clin. Invest., *24*, 332, 1945.

8. CASE, R. B., BERGLUND, E. and SARNOFF, S. J.: Changes in Coronary Resistance and Ventricular Function Resulting from Acutely Induced Anemia and the Effect Thereon of Coronary Stenosis, Am. J. Med., *18*, 397, 1955.

12. FÖLDI, M., KORÁNYI, A. and SZABÓ, G.: Über die Entstehung anämischer Ödeme, Acta med. scandinav., *129*, 486, 1948.

14. HUNTER, A.: The Heart in Anæmia, Quart. J. Med., *15*, 107, 1946.

19. MARSHALL, R. A.: A Review of Lesions in the Optic Fundus in Various Diseases of the Blood, Blood, *14*, 882, 1959.

20. McILROY, M. B., ELDRIDGE, F. L. and STONE, R. W.: The Mechanical Properties of the Lungs in Anoxia, Anaemia and Thyrotoxicosis, Clin. Sc., *15*, 353, 1956.

22. PASCHER, F. and KEEN, R.: Chronic Ulcers of the Leg Associated with Blood Dyscrasias, Arch. Dermat. & Syph., *66*, 478, 1952.

23. PICKERING, G. W. and WAYNE, E. J.: Observations on Angina Pectoris and Intermittent Claudication in Anemia, Clin. Sci., *1*, 305, 1933.

24. RODMAN, T., CLOSE, H. P. and PURCELL, MAY K.: The Oxyhemoglobin Dissociation Curve in Anemia, Ann. Int. Med., *52*, 295, 1960.

25. ROMANO, J. and EVANS, J. W.: Symptomatic Psychosis in a Case of Secondary Anemia, Arch. Neurol. & Psychiat., *39*, 1294, 1938.

26. RYAN, J. M. and HICKAM, J. B.: The Alveolar-Arterial Oxygen Pressure Gradient in Anemia, J. Clin. Invest., *31*, 188, 1952.

27. SHARPEY-SCHAFER, E. P.: Transfusion and the Anemic Heart, Lancet, *2*, 296, 1945.

28. SPROULE, B. J., MITCHELL, J. H. and MILLER, W. F.: Cardiopulmonary Physiological Responses to Heavy Exercise in Patients with Anemia, J. Clin. Invest., *39*, 378, 1960.

30. WHITAKER, W.: Some Effects of Severe Chronic Anaemia on the Circulatory System, Quart. J. Med., *25*, 175, 1956.

31. WINTROBE, M. M.: Anemia: Classification and Treatment on the Basis of Differences in the Average Volume and Hemoglobin Content of the Red Corpuscles, Arch. Int. Med., *54*, 256, 1934.

32. ——— The Cardiovascular System in Anemia, Blood, *1*, 121, 1946.

33. WINTROBE, M. M., CARTWRIGHT, G. E., PALMER, J. G., KUHNS, W. J. and SAMUELS. L. T.: Effect of Corticotrophin and Cortisone on the Blood in Various Disorders in Man, Arch. Int. Med., *88*, 310, 1951.

34. WINTROBE, M. M. and MILLER, M. W.: Normal Blood Determinations in the South, Arch. Int. Med., *43*, 96, 1929.

35. WITTS, L. J.: The Pathology and Treatment of Anemia, Lancet, *1*, 495, 549, 106, 653, 1932.

Antipernicious Anemia Principle

52. ADAMS, W. S. and LAWRENCE, J. S.: Folic Acid Therapy, Am. J. Med. Sc., *215*, 487, 1948.

53. ALLIN, R. N. and MEYER, O. O.: The Development of Eosinophilia Following Liver Therapy, J. Lab. & Clin. Med., *26*, 457, 1940.

54. BEEBE, R. T. and LEWIS, G. E.: Maintenance Dose of Potent Material in Pernicious Anemia, Am. J. Med. Sc., *181*, 796, 1931.

55. BERK, L., DENNY-BROWN, D., FINLAND, M. and CASTLE, W. B.: Effectiveness of Vitamin B₁₂ in Combined System Disease. Rapid Regression of Neurologic Manifestations and Absence of Allergic Reactions in a Patient Sensitive to Injectable Liver Extracts, New England J. Med., *239*, 328, 1948.

56. BETHELL, F. H.: Relation Between Total Reticulocyte Production and Degree of Bone Marrow Involvement in Pernicious Anemia, Am. J. Med. Sc., *188*, 476, 1934.

57. BETHELL, F. H., CASTLE, W. B., CONLEY, C. L. and LONDON, I. M.: Present Status of Treatment of Pernicious Anemia, J. A. M. A., *171*, 2092, 1959.

58. BETHELL, F. H., MEYERS, M. C. and Neligh, R. B.: Vitamin B₁₂ in Pernicious Anemia and Puerperal Macrocytic Anemia, J. Lab. & Clin. Med., *33*, 1477, 1948.

59. BLACKBURN, E. K. *et al.*: Oral Treatment of Pernicious Anaemia with Vitamin B₁₂ and Desiccated Hog Duodenal Extract, Brit. M. J., *2*, 535, 1959.

59a. BLACKBURN, E. K., SWAN, H. T., TUDHOPE, G. R. and WILSON, G. M.: Haemopoietic

Activity of Analogues of Vitamin B_{12} (Cyanocobalamin), Brit. J. Haemat., *3*, 429, 1957.

60. BRODY, E. A., ESTREN, S. and WASSERMAN, L. R.: Treatment of Pernicious Anemia by Oral Administration of Vitamin B_{12} without Added Intrinsic Factor, New England J. Med., *260*, 361, 1959.

61. CASTLE, W. B. and STRAUSS, M. B.: Effect of Autolysis on Potency of Liver in Treatment of Pernicious Anemia, J.A.M.A., *104*, 798, 1935.

62. CHALMERS, J. N. M. and SHINTON, N. K.: Absorption of Orally Administered Vitamin B_{12} in Pernicious Anemia, Lancet, *2*, 1298, 1958.

63. CONLEY, C. L., GREEN, T. W., HARTMAN, R. C. and KREVANS, J. R.: Prolonged Treatment of Pernicious Anemia with Vitamin B_{12}, Am. J. Med., *13*, 284, 1952.

64. COWAN, G. A. B.: Folic Acid in Severe Nutritional Anæmia: A Report of Five Cases, Trans. Roy. Soc. Trop. Med. & Hyg., *41*, 525, 1948.

65. DARBY, W. J., JONES, E., WARDEN, H. F. and KASER, M. M.: The Influence of Pteroylglutamic Acid (A Member of the Vitamin M Group) on Gastro-intestinal Defects in Sprue. A Study of Interrelationships of Dietary Essentials, J. Nutrition, *34*, 645, 1947.

66. DAVIDSON, L. S. P.: Treatment of Pernicious Anemia With Fish-liver Extract, Brit. M. J., *2*, 347, 1932.

67. ———— Pteroylglutamic Acid (Folic Acid). Therapeutic Indications and Limitations, Edinburgh Med. J., *55*, 400, 1948.

68. DAVIDSON, L. S. P., DAVIS, L. J. and INNES, J.: The Effect of Liver Therapy on Erythropoiesis as Observed by Serial Sternal Punctures in Twelve Cases of Pernicious Anæmia, Quart. J. Med., *11*, 19, 1942.

68a. DAVIS, L. J., DAVIDSON, L. S. P., RIDING, D. and SHAW, G. E.: Treatment of Pernicious Anæmia With an Experimental Proteolysed Liver Preparation, Brit. M. J., *1*, 655, 1943; Quart. J. Med., *13*, 53, 1944.

69. DAVISON, C.: Subacute Combined Degeneration of Cord, Arch. Neurol. & Psychiat., *26*, 1195, 1931; Arch. Int. Med., *67*, 473, 1941.

69a. DELLA VIDA, B. L.: Maximal Response to Liver Therapy in Pernicious Anæmia, Lancet, *2*, 275, 1942.

70. DOBRINER, K. and RHOADS, C. P.: The Metabolism of Blood Pigments in Pernicious Anemia, J. Clin. Invest., *17*, 95, 1938.

70a. DYKE, S. C., DELLA VIDA, B. L., DELIKAT, E.: Vitamin C Deficiency in "Irresponsive" Pernicious Anæmia, Lancet, *2*, 278, 1942.

71. ERCKLENTZ, B. W.: Leukämoide Reaktion bei Leberremission einer Anæmia perniciosa, Folia hæmatol., *53*, 382, 1935.

72. FARQUHARSON, R. F., BORSOOK, H. and GOULDING, A. M.: Pigment Metabolism and Destruction of Blood in Addison's (Pernicious) Anemia, Arch. Int. Med., *48*, 1156, 1931.

72a. FEINBERG, S. M., ALT, H. L. and YOUNG, R. H.: Allergy to Injectable Liver Extracts; Clinical and Immunological Observations, Ann. Int. Med., *18*, 311, 1943.

73. FOX, H. J.: A Comparison of Pteroylglutamic Acid and Liver Extract Maintenance Therapy in Sprue, New England J. Med., *240*, 801, 1949.

74. GLASS, G. B. J., BOYD, L. J. and GELLIN, G. A.: Surface Scintillation Measurements in Humans of the Uptake of Parenterally Administered Radioactive Vitamin B_{12}, Blood, *10*, 95, 1955.

75. HARRIS, J. W.: Aggravation of Clinical Manifestations of Folic Acid Deficiency by Small Daily Doses of Vitamin B_{12}, Am. J. Med., *21*, 461, 1956.

76. HARVEY, E. A., HOWARD, I. and MURPHY, W. P.: Absence of a Toxic Effect of Folic Acid on the Central Nervous System of Persons without Pernicious Anemia, New England J. Med., *242*, 446, 1950.

77. HAWKINS, C. F.: Value of Serum Iron Levels in Assessing Effect of Hæmatinics in the Macrocytic Anæmias, Brit. M. J., *1*, 383, 1955.

78. HAY, J. D.: Folic Acid in Coeliac Disease, Arch. Dis. Child., *23*, 220, 1948.

79. HEILMEYER, L.: Blutfarbstoffwechselstudien; die Regenerations- und Farbstoffwechselvorgänge beim Morbus Biermer sowie bei einer Botriocephalusanämie vor und nach Leberbehandlung, Deutsch. Arch. klin. Med., *173*, 128, 1932.

80. HEINLE, R. W., DINGLE, J. T. and WEISBERGER, A. S.: Folic Acid in the Maintenance of Pernicious Anemia, J. Lab. & Clin. Med., *32*, 970, 1947.

82. ISAACS, R., BETHELL, F. H., RIDDLE, M. C. and FRIEDMAN, A.: Standards for Red Blood Cell Increase After Liver and Stomach Therapy in Pernicious Anemia, J.A.M. A., *111*, 2291, 1938.

83. ISAACS, R. and FRIEDMAN, A.: Standards for Maximum Reticulocyte Percentage After Intramuscular Liver Therapy in Pernicious Anemia, Am. J. Med. Sc., *196*, 718, 1938.

85. JONES, E., DARBY, W. and TOTTER, J. R.: Pernicious Anemia and Related Anemias Treated with Vitamin B_{12}, Blood, *4*, 827, 1949.

86. LEAR, A. A. and CASTLE, W. B.: Supplemental Folic Acid Therapy in Pernicious Anemia, J. Lab. & Clin. Med., 47, 88, 1956.

87. LIMARZI, L. R. and LEVINSON, S. A.: An Undescribed Type of Erythropoiesis Observed in Human Sternal Marrow, Arch. Path., 36, 127, 1943.

88. LUHBY, A. L. and WHEELER, W. E.: Megaloblastic Anemia of Infancy: II. Failure of Response to Vitamin B₁₂ and the Metabolic Rôle of Folic Acid and Vitamin C, Health Center Jour.—Ohio State Univ., 3, 1, 1949.

89. MARSHALL, R. A. and JANDL, J. H.: Responses to "Physiologic" Doses of Folic Acid in the Megaloblastic Anemias, A. M. A. Arch. Int. Med., 105, 352, 1960.

89a. McINTYRE, PATRICIA A., HAHN, ROZELLE, MASTERS, J. M. and KREVANS, J. R.: Treatment of Pernicious Anemia with Orally Administered Cyanocobalamin (Vitamin B₁₂), A. M. A. Arch. Int. Med., 106, 280, 1960.

90. McPHERSON, A. Z., JONSSON, U. and RUNDLES, R. W.: Vitamin B₁₂ Therapy in Megaloblastic Anemia of Infancy, J. Pediat., 34, 529, 1949.

91. McSORLEY, J. G. and DAVIDSON, L. S. P.: Sensitivity to Liver Extract, Brit. M. J., 1, 714, 1944.

92. MEULENGRACHT, E. and HOLM, S.: Eosinophilia in Liver Diet, Am. J. Med. Sc., 179, 199, 1930.

93. MINOT, G. R. and CASTLE, W. B.: The Interpretation of Reticulocyte Reactions: Their Value in Determining the Potency of Therapeutic Materials, Especially in Pernicious Anæmia, Lancet, 2, 319, 1935.

94. MINOT, G. R. and MURPHY, W. P.: Treatment of Pernicious Anemia by a Special Diet, J.A.M.A., 87, 470, 1926.

95. MITCHELL, D. C., VILTER, R. W. and VILTER, C. F.: Hypersensitivity to Folic Acid, Ann. Int. Med., 31, 1102, 1949.

96. MOLLIN, D. L.: Relapse of Pernicious Anæmia During Maintenance Therapy with Folic Acid, Lancet, 2, 928, 1948.

97. MOLLIN, D. L. and ROSS, G. I. M.: Serum Vitamin B₁₂ Concentrations of Patients with Megaloblastic Anæmia After Treatment with Vitamin B₁₂, Folic Acid, or Folinic Acid, Brit. M. J., 2, 640, 1953; J. Clin. Path., 6, 54, 1953.

97a. MONTO, R. W. and REBUCK, J. W.: Nasal Instillation and Inhalation of Crystalline Vitamin B₁₂ in Pernicious Anemia, Arch. Int. Med., 93, 219, 1954; Blood, 10, 1151, 1955.

98. MOORE, C. V., BIERBAUM, O. S., WELCH, A.

D. and WRIGHT, L. D.: The Activity of Synthetic Lactobacillus casei Factor ("Folic Acid") as an Antipernicious Anemia Substance, J. Lab. & Clin. Med., 30, 1056, 1945.

99. MOOSNICK, F. B., SCHLEICHER, E. M. and PETERSON, W. E.: Progressive Addisonian Pernicious Anemia, Successfully Treated With Intravenous Choline Chloride, J. Clin. Invest., 24, 278, 1945.

100. MORGANS, M. E., RIMINGTON, C. and WHITTAKER, N.: Folic Acid in Megaloblastic Anæmia After Total Gastrectomy, Lancet, 2, 128, 1947.

101. MUELLER, J. F. and WILL, J. J.: Interrelationships of Folic Acid, Vitamin B₁₂ and Ascorbic Acid in Patients with Megaloblastic Anemia, Am. J. Clin. Nutrition, 3, 30, 1955.

102. NITTIS, S.: Blood Platelets in Pernicious Anemia After Liver Therapy, Ann. Int. Med., 4, 931, 1931.

103. ÖSTLING, G., NYBERG, W. and GORDIN, R.: Antianemic Activity of Alkali-Treated Crude Liver Extract, Acta med. scandinav., 145, 40, 1953.

104. PATEL, J. C.: Crystalline Anti-Pernicious-Anæmia Factor in Treatment of Two Cases of Tropical Macrocytic Anæmia, Brit. M. J., 2, 934, 1948.

105. PORTER, W. B., WILLIAMS, J. P., FORBES, J. C. and IRVING, H.: Aqueous Extract of Liver, J.A.M.A., 93, 176, 1929.

106. PRICE-JONES, C.: Red Cell Diameters in One Hundred Healthy Persons and in Pernicious Anemia: Effect of Liver Treatment, J. Path. & Bact., 32, 479, 1929.

107. RAMALINGASWAMI, V. and MENON, P. S.: Folic Acid in Nutritional Macrocytic Anaemia, Ind. J. Med. Res., 37, 471, 1949.

111. RIDDLE, M. C.: Endogenous Uric Acid Metabolism in Pernicious Anemia, J. Clin. Invest., 8, 69, 1929.

112. ——— Pernicious Anemia, Blood Regeneration During Early Remission, Arch. Int. Med., 46, 417, 1930.

113. ——— Pernicious Anemia, the Erythrocyte Response to Treatment, Am. J. Med. Sc., 200, 145, 1940.

114. ROSS, J. F., BELDING, H. and PAEGEL, B. L.: The Development and Progression of Subacute Combined Degeneration of the Spinal Cord in Patients with Pernicious Anemia Treated with Synthetic Pteroylglutamic (Folic) Acid, Blood, 3, 68, 1948; ibid., 6, 1213, 1951.

115. RYNES, S. E. and TOCANTINS, L. M.: Arthus Type of Sensitivity to Liver Extract, J. Allergy, 15, 173, 1944.

116. Schieve, J. F. and Rundles, R. W.: Response of Lingual Manifestations of Pernicious Anemia to Pteroylglutamic Acid and Vitamin B₁₂, J. Lab. & Clin. Med., *34*, 439, 1949.

117. Sharp, E. A.: An Anti-anemic Factor in Desiccated Stomach, J.A.M.A., *93*, 749, 1929.

118. Sharp, E. A., Schleicher, E. M. and Wolter, J. W.: The Myeloid Pattern in Pernicious Anemia, Am. J. Clin. Path., *9*, 189, 1939.

119. Stasney, J. and Pizzolato, P.: Serial Bone Marrow Studies in Pernicious Anemia, Proc. Soc. Exper. Biol. & Med., *51*, 335, 338 and 340, 1943.

120. Sturgeon, P. and Carpenter, G.: Megaloblastic Anemia of Infancy. Response to Vitamin B₁₂, Blood, *5*, 458, 1950.

121. Sturgis, C. C. and Isaacs, R.: Treatment of Pernicious Anemia With Desiccated Defatted Stomach, Am. J. Med. Sc., *180*, 597, 1930.

122. Suárez, R. M., Spies, T. D., Hernandez-Morales, F. and Perez, E.: A Note on the Effectiveness of Vitamin B₁₂ in the Treatment of Tropical Sprue in Relapse, Blood, *4*, 1124, 1949.

123. Suárez, R. M., Spies, T. D. and Suárez, R. M., Jr.: The Use of Folic Acid in Sprue, Ann. Int. Med., *26*, 643, 1947.

123a.Suárez, R. M., Sr., Suárez, R. M., Jr., Buso, R. and Sabater, J.: The Effect of Orally Administered Folinic Acid in the Treatment of Tropical Sprue, Blood, *9*, 489, 1954.

124. Suhrland, L. G., Rubin, D., Weisberger, A. S. and Meacham, G. C.: Failure of Oral Therapy in the Maintenance of Pernicious Anemia, A. M. A. Arch. Int. Med., *104*, 411, 1959.

125. Thomson, M. L., Dalton, H. W. and Wilson, V. K.: Megaloblastic Anæmia in Coeliac Disease Treated with Folic Acid, Lancet, 2, 238, 1949.

126. Ungley, C. C.: Vitamin B₁₂ in Pernicious Anæmia: Parenteral Administration, Brit. M. J., 2, 1379, 1949.

127. ———— Subacute Combined Degeneration of the Cord, Brain, 72, 382, 1949.

128. Vilter, C. F., Vilter, R. W. and Spies, T. D.: The Treatment of Pernicious and Related Anemias with Synthetic Folic Acid, J. Lab. & Clin. Med., *32*, 262, 1947.

129. Wagley, P. F.: Neurologic Disturbances with Folic Acid Therapy, New England J. Med., *238*, 11, 1948.

129a.Walker, W. and Hunter, R. B.: Single Massive Dose of Vitamin B₁₂ in Untreated Pernicious Anæmia, Brit. M. J., 2, 593, 1952.

129b.Watson, R. J., Lichtman, H. C., Messite, J., Ellison, R. R., Conrad, H. and Ginsberg, V.: Clinical Studies with the Citrovorum Factor in Megaloblastic Anemia, Am. J. Med., *17*, 17, 1954.

129c.Weissberg, J., McGavack, T. H., Vogel, M. and Kenigsberg, S.: The Effect of Folic Acid on the Central Nervous System of Normal Subjects and Subjects with Anemia Other than Pernicious Anemia, Blood, *5*, 148, 1950.

130. West, R. and Reisner, E. H., Jr.: Treatment of Pernicious Anemia with Crystalline Vitamin B₁₂, Am. J. Med., *6*, 643, 1949.

131. Wilkinson, J. F. and Israëls, M. C. G.: Pteroyl-Polyglutamic Acids in the Treatment of Pernicious Anæmia, Lancet, 2, 689, 1949.

131a.Will, J. J. et al.: Folic Acid and Vitamin B₁₂ in Pernicious Anemia, J. Lab. & Clin. Med., *53*, 22, 1959.

132. Wills, L.: Nature of Hæmopoietic Factor in Marmite, Lancet, *1*, 1283, 1933.

133. Wintrobe, M. M.: Hemoglobin Content, Volume and Thickness of Erythrocyte in Pernicious Anemia and Sprue and Changes Produced by Liver Therapy, Am. J. Med. Sc., *181*, 217, 1931.

134. ———— Relation of Variations in Mean Corpuscular Volume to Number of Reticulocytes in Pernicious Anemia, J. Clin. Invest., *13*, 669, 1934.

135. ———— The Antianemic Effect of Yeast in Pernicious Anemia, Am. J. Med. Sc., *197*, 286, 1939.

136. Woodruff, C. W., Ripy, H. W., Peterson, J. C. and Darby, W. J.: Variable Response to Vitamin B₁₂ of Megaloblastic Anemia of Infancy, Pediatrics, *4*, 723, 1949.

Iron and Accessory Substances

137. Badenoch, J. and Callender, Sheila T.: Iron Metabolism in Steatorrhea, Blood, *9*, 123, 1954.

138. Bronson, W. R. and Sisson, T. R. C.: Studies on Acute Iron Poisoning, A. M. A. J. Dis. Child., *99*, 18, 1960.

139. Brown, E. B., Moore, C. V., Reynafarje, C. and Smith, D. E.: Intravenously Administered Saccharated Iron Oxide in the Treatment of Hypochromic Anemia, J.A.M.A., *144*, 1084, 1950.

140. Brown, E. B. and Moore, C. V.: Parenterally Administered Iron in the Treatment of Hypochromic Anemia, *in Progress in Hematology*, New York City, Grune & Stratton, 1956, p. 22.

30

142. GOETSCH, A. T., MOORE, C. V. and MINNICH, V.: Observations on the Effect of Massive Doses of Iron Given Intravenously to Patients With Hypochronic Anemia, Blood, 1, 129, 1946.

143. HADEN, R. L.: Historical Aspects of Iron Therapy in Anemia, J.A.M.A., 111, 1059, 1938.

144. HADDOW, A. and HORNING, E. S.: On the Carcinogenicity of an Iron-Dextran Complex, J. Nat. Cancer Inst., 24, 109, 1960.

145. HURST, A. F.: A Case of Iron Encephalopathy, Guy's Hosp. Rep., 81, 243, 1931.

146. KARLEFORS, T. and NORDÉN, A.: Studies on Iron-Dextran Complex, Acta med. scandinav.(suppl. 342), 163, 7, 1958.

147. KERR, D. N. S. and DAVIDSON, S.: Gastrointestinal Intolerance to Oral Iron Preparations, Lancet, 2, 489, 1958.

148. LIMARZI, L. R.: The Effect of Arsenic (Fowler's Solution) on Erythropoiesis, Am. J. Med. Sc., 206, 339, 1943.

149. LUONGO, M. A. and BJORNSON, S. S.: The Liver in Ferrous Sulfate Poisoning, New England J. Med., 251, 995, 1954.

150. MINOT, G. R. and HEATH, C. W.: The Response of the Reticulocytes to Iron, Am. J. Med. Sc., 183, 110, 1932.

151. MOORE, C. V., DUBACH, R., MINNICH, V. and ROBERTS, H. K.: Absorption of Ferrous and Ferric Radioactive Iron by Human Subjects and by Dogs. J. Clin. Invest., 23, 755, 1944.

152. NISSIM, J. A.: Intravenous Administration of Iron, Lancet, 2, 49, 1947; Brit. Med. J., 1, 352, 1954.

152a. O'SULLIVAN, D. J., HIGGINS, P. G. and WILKINSON, J. F.: Oral Iron Compounds, Lancet, 2, 482, 1955.

153. POHLE, F. J. and HEATH, C. W.: The Influence of Acid and Alkaline Salts Upon the Blood in Hypochromic Anemia Treated by Iron Parenterally, Am. J. Med. Sc., 197, 437, 1939.

154. REISSMANN, K. R., COLEMAN, T. J., BUDAI, B. S. and MORIARTY, L. R.: Acute Intestinal Iron Intoxication, Blood, 10, 35, 1955.

155. SIMPSON, K. and BLUNT, A.: Acute Ferrous Sulphate Poisoning Treated with Edathamil Calcium-Disodium, Lancet, 2, 1120, 1960.

156. SJÖBERG, H.: Symptoms of Ileus From Retention of Iron in Cecum Following the Administration of Large Doses of Iron, Acta med. scandinav., 85, 129, 1935.

157. SWAN, H. T. and JOWETT, G. H.: Treatment of Iron Deficiency with Ferrous Fumarate, Brit. M. J., 2, 782, 1959.

158. WATSON, C. J., GRINSTEIN, M. and HAWKINSON, V.: Studies of Protoporphyrin: IV. A Comparison of the Erythrocyte Protoporphyrin Concentration With the Reticulocyte Percentage Under Experimental and Clinical Conditions, J. Clin. Invest., 23, 69, 1944.

159. WHIPPLE, G. H., ROBSCHEIT-ROBBINS, F. S. and WALDEN, G. B.: Blood Regeneration in Severe Anemia, Am. J. Med. Sc., 179, 628, 1930.

Chapter 10

Pernicious Anemia and Related Macrocytic Anemias

PERNICIOUS ANEMIA

Synonyms and Definition.—This is a chronic disease characterized by the presence of achylia gastrica, an insidious onset and the development of macrocytic anemia, certain gastrointestinal and neurologic disturbances and evidences of increased blood destruction. Before the discovery of liver therapy, its course, even though interrupted by periods of remission and relapse, was eventually fatal. Thus arose the term "pernicious," which is no longer appropriate. The response to specific treatment is so characteristic that in the absence of such a response the diagnosis may be questioned. The disease is also known by the names of the physicians who first clearly described it, Addison and Biermer, or as "primary" anemia. The condition is now generally regarded as being produced by a permanent gastric defect associated with atrophy in which the failure to secrete an "intrinsic factor" necessary for the absorption of vitamin B_{12} is the crucial fault.

History.—The clinical features of pernicious anemia were fully described by Addison in 1855, but it is noteworthy that cases of what would now be called pernicious anemia were recorded in 1823 by Combe and by Andral, and in 1837 by Marshall Hall.[24] Biermer,[15] apparently without knowledge of Addison's account, wrote a still more comprehensive description in 1872. At this time W. Pepper and J. Cohnheim discovered the changes in the bone marrow, and the histologic changes in the blood were described by Ehrlich shortly afterwards. The possible primary rôle of the stomach in the etiology of pernicious anemia was suggested by Fenwick (1880). Lichtheim called attention to the changes in the spinal cord in 1887. The hemolytic concept of pernicious anemia is based on the results of William Hunter's researches (1888) upon the iron in the liver and other organs.

Although the concept that food bears a relationship to anemia had been expressed for centuries, and it was recognized by Manson in 1883 that liver feeding could benefit patients with sprue and pellagra, it remained for Whipple to demonstrate in scientific experiments the value of liver and other foods in the relief of anemia from blood loss in dogs. In 1922 he expressed the view that there might be in pernicious anemia a scarcity of material from which the stroma of red cells is formed. Although others had given high calorie diets and even liver in the treatment of this disease, it remained for Minot and Murphy, in 1926, to demonstrate conclusively the value of

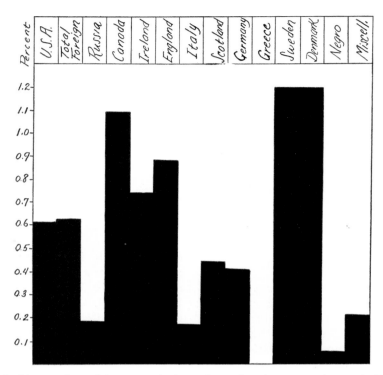

FIG. 10–1.—Incidence of pernicious anemia in natives of various countries, as indicated by 500 admissions from 1913 to 1932 to the Peter Bent Brigham Hospital, Boston. The values in per cent indicate the proportion of cases of pernicious anemia among the total admissions from the various countries. (Friedlander, Am. J. Med. Sc.)

liver therapy. Castle's experiments, which followed shortly afterwards, clarified the relationship between achylia gastrica and the hematopoietic effectiveness of liver.

Etiology. — Geographic Distribution and Race.—Pernicious anemia is a disease chiefly of the temperate zone and the white race. It is much more common in persons from the Scandinavian countries as well as from England, Ireland, and Canada than in Russians or Italians[38] (Fig. 10–1). It is relatively uncommon in Jews and rare in Orientals.[78,83a,97d] It has been said to occur seldom, if ever, in full blooded negroes but its rarity in this race has been overemphasized. Thus, of 329 cases of pernicious anemia admitted between the years 1925 and 1940 to the wards of the Johns Hopkins Hospital, where the admission of white and colored patients was about 3 to 1, 33 were negroes (Fig. 10–2). The ratio

at the Charity Hospital in New Orleans, Louisiana, where 45 per cent of the patients are colored, was 1 colored to 7 white patients.[64] In a study at the Cook County Hospital, Chicago, pernicious anemia was found in 36 negroes as compared with 170 Caucasians, per 100,000 hospital admissions.[97a] Some of the negro patients the writer has seen have shown the deep pigmentation and features of fullblooded negroes although many have obviously been of mixed blood. Pernicious anemia has been seen in the South African Bantu[74b] and is encountered in the tropics,[125b] although, no doubt, the majority of tropical cases of megaloblastic anemia are related to nutritional deficiency and to sprue.

There are few data regarding the incidence of the disease in various localities in the same country. Statistics for Sweden suggested a greater frequency in

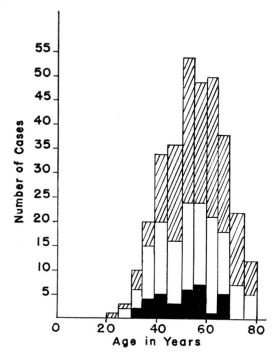

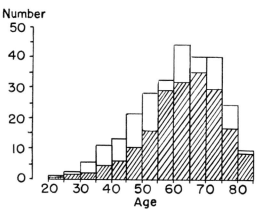

FIG. 10–3.—Incidence of pernicious anemia at various ages, calculated according to number of cases per 100,000 population. Females, hatched columns; males, open columns. (From data for Sweden collected by Nordenson et al., Acta med. scandinav.)

FIG. 10–2.—Age, sex and race of 329 cases of pernicious anemia admitted to the Johns Hopkins Hospital from 1925 to 1940. Negro patients of both sexes are represented together in the black portion of each column; white men are indicated by the hatched portion of each column; white women by the open portion. The height of each column represents the total number of patients of each age group. There were 171 white men, 125 white women and a total of 33 negroes, of which 20 were men, 13 women. The ratio of all white to negro admissions at this hospital was about 3 to 1.

the central part of the country.[82] In North America, the incidence in Canada, the Great Lakes region and in the New England states is higher than in the Southern states. It once was suggested that these variations might be related to differences in soil[77] or solar radiation,[100] but racial and hereditary influences appear to be of chief importance.

Age. — Pernicious anemia is a disease of late adult life, being most frequent after forty years of age and increasing in frequency as age advances (Fig. 10–3). It is rare under thirty years of age and extremely unusual in children. Of a total of 1,532 cases of pernicious anemia

derived from six large surveys, only 4 cases were below the age of twenty years.[26a] Some reported cases of macrocytic anemia in infants and in children[26a] are not readily acceptable as cases of true pernicious anemia because of lack of conclusive evidence but there are highly suggestive accounts in children ranging from nine months[27a] to fourteen years of age.[26b,48b,62a,84a] It was pointed out that in some of the reported cases of megaloblastic anemia in childhood latent forms of steatorrhea were not excluded.[67b] However, even on the basis of the most rigid criteria, which would also include demonstration of specific inability to absorb labelled vitamin B_{12} unless intrinsic factor was supplied, the diagnosis of juvenile pernicious anemia can be considered as having been established in 12 children ranging from eight months to 16 years of age.[13a,22,67b,69,76,88] This includes two Negro children two and two and a half years of age, respectively.[69]

Significant features of these cases in children were the presence of symptoms such as anorexia, vomiting and diarrhea, some evidence of glossitis, minimal or no abnormalities in the nervous system and a high familial incidence. The cases include two pairs of sibs. The father of one of the juvenile patients himself had pernicious anemia and the patient's parents were first cousins.[76] Especially noteworthy is the fact that the intrinsic factor deficiency could be demonstrated to be an isolated abnormality, unaccompanied by reduced secretion of acid or pepsin or by histologically abnormal gastric mucosa.[22,67b,76] In several instances, however, temporary loss of acid secretion was observed during relapse of the anemia and, in one child, a malabsorption syndrome disappeared after treatment with vitamin B_{12}.[67b]

Sex.—In the United States (Fig. 10–2) and in England males have been more frequently the victims of this disease, but in Germany and the Scandinavian countries the opposite has been recorded. In Sweden pernicious anemia was found to be half again as common in women as compared with men[82] (Fig. 10–3).

Heredity, Family Predisposition. —Every student of this disease has been impressed with the frequency with which several members of a family,[6,71] either in one generation or in several, have been affected. In one study of 48 families,[66] comprising 168 persons, multiple occurrences of pernicious anemia were found in 8 families (16.7 per cent). In another series of 645 cases, the percentage of familial incidence was 7.9.[103] In a series in which data were available for 3 generations, and included persons in the older age groups, the familial incidence was 30 per cent.[78a]

Pernicious anemia has been described in identical male and female Caucasian twins and even in Negro twins. In the latter the disease developed in both at the age of seventy-two.

Achlorhydria occurs more commonly among relatives of patients known to have pernicious anemia than in the general population,[6,78a] especially after middle age.[19a] In addition, macrocytosis, low uropepsinogen excretion, gastric atrophy, poor absorption of vitamin B_{12}

which could be corrected by intrinsic factor and low or low normal serum vitamin B_{12} levels were observed. Low absorption of vitamin B_{12} occurs in the families of pernicious anemia subjects even in the absence of achlorhydria.[74a]

There is considerable evidence to indicate that the dominant factor in the development of pernicious anemia is a significantly reduced capacity to absorb vitamin B_{12} from the gastrointestinal tract. It appears, however, that this is a latent state which may persist throughout life without pernicious anemia developing.[74a] Accessory factors are necessary to cause the disease to appear. Age, in some manner, may be one of these and perhaps diet and the size of the vitamin B_{12} stores in the tissues. Other factors may be involved which influence the requirement for the vitamin. There is no clear evidence that achlorhydria, *per se*, is one of the modifying factors.

While much more needs to be learned concerning the genetic aspects of pernicious anemia, present evidence is consistent with the view that low vitamin B_{12} absorption depends on the presence of a heterozygous gene which is a necessary but, alone, not sufficient precondition for pernicious anemia. A single dominant autosomal gene may be responsible for the abnormality of the gastric mucosa which brings about this functional defect.[74a]

In the first description of pernicious anemia Addison noted that "the disease occurs in patients of a somewhat large and bulky frame and with a distinct tendency to fat formation." Although exceptions are encountered it is true that the victims of this disease often possess a short, broad face, with the eyes set far apart, long ears, a short, deep chest with wide costal angle, gray or white hair which has turned so prematurely, and blue or light-colored eyes. Males may show a eunuchoid broad pelvis and abnormal distribution of hair. The frequency of blood group A has been observed to be higher in pernicious anemia victims than in the average population,[1a,24b] but this is true of their normal relatives also.[74a]

The constitutional features which have been described are characteristic of the North European populations among whom pernicious anemia is common. Thus these associations seem to be ethnic rather than concerned with close genetic linkage or pleiotropy.[74a]

If the development of pernicious anemia depends on the inheritance of a genetic factor it is to be expected that this should be a disease which makes no distinction between rich and poor, city or country dweller, luxury or filth, occupation, overexertion or similar factors which are so important in the incidence of certain other diseases.

Association with Other Diseases. —In dealing with a chronic disease of adult or late life, such as pernicious anemia, it is to be expected that it may be found to be associated with other disorders.[80] The nature of these conditions has received attention because of the bearing they may have on the development or the course of pernicious anemia.

In one series of 370 cases of pernicious anemia,[119] concomitant diseases were found in 23.2 per cent of the patients. The associated diseases included asthma and bronchitis, pneumonia, hypertension, exophthalmic goiter, simple thyroid adenoma, myxedema, diabetes, syphilis, cystitis, and various dermatoses. In another series of cases, chronic arthritis was found in 5 per cent. Tuberculosis, on the other hand, was very rarely found in cases of pernicious anemia.[11] Tuberculous stricture of the small intestine, however, may be associated with macrocytic anemia (p. 515), and simultaneous tuberculosis and carcinoma of the stomach in a case of pernicious anemia has been reported.[117a] Iron deficiency anemia may sometimes be associated with pernicious anemia (p. 457), but other disorders of the blood are rarely encountered. Association

with the sickle cell trait and with thalassemia has been reported.[38a] Before diagnosis became more exact, cases of leukemia with severe anemia and cases of pernicious anemia with a leukemoid leukocytic picture were sometimes referred to as "leukanemia." A true association of pernicious anemia and leukemia is unusual. In four instances pernicious anemia was known to precede the onset of acute myeloblastic leukemia by several years[103a,109b,124b] and, in one case, polycythemia vera and, ultimately, acute myeloblastic leukemia developed.[125a] Both chronic myelocytic[16a,55,78b,109c] and chronic lymphocytic[89] leukemia have been known to develop in patients with pernicious anemia but this is rare and there is no clear evidence for a common predisposition to pernicious anemia and leukemia.[78a] One or two instances of the development of polycythemia vera in a patient with pernicious anemia have been recorded.[39]

The majority of the diseases mentioned above are no doubt unrelated etiologically to pernicious anemia and they are of importance chiefly on account of the bearing they have on the course of the disease. Thus, infections of various kinds, and arteriosclerosis tend to impair the response to therapy (p. 448). Diabetes is of interest because symptoms such as atrophic tongue, diarrhea, and neurological disturbances are common to both disorders[93] and thus errors in diagnosis may occur. The same is true of myxedema, in which condition macrocytic anemia may also be found (see p. 519). Hyperthryoidism and pernicious anemia have been reported as occurring in the same individual in 78 instances.[4,17a,36] The association may be entirely fortuitous but the possibility of a metabolic relationship has been considered. The association of pernicious anemia with hyperthyroidism and with pituitary disease (p. 581) led to the suggestion that a hormonal mechanism may lead to degeneration of the cells which secrete "intrinsic factor." The concurrence of Addison's disease and Addisonian anemia, reported several times,[13b,17] is at least of historical interest.

Gastric secretory dysfunction is a characteristic finding in pernicious anemia (p. 483). It is not surprising, therefore, to find in association with this disease conditions which, like pernicious anemia, are frequently associated with achlorhydria. Evidence of gallbladder dysfunction was noted in 22.5 per cent of one series of cases[14] and in 42 per cent in another.[17b] Cholecystitis and cholelithiasis were found in 16 per cent of 151 autopsied cases.[19] The frequency of arthritis and of exophthalmic goiter, two diseases in which there is a high incidence of achlorhydria, has been mentioned. It is also noteworthy that, whereas in a series of 840 cases of pernicious anemia no peptic ulcer was found,[63] the incidence of **carcinoma of the stomach** is greater among patients with pernicious anemia as well as in their relatives.[78a] In a few instances macrocytic anemia and carcinoma of the stomach have been described at the same time,[119] a fact which brings up the possibility that the gastric neoplasm interfered with the normal secretory functions of the stomach;[42] in most cases,[92] however, carcinoma of the stomach developed some time after the anemia was recognized and successfully treated. In a series of 23,231 autopsies at the University of Minnesota[65] on individuals forty-five years of age or over, there were 293 cases of pernicious anemia. Of these, 36 (12.3 per cent) also had carcinoma of the stomach, an incidence more than three times as great as in the remainder of the autopsied cases. In roentgen studies of 259 patients having pernicious anemia, the same investigators found carcinoma of the stomach in 6.9 per cent and benign polyps in 6.6 per cent.[92] Noteworthy in this series was the lack of symptoms even

when large lesions existed, the rapid change from a benign polyp to cancer, the presence of both benign and malignant tumors side by side and the rapid change from a small, barely detectable lesion to an extensive, inoperable carcinoma.

A survey of other reports in the literature reveals wide differences in the incidence of carcinoma of the stomach in pernicious anemia, figures as low as 1.7 per cent being cited.[81b] Some of these differences depend on the samples selected. A compilation of findings derived from 8,492 living and dead patients with pernicious anemia reported by 20 authors since 1923 yielded an over-all prevalence of gastric cancer of 2.04 per cent.[125] A much higher figure, approximately 10 per cent, is obtained when autopsied cases are reviewed.

Such a high incidence of gastric carcinoma warrants the routine use of screening tests. Of these the cytological test has many advantages. The simplest procedure[125] consists in the collection of cells from the stomach by forcibly injecting a small quantity of saline solution through an ordinary stomach tube, withdrawing and reinjecting this several times. The collected aspirate is promptly centrifuged at high speed for twenty or thirty minutes and smears of the sediment are fixed immediately in equal parts of 95 per cent ethanol and anesthetic ether. The fixed slides are then examined for malignant cells in the usual manner. The cytological studies, which should be made at intervals of, say three to six months, can be supplemented with stool examinations for occult blood and, in suspicious cases, with roentgen and gastroscopic studies.

There are conflicting reports concerning the most frequent location of carcinoma of the stomach in patients with pernicious anemia. In one series[78c] it was noted that the carcinoma did not tend to develop in the fundus or upper part of the body of the stomach where the pathological changes characteristic of pernicious anemia are localized. In another[96] it was found that they tended to be fundic or cardiac in origin, and were also polypoid and multicentric.

Symptomatology.—Mode of Onset and Initial Symptoms.—The onset of pernicious anemia is characteristically insidious and, by the time the patient seeks medical attention, the anemia may be moderately severe. It is common in this disease to discover a degree of anemia which is much greater than the appearance of the patient or the severity of his symptoms would suggest. The chief exceptions to this rule are those cases in which symptoms referable to the nervous system appear early and progress rapidly before anemia has become severe or has even developed. Sometimes soreness of the tongue may appear early, before much anemia has developed.

The diagnostic triad, weakness, sore tongue, and numbness or tingling of the extremities, are common initial complaints but the initial symptoms may be very varied. Not infrequently they suggest the presence of some digestive disorder, or cardiac, renal or genito-urinary disease, mental aberration, or obscure infection. In such instances, the underlying disease may not be suspected until the blood has been examined.

Initial complaints, in order of frequency, are fatigability, weakness and faintness, numbness, tingling and stiffness, headache, nausea, lack of appetite, vomiting, dizziness, shortness of breath, palpitation, diarrhea, loss of weight, pallor, abdominal pain, and sore tongue. These will be found to have been present for a number of months, rarely for several years and, characteristically, have varied in their intensity from one time to another.

Outward Appearance of the Patient.—Addison, in the first adequate description of this disease (1855), wrote as follows: "The countenance gets pale, the whites of the eyes become pearly, the general frame flabby rather than wasted; the pulse perhaps large but remarkably soft and compressible, and occasionally with a slight jerk, especially under the slightest excitement. There is an increasing indisposition to exertion with an uncomfortable feeling of faintness or breathlessness on attempting it; the heart is readily made to palpitate; the whole surface presents a blanched, smooth and waxy appearance; the lips, gums and tongue seem bloodless; the flabbiness of the solids increases; the appetite fails, extreme languor and faintness supervene, breathlessness and palpitation being produced by the most trifling exertion or emotion; some slight edema is probably perceived about the ankles. The debility becomes extreme; the patient can no longer arise from his bed; the mind occasionally wanders; he falls into a prostrate and half torpid state, and at length expires. Nevertheless, to the very last, and after a sickness of perhaps several months' duration, the bulkiness of the general frame and the obesity often present a most striking contrast to the failure and exhaustion observable in every other respect."

When the anemia is severe, the skin presents a delicate lemon or grapefruit tint. The sclerae may show a yellowish tint, but often the increased bilirubinemia detectable in the blood is scarcely noticeable clinically. There may be brownish pigmentation which is diffuse or blotchy. Interspersed with this, patches of leucoderma (vitiligo) may be found. The skin may be dry but is often peculiarly velvety and smooth, yet inelastic. Petechiae in the skin are unusual.

It is remarkable how frequently patients suffering from this disease have blond or prematurely gray hair and light-colored eyes. Often the face is wide and the chest is broad with a wide costal angle.[29] It must be stated, how-

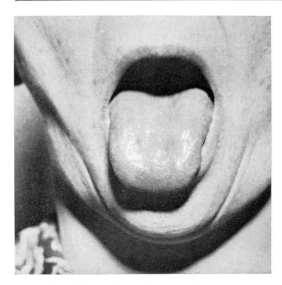

Fig. 10–4.—Smooth tongue in a case
of pernicious anemia.

dorsum of the tongue may be involved, or there may be red patches at the margins or on the dorsum. In some instances shallow white ulcers like those of aphthous stomatitis may be found, and even inflamed vesicles, sometimes large and even hemorrhagic, have been observed. Occasionally the entire mouth and throat may be involved, causing the patient to complain of burning and pain on swallowing. More frequently there is simply burning or soreness, particularly of the anterior half of the tongue.

The intensity of the glossitis usually subsides after several days but the sore tongue often recurs at intervals of varying length. Between attacks the epithelium of the tongue is left devoid of papillae, thus producing the smooth, glazed tongue which is characteristic of pernicious anemia (Fig. 10–4). Partial loss of taste may ensue. Some patients whose tongue is quite smooth deny even having had soreness of the tongue. Some restoration of the papillae is often associated with adequate therapy.[83]

ever, that there are many exceptions to the rule.

Weight loss, while often slight, may be considerable in many instances.[60] Actual emaciation, however, is rare.

Body Temperature.—Fever of several degrees is common when the anemia is severe and may have no connection with infection. Such fever disappears promptly after effective treatment with liver. Knowledge of this fact, however, should not cause one to overlook cystitis or some other inflammatory condition which impairs the response to therapy.

Alimentary System.—Sore tongue and diarrhea are the two most common complaints referable to this system. Sore tongue occurs at some time in at least 50 per cent of cases of pernicious anemia. As already mentioned, **glossitis** may be the first symptom and may appear when there is little or no anemia. The reappearance of tongue symptoms portends a relapse and, in patients under treatment, is an indication of inadequate therapy.

When glossitis is at its height, the tongue is very sore and painful and "beefy" red in color. The whole of the

Diarrhea likewise occurs at some time in about 50 per cent of the cases. Even when frank diarrhea has not occurred, direct questioning frequently will bring out the fact that there is a semi-solid bowel movement immediately on arising and another one or two stools later in the day. This type of bowel habit, according to the writer's observation, is often associated with achlorhydria.

Less frequently complaints referred to the gastrointestinal tract may suggest the presence of a large variety of diseases, including gallbladder or malignant disease and peptic ulcer. Pseudotumors caused by hypertrophy of the musculature of the pylorus have been described.[12,81a] There may be anorexia, nausea, "gas," a sense of fulness and epigastric discomfort, heartburn, vomiting, and irregular abdominal pain which varies in intensity. Attacks of paroxysmal pain resembling the gastric crises of tabes dorsalis sometimes occur.[7] Such an attack may be associated with vomiting and some abdominal rigidity. It is rare, however, to observe attacks as severe as are often seen in sickle cell anemia or in hereditary spherocytosis. In pernicious anemia the pain may be symptomatic of changes in the spinal cord.

The **liver** may be found to be slightly enlarged. When there is congestive heart failure in association with the anemia, this organ may be greatly enlarged and tender. The **spleen** is moderately increased in size in relapse. It is found enlarged in practically all cases at autopsy but there is no agreement as to how often the spleen is palpable clinically. Various statistics range from 3 to 40 per cent.[16] Decided enlargement is unusual. With adequate treatment, the liver and spleen recede beneath the costal borders.

Circulatory System.—The symptoms referable to this system may be so pronounced as to lead to a mistaken diagnosis of primary cardiovascular disease. Dyspnea, palpitation, sensations of extra beats, excessive weakness, vertigo, and tinnitus may be associated with signs of congestive cardiac failure, including well-marked edema and cardiac and hepatic enlargement. In other cases angina pectoris may develop.[102] Systolic murmurs at the base of the heart and even at the apex are often heard and occasionally a diastolic murmur at the aortic area, possibly due to dilatation of the aortic ring, may be found. Cardiac irregularity seldom occurs but tachycardia is common. The vessels in the neck may be seen to pulsate if the anemia is severe and a loud venous "hum" may be present. The blood pressure is more commonly low in pernicious anemia than in tuberculosis.[69a] Electrocardiographic changes may be associated with the anemia (p. 437).

Since the age incidence of pernicious anemia and of degenerative cardiac disease is approximately the same, many instances of cardiac failure in this disease may be attributed in large part to degenerative changes not due directly to the anemia. The anoxemia associated with anemia often plays an important rôle, nevertheless, for it is common to find partial or complete relief of anginal symptoms or of intermittent claudication and maintenance of compensation when the anemia has been treated successfully. It is significant in indicating the rôle of anemia in producing symptoms of angina that, contrary to the findings in cases of angina associated with organic heart disease, such symptoms in cases of anemia are as frequent, or more so, in women than in men.[19b] Furthermore, the mortality from angina in anemic patients is comparatively low. The cardiovascular adjustments to anemia were discussed in an earlier chapter (p. 436). Many of these physiologic studies were carried out in cases of pernicious anemia.[104]

Genito-urinary System. — Occasionally the clinical picture of chronic nephritis may be simulated in pernicious anemia. The renal function, as measured by fixation of the specific gravity of the urine, may be impaired and small amounts of albumin and casts are commonly found.[21] Phenolsulfonphthalein excretion, however, is rarely decreased and the non-protein nitrogen is not often elevated above 50 mgm. per 100 ml. The renal functional defects generally decrease with subsidence of anemia.

Pyelitis and, particularly in female patients, cystitis are frequent complications, especially if there are neurological disturbances.

Nervous System.—Complaints referable to the nervous system at one time were encountered in 70[46] to 95 per cent[43,101] of cases of pernicious anemia. In 25 per cent, or more, of cases such symptoms were the first to attract attention. Well-marked signs of neurological involvement were found in about 30 per cent of cases,[101] and in perhaps 10 per cent of all cases with nervous symptoms the changes may be very severe.[46] In such cases sphincter disturbances, contractions, and decubitus occurred and these presented a most difficult problem. The clinical picture of the presenting case of pernicious anemia has changed somewhat, however, as facilities for diagnosis and treatment have improved. Serious manifestations are less common than they once were,[26] except in cases in which the anemia has been masked by taking folic acid in multivitamin capsules.[30] In such individuals striking changes in the nervous system have been known to develop in the absence of anemia.

Subjective sensory disturbances constitute the earliest and most frequent evidence of involvement of the nervous system.[115a] Common complaints are weakness, numbness and tingling in the extremities, difficulty in walking, stiffness of the limbs, irritability, lack of concentrating power, dulness, drowsiness, and depression. Less frequent are delayed sensation, bladder disturbances, headache, tinnitus, blurring of vision, girdle sensations and loss of sexual power. Lightning pains and abdominal crises such as are met with in tabes dorsalis are unusual.

It was originally assumed that the neurologic lesions in pernicious anemia are confined to the spinal cord but later studies demonstrated that **peripheral nerve degeneration** also occurs in this disease.[44,48,114] Numbness may result from peripheral nerve change. Impaired sensation of the "stocking" type as well as hyperesthesia of the soles of the feet may develop from the same cause. Changes in peripheral motor nerves, however, with resulting motor paralysis and muscular atrophy are unusual although they do occur.[112]

Signs referable to changes in the spinal cord may be mainly those characteristic of degeneration in the posterior funiculi, such as absent reflexes, hypotonicity, disturbance in sense of position, and incoördination and loss of vibratory sense as well as difficulty in walking; or the lateral funiculi may be chiefly involved with resulting spasticity, exaggerated reflexes, hypertonicity and positive Babinski response. Most often the neurological signs indicate involvement of peripheral nerves and of both the posterior and the lateral funiculi. Physical signs, in order of frequency, are impaired vibratory sensation, ataxia, positive Romberg's sign, disturbed position sense, plantar extensor response (Babinski), spasticity, diminished reflexes, increased reflexes, disturbed cutaneous sensibility, and sphincter disturbance.[8]

Physical signs are usually found bilaterally but they may not be of equal degree or extent on the two sides.[43] They are more common in the lower than in the upper extremities. Loss of vibratory sensation is usually most marked in the legs and may be less pronounced at the anterior superior spines, the crest of the ilium and the sacrum. It is unusual for vibratory sensation to be lost from the thoracic cage.

If minor manifestations are included, *mental disturbances* may be considered to be common in pernicious anemia in relapse. The first manifestations may be mental.[86] In one series,[43] irritability, memory disturbances and mild depression were found in two-thirds of the cases. In another,[95a] in 13 out of 14 patients with red cell counts of 2 million per c.mm. or less there was a clinically demonstrable reduction in the level of consciousness, justifying the diagnosis of delirium. In this study the most valuable single test was the serial subtraction of numbers, such as 3 from 100. Electroencephalograms showed slowing in frequency of the waves. Therapy was associated with improvement in the level of awareness and in the behavioral disturbances consequent to the reduced awareness. The abnormal electroencephalograms were reversed in most instances. Since improvement has been observed to take place about the time the reticulocyte response begins, it seems likely that the cerebral involvement is a metabolic one and not secondary to the anemia.

More serious changes, as indicated by delusions, hallucinations, maniacal outbursts, and paranoid and schizophrenic states are much less common.[54] In such instances it is frequently difficult to determine the rôle played by the anemia itself, the effect of a debilitating disease, and the mental changes caused by associated conditions such as senility, arteriosclerosis, diabetes, and other disorders which occur in persons of advanced years.[18]

Disturbances of the *special senses* may occur in the form of tinnitus and visual defects. These are usually the result of anemia or of retinal hemorrhages (Fig. 10–11). Actual optic atrophy has been observed, however, and may even be the presenting symptom.[48a] Tobacco amblyopia has been observed in vitamin B_{12} deficiency.[50a]

LABORATORY FINDINGS

The Anemia.—Macrocytosis is the chief characteristic of the blood in cases of pernicious anemia. This does not affect all of the cells but involves the majority. It can be perceived microscopically in blood smears (Fig. 10–5) or wet films of blood. It should be pointed out, however, that persons who do not examine blood daily should make actual comparison with normal blood and should not rely on their memory for the recognition of macrocytosis. It is all too common for physicians and technicians not adequately trained to pass up as normal the blood of a patient with only a moderate degree of macrocytosis or to mistake the occasional macrocytes found in hypochromic microcytic anemia for the macrocytosis of pernicious anemia.

In general, the greater the anemia, the more macrocytes in the blood. When there is relatively little anemia, although most of the cells may be larger than normal, this is difficult to appreciate except by comparison with the cells of normal blood. However, careful examination will reveal occasional exceptionally large cells, half again as large as the rest. These may be circular or oval in shape and may have a grayish-blue hue (diffuse basophilia). Such cells are the products of the pernicious anemia megaloblasts.

Poikilocytosis is another characteristic of the blood in pernicious anemia but it is found only when the anemia is advanced. The most bizarre shapes may be seen: cells in the form of dumbbells, anvils, cocked hats, hand mirrors, and so on. Many of these structures are smaller in diameter than the cells of normal blood.

With few exceptions, the red corpuscles whether large, small, or bizarre in shape, are *well filled with hemoglobin* and do not show the central achromia or the "ring-like," "pessary" forms of hypochromic microcytic anemia. Marked hypochromia is seen in pernicious anemia only when iron deficiency is associated, a combination of deficiencies which is uncommon. It should be pointed out that in doubtful cases more than one blood smear should be examined, for sometimes artefacts may be produced in preparing blood smears which give a false impression of central pallor in the red corpuscles.

In cases of advanced anemia, almost all the abnormalities of red corpuscles which have ever been described, except hypochromia, may be found. There may be many diffusely polychromatophilic cells and others which show punctate basophilia. The stippling may be fine or coarse. In occasional cells, still larger,

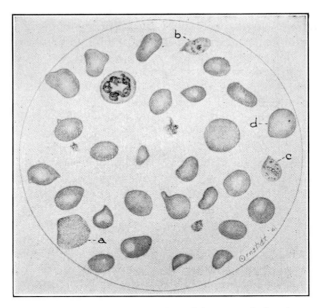

Fig. 10–5.—Drawing of blood smear from a case of pernicious anemia in relapse. From a preparation stained with Wright's and magnified, × 960. Note the extreme variation in the size and shape of the red corpuscles, the large polychromatophilic red corpuscle (*a*), the cells containing nuclear remnants and Howell-Jolly bodies (*b* and *c*) and a Cabot "ring" (*c*), the "granule red corpuscle" (*d*), and the multi-segmented polymorphonuclear leukocyte.

blue or reddish particles, usually circular in shape (chromatin particles, Howell-Jolly bodies) and acidophilic rings of various shapes (Cabot's rings) may be seen. In addition, nucleated red cells may be found. The diameters of these cells are greater than those of the majority of the non-nucleated corpuscles. Their cytoplasm may be acidophilic, poly-chromatic or basophilic. The chromatin structure of the nuclei may be very fine so that they are readily recognized as megaloblasts or, as the nucleus approaches pyknosis, it is found to be coarse (Fig. 2–1, p. 87 and Plate V, p. 94).

At one time a diagnosis of pernicious anemia would not be made until all the abnormalities already mentioned, includ-ing megaloblasts, could be demonstrated. Since these can be found only when the anemia is very severe, it is important to learn to recognize pernicious anemia before the blood changes have advanced

to this stage. This can be done with the aid of red cell measurements and by careful study of the blood smear.

The macrocytosis of pernicious anemia can be demonstrated by the measurement of the diameters or the mean volume of the red corpuscles. If the *diameters* are measured (p. 401) and the results plotted in the form of a frequency curve (Fig. 10–6), quantitative expression can be given to what can be observed on careful examination of the blood smear; namely, there is much greater variation in the diameters than is normal and the majority of the cells are larger than normal. As Price-Jones termed it, the curve has a broad base and is swung to the right. The extent of these changes varies roughly with the degree of anemia. An excessive variability is more constant in pernicious anemia than a high mean diameter.[87]

The measurement of red cell diameters

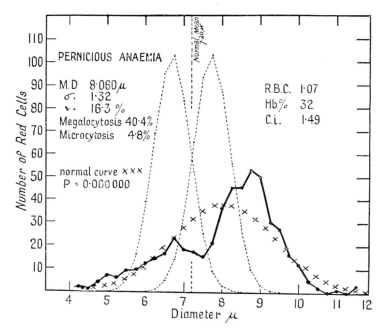

Fig. 10–6.—The variation in the diameters of the red corpuscles in a case of pernicious anemia in relapse (continuous line) compared with the variation in health. The curves set out by the interrupted lines define the limits of normality as represented by ± three times the standard deviation of the mean diameter in the healthy adult. The degree of megalocytosis and microcytosis was estimated by counting the number of cells outside these boundaries. The skewness of the pernicious anemia curve is emphasized by comparison with the normal distribution curve (marked by crosses) for cells of this mean diameter. (Price-Jones, Red Blood Cell Diameters, courtesy of Oxford University Press.)

is a tedious and time-consuming procedure and it has been superseded by the measurement of *mean corpuscular volume* (p. 402). The latter can be done simply by dividing the red cell count into the volume of packed red cells as determined in the hematocrit. The sole disadvantage of this method, as compared with cell diameter measurement, is that it gives information regarding only the average size of the cells. An advantage in the method, in addition to its simplicity is derived from the fact that, since variations in all the dimensions of the red corpuscles affect mean corpuscular volume, smaller differences in size can be recognized by this means than by the measurement of mean diameter. Thus, whereas mean diameter in pernicious anemia may be little, or not at all greater

than normal when the anemia is moderate in degree, mean corpuscular volume is almost invariably increased as long as any anemia is present (Fig. 8–13, p. 406). Consequently it is possible to recognize macrocytosis before anemia has advanced to a great extent. The variability in cell diameter which the frequency curve demonstrates can be recognized by careful examination of the blood smear.[123]

The increase in mean corpuscular volume is to a large extent directly proportional to the degree of anemia, but other factors, such as the number of immature red corpuscles, are also important (Fig. 2–2, p. 91).[124] When the anemia is slight or moderate in degree, values of 95 to 110 c.μ are common (normal 82 to 92 c.μ); where it is more severe the mean corpuscular volume may be 110 to even 160 c. μ and generally is found to range between 110 and 130 c. μ. Similar increases are found in the "volume index" (p. 402).

The *hemoglobin content* of the red corpuscles in pernicious anemia is, on the whole, increased proportionately to the increase in their size. The values for mean corpuscular hemoglobin will be found generally to range from 33 to 38 $\gamma\gamma$ (normal 27 to 31 $\gamma\gamma$) when the anemia is moderate and from 33 to even 56$\gamma\gamma$ when it is more severe. The "color index," which measures the quantity of hemoglobin in the red corpuscles in relation to an arbitrary normal, is also increased.

It is an error to assume that the red corpuscles in pernicious anemia are supersaturated with hemoglobin. Their well-filled and even dark appearance in stained smears is due to their greater thickness, which allows less light to pass through them than is the case with normal cells. The concentration of hemoglobin in these cells, the ratio of the weight of hemoglobin to their size (mean corpuscular hemoglobin concentration) is the same as in normal blood (32 to 36 per cent).

The increased corpuscular size and hemoglobin content explain the well recognized fact that in pernicious anemia the diminution in red cell count is greater than the decrease in the quantity of hemoglobin or the volume of packed red cells per 100 ml. of blood. The red cell count is often found to be lower than the appearance of the patient suggests and in this disease there have been recorded counts so low that it is hard to believe that life could have been maintained in the presence of such severe anemia. Thus, Naegeli[81] found a count of 138,000 per c.mm. in one of his patients and Zadek[124c] recorded 86,000 (!). Were the anemia other than macrocytic and the hemoglobin proportionately reduced, this surely would have been impossible.

Leukocytes.—The most constant ab-

normality in the leukocytes is the presence of polymorphonuclear neutrophilic leukocytes which are usually multisegmented and are often exceptionally large (*macropolycytes*). These cells may have 8, 10 or more lobes.[61] The lobes are often bizarre in shape, vary greatly in size and may have peculiar bridges of connecting chromatin strands. The chromatin arrangement is less compact than in the normal neutrophil and the granules of the cytoplasm are larger and more acidophilic. These changes in the neutrophil usually precede pronounced alterations in the red cells and, therefore, are of importance in recognizing pernicious and the related forms of anemia.

At the same time there may be found *immature cells* of the myeloid series, such as myelocytes or even younger forms. These cells rarely constitute more than 0.5 to 1.5 per cent of all the leukocytes but very occasionally their number may be so great as to suggest a diagnosis of myelocytic leukemia.[51,99] In spite of the "shift to the right" and to the left in pernicious anemia the *total number* of cells of the myeloid series is reduced during relapse. There is absolute neutropenia, and also leukopenia (3000 to 5000 leukocytes per c.mm.) as well as relative lymphocytosis.

Following the introduction of liver therapy much attention was given to the occurrence of eosinophilia. This was frequently observed following the ingestion of raw liver but may occur after cooked liver, liver extract or stomach therapy (p. 454). It should be noted that eosinophilia, even as great as 15 to 28 per cent was observed in the blood of cases of pernicious anemia before the introduction of liver therapy.[70]

Platelets.—The platelets are generally reduced in number in relapse, particularly when the red cell count is lower than 2,000,000 per c.mm. The platelet count may then be less than 100,000 per c.mm.[84] Bizarre forms, including giant platelets, may be found.[5] At the same time *bleeding time* may be prolonged, the blood clot retracts poorly, and purpura as well as retinal hemorrhages may occur. *Coagulation time* is usually normal or only slightly delayed.

Red Cell Resistance.—The resistance of the red cells to hypotonic saline solutions is not significantly altered in this disease. Their permeability to glucose, however, and to malonamid and thiourea has been found increased during relapse while permeability to glycerin is normal.[10] It was reported that the red cell resistance to hemolysis by the exotoxins of the intestinal flora of individuals with pernicious anemia is lowered[110] and the resistance to saponin hemolysis was also found to be greatly decreased.[85] These observations suggest that the structure or the function of the cell membrane is of a peculiar quality in pernicious anemia.

Total Blood Volume.—The total blood volume is reduced, but the reduction is due to the decrease of cells. The total plasma volume may actually be increased. This was observed in measurements by the Evans' blue dye method[40] and by the carbon monoxide method[47b] but, by the Cr^{51} method, plasma volume was also low.[73a] Treatment is followed by a rapid increase in blood volume but, in the first week, a disproportionate increase in plasma volume may mask the rise in red cell volume.[2,73]

Serum Bilirubin and Urine and Stool Urobilinogen.—A slight and sometimes moderate increase in serum bilirubin is present in relapse. This is indicated by the color of the plasma (Plate I) and the icterus index, which is usually greater than 8 (normal 5 to 7) and may be as high as 20 units. In iron deficiency anemia, in simple chronic anemia and in aplastic anemia, the color of the plasma is, in contrast, normal or paler than normal. The van den Bergh reaction is indirect. In a series of 85 cases the quantity of serum bilirubin was

0.98 ± 0.06 mg.[76] The return to normal following specific therapy was described earlier (p. 456).

The excretion of urobilinogen in the urine and stools is greatly increased during relapse and may be several times the normal values.[52] The significance of these findings will be discussed shortly (p. 482).

The Bone Marrow.—During relapse the morphology of the bone marrow in pernicious anemia is characteristic. There is well-marked hyperplasia, due particularly to the presence of great numbers of cells of the erythrocyte series; moreover, characteristic types of nucleated red corpuscles and leukocytes are to be found. These changes can be demonstrated in specimens of sternal marrow obtained by sternal puncture or by biopsy.

Cells of the red series may make up 30 to 50 per cent of all the nucleated cells, instead of approximately 20 per cent, as is found in normal marrow. Active erythropoiesis, however, occurs in the marrow in many types of anemia. What is characteristic of the marrow in pernicious anemia and in the related anemias is the preponderance of nucleated red cells of a special type, the *megaloblast* (Chapter 2). These cells are distinguished by their large size and the delicate nuclear chromatin which resembles fine scroll work (Fig. 2–1, p. 87 and Plate V, p. 94). Their cytoplasm may be so deeply basophilic ("promegaloblasts") that it is difficult to recognize them as members of the erythroblastic series. Other cells, possessing the same type of nucleus and often lying in close proximity to the promegaloblasts, present lighter areas in the cytoplasm or even pink cytoplasm (polychromatophilic and acidophilic megaloblasts) so that they are easily classified in the red series. Even in smears of marrow material these cells are often found in small groups of 3 to 6 or 7, suggesting a common origin or a close relationship. Jones[62] found pro-

31

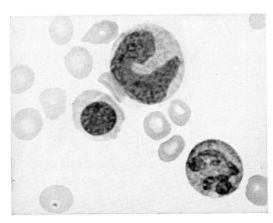

Fig. 10–7.—Photomicrograph of material obtained by sternal puncture in a case of pernicious anemia in relapse. Wright's stain. × 1050. Note the giant metamyelocyte, the large nucleated red cell below it, and the "macropolycyte" at the lower right.

megaloblasts and basophilic megaloblasts to constitute 6 per cent of the marrow cells in his series of cases of pernicious anemia in relapse and polychromatophilic and orthochromatic megaloblasts formed 24 per cent. An unusually large number of mitotic figures is to be found among these cells. They have been studied in great detail by Fieschi.[33] Normoblasts are few in number in comparison to the megaloblasts.

At the same time there is evidence of active and of **abnormal leukopoiesis.** There is often an obvious increase in the number of myeloid leukocytes even though their actual percentage, because of the higher proportion of nucleated red cells, may be lower than normal. Furthermore, striking qualitative changes in these cells occur. In addition to myeloid leukocytes of normal appearance, almost as many extraordinarily large (30 μ) leukocytes will be found. These monstrosities of cellular development may occur at any stage in the myeloid series but they are particularly common among the metamyelocytes. The nucleus of such cells is increased both relatively and

absolutely in size, it may be bizarre in shape and in chromatin structure or in staining properties (Fig. 10–7). The nucleus may be unusually irregular in shape or have the form of a doughnut, it may contain vacuoles and it may stain poorly. The cytoplasm may appear to have developed at a slower rate than the nucleus for it may be basophilic or it may be light blue and contain very few granules, thus suggesting the type of cytoplasm found in early, undifferentiated myelocytes. The macropolycyte of pernicious anemia is probably derived from these cells.[61]

In addition to these characteristic changes, it may be observed that "reticulum" or "Ferrata" cells, and lymphocytes are more numerous than usual,[25,111] and the megakaryocytes may be reduced in number and may be abnormal.[30a, 62] Schleicher,[97e] in fact, regarded pernicious anemia as fundamentally affecting the reticulum, the latter being pathologically activated.

The degree of abnormality of the bone marrow in pernicious anemia appears to be related to the presence or imminence of relapse rather than to the red cell count. Thus, it has been observed that following institution of effective treatment there is rapid replacement of megaloblasts by macroblasts and normoblasts (see p. 455). The bone marrow in such cases may be found to consist of relatively fewer megaloblasts and giant metamyelocytes than that of an *untreated* patient even though the erythrocyte count of the latter is actually higher than in the former.[25]

It has been observed that, when a complication sets in, the bone marrow picture changes and may be no longer typical of pernicious anemia. In the presence of infection a leukemoid picture may develop.[106a]

Erythrocyte Life Span and Erythrokinetics.—Red cell survival studies have shown an average destruction rate of three times normal.[99a] This may be the consequence of faulty construction. However, it has also been shown that normal adult erythrocytes, transfused to untreated patients with pernicious anemia, are destroyed at random, irrespective of their ages.[48c] The slow disappearance curve could be differentiated from the rapid curves of disappearance due to isoimmunization. Furthermore, plasma of untreated patients in contact with normal erythrocytes so affected them that they had a shortened survival time when transfused to normal persons. The random destruction did not occur after the patients had been treated. In contrast, the erythrocytes of untreated patients were destroyed in the circulation of a normal subject at the same rate as normal tranfused adult erythrocytes. These observations imply that vitamin B_{12} deficiency exerts a noxious influence on normal adult erythrocytes in the circulation.

As already indicated, the bone marrow in untreated pernicious anemia shows striking erythroid hyperplasia and the excretion of urobilinogen in the urine and stools is greatly increased. Measurements of plasma iron turnover have also given evidence of greatly increased erythroid marrow activity.[56c,117] However, it has been observed that these measures of heme turnover, which are assumed to represent *total erythropoiesis*, are not reflected in *effective erythropoiesis*, as represented by reticulocyte count, red cell utilization of radioiron and cell survival studies.[34]

These findings have led to the concept that a "shunt" in erythropoiesis is present during relapse, a certain proportion of the product going to waste. Consistent with this view is the observation that as much as 40 per cent of the fecal urobilinogen in untreated pernicious anemia is not derived from the circulating red cell mass.[70a] It is assumed that red cell destruction occurs in the marrow. *In vivo*

counting over sacrum, sternum and liver and direct counting of blood showed sustained levels of radioiron in marrow and liver with only a small proportion appearing in the circulating red cells.[34] It was also found that, following administration of vitamin B_{12}, available iron moved from tissues and marrow into red cells whereas plasma iron turnover remained the same or decreased. Thus it was shown that *total* erythropoiesis is not increased by therapy whereas *effective* erythropoiesis is restored to normal.

Gastrointestinal Secretions. — Failure to secrete free hydrochloric acid after maximal stimulation with histamine is so characteristic of pernicious anemia that in the absence of this finding a diagnosis of Addisonian anemia must be made with much hesitation. Furthermore, there is not only achlorhydria but the total amount of secretion is greatly reduced, the pH of the gastric contents is high, pepsin and rennin are almost entirely deficient, and only a few cubic centimeters of mucoid material is the usual reward of gastric analysis.[49,53,72a,260] It has been observed in some instances that the achlorhydria preceded by many years the development of symptoms.[118] The gastric secretory deficiency is usually permanent and uninfluenced by treatment.[94]

A total of 36[35] to 47[6a,13] instances have been described in which free hydrochloric acid was found in the gastric secretion of otherwise more or less typical cases of pernicious anemia. In three cases free hydrochloric acid was discovered in the gastric secretion following treatment of patients who formerly had had achlorhydria.[20,23,25b] This is not surprising since the fundamental defect, as stated earlier (p. 467), is a failure to secrete intrinsic factor. From a practical standpoint, however, it is a good working rule to question a diagnosis of pernicious anemia if hydrochloric acid is found on gastric analysis unless the Schilling test

(p. 490) gives evidence of intrinsic factor deficiency.

The secretion of *uropepsinogen* in the urine is greatly reduced but this is related to the achlorhydria itself and is not a dependable test for pernicious anemia.[56b]

Gastroscopic examination of the stomach during relapse reveals atrophy. The mucosa is grayish-yellow or grayish-green, rather than red, and the blood vessels are sharply outlined through the thin and atrophic mucous membrane. Such changes may affect the mucosa of the whole stomach or they may be patchy and involve only parts of the antrum and body, or the body alone. In some instances a superficial gastritis has been observed. Polyps are common and large rugae may be found on gastroscopy or by roentgenography.[59] Following specific therapy, the mucosa may resume a normal appearance but in many instances generalized or patchy atrophy has been observed to persist. Cells obtained from the stomach by gastric lavage are illustrated in Figure 10–9.

The gastric juice of patients suffering from pernicious anemia contains blood group specific substances at least in the same large amounts as normal gastric juice.[124a] A reduction in the secretion of **saliva** has been noted in pernicious anemia.[32]

Pancreatic enzymes have been found present in cases of pernicious anemia but tryptic activity has been observed to be decreased in a number of cases in which there was moderate or advanced nervous system involvement.[53]

The **stools** are often soft and, when frequent movements occur, they may contain a considerable quantity of mucus. This may sometimes be so great as to suggest mucous colitis. The stools may be brownish-yellow in color and generally are found to contain excessive quantities of urobilinogen.

Attempts to assay the *absorptive capacity of the gastrointestinal tract* by measuring the absorption of glucose,[47] xylose,[53] potassium iodide[50] or glycine[31,50] have given variable results.

Urine.—The specific gravity is usually low and may be fixed. The color may be pale but at times of excessive hemolysis it is brown. Small amounts of albumin and a few hyaline and granular casts are often present and there may be an increase of the night over the day volume of urine.[105]

Because of such findings, and particularly when some edema has also been present, cases of pernicious anemia have been mistaken for chronic nephritis. However, phenolsulfonphthalein excretion is not altered as a rule, nor is the non-protein-nitrogen of the blood usually greater than 50 mg. per 100 ml. nor is the blood urea nitrogen increased. The disturbance in specific gravity of the urine appears to be circulatory in origin. It was suggested that deposition of iron pigment in the kidney tubules produces renal damage.[105]

Chemical and Other Evidences of Disturbed Metabolism. — A well-marked disturbance in metabolism is demonstrable in the severe relapse of pernicious anemia. There is a negative **nitrogen balance,**[3] the **total protein** and the **colloid osmotic pressure** of the plasma are somewhat reduced, and there is some **water retention.**[75] There may be a slight increase in **basal metabolic rate.**[115] The **iron content of the serum** is abnormally high[77a] unless iron deficiency is present in addition, erythrocyte coproporphyrin is absent[95] and the free **protoporphyrin** content of the erythrocytes is normal or slightly low. The rate of excretion of **coproporphyrin I** is increased.[28] A mild **aminoaciduria** takes place.[112a] The finding of increased blood phenol levels, reduced urinary levels of the volatile phenols and increased urinary excretion of total phenolic compounds[109a] suggests aberrant **tyrosine metabolism** (see p. 133). Enzyme abnormalities in leukocytes and erythrocytes suggesting "pyrimidine starvation" have been reported.[100a]

During remission striking changes occur in these as well as in other metabolites. Alterations in plasma iron and in porphyrins were described elsewhere (p. 456). There is a well-marked retention of nitrogen and the nitrogen balance becomes positive.[9] At the same time the oxygen consumption, as measured by the basal metabolic rate, decreases in an orderly and gradual manner.[9] This may be preceded by a preliminary increase and fever may develop.[37] In other cases the basal metabolic rate has decreased in spite of the increased oxygen requirement of the newly liberated reticulocytes and the changes in uric acid metabolism.[3] The excretion of tyrosine metabolites is restored to normal.[1] This sometimes precedes the reticulocytosis.

The **serum uric acid,** which varies greatly during relapse but is usually normal or lower than normal in amount, increases very promptly during remission. This change may occur within twenty-four hours of the administration of an effective therapeutic agent and is soon followed by an increased urinary excretion of uric acid. The maximum increase in serum uric acid characteristically occurs twenty-four hours before the maximal increase in reticulocytes and subsequent variations in serum and urine uric acid tend to parallel the changes in the percentage of reticulocytes.[90]

Urinary phosphorus decreases rapidly after administration of vitamin B_{12}, increases during reticulocytosis and then returns gradually to normal values.[58] It seems likely that these changes are related to increased phosphorus uptake in association with the formation of increasing quantities of cellular nucleotides and polynucleotides, with subsequent formation of globin in response to specific therapy. At the same time, changes in nucleoprotein metabolism and disappearance of nuclear material from the normoblast are reflected in the elevation of serum and urinary uric acid.

The diffuse, barely discernible edema of the skin and subcutaneous tissues of patients in relapse may become more marked at the height of the reticulocyte response, when water retention may develop. This is followed by increased excretion of urine and loss of edema but, if the patient has been confined to bed, the edema may be noticed for the first time only after the patient has been allowed out of bed.[75,115] Decreased colloid osmotic pressure of the plasma is probably a factor in the development of edema but dilatation of the heart and increased permeability of the capillaries probably also influence water retention. It is well recognized that weight gain usually occurs during remission in pernicious anemia, and at times it may be very marked. Water retention accounts in part for the initial weight gain but an increased caloric intake associated with the general improvement is, no doubt, responsible for the later gain in weight.

Liver therapy is followed by a decrease in the **blood sugar** values which is most marked during the peak of the reticulocyte response and may be so pronounced as to be associated with hunger symptoms.[41,91] The fall in fasting blood-sugar values is probably related to the metabolic adjustment accompanying early remission. As judged by the changes in the plasma 17-hydroxycorticosteroids after ACTH administration, *adrenocortical function* is not impaired in patients with pernicious anemia in relapse.[95b]

Fat Metabolism.—Well-marked alterations in fat metabolism have also been described. In relapse the serum cholesterol is low and the lecithin phosphorus is also usually decreased, although this is not so constant as the reduction in cholesterol.[79] The red corpuscles contain excessive amounts of cholesterol esters and they are deficient in phospholipid and free cholesterol.[67,122] At the onset of remission there is a sudden rise in the serum cholesterol which is concomitant with the response of the reticulocytes and as a rule is proportional to the intensity of the remission. Similar changes in lecithin-phosphorus take place. The ether-insoluble phosphatide of the plasma increases two to four weeks following the onset of remission.[67] When remission is complete the chemical composition of the erythrocytes is found to be normal. The total fatty acids of the blood vary within limits in relapse and remission, and no consistent changes have been found to occur in the lecithin, cephalin, and cerebroside concentrations of the plasma. The significance of these alterations in the fat constituents of the plasma and red cells is not clear but it has been suggested that they may be related to alterations in the sensitivity of the red corpuscles to hemolysis.[79] They may also have some significance in relation to degenerative changes in the nervous system.[67]

Liver Function.—Although one or more liver function tests is frequently abnormal in cases of pernicious anemia in relapse, no consistent pattern of hepatic dysfunction has been found.[96a] The **plasma prothrombin** measured by Quick's method is generally normal.[96a] In contrast to the normal findings in other types of anemia, reduced prothrombin levels were demonstrated by Owren's method in 75 per cent of cases of pernicious anemia.[43a] Administration of vitamin K had no effect on the plasma prothrombin and the effect of vitamin B_{12} was only transient; the administration of liver extract, however, led to a return to normal which persisted.[43a] It was postulated that the prothrombin deficiency was due to the lack of a "protein synthesis factor" which is present in liver and is neither vitamin B_{12} or folic acid.[83b]

Vitamin A, B Complex and Ascorbic Acid. —Levels of plasma vitamin A, carotene and ascorbic acid have been found to be normal in pernicious anemia[19c] and no deficiency of thiamin was demonstrated even when there was involvement of the nervous system.[94a] No evidence of impaired absorption of riboflavin, pantothenic acid[75a] or folic acid[21a] has been demonstrated. The reported relief of glossitis by the administration of calcium pantothenate, niacin, riboflavin or folic acid in several cases of pernicious anemia[18a] probably is attributable to the existence of associated deficiencies of these substances.[19c]

Microbiological assays have demonstrated an absence of free *vitamin* B_{12} and low total vitamin B_{12} concentrations in the serum of patients with pernicious anemia in relapse (p. 132).

The *cholineesterase* activity of the whole blood, red corpuscles and plasma are below normal levels in relapse.[75b] With therapy a rise in activity takes place first in the red cells. Similar alterations have not been found in other hemopoietic disorders, with the possible exception of myeloid leukemia.

Diagnosis.—In the average case the recognition of pernicious anemia is simple. The diagnostic triad of sore tongue, numbness and tingling, and weakness, together with macrocytic anemia and achlorhydria, forms a clinical picture which is well known. It is noteworthy, however, that the chief complaints may differ from the classical ones and, unless the blood is carefully examined, the presence of pernicious anemia may not be suspected.

The presenting complaints may suggest heart disease, malignancy, chronic nephritis, myxedema, tuberculosis, subacute bacterial endocarditis, or various fevers, as well as nervous disturbances such as tabes dorsalis, disseminated sclerosis, or psychotic states. It must be kept in mind that weight loss may be great in pernicious anemia, that fever is usual in the stage of relapse, and that gastrointestinal disturbances of great variety are common. A history of sore tongue or paresthesias may be elicited only on direct questioning. The absence of a smooth tongue or of neurological changes does not rule out pernicious anemia. It has been pointed out that the onset of symptoms may be acute and may be associated with manifestations suggesting heart disease and fever which are so prominent that the diagnosis is easily missed.[97b] This is especially true if the patients are young and of the negro race, and when neurologic complaints are lacking.

If the blood is examined, macrocytic anemia should be demonstrable. The mean corpuscular volume will be greater than normal, and the mean corpuscular hemoglobin will also be increased if the method for hemoglobin determination is an accurate one. Determinations of the size and hemoglobin content of the red corpuscles must always be checked by examination of the blood smear, for errors in counting or calculation are all too common. The smear will show large, often slightly oval, and well-filled red corpuscles in varying numbers according to the severity of the anemia and, when the latter is well marked, also small and misshapen red cells, as well as diffuse and punctate basophilia, and possibly occasional nucleated red cells (macroblasts and megaloblasts). The reticulocytes are not as a rule increased in pernicious anemia except during the time of response to therapy. The leukocyte count may be somewhat low, there may be relative lymphocytosis, and multisegmented neutrophilic leukocytes will be found. The blood plasma is usually deeper in color than is normal.

When blood examination reveals macrocytic anemia, unless the signs of some other disease are obvious, the most probable diagnosis is pernicious anemia. It is not generally realized, however, that macrocytic anemia may develop in various types of acute and chronic hemolytic anemia. It is also encountered in various forms of aplastic anemia, in myelophthisic anemia, aleukemic leukemia, and even in Hodgkin's disease. In the hemolytic anemias, a degree of blood destruction which is exceptional for pernicious anemia, well-marked reticulocytosis unrelated to therapy, sickling or increased fragility of the red corpuscles, normal gastric secretion, as well as the clinical history and physical findings, help to rule out pernicious anemia as the cause of the macrocytic anemia. In aplastic and myelophthisic anemias, leukopenia and thrombocytopenia are often more pronounced than in pernicious anemia, the anemia if macrocytic is not strikingly so, and there is usually little or no evidence of increased blood destruction. Furthermore, when the red cell count is below about 2.5 million cells per c.mm., the degree of anisocytosis in pernicious anemia is usually quite pronounced, whereas in other types of macrocytic anemia it is rarely so striking.[24c] Bone marrow puncture or biopsy may be required in some instances to rule out pernicious anemia.

The writer has studied several cases of pernicious anemia in which there was *no increase in mean corpuscular volume above normal.* Out of a series of well over 200 cases of pernicious anemia, the mean corpuscular volume was normal or low in 5. One patient known to have pernicious anemia and successfully treated previously, returned because of abdominal pain and weight loss. The red cell count was 3.1 million per c.mm., the M.C.V. 86 c.μ, M.C.H.C. 27 per cent. Carcinoma of the stomach was demonstrated. Another who gave a typical past history of pernicious anemia with successful treatment, came to the hospital because of menorrhagia. The red cell count was 4.07, M.C.V. 67 c.μ, M.C.H.C. 29 per cent. Adenocarcinoma of the uterus was found, hysterectomy was done

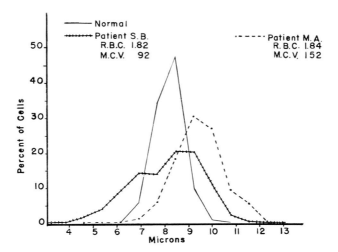

Fig. 10–8.—Diameters of red cells in the blood of a case of pernicious anemia with normocytic anemia (patient S. B.) compared with those of another case of pernicious anemia with typical macrocytic anemia (patient M. A.). The red cell count of patient S. B. was 1.82 million, the M.C.V. 92 c.μ. The corresponding values for M. A. were 1.84 million and 152 c.μ., respectively. The "double population" of (1) macrocytes resulting from vitamin B_{12} deficiency and (2) microcytes formed as a consequence of iron deficiency, is indicated by the curve for S. B.

and iron therapy given. The red cells increased, the red cell count becoming 3.55, M.C.V. 101 c.μ. Liver therapy caused a change to normal values. Two other patients, whose history and physical signs suggested pernicious anemia, were found to have normocytic anemia. One was treated successfully with iron and yeast and the other required liver extract parenterally. The fifth patient, who was seen in several relapses, had macrocytic anemia only when very anemic. When the red cell count was greater than 3.0 million per c.mm., the mean corpuscular volume was normal or below normal. This patient had menorrhagia and moderate hypothyroidism.

As would be expected, the red corpuscles in these cases showed an extreme degree of anisocytosis, well-marked poikilocytosis, and hypochromia in some of the cells. The two "populations" of red corpuscles are indicated by the double peak of the diameter frequency curve for the blood of S. B. (Fig. 10–8). This type of anemia has been referred to as "*dimorphic*".[226b]

Achlorhydria persisting even after the injection of histamine is the most constant finding in pernicious anemia. The augmented histamine test (0.04 mg. histamine acid phosphate per Kg. body weight together with an antihistaminic drug, given intramuscularly)[66a] should be employed or, if this is inconvenient, use can be made of the action of a cationic resin such as azuresin (Diagnex) which is acted upon by the HCl of the gastric juice with the release of an indicator substance detectable in the urine. If free hydrochloric acid is demonstrated, a diagnosis of pernicious anemia cannot be accepted unless absence of intrinsic factor can be demonstrated (p. 490).

It is rarely essential to examine the bone marrow if adequate physical and blood examinations have been made but, in doubtful cases, the demonstration of megaloblasts and of giant metamyelocytes and multisegmented neutrophils is very helpful. The leukocyte abnormalities may sometimes be more clearly discernible than the red cell changes in cases with little anemia. In equivocal cases, the demonstration of low serum vitamin B_{12} levels has been found helpful.[67a]

The separation of pernicious anemia from other forms of megaloblastic macrocytic anemia may be extremely difficult. In tropical, sub-tropical and even occasionally in temperate climates, the differentiation of sprue and pernicious anemia is frequently very difficult, because diarrhea may be severe in pernicious anemia. The passage of bulky, foamy and fatty stools suggests sprue. Paresthesias may be present in this disease but objective signs of neurological changes are unusual. Furthermore, achlorhydria occurs in only half of the cases of sprue. The blood picture of the two conditions is identical. The finding of a low plasma iron level suggests that one is dealing either with combined iron deficiency and pernicious anemia or with one of the related macrocytic anemias of nutritional origin such as sprue or macrocytic anemia of dietary origin (p. 508).

Diagnosis is now facilitated by therapeutic test. The administration of vitamin B_{12} should be followed in several days by a characteristic reticulocyte response and rapid relief of symptoms, and soon by a rise in the red cell count unless there is some complicating disease. If the parenteral administration of vitamin B_{12} is not followed within ten to fourteen days by definite signs of response, the diagnosis of pernicious anemia must be seriously questioned. However, since a diagnosis of pernicious anemia once made condemns the patient to treatment for life, a therapeutic trial should be the *last* resort rather than the first. There is but one exception to this statement. The patient with severe anemia and a classical picture should not be subjected to exhaustive investigation taking considerable time before treatment is given. In one or two days the crucial studies can be made. Roentgenography, for example, should be done later. If carcinoma is the cause of so severe an anemia, delay of a week or two will make little difference in the outlook.

Real difficulty in diagnosis is encountered in (1) patients who fail to respond adequately to treatment, possibly because of infection, arteriosclerosis, or other disease; (2) those in whom nervous or mental symptoms and signs are found in the absence of well-marked changes in the blood; and (3) patients who have received treatment recently and in whom it is necessary, for one reason or another, to confirm or disprove the diagnosis.

In the first mentioned group, exhaustive studies and examinations may be necessary. If macrocytic anemia, moderate bilirubinemia and achlorhydria are present, chance favors the probability of pernicious anemia. The same diagnostic triad should be looked for in obscure neurological or mental disorders. In many instances of pernicious anemia of the latter type, failure to make the diagnosis is more often due to the fact that this disease has not been considered rather than because it cannot be demonstrated. Even when anemia is slight or moderate, careful study of the blood smear and determination of mean corpuscular volume will usually reveal macrocytosis. Bone marrow examination may be helpful although, when anemia is slight, megaloblasts may not be readily recognizable. In such cases the typical giant metamyelocytes and macropolycytes of pernicious anemia may nevertheless be found.

In the patient who has been treated recently and whose clinical picture at the time of examination is nearly normal, it may still be possible to demonstrate slight macrocytosis and bilirubinemia in addition to achlorhydria. Such findings strongly favor the diagnosis of pernicious anemia. It is more conclusive to test the ability of the gastrointestinal tract to absorb vitamin B_{12} by the use of vitamin B_{12} labelled with radioactive cobalt.

Use of Radioactive Vitamin B$_{12}$ in Diagnosis.—Co^{60}, which has a half-life of five years,[75c] is most commonly used although some prefer Co^{56} and Co^{58}, which have a half-life of 72 days.[75c] As a rule, material of specific activity of 0.1 to 1.0 μc/μg. is employed. The absorption of radioactive vitamin B$_{12}$ can be measured in any one of four ways:

(1) *Urinary Excretion (Schilling Test).*[295] —When a small dose of radioactive B$_{12}$ is given by mouth to a normal person, no radioactivity can be detected in the urine unless the test dose is "flushed out" by a large parenteral injection of non-radioactive B$_{12}$ (1000 μg.). If this is done one to three hours after the oral dose has been taken, control subjects will excrete, on the average, 26 to 11 per cent of the oral dose in the next 24 hours, depending on the size of the dose (0.5 to 2.0 μg.). The greatest percentage is passed when the smallest dose is used.[75c] Patients with pernicious anemia will excrete little or no radioactive material unless the radioactive B$_{12}$ is given with intrinsic factor. In other types of impaired absorption, such as occurs in some cases of sprue, the excretion of labelled vitamin B$_{12}$ is poor, even after mixture with intrinsic factor.[151] The excretion of the radiovitamin is also impaired in the presence of renal disease, being both delayed and diminished. This is observed even in cases in which the urinary volume is normal and clinical signs of uremia are absent.[87a]

Details of the procedure used vary.[84b] It is always important for the laboratory where the test is made to check its procedure in control subjects and to test the potency of the intrinsic factor preparation which is being used.[113] When 0.1 μc of Co^{60}-labelled vitamin B$_{12}$, made up to a total of 0.5 μg., was employed and a flushing dose of 1 mg. non-radioactive B$_{12}$ was given intravenously 30 minutes later, the subsequent 24 hour specimen of urine contained 8.4 to 28.0 per cent of the administered oral dose, with an average of 15.3 per cent.[87a] In patients with pernicious anemia 0 to 6.9 per cent of the oral dose was excreted, the average being 1.8 per cent. In other studies excretion in normal persons ranged from 7 to 22 per cent, averaging 14.2 per cent, as compared with 0 to 7.3 per cent (average 0.6 per cent) in cases of pernicious anemia.[295] In the latter, with the simultaneous administration of intrinsic factor and radioactive B$_{12}$ 3.1 to 30 per cent (average 9.8 per cent) of the dose was excreted. The response of totally gastrectomized subjects was the same as that of patients with pernicious anemia. Achlorhydric subjects without evidence or previous history of pernicious anemia excreted 2.2 to 29 per cent of the radioactivity.[71a,295]

(2) *Fecal Excretion.*[240a]—An oral dose of radioactive B$_{12}$ is given to the fasting subject and the fecal excretion of radioactivity is measured. Whereas normally only about 30 per cent of a 0.5 μg. oral dose of radioactive B$_{12}$ can be recovered in the feces, in patients with pernicious anemia, even in remission, almost three times this amount is found. A parasympathetic stimulant ("carbachol") has been used in a modified procedure to increase secretion of intrinsic factor and other improvements have been introduced[75c] but the test has the serious disadvantage that seven days are required to complete it.

(3) *Hepatic Uptake.*[40a]—When Co-60 B$_{12}$ is given by mouth to control subjects, radioactive material accumulates in the liver, reaching a peak during the first week. This can be measured with a scintillation counter.

(4) *Blood and Plasma Radioactivity.*[28a]— If the radioactive B$_{12}$ is of sufficiently high specific activity, the amount appearing in the blood after its ingestion, with or without intrinsic factor, can be measured.

The difficulties encountered in making the diagnosis of pernicious anemia in patients previously treated emphasize the importance of accuracy in the original diagnosis. The confirmatory value of a clear-cut therapeutic response to vitamin B_{12} makes evident why it is important to avoid the use of therapeutic preparations of a mixed nature, containing folic acid, iron, and other substances, in a disease in which treatment must be continued for life and in which cessation of therapy may be followed by crippling alterations in the nervous system. It is essential for the treatment of this disease that the physician as well as the patient have full confidence in the accuracy of the diagnosis so that adequate therapy can be continued with the assurance that time, effort, and funds are not being wasted.

Complications.—When the anemia is severe, heart failure with symptoms of angina or of congestive failure may develop, or renal insufficiency may ensue. Such complications are very unusual in young persons with pernicious anemia, however, and therefore it may be assumed that oxygen want may precipitate functional collapse in a person in whom degenerative changes in the cardiovascular system are already present. Fever, if present, usually disappears as the anemia is relieved but the writer has observed it to persist in mild degree in some instances after the blood count had already risen substantially. Severe diarrhea and even vomiting may occur but these symptoms are usually readily controlled by vitamin B_{12} therapy.

When changes in the nervous system are present, infections such as cystitis, and bed sores, may cause great difficulty in treatment for they may not only be intractable in themselves but the response to therapy is impaired by their presence.

In a chronic ailment like pernicious anemia, other diseases may develop in the course of time. These have been discussed already (p. 471).

Treatment.—In the preceding chapter the treatment of anemia was fully discussed (p. 438). The principles of therapy by means of vitamin B_{12} as well as the general measures for the management of anemia which were outlined, should be followed.

Transfusion is now rarely required in pernicious anemia. Even when the anemia is severe, the possibility of obtaining a physiological response in forty-eight to seventy-two hours when specific therapy is given parenterally makes it unnecessary to subject the patient to the risks, discomfort, and expense of blood transfusion. Only when circulatory collapse is present or imminent (and this is very unusual), need transfusion be considered. The effect of rapidly repeated *blood transfusions* on erythropoiesis was found in five patients with pernicious anemia in relapse to produce no striking clinical improvement. The leukocyte and platelet counts did not rise but the bone marrow megaloblasts disappeared. Reticulocyte responses to subsequent liver extract injections occurred only in those patients whose red cell counts were below 5 million per c.mm. In one case the writer observed a similar change in bone marrow morphology but a reticulocyte response of 20 per cent took place when the red cell count had been raised by transfusion to 4 million cells per c.mm. In another study[72b] the bone marrow megaloblasts were noted to become more mature and the absolute reticulocyte count decreased but a megaloblastic picture persisted until vitamin B_{12} was given. It was concluded that the multiple transfusions of erythrocytes decreased erythropoiesis but did not cause any basic change in the type of erythrocyte maturation.

There is no need for iron therapy in pernicious anemia unless there is evidence of associated iron deficiency (Fig. 10–8, p. 488) or reason to expect that tissue iron reserves are not abundant; as, for example, in women of early middle age who may have had heavy menstrual losses or several pregnancies. Arsenic, and splenectomy, once popular in the treatment of pernicious anemia, no longer have a place.

There is nothing to be gained from the administration of hydrochloric acid in pernicious anemia unless the gastro-intestinal complaints fail to be relieved by vitamin B_{12} therapy. In such cases it will usually be found that 4 to 8 ml. of the "dilute hydrochloric acid," U.S.P., given three times a day with meals, brings prompt relief. The acid may be taken in water or in fruit juices, prefer-ably through a glass "straw."

When neurological involvement is pres-ent, vitamin B_{12} therapy offers as much as liver extract or whole liver. Especially when the nervous system is involved, confinement to bed should be as brief as possible and the patient should be en-couraged at least to move the limbs about in bed. In addition, passive movement, massage, and dry heat are valuable for improving the tone of the muscles, the circulation and the sense of well-being. As soon as possible, coördination exer-cises[47a] should be instituted and, begin-ning with slow, rhythmic sliding move-ments of the legs with the patient recum-bent, they are gradually made more com-plex. Exercises should be prescribed specifically and repeated three or four times every few hours. Even when advanced changes in the nervous system are present, it is remarkable how much can be accomplished by encouragement and reëducation. The furniture should be so arranged that the patient will have support enough to get out of bed and to move about. Small house rugs should be removed so that accidents which may discourage the patient may be prevented. A most useful mechanical device is a semicircular frame on wheels which gives the patient grips for his hands and sup-port under the axillae, allowing him to walk even though strength and coördina-tion are poor.

In view of the high incidence of car-cinoma of the stomach in cases of perni-cious anemia (p. 472) some recommend that roentgenographic examination of the stomach be made once a year.

Prognosis.—Prior to the introduction of liver therapy the outcome in a case of pernicious anemia was fatal. In the majority of patients the course of the disease was one of remissions and relapses of varying severity and duration until death occurred in one to three years.[109] Rarely, progress was more rapid. Some patients were known to live for as long as fourteen years, or even twenty years.[106] In Cabot's large series, **remissions** occurred in 86 per cent, and in 15 per cent of the cases there were more than two remissions. Some of these remissions followed blood transfusion, the adminis-tration of arsenic, or splenectomy and probably some patients unwittingly took liver or other substances now known to have real therapeutic value. Competent clincans insist[166] that spontaneous remis-sions did occur in the pre-liver era which were not the result of the inadvertent ingestion of anti-anemic material. In any event, remission was rarely complete, achylia gastrica persisted, and neuro-logical involvement increased. In the very few cases reported as recovered, the diagnosis must be held in doubt.

Present methods of treatment have completely changed the outlook in perni-cious anemia. Only in some cases with extreme neurological involvement and secondary infection is death from this disease not preventable. Since 1926 there has been a striking decrease in mortality from pernicious anemia in various countries.[74,98,108,109] All ages and both sexes have shown lower mortal-ity although the reduction in death rate has been most marked at younger ages.

The chief dangers to patients at present lie in inadequate dosage, intercurrent infections interfering with the utilization of the specific anti-anemic agent, and complications arising from neurological involvement.[109] Signs of degeneration in the nervous system may appear for the first time during folic acid therapy as has been discussed elsewhere (p. 450). If adequate amounts of vitamin B_{12} are given and maintained, cord degeneration can be prevented from developing or, having appeared, may be completely arrested. Study of reports which contradict this statement reveals that truly normal erythrocyte counts and restitution of cell size to normal were never attained. Of other possible complications, the high incidence of carcinoma of the stomach has been discussed already (p. 472).

An important source of trouble is the patient's reluctance to continue treatment for life and his readiness when new complaints develop to attribute them to the treatment. It is common to find that a relapse followed the onset of some intercurrent disease or that the need for some surgical measure distracted attention from anti-anemic therapy and caused neglect at a time when it was most needed. "Aplastic" forms of pernicious anemia which fail to respond to therapy are sometimes mentioned. Such cases must be rare. The writer has not encountered a single case in which at autopsy there was neither evidence to disprove the diagnosis nor some explanation of the failure to respond to treatment. Refractory megaloblastic and achrestic anemia will be discussed later (p. 510).

How soon **relapse** will occur once therapy has been stopped, is unpredictable in the individual case. This depends not only on the development of intercurrent diseases but also, in addition to possible unknown factors, on the quantity of vitamin B_{12} which is stored within the body, the inadvertent consumption of food factors having therapeutic value in pernicious anemia and the degree of intrinsic factor deficiency. It has been reported that the lack of intrinsic factor is not absolute and differs in various cases.[260] In one study of 54 cases,[97c] relapses developed at intervals varying from two to thirty-eight months. In a third of the cases these appeared during the first six months and in 36 per cent during the second six months. In 24 per cent of the cases relapse did not develop until the second year after treatment had ceased. Following withdrawal of liver extract in another group of 12 patients, 6 failed to show hematologic relapse in 26 to 29 months and in the remainder relapse developed in 8 to 18 months.[59a] Remission lasted 42 to 78 months in four patients. In none did neurologic manifestations appear. It is probable that the time of recurrence of relapse will not always be the same even in the same patient.

Pathology.—The characteristic morbid anatomy of this disease is now rarely encountered in the autopsy room. In the typical case in relapse, the pathologist noted the yellowish appearance of the skin, the lack of wasting, the dilated and flabby heart, as well as fatty changes in the parenchymatous viscera, especially the liver, heart and kidneys. Sections of the liver, as well as of the spleen and kidneys, when treated with a weak solution of ferrocyanide and then washed in a weak aqueous solution of hydrochloric acid, assumed a strikingly beautiful blue color. In this way the heavy deposit of iron was demonstrated. The red bone marrow was found to be strikingly deepened in color and the yellow marrow of the long bones was transformed into a deep red gelatinous substance which was likened to currant jelly. The details of the morphology of the bone marrow in pernicious anemia have been described already (p. 481). In the spleen and liver, foci of extramedullary blood formation were regularly found.

These changes are absent in patients dying as a result of intercurrent disease during liver-induced remission. In such cases, however, as well as in those dying

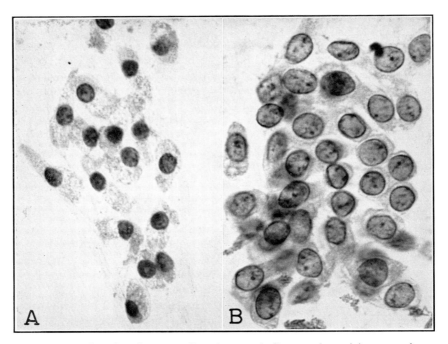

FIG. 10–9.—Gastric columnar cells: *A*, normal; *B*, treated pernicious anemia. Magnification 750 ×. (Courtesy of Dr. Cyrus E. Rubin.)

in relapse, morphological abnormalities are found in the gastrointestinal tract and in the nervous system.

The mucosa of the tongue is usually atrophied. The changes in the *stomach* [24a,72] are striking in tissue fixed soon after death. Severe atrophy of the upper two-thirds of the stomach is evident even to the naked eye, this area being reduced to the thinness of parchment. At the junction of the body with the pyloric mucosa the transition to the normal thickness of the stomach wall is usually abrupt. Microscopically, in the mucosa of the fundus and body of the stomach all that remain are the surface epithelium and a few scattered glands lined by mucus-producing cells. The specialized oxyntic and peptic cells are not seen. At the same time there is no fibrosis, cellular infiltration or other evidence of past inflammation. The muscle coat likewise shows atrophy. No evidence of a reduction in the number of argentaffin cells, at one time proposed as the source of

intrinsic factor,[57] has been found.[72,271b] No regeneration of the mucosa follows intensive therapy.[72,253a]

Gastric biopsy has shown mucosal atrophy, usually complete, often with a moderate degree of infiltration with inflammatory cells.[121] No lesions pathognomonic of pernicious anemia were noted.

The examination of cells obtained from the stomach by gastric lavage and abrasion has revealed groups of columnar cells which differ from normal ones chiefly in size.[73] Approximately twice normal in size, their nuclear membrane may be creased or folded in appearance and small aggregates of chromatin stand out on the relatively empty background of the nucleus. The cytoplasm, as well as the nucleus, is enlarged and has a more vacuolated and granular appearance than is normal (Fig. 10–9). The nuclei of cells from the buccal mucosa show similar enlargement.[16c]

Changes in the central nervous system

vary in extent. Myelin degeneration and loss of nerve fibers in the dorsal and lateral tracts of the cord, and degenerative changes in the dorsal root ganglia are commonly found. Following liver therapy an increase in gliosis has been reported.[27] Degenerate changes are not infrequent in peripheral nerves[44,48,114] and degeneration of the celiac ganglia, Auerbach's and Meissner's plexuses as well as lesions in the lateral horns of the spinal cord have been described.[19] Changes similar to those found in the spinal cord have been observed in the brain.[56a] The rarity of optic atrophy has been mentioned.[65] Changes in other cranial nerves have not been described.

SPRUE, IDIOPATHIC STEATORRHEA AND CELIAC DISEASE

Next to pernicious anemia, sprue is the most common condition in which macrocytic megaloblastic anemia is encountered. It will be convenient to discuss at the same time two other conditions in which macrocytic anemia may occur, namely, idiopathic steatorrhea, a disease found in non-tropical countries, and celiac disease, an affection of infants and children.

Definitions, Synonyms and History.—The term sprue originally referred to a chronic, wasting disorder which occurs in tropical countries and is characterized by glossitis, diarrhea, and the passage of light-colored, bulky and frothy stools. This condition was first described in 1669 by Vincent Ketelaer and later by William Hillary in Barbados in 1759,[157] but for many years it was confused with dysentery and other intestinal affections. Many names have been given the disease, including Indische Spruw (Dutch), Psilosis (British), Aphthae tropicae, and Tisis intestinal. Sir Patrick Manson, in 1880, published a clear description and suggested the present name.

A condition similar to sprue occurs in individuals who have never been to the tropics. This fact, as well as the relationship of sprue, idiopathic steatorrhea, and celiac disease, has been emphasized by the work of many recent investigators, but it is noteworthy that descriptions of non-tropical disorders resembling sprue can be found in the writings of Gee[137a] ("The Coeliac Affection," 1888) and Herter (1908) ("Gee-Herter disease"). The term "idiopathic steatorrhea" is used synonymously with "non-tropical sprue" and is qualified in order to distinguish the condition from steatorrhea resulting from insufficiency of pancreatic or biliary secretions, or other causes.[160] In addition to symptoms characteristic of tropical sprue, tetany due to calcium deficiency, as well as osteoporosis and osteomalacia, are often found in idiopathic steatorrhea.

Celiac disease is the name given to a similar disorder occurring in infants.[125c, 134d] In all of these diseases anemia is found frequently.

Etiology. — Geographic Distribution and Climate.—Sprue is endemic in the Far East, India[127b] and the Caribbean area.[137] However, the distribution of the disease is curious. It is rarely seen in Africa or in Brazil and, while common in Hong Kong it is rare in Singapore. Again, although common in Puerto Rico and Cuba it is not observed in Jamaica. In the United States, it was common in the South.

The non-tropical disorder is well known in the British Isles and a large number of cases were studied there during World War II.[134b] A large number of cases have been reported from the Scandinavian countries and Switzerland and it is seen in the United States but no useful comparative statistical data are available.

Race.—It has been observed frequently that European personnel moving to endemic zones are likely to develop sprue. The same was noted in American military personnel in Puerto Rico.[137] Yet sprue was not a problem among the prisoners of war in Japanese camps. Sprue seems to be rare in full-blooded Negroes or in Chinese. In a series of 100 cases in Puerto Rico, 87 were white and 13 colored, two being "full-blooded" Negroes. All but two were natives of the island.[155]

Age.—The tropical condition occurs at all ages. The non-tropical disorder has been called celiac disease when occurring in the first few years of life. The onset of celiac disease is between six and twenty-one months of age, and even earlier.[125c,140] "Idiopathic steatorrhea" is found in adolescents and adults. In many instances, however, it is apparent that symptoms suggestive of the disorder commenced in early childhood.[133b]

Sex.—The disease, as recorded, is slightly more common in females than males.

Heredity. Familial Predisposition.—A few instances of celiac disease[125c] and idiopathic steatorrhea in the same family have been recorded from time to time.[142] In the United Kingdom, two or more relatives were found to be affected in a number of instances but no evidence was obtained to indicate whether the cause was environmental or genetic.[133b,134b]

Personal Factors. Individual Susceptibility.—In Puerto Rico, Ashford observed that sprue was more common among the well-to-do than among the poor[126] and was much more often seen in the cities and towns than in rural districts. He noted the condition in northerners who lived on canned foods, and sweets, in those whose life was a sedentary one and in persons of a "naturally weak constitution." The cases studied by Rodriguez-Molina,[155] on the other hand, were of the indigent or underprivileged class with very few exceptions.

Association With Other Diseases.—In the tropics the disease is often associated with dysentery, malaria, chronic alcoholism, and various chronic infections. In Italian prisoners of war, many of whom developed sprue in a camp in South-East India, *dietary deficiency*, especially a lack of animal protein, appeared to be a significant factor in the pathogenesis of the disorder, in addition to climatic and seasonal factors.[158] However, this could not be said of the American military personnel in Puerto Rico.[137]

Symptomatology.—Mode of Onset.—This varies greatly. In some cases of sprue the onset may be relatively sudden with diarrhea and rapidly developing loss of weight and strength, palpitation, pallor and exhaustion. In troops in India, sudden onset of diarrhea was common and this was accompanied by extreme asthenia and meteorism.[158] In other instances, fatigue and asthenia may be the initial complaints and there may be no diarrhea but the passage of one or two daily large bulky stools. Such symptoms may be intermittent and remissions may occur. This "early phase" [137,158] is followed by a second stage or "deficiency phase" which develops when the prolonged small bowel malabsorption has resulted in depletion of nutrients. Weight loss, glossitis, stomatitis, cheilosis and hyperkeratosis are superimposed, in varying degrees, on the asthenia resulting from the depletion of sodium and cellular potassium which characterize the first stage. Iron deficiency may develop.[127] Finally, in the third stage, with progression of defective vitamin absorption the bone marrow becomes megaloblastic and the picture of the disease is fully developed.

In idiopathic steatorrhea, on the other hand, there is often a period of months or years of "chronic indigestion," flatulence, excess of intestinal gas, constipation with occasional loose bowels, anorexia, usual sensitivity of the tongue, loss of weight and strength, increasing psychic

Table 10–1—Diagrammatic Representation of Frequency of Various Symptoms in Pernicious Anemia, Nutritional Macrocytic Anemia, Sprue, Idiopathic Steatorrhea and Celiac Disease

	Pernicious anemia	Nutritional macrocytic anemia	Sprue	Idiopathic steatorrhea	Celiac disease
Psychoses	+	++	..	..	..
Neurologic involvement	++	+	+	..	..
Absence of intrinsic factor	+++	+	+	..	..
Achlorhydria	+++	++	+	+	..
Macrocytic anemia	+++	+++	++	+	..
Glossitis	++	+++	+++	+	..
Esophagitis, proctitis, vaginitis	..	+++	+++	+	..
Diarrhea	+	++	+++	++	++
Weight loss	+	++	+++	+++	+++
Skin changes (pigmentation, etc.)	+	+++	++	++	++
Anasarca	+	+	+	+	++
Steatorrhea	..	+	+++	+++	+++
Abdominal distention and dilatation of colon	..	+	+++	+++	+++
Flat blood sugar curve	..	..	++	+++	+++
Low serum Ca++ and tetany	..	..	+	+++	+++
Hypochromic anemia	..	++	+	++	+++
Onset in childhood	..	..	+	++	+++
Bone deformities	..	..	..	+++	+++
Infantilism	..	..	..	+++	+++
Erythroblastic anemia	..	..	..	+	+

depression, and nervous irritability and asthenia. The tongue may become sore and there may be a sense of irritation in the esophagus or rectum. Diarrhea may not occur but calcium deficiency, produced by calcium lost with the excessive amounts of fat passed in the stool, may cause bone pains and deformities which thus become the initial complaints; or the symptoms of tetany may be the first to attract serious attention.

Comparison of Clinical Picture With That of Pernicious Anemia.— In pernicious anemia, nutritional macrocytic anemia, sprue, idiopathic steatorrhea and celiac disease, certain symptoms are encountered which are common to all these disorders.[126,140] When the various forms in which each condition may be encountered are considered, it is evident that the clinical picture of one shades off to the other, the chief difference being one of emphasis on one symptom or group of complaints, or on another.

If the symptoms and signs which are found in these disorders are tabulated (Table 10–1), the relation between these variations of the clinical picture can be appreciated. At one extreme there is the well-preserved person of middle age or older with little or no anemia suffering from the effects of degeneration in the spinal cord; at the other is the thin, pale infant, a skeleton but for the distended abdomen, who passes frequent voluminous stools. Between these widely different clinical pictures can be set cases with less of one complaint and more of another which seem to link the two extremes. Cases of pernicious anemia are seen in which the glossitis and diarrhea are so prominent that the differentiation from sprue is difficult if not impossible. Examples of tropical sprue are found in which some degree of mineral deficiency has developed. Many instances of idiopathic steatorrhea in adults

32

are found on inquiry to have had their beginnings in childhood.

Alimentary System.—In sprue the chief complaints are referable to this system. The appearance of small aphthae in the **buccal cavity** or on the tip and edges of the tongue is followed by a reddening of the entire tongue. In early sprue, a "strawberry" appearance of the tongue may be produced by the general reddening and the swelling of some papillae at the same time as there is atrophy of others. The lingual symptoms characteristically recede and recrudesce, leaving eventually the total papillary atrophy of the advanced condition. At the same time there may be painful deglutition, burning in the rectum and anus, and even in the vagina, due to involvement of these parts. Cheilitis is rather uncommon.[155]

In the majority of cases of sprue, diarrhea is the most prominent symptom. There may be as many as 30 or more stools in twenty-four hours.[126] In some instances diarrhea may be intermittent with variable periods of constipation. Constipation without diarrhea was present in 5 out of 100 cases in Puerto Rico.[155] Abdominal distention, epigastric distress and heartburn are common complaints. Abdominal discomfort and pain following ingestion of food are often found and carbohydrate and fat intolerance are characteristic symptoms. Starchy and sweet foods, mistakenly regarded as "bland," merely aggravate the abdominal distress and diarrhea. Anorexia may be present or there is fear of eating because of the bowel movements which follow. As a rule there is no tenesmus, or blood or mucus in the stools but these features may be encountered in otherwise typical cases.[155]

In the non-tropical disorders, the symptoms may be like those above described but generally the glossitis is not so severe, or may be absent, and diarrhea may not be so pronounced. In those cases in which there are few bowel movements or only one bulky, pale stool each day, a history of recurrent diarrhea is usually obtainable and on roentgenologic examination a megacolon is found.

Roentgenographic examination of the intestines reveals a characteristic picture. There is a striking variation in the caliber and contour of the intestinal lumen and a distortion of the mucosal pattern. Instead of the normal delicate feathery appearance produced by the valvulae conniventes in the distal duodenum and upper half of the jejunum there is a coarser outline (Fig. 10–10). If the condition is severe the obliteration of the valvulae conniventes may be so complete that the roentgen appearance of the bowel "resembles a tube into which wax has been poured and allowed to harden" ("moulage sign").[143] The small intestine may be dilated to such a degree that the diameter is almost as great as that of the large bowel. This is usually most prominent in the mid- and distal jejunum.[146a] Segmentation occurs, probably as the result of irregularity of movement, with the production of smooth, sausage-like areas. The long, barium-filled loops of ileum are characteristically divided, instead of continuous. These changes in the small intestine are best brought out by giving two to four ounces of barium sulfate to the fasting patient. Roentgenograms are then taken every hour until the head of the barium meal has reached the colon. Dilatation of the colon is often present, especially in idiopathic steatorrhea, but this will not be demonstrated unless large amounts of opaque medium are given.[146]

It has been suggested that the segmentation pattern of the small intestine is the result of nutritional deficiency or disordered motor function. In regard to the latter, it is noteworthy that records of the small intestinal motor activity, made with small balloons, showed the bowel to lack the usual resistance to

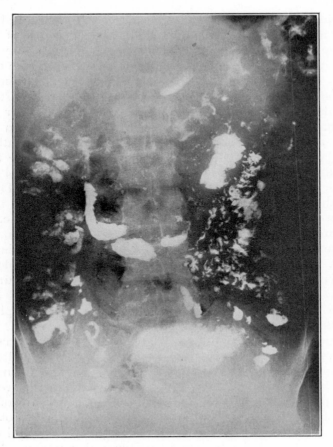

Fig. 10–10.—Roentgenogram showing gastrointestinal tract in a case of sprue two hours following a barium meal. The stomach is almost completely empty. The barium is distributed throughout the small intestine and has reached as far as the splenic flexure of the large intestine. The small bowel shows the characteristic "moulage" sign. The pattern of an irritative lesion in the jejunum is shown by the many small irregular collections of barium on the left side of the abdomen.

distention exhibited by the normal intestine.[142a] Since injections of acetyl-beta-methylcholine chloride stimulated the intestinal motility whereas prostigmine was without effect, it was suggested that the primary defect in sprue is the inability of the intestinal autonomic nervous system to liberate acetylcholine. However, it has been shown[136b] that the segmental pattern can be induced in normal individuals by the addition of fatty acids or hypertonic solutions to the barium suspension and that the latter is flocculated by mucous secretions. Thus, the segmentation pattern is not necessarily an index of vitamin deficiencies or disturbed motor function.

Skeletal System.—Skeletal abnormalities are common in idiopathic steatorrhea and in celiac disease. These include osteoporosis,[133b] infantilism and stunting of growth, scurvy,[140] spontaneous fractures and skeletal deformities (genu valgum, genu varum, bending and bowing of bones, beading of ribs, bossing of wrists and ankles, clubbing of fingers and toes, pelvic deformities). Stunting of growth is common in tropical sprue when it begins in childhood and scoliosis and kyphosis are found in adults, but the severe deformities found in the non-tropical disorders are unusual. There may be vague pains in the bones and joints.

Nervous System.—Nervous instability and irritability, mental depression, and asthenia have been mentioned already. These symptoms are found in the tropical as well as the non-tropical forms of the disorder and occur at all ages. In sprue tetanoid contraction of the muscles of the leg or forearm is found and in the non-tropical groups of cases true tetany, latent or manifest, is frequently found and may be the presenting complaint. A history of attacks of cramps or muscular spasm may be given. In such cases positive Chvostek and Trousseau signs may be found.

There may be numbness and tingling in the extremities or neuritic manifestations[161] but spinal cord involvement of the type encountered in pernicious anemia is rare.[142]

Outward Appearance of the Patient.—In the fully developed condition the clinical picture is characteristic. There is striking emaciation which the distended abdomen makes all the more apparent. As much as 50 per cent of the body weight may have been lost. Pallor is usual and the skin is dry and inelastic. Brownish pigmentation may be generalized and may closely resemble that of Addison's disease, or it may be irregular in distribution.[133b] Together with roughening of the skin it is likely to be found on the forehead, cheeks, neck, the extensor surface of the forearms and the anterior surface of the legs. The skin may become parchment-like and there may be a scaly and eczematoid eruption but the erythema and ulceration of pellagra are unusual.[155] The nails may be brittle and spoonshaped. Clubbing of the fingers of various degrees has been observed both in idiopathic steatorrhea[133b]

and in celiac disease.[140] The hair is lusterless. In advanced cases petechiae and even bleeding of the gums and extensive purpura may develop. The facial expression of the child with celiac disease has been described as "mournful, querulous and pessimistic." The child appears much younger than his stated age and this is often true of adults suffering from idiopathic steatorrhea. The appearance of the tongue has been described already (p. 498) and so have the bone deformities. There is no general glandular enlargement nor is the spleen or liver usually palpable. The distended bowel may be easily made out through the atrophied abdominal musculature. Peristalsis may be visible. Ascites is uncommon but may occur.[140] A number of authors have called attention to the marked degree of atrophy of the gluteal muscles which is to be found.[140,142] Hypogenitalism may occur. The lower extremities may be edematous. Hypotension is a frequent finding.

Lenticular opacities were demonstrated by the slit lamp in 6 of the 15 cases of idiopathic steatorrhea of Bennett et al.[130] These opacities resembled those found in postoperative tetany. Moderate remittent fever may be present.

Laboratory Findings.—The Blood and Bone Marrow.—In *tropical sprue* macrocytic anemia is usually found[123] but sometimes it is hypochromic microcytic in type[132] and rarely it is normocytic[155] or is absent altogether. The macrocytic anemia is identical with that found in pernicious anemia and is often accompanied by leukopenia and relative lymphocytosis, as well as by changes in the bone marrow[142] resembling those described in the section on pernicious anemia. Alterations in erythrokinetics[156c] are similar to those found in pernicious anemia (p. 482). Macropolycytes and giant metamyelocytes with broad, tortuous, vacuolated nuclei like those seen in pernicious anemia have been observed.

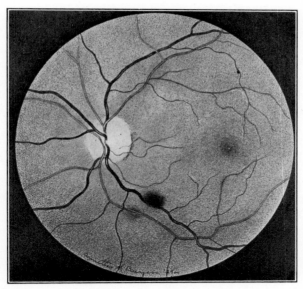

Fig. 10–11.—Hemorrhages in the fundus oculi in a case of very severe macrocytic anemia with thrombocytopenia. There was a multiple nutritional deficiency and tetany as well as temporary achlorhydria. Prompt improvement followed parenternal liver therapy. (Photograph by courtesy of Dr. Alan C. Woods.)

The hypochromic microcytic anemia is the same as that which will be described under that heading (Chapter 14).

In *idiopathic steatorrhea*[133b] and in *celiac disease*,[140] severe degrees of anemia are less common than in pernicious anemia. The anemia may be macrocytic (Fig. 10–12), normocytic or hypochromic microcytic. In idiopathic steatorrhea macrocytic anemia is more common than hypochromic microcytic anemia; in celiac disease the reverse is the case. In these two disorders, and particularly in celiac disease, the anemia may be associated with the presence in the blood of great numbers of normoblasts ("erythroblastic anemia"[130]). When the anemia is macrocytic, the bone marrow is usually megaloblastic;[133b] when it is hypochromic microcytic, there is a striking preponderance of normoblasts.[142b] When the mean corpuscular volume is normal, the bone marrow picture may be mixed.

Deficiencies of iron in addition to folic acid and vitamin B_{12} are more often encountered in sprue and in the non-tropical steatorrheas than in pernicious anemia. As a result, macrocytosis is common and there may be extreme variability in the size and coloring of the red corpuscles; yet the mean corpuscular volume may be essentially normal. In these cases of mixed anemia, as relapse occurs a hypochromic microcytic anemia may change to a macrocytic form, or well-marked microcytosis may develop as macrocytic anemia is relieved by appropriate therapy.

It has been stated that aplastic and hypoplastic anemia which fails to respond to any form of treatment may be found in sprue. Just as an "aplastic stage" seems to be more hypothetical than real in pernicious anemia, so it probably is in sprue. With the development of liver extracts for parenteral use and with better knowledge regarding the rôle of infections and other conditions inhibiting the therapeutic response, it became apparent that in most instances at least,

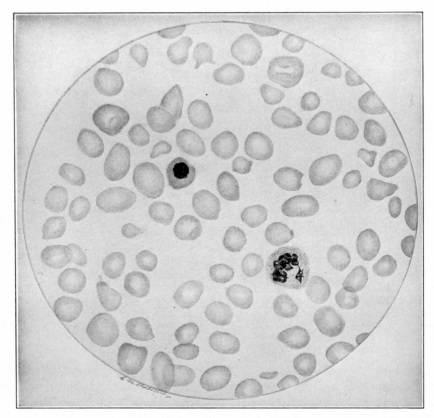

FIG. 10–12.—Blood smear from a case of idiopathic steatorrhea (non-tropical sprue) with macrocytic anemia. In the field is a macroblast and a macropolycyte (multilobed neutrophil).

failure to respond was not due to a lack of active marrow. Early reports describing fatty marrow in this disease can be accounted for by the fact that the marrow of long bones was examined rather than locations such as the sternum where active marrow is to be found.[152]

When there is severe folic acid or vitamin B[12] deficiency, some *thrombocytopenia* may be encountered. *Hemorrhagic manifestations* occurring in the skin and in the urinary and intestinal tracts[133b] may, however, be related to associated ascorbic acid[142] or to vitamin K deficiency.[129,144]

The **icterus index** may be increased,[133a] normal or low.[132] In tropical sprue it may be elevated, as in pernicious anemia. In idiopathic steatorrhea it is usually normal. When the anemia is hypochromic and microcytic the icterus index may be actually reduced below normal. The **fragility** of the red corpuscles to hypotonic saline solutions is normal, or decreased.[133a]

Gastrointestinal Secretions and Stool. — Free hydrochloric acid is more often present than absent (82 per cent in one series,[155] 69 per cent in another,[132] examined after histamine injection) and, if absent, may return[130] during treatment. In a few cases clinically suggestive of sprue, "intrinsic factor" could not be demonstrated in the gastric secretion. Such cases emphasize the difficulty of sharply differentiating some cases of sprue and pernicious anemia. The pepsin content of the gastric juice in general parallels the content of free hydrochloric acid.[132]

Of 11 children with celiac disease who were examined, 4 were found to have achlorhydria.[140]

Pancreatic and biliary secretion is normal[132b,157] or only slightly reduced[126] in the tropical and non-tropical forms of sprue and this finding serves to differentiate these conditions from steatorrhea resulting from a deficiency or lack of such secretions.

The **stools** may be soft, mushy or watery and are characteristically voluminous and light in color, grayish-white or bright yellow. Rodriguez-Molina[155] found, however, in his series of cases in Puerto Rico, that the stools were often small in size and light yellow, golden or brown in color. They contained variable amounts of foam. A sickening, sour-sweetish pungent odor is characteristic. The frothy character of the stool of tropical sprue is usually absent in the non-tropical conditions. Blood and mucus are usually absent. There is an excess of fat which, unlike that in pancreatogenous diarrhea, is chiefly in the form of needles of fatty acids rather than neutral fat.

No characteristic abnormalities have been described in the **urine.** There may be some increased excretion of urobilinogen and urobilin but this is rarely of the degree seen in pernicious anemia.

Absorption of Foodstuffs, Vitamins and Minerals, Tolerance Tests. —The **fat** content of the stool varies considerably but it is always excessive except in some patients in the early phase of tropical sprue[137] or when the fat content of the diet is greatly reduced.[129] Fatty acids make up the major portion of the fatty substance of the stool and long-chain, saturated fatty acids, such as those of mutton or beef fat, are tolerated especially poorly. Volatile, short-chain fatty acids are also increased in the stool.

Microscopic examination of the feces is an unreliable method of detecting the *abnormal fat absorption.* This is best demonstrated by chemical examination of the stools of subjects receiving a measured quantity of dietary fat over a period of five to twelve days, the periods being marked by feeding charcoal or carmine at their beginning and end.[135b] Normally 95 per cent of the dietary fat is absorbed. In sprue only 50 to 85 per cent is absorbed.[129,136] The absorption of fat can also be measured by determining the radioactivity in blood and feces following the administration of a test dose of I^{131}-labelled fat (triolein).[139,143a, 145a] The defect remains the same in degree even when the quantity of fat in the diet is substantially increased.

The administration of a fat meal is not followed by a normal rise in the blood fat curve but a flat curve is obtained instead,[128] and there is no increase in the number of chylomicrons in the blood.[136] Neither does the plasma vitamin A rise as in normals when patients with steatorrhea are given unemulsified vitamin A [135c,147] and the same is true in regard to plasma tocopherol levels.[134a] Low values for fasting serum carotenoids due to nutritional deficiency can be differentiated from those attributable to faulty absorption by failure of the blood levels to rise when carotene-in-oil is given.[100a]

The *serum choleserol* is usually reduced[136,157] as is the blood phospholipid.

By passing a Miller-Abbott tube into the small intestine and examining samples of intestinal contents before and after the administration of fat, it has been possible to show that hydrolysis and initial emulsification in the upper part of the small intestine are within normal limits.[136] All the usual enzymes are present in approximately normal concentrations but exceptionally large numbers of bacteria are found in the upper intestine.

The glucose tolerance test is an unreliable measure of the impairment in *absorption of* **carbohydrates**.[137] Much better is the five-hour measurement of blood levels and urinary excretion following a 25 Gm. oral dose of *d-xylose*.[53,135a] In the absence of renal disease, this procedure is considered to provide the best "screening" test for small bowel absorption now available.[137] In patients with pancreatic disease the xylose test is normal although fat absorption may be abnormal. In idiopathic steatorrhea it is consistently abnormal.[133]

In cases with severe cachexia the *plasma* **proteins** are usually decreased and the albumin-globulin ratio is reversed.[157] Fecal losses of *nitrogen* may be excessive in idiopathic steatorrhea but positive nitrogen balance can be maintained by a high intake of nitrogen except during acute exacerbations.[133a] Glycine absorption from the gastrointestinal tract has been found to be delayed[31] and evidence of deranged tyrosine metabolism together with ascorbic acid inadequacy has been presented.[130a] There is some evidence of an abnormality in sprue of the enzyme which converts to glutamic acid formimino glutamic acid (FIGLU), a compound which has been found in the urine of folic acid deficient animals and of humans receiving folic acid antagonists.[131]

The *folic acid* excretion test, which consists of the intramuscular injection of sufficient folic acid to saturate tissue stores and the administration 48 hours later of an oral dose of 5 mg., has provided evidence of impaired absorption of folic acid in sprue[137] and in idiopathic steatorrhea.[134] In many cases the absorption of *vitamin B_{12}* is also impaired.[150a] In one series of non-tropical cases of malabsorption of the sprue type, folic acid absorption was found to be impaired in 83 per cent of the cases and cyanocobalamin absorption was impaired in 40 per cent[134c]

Depletion of *sodium, potassium* and water of some degree occurs in all cases and an increase of bowel movements may result in critical losses. *Hypokaliemia* of moderate degree may be associated with loss of weight, weakness, "heaviness" of the limbs and mental apathy; in more severe cases hypotension, absence of reflexes, profound muscle weakness, abdominal distention, vomiting and personality changes have been described.[133b]

As already stated, the absorption of *iron* is impaired.[127]

Calcium deficiency, ranging from a slight lowering of the serum calcium to marked deficiency with osteoporosis and severe tetany, is found in idiopathic steatorrhea and in celiac disease and, rarely, in tropical sprue. The serum calcium is usually 8 to 10 mg. per 100 ml. but may be as low as 5 or even 4 mg.[140] Plasma *phosphorus* is more variable and is often somewhat low (below 3.5 mg. per cent) but has been recorded above 5 mg. per cent. In idiopathic steatorrhea the alkaline *phosphatase* is usually normal[157] but may be increased.[130] In celiac disease it has been found low. Calcium balance studies have shown an increased calcium output in the stool[133a] and low[140] urinary output. The *hypocalcemia* has been attributed to two factors; namely, impaired absorption of vitamin D with secondary failure to absorb calcium and, in addition, combination of calcium with unabsorbed fatty acids in the alimentary tract to form soaps, thus preventing its absorption.[127a,129]

Diagnosis. — In the early stages, tropical sprue is likely to be mistaken for some form of dysentery if diarrhea is prominent, or it may be attributed to food intolerance or functional disorders of one kind or another. In the sprue syndromes abdominal distention out of proportion to tympany and without a fluid wave or shifting dullness is found; in functional disorders, if abdominal distention occurs the tympany is usually striking.[148]

Early diagnosis and prompt treatment are important since the pathological process in sprue can be reversed if recognized early.[137] Idiopathic steatorrhea or celiac disease are more likely than sprue to be misdiagnosed for a long time since diarrhea may not be prominent or may be totally absent.[142] Steatorrhea is suggested by the passage of voluminous stools and may be suspected if signs of calcium deficiency are present. All three of these disorders are ultimately accompanied by more or less pronounced signs of nutritional deficiency, such as muscle wasting, glossitis, cheilitis,[132a] macrocytic or hypochromic microcytic anemia and purpuric manifestations. Xerophthalmia and disturbance of vision due to vitamin A deficiency have been described.[134c,154] Lack of vitamin D probably plays a role in the osteoporosis which develops in nontropical sprue.[129] Bleeding may be the result of vitamin K deficiency[129,144] and purpura may be a manifestation of scurvy.[142] Of the various tests, mentioned above which have been used to demonstrate malabsorption, the excretion of d-xylose, the daily fecal fat excretion and the absorption of vitamin A are among the most useful. From one case to another, however, some variation in the results of various absorption tests can be expected.

Obviously, it is always necessary to exclude various conditions which may produce symptoms and signs like those found in sprue, idiopathic steatorrhea or celiac disease.[160] If diarrhea is prominent, that caused by bacterial or protozoal agents or by malignancy must be ruled out. The lack of such symptoms as fever, pain, tenesmus and small frequent stools and the absence of blood, mucus or pathogenic agents in the stool, favor sprue, idiopathic steatorrhea or celiac disease.

Roentgenographic and proctoscopic examinations will help to rule out such causes of steatorrhea as metastatic malig-

nancy in the retro-peritoneal nodes, carcinoma of the pancreas, and stone or tumor of Wirsung's duct, all of which conditions may interfere with pancreatic function. In pancreatogenous steatorrhea the stool contains neutral fats rather than fatty acids and fecal nitrogen loss is usually much greater than in the idiopathic form.[135b]

A syndrome closely simulating sprue or idiopathic steatorrhea may be produced by lymphosarcoma,[159] reticulum cell sarcoma, lymphogranulomatosis and other diseases involving the small intestine[160] and has been observed in association with ulcerogenic tumor of the pancreas,[149] functioning islet-cell adenoma of the pancreas[156a] and thrombosis of the mesenteric arteries.[156b] Intestinal strictures and resection, anastomoses and gastro-jejuno-colic fistulas may be associated with macrocytic anemia and a clinical picture identical with that of sprue (p. 515).

A rare disorder which closely simulates sprue is *intestinal lipodystrophy* or Whipple's disease,[135,138] a condition characterized by the presence of Schiff-positive macrophages in the mesenteric and, occasionally, peripheral lymph nodes. Antecedent polyarthralgia, generalized lymphadenopathy, sometimes a febrile course and signs of malabsorption suggest such conditions as idiopathic steatorrhea, lymphoma, sarcoidosis and Addison's disease. The condition has been seen most often in middle-aged men. An upper abdominal mass may be felt and there may be radiological evidence of gastric or duodenal displacement.

Addison's disease may be suggested by the asthenia, hypotension and pigmentation seen in sprue and in idiopathic steatorrhea. Still other disorders may be suggested by various other manifestations, especially if the intestinal complaints are not prominent.

As discussed earlier (p. 497), the differentiation of sprue and pernicious anemia is sometimes difficult. The absence of free hydrochloric acid and the presence of neurological involvement favor pernicious anemia. Reduced excretion of radioactive vitamin B_{12} (p. 490) which is not enhanced by intrinsic factor has been observed in sprue.[151] Differentiation is important since folic acid is so valuable in sprue but may be harmful in pernicious anemia.

The sprue syndromes themselves should be differentiated. In tropical sprue folic acid is an extremely important remedy and recovery is frequent, especially on return to a temperate climate. Idiopathic steatorrhea and celiac disease are not as consistently responsive to such therapy and long term dietetic management is usually required. Further, some patients do well on a gluten-free diet whereas others respond well to antibiotics (see p. 528).

Treatment.—Folic acid was found to be the treatment of choice for tropical sprue in Puerto Rico.[137] The beneficial effect was manifested at all stages and controlled diarrhea as well as anemia. In earlier stages the oral tolerance tests, dietary fat balance and X-ray pattern of the bowel returned to normal. Only in the late stage was the impaired intestinal absorption irreversible. Usually 5 mg. folic acid thrice daily for a week followed by 5 mg. daily thereafter was used. These observations are consistent with the practice of native doctors in Ceylon who for centuries used liver soup successfully in the treatment of sprue.

The experience elsewhere has, in general, been similar,[158] folic acid having a beneficial effect even in the absence of anemia. In southern India, however, results have not been so fortunate, folic acid or vitamin B_{12} being helpful only in the relief of macrocytic anemia.[127b] This may be explained, perhaps, on the ground of different degrees and greater duration of the pathological process. The Indian experience more nearly approaches

the course of non-tropical, idiopathic steatorrhea which is a much more chronic disorder than may be the case in many instances of sprue.

The sprue syndromes have been classified according to therapeutic response to include (1) cases responding dramatically to folic acid, like those in Puerto Rico;[137] (2) those responding to a gluten-free diet; and (3) those helped by treatment with sulfonamides and antibiotics.[136a] The cases responding to chemotherapy have usually been examples of tropical sprue[136c] but, no doubt, active growth of intestinal flora may be responsible for many of the characteristics of the steatorrheic stool and their elimination for a time might be expected to be helpful. Some patients seem to have been cured by chemotherapy.[136c]

The group of patients who appear to be sensitive to wheat gluten differ from the rest. All symptoms disappear on a gluten-free regimen but relapse occurs when wheat gluten is given again.[136c] Such patients must be maintained on an appropriate dietary regimen.[150] They include most cases of celiac disease and many instances of idiopathic steatorrhea in adults.[137b]

Diet for the sprue patient must be low in fat and high in proteins and minerals. Intolerance for starches and sweets may be as great as for fats. Sugar and anything that may contain it, such as preserved and sweetened canned fruits, raisins, dried prunes, chocolate, and soft drinks, as well as cereals and starchy foods, such as bread, cakes, biscuits, crackers, pastry, rice, corn flakes, potatoes, and beans, must be avoided. Sweetening should be done with saccharin instead of sugar. Since the carbohydrate intolerance is often limited to the polysaccharides, monosaccharides such as glucose may be allowed. Likewise, vegetable oil such as olive oil may be tolerated when fats of animal origin cause diarrhea. The absorption of food lipids may be enhanced by the use of emulsifying agents.[142d,147]

Additions to the diet should be made cautiously and only one at a time and in small amounts. As the patient's condition permits, various meats, eggs (especially the whites of eggs), cottage cheese, fresh fruit and finally vegetables may be allowed. Meals should be small and frequent. Meats must be lean. Chicken, liver and fresh fish may be taken. These should be boiled, broiled, baked or roasted but not fried. Fruits which are well tolerated include bananas, strawberries and apples. Apple juice, orange juice and tomato juice may be given. Vegetables should be baked or boiled at first but later salads should be eaten in abundance. Hot bouillon or skimmed chicken broth, gelatin (Jell-O), tea and coffee may be taken. Lard, mayonnaise and ice cream are prohibited. Fruit ices and sherbets, plain cake and cookies, puddings made of skimmed milk, butter, American cheese and even candy may be tolerated in time. White bread, rice, sugar, ice cream, nuts, pies, pastries, pancakes, waffles or grease may cause a recurrence of diarrhea.

Treatment must, in essence, be tailored to the individual patient. It is rarely necessary to use measures directed specifically to the control of diarrhea, such as bismuth subnitrate (8 Gm. several times a day) or paregoric (4 ml. after every two bowel movements). In severe cachexia prolonged parenteral supplementation may be necessary. Skimmed milk, ground meat and bananas to the exclusion of every other food may be necessary for a time. If calories are badly needed, fats may be given more liberally than they would otherwise since a larger amount of dietary fat yields greater net absorption of fat than would a low fat intake.

To protect the patient with chronic steatorrhea from hypoprothrombinemia, daily oral water-soluble vitamin K de-rivatives are required, such as menadione, 5 to 10 mg. Other vitamins should be given if a liberal, well-rounded diet cannot be taken.

To protect against osteomalacia calcium lactate or calcium gluconate, 5 to 15 Gm. daily, should be given as well as vitamin D (25,000 to 600,000 units daily by mouth). The appearance of tetany will require intravenous administration of calcium gluconate.

When iron deficiency is present, *iron* should be prescribed (p. 457). It is only rarely necessary to resort to parenteral therapy.[127]

As the result of therapy, weight may be gained at a rate which is surprising in view of the restriction of carbohydrate and fats. However, blood regeneration may not be as rapid as in pernicious anemia[132] and improvement in fat absorption usually is less marked in idiopathic steatorrhea[130] and in celiac disease than in tropical sprue.[128]

In very acute or resistant chronic states the administration of steroid drugs may be very valuable[145] and occasionally produces dramatic results.[160]

Prognosis and Maintenance Therapy.—In tropical sprue complete recovery has been described in 70 per cent[137] or more[158] of cases. In some cases,[127b] however, and in essentially all cases of idiopathic steatorrhea and celiac disease,[125c] recovery is incomplete even though symptoms may subside. In celiac disease the maintenance of a diet free of wheat gluten until full maturity seems desirable. In idiopathic steatorrhea some permanent degree of dietary restriction is often necessary[137b] although folic acid therapy now permits much greater dietary liberties than was once possible.

Pathology.—In patients dying in relapse there is striking absence of fat throughout the body, the tongue is atrophic and the bone marrow is hyperplastic.[152] There may be fatty degenera-

developing during pregnancy and the puerperium which are distinct from the common, "physiological" anemia of pregnancy (p. 575) and simple hypochromic, microcytic anemia due to iron deficiency (p. 734). The condition has been observed most frequently in women of the poorer economic level whose diet has been deficient;[172,181c] yet it has been encountered sufficiently often in well-to-do women whose diet seemed to be satisfactory to raise doubt as to its dietary origin.[181b] Affected women have been under thirty-five years of age, as a rule, more often multiparae than primiparae. The onset is most often in the third trimester of pregnancy and may be insidious or sudden. In addition to symptoms of anemia, gastro-intestinal complaints such as vomiting and diarrhea may be prominent and the tongue may be sore.[199a] Fever is common. In a certain number of cases infections or toxemia are found, appearing to precipitate the development of the severe anemia.[172] Slight edema is common; occasionally it is marked. In other cases the predominating symptoms were those of pre-eclamptic toxemia: edema, hypertension and albuminuria.[216a] The spleen has been palpable in about a third of the reported cases and the liver is sometimes enlarged. Purpura may occasionally develop as well as hemorrhages from mucous membranes.

The blood picture may be quite similar to that found in Addisonian pernicious anemia but it has been emphasized that this is frequently not the case.[233b] There may be little variation in the size or shape of the red corpuscles and the Price-Jones curve may not have a broad base and be shifted to the right as occurs in pernicious anemia.[172] The mean corpuscular volume may be greatly increased or it may be normal and in certain cases the anemia has been microcytic and hypochromic.[216a] There may or may not be an increase in reticulocytes but,

generally, nucleated red cells, identified as megaloblasts,[172] are found in the peripheral blood if the anemia is severe. The leukocyte count is also very variable, values from 1000 to 12,000 per c.mm., and much higher figures, having been recorded. Leukopenia is more frequent than leukocytosis, however. Often a few immature forms are found, as well as multi-segmented neutrophils. Some thrombocytopenia may be present.

In spite of the variability of the peripheral blood picture, that of the marrow appears to be consistent in that a megaloblastic hyperplasia like that seen in pernicious anemia is found.[172] A normoblastic reaction may co-exist, however, side by side with the megaloblastic picture. Pathological leukocytes resembling those seen in the bone marrow of pernicious anemia are also found.[199a] The changes associated with successful treatment are like those occurring in pernicious anemia.

Bilirubinemia may be so pronounced as to at once suggest a hemolytic anemia;[216a] yet in other cases normal values for plasma bilirubin have been found.[172] In the few cases in which serum iron determinations have been reported, the values have been within the normal range or increased. Free hydrochloric acid is more often present in the gastric juice than absent (about 3:1).

If the cases of "tropical" macrocytic anemia associated with pregnancy (p. 508) are excluded, macrocytic anemia is relatively rare in pregnancy. The condition appears to be less rare in Great Britain[172,181b] than in the United States. A number of cases have been reported from Canada[199a] and Venezuela.[161c]

Some degree of refractoriness to therapy during pregnancy seems to be characteristic of many of the cases of "pernicious anemia of pregnancy." This was noted when only liver or liver extract were available and has been true to some extent since folic acid and vitamin B_{12}

have been in use.[194b] This may take the form of a slow and protracted reticulocyte response with delayed and incomplete relief of anemia. In some cases the delayed response could be attributed to a complicating infection[172] but this has not always been true. There have been a few observations of failure to respond to concentrated liver extracts given parenterally with good response to liver extracts given by mouth.[228a]

In the majority of cases, however, folic acid therapy has been effective[181b,192] (p. 451), thereby changing the prognosis of this disorder, which was poor at one time (mortality 50 to 75 per cent). As a rule a more complete response has followed the oral administration of 20 mg. folic acid per day than following the administration of vitamin B_{12}.[161b,174,199a] Folinic acid in large doses (50 mg. initially) has also been effective.[216a]

A characteristic feature of pernicious anemia of pregnancy, which distinguishes it from true pernicious anemia and serves to differentiate it from pregnancy occurring in a person who has true pernicious anemia, is the disappearance of the anemia spontaneously on interruption or termination of the pregnancy and its failure to return even though folic acid therapy is not continued. However, recurrences of this type of anemia in subsequent pregnancies have been about twice as common as non-recurrences. Occasionally relapse of anemia has been observed to occur in the absence of pregnancy.[172]

The etiology of this disorder is obscure. In one study the serum vitamin B_{12} levels of normal pregnant women were found to be lower than those of non-pregnant women and were observed to decrease during pregnancy and progressively increase during the early weeks of the postpartum period.[199a] There was no alteration in the capacity of the serum to bind B_{12}. In some pregnant patients with megaloblastic anemia, se-

rum vitamin B_{12} levels as low as those in pernicious anemia were observed.[199a] Folic acid excretion was not abnormal. In other cases, however, normal serum B_{12} concentrations have been reported.[161c, 194b]

Reference has been made to the poor diet of some of the patients.[181b,199a] In others impaired intestinal absorption was demonstrable and in still others toxemia and infection were present.[163a] A comparison of vitamin B_{12} and folic acid serum levels of mothers and infants showed substantially lower levels in the mothers.[163b] Yet, in a series of cases in South Africa, no evidence of malabsorption of vitamin B_{12} could be demonstrated.[201a]

It was shown some years ago that, as the fetus develops the number of erythrocytes increases and their size decreases in a manner similar to that seen in pernicious anemia following liver therapy.[328] It was suggested that these changes might be produced by antianemic liver principle derived from the mother.[323,324] When the effect of antianemic substances on the first or prehepatic generation of cells in yolk sac blood (Fig. 2–1, p. 87) was studied in the eleven-day rat embryo, it was observed that maturation of these cells was accelerated by the administration of either liver extract or folic acid.[270] Assays of the antianemic potency of the livers of pig fetuses failed to demonstrate activity[324] except in slight degree in the liver of the last third of the gestation period.[323] Desiccated fetal pig stomach, however, does contain a significant amount of antipernicious anemia principle. Presumably the requirements of the fetus for hemopoietic factors are met from the stores of the mother. That these demands can exhaust her supplies and thereby lead to the development of megaloblastic anemia seems highly probable.[187a]

Consideration of the variety of observations which have been made in connce-

33

tion with the macrocytic anemia of pregnancy, some of which are quite contradictory, forces the conclusion that megaloblastic anemia may develop in pregnancy as the effect of many factors, which include deficient diet, impaired intestinal absorption, defective utilization and increased demands as the result of the needs of the fetus and in consequence of hemorrhage and rapidly repeated pregnancies. Furthermore, in some cases, none of these factors seems to have been responsible. No evidence has been presented to support the suggestion that the anemia is due to some abnormal metabolite which acts as an anti-vitamin but this possibility has not been excluded. This topic will be discussed further shortly.

MACROCYTIC ANEMIA IN ASSOCIATION WITH SURGICAL PROCEDURES OR ORGANIC DISEASE IN THE GASTROINTESTINAL TRACT

Carcinoma of the Stomach.—It was often mentioned that macrocytic anemia may be caused by carcinoma of the stomach. This is a very rare occurrence, however, very few well-studied cases having been recorded.[173a,184,204] The development of carcinoma of the stomach in treated cases of pernicious anemia is not so unusual (p. 472). It has also been stated that syphilis may produce the blood picture of pernicious anemia. In a series of 4800 cases of syphilis studied by Foucar and Stokes,[180] anemia was present in only 0.5 per cent and in no instance was it found that there was incontestable evidence that macrocytic anemia and syphilis were etiologically connected. A similar conclusion can be drawn from other studies.[213] It is of interest, however, that macrocytic anemia responding to vitamin B_{12} therapy has been observed in association with *linitis plastica* of neither neoplastic nor

luetic origin.[166] **Gastric polyposis** was reported as causing macrocytic anemia in one case[223] and, in another, this type of anemia developed following **corrosion of the stomach with nitric acid.**[162] Again, as in connection with carcinoma of the stomach, it is more common for gastric polyposis to develop in cases of pernicious anemia than to precede the anemia and lead to its development.

Gastrectomy and Gastroenterostomy.—It is now quite clear that, following *total gastrectomy*, deficiency of vitamin B_{12} develops. At least 73 cases of megaloblastic anemia following total gastrectomy have been reported.[190,201] Since about 1000 to 2000 μg. of vitamin B_{12} are stored in the body[259] and since the daily requirement for B_{12} is probably less than 1 μg., it is not surprising that evidence of deficiency is slow to appear. The first sign observed in a series of 28 cases was macrocytosis, which was noted within six months to seven years (average 2.5 years) after operation.[190] Anemia (volume of packed red cells 37 per cent or less) developed in six months to nine years (average four years). Ultimately megaloblasts were demonstrated in the bone marrow (two to ten years, average 4.5 years). In three patients signs of spinal cord degeneration were found six to eight years after operation. It has been shown that the absorption of vitamin B_{12} is impaired in such patients[190] and that the serum vitamin B_{12} concentration decreases progressively after operation.[208a]

Following *partial gastrectomy* the incidence of megaloblastic anemia is much lower. Only 20 cases following partial gastrectomy have been reported and 15 following gastroenterostomy.[185a,189,197,200,201,211,219] In relation to the number of such operations which have been performed, the proportion is very small. Whether or not megaloblastic anemia will develop may depend on the portion removed. Impaired absorption of vitamin B_{12} and megaloblastic anemia were observed when the proximal portion of the stomach was resected whereas after the distal two-thirds or three-fourths was removed megaloblastic anemia was infrequent.[201] Iron deficiency anemia, on the other hand, is relatively common (p. 733).

Intestinal Strictures and Anastomoses.—The association of a clinical picture of pernicious anemia with intestinal stricture was first noted in 1897 by Faber. By 1949, 61 cases of megaloblastic anemia associated with anatomic lesions in the small intestine had been collected.[172a] Since then at least 20 more have been reported[161d,171b,208,209a,217,219a, 226a,227a] and the writer has observed one case. In 43 instances strictures were present, in 34 there were various types of anastomoses with or without bowel resections, and in six diverticula of the small bowel were present. The strictures have been single or multiple. The majority were in the small intestine, usually in the ileum. Somewhat more than a third were tuberculous in origin. The anastomoses were chiefly entero-enterostomies and entero-colostomies, but there were eight instances of gastro-jejuno-colic fistula or gastro-colic fistula and three esophago-jejunostomies. The diverticula were all in the small intestine. Our patient had tuberculous stricture of the small bowel.

In a number of the cases the symptoms consisted of indefinite dyspepsia of several years' duration, followed eventually by pain, intermittent diarrhea, abdominal distention and, less often, nausea and vomiting. Abdominal fulness and tenderness, especially in the right lower quadrant, visible intestinal peristalsis and audible borborygmi were frequently present. In those cases in which an operation had been performed, there were initially the symptoms of the abdominal condition which led to surgery, followed by a period of variable duration before diarrhea and the other symptoms above mentioned developed.

In the fully developed disorder, the symptoms in many respects often have been like those of pernicious anemia or sprue. Progressive weakness and loss of weight have been constant complaints and in a number of instances there was glossitis. Icterus was observed in half the cases.[172a] Paresthesias in the extremities, and objective signs of disease of the nervous system[229b] have been less common than in pernicious anemia.

The blood picture is identical with that of pernicious anemia both in regard to morphology and degree of reduction in the red cell count. As in the latter condition, leukopenia is common. The bone marrow, in the cases which were studied adequately, was found to be hyperplastic and megaloblastic. In contradistinction to pernicious anemia, free hydrochloric acid was found on gastric analysis in about half of the cases examined and this incidence of normal hydrochloric acid secretion would probably have been higher had histamine been used more often to stimulate secretion.

In addition to the normal secretion of free hydrochloric acid in many cases, it was possible to demonstrate intrinsic factor in the gastric juice in one case.[215] and impaired absorption of vitamin B_{12} which could not be corrected by giving intrinsic factor was demonstrated in several.[209a,217] Low serum vitamin B_{12} levels have also been observed.[226a] A number of the patients described were much younger than persons with pernicious anemia. Still more significant is the fact that in several instances the anemia, as well as the gastrointestinal complaints, were relieved when the intestinal disorder was corrected surgically.[165,172a,209a,227a]

The intimate relationship of these cases to pernicious anemia is indicated by the demonstrated effectiveness of liver extracts in the relief of the macrocytic anemia whether surgical measures were employed or not. In other cases vitamin B_{12} had little effect and a good response followed folic acid therapy,[228] but in a number vitamin B_{12} therapy was satisfactory.[226a] Of special interest is the fact that good hemopoietic responses were observed after administration of tetracyclines.[219b,227a,228] This makes plausible the thesis that the anemia is caused by the colonization of the small intestine by abnormal bacteria which in some way divert folic acid or vitamin B_{12} from the host.[228] This topic will be discussed further shortly (p. 527).

Chronic Dysentery. Regional Ileitis. Chronic Pancreatic Disease and Resection of Small Intestine.—Macrocytic anemia may also be encountered in other instances in which the function of the alimentary system is disturbed. This type of anemia has been described in cases of chronic dysentery,[194c] in regional ileitis,[208b] in jejunal diverticulosis[209] and in chronic pancreatic disease.[171] A clinical picture typical of sprue with macrocytic anemia was present in one of our patients in whom 316 cm. of small intestine had been removed five years before. The anemia responded to liver therapy and the diarrhea decreased on a high protein, low fat diet. Six years following the first operation, an exploratory operation revealed that only 560 cm. of small intestine remained and a blind loop of intestine, 12 cm. long, was found. The latter was removed but the symptoms were relieved only temporarily, and the high protein, low fat diet as well as liver therapy had to be resumed. In another patient, 300 cm. of small intestine had been resected and an ileocolostomy performed. When she died, five years later, a blind loop of ileum 135 cm. in length and a blind loop of colon 20 cm. long, as well as chronic ulcerative colitis and an extremely fatty liver, were found. One

case has been reported in which extensive ileal resections for Crohn's disease and impaired absorption of vitamin B_{12} uninfluenced by intrinsic factor or a course of chlortetracycline were followed by the development of subacute combined degeneration of the spinal cord.[165a]

It would be of great interest to know in what proportion of cases of intestinal disorder of the various types discussed, macrocytic anemia develops. Adequate data to answer this question have not been published.

MACROCYTIC ANEMIA IN DISEASE OF THE LIVER

Anemia may or may not be associated with liver disease and when it is found may be of several varieties. In a series of 132 cases of liver disease of various types, the writer found no anemia in 22.7 per cent, macrocytic anemia in 32.6 per cent, normocytic anemia in 30.3 per cent, and microcytic anemia in 14.4 per cent.[232] The last named type of anemia could be attributed in most instances to chronic loss of blood. Macrocytic anemia was found only in cases of hepatic disease of long duration and of wide extent. It was most common in cases of cirrhosis of the liver and often was present when malignancy and cirrhosis were associated. It was not found in cases of acute necrosis or when the liver damage was only slight or moderate.

There are great differences in the reported frequency of macrocytosis in hepatic disease,[167a,202] some of which may be attributable to technical factors but in other instances differences in the types of hepatic disease included in the study were probably important. The macrocytosis which may be encountered has been characterized from blood film examination as consisting mainly of "thin macrocytes," cells with increased diameter, decreased thickness and normal volume; "target macrocytes," the film consisting essentially of numerous target cells (p. 100); and "thick macrocytosis."[167a] Probably only the latter should be referred to as true macrocytosis. In such cases the mean corpuscular volume is substantially increased and the blood film resembles that of pernicious anemia in partial remission. Oval macrocytes are found but poikilocytosis, polychromatophilia and nucleated red corpuscles are rare. Mean corpuscular hemoglobin concentration is usually normal and erythrocyte fragility is normal. The leukocytes and platelets show no abnormality as a rule. In a small proportion of cases megaloblasts have been described in the bone marrow.[193a,195, 195b,205]

On the basis of current knowledge it is difficult to find a single pathogenetic factor or mechanism common to all instances of anemia associated with liver disease. First of all, the degree of anemia varies. In fact, it has been claimed that true anemia is less common in liver disease than would be assumed from hemoglobin or hematocrit determinations,[188a] since plasma volume may be increased. This has been noted particularly in patients with esophageal varices.[176a] Even increased red cell mass has been found in cirrhosis.[188a]

Studies of erythrocyte dynamics in patients with chronic liver disease who had been receiving good diets for at least two weeks and were in a relatively steady state showed the mean life span of the erythrocytes to be shortened.[188a] In another series the red cell life-span, as measured by Cr[51], was found to be shortened in approximately half the cases.[161e] The survival of normal erythrocytes transfused into patients with chronic liver disease has also been found to be reduced.[193a] The shortened survival of the red cells of patients with chronic liver disease appears to be the result of two processes; namely, increased senescence from inherent cell defects and increased

random cell destruction.[188a] In many instances, however, erythropoiesis was found to be increased sufficiently to compensate for the increased cell destruction.

Other factors include blood loss, poor diet,[167] the non-specific effect of chronic disease, sequestration and local destruction in the spleen,[193a] and factors related to the metabolism of folic acid and vitamin B_{12}. It is conceivable that the requirement for these substances may be increased[193a] or their storage or utilization may be impaired. In some cases parenteral liver therapy was associated with reticulocyte responses.[183,205,232,233] The concept of faulty storage was suggested by the observation that the liver of a patient with macrocytic anemia who died of cirrhosis was found to be ineffective in the treatment of a case of pernicious anemia whereas the liver of a patient who died of acute yellow atrophy contained the active hemopoietic principle.[185] However, other investigators were able to demonstrate active hemopoietic factor in the livers of patients dying of extensive hepatic disease.[214] That alcohol itself may inhibit hemopoietic activity is suggested by the reticulocytosis which developed in patients when alcohol intake was stopped, even when they continued to be fed diets low in known hemopoietic factors.[193a]

INFESTATION WITH FISH TAPEWORM

A clinical picture resembling pernicious anemia in all respects, including such symptoms as glossitis, diarrhea, paresthesias and even ataxia,[168a] as well as the classical blood picture, may be found in persons harboring the fish tapeworm, Diphyllobothrium latum.[168] The onset of "Bothriocephalus anemia" is said to be somewhat more acute than that of cryptogenic pernicious anemia, its age incidence is somewhat earlier, the course of the anemia is more rapidly progressive and remissions are less frequent. Free hydrochloric acid has been found in as many as 16 per cent of cases of tapeworm anemia.[168] The bone marrow is megaloblastic, as in pernicious anemia. Expulsion of the worm has been reported to result in improvement or complete relief of the anemia, even with remission of the neurological manifestations.[168a] Liver therapy and vitamin B_{12} effectively relieve the anemia, the response to treatment being exactly like that seen in pernicious anemia. This will occur even when the worm is not expelled. Folic acid may produce a hemopoietic response but, as in pernicious anemia, neurological relapse may develop.[168a]

The parasite is common in the countries along the shores of the Baltic Sea and in the section of Switzerland bordering France, whence it has been distributed to neighboring countries. In the large lakes of the north central United States and the adjacent provinces of Canada, the pickerel or great northern pike, the wall-eyed pike, and the perch have been found to act as intermediate hosts, transmitting the parasites from infested immigrant Europeans to native inhabitants of these regions. Contrary to earlier statements, the parasite is rare in Japan.[207a]

Macrocytic anemia, however, is only rarely encountered when there is infestation with the fish tapeworm. In Finland, where infestation is heaviest, it has been estimated that 1.9 to 3.0 per cent of persons harboring the parasite develop definite anemia.[207a] It is noteworthy, furthermore, that cryptogenic pernicious anemia is not rare in Finland. In Japan, where infestation is also very heavy, but where pernicious anemia is very uncommon, only 2 cases with macrocytic anemia have been described.

These and similar observations led to the view that the anemia represents the accidental occurrence of tapeworm infestation and pernicious anemia in the same individuals, or that at least a constitutional predisposition to anemia is necessary. Schauman, an early student of the disease, held this opinion[168] and pointed out that in a household in which all the members were infested, macrocytic anemia would be found in related persons and not among the servants. He and others observed true pernicious anemia in relatives of patients considered to have tapeworm anemia.

It has been observed that the tapeworm lodges in the ileum in tapeworm carriers without anemia, whereas in those who have tapeworm anemia it is found as high as the jejunum.[170] The tapeworm itself has been shown to contain considerable amounts of vitamin B_{12}.[168a,170] It has been postulated, therefore, that, depending on its situation in the intestine, the tapeworm is capable of interfering with the assimilation of vitamin B_{12} and thereby producing a deficiency. In two cases of tapeworm anemia there was no hepatic uptake of vitamin B_{12} but marked and persistent radioactivity was noted over the left lower region of the abdomen.[170b] In another study, it was found by the fecal excretion test (p. 490) that 55 per cent less B_{12} was absorbed by tapeworm carriers than by normal subjects.[207a] Urinary excretion of radioactive vitamin B_{12} was significantly less in both anemic and non-anemic worm carriers than in normal subjects and increased significantly after the expulsion of the worm.[207a] Serum vitamin B_{12} levels below $100\mu\mu g./ml.$ were found in more than 50 per cent of the worm carriers.

Thus it seems that the tapeworm competes with the host for vitamin B_{12}. The worm is able to take up free vitamin B_{12} in the intestinal tract but it is uncertain whether or not the worm is able to break down the interaction product between intrinsic factor and vitamin B_{12} or prevents the intestinal wall from accepting the vitamin from the intestinal contents.[170b,207a] Some studies indicate that the worm may interfere with the secretion of intrinsic factor.[170,219a]

It has been suggested that the tapeworm associated with the development of megaloblastic anemia in the Baltic area is not of the same species as that found in those parts of the world where infestation is heavy but the anemia is rare. An alternative explanation is that constitutional predisposition is necessary before serious deficiency of vitamin B$_{12}$ will develop.[168]

No evidence has been presented to support the theory that the tapeworm produces a hemolysin, as Tallqvist suggested,[168] or that the anemia is the result of an allergic reaction to the tapeworm.[225]

There is no evidence that other parasites play any role in the development of macrocytic anemia. Two cases of macrocytic anemia have been observed in association with infestation with the beef tapeworm, *Taenia saginata*, and one in association with the round worm, *Ascaris lumbricoides*.[164]

MACROCYTIC ANEMIA IN HYPOTHYROIDISM

Pallor is common in hypothyroidism and true anemia may be present. In some instances the clinical picture may strongly suggest pernicious anemia, not only because of the yellowish pallor, the fatigability, and the absence of weight loss, but because there may also be paresthesias, difficulty in walking, and glossitis. Achlorhydria occurs in 53 per cent of cases of myxedema,[199] and there may be macrocytic anemia. Even the blood plasma may suggest slight icterus, possibly as the result of carotinemia.[169]

It was found in one series of 52 cases that the red cell count was lower than 4,000,000 in 60 per cent of the cases.[199] Anemia was observed more frequently when achlorhydria was present. In another series anemia was present only in 31 per cent of 116 cases.[226c] Anemia in cases of myxedema is rarely severe and is usually normocytic or macrocytic but it may be hypochromic.[198] Associated iron deficiency is the cause of the hypochromic anemia. It has been mentioned already that true pernicious anemia and myxedema may occur in the same individual (p. 471) and that the presence of hypothyroidism may inhibit the response to therapy. In occasional cases, defective gastric secretion, which is so common in myxedema, and perhaps loss of appetite, may possibly lead to a true deficiency of vitamin B$_{12}$ or of iron. In such cases the administration of the deficient antianemic substance, together with desiccated thyroid is followed by a reticulocyte response and prompt relief of the anemia. Defective intestinal absorption of vitamin B$_{12}$, uninfluenced by intrinsic factor, has been demonstrated in some cases of myxedema but not in other instances.[226c]

There is a true anemia of hypothyroidism, however, for it is observed not only in cases of spontaneous hypothyroidism but develops after total ablation of the thyroid in man[222] and in experimental animals.[196,218] The red cell count is rarely lower than 3,500,000 and the mean corpuscular volume may be 95 to 120 c.μ, while the mean corpuscular hemoglobin concentration is normal. There is little anisocytosis, the red corpuscles being uniformly larger than normal cells and the frequency (Price-Jones) curve of red cell diameters is similar in shape to the normal curve but swung to right.[169] There is no poikilocytosis nor evidence of active blood regeneration. The bone marrow may be hypoplastic.[169,194,196] Plasma and total blood volume are reduced but, according to the majority of reports, red cell survival is normal.[226c] The administration of thyroid is followed by a slow restoration of the blood to normal (Fig. 10–14). This may take three to nine months to occur, in spite of the fact that the anemia is not

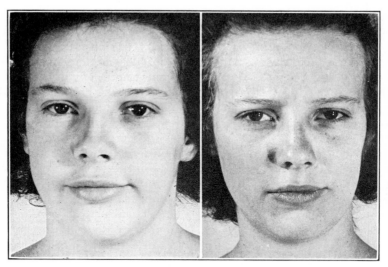

Fig. 10-13.—Photographs of a girl of fifteen years with "refractory" anemia, before and four months after therapy with desiccated thyroid. Note the pale, puffy, pasty appearance before therapy.

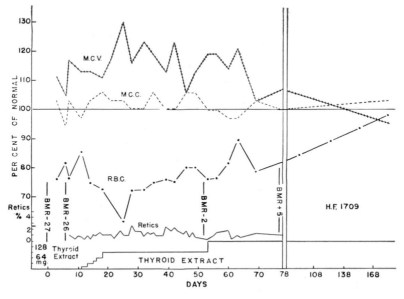

Fig. 10-14.—Gradual relief of anemia and disappearance of macrocytosis following thyroid therapy in a case of myxedema previously treated unsuccessfully with liver extract and iron. On admission R.B.C. was 4,120,000, M.C.V. 102 c.μ.

very severe at any time. It has been reported[174b] that the addition of testosterone to the therapeutic regimen results in a prompt erythropoietic response.

MEGALOBLASTIC ANEMIA ASSOCIATED WITH ANTIMETABOLITES AND INCREASED DEMANDS FOR HEMOPOIETIC FACTORS

Macrocytic megaloblastic anemia is known to develop in patients under treatment with folic acid antagonists, such as amethopterin, in those receiving 6-mercaptopurine (p. 981) or 5-fluorouracil, an inhibitor of thymine synthesis.[170c]

Such anemia has also been observed in patients receiving *anticonvulsant drugs*.[173, 179,233d] A total of 58 cases have been reported. The drugs have included diphenylhydantoin sodium (Dilantin), primidone (Mysoline) and barbital derivatives (methophenobarbital, amylobarbitone sodium and quinalbarbitone sodium). One case has been reported in which phenylbutazone seemed to be offending drug.[211a] The majority of the reported cases have been from the British Isles. Temporary remissions have been observed following withdrawal of the associated drug[190b] but striking response followed the administration of folic acid. In some cases vitamin B_{12} was effective in relieving the anemia but this was not always true. There is no report of a treatment failure when folic acid was given.[179]

The number of cases reported is very small when one considers the countless patients receiving these agents. It had been suggested that the offending drugs may act as folic acid antagonists since there is structural similarity between their pyrimidine and hydantoin rings and the pterodyl portion of folic acid. However, the addition of these drugs to microbiological systems has provided no evidence of inhibition of folic acid metabolism. This fact, together with the small percentage of cases in which megaloblastic anemia is found, has led to the suggestion that some predisposing factor must be involved as well. Of those considered, associated folic acid deficiency secondary to inadequate diet seems to be the most plausible.[188] Slight but significant macrocytosis, without anemia, was reported in about one-third of patients receiving these drugs.[190b] This could be corrected by giving folic acid. In cases appropriately studied no evidence of intestinal malabsorption or faulty intrinsic factor secretion could be demonstrated.[179]

Megaloblastic anemia has been reported occasionally *in association with certain hemopoietic disorders*, especially hemolytic anemias.[194a] In some instances, at least, it is likely that some degree of nutritional deficiency was associated. It is intriguing to speculate whether folic acid or other hemopoietic factors may be required in such increased amounts when erythropoiesis is very active that a relative deficiency may result, particularly in patients whose stores of these substances are marginal.

PATHOGENESIS OF PERNICIOUS ANEMIA AND RELATED FORMS OF MACROCYTIC ANEMIA

The discovery of the value of liver therapy[281] in pernicious anemia marked an important shift in popular views regarding hematopoiesis in general, and pernicious anemia in particular. Flint, in 1860, and Fenwick, twenty years later,[248] as well as others, had suggested that inadequate assimilation of food was the underlying cause of pernicious anemia. In spite of this, the concepts most widely accepted until 1926 were the view that the anemia is fundamentally a *hemolytic* one, and the *theory* that a *bacterial agent* is responsible. William Hunter,[267] in 1888, called attention to the hemolytic character of pernicious anemia and suggested that oral sepsis is the cause. Others attempted to incriminate Bacillus welchii, Bacillus coli, streptococci and other organisms.[248,284] Recognition of the fact that achylia gastrica is almost uniformly present and often long precedes the onset of anemia led to the hypothesis that the absence of acid permits the entrance and growth of organisms in the small bowel with the production and absorption of a hemotoxin and a neurotoxin.[268] These theories were never satisfactorily substantiated.

With the discovery of the value of liver therapy, these uncertainties concerning the pathogenesis of pernicious anemia were essentially resolved. Impressive evidence that the fundamental defect in pernicious anemia is faulty blood construction because of deficiency of some essential substance was provided by the striking effect on the blood in cases of pernicious anemia and the general improvement which took place following the administration of liver or certain extracts of liver, the quantitative relationship of the response to the amount of active material given, the continuance of remission when treatment was pursued, and the occurrence of relapse on cessation of therapy. The fact that in relapse the bone marrow is hyperplastic and megaloblastic, whereas following effective treatment the overactive marrow is replaced by normoblastic tissue of normal amount suggested that the deficient substance is one without which normal maturation of red cells cannot take place.

Role of Achylia Gastrica.—The relationship of the characteristic achylia gastrica and the postulated nutritional deficiency of pernicious anemia was clarified by the ingenious, yet simple experiments of Castle and his associates[245] who showed that patients with this disease "starve in the midst of plenty." It was postulated that, by substituting some digestive process of the normal stomach one might affect the patient's disease favorably. This was done by feeding daily by stomach tube to patients with pernicious anemia the liquefied stomach contents of a normal person removed an hour after ingestion of 300 Gm. of lean beef muscle. A clear-cut hemopoietic response followed whereas, in a preceding ten-day control period during which the patients were fed a corresponding amount of beef muscle without preliminary digestion in the stomach of a normal person, no reticulocyte response, rise in red cell count or clinical improvement took place. It was demonstrated, moreover, that normal human gastric juice is without effect when given alone, as is beef muscle even after complete digestion with pig pepsin. It was also found that the antianemic value of a mixture of normal gastric juice and beef muscle is destroyed by procedures, such as heating, which were employed in the manufacture of liver extract.[255] The significance of the observation that a parenterally effective substance ("haemopoietin") could be obtained from the product of incubation of hog's stomach and beef muscle[271] was not fully appreciated. This demonstration of the hemopoietic effectiveness of beef muscle when administered parenterally was confirmed only later.[257] In the interval it was generally assumed that food contains an essential "extrinsic factor" which requires a gastric "intrinsic factor" for the production of an antianemic principle which is stored in the liver.

It is now quite clear that the extrinsic factor and the antianemic principle are one and the same, the role of the intrinsic factor being to permit its assimilation[242] rather than to transform it into a hemopoietic substance.[244] Vitamin B_{12} has been shown to be the remarkably potent dietary factor which depends on an endogenous substance for its absorption. Unlike vitamin B_{12}, the hemopoietic effectiveness of orally administered folic acid is not enhanced by incubation with normal human gastric juice.[257]

The chemical nature of vitamin B_{12} and its distribution in various foods were discussed in an earlier chapter (p. 131). It is now known that this substance is generally essential to animal nutrition and can be synthesized only by certain bacteria and algae, not by the higher plants. Cobalt is an essential constituent and, when this mineral is present in the forage, the bacterial production of vitamin B_{12} in the rumen of herbivorous animals is large. Non-ruminant animals, including man, derive vitamin B_{12} largely from animal food (thus the term "animal protein factor," p. 131). Although large amounts of vitamin B_{12} are synthesized by bacteria in the cecum and colon,[238,240] the amount derived from this source is uncertain. In certain species, coprophagy is probably a good source of vitamin B_{12}.

In pernicious anemia the total volume of gastric secretion is greatly reduced. For this reason the term "achylia gastrica," in contrast to "achlorhydria," is used. It has been widely assumed that gastric atrophy is the primary defect in pernicious anemia and that this ultimately leads to intrinsic factor deficiency. However, observations in cases of pernicious anemia in childhood (p. 469), as well as pathological studies[72] indicate that the reverse more probably is the true sequence of events.[67b] Intrinsic factor has been shown to be lacking in the rare instances of pernicious anemia in adults in which secretion of hydrochloric acid could be demonstrated;[76,245] it has not necessarily been absent from the gastric secretion whenever hydrochloric acid was lacking.[245] Saliva and normal duodenal contents collected without admixture with gastric juice are not sources of intrinsic factor.

The exact nature of the intrinsic factor is obscure. What is known of its nature, secretion and action was reviewed earlier (p. 132).

The metabolic functions of vitamin B_{12} were discussed in an earlier chapter (p. 133). These are poorly understood but, in any event, it appears that, when this vitamin is lacking, many of the body cells are unable to divide to form new cells at the usual rate. Consequently, they grow large. This is most apparent where the production of new cells is normally rapid, such as the bone marrow and the intestinal tract. The megaloblasts, the macrocytes, the "giant" juvenile metamyelocytes, the multisegmented polymorphonuclear neutrophils and even the thrombocytopenia of pernicious anemia reflect the lowered rate of cell division in the bone marrow. The smooth tongue has been attributed to the "too leisurely division of its epithelial cells."[242] The same phenomenon may be responsible for the large epithelial cells found in the gastric washings[73] and vaginal scrapings[261] of patients with pernicious anemia. The spinal cord degeneration has been attributed to defective ribose nucleic acid synthesis which affects especially the long axones of nerve cells in the spinal cord.[282]

Relationship of Vitamin B_{12} and Folic Acid.—The metabolic interrelationships of vitamin B_{12} and folic acid were discussed in Chapter 3 (p. 133). Assays[259a] of vitamin B_{12} and folic acid blood levels in various disorders characterized by megaloblastic anemia showed that in pernicious anemia in relapse the vitamin B_{12} content of the serum was low whereas the results of folic acid assays were variable.[282] Following the injection of vitamin B_{12}, when the folic acid level was normal, a rapid fall occurred, sometimes within two hours. In the next 72 hours a rise took place. When folic acid was given to cases of pernicious anemia in relapse, a decrease in the serum vitamin B_{12} activity accompanied the hemopoietic response.[239] The opposite effect has also been observed; namely, the appearance of severe painful glossitis and cheilosis, presumably signs of folic acid deficiency, during the administration of daily doses of vitamin B_{12}.[262]

In nutritional macrocytic anemia, on the other hand, vitamin B_{12} values were within normal limits or higher than normal and the folic acid activity of the blood was lower than normal. In a case of sprue, low values for both vitamin B_{12} and folic acid were found and in this case the bone marrow remained megaloblastic until both substances were administered. In another case serum vitamin B_{12} levels were high. In a case of megaloblastic anemia of pregnancy, high serum levels of vitamin B_{12} were found which decreased following folic acid therapy. In such patients a close correlation was found between serum vitamin B_{12} levels and the urinary excretion of folic acid following the subcutaneous administration of 5 mg. of the latter.[304]

It must be assumed from these and similar studies that the metabolic roles of vitamin B_{12} and folic acid are very closely related. The balance between folic acid and vitamin B_{12} is a finely adjusted one; as a deficiency of vitamin B_{12} becomes more pronounced the requirement for folic acid may increase.

Pathogenesis of Various Forms of Megaloblastic Anemia.—Up to this point it has been shown that there is a close interrelationship between vitamin B_{12} and folic acid and that the expression of serious deficiency of these substances is the development of megaloblastic anemia. It is assumed that pernicious anemia is attributable to pure vitamin B_{12} deficiency and that the megaloblastic anemia which may develop following total gastrectomy is due to the same cause. Nevertheless it would be of interest to know that no deficiency, whatsoever, of folic acid is associated with the lack of vitamin B_{12}. Measurement of serum *Lactobacillus casei* activity and urine formiminoglutamic acid (FIGLU) excretion may help answer this question. (Blood, *17*, 368, 1961). It

may be noted that evidence has been presented that a dietary deficiency of folic acid may be present in certain cases of pernicious anemia.[203,322] In addition, it has been postulated that vitamin B_{12} in some manner influences the storage, absorption[282] and utilization[299] of folic acid and that, when vitamin B_{12} is deficient, these functions are impaired. It may be significant that in the vegans whose diet was totally lacking in foods of animal origin and presumably was very deficient in vitamin B_{12}, little or no anemia was found and only an increase in mean corpuscular volume above the normal was mentioned.[233a] The failure to produce megaloblastic anemia in swine on a vitamin B_{12} deficient regimen when folic acid was supplied should also be noted.[241]

In practically all other forms of megaloblastic anemia folic acid deficiency has been present, with or without accompanying vitamin B_{12} deficiency. A wide variety of circumstances and factors appear to be concerned in the development of these deficiencies. With a few exceptions, dietary deficiency has not often been the sole factor in the development of serious deficiency of these vitamins. Dietary deficiency of folic acid with or without associated B_{12} deficiency may be seen occasionally in single cases in the temperate zones, but the more common examples of nutritional deficiency which are found throughout the world, and especially in the tropics, are often complicated by intestinal malabsorption, intestinal and other infections, and increased requirements. Such appears to be the explanation of "tropical" macrocytic anemia (p. 508) and probably is true in most cases of pernicious anemia of pregnancy as seen in the tropics (p. 511).

In the sprue syndromes, dietary deficiency rarely, if ever, constitutes the primary cause of these disorders, as will be discussed below. Here, however, deficiency of folic acid and sometimes of vitamin B_{12} is responsible for many of the clinical manifestations, especially megaloblastic anemia.

In the cases of megaloblastic anemia in patients who receive anticonvulsant drugs (p. 521) both metabolic impairment and nutritional deficiency may play a role. The anemia of liver disease (p. 516) is probably also the effect of a multiplicity of factors, but these probably do not include faulty storage or utilization (p. 517). In the case of tapeworm anemia (p. 517) competition by the worm with the host for vitamin B_{12} appears to be an important factor.

There is reason to suspect that deficiencies of other substances related to the metabolism of folic acid and vitamin B_{12}, especially ascorbic acid (p. 138), are important in the development of certain instances of megaloblastic anemia; for example, megaloblastic anemia of infancy (p. 768). It is also possible that in rare instances (p. 133) disturbances in the metabolic pathways of pyrimidine metabolism may result in megaloblastic anemia. A case has been reported in which a metabolic defect in the utilization of folinic acid seemed to be present which could only be corrected by the administration of massive doses of vitamin B_{12}, by folinic acid or by a combination of ascorbic acid and folic acid.[190a]

Yet these explanations are not adequate for all known examples of megaloblastic anemia. Thus, in some cases of pregnancy macrocytic anemia dietary intake had been good and it would be difficult to postulate nutritional deficiency as a factor. Nor could intestinal malabsorption be incriminated in certain cases. For this reason, the effect of some "toxin" or the action of an antimetabolite has been considered. Finally the pathogenesis of the anemia associated with intestinal strictures and blind loops is not entirely settled, as will be indicated shortly.

Experimental Production of Pernicious Anemia and Related Disorders. —It has not been possible to produce in an experimental animal a condition identical in every respect with pernicious anemia. Although total gastrectomy in man, as already discussed (p. 514) has been followed by the development of macrocytic anemia in persons who have survived the operation for a period of time presumably long enough to deplete the body of stores of anti-anemic substances, it has not been possible to produce macrocytic anemia in animals by this means.[241,286] A variety of animals have been used (monkeys, pigs, dogs, cats, rats) and some of the observations have been carried on for almost three years. Only in rare and isolated exceptions has macrocytic anemia been noted.[236,298] The failure of gastrectomy to produce this type of anemia is all the more puzzling since loss of anti-anemic potency of the livers of gastrectomized animals has been reported.[236,241,258,286] Furthermore, extensive degenerative changes developed in the nervous systems of dogs and swine following gastrectomy and other operations on the gastrointestinal tract.[286,287] The curious observation was made that, whereas even after removal merely of the fundus of the pig's stomach its liver loses anti-anemic potency, this loss of anti-anemic material did not occur if the pig was given nicotinic acid.[286] The vitamin did not have this effect in totally gastrectomized pigs.

This failure to produce macrocytic anemia in animals is not easily accounted for by assuming that the formation of intrinsic factor is not limited to the stomach. Castle and his co-workers[252] showed that the anti-anemic activity of the intestine is lost if the bowel is first thoroughly washed. Thus, the reports that the whole of the small intestine[311] and the colon[294] possess anti-anemic activity lose their significance. It appears that the observed hematopoietic effect, except possibly in the case of the duodenum,[307] could be accounted for by the passive adsorption of intrinsic factor of gastric origin. Furthermore, subtotal[235] and total[258] gastrectomy, even when combined with duodenectomy and partial jejunectomy, or resection of a large part of the small intestine[287] have failed to produce pernicious anemia in animals.

Attempts to produce macrocytic anemia by feeding diets deficient in extrinsic factor have been somewhat more successful. Wills and Bilimoria[320] fed monkeys a diet similar to that taken by the Mohammedan women who were found to have this type of anemia. Macrocytic anemia as well as megaloblastic bone marrow hyperplasia developed, but this anemia, although it responded to yeast and crude liver extracts given by mouth, was not relieved by purified liver extracts potent in pernicious anemia.[321] A prompt response follows the administration of folic acid. Oral mucous membrane lesions, achylia and loss of anti-anemic potency of the gastric juice and livers of swine fed a modified canine-black-tongue producing diet have been reported,[279] but the anemia was not consistently similar to that seen in pernicious anemia. A syndrome resembling sprue has been reported in dogs fed a low protein, high fat diet deficient in the vitamin B complex,[277] and in rats raised on goat's milk.[292] Other workers reported failure to produce macrocytic anemia by giving a deficient diet to gastrectomized dogs.[275]

The nearest approach to pernicious anemia which has been observed in experimental animals is the anemia developing in swine fed a diet from which pteroylglutamic acid and vitamin B_{12} were omitted and to which succinylsulfathiazole and a crude folic acid antagonist were added (p. 132). In such animals the combined deficiency of folic acid and vitamin B_{12} produced bone marrow changes more closely simulating those seen in pernicious anemia than occurred in folic acid deficiency alone.[241] Both agents were required to relieve the anemia. However, even in such animals no changes in the nervous system took place. One can only assume that the deficiency of vitamin B_{12} was not so severe as to impair the nervous system. It has been shown that total gastrectomy in rats rapidly reduces their serum vitamin B_{12} levels.[170a] However, in the swine fed deficient diets, attempts to further reduce the quantity of available vitamin B_{12} by performing gastrectomies were unsuccessful, perhaps because of the difficulty of preventing early death. It is also possible that an additional problem arises from the fact that ascorbic acid is related to the metabolism of folic acid and vitamin B_{12} and the pig does not require an exogenous source of this vitamin. The sensory neuron degeneration developing in animals fed diets lacking pyridoxine and pantothenic acid[254] does not now appear to be related to the changes observed in pernicious anemia although room must be left for another interpretation since greater protection against the development of these changes was afforded by the extract of liver effective anti-anemically in pernicious anemia than by other fractions of liver.[326,327]

Possible Role of Toxins.—The difficulties encountered in the experimental production of macrocytic anemia, as well as the well-marked signs of increased blood destruction which are found in pernicious anemia, have led from time to time to a revival of theories involving toxins as a cause of this disorder.[253] It has been suggested that hemolysis is a primary cause of the anemia rather than the secondary effect of faulty blood construction. It has been pointed out that the deficiency theory fails to explain adequately the spontaneous remissions occurring in the absence of liver or other antianemic factors in the diet.[16b] According to this view the action of liver is an antitoxic effect. Liver extract was found to protect animals against the anemia which developed when they were fed indol or amidopyrine together with a black-tongue producing diet.[289] The urine in cases of pernicious anemia was reported to contain a toxic factor.[313] Again, the red corpuscles from untreated cases of pernicious anemia were reported to be abnormally susceptible to the hemolytic action of lipemic serum.[269] This excessive sensitivity, it was claimed, leads to their destruction by the digestion products of fat. This was proposed as only one manifestation of a general disturbance of fat metabolism in pernicious anemia, other manifestations being the striking variations in cholesterol and related constituents of the blood in pernicious anemia (p. 485), and the changes in the nervous system.

The toxic theory was revived by *in vitro* studies which were interpreted as indicating that the serum of patients with untreated pernicious anemia contains a factor which inhibits the ripening of megaloblasts to normoblasts in bone marrow cultures.[272,308] The macrocytic anemia occurring in association with intestinal strictures and blind loops of various types (p. 515) also brought adherents to the toxin theory. It was suggested that such anemia might be caused by toxins produced in the partially obstructed intestines, possibly by the action of bacteria.[165] It is noteworthy in this connection that macrocytic anemia was described in 1924 in animals in which intestinal strictures were produced.[297] This anemia, as well as that of several patients with pernicious anemia, was said to be relieved by ileostomy. Since then it has been reported that the formation of a *blind intestinal loop* in the rat causes a macrocytic anemia and it has been observed that the anemia depends on dilatation of the blind loop, with

accumulation within it of intestinal contents[314] and does not develop when aureomycin is administered.[309] The anemia is hemolytic and is accompanied by hemosiderosis in the spleen. While a hematological remission could be induced in some of the animals by the administration of purified liver extracts or vitamin B_{12}, a greater proportion responded to folic acid.[314] The decisive event in the development of anemia in such animals was postulated as being a change in the flora of the loop or of the small intestine. This change might involve the disappearance of an organism which synthesizes hemopoietic material, or the emergence of an organism which interferes with the absorption or utilization of hemopoietic material. More complicated theories involving the interaction of toxic and nutritional factors have also been proposed.[310]

Possible Causes of Faulty Gastrointestinal Function in Pernicious Anemia, Sprue and Related Disorders.—As discussed earlier (p. 470), achylia gastrica is a characteristic feature of *pernicious anemia*. This may be the consequence of the intrinsic factor deficiency (p. 523) which is the primary fault in this disease. Considerable evidence indicates that the abnormality is inherited (p. 470). There is nothing to suggest that deficient diet leads to the development of the gastric defect.

A considerable body of evidence also suggests that dietary deficiency is not the primary defect in *sprue* or in idiopathic steatorrhea.[137] In spite of the fact that in certain cases of tropical sprue dietary deficiency appears to have been a significant etiologic factor,[158] it must be recognized that this disease may develop in persons consuming bountiful and mixed diets and does not usually affect both husband and wife even though they consume the same diet. The peculiar distribution of sprue in certain parts of the world and its absence elsewhere where similar dietary conditions exist, already alluded to (p. 495), is also significant. It is evident, however, that many of the manifestations of tropical sprue are attributable to nutritional deficiencies, especially to lack of folic acid.

The nature of the underlying disorder is quite obscure, however. In spite of repeated attempts to find a bacterial, fungal[126] or parasitic agent, none has been incriminated. This possibility is not necessarily closed, as reports such as that which recorded cures following the use of sulfonamides and antibiotics continue to suggest.[136c] There is no doubt that transient infections may hasten or accentuate the bowel malabsorption defect. The cephalad extension of abnormal intestinal flora has been postulated as making possible bacterial competition with the host for vital nutritional factors. Diet may play a role through providing the medium for the development of altered bacterial flora. The early appearance of changes in the small bowel which intraluminal biopsy has made it possible to demonstrate, raises the possibility that the application of histochemical technics may help to provide an answer.[137] Biochemical abnormalities of the intestinal mucosal cells may be the primary factor in the pathogenesis of the sprue syndromes. An underlying constitutional factor may be involved.

In idiopathic steatorrhea and celiac disease, in contrast to tropical sprue, gluten sensitivity is significant in many instances[136] (p. 506). The role of fat in the diet in the pathogenesis of the sprue syndromes also requires further elucidation. It has been observed that unsaturated fats predominate in the diet in tropical areas where sprue is endemic. Frazer,[136] whose "partition hypothesis" of fat digestion and absorption has re-received wide acceptance, considers interference with particulate absorption to be the main defect in sprue. The more

unsaturated, long-chain fatty acids appear to be absorbed but the more saturated ones are excreted. The latter may be related to the excessive quantities of mucus in the bowel which, in turn, interfere with particulate absorption and also produce the characteristic radiographic pattern of the small intestine, as previously mentioned. The diarrhea is attributed to the action of the long-chain fatty acids derived from fat breakdown as well as to the short-chain fatty acids arising from starch fermentation. The intermittent characteristics of the diarrhea are attributed to the growth of bacteria high in the intestinal tract.

BIBLIOGRAPHY

Pernicious Anemia

1. ABBOTT, L. D., JR. and JAMES, G. W.: Effect of Vitamin B_{12} on the Urinary Phenol Fractions in Pernicious Anemia, J. Lab. & Clin. Med., *35*, 35, 1950.
   Fractions in Pernicious Anemia, Jour. Lab. and Clin. Med., *35*, 35, 1950.
1a. AIRD, I. *et al.*: An Association between Blood Group A and Pernicious Anaemia, Brit. M. J., *2*, 723, 1956.
2. ALLINGTON, M. J. and TAYLOR, W. H.: Changes of Plasma Volume and Their Effect on the Red-Cell Count during the Treatment of Pernicious Anæmia, Brit. J. Hæmat., *1*, 241, 1955.
3. ALT, H. L.: Metabolism in Pernicious Anemia, Arch. Int. Med., *43*, 488, 1929.
4. ANDRUS, E. C. and WINTROBE, M. M.: Hyperthyroidism and Pernicious Anemia, Bull. Johns Hopkins Hosp., *59*, 291, 1936.
5. ARNETH, J.: Über das qualitative Verhalten der Blutplättchen bei der Perniciösa, Folia hæmatol., *57*, 1, 1937.
6. ASKEY, J. M.: Prevention of Pernicious Anemia, Ann. Int. Med., *14*, 593, 1940.
6a. ——— Addisonian Pernicious Anemia Without Achlorhydria: Does It Exist? Gastroenterology, *2*, 1, 1944.
7. BAILEY, H.: Abdominal Crisis of Pernicious Anemia, Brit. M. J., *2*, 554, 1926.
8. BAKER, B. M., JR., BORDLEY, J. and LONGCOPE, W. T.: Effect of Liver Therapy on Neurologic Manifestations of Pernicious Anemia, Am. J. M. Sc., *184*, 1, 1932.
9. BALDRIDGE, C. W. and BARER, A.: Studies on Relationship Between Oxygen Consump-

tion and Nitrogen Metabolism in Pernicious Anemia, J. Clin. Invest., *10*, 529, 1931.

10. BANG, O. and ØRSKOV, S. L.: Variations in the Permeability of the Red Cells in Man, With Particular Reference to the Conditions Obtaining in Pernicious Anemia, J. Clin. Invest., *16*, 279, 1937.

11. BARRON, M.: Pernicious Anemia and Tuberculosis: Is There an Antagonism? J.A.M.A., *100*, 1590, 1933.

12. BÄSTECKÝ, J. and VÁRADI, ST.: Les pseudotumeurs de l'estomac dans l'anémie pernicieuse, Sang, *9*, 41, 1935.

13. BEEBE, R. T. and WINTROBE, M. M.: Diagnosis of Obscure Cases of Pernicious Anemia, Arch. Int. Med., *51*, 630, 1933.

13a. BENJAMIN, B.: Infantile Form of Pernicious Anemia, Am. J. Dis. Child., *75*, 143, 1948.

13b. BERLIN, R.: Addison's Disease: Familial Incidence and Occurrence in Association with Pernicious Anemia, Acta med. scandinav., *144*, 1, 1952.

14. BETHELL, F. H. and HARRINGTON, B. D.: Incidence and Significance of Disease of Gall Bladder and Liver in Pernicious Anemia, Am. J. Digest. Dis., *1*, 256, 1934.

15. BIERMER, A.: Über progressive perniciöse Anämie, Korresp. f. schweiz. Aerzte, *2*, 15, 1872.

16. BIGG, E.: Spleen Size in Pernicious Anemia, Ann. Int. Med., *14*, 277, 1940.

16a. BLACKBURN, E. K.: Pernicious Anaemia Complicated by Granulocytic Leukaemia, J. Clin. Path., *10*, 258, 1957.

16b. BLOOMFIELD, A. L.: The Spontaneous Remission of Pernicious Anemia, Stanford Med. Bull., *2*, 5, 1944.

16c. BODDINGTON, M. M.: Changes in Buccal Cells in the Anaemias, J. Clin. Path., *12*, 222 and 228, 1959.

17. BOENHEIM, F.: Addison's Disease and Pernicious Anemia, Endokrinologie, *28*, 140, 1951.

17a. BOENHEIM, F., SCHWIMMER, D. and McGAVACK, T. H.: The Combination of Hyperthyroidism and Pernicious Anemia, Ann. Int. Med., *27*, 869, 1945.

17b. BOYDEN, E. A. and LAYNE, J. A.: The Gall Bladder in Patients With Pernicious Anemia: A Study of Non-Visualization and Rate of Emptying, Gastroenterology, *4*, 121, 1945.

18. BOWMAN, K. M.: Psychoses With Pernicious Anemia, Am. J. Psychiat., *92*, 371, 1935.

18a. BROWN, A.: Glossitis in Addisonian Pernicious Anaemia, Brit. M. J., *1*, 704, 1949.

19. BROWN, M. R.: The Pathology of the Gastro-Intestinal Tract in Pernicious Anemia and Subacute Combined Degeneration of the Spinal Cord, New England J. Med., *210*, 473, 1934.

19a. CALLENDER, SHEILA T. and DENBOROUGH, M. A.: A Family Study of Pernicious Anaemia, Brit. J. Haemat., *3*, 88, 1957.

19b. CARTER, J. B. and TRAUT, E. F.: Cardiovascular Manifestations in Pernicious Anemia, Arch. Int. Med., *72*, 757, 1943.

19c. CAYER, D., RUFFIN, J. M. and PERLZWEIG, W. A.: Vitamin Levels in Pernicious Anemia, Am. J. M. Sc., *212*, 179, 1946.

20. CHEVALLIER, P., GUTMANN, R. A., SALMON, A. R. and FIEHRER, A.: Sur la reprise très rapide de la sécrétion gastrique dans la maladie de biermer traitée par le foie, Sang, *7*, 756, 1933.

21. CHRISTIAN, H. A.: Renal Function in Pernicious Anemia, Arch. Int. Med., *18*, 429, 1916.

21a. CLARK, S. L.: Oral Folic Acid Tolerance Test in Normal Human Subjects and Patients with Pernicious Anemia, Proc. Soc. Exper. Biol. & Med., *82*, 25, 1953.

22. CLEMENT, D. H., NICHOL, C. A. and WELCH, A. D.: A Case of Juvenile Pernicious Anemia: Study of the Effects of Folic Acid and Vitamin B$_{12}$, Blood, *17*, 618, 1961.

23. CONNERY, J. E. and JOLLIFFE, N.: Studies on "Acid Deficit" in Pernicious Anemia, Am. J. M. Sc., *181*, 830, 1931.

24. CORNELL, B. S.: *Pernicious Anemia*, Durham, N. C., Duke University Press, 1927 (Bibliography).

24a. COX, A. J.: The Stomach in Pernicious Anemia, Am. J. Path., *19*, 491, 1943.

24b. CREGER, W. P. and SORTOR, A. T.: The Incidence of Blood Group A in Pernicious Anemia, A. M. A. Arch. Int. Med., *98*, 136, 1956.

24c. DALAND, G. A., HEATH, C. W. and MINOT, G. R.: Differentiation of Pernicious Anemia and Certain Other Macrocytic Anemias by the Distribution of Red Blood Cell Diameters, Blood, *1*, 6, 1946.

25. DAMESHEK, W. and VALENTINE, E.: The Sternal Marrow in Pernicious Anemia, Arch. Path., *23*, 159, 1937.

25a. DAVIDSON, C. S., MURPHY, J. C., WATSON, R. J. and CASTLE, W. B.: Comparison of the Effects of Massive Blood Transfusions and of Liver Extract in Pernicious Anemia, J. Clin. Invest., *25*, 858, 1946.

25b. DAVIDSON, L. S. P.: Pernicious Anemia With Return of Hydrochloric Acid and Ferments After Treatment, Brit. M. J., *1*, 182, 1933.

26. DAVIDSON, S.: Clinical Picture of Pernicious Anaemia Prior to Introduction of Liver Therapy in 1926 and in Edinburgh Subsequent to 1944, Brit. M. J., *1*, 241, 1957.

34

26a.DAVIS, L. J.: Macrocytic Anæmia in Children, Arch. Dis. Child., *19*, 147, 1944.

26b.DAVIS, R. W., CHRISTINA, R. M., ERVIN, D. M. and YOUNG, L. E.: Pernicious Anemia in Childhood, Blood, *4*, 1361, 1949.

27. DAVISON, C.: Subacute Combined Degeneration of Cord, Arch. Neurol. & Psychiat., *26*, 1195, 1931; Arch. Int. Med., *67*, 473, 1941.

27a.DEDICHEN, I.: Anémie à type pernicieux chez un enfant de 9 mois, Acta med. scandinav., *111*, 90, 1942.

28. DOBRINER, K. and RHOADS, C. P.: The Metabolism of Blood Pigments in Pernicious Anemia, J. Clin. Invest., *17*, 95, 1938.

28a.DOSCHERHOLMEN, A. and HAGEN, P. S.: Radioactive Vitamin B_{12} Absorption Studies: Results of Direct Measurement of Radioactivity in the Blood, Blood, *12*, 336, 1957; J. Clin. Invest., *36*, 1551, 1957; J. Lab. & Clin. Med., *54*, 434, 1959; *ibid.*, *56*, 547, 1960.

29. DRAPER, G.: *Human Constitution: A Consideration of Its Relationship to Disease*, Philadelphia and London, W. B. Saunders Company, 1924.

30. ELLISON, A. B. C.: Pernicious Anemia Masked by Multivitamins Containing Folic Acid, J.A.M.A., *173*, 240, 1960.

30a.EPSTEIN, R. D.: Cells of the Megakaryocyte Series in Pernicious Anemia, Am. J. Path., *25*, 239, 1949.

31. ERF, L. A. and RHOADS, C. P.: The Glycine Tolerance Test in Sprue and Pernicious Anemia, J. Clin. Invest., *19*, 409, 1940.

32. FABIAN, G.: Secretion of Saliva, Ztschr. klin. Med., *131*, 161, 1937.

32. FABIAN, G.: Secretion of Saliva, Ztschr. klin. Med., *131*, 161, 1937.

33. FIESCHI, A.: Semeiologia del midollo osseo: VI. Biblioteca "Hæmatologica," Pavia, Tipografia gia Cooperativa, 1938.

34. FINCH, C. A. *et al.*: Erythrokinetics in Pernicious Anemia, Blood, *11*, 807, 1956.

35. FINNEY, J. O.: Pernicious Anemia Unassociated With Achlorhydria, Ann. Int. Med., *12*, 1521, 1939.

36. FORSSELL, J. and HALONEN, P. I.: Thyroid Function and Pernicious Anaemia, Acta med. scandinav., *162*, 61, 1958.

37. FOWLER, W. M.: Fever Accompanying the Induced Reticulocyte Crisis of Pernicious Anemia, J. Lab. & Clin. Med., *22*, 155, 1936.

38. FRIEDLANDER, R. D.: Racial Factor in Pernicious Anemia, Am. J. M. Sc., *187*, 634, 1934.

38a.FUSCO, F. A. and BOURONCLE, BERTHA A.: The Coincidence of Sickle Cell Trait and Pernicious Anemia, Acta haemat., *20*, 383, 1958.

39. GALT, J., HUNTER, R. B. and HILL, J. M.: Pernicious Anemia Superseded by Polycythemia Vera, Am. J. M. Sc., *223*, 61, 1952.

40. GIBSON, J. G., II: Clinical Studies of the Blood Volume, J. Clin. Inves., *18*, 401, 1939.

40a.GLASS, G. B. J., BOYD, L. J., GELLIN, G. A. and STEPHANSON, L.: Uptake of Radioactive Vitamin B_{12} by the Liver in Humans, Arch. Biochem., *51*, 251, 1954; Ann. Int. Med., *47*, 274, 1957; Proc. Soc. Exper. Biol. & Med., *95*, 325, 1957.

41. GOLDHAMER, S. M.: The Effect of Ventriculin on the Blood Sugar Level in Patients With Pernicious Anemia, J. Clin. Invest., *11*, 641, 1932.

42. ———— Macrocytic Anemia in Cancer of the Stomach, Apparently Due to Lack of Intrinsic Factor, Am. J. M. Sc., *195*, 17, 1938.

43. GOLDHAMER, S. M., BETHELL, F. H., ISAACS, R. and STURGIS, C. C.: Occurrence and Treatment of Neurologic Changes in Pernicious Anemia, J.A.M.A., *103*, 1663, 1934.

43a.GORDIN, R.: Prothrombin in Cryptogenetic Pernicious Anemia and Pernicious Tapeworm Anemia and Its Response to Treatment, Acta med. scandinav., *149*, 1, 1954.

44. GREENFIELD, J. G. and CARMICHAEL, E. A.: The Peripheral Nerves in Cases of Subacute Combined Degeneration of the Cord, Brain, *58*, 483, 1935.

46. GRINKER, R. R. and KANDEL, E.: Pernicious Anemia: Results of Treatment of Neurologic Complications, Arch. Int. Med., *54*, 851, 1934.

47. GROEN, J.: The Absorption of Glucose From the Small Intestine in Deficiency Disease, New England J. Med., *218*, 247, 1938.

47a.HALL, B. E., KNISEN, F. H. and WOLTMAN, H. W.: Vitamin B_{12} and Coördination Exercises for Combined Degeneration of the Spinal Cord in Pernicious Anemia, J. A. M. A., *141*, 257, 1949.

47b.HALLBERG, L.: Blood Volume, Hemolysis and Regeneration of Blood in Pernicious Anemia, Scandinav. J. Clin. & Lab. Invest., 7 Supp. 16, 1955.

48. HAMILTON, A. S. and NIXON, C. E.: Sensory Changes in the Subacute Combined Degeneration of Pernicious Anemia, Arch. Neurol. & Pschyiat., *6*, 1, 1921.

48a.HAMILTON, H. E., ELLIS, P. P. and SHEETS, R. F.: Visual Impairment Due to Optic Neuropathy in Pernicious Anemia, Blood, *14*, 378, 1959.

48b.HAMILTON, H. E. and FOWLER, W. M.: Pernicious Anemia in Early Adolescence, Arch. Int. Med., *84*, 445, 1948.

48c.HAMILTON, H. E., DeGowin, E. L., Sheets, R. F., Janney, D. C. and Ellis, J. A.: Accelerated Destruction of Normal Adult Erythrocytes in Pernicious Anemia; Contribution of Hemolysis to the Oligocythemia, J. Clin. Invest., *33*, 191, 1954; J. L b. & Clin. Med., *46*, 821, 1955, ibid., *51*, 942, 1958.

49. Hartfall, S. J.: Secretion of Gastric Juice in Response to Histamine in Addisonian Anemia, Guy's Hosp. Rep., *83*, 37, 1933.

50. Heath, C. W. and Fullerton, H. W.: The Rate of Absorption of Iodide and Glycine From the Gastrointestinal Tract in Normal Persons and in Disease Conditions, J. Clin. Invest., *14*, 475, 1935.

50a.Heaton, J. M., McCormick, A. J. A. and Freeman, A. G.: Tobacco Amblyopia: A Clinical Manifestation of Vitamin-B_{12} Deficiency, Lancet, *2*, 286, 1958.

51. Heck, F. J.: Myeloid Immaturity in Pernicious Anemia, Am. J. Clin. Path., *2*, 443, 1932.

52. Heilmeyer, L.: Blutfarbstoffwechselstudien; die Regenerations- und Farbstoffwechselvorgänge beim Morbus Biermer sowie bei einer Bothriocephalusanämie vor und nach Leberbehandlung, Deutsch. Arch. kiln. Med., *173*, 128, 1932.

53. Helmer, O. M. and Fouts, P. J.: Gastro-intestinal Studies: VII. The Excretion of Xylose in Pernicious Anemia, J. Clin. Invest., *16*, 343, 1937.

54. Herman, M., Most, H. and Jolliffe, N.: Psychoses Associated With Pernicious Anemia, J.A.M.A., *109*, 1075, 1937.

55. Hitzenberger, G.: Gleichzeitiges Bestehen von perniziöser Anämie und chronischer Myelose, Folia haemat., *2*, 203, 1958.

56. Holly, P. B., Felts, W. R. and Rheingold, J. J.: Pernicious Anemia Occurring Simultaneously in Identical Negro Twins, Arch. Int. Med., *90*, 707, 1952.

56a.Holmes, J. MacD.: Cerebral Manifestations of Vitamin-B_{12} Deficiency, Brit. M. J., *2*, 1394, 1956.

56b.Høstrup, H. and Bastrup-Madsen, P.: Uropepsinogen Excretion in Patients with Pernicious Anaemia and in Subjects with Simple Achlorhydria, Acta med. scandinav., *158*, 193, 1957.

56c.Huff, R. L. et al.: Plasma and Red Cell Iron Turnover in Normal Subjects and in Patients Having Various Hemopoietic Disorders, J. Clin. Invest., *29*, 1041, 1950.

57. Jacobson, W.: The Argentaffine Cells and Pernicious Anaemia, J. Path. & Bacteriol., *49*, 1, 1939; Ibid., *57*, 101, 1945; Biochem. J., *40*, 3, 1946.

58. James, G. W., III, and Abbott, L. D., Jr.:

Nitrogen and Phosphorus Metabolism during Vitamin B_{12}-Induced Remission, Metabolism, *1*, 259, 1952.

59. Jones, C. M., Benedict, E. B. and Hampton, A. O.: Variations in the Gastric Mucosa in Pernicious Anemia: Gastroscopic, Surgical and Roentgenologic Observations, Am. J. M. Sc., *190*, 596, 1935.

59a.Jones, E., Tillman, C. C. and Darby, W. J.: Observations on Relapses in Pernicious Anemia, Ann. Int. Med., *30*, 374, 1949; Am. J. Clin. Nutrition, *6*, 513, 1958.

60. Jones, E.: Observations on Seventy-eight Cases of Pernicious Anemia With Special Reference to Weight Changes, Am. J. M. Sc., *195*, 150, 1938.

61. Jones, O. P.: Origin of Neutrophils in Pernicious Anemia (Cooke's Macropolycytes), Arch. Int. Med., *60*, 1002, 1937.

62. ———— Nature of the Reticulocytosis in Pernicious Anemia Following Liver Therapy, Proc. Soc. Exper. Biol. and Med., *38*, 222, 1938; Arch. Path., *35*, 752, 1943.

62a.Kade, H.: Pernicious Anemia During Childhood, Ztschr. Kinderheilk., *65*, 47, 1947.

63. Kahn, J. R.: Absence of Peptic Ulcer in Pernicious Anemia, Am. J. M. Sc., *194*, 463, 1937.

64. Kampmeier, R. H. and Cameron, P. B.: Pernicious Anemia in the Negro, Am. J. M. Sc., *192*, 751, 1936.

65. Kaplan, H. S. and Rigler, L. G.: Pernicious Anemia and Carcinoma of the Stomach—Autopsy Studies Concerning Their Interrelationship, Am. J. M. Sc., *209*, 339, 1945.

66. Kaufmann, O. and Thiessen, K.: Hereditary Biology of Pernicious Anemia, Ztschr. klin. Med., *136*, 474, 1939.

66a.Kay, A. W.: Effect of Large Doses of Histamine on Gastric Secretion of HCl and an Augmented Histamine Test, Brit. M. J., *2*, 77, 1953.

67. Kirk, E.: The Concentration of the Individual Phosphatides (Lecithin, Kephalin, Ether-Insoluble Phosphatide) and of Cerebrosides in Plasma and Red Blood Cells in Pernicious Anemia Before and During Liver Treatment, Am. J. M. Sc., *196*, 648, 1938.

67a.Kristensen, H. P. O. and Gormsen, H.: Vitamin B_{12} Deficiency in Uncharacteristic Macrocytic Anaemia, Acta med. scandinav., *162*, 415, 1958.

67b.Lambert, H. P., Prankerd, T. A. J. and Smellie, Jean M.: Pernicious Anaemia in Childhood, Quart. J. Med., *30*, 71, 1961.

68. Lear, A. A., Harris, J. W., Castle, W. B. and Fleming, E. M.: The Serum Vitamin B_{12} Concentration in Pernicious Anemia, J. Lab. & Clin. Med., *44*, 715, 1954.

69. LEIKIN, S. L.: Pernicious Anemia in Childhood, Pediatrics, *25*, 91, 1960.

69a. LERMAN, J. and MEANS, J. H.: Blood Pressure in Pernicious Anemia, Am. J. M. Sc., *175*, 777, 1928.

70. LEVINE, S. A. and LADD, W. S.: Pernicious Anemia: Clinical Study of One Hundred and Fifty Consecutive Cases With Special Reference to Gastric Anacidity, Bull. Johns Hopkins Hosp., *32*, 254, 1921.

70a. LONDON, I. M., SHEMIN, D., WEST, R. and RITTENBERG, D.: Heme Synthesis and Red Blood Dynamics in Normal Humans and in Subjects with Polycythemia Vera, Sickle-Cell Anemia and Pernicious Anemia, J. Biol. Chem., *179*, 463, 1949.

71. MACLACHLAN, W. W. G. and KLINE, F. M.: Occurrence of Anemia in Four Generations, Am. J. M. Sc., *172*, 533, 1926.

71a. MACLEAN, L. D.: The Differentiation of Achylia Gastrica and Achlorhydria by Means of Radioactive Vitamin B_{12}, Gastroenterology, *29*, 653, 1955.

72. MAGNUS, H. A. and UNGLEY, C. C.: The Gastric Lesion in Pernicious Anemia, Lancet, *1*, 420, 1938; *Modern Trends in Gastroenterology*, 1952, Butterworth & Co., Ltd., London; J. Clin. Path., *11*, 289, 1958.

72a. MALTBY, E. J.: Digestion of Beef Proteins in Human Stomach, J. Clin. Invest., *13*, 193, 1934.

72b. MASON, J. D., JR. and LEAVELL, B. S.: The Effect of Transfusions of Erythrocytes on Untreated Pernicious Anemia, Blood, *11*, 632, 1956.

73 MASSEY, B. W. and RUBIN, C. E.: The Stomach in Pernicious Anemia, Am. J. M. Sc., *227*, 481, 1954; *ibid.*, *230*, 506, 1955; Gastroenterology, *29*, 563, 1955

73a. MASSIE, R. W.: Relationship between Red Cell and Plasma Volume during Recovery from Pernicious Anemia, A. M. A. Arch. Int. Med., *103*, 593, 1959.

74. McKINLAY, P. L.: Influence of Liver Treatment on Mortality From Pernicious Anemia, Lancet, *2*, 1086, 1929.

74a. McINTYRE, PATRICIA A., HAHN, ROZELLE, CONLEY, C. L. and GLASS, B.: Genetic Factors in Predisposition to Pernicious Anemia, Bull. Johns Hopkins Hosp., *104*, 309, 1959.

74b. METZ, J., CASSEL, R. and LEWIS, S. M.: Pernicious Anaemia in the South African Bantu, South African M. J., *31*, 190, 1958.

75. MEULENGRACHT, E., IVERSEN, P. and NAKAZAWA, F.: Pernicious Anemia, Arch. Int. Med., *42*, 425, 1928.

75a. MEYER, C. E., BURTON, I. F. and STURGIS, C. C.: Riboflavin Absorption in Pernicious Anemia, Proc. Soc. Exper. Biol. & Med., *50*, 251, 1942.

75b. MEYER, L. M., SAWITSKY, A., RITZ, N. D. and FITCH, H. M.: A Study of Cholinesterase Activity of the Blood of Patients with Pernicious Anemia, J. Lab. & Clin. Med. *33*, 189, 1948.

75c. MOLLIN, D. L.: Radioactive Vitamin B_{12} in the Study of Blood Diseases, Brit. M. Bull., *15*, 8, 1959.

76. MOLLIN, D. L., BAKER, S. J. and DONIACH, I.: Addisonian Pernicious Anæmia without Gastric Atrophy in a Young Man, Brit. J. Hæmat., *1*, 278, 1955.

77. MONTGOMERY, E. W.: Studies in Pernicious Anemia; Outstanding Clinical Problem and Geographical Distribution in Western Canada, Canad. M. A. J., *16*, 244, 1926.

77a. MOORE, C. V., DOAN, C. A. and ARROWSMITH, W. R.: The Mechanism of Iron Transportation: Its Significance in Iron Utilization in Anemic States of Varied Etiology, J. Clin. Invest., *16*, 627, 1937.

78. MORRIS, H. H.: Anemias in China, Chinese M. J., *43*, 768, 1929.

78a. MOSBECH, J.: *Heredity in Pernicious Anaemia*, Copenhagen, Ejnar Munksgaard, 1953.

78b. MOSBECH, J.: Pernicious Anaemia and Myeloid Leukaemia, Folia haemat., *76*, 487, 1959.

78c. MOSBECH, J. and VIDEBAEK, A.: Mortality from and Risk of Gastric Carcinoma Among Patients with Pernicious Anæmia, Brit. M. J., *2*, 390, 1950.

79. MULLER, G. L.: Relation of Cholesterol Lecithin, Phosphorus and Fatty Acids to Remission of Pernicious Anemia, Am. J. M. Sc., *179*, 316, 1930.

80. MURPHY, W. P. and HOWARD, I.: An Analysis of the Complications Occurring in a Series of Patients With Pernicious Anemia, Rev. Gastroenterology, *3*, 98, 1936.

81. NAEGELI, O.: *Blutkrankheiten und Blutdiagnostik*, 5th ed., Berlin, Julius Springer, 1931.

81a. NELSON, R. S. and SALVADOR, D. S. J.: Pseudotumors of Gastric Antrum in Pernicious Anemia, J.A.M.A., *67*, 1487, 1958.

81b. NORCROSS, J. W., MONROE, S. E. and GRIFFIN B. G.: The Development of Gastric Carcinoma in Pernicious Anemia, Ann. Int Med., *37*, 338, 1952.

82. NORDENSON, N. G., SEGERDAHL, E., STRANDELL, B. and WALLMAN-CARLSSON, C. Die Frequenz und geographische Verbreitung der perniziösen Anämie in Schweden, Acta med. scandinav., *97*, 222, 1938.

83. OATWAY, W. H. and MIDDLETON, W. S. Correlation of Lingual Changes With

Other Clinical Data, Arch. Int. Med., *49*, 860, 1932.

83a. OTSUKA, S., KOSHIISHI, Y., NARUTO, K. and KUMAI, K.: Die Anaemia perniciosa in Japan (Statistik), Acta haemat., *16*, 199, 1956.

83b. OWREN, P. A.: A Protein Synthesis Liver Factor Lacking in Pernicious Anemia and Related Macrocytic Anemias, Scand. J. Clin. & Lab. Invest., 2, 241, 1950.

84. PADDOCK, F. K. and SMITH, K. E.: The Platelets in Pernicious Anemia, Am. J. M. Sc., *198*, 372, 1939.

84a. PETERSON, J. C. and DUNN, S. C.: Pernicious Anemia in Childhood, Am. J. Dis. Child., *73*, 578, 1947.

84b. PITNEY, W. R. and STOKES, J. B.: Diagnostic Value of Radioactive Vitamin B_{12}, Australasian Ann. Med., *7*, 126, 1958.

85. PONDER, E. and RHOADS, C. P.: Red Cell Resistance to Lysins in Pernicious Anemia, Proc. Soc. Exper. Biol. & Med., *38*, 540, 1938.

86. PREU, P. W. and GEIGER, A. J.: Symptomatic Psychoses in Pernicious Anemia, Ann. Int. Med., *9*, 766, 1935.

87. PRICE-JONES, C.: Red Cell Diameters in One Hundred Healthy Persons and in Pernicious Anemia: Effect of Liver Treatment, J. Path. & Bact., *32*, 479, 1929.

87a. RATH, C. E., MCCURDY, P. R. and DUFFY, B. J., JR.: Effect of Renal Disease on the Schilling Test, New England J. Med., *256*, 111, 1957.

88. REISNER, E. H., JR., WOLFF, J. A., MCKAY, R. J., JR. and DOYLE, E. F.: Juvenile Pernicious Anemia, Pediatrics, *8*, 88, 1951; Ann. Int. Med., *43*, 1116, 1955.

89. RICH, M. L. and SCHIFF, L.: A Case of Pernicious Anemia and Chronic Lymphatic Leukemia, Ann. Int. Med., *10*, 252, 1936.

90. RIDDLE, M. C.: Endogenous Uric Acid Metabolism in Pernicious Anemia, J. Clin. Invest., *8*, 69, 1929.

91. ———— Blood Sugar During Remission in Pernicious Anemia, Ann. Int. Med., *3*, 1097, 1930.

92. RIGLER, L. G., KAPLAN, H. S. and FINK, D. L.: Pernicious Anemia and the Early Diagnosis of Tumors of the Stomach, J.A.M.A., *128*, 426, 1945; J. Lab. & Clin. Med., *32*, 644, 1947.

93. ROOT, H. F.: Diabetes and Pernicious Anemia, J.A.M.A., *96*, 928, 1931.

94. ROZENDAAL, H. M. and WASHBURN, R. N.: Gastric Secretion in Cases of Pernicious Anemia, Ann. Int. Med., *11*, 1834, 1938.

94a. ROWLANDS, E. N. and WILKINSON, J. F.: The Clinical Significance and Estimation of Blood Vitamin B_1, Brit. M. J., *2*, 878, 1938.

95. SAITA, G., MOREO, L. and PERINI, A.: Contributo allo studio delle porfirine libere eritrocitarie nell'anemia di Biermer, Haematologica, *43*, 51, 1958.

95a. SAMSON, D. C., SWISHER, S. N., CHRISTIAN, R. M. and ENGEL, G. L.: Cerebral Metabolic Disturbance and Delirium in Pernicious Anemia, Arch. Int. Med., *90*, 4, 1952.

95b. SANDBERG, A. A., EIK-NES, K., NELSON, D. H., PALMER, J. G., CARTWRIGHT, G. E. and WINTROBE, M. M.: Adrenocortical Function and Metabolism of 17-Hydroxycorticosteroids in Pernicious Anemia, New England J. Med., *251*, 169, 1954.

96. SCHELL, R. F., DOCKERTY, M. B. and COMFORT, M. W.: Carcinoma of the Stomach Associated with Pernicious Anemia, Surg., Gynec. & Obst., *98*, 710, 1954.

96a. SCHILLING, R. F., HARRIS, J. W.: Liver Function in Untreated Addisonian Pernicious Anemia, J. Lab. & Clin. Med., *40*, 718, 1952.

97a. SCHWARTZ, S. O. and GORE, M.: Pernicious Anemia in Negroes, Arch. Int. Med. *72*, 782, 1943.

97b. SCHWARTZ, S. O. and LEGERE, H.: Atypical Pernicious Anemia of Young Adults, Am. J. M. Sc., *206*, 1, 1943.

97c. ———— Relapses in Pernicious Anemia, J.A.M.A., *124*, 637, 1944.

97d. SCHWARTZ, S. O. and RAPPOLT, Z. A.: Pernicious Anemia in Chinese, Arch. Int. Med., *75*, 404, 1945; *ibid.*, *76*, 130, 1945.

97e. SCHLEICHER, E. M.: The Morphology of the Erythrogenic Reticulum of the Bone Marrow in Addison-Biermer's Disease in Relapse and Early Remission as Seen by the Imprint Method, J. Lab. & Clin. Med., *30*, 928, 1945.

98. SELLERS, A. H.: Study of the Objective Efficacy of Liver Therapy in Pernicious Anemia Based on Recorded Mortality Data, Am. J. Hyg., *25*, 259, 1937.

99. SHARP, E. A., SCHLEICHER, E. M. and WOLTER, J. W.: The Myeloid Pattern in Pernicious Anemia, Am. J. Clin. Path., *9*, 189, 1939.

99a. SINGER, K., KING, J. C. and ROBIN, S.: The Life Span of the Megalocyte and the Hemolytic Syndrome of Pernicious Anemia, J. Lab. & Clin. Med., *33*, 1068, 1948.

100. SMITH, J. H.: Relation Between Deficiency of Solar Radiation and Mortality Due to Pernicious Anemia in United States, Am. J. M. Sc., *188*, 200, 1934.

100a. SMITH, L. H., JR. and BAKER, FAITH A.:

Pyrimidine Metabolism in Man, J. Clin. Invest., *39*, 15, 1960.

101. SMITHBURN, K. C. and ZERFAS, L. G.: The Neural Symptoms and Signs in Pernicious Anemia, Arch. Neu ol. & Psychiat., *25*, 1110, 1931.

102. STALKER, H.: Angina Pectoris and Pernicious Anemia (Old Terminology): A Résumé of the Literature, With a Case Report, Ann. Int. Med., *10*, 1172, 1937.

103. STAMOS, H. F.: Heredity in Pernicious Anemia, Am. J. M. Sc., *200*, 586, 1940.

103a. STERNE, E. H., JR., SCHIRO, H. and MOLLE, W.: Pernicious Anemia Complicated by Myelogenous Leukemia, Am. J. M. Sc., *202*, 167, 1941.

104. STEWART, H. J., CRANE, N. F. and DEITRICK, J. E.: Studies of the Circulation in Pernicious Anemia, J. Clin. Invest., *16*, 431, 1937.

105. STIEGLITZ, E. J.: Disturbances of Renal Function in Pernicious Anemia, Arch. Int. Med., *33*, 58, 1924.

106. STOCKTON, C. G.: Long Duration of Remission in Pernicious Anemia, Am. J. M. Sc., *158*, 471, 1919.

106a. STRAUSS, M. B., BROKAW, R. and CHAPMAN, C. B.: Leukemoid Bone Marrow in Pernicious Anemia, Am. J. M. Sc., *223*, 54, 1952.

108. STUB, O.: The Death Rate From Pernicious Anemia in Norway, Acta med. scandinav., *81*, 535, 1934.

109. STURGIS, C. C.: An Analysis of the Causes of Death in 150 Fatal Cases of Pernicious Anemia Observed Since 1927, Trans. A. Am. Physicians, *54*, 46, 1939.

109a. SWENDSEID, M. E., BURTON, I. F. and BETHELL, F. H.: Excretion of Keto Acids and Hydroxyphenyl Compounds in Pernicious Anemia, Proc. Soc. Exper. Biol. & Med., *52*, 202, 1943; J. Lab. & Clin. Med., *32*, 1242, 1947.

109b. TALLEY, R. W., DOHERTY, J. E. and SHUKERS, C. F.: Pernicious Anemia Complicated by Acute Granulocytic Leukemia, South. M. J., *45*, 559, 1952.

109c. TAWAST, M. and SIURALA, M.: Transition of Pernicious Anaemia into Chronic Myeloid Leukaemia, Acta med. scandinav., *154*, 211, 1956.

110. TEMPKA and BRAUN, B.: Zur Frage des Mechanismus der gesteigerten Hämolyse und der antihämolytischen Leberwirkung im Verlaufe der perniziösen Anämie, Folia hæmatol., *45*, 269, 1931.

111. ———— Das morphologische Verhalten des Sternumpunktates in verschiedenen Stadien der perniziösen Anämie und seine Wandlungen unter dem Einflusse der Therapie, Folia hæmatol., *48*, 355, 1932.

112. THADDEA, S. and SAUERBRUCH, F.: Über besondere Verlaufsformen der perniziösen Anämie, Folia hæmatol., *61*, 289, 1939.

112a. TODD, D.: Observations on the Amino-Aciduria in Megaloblastic Anaemia, J. Clin. Path., *12*, 238, 1959.

113. TOPOREK, M., BISHOP, R. C., NELSON, N. A. and BETHELL, F. H.: Urinary Excretion of Co^{60} Vitamin B$_{12}$ As a Test for Effectiveness of Intrinsic Factor Preparations, J. Lab. & Clin. Med., *46*, 665, 1955.

114. VAN DER SCHEER, W. M. and KOEK, H. C.: Peripheral Nerve Lesions in Cases of Pernicious Anemia, Acta psychiat. et neurol., *13*, 61, 1938.

115. VAUGHAN, J. M.: Gain in Body Weight Associated With Remissions in Pernicious Anemia, Arch. Int. Med., *47*, 688, 1931.

115a. VICTOR, M. and LEAR, A. A.: Subacute Combined Degeneration of the Spinal Cord, A m. J. Med., *20*, 896, 1956.

116. VILTER, R. W., HORRIGAN, D., MUELLER, J. F., JARROLD, T., VILTER, C. F., HAWKINS, V. and SEAMAN, A.: Studies on the Relationships of Vitamin B$_{12}$, Folic Acid, Thymine, Uracil and Methyl Group Donors in Persons with Pernicious Anemia and Related Megaloblastic Anemias, Blood, *5*, 695, 1950.

117. WASSERMAN, L. R. et al.: Rate of Removal of Radioactive Iron from Plasma-Index of Erythropoiesis, J. Clin. Invest., *31*, 32, 1952.

117a. WHITE, R. R.: Simultaneous Carcinoma and Tuberculosis of the Stomach in a Case of Pernicious Anemia, Staff Meet. Mayo Clin., *18*, 165, 1943.

118. WILKINSON, J. F.: Gastric Secretion in Pernicious Anaemia, Quart. J. Med., *1*, 361, 1932.

119. ———— Diseases Associated With Pernicious Anaemia, Quart. J. Med., *2*, 281, 1933.

121. WILLIAMS, A. W., COGHILL, N. F. and EDWARDS, FELICITY: The Gastric Mucosa in Pernicious Anaemia: Biopsy Studies, Brit. J. Haemat., *4*, 457, 1958.

122. WILLIAMS, H. H., ERICKSON, B. N., BERNSTEIN, S., HUMMEL, F. C. and MACY, I. G.: The Lipid and Mineral Distribution of the Serum and Erythrocytes in Pernicious Anemia, J. Biol. Chem., *118*, 599, 1937; Proc. Soc. Biol. & Med., *45*, 151, 1940.

123. WINTROBE, M. M.: Hemoglobin Content Volume and Thickness of Erythrocyte in Pernicious Anemia and Sprue and Change

Produced by Liver Therapy, Am. J. M. Sc., *181*, 217, 1931.

124. ———— Relation of Variations in Mean Corpuscular Volume to Number of Reticulocytes in Pernicious Anemia, J. Clin. Invest., *13*, 669, 1934.

124a. WITEBSKY, E., KLENDSHOJ, N. C. and VAUGHAN, S. L.: Occurrence of Blood Group Specific Substances in Gastric Juice of Patients With Pernicious Anemia, Proc. Soc. Exper. Biol. & Med., *49*, 633, 1942.

124b. WOOLLEY, P. B.: Myelogenous Leukemia Complicating Pernicious Anemia, Lancet, *1*, 85, 1944.

124c. ZADEK, I.: Pathogenesis of Pernicious Anemia: Result of Postmortem Examination of Patients Who Died During Remission, Klin. Wchnschr., *8*, 1527, 1929.

125. ZAMCHECK, N., GRABLE, E., LEY, A. and NORMAN, L.: Occurrence of Gastric Cancer Among Patients with Pernicious Anemia at the Boston City Hospital, New England J. Med., *252*, 1103, 1955.

125a. ZARAFONETIS, C. J. D., OVERMAN, R. L. and MOLTHAN, L.: Unique Sequence of Pernicious Anemia, Polycythemia, and Acute Leukemia, Blood, *12*, 1011, 1957.

125b. ZIMMERMAN, S. P. and DUGGER, S.: Pernicious Anemia in the Tropical Negro, Arch. Int. Med., *82*, 184, 1948.

Sprue, Idiopathic Steatorrhea and Celiac Disease

125c. ANDERSON, D. H.: Celiac Syndrome, J. Pediat., *30*, 564, 1947; Pediatrics, *11*, 207 and 224, 1953.

126. ASHFORD, B. K.: Sprue, *Tice's Practice of Medicine*, Hagerstown, Md., W. F. Prior Company, Inc., *4*, 173.

127. BADENOCH, J. and CALLENDER, S. T.: Iron Metabolism in Steatorrhea, Blood, *9*, 123, 1954; Lancet, *1*, 192, 1960.

127a. BADENOCH, J. and FOURMAN, P.: Osteomalacia in Steatorrhoea, Quart. J. Med., *23*, 165, 1954.

127b. BAKER, S. J.: Idiopathic Tropical Steatorrhea, Indian J. M. Sc., *11*, 687, 1957.

128. BARKER, W. H. and RHOADS, C. P.: The Effect of Liver Extract on the Absorption of Fat in Sprue, Am. J. M. Sc., *194*, 804, 1937.

129. BASSETT, S. H., KEUTMANN, E. H., HYDE, H. van Z., VAN ALSTINE, H. E. and RUSS, E.: Metabolism in Idiopathic Steatorrhea, J. Clin. Invest., *18*, 101 and 121, 1939

130. BENNETT, T. I., HUNTER, D. and VAUGHAN, J. M.: Idiopathic Steatorrhœa, Quart. J. Med., *1*, 603, 1932 (Bibliography).

130a. BOSCOTT, R. J. and COOKE, W. T.: Ascorbic Acid Requirements and Urinary Excretion of p-Hydroxyphenylacetic Acid in Steatorrhœa and Macrocytic Anæmia, Quart. J. Med., *23*, 307, 1954.

131. BUTTERWORTH, C. E., JR., SOLER, J., SANTINI, R., JR. and PEREZ-SANTIAGO, E.: Certain Aspects of Glycine and Histidine Metabolism in Patients with Sprue, Blood, *15*, 60, 1960.

131a. BUTTERWORTH, C. E., JR. and PEREZ-SANTIAGO, E.: Jejunal Biopsies in Sprue, Ann. Int. Med., *48*, 8, 1958.

132. CASTLE, W. B., RHOADS, C. P., LAWSON, H. A. and PAYNE, G. C.: Etiology and Treatment of Sprue, Arch. Int. Med., *56*, 627, 1935.

132a. CAYER, D., RUFFIN, J. and PERLZWEIG, W. A.: Vitamin Levels in Sprue, Am. J. M. Sc., *210*, 200, 1945.

132b. CHILDS, A. and DICK, G. F.: Pancreatic Function in a Case of Non-Tropical Sprue, Arch. Int. Med., *66*, 833, 1940.

133. CHRISTIANSEN, P. A., KIRSNER, J. B. and ABLAZA, JEAN: D-Xylose and Its Use in the Diagnosis of Malabsorptive States, Am. J. Med., *27*, 443, 1959.

133a. COMFORT, M. W., WOLLAEGER, E. E., TAYLOR, A. B. and POWER, M. H.: Nontropical Sprue: Observations on Absorption and Metabolism, Gastroenterology, *23*, 155, 1953.

133b. COOKE, W. T., PEENEY, A. L. P. and HAWKINS, C. F.: Symptoms, Signs, and Diagnostic Features of Idiopathic Steatorrhœa, Quart. J. Med., *22*, 59, 1953.

134. COX, E. V., MEYNELL, M. J., COOKE, W. T. and GADDIE, R.: The Folic Acid Excretion Test in the Steatorrhea Syndrome, Gastroenterology, *35*, 390, 1958.

134a. DARBY, W. J., CHERRINGTON, M. E. and RUFFIN, J. M.: Plasma Tocopherol Levels in Sprue, Proc. Soc. Exper. Biol. & Med., *63*, 310, 1946.

134b. DAVIDSON, L. S. P. and FOUNTAIN, J. R.: Incidence of the Sprue Syndrome, Brit. M. J., *1*, 1157, 1950.

134c. DOIG, A. and GIRDWOOD, R. H.: The Absorption of Folic Acid and Labelled Cyanocobalamin in Intestinal Malabsorption, Quart. J. Med., *29*, 333, 1960.

134d. FANCONI, G.: Der intestinale infantilismus und ähnliche Formen der chronischen Verdauungsstorung, Abh. a. d. Kinderhk., *21*, 1, 1928 (Bibliography).

135. FARNAN, P.: Whipple's Disease, Quart. J. Med., *28*, 163, 1959.

135a. FOURMAN, L. P. R.: The Absorption of Xylose in Steatorrhœa, Clin. Sc., 6, 289, 1948.

135b. FOURMAN, L. P. R., HIGGINS, G., QUELCH, P., O'BRIEN, J. R. P. and WITTS, L. J.: The Investigation and Diagnosis of Steatorrhœa, Clin. Sc., 7, 121, 1948.

135c. FOX, H. J.: Absorption of Unemulsified and Emulsified Vitamin A in Sprue, J. Lab. & Clin. Med., 34, 1140, 1949.

136. FRAZER, A. C.: Fat Metabolism and the Sprue Syndrome, Brit. M. J., 2, 669, 1949; Trans. Roy Soc. Trop. Med. & Hyg., 46, 576, 1952.

136a. FRAZER, A. C.: Pathogenetic Concepts of the Malabsorption Syndrome, in Proc. World Congress Gastroenterol., Baltimore, The Williams & Wilkins Co., 1958, p. 619.

136b. FRAZER, A. C., FRENCH, J. M. and THOMPSON, M. D.: Radiographic Studies Showing the Induction of a Segmentation Pattern in the Small Intestine in Normal Human Subjects, Brit. J. Radiol., 22, 123, 1949.

136c. FRENCH, J. M., GADDIE, R. and SMITH, NADYA, M.: Tropical Sprue, Quart. J. Med., 25, 333, 1956.

137. GARDNER, F. H.: Tropical Sprue, New England J. Med., 258, 791 and 835, 1958.

137a. GEE, S.: On the Cœliac Affection, St. Bartholomew Hosp. Rep., 24, 17, 1888.

137b. GREEN, P. A., WOLLAEGER, E. E., SCUDAMORE, H. H. and POWER, MARSCHELLE H.: Nontropical Sprue, J. A. M. A., 171, 2157, 1959.

138. GROSS, J. B. et al.: Whipple's Disease, Gastroenterology, 36, 65, 1959.

139. GROSSMAN, M. I. and JORDAN, P. H., JR.: The Radio-iodinated Triolein Test for Steatorrhea, Gastroenterology, 34, 892, 1958.

140. HARDWICK, C.: Prognosis in Celiac Disease, Arch. Dis. Child., 14, 279, 1939.

142. HOTZ, H. W. and ROHR, K.: Die einheimische Sprue, Ergebn. inn. Med. u. Kinderh., 54, 174, 1938 (Bibliography).

142a. INGELFINGER, F. J. and MOSS, R. E.: The Motility of the Small Intestine in Sprue, J. Clin. Invest., 22, 345, 1943.

142b. INNES, E. M.: The Blood and Bone Marrow in the Sprue Syndrome, Edinburgh M. J., 55, 282, 1948.

142c. JACOBSON, E. D., PRIOR, J. T. and FALOON, W. W.: Malabsorptive Syndrome Induced by Neomycin: Morphologic Alterations in the Jejunal Mucosa, J. Lab. & Clin. Med., 56, 245, 1960.

142d. JONES, C. M., CULVER, P. J., DRUMMEY, G. D. and RYAN, A. E.: Modification of Fat Absorption in the Digestive Tract by the Use of an Emulsifying Agent, Ann. Int. Med., 29, 1, 1948.

143. KANTOR, J. L.: The Roentgen Diagnosis of Idiopathic Steatorrhea and Allied Conditions. Am. J. Roentgenol., 41, 758, 1939; Arch. Int. Med., 65, 988, 1940.

143a. KAPLAN, E., EDIDIN, B. D., FRUIN, R. C. and BAKER, L. A.: Intestinal Absorption of Iodine[131]-labeled Triolein and Oleic Acid in Normal Subjects and in Steatorrhea, Gastroenterology, 34, 901, 1958.

144. KARK, R., SOUTER, A. W. and HAYWARD, J. C.: A Hæmorrhagic Diathesis in Idiopathic Steatorrhœa: Observations on Its Association With Vitamin K Deficiency, Quart. J. Med., 9, 247, 1940.

145. LEPORE, M. J.: Long-term or Maintenance Adrenal Steroid Therapy in Non-tropical Sprue, Am. J. Med., 25, 381, 1958.

145a. LUBRAN, M. and PEARSON, J. D.: A Screening Test for Steatorrhoea Using ^{131}I-labelled Triolein, J. Clin. Path., 11, 165, 1958.

146. MACKIE, T. T., MILLER, D. K. and RHOADS, C. P.: Sprue: Roentgenologic Changes in Small Intestine, Am. J. Trop. Med., 15, 571, 1935.

146a. MARSHAK, R. H., WOLF, B. S. and ADLERSBERG, D.: Roentgen Studies of the Small Intestine in Sprue, Am. J. Roentgenol., 72, 380, 1954.

147. MAY, C. D. and LOWE, C. U.: The Absorption of Orally Administered Emulsified Lipid in Normal Children and in Children with Steatorrhea, J. Clin. Invest., 27, 226, 1948.

148. MELLINKOFF, S. M.: A Physical Sign in Sprue, Am. J. Digest. Dis., 3, 408, 1958.

149. MAYNARD, E. P., III and POINT, W. W.: Steatorrhea Associated with Ulcerogenic Tumor of the Pancreas, Am. J. Med., 25, 456, 1958.

150. MIKE, EMMA M.: Practical Dietary Management of Patients with the Celiac Syndrome, Am. J. Clin. Nutrition, 7, 463, 1959.

150a. OXENHORN, S., ESTREN, S., WASSERMAN, L. R. and ADLERSBERG, D.: Malabsorption Syndrome: Intestinal Absorption of Vitamin B₁₂, Ann. Int. Med., 48, 30, 1958.

151. REISNER, E. H., JR., GILBERT, J. P., ROSENBLUM, C. and MORGAN, M. C.: Applications of the Urinary Tracer Test (of Schilling) as an Index of Vitamin B₁₂ Absorption, Am. J. Clin. Nutrition, 4, 134, 1956.

152. RHOADS, C. P. and CASTLE, W. B.: The Pathology of the Bone Marrow in Sprue Anemia, Am. J. Path., 9, 813, 1933.

154. RIDDELL, W. J. B.: Cœliac Disease Associated With Night Blindness and Xerosis Conjunctivæ, Trans. Ophth. Soc. United Kingdom, 53, 295, 1933.

155. Rodriguez-Molina, R.: Hematology of
Sprue, Puerto Rico J. Pub. Health & Trop.
Med., *15*, 89, 1939; *Ibid.*, *17*, 134, 1941;
Ann. Int. Med., *40*, 33, 1954.

156. Salvesen, H. A. and Skogrand, A.: The
Pathology of Steatorrhoea Idiopathica,
Acta med. scandinav., *159*, 389, 1957.

156a. Scudamore, H. H., McConahey, W. M.
and Priestley, J. T.: Nontropical Sprue
and Functioning Islet-cell Adenoma of the
Pancreas, Ann. Int. Med., *49*, 909, 1958.

156b. Shaw, R. S. and Maynard, E. P., III: Acute
and Chronic Thrombosis of the Mesenteric
Arteries Associated with Malabsorption,
New England J. Med., *258*, 874, 1958.

156c. Sheehy, T. W., Rubini, M. E., Baco-Da-
pena, R. and Perez-Santiago, E.: Erythrokinetics in the Megaloblastic Anemia
of Tropical Sprue, Blood, *15*, 761, 1960.

157. Snell, A. M.: Tropical and Nontropical
Sprue (Chronic Idiopathic Steatorrhea),
Ann. Int. Med., *12*, 1632, 1939.

158. Stefanini, M.: Clinical Features and Pathogenesis of Tropical Sprue, Medicine, *27*,
379, 1948 (Bibliography).

158a. Thurlbeck, W. M., Benson, J. A., Jr. and
Dudley, H. R., Jr.: The Histopathologic
Changes of Sprue and Their Significance,
Am. J. Clin. Path., *34*, 108, 1960.

159. Upshaw, C. B., Jr. and Pollard, H. M.:
The Sprue Syndrome Associated with
Intra-abdominal Lymphoblastoma, Gas-
troenterology, *33*, 104, 1957.

160. Volwiler, W.: Gastrointestinal Malabsorptive Syndromes, Am. J. Med., *23*, 250,
1957.

160a. Wenger, J., Kirsner, J. B. and Palmer,
W. L.: Blood Carotene in Steatorrhea and
the Malabsorptive Syndromes, Am. J.
Med., *22*, 373, 1957.

161. Woltman, H. W. and Heck, F. J.: Funicular
Degeneration of the Spinal Cord Without
Pernicious Anemia: Neurologic Aspects of
Sprue, Nontropical Sprue and Idiopathic
Steatorrhea, Arch. Int. Med., *60*, 272,
1937.

161a. Zetterqvist, H. and Hendrix, T. R.: A
Preliminary Note on an Ultrastructural
Abnormality of the Intestinal Epithelium
in Adult Celiac Disease (Nontropical
Sprue) Which Is Reversed by a Gluten
Free Diet, Bull. Johns Hopkins Hosp.,
106, 240, 1960.

Miscellaneous Macrocytic Anemias

161b. Adams, E. B.: Treatment of Megaloblastic
Anaemia of Pregnancy and the Puerperium with Vitamin B₁₂, Brit. M. J., *2*,

398, 1956; South African J. Lab. & Clin.
Med., *3*, 291, 1957.

161c. Agüero, O. and Layrisse, M.: Megaloblastic Anemia of Pregnancy in Venezuela,
Am. J. Obst. & Gynec., *76*, 903, 1958.

161d. Alexeieff, G.: Sur le problème des "anémies
chirurgicales," Sang, *28*, 305, 1957.

161e. Allen, Frances A., Carr, Marie H. and
Klotz, A. P.: Decreased Red Blood Cell-
Survival Time in Patients with Portal Cir-
rhosis, J. A. M. A., *164*, 955, 1957.

162. Alsted, G.: Pernicious Anæmia After Nitric
Acid Corrosion of the Stomach, Lancet, *1*,
76, 1937.

163. ——— Exogenous Pernicious Anemia,
Am. J. M. Sc., *197*, 741, 1939.

163a. Badenoch, J., Callender, S. T., Evans, J.
R., Turnbull, A. L. and Witts, L. J.:
Megaloblastic Anæmia of Pregnancy and
the Puerperium, Brit. M. J., *1*, 1245, 1955.

163b. Baker, H., Ziffer, H., Pasher, Inez and
Sobotka, H.: A Comparison of Maternal
and Foetal Folic Acid and Vitamin B₁₂ at
Parturition, Brit. M. J., *1*, 978, 1958.

163c. Baker, S. J.: Tropical Megaloblastic Anaemia
in South India, Indian J. Path. & Bact.,
1, 11, 1958.

164. Bardenwerper, H. W.: Ascaris Lumbricoides Infestation With Extreme Anemia,
J.A.M.A., *91*, 1037, 1928.

165. Barker, W. H. and Hummel, L. E.: Macrocytic Anemia in Association With Intestinal
Strictures and Anastomoses, Bull. Johns
Hopkins Hosp., *64*, 215, 1939 (Bibliography).

165a. Best, C. N.: Subacute Combined Degeneration of Spinal Cord after Extensive Resection of Ileum in Crohn's Disease, Brit.
M. J., *2*, 862, 1959.

166. Beyers, M. R., Diefenbach, W. C. L., Mark,
H. and Meyer, L. M.: Interrelationship of
Folic Acid and Vitamin B₁₂ in Macrocytic
Anemia Associated with Linitis Plastica,
Acta med. scandinav., *142*, 351, 1952.

167. Bianco, A. and Jolliffe, N.: The Anemia of
Alcohol Addicts, Am. J. M. Sc., *196*, 414,
1938.

167a. Bingham, J.: The Macrocytosis of Hepatic
Disease, Blood, *14*, 694, 1959.

168. Birkeland, I. W.: "Bothriocephalus Anemia," Medicine, *11*, 1, 1932 (Bibliography).

168a. Bjorkenheim, G.: Neurological Changes in
Pernicious Tapeworm Anæmia, Acta med.
scandinav., Supp. 260, 1951; *Ibid.*, *145*,
406, 1953; Acta med. scandinav., *159*,
433, 1957.

169. Bomford, R.: Anæmia in Myxœdema,
Quart. J. Med., *7*, 495, 1938.

170. von Bonsdorff, B.: Pernicious Anemia

Caused by Diphyllobothrium Latum, in the Light of Recent Investigations, Blood, 3, 91, 1948; Acta med. scandinav., 144, 263, 1953; Exper. Parasitol., 5, 207, 1956.

170a. BOOTH, MAUREEN A. and SPRAY, G. H.: Vitamin B$_{12}$ Activity in the Serum and Liver of Rats After Total Gastrectomy, Brit. J. Haemat., 6, 288, 1960.

170.b BRANTE, G. and ERNBERG, T.: The Mechanism of Pernicious Tapeworm Anemia Studied with ^{60}Co-labelled Vitamin B$_{12}$, Acta med. scandinav., 160, 91, 1958; Scandinav. J. Clin. & Lab. Invest., 9, 313, 1957.

170c. BRENNAN, M. J., VAITKEVICIUS, V. K. and REBUCK, J. W.: Megaloblastic Anemia Associated with Inhibition of Thymine Synthesis, Blood, 16, 1535, 1960.

171. BRUGSCH, H.: Hyperchromic Anemia in Chronic Disorders of Pancreas, Deutsch. Arch. klin. Med., 173, 199, 1932.

171a. BUSÓ, R., OLAVARRIETA, S. T. and SUÁREZ, R. M.: Studies on the Pathogenesis of the Anemia of Hypothyroidism, J. Clin. Endocrinol., 18, 501, 1958.

171b. BUSSI, L.: Anémie mégaloblastique à la suite d'une oesophago-jejunotomie, Sang, 29, 248, 1958.

172. CALLENDER, S. T. E.: A Critical Review of Pernicious Anæmia of Pregnancy, Quart. J. Med., 13, 75, 1944.

172a. CAMERON, D. G., WATSON, G. M. and WITTS, L. J.: The Clinical Association of Macrocytic Anemia with Intestinal Stricture and Anastomosis, Blood, 4, 793, 1949.

173. CHANARIN, I., ELMES, P. C. and MOLLIN, D. L.: Folic-acid Studies in Megaloblastic Anæmia Due to Primidone, Brit. M. J., 2, 80, 1958; ibid., 1, 1099, 1960.

173a. CONNER, H. M. and BIRKELAND, I. W.: Coexistence of Pernicious Anemia and Lesions of the Gastrointestinal Tract, Ann. Int. Med., 7, 89, 1933.

174. DAS GUPTA, C. R., CHATTERJEA, J. B. and BASU, P.: Vitamin B$_{12}$ in Macrocytic Anæmia in Pregnancy, Indian M. Gaz., 88, 1, 1953; Ind. J. M. Res., 42, 411, 1954.

174a. ——— Vitamin B$_{12}$ in Nutritional Macrocytic Anæmia, Brit. M. J., 2, 645, 1953.

174b. DAUGHADAY, W. H., WILLIAMS, R. H. and DALAND, G. A.: The Effect of Endocrinopathies on the Blood, Blood, 3, 1342, 1948.

175. DAVIDSON, L. S. P.: Refractory Megaloblastic Anemia, Blood, 3, 107, 1948.

176. DAVIES, J. N. P.: The Essential Pathology of Kwashiorkor, Lancet, 1, 317, 1948.

176a. EISENBERG, S.: Blood Volume in Patients with Laennec's Cirrhosis of the Liver as Determined by Radioactive Chromium-

Tagged Red Cells, Am. J. Med., 20, 189, 1956.

177. FAIRLEY, N. H.: Tropical Macrocytic Anæmia in an Indian Treated With Anahæmin, Lancet, 1, 1118, 1940.

178. FAIRLEY, N. H., BROMFIELD, R. J., FOY, H. and KONDI, A.: Nutritional Macrocytic Anæmia in Macedonia, Trans. Roy. Soc. Trop. Med. & Hyg., 32, 132, 1938.

179. FLEXNER, J. M. and HARTMANN, R. C.: Megaloblastic Anemia Associated with Anticonvulsant Drugs, Am. J. Med., 28, 386, 1960.

180. FOUGAR, H. O. and STOKES, J. H.: Effect of Treatment for Syphilis on Severe Anemias, Am. J. M. Sc., 162, 633, 1921.

181. FOY, H. and KONDI, A.: Response of Nutritional Macrocytic Anæmia to Anahæmin, Lancet, 2, 360, 1939.

181a. ——— Treatment of Megaloblastic Anæmias, Relation of Penicillin to Vitamin B$_{12}$, Lancet, 2, 1280, 1953; ibid., 2, 693, 1955.

181b. GATENBY, P. B. B. and LILLIE, E. W.: Clinical Analysis of 100 Cases of Severe Megaloblastic Anaemia of Pregnancy, Brit. M. J., 2, 1111, 1960.

181c. GILES, C. and SHUTTLEWORTH, EILEEN M.: Megaloblastic Anaemia of Pregnancy and the Puerperium, Lancet, 2, 1341, 1958.

183. GOLDHAMER, S. M.: Liver Extract Therapy in Cirrhosis of the Liver, Arch. Int. Med., 53, 54, 1934.

184. ——— Macrocytic Anemia in Cancer of the Stomach, Am. J. M. Sc., 195, 17, 1938.

185. GOLDHAMER, S. M., ISAACS, R. and STURGIS, C. C.: The Rôle of the Liver in Hematopoiesis, Am. J. M. Sc., 188, 193, 1934.

185a. GORDON, N. S. and JAPA, J.: Macrocytic Anæmia Following Gastro-Enterostomy, Brit. M. J., 2, 769, 1941.

186. GRÄSBECK, R.: Familial Selective Vitamin B$_{12}$ Malabsorption with Proteinuria, Nord. med., 63, 322, 1960.

187. GROEN, J. and SNAPPER, I.: Dietary Deficiency as a Cause of Macrocytic Anemia, Am. J. M. Sc., 193, 633, 1937.

187a. GROSSOWICZ, N. et al.: Folic and Folinic Acid in Maternal and Foetal Blood, Brit. J. Haemat., 6, 296, 1960.

188. GYDELL, K.: Megaloblastic Anaemia in Patients Treated with Diphenylhydantoin and Primidone, Acta haemat., 17, 1, 1957.

188a. HALL, C. A.: Erythrocyte Dynamics in Liver Disease, Am. J. Med., 28, 541, 1960.

189. HARTMAN, H. R. and EUSTERMAN, G. B.: Anemia Following Operations on the Stomach, Am. J. Digest. Dis., 1, 829, 1935.

190. HARVEY, J. C.: The Vitamin B$_{12}$ Deficiency State Engendered by Total Gastrectomy, Surgery, 40, 977, 1956.

190a.HAURANI, F. I., WANG, G. and TOCANTINS, L. M.: Megaloblastic Anemia Probably Caused by Defective Utilization of Folinic Acid, Blood, *16*, 1546, 1960.

190b.HAWKINS, C. F. and MEYNELL, M. J.: Macrocytosis and Macrocytic Anaemia Caused by Anticonvulsant Drugs, Quart. J. Med., *27*, 45, 1958.

191. HOLMES, E. G.: Observations on Œdema Occurring During the Course of Macrocytic Anaemia, Brit. M. J., *2*, 561, 1945.

191a.HORRIGAN, D. L. and HEINLE, R. W.: Refractory Macrocytic Anemia with Defect in Vitamin B_{12} Binding and with Response to Normal Plasma, J. Lab. & Clin. Med., *40*, 811, 1952 (abstract-Proc. Central Soc. Clin. Res., Chicago, Nov. 7, 8, 1952).

191b.HUGULEY, C. M., JR., BAIN, J. A., RIVERS, SHIRLEY L. and SCOGGINS, R. B.: Refractory Megaloblastic Anemia Associated with Excretion of Orotic Acid, Blood, *14*, 615, 1959.

192. ISRÄELS, M. C. G. and DA CUNHA, F. A. L.: Megaloblastic Anæmia of Pregnancy, Lancet, *2*, 214, 1952.

193. ISRÄELS, M. C. G. and WILKINSON, J. F.: Achrestic Anaemia, Quart. J. Med., *5*, 69, 1936; *Ibid.*, *9*, 163, 1940.

193a.JANDL, J. H.: The Anemia of Liver Disease: Observations on its Mechanism, J. Clin. Invest., *34*, 390, 1955; Ann. Int. Med., *45*, 1027, 1956.

194. JONES, R. M.: Human Sternal Marrow in Hyperthyroid and Myxedematous States, Am. J. M. Sc., *200*, 211, 1940.

194a.JONSSON, U., ROATH, O. S. and KIRKPATRICK, CHARLOTTE I. F.: Nutritional Megaloblastic Anemia Associated with Sickle Cell States, Blood, *14*, 535, 1959.

194b.KILLANDER, A.: Megaloblastic Anaemia Associated with Pregnancy or Puerperium, Acta haemat., *19*, 9, 1958.

194c.KEEFER, C. S., HUANG, K. K. and YANG, C. S.: Anemia Associated With Chronic Dysentery, Arch. Int. Med., *47*, 436, 1931.

195. KOSZEWSKI, B. J.: The Occurrence of Megaloblastic Erythropoiesis in Patients with Hemochromatosis, Blood, *7*, 1182, 1952.

195a.KOTHARI, B. V. and BHENDE, Y. M.: Nutritional Megaloblastic Anæmia, Indian J. M. Res., *37*, 347, 1949.

195b.KRASNOW, S. E., WALSH, J. R., ZIMMERMAN, H. J. and HELLER, P.: Megaloblastic Anemia in "Alcoholic" Cirrhosis, A. M. A. Arch. Int. Med., *100*, 870, 1957.

196. KUNDE, M. M., GREEN, M. F. and BURNS, G.: Blood Changes in Experimental Hypo- and Hyper-thyroidism (Rabbit), Am. J. Physiol., *99*, 469, 1931–1932.

197. LARSEN, T. H.: On the Presence of Anemia After Ventricle Operations, Acta med. scandinav., *83*, 110, 1934.

198. LARSSON, S. O.: Anemia and Iron Metabolism in Hypothyroidism, Acta med. scandinav., *157*, 349, 1957.

198a.LEITHOLD, S. L., DAVID, D. and BEST, W. R.: Hypothyroidism with Anemia Demonstrating Abnormal Vitamin B_{12} Absorption, Am. J. Med., *24*, 535, 1958.

199. LERMAN, J. and MEANS, J. H.: Treatment of the Anemia of Myxœdema, Endocrinology, *16*, 533, 1932.

199a.LOWENSTEIN, L., PICK, C. and PHILPOTT, N.: Megaloblastic Anemia of Pregnancy and the Puerperium, Am. J. Obst. & Gynec., *70*, 1309, 1955; Am. J. Clin. Nutrition, *8*, 265, 1960.

200. LUBLIN, H.: On the Anemia Following Gastric Operations, Am. J. Digest. Dis., *3*, 8, 1936.

201. MacLEAN, L. D.: Megaloblastic Anemia Following Total and Subtotal Gastrectomy, Surg. Gynec. & Obst., *106*, 415, 1958.

201a.METZ, J., LEWIS, S. M., KEELEY, K. J. and HART, D.: The Absorption of Vitamin B_{12} in Megaloblastic Anaemia Associated with Pregnancy, J. Clin. Path., *13*, 394, 1960.

202. MEULENGRACHT, E. and GORMSEN, H.: Blood and Bone Marrow in Infective Subacute and Chronic Atrophy of the Liver, Blood, *3*, 1416, 1948.

203. MOORE, C. V., VILTER, R., MINNICH, V. and SPIES, T. D.: Nutritional Macrocytic Anemia in Patients With Pellagra or Deficiency of the Vitamin B Complex, J. Lab. & Clin. Med., *29*, 1226, 1944.

204. MORGENSEN, E.: The Anemia of Gastric Cancer, Folia hæmatol., *56*, 206, 1936.

205. MOVITT, E. R.: Megaloblastic Bone Marrow in Liver Disease, Am. J. Med., *7*, 145, 1949; Blood, *5*, 468, 1950.

205a.MUELLER, J. F., HAWKINS, V. R. and VILTER, R. W.: Liver Extract Refractory Megaloblastic Anemia, Blood, *4*, 1117, 1949.

206. NAPIER, L. E., *et al.*: Tropical Macrocytic Anæmia, Indian M. Gaz., *73*, 385, 1938; *Ibid.*, *74*, 1, 1939.

207. NICOL, W. A.: Non-addisonian Megaloblastic Anaemia, Complicated by Subacute Combined Degeneration of the Cord, Brit. M. J., *1*, 322, 1960.

207a.NYBERG, W.: Absorption and Excretion of Vitamin B_{12} in Subjects Infected with Diphyllobothrium latum and in Non-infected Subjects Following Oral Administration of Radioactive B_{12}, Acta haemat., *19*, 90, 1958; New England J. Med., *259*, 216, 1958; Am. J. Clin. Nutrition, *9*, 606, 1961.

208. PATERSON, D., PIERCE, M. and PECK, E.: The Treatment of Coeliac Disease with Vitamin

B Complex and Concentrated Liver, Arch. Dis. Childhood, *19*, 99, 1944.

208a.PITNEY, W. R. and BEARD, M. F.: Vitamin B₁₂ Deficiency Following Total Gastrectomy, Arch. Int. Med., *95*, 591, 1955.

208b.PLUM, P. and WARBURG, E.: Hematological Changes, Especially Megalocytic Anemia in Regional Ileitis, Acta med. scandinav., *102*, 449, 1939.

209. POLACHEK, A. A., PIJANOWSKI, W. J. and Miller, J. M.: Diverticulosis of the Jejunum with Macrocytic Anemia and Steatorrhea, Ann. Int. Med., *54*, 636, 1961.

209a.QUINBY, W. C., JR. and McGOVERN, J. J.: Surgical Correction of Defective Absorption of Vitamin B₁₂ in a Child, New England J. Med., *259*, 755, 1958.

210. RICHMOND, J. and DAVIDSON, S.: Subacute Combined Degeneration of the Spinal Cord in Non-addisonian Megaloblastic Anaemia, Quart. J. Med., *27*, 517, 1958.

211. RICHTER, O., MEYER, A. E. and IVY, A. C.: One Case of Pernicious Anemia Following Gastrectomy, Ann. Int. Med., *7*, 353, 1933.

211a.ROBSON, H. N. and LAWRENCE, J. R.: Megaloblastic Anaemia Induced by Phenylbutazone, Brit. M. J., *2*, 475, 1959.

212. RODRIGUEZ-MOLINA, R.: Tropical Macrocytic Anemia in Puerto Rico, Puerto Rico J. Pub. Health & Trop. Med., *15*, 177, 1939.

212a.ROELSEN, E. and OHLSEN, A. S.: Achrestic Anemia, Acta med. scandinav., *150*, 17, 1954.

213. ROSAHN, P. D. and PEARCE, L.: Blood Cytology in Untreated and Treated Syphilis, Am. J. M. Sc., *187*, 88, 1934.

214. SCHIFF, L., RICH, M. L. and SIMON, S. D.: The "Hæmatopoietic Principle" in the Diseased Human Liver, Am. J. M. Sc., *196*, 313, 1938.

215. SCHLESINGER, A.: Demonstration of Antipernicious Anemia Principle in Gastric Juice of Patient With Stenosis of Small Intestine and With Blood Picture of Pernicious Anemia, Klin. Wchnschr., *12*, 298, 1933.

216. SCLARE, G. and CRAGG, J.: A Leukaemoid Blood Picture in Megaloblastic Anaemia of the Puerperium, J. Clin. Path., *11*, 45, 1958.

216a.SCOTT, J. M. and GOVAN, A. D. T.: Anæmia Simulating Pre-Eclamptic Toxaemia, J. Obst. & Gynec. Brit. Emp., *56*, 27, 1949; Brit. M. J., *2*, 270, 1957.

217. SCUDAMORE, H. H., HAGEDORN, A. B., WOLLAEGER, E. E. and OWEN, C. A., JR.: Diverticulosis of the Small Intestine and Macrocytic Anemia with Radioactive Vitamin B₁₂ Absorption Studies, Gastroenterology, *34*, 66, 1958.

218. SHARPE, J. C. and BISGARD, J. D.: The Relation of the Thyroid Gland to Hematopoiesis, J. Lab. & Clin. Med., *21*, 347, 1936.

219. SINGER, H. A. and STEIGMANN, F.: Pernicious Anemia Following Resection for Gastric Syphilis, Am. J. Syph., *18*, 444, 1934.

219a.SIURALA, M.: Gastric Lesion in Some Megaloblastic Anemias, Acta med. scandinav., *154*, 337, 1956; ibid., *157*, 435, 1957.

219b.SIURALA, M. and KAIPAINEN, W. J.: Intestinal Megaloblastic Anaemia, Treated with Aureomycin and Terramycin, Acta med. scandinav., *147*, 197, 1953.

220. SPIES, T. D., BEAN, W. B. and ASHE, W. F.: Recent Advances in the Treatment of Pellagra and Associated Deficiencies, Ann. Int. Med., *12*, 1830, 1939.

221. SPIES, T. D. and CHINN, A. B.: Studies on the Anemia of Pellagra, J. Clin. Invest., *14*, 941, 1935.

222. STERN, B. and ALTSCHULE, M. D.: Hematological Studies in Hypothyroidism Following Total Thyroidectomy, J. Clin. Invest., *15*, 633, 1936.

223. STRAUSS, A. A., MEYER, J. and BLOOM, A.: Gastric Polyposis, Am. J. M. Sc., *176*, 681, 1928.

224. SYDENSTRICKER, V. P., SCHMIDT, H. L., JR., GEESLIN, L. E. and WEAVER, J. W.: The Liver in Pellagra, Am. J. M. Sc., *197*, 755, 1939.

224a.TALBOT, T. R., JR. and TETREAULT, A. F.: Probable Deficiency of Vitamin B₁₂ with "Pernicious Anemia" in Two Patients with Normal Schilling Test, Ann. Int. Med., *47*, 338, 1957.

224b.TAYLOR, G. F. and CHHUTTAINI, P. N.: Nutritional Macrocytic Anæmia and the Animal Protein of Diet, Brit. M. J., *1*, 800, 1945.

225. TÖTTERMAN, G.: Über die Pathogenese der Wurmanämie, Acta med. scandinav., *96*, 268, 1938; Ibid., *118*, 422, 1944; Scandinav. J. Clin. & Lab. Invest., *6*, 33 and 85, 1954; Acta med. scandinav., *153*, 421, 1956.

226. TOWNSEND, S. R. and BEGOR, F. B.: Pernicious Anæmia Due to Deficiency of Extrinsic Factor, Canad. M. A. J., *47*, 352, 1942.

226a.TOWNSEND, S. R. and CAMERON, D. G.: Megaloblastic Anemia Associated with Diverticula of the Small Bowel, Am. J. Med., *23*, 668, 1957.

226b.TROWELL, H. C.: Dimorphic Anæmia: Deficiency of Iron Associated With Nutritional Macrocytic Anemia, Trans. Roy. Soc. Trop. Med. & Hyg., *37*, 19, 1943.

226c.TUDHOPE, G. R. and WILSON, G. M.: Anæmia in Hypothyroidism, Quart. J. Med., *29*, 513, 1960.

227. TURNER, R. H. and SHELTON, E.: Erythrocytes in Pellagra, Am. J. M. Sc., *185*, 381, 1933.

227a. WATKINSON, G., FEATHER, D. B., MARSON, F. G. W. and DOSSETT, J. A.: Massive Jejunal Diverticulosis with Steatorrhoea and Megaloblastic Anaemia Improved by Excision of Diverticula, Brit. M. J., *2*, 58, 1959.

228. WATSON, G. M. and WITTS, L. J.: Intestinal Macrocytic Anæmia, Brit. M. J., *1*, 13, 1952.

228a. WATSON, J. and CASTLE, W. B.: Nutritional Macrocytic Anemia Especially in Pregnancy. Response to a Substance Other Than That Effective in Pernicious Anemia, Am. J. M. Sc., *211*, 513, 1946.

229. WELLS, R.: Nutritional Vitamin B_{12} Deficiency, J. Trop. Med., *61*, 81, 1958.

229a. WILKINSON, J. F.: Megaloctyic Anæmias, Lancet, *1*, 249, 336, 1949.

229b. WILKINSON, R. W.: Subacute Combined Degeneration of the Spinal Cord, Lancet, *1*, 74, 1955.

230. WILLS, L. and EVANS, B. D. F.: Tropical Macrocytic Anæmia: Its Relation to Pernicious Anæmia, Lancet, *2*, 416, 1938; Blood, *3*, 36, 1948.

231. WILLS, L., MEHTA, M. M., TALPADE, S. N. and BILIMORIA, H. S.: Studies in Pernicious Anemia of Pregnancy, Indian J. M. Res., *17*, 777, 1930; *Ibid.*, *18*, 283, 1930; *Ibid.*, *20*, 391, 1932; *Ibid.*, *21*, 669, 1934.

232. WINTROBE, M. M.: The Relation of Disease of Liver to Anemia, Arch. Int. Med., *57*, 289, 1936.

233. WINTROBE, M. M. and SHUMACKER, H. B., JR.: Occurrence of Macrocytic Anemia in Association With Disorder of Liver, Bull. Johns Hopkins Hosp., *52*, 387, 1933.

233a. WOKES, F., BADENOCH, J. and SINCLAIR, H. M.: Human Dietary Deficiency of Vitamin B_{12}, Voeding, *16*, 590, 1955; Am. J. Clin. Nutrition, *3*, 375, 1955.

233b. WOLFF, J. R. and LIMARZI, L. R.: Anemia in Pregnancy, J.A.M.A., *128*, 482, 1945.

233c. WOODRUFF, A. W.: The Natural History of Anæmia Associated with Protein Malnutrition, Brit. M. J., *1*, 1297, 1955.

233d. ZBINDEN, J.: Megaloblastäre Anämie mit Vitamin-B_{12}-Defizit bei antiepileptischer Therapie, Schweiz. med. Wchnschr., *89*, 1072, 1959.

Pathogenesis of Pernicious Anemia and Related Anemias

235. BACHRACH, W. H. and FOGELSON, S. J.: The Rôle of the Upper Gastro-intestinal Tract in the Etiology of Pernicious Anemia, J. Lab. & Clin. Med., *24*, 249, 1938.

236. BENCE, J.: Die Beziehungen der experimentellen agastrischen Anämie zur Perniciosa, Ztschr. klin. Med., *130*, 275, 1936.

237. BENNETT, T. I. and HARDWICK, C.: Chronic Jejuno-ileal Insufficiency, Lancet, *2*, 381, 1940.

238. BETHELL, F. H., MEYERS, M. C. and NELIGH, R. B.: Vitamin B_{12} in Pernicious Anemia and Puerperal Macrocytic Anemia, J. Lab. & Clin. Med., *33*, 1477, 1948. *See also* Blood, *5*, 1009, 1950.

239. BOK, J. *et al.*: The Effect of Pteroylglutamic Acid Administration on the Serum Vitamin B_{12} Concentration in Pernicious Anemia in Relapse, J. Lab. & Clin. Med., *51*, 667, 1958.

240. CALLENDER, S. T. E., MALLETT, B. J., SPRAY, G. H. and SHAW, G. E.: Anti-Anæmia Activity of Fæcal Extract from Pernicious Anæmia Patient, Lancet, *2*, 57, 1949.

240a. CALLENDER, S. T., TURNBULL, A. and WAKISAKA, G.: Estimation of Intrinsic Factor of Castle by Use of Radioactive Vitamin B_{12}, Brit. M. J., *1*, 10, 1954; Clin. Sci., *14*, 387, 1955.

241. CARTWRIGHT, G. E., PALMER, J. G., TATTING, B., ASHENBRUCKER, H. and WINTROBE, M. M.: Experimental Production of Nutritional Macrocytic Anemia in Swine, J. Lab. & Clin. Med., *36*, 675, 1950; Blood, *6*, 867, 1951; *ibid.*, *7*, 992, 1952.

242. CASTLE, W. B.: Development of Knowledge Concerning the Gastric Intrinsic Factor and Its Relation to Pernicious Anemia, New England J. Med., *249*, 603, 1953.

244. CASTLE, W. B., HEATH, C. W., STRAUSS, M. B. and HEINLE, R. W.: VI. The Site of the Interaction of Food (Extrinsic) and Gastric (Intrinsic) Factors, Am. J. M. Sc., *194*, 618, 1937.

245. CASTLE, W. B., TOWNSEND, W. C., HEATH, C. W. and STRAUSS, M. B.: Observations on the Etiologic Relationship of Achylia Gastrica to Pernicious Anemia, I–IV, Am. J. M. Sc., *178*, 748, and 764, 1929; *Ibid.*, *180*, 305, 1930; *Ibid.*, *182*, 741, 1931.

248. CORNELL, B. S.: Etiology of Pernicious Anemia, Medicine, *6*, 375, 1927 (Bibliography).

250. COX, E. V. *et al.*: Cyanocobalamin, Ascorbic Acid and Pteroylglutamates in Normal and Megaloblastic Bone Marrow, Blood, *15*, 376, 1960.

252. DEXTER, S. O., HEINLE, R. W., FOX, H. J. and CASTLE, W. B.: Basis of the Hematopoietic Activity in Pernicious Anemia of Desiccated Hog Ileum, J. Clin. Invest., *18*, 473, 1939.

253. DOCK, W.: The Ebb and Flow of Theories About Pernicious Anemia, Am. J. Clin. Path., *8*, 620, 1938.

253a. FINCKH, E. S. and WOOD, I. J.: Failure of Vitamin B$_{12}$ Therapy to Improve Gastric Atrophy in Pernicious Anemia, Gastroenterology, 25, 48, 1953.

254. FOLLIS, R. H., JR. and WINTROBE, M. M.: A Comparison of the Effects of Pyridoxine and Pantothenic Acid Deficiencies on the Nervous Tissues of Swine, J. Exper. Med., 81, 539, 1945.

255. FORMIJNE, P.: Experiments on the Properties of the Extrinsic Factor and on the Reaction of Castle, Arch. Int. Med., 66, 1191, 1940.

257. GARDNER, F. H., HARRIS, J. W., SCHILLING, R. F. and CASTLE, W. B.: Hematopoietic Activity in Pernicious Anemia of a Beef Muscle Extract Containing Food (Extrinsic) Factor upon Intravenous Injection without Contact with Gastric (Intrinsic) Factor, J. Lab. & Clin. Med., 34, 1502, 1949.

258. GEIGER, A. J., GOODMAN, L. S. and CLAIBORN, L. N.: Effects of Gastro-intestinal Resections in Swine on the Anti-anemia Potency of the Liver, Yale J. Biol. & Med., 13, 259, 1940.

259. GIRDWOOD, R. H.: The Occurrence of Growth Factors for *Lactobacillus leichmannii*, *Streptococcus fæcalis* and *Leuconostoc citrovorum* in the Tissues of Pernicious Anæmia Patients and Controls, Biochem. J., 52, 58, 1952.

259a. GIRDWOOD, R. H.: Microbiological Methods of Assay in Clinical Medicine with Particular Reference to the Investigation of Deficiency of Vitamin B$_{12}$ and Folic Acid, Scottish M. J., 5, 10, 1960.

260. GOLDHAMER, S. M.: The Presence of the Intrinsic Factor of Castle in the Gastric Juice of Patients With Pernicious Anemia, Am. J. M. Sc., 191, 405, 1936; *Ibid.*, 193, 23, 1937.

261. GRAHAM, R. M. and RHEAULT, M. H.: Characteristic Cellular Changes in Cells of Nonhemopoietic Origin in Pernicious Anemia, J. Lab. & Clin. Med., 43, 235, 1954.

262. HARRIS, J. W.: Aggravation of Clinical Manifestionations of Folic Acid Deficiency by Small Daily Doses of Vitamin B$_{12}$, Am. J. Med., 21, 461, 1956.

267. HUNTER, W.: Specific Infective Nature of Addison's Anemia: Its Course and Treatment, Brit. M. J., 2, 1299, 1907.

268. HURST, A. F. and BELL, J. R.: The Pathogenesis of Subacute Combined Degeneration of the Spinal Cord, Brain, 45, 266, 1922.

269. JOHNSON, V., FREEMAN, L. W. and LONGINI, J.: Erythrocyte Damage by Lipemic Serum in Normal Man and in Pernicious Anemia, J.A.M.A., 124, 1250, 1944.

270. JONES, O. P.: Transmission of Antianemic Principle Across the Placenta and Its Influence on Embryonic Erythropoiesis, Arch. Int. Med., 68, 476, 1941; Anat. Rec., 85, 321, 1943; Blood, 5, 499, 1950; Rev. hémat., 5, 618, 1950.

271. KLEIN, L. and WILKINSON, J. F.: Investigations on the Nature of Haemopoietin, Biochem. J., 28, 1684, 1934: Quart. J. Med., 7, 555, 1938.

272. LAJTHA, L. G.: An Inhibitory Factor in Pernicious Anæmia Serum, Clin. Sci., 9 287, 1950.

273. LANDBOE-CHRISTENSEN, E. and PLUM, C. M.: Experimental Study on the Localization of Castle's Intrinsic Factor in the Human Stomach. Anti-Anemic Effect of Powdered Human Fundus and Pylorus, Am. J. M. Sc., 215, 17, 1948; *ibid.*, 224, 1, 1952; Acta med. scandinav., 144, 467, 1953; *ibid.*, 150, 369, 1954.

275. METTIER, S. R. and PURVIANCE, K.: Effect of Artificial Achylia Gastrica and a Diet Restricted in Vitamin B$_2$ (G) on Hematopoiesis, Proc. Soc. Exper. Biol. & Med., 36, 429, 1937.

277. MILLER, D. K. and RHOADS, C. P.: Production in Dogs of a Syndrome Similar to Sprue by Diets Deficient in Vitamin B$_2$, Proc. Soc. Exper. Biol. & Med., 30, 540, 1933.

279. ————The Experimental Production of Loss of Hematopoietic Elements of the Gastric Secretion and of the Liver in Swine With Achlorhydria and Anemia, J. Clin. Invest., 14, 153, 1935.

281. MINOT, G. R.: The Development of Liver Therapy in Pernicious Anemia, Lancet, 1, 361, 1935.

282. NIEWEG, H. O., FABER, J. G., deVRIES, J. A. and KROESE, W. F. S.: The Relationship of Vitamin B$_{12}$ and Folic Acid in Megaloblastic Anemias, J. Lab. & Clin. Med., 44, 118, 1954.

284. NYE, R. N.: Investigation Relative to B. Welchii Infection of Intestinal Tract as Etiological Factor in Pernicious Anemia. J. Clin. Invest., 4, 71, 1927.

286. PETRI, S., NØRGAARD, F. and BING, J.: Pathological Changes Produced by Gastrectomy in Young Swine, Am. J. M. Sc., 195, 717, 1938; *Ibid.*, 104, 245, 1940; *Ibid.*, 109, 59, 1941; *Ibid.*, 114, 184, 1943; *Ibid.*, 116, 273, 1944; *Ibid.*, 119, 103 and 356, 1944.

287. PETRI, S. and JENSENIUS, H.: Experimental Studies on Production of Pernicious Anemia by Operation on the Digestive Tract.

Acta med. scandinav., *106*, 274, 1941; *Ibid.*, *107*, 506 and 532, 1941; *Ibid.*, *111*, 75 and 116, 1942; *Ibid.*, *117*, 90, 1944.

289. RHOADS, C. P. and MILLER, D. K.: Induced Susceptibility of the Blood to Indol, J. Exper. Med., *67*, 273, 1938.

292. ROMINGER, E. and BOMSKOV, C.: Untersuchungen an hyperchromen Anämien bei experimentell Erzeugten sprueartigen Erkrankungen, Klin. Wchnschr., *14*, 148, 1935.

294. SCHEMENSKY, W.: Pathology of Pernicious Anemia: Therapeutic Results With Oral Administration of Powder From Colon of Hogs, Ztschr. klin. Med., *128*, 428, 1935.

295. SCHILLING, R. F.: The Effect of Gastric Juice on the Urinary Excretion of Radioactivity after the Oral Administration of Radioactive Vitamin B_{12}, J. Lab. & Clin. Med., *42*, 860, 1953; *ibid.*, *45*, 926, 1955.

297. SEYDERHELM, R., LEHMANN, W. and WICHELS, P.: Experimental Pernicious Anemia, Klin. Wchnschr., *3*, 1439, 1924.

298. SHUMACKER, H. B., JR. and WINTROBE, M. M.: Morphologic Changes in the Blood Associated With Experimentally Produced Hepatic Damage, Bull. Johns Hopkins Hosp., *58*, 343, 1936.

299. SPRAY, G. H. and WITTS, L. J.: The Utilization of Folic Acid Given by Mouth, Clin. Sc., *2*, 273, 1952.

299a. STANNUS, H. S.: Sprue, Trans. Roy. Soc. Trop. Med. & Hyg., *36*, 123, 1942.

304. TASKER, P. W. G.: Correlation of Serum-Vitamin B_{12} Levels and Urinary Folic Acid in Nutritional Megaloblastic Anæmia, Lancet, *2*, 61, 1955.

307. THOMPSON, J. C.: The Hematopoietic Response Following Oral Administration of Desiccated Duodenal Mucosa, Ann. Int. Med., *2*, 39, 1937.

308. THOMPSON, R. B.: Addisonian Pernicious Anæmia. Confirmatory Evidence of a Factor Inhibiting Erythropoiesis, Clin. Sci., *9*, 281, 1950.

309. TOON, R. W. and WANGENSTEEN, O. W.: Anemia Associated with Blind Intestinal Segments and Its Prevention With Aureomycin, Proc. Soc. Exper. Biol. & Med., *75*, 762, 1950.

310. ————The Pathogenesis of Megaloblastic Anæmias and the Value of Vitamin B_{12}, Brit. J. Nutrition, *6*, 299, 1952.

311. UOTILA, U.: On the Antianemic Function of the Small Intestine, Acta med. scandinav., *95*, 415, 1938.

313. WAKERLIN, G. E. and BRUNER, H. D.: Further Evidence for the Presence of a Toxic Factor in Pernicious Anemia, Science, *82*, 494, 1935.

314. WATSON, G. M., CAMERON, D. G. and WITTS, L. J.: Experimental Macrocytic Anæmia in the Rat, Lancet, *2*, 404, 1948; Nature, *164*, 188, 1949.

320. WILLS, L. and BILIMORIA, H. S.: Production of a Macrocytic Anæmia in Monkeys by Deficient Feeding, Indian J. M. Res., *20*, 391, 1932.

321. WILLS, L., CLUTTERBUCK, P. W. and EVANS, B. D. F.: A New Factor in the Production and Cure of Macrocytic Anæmias and Its Relation to Other Hæmopoietic Principles Curative in Pernicious Anæmia, Biochem. J., *31*, 2136, 1937.

322. WINTROBE, M. M.: Antianemic Effect of Yeast in Pernicious Anemia, Am. J. M. Sc., *197*, 286, 1939.

323. WINTROBE, M. M., CLARK, D., TRAGER, W. and DANZIGER, L.: Studies of Blood Formation in the Fetus and Newborn, IV, J. Clin. Invest., *16*, 667, 1937.

324. WINTROBE, M. M., KINSEY, R. E., BLOUNT, R. C. and TRAGER, W.: Studies of Blood Formation in the Fetus and Newborn, III, Am. J. M. Sc., *193*, 449, 1937.

326. WINTROBE, M. M., MILLER, M. H., FOLLIS, R. H., JR., STEIN, H. J., MUSHATT, C. and HUMPHREYS, S.: Sensory Neuron Degeneration in Pigs. IV. Protection Afforded by Calcium Pantothenate and Pyridoxine, J. Nutrition, *24*, 345, 1942.

327. WINTROBE, M. M., MUSHATT, C., MILLER, J. L., JR., KOLB, L. C. and STEIN, H.: Sensory Neuron Degeneration in Young Pigs, J. Clin. Invest., *21*, 71, 1942.

328. WINTROBE, M. M. and SHUMACKER, H. B., JR.: Comparison of Hematopoiesis in the Fetus and During Recovery From Pernicious Anemia, J. Clin. Invest., *14*, 837, 1935.

Chapter 11

The Normocytic Anemias

General Considerations. — Normocytic anemia may be *defined* as that type of anemia in which there is no significant deviation from the normal in the mean volume and hemoglobin content of the red corpuscles, no matter how severe the anemia may be. The mean corpuscular volume ranges from 82 to 92 c. μ and the mean corpuscular hemoglobin concentration from 32 to 36 per cent.

This does not necessarily mean that the individual red corpuscles are uniform in size or in hemoglobin content. It is generally true, however, that in most instances of true normocytic anemia the degree of anisocytosis, poikilocytosis, and achromia is relatively slight. When marked variations in the morphology of the red corpuscles in the blood smear are found, it is wise to suspect an error in the determination of cell size or hemoglobin content or to consider the possibility of a combined deficiency of vitamin B_{12} or folic acid and of iron. In the latter case, the two types of deficiency, by producing macrocytosis and microcytosis, respectively, may be so balanced as to produce normocytic anemia (p. 487). Such cases, however, are very rare and it is much more common when there is deficiency of vitamin B_{12} or folic acid, to find macrocytic anemia even when iron deficiency is also present. The need for iron only becomes apparent after a certain amount of blood regeneration has occurred in response to appropriate therapy.

As already stated (Chpater 9), normocytic anemia may be found (1) when there has been **sudden loss of blood;** (2) when there has been **increased destruction of blood.** In both of these circumstances the cells remaining in circulation are normal. A third cause of normocytic anemia is (3) **decreased blood formation.** Here we refer to the anemia which develops (*a*) when the bone marrow has become fatty ("aplastic anemia") or even in the absence of fatty marrow ("pseudo-aplastic," "refractory" anemias); (*b*) when, in association with various types of infection or chronic disease, hematopoietic activity is disturbed ("simple chronic anemia"); or (*c*) when erythropoiesis is disturbed, as in conditions characterized by abnormal leukocyte formation or by marrow infiltration with neoplastic growths. A fourth (4) possible cause of normocytic anemia is not a true anemia but is only an apparent one, being produced by an increase in the amount of plasma without alteration in the total quantity of red corpuscles **(hydremia).**

Certain exceptions to the above outline must be noted. It is important to recognize the fact that the composition of the blood is not necessarily constant and thus, although the immediate effect of sudden blood loss or blood destruction is the production of a normocytic anemia, the character of the anemia will be influenced by the response of the tissues to the anemia. When blood formation is stimulated, immature erythrocytes are liberated. These are larger than their fellow, mature corpuscles (p. 90) and if liberated in sufficient numbers, they may cause an increase in the mean corpuscular volume above normal.

In acute posthemorrhagic anemia macrocytosis is usually not great. If it occurs at all, it is usually of very brief duration and the cause of the anemia is obvious. On the other hand, if blood loss is frequently repeated and the ability of the patient to restore the blood is taxed beyond his capacity, iron deficiency eventually ensues and microcytic hypochromic anemia develops. For this to occur, however, much time is required. A diet which is poor in iron content and impaired absorption of iron from the gastrointestinal tract often contribute to the development of iron deficiency anemia.

Again, acute blood destruction characteristically stimulates active red cell regeneration. In the acute hemolytic anemias or after hemolytic crises in chronic hemolytic anemias, macrocytic anemia may develop. In some forms of aplastic anemia the anemia may be macrocytic rather than normocytic. The anemia caused by "internal radiation" from alpha particles of radium which was observed in dial painters was described as macrocytic.

Further exceptions to the description of the morphology of the normocytic anemias which was given above are found in sickle cell anemia and in familial hemolytic jaundice. The former disease is an exception to the rule that anisocytosis and poikilocytosis are slight in normocytic anemias as compared with the macrocytic and the hypochromic microcytic anemias. In hereditary spherocytosis the number of spherocytes may be so great that the mean corpuscular volume

is reduced below normal, producing microcytic anemia without hypochromia. On the other hand, when there is marked reticulocytosis following a hemolytic crisis, these large and often basophilic corpuscles contrast with the tiny spherocytes so that there is pronounced anisocytosis

These exceptions will be discussed more fully in the following pages. When enumerated as is done here they appear so numerous as to arouse doubt regarding the value of a classification of anemia on morphological grounds. In answer to this, it must be pointed out that cases of macrocytic anemia resulting from vitamin B_{12} or folic acid deficiency are more commonly encountered than cases of macrocytic anemia due to acute blood destruction, faulty blood formation, or acute blood loss. Such cases are too few to constitute an important objection to this method of classification. They must be kept in mind, however, as otherwise an error in diagnosis could result. They serve to emphasize the importance of a well-established principle of clinical medicine; namely, that the patient must be considered as a whole. No single criterion, whether obtained by physical examination or by laboratory diagnostic methods, is a diagnostic index to which there are no exceptions.

ACUTE POSTHEMORRHAGIC ANEMIA

The anemia caused by the more or less sudden and rapid loss of blood may result from a large variety of causes, such as trauma or the rupture of a peptic ulcer; it may be a complication of such unrelated disorders as ectopic gestation and typhoid fever; or it may be a symptom of one of the blood disorders such as hemophilia, purpura hemorrhagica, acute leukemia, or aplastic anemia.

Symptomatology. — Although the clinical picture will differ according to the nature of the underlying disorder, if

35

any, the symptoms caused by the acute blood loss will be essentially the same. The appearance of symptoms from this cause depends on the size of the hemorrhage, its rapidity, and whether it is external or occult. An individual can withstand the loss of even as much as 50 per cent of his blood if the hemorrhage has been prolonged over twenty-four hours or longer, but death may result from a loss of 33 per cent, or 1500 to 2000 ml. of blood, if it is very rapid. If the patient is unconscious at the time the hemorrhage occurs, or if it is otherwise unrecognized by him, symptoms are likely to be less pronounced than when the blood loss is apparent. In the latter instance, and particularly in a high-strung individual, the amount of blood lost is likely to be greatly exaggerated.

The classical signs of acute hemorrhage are prostration, restlessness, thirst, sweating, rapid shallow breathing, a rapid thready pulse and low blood and pulse pressures. A controlled study[2a] in which 500 to 1200 ml. of blood was removed from young healthy adult males showed, however, that *rapid pulse and low blood pressure are unreliable criteria of hemorrhage.* It was found that the withdrawal of 500 ml. of blood was associated with no symptoms at rest and the pulse rate and blood pressure were within normal limits. Only on arising did the pulse rate accelerate unduly and the blood pressure tend to fall, a feeling of weakness and dyspnea on exertion being associated. Even with larger losses of blood no noteworthy abnormalities were observed as long as the subject remained recumbent and at rest; on sitting up, faintness and syncope, accompanied by *bradycardia* and reduced cardiac output, developed. Only when very large amounts were removed did acute symptoms appear when the subject was recumbent. Diminished blood pressure, marked bradycardia and reduced cardiac output, pallor, sweating, hyperpnea and restlessness then supervened. These symptoms were followed by coldness of the extremities, nausea, dizziness, faintness and even loss of consciousness. If acute circulatory collapse occurs, pallor, profuse sweating and a marked fall in arterial pressure and peripheral resistance develop.[10] In view of these studies it seems plausible to assume that tachycardia develops not as the result of blood loss alone but because of the trauma or reflex factors which may be associated with hemorrhage or, if developing some time after the bleeding, it may represent one of the manifestations of the physiologic adjustments to anemia which have been discussed already (p. 436).

The severity of the hemorrhage cannot be gauged immediately by the blood count because vasoconstriction on the one hand, and continuing dilution of the blood as fluids pass into the vessels from the tissues on the other, produce misleading high and low counts, respectively. If the hemorrhage has occurred in the intestinal tract, the blood urea nitrogen will rise ("alimentary azotemia"[1a]). Its degree is a useful index of the amount of blood lost and of the prognosis, values of 50 mg. per 100 ml., or higher, being of grave importance. A method employing Cr^{51} has been described whereby the amount of blood lost in the feces can be measured.[3] If the blood passes into one of the body cavities or into a cyst, the reabsorbed products of hemoglobin breakdown may produce icterus. Moderate fever may accompany gastro-intestinal hemorrhage and a more pronounced rise occurs when blood escapes into muscles, organs, or body cavities.

Blood Findings.—The earliest effect on the blood is an increase in the platelet count, which may reach 1,000,000 per c.mm., and a shortening of the coagulation time. These changes may occur within the first hour. Polymorphonuclear leukocytosis, usually 10,000 to 20,000, follows and may be maximal in two to

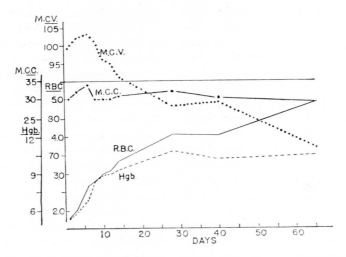

FIG. 11-1.—Temporary increase in mean corpuscular volume in a case of acute posthemorrhagic anemia.

five hours. Counts as high as 35,000 per c.mm. have been observed. There is a shift to the left in the myeloid series and myelocytes, even very occasional myeloblasts, may make their appearance. An increase in reticulocytes does not commence until twenty-four to forty-eight hours have elapsed. The maximal number, which is usually 5 to 15 per cent but may be higher, is found between four and seven days following the hemorrhage.[2c] The *plasma iron* falls gradually after acute blood loss.[1]

The red cell count, hemoglobin and volume of packed red cells, at first misleadingly high as the result of vasoconstriction and of redistribution of corpuscles, decrease and may continue to fall for several days even though hemorrhage has ceased. This is due to readjustment of the blood volume and dilution of the blood by tissue fluids.[2a, 6a] Normoblasts and polychromatophilia only appear after several days if the hemorrhage has been very severe.[6] The red corpuscles in general are normal in appearance and the anemia is usually normocytic. When the hemorrhage has been very profuse and the bone marrow stimulation has been unusually great,

slight macrocytosis (mean corpuscular volume as high as 105 c. μ) may develop for several days during the time of maximal reticulocytosis (Fig. 11–1). In the otherwise normal individual whose diet has been satisfactory and whose stores of blood building substances are adequate, significant microcytosis does not develop.[11] The finding of hypochromia should arouse suspicion of previous hemorrhages.

In animals in which anemia has been produced experimentally by withdrawing blood, areas of fatty *marrow* adjacent to the normally active regions show a replacement of fat by diffuse gelatinous tissue in which blood formation is taking place.[4] There is an increased number of normoblasts and myelocytes. The degree of change is small in comparison to the effects of anemia caused by increased red cell destruction but, presumably, this depends on the demand and the availability of materials required to meet the demand.[9]

In the otherwise healthy individual, blood regeneration is rapid and will occur without treatment of any kind. Schiødt[7] found that, no matter how great the blood loss had been the rate of erythrocyte regeneration was such that a level of about 4,500,000 red corpuscles was reached in about thirty-three days, the curve of regeneration rising more sharply in the more severe cases of anemia. The red cell count was usually entirely restored to normal in four to six weeks, although the hemoglobin lagged behind, reaching normal only after six to eight weeks. In blood donors from whom an average of 555 ml. of blood had been removed, Fowler and Barer[2b] observed an average drop in hemoglobin of 2.3 Gm., an amount which required fifty days to replace.

After ten to fourteen days there should be no morphological evidence of active red cell regeneration. The leukocyte count should be normal after three or four days. Continued bleeding is suggested by a maintained high level of reticulocytes. Persistent leukocytosis may result from the same cause or may be due to hemorrhage into body cavities or to complications. The latter, particularly infections, tend to delay the hematopoietic response.

Diagnosis.—The sudden onset of severe anemia, when not due to an obvious cause, should direct suspicion to the gastro-intestinal tract or, if the patient is a female, to the reproductive organs as sites of a hemorrhage. Acute hemolytic anemia is rare and is accompanied by bilirubinemia, hemoglobinemia, and other signs (Chapter 12). As already mentioned, hemorrhage into one of the body cavities, or into a cyst, may be followed by icterus as the blood is absorbed.

Acute blood loss may be a symptom of one of the blood disorders. In purpura hemorrhagica, the platelets are reduced in number, the bleeding time is prolonged and the clot is non-retractile. The character of the anemia is the same as that of acute blood loss from any other cause and a similar leukocytosis may occur. In aplastic anemia, on the other hand, there is not only anemia and thrombocytopenia but leukopenia is also found.

In hemophilia, the blood picture is that of acute posthemorrhagic anemia except for the prolonged coagulation time and other related changes (p. 867).

Treatment.—The immediate indications in the treatment of acute blood loss are to stop the bleeding, restore blood volume, and treat shock. Fluids must be given at once. When the hemorrhage has been severe, it is of utmost importance to restore the blood volume and for this purpose blood transfusion is by far the most valuable method. This subject has been fully discussed already (Chapter 9). The system of blood banks, making large quantities of blood easily available, makes it unnecessary to resort to substitutes for transfusions. These have not been found as effective as whole blood.

Once the emergency has been met, treatment of the acute posthemorrhagic anemia is simple. A diet of high protein, vitamin and mineral content, as described in Chapter 9, should be given as soon as possible. By the use of puréed foods,[5] this can be done with safety even when the hemorrhage has occurred in the gastro-intestinal tract. Liver extracts, vitamin B_{12} or folic acid are unnecessary. The agents effective in pernicious anemia are valueless in the anemia due to blood loss. The limiting factor in the rate of blood production in response to blood loss is the amount of available iron.[2] The normal available iron store has been estimated to be approximately 1.2 to 1.5 Gm. (p. 143). Recovery times from a 500 ml. phlebotomy have been found to vary from 2 to 3 weeks to 3 or 4 months.[2] When supplementary iron was given it was found that phlebotomies could be performed every two weeks without the production of significant anemia.

ANEMIAS CHARACTERIZED CHIEFLY BY LACK OF SIGNS OF ACTIVE BLOOD FORMATION

General Considerations.—The anemias to be considered under this heading form a much less well-defined group than those which have been described in the preceding pages. The macrocytic anemias due to deficiency of vitamin B_{12} or folic acid present a rather characteristic clinical picture and are distinguished by a typical response to specific therapy. Anemia due to acute blood loss needs no description. Anemias in which excessive blood destruction is the major etiological factor can be recognized by certain anamnestic, physical and laboratory findings. So also the anemias due to iron deficiency, which are yet to be discussed, present a homogeneous group with a characteristic blood picture and response to therapy. The remaining anemias, which include that associated with a great variety of chronic diseases and infections as well as the "refractory anemias" and myelophthisic anemia, do not fall into so uniform and clearly definable a class.

The anemias found in association with various chronic diseases and infections are referred to as anemias characterized chiefly by lack of signs of active blood formation because they generally present the picture which, in more extreme form, is found in what is known as aplastic anemia. The anemia is usually normocytic; that is, there is usually no significant alteration from the normal in the average size or hemoglobin content of the red corpuscles. In fact, even the *individual* corpuscles ordinarily vary little in their size, shape, or hemoglobin content. At the same time leukocytes of bone marrow origin may be somewhat decreased in number and even the platelet count may be low, although usually these features resembling aplastic anemia are not to be found. There is no evidence of excessive blood destruction nor of erythrocyte regeneration, such as an increase in the reticulocyte count or the presence in the smear of polychromatophilic or nucleated red corpuscles. Furthermore, the use of specific anti-anemic substances such as

vitamin B_{12} or iron is of no value in relieving the anemia. Although macrocytic and hypochromic microcytic anemias due to nutritional deficiency are also in a sense anemias due to lack of blood formation, the regenerative failure is more apparent than real for the bone marrow is actually hyperplastic and the administration of the deficient substance is followed by a prompt response.

The Pancytopenias. — The term, pancytopenia, may be introduced at this point. This refers to a reduction in all three formed elements of the blood, the red corpuscles, the leukocytes and the platelets. The leukopenia is usually due to an absolute reduction in the cells of the myeloid series and there is often a relative lymphocytosis. However, if the reduction is sufficiently great, lymphocytopenia is found as well.

Pancytopenia is not a disease entity but rather a triad which is found under a number of different circumstances (Table 11–1). While its causes are numerous, its recognition is useful since certain simple details will often rule out some disorders while other findings will make other conditions quite likely. Thus, the presence of marked splenic enlargement calls attention to the possibility of leukemia, the lymph node disorders, myelosclerosis (p. 581), Gaucher's disease (p. 772), congestive splenomegaly (p. 1060), kala-azar and "primary splenic panhematopenia" (p. 1052). The finding of enlarged lymph nodes will support the possibility that leukemia or Hodgkin's disease, for example, may be the cause of the pancytopenia. On the other hand, lack of these signs and the absence of evidence to suggest the deficiency anemias permit the consideration of certain types of myelophthisic anemia and the "refractory anemias." Myelophthisic anemias, however, are often characterized by the presence of immature cells of the red and white series in the blood and thus they can be distinguished

Table 11–1—Causes of Pancytopenia

1. "Aleukemic," leukopenic or subleukemic leukemia

2. Primary refractory anemias
    (a) "Aplastic anemias" due to
        (1) chemical agents: benzol, organic arsenicals, gold compounds, anticonvulsants, *etc.* (Table 11–3, p. 553).
        (2) Physical agents: ionizing radiation
    (b) "Idiopathic aplastic anemia," including the familial type ("Fanconi syndrome")

3. Myelophthisic anemia
    (a) metastatic carcinoma in bone marrow
    (b) multiple myeloma
    (c) myelofibrosis, myelosclerosis, chronic non-leukemic myelosis, "agnogenic myeloid metaplasia"
    (d) marble bone disease, osteopetrosis

4. Disorders involving the spleen—"hypersplenism"
    (a) congestive splenomegaly
    (b) lymph node disorders: lymphosarcoma, reticulum cell sarcoma, Hodgkin's disease, giant follicular lymphoma
    (c) infiltrative disorders: Gaucher's disease, Niemann-Pick's, Letterer-Siwe disease
    (d) infectious diseases: kala-azar, miliary tuberculosis, sarcoid, syphilis
    (e) "primary splenic panhematopenia"

5. Deficiency anemias: pernicious anemia and other megaloblastic macrocytic anemias

6. Paroxysmal nocturnal hemoglobinuria (rarely)

from the "refractory anemias" where such signs are usually lacking.

Examination of the bone marrow is often extremely valuable in such cases. This may offer such crucial evidence as a picture typical of leukemia or of the megaloblastic macrocytic anemias, or Gaucher cells, tumor cells or leishmania may be found; or, instead, the marrow may seem gritty and may yield little or nothing.

Difficulty arises when one of these clearly defined syndromes cannot be demonstrated and one is forced, by exclusion, to consider other possibilities. Furthermore, conditions falling in this category are not always consistent with the average or classical picture. Thus, as will be shown in the next section, in "aplastic anemia" the bone marrow may not always be aplastic; in fact, in cases otherwise fitting this category even hyperplastic bone marrow has been found. Again, the effects of exposure to benzol range from the production of an aplastic to a regenerative and even a leukemic

picture. The same can be said to some extent of the action of ionizing radiation. Finally, myelosclerosis may present a picture which is most difficult to distinguish from that of leukemia.

As will be indicated in subsequent sections, observations concerning the effects of agents such as benzol and ionizing radiation as well as studies of the pathogenesis of myelosclerosis suggest that a range of variation from complete aplasia of the bone marrow without any signs of regeneration whatever, to one of myelofibrosis with extramedullary blood formation in the spleen, as well as a picture closely resembling if not identical with that of leukemia, may be expected to develop according, probably, to the operation of a number of factors: the nature of the toxic agent, the dose, the number of exposures and the length of the intervening intervals between exposures, the condition of the affected individual, the capacity of his tissues to regenerate or, instead, to form "scar tissue," the appearance of intercurrent factors such as infection and malnutrition and the effect of other, as yet obscure, influences.

PRIMARY REFRACTORY ANEMIAS

Definition and Classification. — This term is applied to cases of anemia characterized clinically by persistent and often severe anemia, accompanied in most instances by granulocytopenia and thrombocytopenia, which are refractory to any treatment other than transfusion of blood and which are not associated with infection, chronic renal or hepatic disease, malignancy, malnutrition or other conditions here classified as "simple chronic anemias" (p. 573). Since these last mentioned anemias, like the "primary" refractory anemias, are in certain respects unresponsive to therapy, they might be regarded as examples of "secondary" refractory anemia.

The concept of "aplastic anemia" was introduced in 1888 by Ehrlich[20] who described a rapidly fatal process occurring most frequently in young adults between the ages of 15 and 30 years and often associated with high fever, bleeding from the mucous membranes, and ulcerated lesions of the pharynx and gums. Ehrlich's observations indicated that the primary defect was one of decreased cell production. There were marked leukopenia and thrombocytopenia as well as severe anemia and acellular bone marrow.

In the course of time the concept of aplastic anemia has been broadened. It was noted that the acute fulminating type of case described by Ehrlich was rare but that a similar pancytopenia with aplastic marrow and not accompanied by lymphadenopathy or splenomegaly which pursued a more chronic course was seen more often. Another important observation was the fact that an identical condition might be associated with exposure to a variety of chemical and physical agents. It was also noted that a similar condition may begin in early childhood, is often familial and is usually associated with a variety of congenital anomalies. Finally it was observed that cases may be encountered in which only the erythropoietic tissue is involved in the aplastic process, the leukocytes and platelets being normal.

To compound the complexity still further, the bone marrow in cases in which the clinical and blood picture were consistent with a diagnosis of aplastic anemia has not always been found to be aplastic. The marrow in some cases has been cellular or even hyperplastic.[13c, 51] In some cases even occasional nucleated red cells as well as polychromatophilia and stippling, rather than the classical "aregenerative" picture were found in the blood.

It is highly probable that the above range of cases does not represent a single disorder. It is evident that bone marrow morphology does not necessarily accurately mirror bone marrow function and that a clinical and blood picture resembling the acute disorder described by Ehrlich or even the more chronic forms will not always be accompanied by fatty marrow. The term "aplastic anemia" should perhaps be reserved for acute and chronic forms of a disorder like that reported by Ehrlich. For the group as a whole, the term "primary refractory anemias" is employed. In refractory anemias the essential feature is bone marrow failure which is not due to a recognized deficiency such as that seen in pernicious anemia and in iron deficiency anemia. A classification of refractory anemias is presented in Table 11–2. The various clinical syndromes will be described in turn. Such terms as *progressive hypocythemia*,[51] *aregeneratory anemia, aleukia haemorrhagica, panmyelophthisis, hypoplastic anemia* and *toxic paralytic anemia* have been used in referring to cases such as those under discussion.

Table 11–2—Classification of Refractory Anemias

A. *Primary Refractory Anemias*

    I. "Aplastic anemias"—Pancytopenia
        (*a*) Acquired: various physical and chemical agents (Table 11–3).
        (*b*) Idiopathic
            (1) without associated anomalies. Acute and chronic forms
            (2) congenital pancytopenia (Fanconi)

    II. Erythrocytic hypoplasia
        (*a*) Acute transitory erythroblastopenia—in hemolytic anemia and in association with various disorders in children
        (*b*) Congenital hypoplastic anemia (Blackfan and Diamond)
        (*c*) Acquired erythrocytic hypoplasia

B. *Simple Chronic Anemias* ("Secondary" Refractory Anemias)
    Anemia associated with infection, renal disease, malignancy, endocrine disorders, etc.

Chemical and Physical Agents Associated with the Development of Pancytopenia.—These can be divided into two main categories (Table 11–3). Certain agents can be expected to produce marrow aplasia whenever a sufficient dose has been given. The effects are more or less predictable and the changes observed in human subjects can be reproduced in experimental animals. Of these agents, benzol and radiation will be discussed here. The mustards, urethane, busulfan and the antimetabolites will be considered in later chapters because their ability to damage the cells of the hemopoietic system has been found to be useful in the treatment of the leukemias and lymphomas.

There is, in addition, an ever increasing number of compounds which are only occasionally associated with bone marrow hypoplasia or aplasia or with granulocytopenia or thrombocytopenia. The great majority of these differ from the mustards and other agents belonging in the preceding category because their deleterious effects are unpredictable. The development of noxious effects has been attributed by various writers to the intermittent, prolonged or excessive usage of these agents or to their administration to individuals who had manifested other signs of sensitivity, either to the same or to other agents. Although in individual cases this argument seems to be plausible, when viewed as a whole no consistent pattern is discernible. Noteworthy, however, is the fact that attempts to reproduce similar hemopoietic changes in experimental animals have been met as a rule with failure. Consequently the development in some manner of drug idiosyncrasy is regarded generally as the probable mechanism.

The different drugs which have been mentioned in various reports as the causative agents in the production of aplastic anemia are listed in Table 11–3. It will be noted that some of these are also listed in the chapters dealing with thrombocytopenia (p. 818) and granulocytopenia (p. 1098). The classification of the drugs according to the number of cases in which they have been suspected as being the causative agents is necessarily an arbitrary one. None of these drugs, in fact, has been incriminated often in comparison to its usage, but adequate statistics are not available. Only for quinacrine are there any reliable data.[16c] For this drug the incidence of aplastic anemia was estimated as being approximately once among 25,000 persons exposed to the risk each year. Obviously, therefore, the fact that drug "idiosyncrasy" may occur does not preclude the use of one of these agents; however, the

Table 11–3—Agents Associated with the Occurrence of Pancytopenia

A. *Agents which regularly produce* marrow hypoplasia and aplasia if a sufficient dose is given:
   (1) Ionizing radiation (roentgen rays, radioactive P, Au, etc.)
   (2) Mustards (sulfur[37] and nitrogen mustards, triethylenemelamine (TEM), etc.)
   (3) Urethane, myleran
   (4) Benzene
   (5) Anti-metabolites (antifolic compounds, 6-mercaptopurine, etc.)
B. *Agents occasionally associated* with hypoplasia or aplasia (drug idiosyncrasy?):

Class of Compound	20 to 100 or more reported cases	Single or very few reports
Anti-microbial agents	Arsenobenzols	Inorganic arsenicals
	Chloramphenicol	Streptomycin[17a]
		Sulfonamides[48]
		Oxytetracycline[52d]
		Chlortetracycline[52d]
Anti-convulsants	Mesantoin (Methyl-	Tridione (trimethadione)
	phenylethylhydantoin)	Nuvarone (methylphenylhydantoin)
Anti-thyroid drugs		Carbimazole (carbethoxythiomethylglyoxaline)[15c]
		Tapazole (methylmercaptoimidazole)[39b]
Anti-histaminics		Pyribenzamine[26]
Insecticides		Chlorophenothane (DDT)[22d]
Miscellaneous agents	Gold preparations	Quinacrine (atabrine)
	Trinitrotoluene	Dinitrophenol[32]
		Phenylbutazone[27c]
		Chlorpromazine[49b] and promazine[48]
		Hair dyes[12d]
		Meprobamate[41b]
		Bismuth[17,49]
		Mercury[30]
		Colloidal Silver[30]
		Carbon tetrachloride[50c]

risk requires discriminating employment of the drug in question. Unfortunately, in a number of fatal instances of aplastic anemia, the indications for the use of the agent involved have often been of a doubtful character or were entirely lacking.

Some of the agents which have been mentioned may now be considered in somewhat more detail.

Benzene.—Benzene has been known as a cause of fatal aplastic anemia since Santesson's description (1897) of 4 cases in workers in a bicycle tire factory.[15] Benzene (C_6H_6) is a hydrocarbon which is obtained as a byproduct in the manufacture of coke. It is also to be found in petroleum distillates, the amount depending in part on the composition of the crude petroleum from which it has been derived. Certain crude petroleums contain significant quantities of benzene.[48] Benzene is used as a solvent for rubber, gum, resins, fats, and alkaloids as well as in the manufacture of drugs, dyes, and explosives. It has been employed in many industries, including the manufacture of artificial leather, natural leather, enamels, rubber, waterproof fabrics, lacquers, shellac, paint removers, bronzing, silvering and gilding liquids, and batteries; in electroplating, lithography and photography, dry cleaning, and feather preparation; in the airplane, linoleum and celluloid industries.[31c] A benzene derivative (cymene) is present in the exhaust gases encountered in the sulfite pulp industry.[15d] Benzene is volatile and consequently is absorbed usually by inhalation in badly ventilated rooms. The maximum allowable vapor concentration for industrial usage has been 100 parts per million[15] but this is probably too high.[48] In spite of its wide recognition as a myelotoxic agent, benzene remains an important cause of hemopoietic damage, even in the home where it is used frequently in cleaning agents.

The classical picture of leukopenia, thrombocytopenia, and severe anemia represents only the severe and fatal form of poisoning by benzene. Among exposed workers the most common abnormality is anemia. Next in frequency are macrocytosis, thrombocytopenia and leukopenia.[25,27] Leukopenia was at one time thought to be the earliest sign of poisoning but recent studies show that it is present in only a small percentage of those exposed.[25] Other manifestations of poisoning which have been observed are lymphocytopenia, elevation of reticulocyte count, eosinophilia, immature marrow elements in the circulating blood, and even leukocytosis.[15] There may also be evidence of increased blood destruction. In one survey serum bilirubin determinations showed elevated values in a third of the cases.[27] Data furnished to support the statement that polycythemia may occur[15] are not convincing.

There are great variations in the susceptibility to benzene poisoning but there is no support for the original view that young people, especially young women, are more susceptible than others.[15] Evidence of poisoning may appear in a few weeks or only after many years of exposure, or it may not be discovered until the onset of infection long after exposure has ceased. Any degree of exposure is dangerous.

Like the blood picture, which may be of the regenerative or the hemolytic type instead of aplastic, the bone marrow may be found to be hyperplastic rather than acellular and this can be the case

even when the blood shows little evidence of regenerative activity. Extramedullary hematopoiesis has been observed[15] and the complete picture of myeloid leukemia has been described in a few cases.[21] More often when extramedullary hematopoiesis has been present, marked splenomegaly and a blood picture of myelophthisic anemia has been found (p. 587).

When a benzene-olive oil mixture is injected in rats, the neutrophilic granulopoietic system is first stimulated.[38] The blood neutrophils have been observed to increase in number and there is hyperplasia of myelocytes in the marrow. This is followed by destruction of these elements. Degenerative changes occur even more rapidly in the lymphatic tissue than in the bone marrow and coincidentally lymphocytopenia occurs. Erythropoietic tissue is more resistant but hemolytic anemia develops when large doses are given. Eventually hypoplasia follows degeneration of stem cells.

When marrow regeneration was studied in benzene intoxicated and in normal rabbits some of whose bone marrow had been extirpated, it was observed that, in the latter, sheets of primitive reticular cells and bone trabeculae, then fat cells and finally myeloid tissue appeared.[50d] In the benzene intoxicated animals, on the other hand, the extirpated marrow regenerated only to the point of formation of primitive reticular cells. It was postulated, therefore, that at least one part of the mechanism whereby benzene induces aplasia of bone marrow is by the inhibition of cell division and maturation past the level of the primitive reticular cell.

Frequent subcutaneous injections of benzene in olive oil have been observed to produce a leukemoid condition in animals.[15]

Trinitrotoluene is another agent used in industry,[31c] especially in war time,[16] which may be associated with the development of aplastic anemia. This agent may also produce hemolytic anemia (p. 609).

Organic Arsenicals.—The administration of organic arsenicals may be followed by thrombocytopenia (p. 828), granulocytopenia (p. 1098), or severe anemia in addition. Approximately half of the reported cases have shown the complete clinical and hematologic picture of aplastic anemia.[35]

There appears to be no relationship between the size of the dose or the duration of treatment and the onset of hematopoietic disturbances. Furthermore, the total number of cases is very small when compared with the once widespread use of organic arsenicals in the treatment of syphilis. Neoarsphenamine has been incriminated most frequently but this is at least partly attributable to its wide use. Actually sulfarsphenamine appears to be the most dangerous drug as regards the production of blood dyscrasias. No harmful hemopoietic effects have been attributed to tryparsamide. Mapharsen was the cause of aplastic anemia in one of our cases and 3 others have been reported.[22b]

Itching; a mild macular, papular, or vesicular rash; prolonged fever or malaise; or ready bruising were thought to be danger signals in patients receiving arsphenamine or one of its modifications.[43] No thorough study of the frequency of blood changes in such patients was carried out, however, nor is it known whether slight changes in the blood may not occur in patients receiving arsenicals who have no symptoms. Very probably, however, if early symptoms of poisoning were given serious consideration fewer severe hematopoietic disturbances would develop. In many reported cases treatment was continued in the face of premonitory warnings.

Since the arsphenamines are formed by the substitution of arsenic in the benzol ring, it has been suggested that the cause of the blood dyscrasias produced is the disintegration of these drugs *in vivo*, thus permitting a benzene-like action to take place. In support of this view it may be said that aplastic anemia has not been observed to follow the use of inorganic arsenic. However, potassium arsenite has a well-known effect in depressing the leukocyte count (see p. 962) and granulocytopenia with anemia in one case,[53] as well as thrombocytopenia in another,[39] have been reported in inorganic arsenic poisoning. In experimental studies, a decreased production of young red cells following the administration of arsenic and arsenious acid has been observed.[33] Consequently no conclusion is justified at this time regarding the mode of action of the arsenicals.

Chloramphenicol, Mesantoin, Gold and Other Compounds.—Once attention was called to the possibility, many reports of aplastic anemia occurring in patients treated with *chloramphenicol* appeared in the literature.[12b,13,49a,49c] From 1949 until 1952, when its use was unrestrained, this antibiotic was the drug most frequently associated with the development of aplastic anemia in the United States.[48] A sharp decrease in the total number of cases seen annually followed public warning of the hazard in 1952. The number of cases is increasing again as the use of this drug increases. Although it would seem that severe marrow depression is most common following prolonged use of chloramphenicol and when large doses have been given,[31] aplastic anemia has been observed also when intermittent therapy was employed[49c] and sometimes even with the first administration.[48] More than half the reported cases have been fatal. In experimental attempts to produce hemopoietic depression with chloramphenicol, slight suppression of erythropoiesis has been observed in ducks[46] and in man when large doses were given.[36b] There is some ground, however, to suspect that even conventional doses may have deleterious effects in man.[47b] Thus, when ferrokinetic studies were carried out, evidence of erythropoietic depression could be demonstrated.[47a] It was also noted that an increase in plasma iron content and an increase in the saturation of iron binding globulin preceded the fall in volume of packed red cells by an appreciable interval when erythropoietic depression was induced by chloramphenicol. From these and other studies it would seem that the nitrobenzene moiety of the chloramphenicol molecule is the factor concerned in producing damage to the bone marrow.

There is no good evidence to incriminate other antibiotics in the etiology of aplastic anemia.[48] *Sulfonamides* may have been associated with the development of aplastic anemia in some cases.[31a] There are reports involving sulfisoxazole (Gantrisin®), carbutamide, tolbutamide,[15a] acetazolamide (Diamox®)[51c] and compounds sharing the sulfonated nitrobenzene nucleus of the sulfonamide compounds, such as thiosemicarbazone.[48]

Of the *anticonvulsants, Mesantoin®* (methyl-phenylethyl-hydantoin)[13c,56a] and Tridione® (trimethadione)[56a] have been reported most frequently in association with the development of aplastic anemia and methylphenyl hydantoin[34] and phenacemide probably have a similar effect.

Antithyroid compounds,[15c,39b] *antihistamines*[26] and *insecticides*[48] have rarely been associated with the development of aplastic anemia. Antihistaminics and antithyroid compounds are more commonly associated with the development of granulocytopenia. Blood dyscrasias were comparatively common in association with the use of *gold compounds* in the treatment of rheumatoid arthritis, and about 50 per cent were examples of aplastic anemia.[56] The use of *atabrine* as an antimalarial in the southwest Pacific[16c] or in the treatment of lupus erythematosus[44b] has been associated in a few instances with the development of aplastic anemia. Other agents which have been named in isolated instances[48] are listed in Table 11–3.

Ionizing Radiation.—Excessive exposure to ionizing radiation may result in severe and even fatal aplastic anemia. Lesser grades of exposure lead to less serious changes in the blood. It will be convenient to consider various aspects of the hematopoietic effects of radiation injury at this point.

Radiation effects may arise from electromagnetic waves such as roentgen and gamma rays, or from particulate matter having mass, such as alpha and beta particles, protons and neutrons. The results of radiation depend, on the one hand, upon the kind of radiation and, on the other, on the susceptibility of the affected cells. Although every kind of ionizing radiation appears to be similar in its clinical action,[44d] the results of a given exposure depend on its physical properties and mode of application (whether external or internal), its intensity and the duration of exposure. Certain types of radiation, such as roentgen and gamma rays and fast and slow neutrons penetrate the body at will while others, such as alpha and beta particles, although highly damaging, are effective only over a range of a fraction of a millimeter to a few millimeters of tissue. Therefore, alpha and beta particles are very harmful to the hemopoietic system only if they are introduced within the body, as in the case of the radium dial workers (see below). In an atomic explosion, on the other hand, gamma rays and neutrons are liberated instantly in large amounts and thus the hemopoietic tissues are reached promptly.

The *susceptibility of tissue* varies greatly, the hemopoietic tissues being the most sensitive, with the germinal epithelium of the testis and ovary, the epithelium of the intestinal crypts, the basal layer of the skin, the connective tissue, bone, liver, pancreas, kidney, nerve and brain following in decreasing order of sensitivity.[52b] There is considerable variation between species in their sensitivity to radiation and significant differences have been observed between individuals.

Histopathological changes associated with radiation[39c] include the changes produced in (1) the cells, (2) the stroma and (3) the blood vessels. Swelling is the first observed stromal effect and this is followed frequently by fibrosis and hyalinization. The initial vascular effect is thrombosis and this may, in turn, be followed by fibrosis, hyalinization and telangiectasia. The cellular effects include cessation of mitosis and this is followed by disorganization of the structure of the cell and swelling. With resumption of mitosis, bizarre mitotic figures appear. In studies of atomic bomb casualties, complete disappearance of all blood-forming elements was observed in the bone marrow in the early period. However, even within the first week there was evidence of proliferative activity on the part of the reticulum cells and plasma cells. After various lengths of time there was renewed differentiation into granulopoietic and erythropoietic tissue. After the sixth week, hyperplasia of myeloid cells was associated with the presence of considerable numbers of reticulum cells, plasma cells and lymphocytes. In the lymphoid tissue, lymphocytes had disappeared by the third day. Although evidence of regeneration appeared by the fifth day, return was slow and at three months lymphocytes were still reduced in number.

The *mechanism* whereby radiation damages the cells of the body is obscure.[37a, 45] Presumably a series of chemical changes takes place following absorption of the ionizing radiation by the molecules of the cells. Enzymes containing sulphhydryl groups are easily inactivated by ionizing radiation.[52b] In addition, irradiation of cells has been observed,[42a] by the use of the ultraviolet photomicrographic technic, to be associated with inhibition of the synthesis of deoxyribonucleic acid in the nuclei.[51d] This probably explains the inhibition of mitosis which occurs promptly following irradiation[27a] and appears to be a fundamental effect of radiation. There is evidence that radiochemical reactions involving free oxygen play a vital role in radiation injuries and that a reduction in oxygen tension reduces the injury.[18a]

The observable **effects of radiation on the blood** picture depend on several factors: (1) the radiosensitivity of the various parent cells; (2) the ability of the tissue to regenerate; and (3) the length of life of the different morphologic elements in the peripheral blood. Storage of granulocytes, platelets and lymphocytes probably plays little or no rôle but storage of red corpuscles is, no doubt, significant in masking the effects of radiation.

There is little evidence to support the concept that the *circulating blood cells* are affected directly by radiation except when this is given in tremendous amounts.[19, 27a, 38a] (p. 559). Morphologic changes have been described in the leukocytes of human subjects exposed to ionizing radiation,[34a] but it is likely that this was the consequence of the damage to the parent cells. Atypical basophils, giant multilobed polymorphonuclear cells and neutrophils and lymphocytes with massing of their nuclear chromatin, have been reported and pyknotic lymphocytes have been described.[34a, 51a] In the blood of personnel associated with a 130-inch cyclotron, lymphocytes with bilobed or double nuclei were observed.[32a] In supravitally stained preparations a striking increase in the number of refractive neutral red bodies was noted in the cytoplasm of the circulating lymphocytes following exposure to ionizing radiation.[17b]

There is some disagreement concerning the *sensitivity of the various components of hemopoietic tissue* to radiation. On the basis of histopathology in animal experiments, the conclusion was reached that

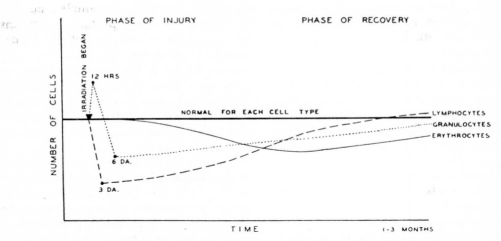

Fig. 11-2.—Graph to show in simplified form the radiolability of three blood cell types and their relative capacity to recover from damage. (From Dunlap,[19] after Minot and Spurling[42].)

lymphocytes are very readily damaged by radiation, that the erythropoietic cells are almost equally sensitive and that the myelopoietic tissue is less sensitive than the erythropoietic.[13a] The monocytes and megakaryocytes were less sensitive than granulocytes, and fat cells, free macrophages and reticular cells, including those lining the sinuses, appeared to be quite radioresistant. Other studies,[52] however, laying emphasis on regenerative capacity and the degree of *functional* impairment, suggest that erythropoietic tissue is significantly less sensitive to radiation injury than is the myelopoietic tissue.

The effects of a single therapeutic dose of x-rays have been carefully studied in patients suffering from ankylosing spondylitis.[15b] A mean surface dose of 300 roentgens was applied to the sacro-iliac joints and the whole length of the spine. The average dose received in the bone marrow was calculated to range from 135 to 285 r. The observed changes correspond to those described by others[19,42] (Fig. 11–2). There was a rise in the neutrophil count within a few hours which was related to the development of radiation sickness. A significant

fall in the lymphocyte count was observed by the end of the first twenty-four hours, which continued thereafter for some days. The total leukocyte count decreased from the first or second post-irradiation day. For the first four or five days this was due mainly to the decrease in the lymphocyte count. A significant fall in the neutrophil count did not occur in the first five post-irradiation days. In more than half the cases the volume of packed red cells began to diminish by the end of the first or second post-irradiation day.

In other studies[19] *anemia* was not observed before four to eight weeks following exposure. Whether or not anemia develops at all, and its time of appearance seem to depend on the amount of radiation. When this is small, little or no anemia will be observed since the impairment of erythropoiesis which takes place[12f] may not be detectable in the blood count. With larger dosage, anemia may appear early as the result of redistribution of intracellular or extracellular fluids.[15b] When doses at or near the median lethal dose have been given to animals, a precipitous drop in red cell mass has been observed.[36] This is due to damage to the capillary wall with resulting diversion of erythrocytes into tissue spaces and lymphatics, and to hemorrhage, but injury of the circulating red cells has also been demonstrated.[50b]

Other than thrombocytopenia, no good evidence for the development of deficiency of other *factors concerned in coagulation* has been demonstrated.[16b] The blood coagulation defect which follows irradiation in the lethal range and the failure to utilize prothrombin can be correlated directly with the platelet deficiency which develops.

Routine radiation therapy seldom produces permanent or dangerous modification in the blood. Although no radiation dosage is so small that no effect is produced and a cumulative effect of small daily increments may be expected,[16a,38a] therapeutic dosage is calculated to produce minimal damage and is ultimately interrupted so that recovery may take place. Leukopenia, due more to lymphocytopenia than neutropenia may occur and a slight decrease in platelets may follow. Anemia is rarely produced. In leukemia and in Hodgkin's disease the number of red corpuscles may actually increase following irradiation if the desired effect on the underlying disease has been produced.

Intense exposure, on the other hand, as in the victims of the atomic explosion,[39a] results in manifestations which depend, in so far as their severity and time of appearance are concerned, on the severity of the injury and the sensitivity of the individual. Pronounced weakness, nausea and vomiting, transient diarrhea which may return in severe form, and hemorrhagic manifestations develop. In the fulminating form of the *acute radiation syndrome*,[52b] prostration, mucosal ulcerations, a step-like rise in fever and rapidly developing infection in the face of severe leukopenia lead rapidly to death. In the hemorrhagic form, bleeding depends on increased vascular fragility and thrombocytopenia. Purpura and petechiae

develop in about four to seven days following the initial injury and these manifestations reach their peak between the sixteenth and the twenty-second day. Severe flash burns and extensive loss of hair from the scalp complete the picture of the acute radiation syndrome. In addition to the fulminating and hemorrhagic forms of the syndrome, just described, a pancytopenic form may be encountered. In such cases, made up of those who survive the 3 to 6 week period during which death may occur from diarrhea and dehydration, infection, hemorrhage or other complications, all three formed elements of the blood are reduced in number and the picture of aplastic anemia is encountered.

The occurrence of leukopenia in individuals receiving local radiation in areas where little or no hemopoietic tissue is located, has led to studies regarding the *"indirect" effects of radiation*. No evidence was found of an effect of radiation on the blood picture of normal cats connected for long intervals of time by carotid anastomoses with irradiated cats at various periods following irradiation.[38b] In fact, non-irradiated marrow of dogs appeared to exert a sparing or maintenance action and such an effect of the marsupialized, non-irradiated spleen has been demonstrated quite convincingly.[34b] Diminished proliferative activity on the part of the circulating leukocytes has been postulated[27a] but the precise mechanism is vague. Changes in lymphoid tissue may depend in part on stimulation of the pituitary-adrenal mechanism (p. 49) as the result of local injury of tissue by radiation,[27b] but this is probably not the complete explanation of the indirect effects of radiation. *In vitro* studies have failed to demonstrate the presence of an antimitotic factor in irradiated plasma.[12c]

As indicated earlier, the *qualitative systemic effects* of all types of radiation are similar. With the use of suitable *isotopes*, changes can be produced in tissues which would not ordinarily be reached by these radiations. However, in contrast to the picture of sudden destruction and subsequent depletion of cells after intense external irradiation, the depletion resulting from the *introduction of radioactive isotopes internally* occurs more gradually. Furthermore, since the irradiation is more continuous and longer lasting, depending on the rate of "decay" or loss of radioactivity of the agent, the effects on the marrow are more persistent. In mice and rats studies have been made[34a] of the effects of the administration of strontium-89, barium-lanthanum-140, phosphorus-32, sodium-24, plutonium (Pu-239), radium and yttrium-91.

The use of *thorium dioxide* as a diagnostic aid in the form of thorotrast has been followed many years later in a few instances by the development of aplastic anemia,[18b,42b] leukemia and primary malignancies in the liver,[43a] the lung and at the site of injection.[39e] The late effects of *radium* and *mesothorium*[12d] are related to changes in the bones (radiation osteitis, neoplasms in or near bone). Only minor degrees of anemia have been observed and rarely aplastic anemia. Acute radium poisoning, like that in the radium dial workers, is accompanied by very striking changes in the blood (*see* below).

In *chronic occupational exposure*, moderate granulocytopenia, relative or absolute lymphocytosis, and varying grades of normocytic or macrocytic anemia as well as leukocytosis, leukemoid reactions, erythrocytosis and thrombocytopenic purpura have been described.[16a] Eosinophilia has been observed as a result of overexposure and in some roentgen-ray and radium workers abnormal and embryonic leukocytes have been found in the circulating blood. A slight relative depression of lymphocytes and a slight elevation of eosinophils have been reported in the surviving victims of the Hiroshima atomic bombing.[50] A high rate of mortality from leukemia (p. 908) and from cancer

has been observed in those exposed to ionizing radiation.

The effects of continuous irradiation were described many years ago in *radium dial workers* by Martland.[40,41] In these individuals, injured by the ingestion of radium through the habit of wetting their brushes by mouth, severe macrocytic anemia with megaloblasts in the circulating blood, leukopenia, and relative lymphocytosis developed. The femur bone marrow was dark red and showed primitive red cells and leukocyte hyperplasia, as well as numerous megakaryocytes. Thrombocytopenia occurred in only one case. In its severity and insidious character the anemia resembled pernicious anemia but bilirubinemia was absent, remissions did not occur, and gastro-intestinal and nervous symptoms were lacking. In a number of cases there were buccal lesions and necrosis of the jaw similar to that found in acute leukemia.[41] Low grade osteitis, replacement fibrosis of the marrow and osteogenic sarcoma were also encountered. In some of the affected workers death occurred as long as four to six years after leaving their occupation. In experimental radium poisoning[47] the first effect of radioactive substances given orally or parenterally was the production of erythrocytosis.[15f] Changes similar to those found in the dial workers followed. It is to be noted that hyperplastic marrow similar to that described by Martland, and macrocytic anemia, have also been seen in human beings and animals subjected only to external roentgen radiation.[19,34a]

The practice of making regular blood counts in persons occupationally exposed to radiation has little to justify it.[42b] Degrees of radiation exposure twenty times greater than the maximal permissible dose may produce a real drop in neutrophils or lymphocytes, but the change is slight and serious aplastic anemia has been seen to occur without necessarily being preceded by much of a decrease in leukocytes.[42d] Regular physical measurement of the doses received by the use of film badges and other methods is a much more practical procedure in most situations.

PANCYTOPENIA IN ASSOCIATION WITH VARIOUS DISORDERS

At one time aplasia of the bone marrow was said to occur in the terminal stage of pernicious anemia, myeloid leukemia, erythremia, myelophthisic anemia, and even in severe chronic posthemorrhagic anemia. Severe overwhelming infections, as in pneumonia, typhoid fever, and diphtheria were also said to cause aplastic anemia. Such effects must be extremely unusual. No cases have been described in recent years. In *miliary tuberculosis*, however, pancytopenia, macrocytosis and severely hypoplastic or aplastic bone marrow, often containing miliary tubercles, may be found.[15g,68,69a] Fever, sweating, loss of weight, splenomegaly and sometimes lymphadenopathy are likely to be present as well. Also infectious in origin is a unique epidemic form of marrow aplasia secondary to the *ingestion of infected grain* which has been observed in Russia and is probably due to a mold.[48,77] "*Equine infectious anemia*" has been claimed to produce in man severe refractory anemia, leukopenia and relative lymphocytosis, without thrombocytopenia.[44c]

Pancytopenia has been observed in association with *pregnancy*[74a] in 12 instances, one of which was the case described by Ehrlich. The anemia was refractory to all types of therapy but in one case gradual recovery occurred following abortion. Aplastic anemia has also been reported in association with sclerosis of the *thyroid gland*[72] and in *Simmonds' disease.*[61a]

FANCONI SYNDROME (CONGENITAL PANCYTOPENIA)

Under the title of "familial, infantile pernicious-like anemia", *Fanconi* described a fatal disorder in three brothers which was characterized by pancytopenia, bone marrow hypoplasia and congenital anomalies. Some 86 cases have been reported[23a,41a,44a,52c] and there are others, no doubt. The writer has observed three cases, two of these being sisters. The anemia is normocytic or slightly macrocytic, and macrocytes and target cells may be present in the blood. Reticulocytes may be slightly increased in number and occasional immature forms of red or white cells have been noted in blood smears but no evidence of a hemolytic process has been published except in one case[16d] which seems more probably to have been one of paroxysmal nocturnal hemoglobinuria. In most cases the leukopenia has been due to neutropenia but in several instances all the varieties of leukocytes were affected equally. The bone marrow has been described as fatty, hypocellular, normally cellular and even hypercellular.

A patchy, brown pigmentation of the skin, due to the deposition of melanin, is a common finding in Fanconi's anemia and other features of the disorder include dwarfism, microcephaly, hypogenitalism, strabismus, anomalies of the thumbs and of the kidneys, mental retardation and microphthalmia. Atrophy of the spleen is common.[23a] Congenital vascular anomalies are unusual.[12a] Somewhat more common in males than in females (2:1) the anemia has generally been detected in the first eight years of life. Out of 66 cases, seven were diagnosed after the age of 12, none after 23 years of age.[23a] There appears to be no racial or geographic preponderance but in a number of instances several siblings have been affected.[52c] Siblings of patients with the complete syndrome have had congenital anomalies without hematologic manifestations. The etiology of the disorder is unknown but it is generally thought to be hereditary, perhaps due to a recessive gene. Sporadic cases may perhaps be due to spontaneous gene mutation. Consanguinity of the parents has been noted a number of times.[23a,52c] Of special interest is the demonstration of a high incidence of leukemia in the families of patients with Fanconi's syndrome.[23a]

"PURE-RED CELL" APLASIA

In hereditary spherocytosis (p. 646) and in other hemolytic anemias (p. 685), and sometimes in children in the course of various infections (p. 755) the erythroblasts may suddenly disappear from the bone marrow for a short time ("*acute erythroblastopenia*"). If this aplastic crisis persists, anemia will develop. Hypoplasia confined to the erythropoietic system is also seen in a rare form of congenital anemia occurring in infancy (*congenital hypoplastic anemia*, p. 765). *Acquired erythrocytic hypoplasia* is the term applied to a similar disorder observed in adults. Approximately 26 cases have been reported, 20 to 67 years of age, with the majority in the fifth, sixth and seventh decades of life.[51b] The anemia is chronic, usually severe and normocytic or slightly macrocytic. Reticulocytes are decreased or absent but the leukocytes and platelets are normal and a normal leukocytic response to pyogenic infections has been observed. The bone marrow has been described as cellular with, however, marked hypoplasia or virtual absence of nucleated cells of the erythroid series. The etiology is obscure. In a few instances the anemia appears to have had its origin in childhood and consequently a relationship to the congenital disorder of infancy, mentioned above, may be suspected.[36a] In a few, exposure to toxic chemical agents was suspected and in

one instance an immune body reaction was postulated.[20a]

This group of cases is probably a heterogeneous one. In five instances, splenomegaly was reported, a finding out of keeping with a diagnosis of "aplastic anemia." More distinct are the 34 cases of refractory anemia which have been associated with *benign thymoma*.[22c,27d,50a] In 27 (including one unreported case of our own) there was selective hypoplasia of erythropoiesis ("*pure-red cell anemia*"), although in three of these leukopenia and/or thrombocytopenia developed later. In five other patients thrombocytopenia was recorded and pancytopenia was found in two. The clinical manifestations were those of anemia, almost always insidious in onset. Myasthenia gravis was noted in six patients. There was no adenopathy but enlargement of the liver and spleen occurred in two patients who had an associated autoimmune hemolytic anemia and in one who had neutropenia.[27d] The tumors varied in size, in three being too small for radiological demonstration. Thymectomy was performed in 15 patients. The microscopic picture of the gland was inconstant. In four cases improvement followed immediately after operation. One can only speculate about the association of the erythroid hypoplasia and the thymic growth since nothing is known.

"SIDEROBLASTIC" REFRACTORY ANEMIAS

Defying satisfactory classification are several groups of cases which have several features in common; namely, refractory anemia, hyperplastic bone marrow and signs of impaired iron utilization (sideroblasts, hemosiderosis). They must be distinguished from the refractory anemias already described, from thalassemia and the hemoglobinopathies (p. 668), from inclusion body anemias (p. 626) and from pyridoxine-responsive anemia (p. 136).

Heilmeyer[29a] called attention to two groups of cases:

(1) "*Anemia hypochromica siderochrestica hereditaria,*" which begins in childhood and has a chronic and benign course. There is slight splenomegaly. The life span of the red cells is normal, osmotic resistance is increased, there are no signs of hyperhemolysis but the bone marrow is hyperplastic and the erythroblasts contain large amounts of iron granules. The serum iron is normal but plasma clearance and iron turnover are accelerated. Red cell protoporphyrin is decreased and coproporphyrin is increased.

(2) "*Anemia refractoria sideroblastica,*" which becomes manifest in older patients and was thought to be an acquired disorder. Leukopenia and occasionally thrombocytopenia occur. The marrow is hyperplastic and there is an increase in non-hemoglobin iron in the erythroblasts. Some megaloblastoid erythroblasts may be present. Protoporphyrin in the red cells is normal or increased, in contrast to the congenital type. There is no hyperhemolysis. Others have reported similar cases.[12,39g] In both of these groups of cases hemosiderosis of the liver has been observed. The acquired disorder was found to change to leukemia in a number of instances.[29a]

There are several reports of cases of refractory anemia resembling the "hereditary sex-linked (?) anemia" described by Rundles and Falls (p. 711) which may be mentioned here. Microcytosis and hypochromia, high serum iron, increased sideroblasts and low free erythrocyte coproporphyrin,[23] shortened red cell life span, hemosiderosis and the presence of a similar disorder in a brother of the patient,[24a] with sideroblasts in the bone marrow,[39f] sometimes moderate splenomegaly[39h] and limitation to the male sex, with possible transmission by the female,[39f] distinguish these cases. They

were not thought to represent thalassemia and did not respond to the administration of pyridoxine in those cases in which this was tested. Another reported case[15e] was thought to differ from these and fro Heilmeyer's case but the differences are not clear. One similar patient was reported to have responded to a crude liver extract.[31b]

SYMPTOMATOLOGY OF THE PRIMARY REFRACTORY ANEMIAS

Some of the special features of each of the syndromes which are grouped among the primary refractory anemias have been described already, in the preceding pages. The onset usually is insidious. The symptoms and their character depend on the rapidity with which the anemia progresses and on the development or absence of complicating infections and hemorrhage. The latter in turn depend in part on the degree of granulocytopenia and thrombocytopenia. If the course is rapid, fever and symptoms attributable to anoxemia arise. If it is slow, progressive weakness and fatigability are the chief complaints until the anemia is well marked, when bleeding from the nose, mouth, or gastro-intestinal tract, menorrhagia, or purpura develops. In general, however, purpura is not the most conspicuous feature of this type of anemia. Ulcerations in the mouth and pharynx or low grade cellulitis in the neck appear late in this disorder, as a rule. In the idiopathic cases the illness is often dated from an attack of some common type of febrile disorder. In the secondary forms, symptoms may develop some weeks or even several months following exposure to the causative agent. The first sign of benzol poisoning may appear with the onset of an infection, long after exposure has ceased.[15]

A waxy pallor is usually well marked by the time attention is drawn to the

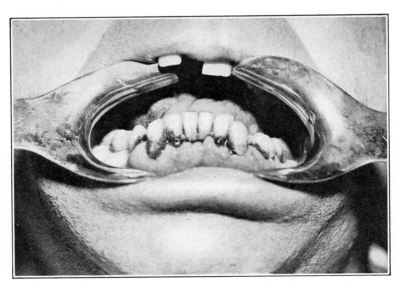

FIG. 11–3.—Bleeding gums in a case of aplastic anemia.

illness. The yellowish tint of pernicious anemia is lacking. Weight loss is unusual. There may be bruises or purpuric spots in the skin but these are often inconspicuous in relation to the degree of thrombocytopenia. Hemorrhages may be found in the eyegrounds. Splenomegaly is so unusual that when the spleen is palpable, "aleukemic" leukemia or some other condition which may simulate aplastic anemia should be looked for. It should be noted, however, that in a few cases of benzol poisoning,[15] as well as in some of the idiopathic cases which were discussed earlier (p. 550), the spleen has been found to be enlarged. The tongue shows no papillary atrophy. Changes in the nervous system are found only when hemorrhage has occurred there, although there may be some complaint of paresthesias in this as in other forms of anemia. The skin may show a brownish pigmentation.[13c] In Fanconi's anemia various congenital anomalies are characteristically present (p. 561).

Blood Changes.—As a rule the red corpuscles are more or less normal in appearance in spite of the severity of the illness. Polychromatophilia, stippling and nucleated red corpuscles are usually not found and the reticulocyte count is low, if not zero. In some instances, however, the anemia has been macrocytic, there has been moderate anisocytosis and poikilocytosis, and immature red cell forms have been present, as mentioned earlier.[51] The finding of young forms, however, suggests an error in diagnosis for even in cases in which the bone marrow was shown to be hyperplastic the circulating blood often gave no sign of regeneration.

The erythrocyte count may be 2,000,000 per c.mm. or lower when the patient is first seen. At the same time there is leukopenia and thrombocytopenia. The leukocytes formed in the bone marrow are affected chiefly and thus the smear may contain as many as 70 to 90 per cent lymphocytes. The leukocyte count may, however, be as low as 1500 per c.mm. or even 150 and thus absolute lymphocytopenia is present as well. In cases in which immature erythrocytic forms have appeared in the circulating blood, occasional immature myeloid leukocytes have been observed. As mentioned earlier, reticulocytes have been found to be moderately increased (6 to 10 per cent) in some of the familial cases. In cases of "pure red cell" aplasia (p. 562), neither leukopenia nor thrombocytopenia accompanies the anemia.

The bleeding time is usually moderately prolonged and the blood clot retracts poorly when thrombocytopenia is present. Coagulation time is generally normal. The fragility of the red corpuscles is normal.

The **plasma iron** is generally increased above normal as is also the free **protoporphyrin** content of the erythrocytes. Ferrokinetic studies in a typical case were illustrated elsewhere (Fig. 3–17, p. 183). Red corpuscles tagged with Cr[51] may show a somewhat shorter survival than is normal[44] but this is not such as to be of significance.

Other laboratory findings are of a negative character. Gastric secretion is not affected significantly. No evidence of increased blood destruction is found in the blood plasma, urine, or stools.

Bone Marrow.—In cases of the classical type, the material obtained on sternal puncture consists chiefly of mature red corpuscles. The majority of the nucleated cells are lymphocytes. The latter may comprise 60 to 100 per cent of the nucleated cells. Such a finding makes it advisable to obtain a larger specimen, by biopsy, in order to be sure that one has obtained actual marrow and also to see how fatty the marrow is.

As has been stated already, however, the marrow may be normally cellular or actually hyperplastic.[13c] In such cases there may be a moderate preponderance of lymphocytes but the differential formula may not be greatly abnormal. In still other cases ("pseudo-aplastic" anemia) the findings have been quite bizarre[42c, 52a] as compared with the marrow picture of the classical disorder. Thus, in some the cytoplasm of many of the normoblasts was found to be poorly formed and contained excessive numbers of large siderotic granules, suggesting thereby impaired maturation and defective hemoglobin formation.[16e] In others, investigators have described megaloblastic-like cells or bizarre chromatin in the normoblasts, sometimes suggesting the di Guglielmo syndrome (p. 941),[52a] as well as mast cell hyperplasia. Even in such cases with hyperplastic bone marrow, however, the large preponderance of myeloblasts or of lymphoblasts which is so characteristic of acute leukemia, was not found.

Biopsy of bone marrow will be discussed under Pathology (p. 570). It is difficult to state the relative numbers of cases with aplastic, hypoplastic, normal or hyperplastic bone marrows. This depends largely on the definitions and criteria used in diagnosis and has varied greatly in different series of cases.

Diagnosis.—From the hematological standpoint, the characteristic triad is anemia, leukopenia and thrombocytopenia. However, as outlined in Table 11–1 (p. 550), the causes of pancytopenia are numerous and these must be ruled out. The finding of adenopathy or splenomegaly makes a diagnosis of primary refractory anemia very unlikely although, as mentioned earlier, slight splenic enlargement has been described in some cases. In addition to a thorough physical examination, which must include rectal examination and careful palpation of all the bones for tenderness, extensive radiographic studies may be required to rule out lesions in bones, or tumors not evident from the physical examination. The urine cannot be overlooked as it may give evidence of multiple myeloma or of renal carcinoma. If fever is present, conditions like Hodgkin's disease must be considered even though fever of slight or even moderate degree may occasionally accompany "aplastic anemia," especially the more fulminating forms. A remote possibility is miliary tuberculosis (p. 561).

The finding of immature forms of the red or white series in the circulating blood is strong evidence against "aplastic anemia," although here again exceptions have been reported. In cases in which the anemia is macrocytic rather than normocytic and in which some signs of red cell regeneration are present, real difficulty may be encountered. Pernicious anemia can be ruled out by the absence of glossitis, achlorhydria, or neural involvement, by the lack of any evidence of increased blood destruction, by the absence of true megaloblasts in the bone marrow, and, if the diagnosis is still in doubt, by the failure of appropriate therapy. Cases of macrocytic megaloblastic anemia not responding to therapy ("achrestic anemia," "refractory megaloblastic anemia") have been discussed already (p. 509). Hemolytic anemias should be excluded; for example, paroxysmal nocturnal hemoglobinuria may be mistaken for primary refractory anemia. In the latter, the leukopenia is characteristically due to neutropenia. If all types of leukocytes are reduced in number or if lymphocytes are reduced to a greater degree than the neutrophilic series, Hodgkin's disease and even disseminated lupus erythematosus must be considered.

Thorough inquiry must be made concerning possible exposure to potentially toxic agents, either at the patient's place of work or at home, in his hobbies or through medication prescribed by his physician. The number of agents which may damage the hemopoietic system is large (Table 11–3).

The absence of neutropenia and thrombocytopenia should cause one seriously to consider the presence of some underlying chronic disease, such as one of the conditions classified under the heading of simple chronic anemia or secondary refractory anemia (p. 573). One that is not rarely mistaken for primary refractory anemia is chronic renal disease because this anemia is notoriously unresponsive to therapy and the manifestations of the renal disease may be insignificant. A diagnosis of "pure red aplasia" (p. 562) must be made with caution for such cases are very rare.

The diagnosis of "aplastic anemia" or primary refractory anemia is one which is made largely by exclusion. Even when bone marrow puncture yields little marrow, the diagnosis is not certain for, in some cases of leukemia or of metastatic disease of the bone marrow, it may be very difficult to withdraw any diagnostic material. It should be pointed out that marrow puncture, even when repeated at several sites, may be misleading; we have demonstrated active marrow by surgical biopsy even when puncture repeatedly yielded very few cells. When, on the other hand, the marrow is not aplastic but cellular material is obtained, the diagnosis of primary refractory anemia is not excluded, as cases with hyperplastic marrow have been described.[52a]

The differentiation of purpura hemorrhagica (p. 816) should cause no difficulty. Although there may be considerable similarity on clinical grounds, any anemia which may be found is only proportional to the degree of blood loss. The leukocyte count should be normal or increased and signs of red cell regeneration may be found if there has been much loss of blood. Likewise "agranulocytic angina" may have to be considered on clinical grounds but in this condition anemia is slight or absent and thrombocytopenia is not found.

The estimation of red cell production by means of ferrokinetic studies (p. 182), provides data which are useful as an indication of decreased erythropoeisis, but this requires considerable time and effort and cannot be regarded as an essential diagnostic tool. Sometimes, however, it is useful to measure red cell survival with Cr^{51} and to determine whether there is excessive destruction in the spleen.

Treatment.—The treatment of refractory anemia consists in (1) discovery of the cause and prohibition of further exposure to the noxious agent; (2) supportive measures, such as blood transfusions and suitable diet; (3) management of complications such as hemorrhage and infection; and (4) consideration of measures designed to stimulate hemopoiesis and to remove possible deleterious effects produced by the spleen.

Although it is obvious that the first requirement is the avoidance of the noxious agent, this is sometimes overlooked or the cause is not recognized. It is essential that a thorough check be made as described above. Ideally, the noxious agent should be removed from the body, but this is usually not possible. However, when the toxic agent is an arsenical, BAL (British anti-lewisite) may at least be tried.

The chief mainstay in the way of supportive measures is blood transfusion. This, however, should be used in moderation. It is impractical and unnecessary to attempt to keep the patient's blood at a normal level by blood transfusion. Usually such a patient can tolerate a volume of packed red cells of, say, 30 to 35 ml. per 100 ml. very satisfactorily. Furthermore, the bone marrow failure may not be complete, in which case it may be found that blood transfusion needs to be given only occasionally in order to maintain the patient in a reasonable state of activity. It is essential that a practical routine be adopted since, with successful management, the patient may be maintained for many years by transfusion alone. In such individuals the ultimate, possible development of hemosiderosis from iron derived from the transfused red corpuscles, as well as the risks of transfusion, especially serum hepatitis, must be kept in mind and therefore the number of transfusions should be kept to a minimum.

The general measures as to rest and diet outlined in Chapter 9 should be followed. As in any chronic disorder, activity should be permitted in accordance with the patient's tolerance. Nothing is gained, in general, from the use of liver extracts, pentnucleotide, folic acid or other vitamins, notwithstanding the interesting report of the successful use of riboflavin in a case of erythrocytic hypoplasia.[22a] Exposure to infections should be avoided, if possible, and prompt antibiotic therapy must be instituted when they develop. There is no good evidence that a person sensitive to the deleterious action of one drug is likely to respond unfavorably to another but drugs should be used with due consideration of the potential risks as well as the gains. However, "prophylactic" antibiotic therapy for the purpose of protecting patients with low leukocyte counts against possible infections is not only unwise; it is unnecessary and, in fact, dangerous since it exposes the patient to fulminating "super-infections" which antibiotic therapy may not be capable of controlling.

When hemorrhage is a problem, blood freshly collected in plastic bags (p. 356) with the object of preserving the platelets is sometimes helpful. Where menorrhagia has been very troublesome, hysterectomy has sometimes been used to advantage.[56]

Of the measures employed to improve marrow function, only cobalt, testosterone and corticosteroids need be considered. *Cobalt* (p. 142) was credited with the recovery of two patients with "pure-red cell aplasia"[22] and was associated with improvement in one case of pancytopenia with a cellular marrow.[50e] In other cases, the use of cobalt met with failure.[48] The oral administration of testosterone proprionate or methyltestosterone in daily doses of 1 or 2 mg./Kg. body weight, together with corticosteroids (8 to 20 mg. triamcinolone) was reported

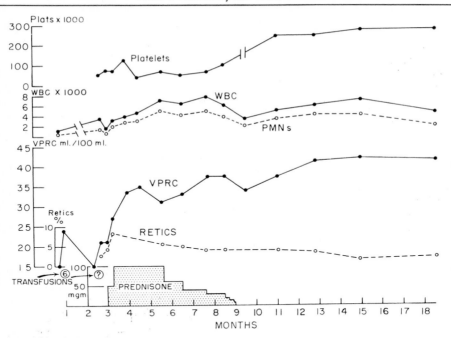

FIG. 11–4.—Blood changes associated with steroid therapy in a case of aplastic anemia secondary to chronic benzene exposure. A modest reticulocytosis and increase in the absolute polymorphonuclear neutrophil count without significant improvement in platelets was observed during prednisone therapy. Transfusions became unnecessary when steroids were administered. (Scott, Cartwright and Wintrobe, courtesy of Medicine[48].)

to produce a sustained remission in nine of 17 children with acquired aplastic anemia treated for periods ranging from two and a half to 15 months, and in six of seven children with congenital pancytopenia (p. 561). In the latter, unlike the former, withdrawal of medication resulted in abrupt relapse.[48b] The use of *corticosteroids* alone has not been very encouraging but, in several cases in our own series a moderate reticulocytosis coincided with such therapy.[48] One no longer required blood transfusion (Fig. 11–4) whereas the need for them was reduced in others. An absolute increase in neutrophils may accompany the erythrocyte response but no significant improvement in platelets has been noted in any of our cases. In our experience improvement, if it will occur at all following corticosteroid therapy, is likely to take place within four or five weeks.

Trial of *splenectomy* has been proposed on two grounds: (1) removal of an inhibitory effect on hemopoiesis; (2) removal of a site where red cells are destroyed. Our own clinical experience,[48] and that of others,[29,39d] has been that the operation is helpful in some cases (Fig. 11-5). It must be admitted, however, that a critical evaluation of the reported results of splenectomy, including our own, did not yield conclusive evidence of benefit from the operation.[48] The selection of cases for operation, the duration of the disease prior to operation and its severity are factors which can prejudice the statistical comparison. The cases which seemed to have benefited might have recovered spontaneously. Further study is required. If shortened red cell survival can be demonstrated and if the spleen appears to be related to this, as judged by isotope studies (p. 630), the operation deserves serious consideration. In many instances, unfortunately, such a positive indication is lacking. In general we have favored splenectomy

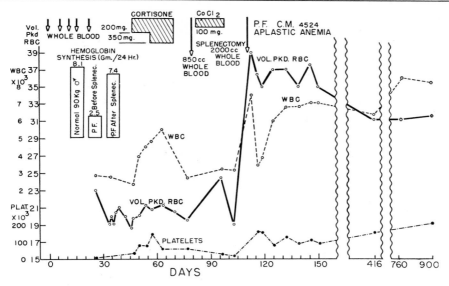

Fig. 11–5.—Effect of splenectomy in a patient with pancytopenia and bone marrow hypoplasia, even on trephine biopsy. Repeated blood transfusions, cortisone administration and cobalt therapy failed to maintain the blood at a level compatible with reasonable activity. Following splenectomy, hemoglobin production as measured by iron turnover rate increased to an almost normal level, the bone marrow appeared to be more cellular and the volume of packed red cells has been maintained for over four years without blood transfusions or other therapy at twice the former level, permitting return to work.

when the condition has been chronic, other measures have failed and no evidence of spontaneous recovery has been apparent, and where it appeared that the operation might reduce the need for, or at least the number and frequency of transfusions. It has been suggested that splenectomy is more likely to be helpful if the bone marrow is not completely aplastic and when the administration of corticosteroids has been associated with some evidence of response.[39d] A return to normal blood levels is unusual, although this occurred in two of our cases. More often a somewhat higher blood level is maintained by the patient than was possible before the operation and this may be such that transfusions are no longer required. The platelets are the slowest of all the corpuscles to increase in number.

The demonstration that lethally radiated rodents can be protected by *injections of bone marrow* has led to considerable interest in the application of these findings to the treatment of marrow depletion in man. This topic will be discussed in some detail later (p. 967). It may be pointed out here, however, that there is as yet no clearly demonstrated instance of successful transplantation of bone marrow in human subjects. Whether or not it will be possible to duplicate the animal experiments in man remains to be seen. The technic is fraught with many difficulties and is under careful study in several centers. The indiscriminate injection of bone marrow in the treatment of aplastic anemia, leukemia and other disorders by physicians outside of the few centers where this procedure is under investigation is to be deplored. The prognosis of primary refractory anemia is by no means always bad and consequently does not justify injudicious attempts and experimentation with human life.

Prognosis.—An adequate discussion of prognosis in a complexity of disorders such as fall under the heading of primary refractory anemia is not possible. Only some general remarks can be made. In

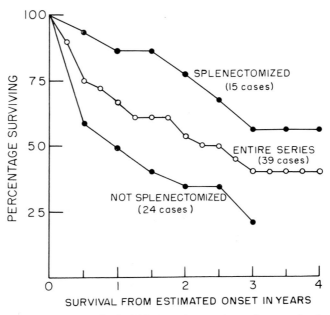

FIG. 11–6.—Percentage survival of 39 cases from estimated onset of aplastic anemia.
(Scott, Cartwright and Wintrobe, courtesy of Medicine[48]).

the classical idiopathic form of aplastic anemia, the course is progressively, inexorably, and more or less rapidly fatal in spite of blood transfusions. Death ensues in the course of a few weeks or life may linger as long as six months. Fortunately, this does not represent the outcome in all cases. There are reports of spontaneous partial or complete recovery in cases of aplastic anemia due to organic arsenicals,[14] gold,[56] benzene[28] and, in our own experience, Mesantoin.® Spontaneous remissions were not uncommon in the cases with partly mature, cellular marrow which Bomford and Rhoads[13c] described. Of our series of 39 cases,[48] 17 were living at the time of the last follow-up. More than half the cases had died as the result of recurrent or resistant infections and repeated bleeding, following a course of steady deterioration. Almost a third recovered to a sufficient degree that medical care was no longer required. The role of therapy in bringing about improvement has been discussed already. Hematological re-

covery was very gradual. Of the entire group (Fig. 11–6), 50 per cent lived for two and a half years and 40 per cent survived four years or longer.

It cannot be said that prognosis is better if the cause is known or suspected. Even if exposure to the offending agent ceases, sufficient damage may have been done already to lead to death. In our experience the outcome in cases associated with chloramphenicol has been especially bad. The severity of the anemia is not necessarily an index of prognosis. It is the writer's impression that improvement is more likely to occur when the anemia is macrocytic, for this is probably an indication of some regenerative capacity. Others have made similar observations.[13c] There is greater hope in those cases in which the marrow is cellular or hypercellular than where it is devoid of cells.

Pathology.—In typical cases only yellowish-white fatty material consisting chiefly of fat, fibrous tissue and lymphocytes is seen in the *marrow* cavities

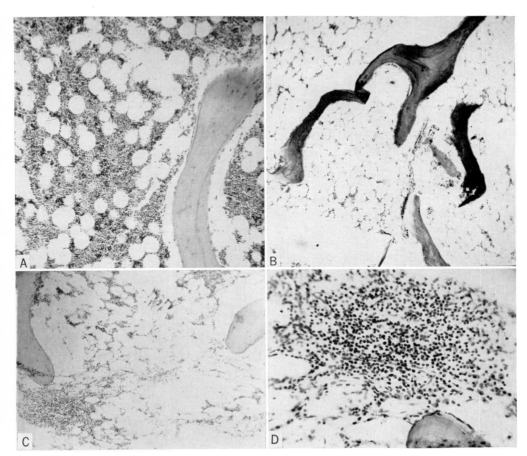

FIG. 11–7.—Sections of bone marrow from cases of aplastic anemia compared with the normal findings.

A, Normal sternal marrow. Note the presence of disseminated erythropoietic foci (small hyperchromatic cells) and several scattered megakaryocytes (large cells with abundant cytoplasm).

B, Marked hypoplasia. Small foci of sparse cellularity, composed of lymphoid or erythropoietic elements, are observed.

C, Moderate hypoplasia. An over-all reduction in cellularity is apparent; the degree of cellular pleomorphism seen in this photograph represents the presence in reduced numbers of both myeloid and erythroid elements in various stages of maturation. A focus of small lymphocytes is present.

D, Higher magnification of the lymphoid follicle present in *C*. Small lymphocytes predominate. The larger cells with more abundant cytoplasm are primitive reticular elements. (Scott, Cartwright and Wintrobe, courtesy of *Medicine*[48].)

(Fig. 11–7). Marrow which is red macroscopically may be found to be composed largely of extravasated blood and to give little evidence of regeneration. However, as already stated, the marrow may be normally cellular or actually hyperplastic. Hyperplasia has been found to be much more common than aplasia in cases of benzol poisoning.[15] In cases resulting from "internal irradiation," bone marrow hyperplasia is the rule rather than the exception. The development of jaw necroses, osteitis and osteogenic sarcoma in these cases has been mentioned.

Atrophy and aplasia may involve lymphoid as well as myeloid tissue. The spleen not infrequently is fibrous, the malpighian corpuscles small and the cells of the pulp scanty. Yet in some cases foci of extramedullary blood formation have been observed in the spleen and liver[15] and such foci have also been produced experimentally[48a] with benzene.

Pathogenesis. — The Fanconi syndrome appears to be due to the inheritance of a recessive gene. There is no evidence that the other disorders included among the primary refractory anemias are genetic in character, although it is noteworthy that congenital hypoplastic anemia of infancy (p. 765) may be due to a metabolic fault. One might speculate about the role of thymoma in the etiology of the cases in which this tumor was demonstrated but there is little to suggest that the remainder of the conditions which come under this heading are related to an abnormality in the victims themselves, except for one fact. Whereas some agents can be counted upon to damage the hemopoietic tissues, it is abundantly evident that only a very small proportion of those persons who are exposed to certain other agents which have been associated with the development of "aplastic anemia" suffer any demonstrable ill effects. This raises the possibility that an underlying abnormality in a detoxifying mechanism, autoimmune factors[24] or deficiency of some factor essential for the sustenance or stimulation of hematopoiesis, is the primary defect.

The studies of Rhoads and his coworkers[11a,13c,18] revealed evidence of hepatic dysfunction and of disturbed pigment metabolism in cases of refractory anemia. In several of their cases disturbances were found in the excretion of glucuronates and sulphates, substances which represent the inactivated forms of aromatic hydrocarbons. Exposure to the latter has been noted frequently in cases of aplastic anemia. These observations led to the suggestion that this disorder is due to a failure of the normal biochemical mechanisms of detoxification. It was postulated that such failure might permit hemolytic substances to circulate and these, in turn, might cause either hemolysis and hyperplastic marrow, or destruction of both circulating and developing cells, thus producing hypoplasia. Unfortunately these and other possibilities are purely speculative since such evidence as has been offered in their support, so far, is unconvincing.[48]

Since an etiologic agent is suspected in some cases of acquired primary refractory anemia, it is tempting to assume that this is the case in all instances of "idiopathic aplastic anemia," the cause being simply undisclosed. It is noteworthy that, in spite of the increasing number of agents which reasonably can be suspected to be of etiologic importance, the majority of cases remain idiopathic. In several recent series, 49, 57 and 44 per cent, respectively, were thus characterized.[48]

It is quite possible, although the opposite may be equally true, that the range of variation in the bone marrow picture which has been described, from total aplasia to hyperplasia, represents a single entity rather than a number of different ones. Benzene poisoning has been found, in experimental investigations, to be capable of producing such a range of changes in the bone marrow, and leukemia as well.[15] It is conceivable that other agents may similarly produce a variety of effects, according to the influence of different factors, such as dose, length and route of exposure, detoxifying capacities of the host and his nutritional status. There is, in fact, evidence of such variations, for many of the agents considered as being capable of causing aplastic anemia are known also to produce thrombocytopenia without anemia or leukopenia, granulocytopenia without damaging the leukopoietic or erythropoietic apparatus, or even hemolytic anemia.

SIMPLE CHRONIC ANEMIA

Definition.—The anemia associated with the majority of infections and chronic systemic diseases may be called "simple," because there is no very radical alteration from the normal blood picture, and "chronic" because it is usually insidious in its inception and frequently slow in repair. The term "secondary anemia" is avoided, because all anemias are essentially "secondary," and because such a designation was originally used to include all types of anemia other than pernicious anemia.

This is perhaps the most common of the various types of anemia. Because the causes are numerous and yet the hematological manifestations have a great deal in common, the clinical features will be considered first and etiology will be discussed later, together with pathogenesis.

Symptomatology.—Often the manifestations of the underlying disorder overshadow those of the anemia. Not infrequently, however, the only symptoms and signs are those common to anemia (p. 433) and the reduction in the hemoglobin level is the first objective evidence of disease which is discovered. This may be the case when the cause of the anemia is malignancy, chronic or subacute infection (*e.g.* subacute bacterial endocarditis), an endocrine disorder such as hypothyroidism or Addison's disease, or chronic renal disease. Other than pallor and the physical signs of the causative disorder, the clinical manifestations are few. Thus, icterus, adenopathy, bone tenderness and splenomegaly are absent, unless they form part of the clinical manifestations of the underlying condition.

Blood Changes.—Frequently the reduction in the number of red corpuscles, quantity of hemoglobin, and volume of packed red cells are equal in degree. The anemia, therefore, is normocytic.

In some instances the decrease in hemoglobin and packed red cells is greater than the decrease in number of corpuscles, so that there is microcytosis without hypochromia ("simple microcytic anemia," p. 432). The anemia is rarely severe. In our cases the red cell counts averaged 3,880,000, although they ranged from 4,790,000 to 2,000,000. The values for hemoglobin and volume of packed red cells were as low as 5 Gm. and 18 ml., respectively, in cases with the most marked grades of anemia, but were usually 9 to 12 Gm. and 25 to 36 ml. per 100 ml. blood, respectively. Values for the corpuscular constants ranged from 70 to 93 c.μ for mean corpuscular volume, 22 to 35 $\gamma\gamma$ for mean corpuscular hemoglobin and 30 to 38 per cent for mean corpuscular hemoglobin concentration. The most severe cases of anemia were found in association with renal dysfunction. When there is nitrogen retention the anemia may be extreme, with hemoglobin levels even as low as 4 or 5 Gm. Then the anemia may be somewhat macrocytic. However, such cases are unusual and the findings in a series of cases of anemia of infection (Fig. 11–8) are more typical of the group as a whole.

There is anisocytosis of moderate degree but poikilocytosis is slight. Few other changes in the red corpuscles are observed as a rule. Evidence of attempted regeneration, in the form of polychromatophilia or nucleated red cells, is conspicuous by its absence. Generally reticulocytes are normal or even reduced in number[66] but sometimes they may be increased.[86] When the anemia is very great, as in severe chronic renal disease, polychromatophilia may be observed and even nucleated red cells may be seen in the blood smear.

In spite of the fact that the survival of the erythrocytes can be shown in some cases to be moderately shortened (p. 557), the usual evidences of increased

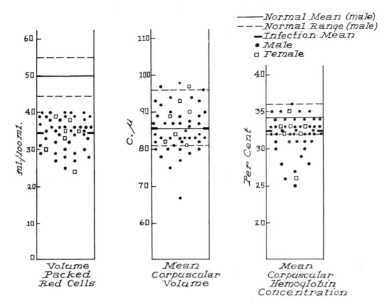

Fig. 11–8.—Degree and type of anemia, as indicated by the volume of packed red cells, the mean corpuscular volume and the mean corpuscular hemoglobin concentration in 50 patients with anemia of infection (Cartwright and Wintrobe, courtesy of Year Book Publishers, Inc.[66a]).

blood destruction, such as increased serum bilirubin and increased urobilinogen excretion, characteristically are absent.[66,86] Total blood volume was found to be reduced below normal in some cases of anemia of infection[66a] whereas in other instances of simple chronic anemia an increase in plasma volume has been noted. Such observations would imply that the hemoglobin or hematocrit may not indicate the true degree of alteration in total hemoglobin. As a rule, however, these have been found to give a satisfactory indication of the degree of anemia.

The leukocytic picture depends on the nature of the causative disorder (see Chapter 4). The platelets are normal in number and function.

Bone Marrow.—Although more thorough investigation is desirable, the available observations[66,86] indicate that there is no hypoplasia of the bone marrow in this type of anemia. In *chronic infection* with anemia there is often found well defined hyperplasia of the leukocytic elements. The erythroid series is plentiful and some observers have reported a qualitative shift to the younger forms, suggesting a red cell maturation arrest.[66a,86] In cases of anemia associated with *renal insufficiency* a decrease in the ratio of nucleated red cells to leukocytes is often seen[80] but this is due to leukocytic and megakaryocytic hyperplasia rather than to a reduction in normoblasts.[65b] Only when the non-protein-nitrogen level was over 150 mg. per cent was definite evidence of quantitative and qualitative hypoplasia of the erythroid tissue observed and in no instance was aplasia found. In addition to a varying degree of "shift to the left" in the myeloid series of leukocytes, an increased number of histiocytes and plasma cells, phagocytic cells and eosinophils are found and there frequently is karyorrhexis of the normoblastic nuclei.[65b]

The bone marrow in the "physiologic anemia" of pregnancy gives no evidence of alteration from the normal in the erythroid series while the leukocytic picture indicates hyperplasia.[96b] The latter is especially marked in the late months of pregnancy, when megakaryocytic hyperplasia may also be found.

Diagnosis.—When the manifestations of the primary condition are not such as to attract attention, errors in diagnosis are common. Here above all it is important to bear in mind that anemia is a *symptom* of disease, not a disease in itself and that its discovery calls for thorough study. Often a careful history and physical examination will yield clues concerning the underlying disorder; for example, a history of weight loss or impaired appetite or of fever, an elevated blood pressure, hemorrhages or other changes in the fundi, cardiac murmurs not attributable to the anemia, a palpable mass in the abdomen or other symptoms or signs too numerous to list. Hypochromic microcytic and macrocytic anemias must be differentiated not only by calculation of the mean red cell size and hemoglobin concentration but also by examination of the blood smear. The leukocytes and platelets must also receive attention since these should be normal in simple chronic anemia unless leukocytosis or, rarely, leukopenia is characteristic of the causative condition. Since this type of anemia is refractory to vitamin B_{12} or iron therapy, it can be designated as refractory but the primary refractory anemias (p. 551) should not be confused with the secondary form. The serum bilirubin and 2-hour urinary urobilinogen test will serve to exclude most instances of hemolytic anemia.

Treatment.—The correction of the anemia lies in the relief of the primary disorder. Blood transfusion may be useful as a temporary measure but the anemia is rarely so severe as to justify the expense, risks and discomforts of transfusion. General measures, as outlined in Chapter 9, should be employed. These include a good, well-balanced diet containing foods of high protein and vitamin content, rest, sometimes alternated with moderate exercise, fresh air and sunshine. Liver extracts, vitamin B_{12} and folic acid are of no value and even iron is of little use. The impaired absorption of iron and the inhibitory effect of inflammation on erythropoiesis were shown to be counteracted by the administration of cobalt in experimental studies.[96a] The oral administration of 300 mg. cobaltous chloride per day was found to have a similar effect in some patients with anemia associated with chronic infections[60] and smaller amounts (100 to 150 mg.) produced increased erythropoiesis in patients with anemia due to renal disease.[70] However, this effect disappeared when the drug was discontinued and, furthermore, has not been observed in all cases. Since the administration of this agent may cause loss of appetite or other gastrointestinal symptoms and the benefits derived, if any, are uncertain, its use cannot be recommended. The rôle of cobalt in hemopoiesis has been discussed already (p. 141).

Prognosis.—This depends on the seriousness of the causative factor. Severe anemia in cases of renal disease is usually a very grave sign. The "physiological anemia" of pregnancy disappears spontaneously after parturition.

Etiology and Pathogenesis.—The claim that anemia of purely *climatic* origin may occur in otherwise healthy persons residing in tropical and semitropical countries has never been confirmed.[95] The most common form of **anemia in pregnancy,** however, has often been considered to be "physiological." Thus, in one large series,[57] in 88 per cent of the women moderate, normocytic anemia was observed. A reduction in blood values below the normal level has been noted by the eighth week of pregnancy.[74] In these subjects, the decrease continued progressively until the 16th to the 22nd week, when the values became stationary at levels of 11 Gm. hemoglobin, 32 to 34 ml. packed red cells and 3.5 to 3.75 million red corpuscles per c.mm. Frequently, a temporary decrease in the severity of the anemia occurred about the 32nd to 34th week. In the puerperium the red cell count and volume of packed red cells increased rapidly but the hemoglobin often rose slowly. Others have made similar observations.[76,96b]

This anemia has been regarded as not being a true anemia since a progressive increase in plasma volume occurs during pregnancy.[60a] Measurements of red cell mass have shown that only a moderate decrease (200 ml.) occurs during the first two months of pregnancy, which is followed by an increase to a peak approximately 270 ml. above normal in the ninth month. In the last month before delivery a decrease occurs, which becomes more marked during delivery and immediately postpartum to reach a level about 200 ml. below normal. The ante- and postpartum changes are accompanied by alterations in plasma volume which exaggerate the "anemia." The total blood volume is adjusted promptly to normal values postpartum but the return of red cell mass to normal levels is slow.

Nevertheless, there are good reasons to believe that the "physiologic" anemia of pregnancy is in part due to iron deficiency. Measurements of serum iron in pregnancy have shown a decrease in the latter part of pregancy together with an increase in iron-binding capacity,[69,93] as occurs in iron deficiency anemia. It is noteworthy that, in pregnant Bantu women, whose diet is habitually high in iron, no significant change in serum iron was observed and no anemia developed.[70a]

In some pregnant women a clearly defined hypochromic microcytic anemia, due to iron deficiency, is observed (p. 734). In this country a reduction in hemoglobin below 10 Gm. per 100 ml. is most often due to this cause.[60b] Sometimes other factors, such as infection and toxemia or protein deficiency play an important part. Macrocytic anemia of pregnancy (p. 511) is rare except where nutritional deficiency and other factors play a role, as in India.

Ferrokinetic studies in pregnancy were reported as indicating decreased plasma and red cell iron turnover rates, reduced uptake of iron in the bone marrow and retarded utilization of iron for hemoglobin synthesis. Other studies, however, showed the reverse; that is, they gave evidence of accelerated rather than retarded erythropoiesis.[82a] It would appear that, under normal circumstances, no important changes take place.

Anemia Associated with Inflammation.—Simple chronic anemia develops in a large variety of subacute and chronic inflammatory conditions and, less often, in acute cases. Only certain infections are associated with hemolytic anemia and this is rare (p. 606). In *rheumatoid arthritis* anemia is common. Sometimes it is accompanied by leukopenia and splenomegaly (p. 1056). In *rheumatic fever* moderate and sometimes severe anemia develops in association with an exacerbation and decreases as the symptoms subside.[71] Anemia is found in two-thirds of cases of *subacute bacterial endocarditis* and in 25 per cent it becomes severe.[78] In *brucellosis* mild anemia occurs.[66] Anemia of moderate severity occurs frequently in *H. influenzae*[87] meningitis but is unusual in meningitis due to the meningococcus. In *tuberculosis* a mild anemia is not uncommon but severe anemia is unusual,[63] except in cases of intestinal involvement with strictures and in the miliary form.[69a] In the last, pancytopenia may develop (p. 561). Moderate anemia may occur in tertiary *syphilis* and severe anemia may be found in the congenital form but otherwise anemia is rare.[85,90] There is no evidence that focal infections produce anemia.

The degree of anemia which is found

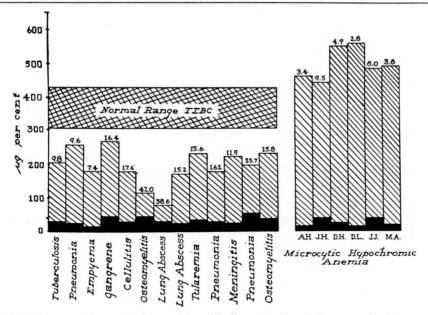

FIG. 11–9.—The serum iron and the total iron-binding capacity of the serum in 13 cases of anemia
associated with infection as compared with the normal and with six cases of iron deficiency anemia.

Solid areas represent serum iron.   Hatched areas represent the unsaturated iron-binding capacity.
The total height of each column represents the total iron-binding capacity of the serum.   The figures
above the columns represent the per cent saturation (SI/TIBC).   (Cartwright and Wintrobe, courtesy
of J. Clin. Invest.)

in association with inflammatory diseases
and its time of appearance vary.   Anemia
tends to be greater in degree in the more
serious and in suppurative infections.
Thus, moderate anemia usually is found
in association with pelvic inflammatory
disease, infections of the genitourinary
tract and bronchiectasis and more severe
anemia is found in osteomyelitis and in
pulmonary abscess.   There is some evidence that the greater the number of
different organisms in a wound, the more
severe the anemia.   There is no clear
evidence that a particular location is
more likely to produce severe anemia
than another.   In most instances, infections of less than a month's duration are
not accompanied by significant anemia.
There is no direct correlation, however,
between duration of infection and severity
of anemia; in general, anemia gradually
progresses while the infection persists but
after a time the degree of anemia becomes
relatively constant.   There are excep-

tions to this pattern, of course.   Sometimes anemia may develop very rapidly
and may continue to progress to become
very severe; this is especially true in
septicemias and in overwhelming sepsis.
Whether in these exceptional instances
the pathogenesis of the anemia is the
same as in the usual cases, is uncertain
but it is plausible to assume that they
represent only an exaggeration of the
disturbances which produce the less
severe anemias of infection.

It seems most likely that the anemia of
infection is the resultant of impaired
erythropoiesis and shortened survival of
the red corpuscles.[66a, 73a]   It is well known
that profound metabolic alterations accompany infection and these have now
been shown to include alterations in iron,
copper and porphyrin metabolism.   The
plasma iron content is markedly lowered,
the serum iron binding capacity is reduced (Fig. 11–9) and iron administered
parenterally is rapidly shunted to the

37

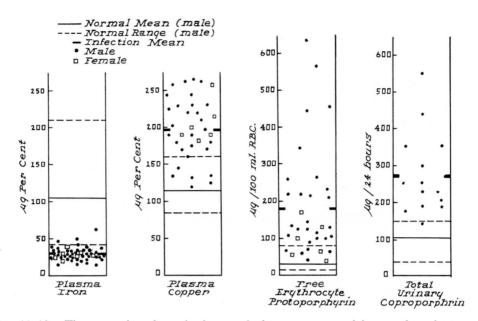

Fig. 11–10.—The severe hypoferremia, increased plasma copper and increased erythrocyte protoporphyrin and urinary coproporphyrin in anemia associated with infection as indicated by a study of 50 cases. (Cartwright and Wintrobe, courtesy of Year Book Publishers, Inc.[66a])

tissues, without influencing the plasma iron level more than temporarily and without relieving the anemia. The serum copper is elevated, the erythrocyte protoporphyrin is increased and the excretion of coproporphyrin is increased (Fig. 11–10). The hypoferremia may develop within forty-eight hours of the onset of infection while the other changes take place more gradually. These abnormalities can be produced experimentally by means of bacterial or sterile abscesses and disappear when the inflammatory process is resolved. Experimental observations also indicate that there is diminished reutilization of iron from senescent, nonviable erythrocytes and that the release of iron from the tissues to the plasma transferrin pool is impaired.[69b] In experimental animals, as well as in man, the incorporation of iron into newly formed erythrocytes is delayed and decreased as compared with the normal.

That there is impaired erythropoiesis is also indicated by the lack of signs of blood regeneration, such as reticulocytosis, and by the failure to respond adequately to the need for a greater rate of erythropoiesis. Although the usual evidences of increased blood destruction, such as increased urobilinogen excretion and elevated serum bilirubin concentration, are lacking in the anemia of infection,[66a] most studies of erythrocyte survival in infection indicate that the erythrocyte life span is shortened. In a group of cases studied in our own laboratory,[65a] this amounted to only 27 per cent, however, a degree of acceleration of destruction which could be easily met by increased erythropoiesis if the bone marrow functional capacity were not impaired. The inhibiting effect of infection on erythropoiesis can be observed in pernicious anemia when an intercurrent infection develops during a hemopoietic response; the rate of blood regeneration slows up and is not restored to normal until the infection has disappeared. A similar inhibitory effect has been demonstrated very clearly in pyridoxine deficient swine in which abscesses were produced[96a] and was shown a number of years ago by Whipple and his co-workers.[83]

The nature of the disturbance in hemoglobin production is not clear but the profound alterations in iron and porphyrin metabolism which have been described above have been interpreted as indicating that there is a quantitative defect in the rate of conversion of proto-porphyrin to hemoglobin.[66]

Observations in *rheumatoid arthritis* have been somewhat contradictory. One investigator observed impairment of erythropoiesis in five out of 18 cases[94] but others reported unimpaired utilization of plasma iron for erythrocyte production in all of their 42 cases.[69c] The latter found that the rate of red cell destruction was increased and that this resulted primarily from a greater random destruction of the red cells. The patients' cells survived normally in a normal individual. Most investigators agree that in rheumatoid arthritis, as in the anemia of infection, anemia results because erythropoiesis fails to increase sufficiently to compensate for a shortened red cell survival.[69c,94] Others, however, were unable to demonstrate an abnormality in erythrocyte survival.[74b]

Renal Insufficiency.—Anemia is observed in most types of renal insufficiency, whether this be due to acute or chronic glomerulonephritis, chronic pyelonephritis, congenital polycystic kidneys or chronic prostatic obstruction, but it is not found in nephrosis or when there is acute suppression of urine. The anemia may be relatively stable or only slowly progressive or it may increase in severity rapidly. Reticulocytes may or may not be increased in number.[65b,72b] Serum iron and free erythrocyte porphyrin values follow no consistent pattern.[66a,75] As noted earlier (p. 574) erythropoiesis in the bone marrow may appear to be normal.

Study of this anemia has been hampered by difficulties in measuring plasma volume in the presence of edema and also because of the alterations in blood volume which myocardial failure may produce. All workers are agreed, however, that erythropoiesis is depressed.[75] Two patterns have been described;[92] namely, one in which the arrest of erythropoiesis is almost complete and rapid falls in red cell mass occur. This was seen in early, type 1 nephritis and in terminal nephritis. In neither condition was there an obvious relationship to the degree of uremia. In the second group, moderate or considerable depression of red cell volume was present and persisted over long periods. Here the anemia appeared to be related to the degree of uremia. This pattern was found in slowly progressive nephritis. It has been stated that severe anemia can be expected when the creatinine rises above 2 mg. per cent and the blood urea nitrogen becomes greater than 70 mg. per cent.[62]

A number of investigators have demonstrated decreased red cell survival.[75] This does not seem to be related to any particular variety of Bright's disease, although a relation to the presence of malignant hypertension has been postulated.[92] Evidence from cross-transfusion experiments indicates that here, as in rheumatoid arthritis, an extracorpuscular factor is responsible for the hemolysis. No evidence of an autoimmune mechanism has been found. Neither is there a clear correlation with any of the recognized products which are retained in renal insufficiency.[62,91] Nevertheless, the observation that hemolytic anemia can be produced in rabbits by bilateral nephrectomy[79a] suggests that the accumulation of some metabolite may be directly responsible. In these studies alterations in red cell metabolism were demonstrated. The relation of the observations concerning the production of erythropoietic serum factor in the kidney (p. 51) to the anemia of renal disease is obscure.[79b]

Malignancy. — Malignancy, *per se*, does not necessarily cause anemia but through its effect on the appetite and, especially if it occurs in the alimentary tract, as the result of interference with gastrointestinal digestion and absorption, or because of blood loss, anemia may become severe. If chronic loss of blood is sufficient in amount, hypochromic microcytic anemia will result. Otherwise normocytic anemia will be found. In rare instances macrocytic anemia may occur,[79] in which case it may be due to nutritional deficiency, failure to secrete "intrinsic factor" (p. 514) or hepatic insufficiency.[80a] When metastases occur and the bone marrow is involved, myelophthisic anemia may develop (p. 587), but metastases may exist without anemia being present.

It is becoming clear that in many instances of anemia associated with advanced neoplastic disease a hemolytic factor is concerned, for the life span of transfused red cells has been shown to be shortened significantly.[71a, 78a, 88a] Measurements of red cell production rate have yielded normal or increased values.[78a] Nevertheless, as in the anemias of infection, arthritis and renal disease, the bone marrow fails to compensate fully for the increased rate of cell destruction, whether the latter is mild or severe, and anemia results. It has been shown repeatedly that this failure cannot be explained by metastases into the bone marrow.[82]

In animal studies, sterile, cell-free extracts of the viable portions of malignant tumors have been found capable of hemolyzing red cells.[88b] It has also been shown that *in vivo* irradiation of normal or carcinomatous tissue can initiate a hemolytic mechanism.[88a] Such observations have led to the suggestion that hemolysins elaborated by the tumor may contribute to the anemia in cancer.

Other studies suggest that vascular injury may be a factor in the pathogenesis of the erythrocyte destruction.[82] According to this hypothesis, red cells are destroyed as the result of leakage into the tumor. Unfortunately, this does not easily explain all the manifestations of the anemia of malignant disease. According to still another study,[70b] malignant cells produce autoantibodies which can be detected by a modified antiglobulin test. Clearly, further investigation is indicated.

The anemia in *leukemia* and in *Hodgkin's disease* and other lymphomas is also of the simple chronic variety, as a rule. It is noteworthy that, when these disorders are treated effectively, the anemia clears spontaneously (pp. 960 and 1034).

In *chronic hepatic disorders* of various types, normocytic and simple microcytic anemia were observed in a third of 132 cases studied by the writer.[96] The pathogenesis of anemia in chronic liver disease has been discussed already (p. 516). In some cases an extracorpuscular hemolytic process may produce normocytic or macrocytic anemia.[72a] A syndrome of hemolysis, fatty liver and hyperlipemia occurring in acute alcoholism may present a difficult diagnostic problem.[96c]

Vitamin Deficiencies.—The role of various vitamins in blood formation was discussed in Chapter 3 (p. 130). The role of nutritional deficiency in the production of macrocytic anemia was discussed in the preceding chapter (p. 508) and hypochromic anemia resulting from iron deficiency will be described shortly (p. 731). Normocytic anemia is observed in many cases of pellagra (p. 509) and may be seen in *kwashiorkor*, but it is difficult to assess the role of protein deficiency in this condition.[57a] Other deficiencies may be associated and megaloblastic or hypochromic microcytic anemia may be found. When these are absent, severe anemia is unusual. The sudden development of "aplastic crises" has been reported.[73b] Normocytic anemia has been observed in *scurvy* (p. 138) and also in *vitamin D intoxication*.[86a] In the latter, the anemia was thought to be due to associated azotemia, although a direct toxic effect on the bone marrow could not be excluded.

Gastrointestinal Disorders. — Faulty absorption is no doubt an important factor in the development of anemia in *chronic dysentery*.[73] This may also be the cause of anemia associated with *biliary fistulae*.[59] Anemia in *chronic pancreatic disease* has been described,[65,67] but requires further study.

Parasite Infestation. — Infestation by parasites, with certain exceptions to be mentioned, does not cause anemia unless nutrition is impaired, blood is lost, or certain organs are invaded. Thus, no evidence was found that trichuris infestation produced anemia.[81] Anemia is found in hookworm infestation, probably as the result of chronic blood loss (p. 739). When anemia is encountered in amebiasis, nutritional disturbance, blood loss, or secondary infection are usually present. The relationship of the fish tapeworm, Diphyllobothrium latum, to macrocytic anemia has been fully considered (p. 517). In Schistosomiasis mansoni, there may be hypochromic microcytic anemia in the intestinal phase, or macrocytic anemia when cirrhosis of the liver develops.[84] The anemia in malaria is hemolytic (p. 606).

Endocrine Disorders.—The anemia of *hypothyroidism* has been discussed (p. 519). It may be normocytic, macrocytic, or hypochromic microcytic but is usually slight in degree. In *Addison's disease*, normocytic anemia of moderate or slight degree is usually found.[58] The true degree of anemia is difficult to estimate because of the markedly contracted blood volume which occurs in untreated Addison's disease.

Following destruction of the *anterior lobe of the pituitary*, as in Simmonds' disease, after a varying interval of time anemia develops and may be moderately severe.[67a] Leukopenia is common and eosinophilia may occur. Aplastic anemia has been described.[61a] The influence of adrenocorticotropic hormone on this anemia has not been clearly demonstrated.[89a] In a few instances, including a case of our own, the administration of "end-organ" hormones, and especially of testosterone, has been associated with relief of the anemia.[67a] A syndrome characterized by hypogonadism, alopecia, achlorhydria and sometimes subacute combined degeneration of the cord, was described[89] in which pituitary disease was associated with anemia, in certain instances macrocytic and responding to liver therapy. It was suggested that there is a hormonal element or mechanism which can lead to the degeneration of the cells which secrete "intrinsic factor." Normocytic anemia was described in women showing signs of hypothyroidism, pituitary failure and hypogonadism.[88] A slight to moderate reduction in erythrocytes and hemoglobin has been found in eunuchoid men.[67a] Such observations, together with the experimental evidence already described (p. 48), support the view that a number of the endocrine organs exert a controlling influence over the hematopoietic system. What relation there is, if any, between such regulatory effects and the signs of endocrine deficiency which may be observed in patients with different forms of anemia, such as sprue and idiopathic steatorrhea (p. 500) and sickle cell anemia (p. 672), is not clear.

Anemia in animals *following nerve resection* has been shown to be due to blood loss as the result of autocannibalism.[61]

MYELOFIBROSIS

Definition and Synonyms.—Also known as myelosclerosis or osteopathia condensans disseminata, this disorder is characterized by an irregular increase of fibrous or bony tissue in the bone marrow, a variety of changes in the blood, splenomegaly and a very slow course.

Etiology.—Occurring most commonly in the later years of life, myelofibrosis has been confused with malignancy, myelocytic leukemia,[104,112,114] and even polycythemia vera and cases have been described under such titles as erythroleukemia, aleukemic leukemia, leukemia with osteosclerosis, leuko-erythroblastosis, megakaryocytic myelosis, and osteosclerotic anemia.[98] Similar but localized changes in bones[110] have been observed in cancer metastases, osteitis associated with absorption of radioactive substances (p. 560), and phosphorus poisoning and have been produced in animals by strontium feeding[98] and by intravenous injection.

Possibly belonging in the same category are cases which have been reported under a confusing array of titles. Under the name of *"aleukemic megakaryocytic myelosis"* a number of cases were described which were characterized by insidious onset, pronounced splenomegaly and moderate anemia.[102,103,107] Polychromatophilia and normoblasts were present in the peripheral blood in spite of the slight degree of anemia. The leukocytes were normal in number or reduced, or a leukemoid picture[100] was present. Atypical platelets and young megakaryocytes were found in the blood in some cases. The bone marrow was sclerotic or myelofibrosis was present.[97,103] The uniform cellularity of leukemic marrow was lacking. Moderate hepatomegaly was present but adenopathy was absent. *"Myeloid megakaryocytic hepato-splenomegaly"*[100] is another name given to this disorder, as well as *"chronic non-leukemic myelosis"*[97] to emphasize the diversity of cell types found in metaplastic organs and in the bone marrow and the absence of characteristic leukemic infiltrations. *"Agnogenic myeloid*

metaplasia"[105] is the title given to still other cases which seem to fall under the same head as far as one can judge by symptoms and signs and the findings in the blood. In some of these cases, however, icterus was present and the disorder was mistaken for hemolytic jaundice. The bone marrow was variously fibrotic, hyperplastic, aplastic or normal, but never leukemic. The spleen showed marked myeloid metaplasia, with scattered foci of immature red and white blood cells and megakaryocytes throughout a slightly or markedly fibrosed organ but the characteristic picture of leukemia was lacking. Hemosiderin in macrophages was sometimes present, often in considerable amount. In a number of the cases a history of exposure to certain industrial solvents, including benzene and carbon tetrachloride was obtained.

The common denominators in all of these cases are the hypoplastic, fibrotic or sclerotic, or at least hypofunctioning bone marrow, the striking splenomegaly, the presence of immature forms of red and white cells in the blood, often out of proportion to the degree of anemia, and myeloid metaplasia in the spleen and liver.[105a] It seems logical to assume that these cases represent instances in which there is a production deficit in the bone marrow with the result that the spleen and liver have attempted to take over the formation of blood. Since these organs lack the regulatory mechanism with which the bone marrow is endowed, cell forms normally present only in the marrow find their way into the circulating blood.

This concept is consistent with the observation that some of these cases followed exposure to a known bone marrow toxin. It is noteworthy that in one large series[118] the suspected etiologic factors corresponded closely with those considered under the head of "refractory anemias" (p. 552). In several cases, acute caseating tuberculosis was present which was thought to be responsible for the bone marrow and generalized fibrosis.[69a,99] As compared with cases of the "idiopathic" type, these patients were younger, there was hyperpyrexia, less splenic but greater lymph node enlargement and a shorter course before death.

Erf and Herbut[101] gathered an imposing list of conditions in which focal or diffuse myelosclerosis had been observed. In addition to those already mentioned, these included osteitis deformans, osteitis fibrosa cystica, osteomalacia, osteogenesis imperfecta cystica, poisoning by fluorine, phosphorus, estrogens, charcoal, anterior pituitary extract, parathyroid extract and irradiated ergosterol and, focally, in Albright's disease, various congenital bone diseases, and in experimentally induced occlusion of nutrient vessels to the marrow by multiple infarction.

Symptomatology.—The symptoms are those of anemia of persistent and refractory nature or complaints associated with splenomegaly, such as a sense of weight, or fullness in the abdomen. Deep pain in the extremities may be encountered and their intensity has been thought to be related to the activity of the process. Sometimes the symptoms are so minimal that they do not cause the patient to seek attention and the splenomegaly is discovered accidentally. Occasionally the presenting manifestations are those of hemolytic anemia or of thrombocytopenic purpura.

In a third to half the cases, roentgenographic changes in the bones can be demonstrated.[106] These appear in the medulla, the cortex being essentially normal. The principal changes involve the spongiosa and are characteristically diffuse. The osteosclerosis is due to thickening of the individual bone trabeculae of the spongiosa and in some cases new trabeculae seem to be formed. These changes are most likely to be found in the ribs, pelvis, vertebrae, clavicles and scapulae (Fig. 11–11). The skull is rarely involved, a point of contrast with marble bone disease (p. 776).

Blood Changes.—Anemia is variable in degree. In some cases of myelosclerosis even moderate polycythemia has been found in the early stages.[116] Frequently the anemia is normocytic but it may be macrocytic. The poikilocytosis, marked by the presence of red cells in the shape of tear drops,[98a] may be so striking as to suggest the diagnosis (Fig. 11–12). Nucleated red cells are usually found in the blood smear as well as an occasional polychromatophilic erythrocyte.

The leukocyte count is normal, reduced or increased and may be so high that leukemia may be suspected. It is rare, however, for it to exceed 50,000 per c.mm. In the differential formula the lymphocytes, in contrast to what occurs in aplastic anemia, do not predominate and the myeloid series maintains its normal proportions. In addition, a variable number of myelocytes and even very occasional myeloblasts will be found. The leukocyte alkaline phosphatase may be normal or decreased but was increased in patients with polycythemia.[106a]

The platelet count may be normal or moderately reduced. Thrombocytopenia may be present even when the leukocytes are normal in number. Some platelets may be particularly large, with pale chromomere and pale-staining hyalomere.[100] Giant platelets, megakaryocytic fragments and megakaryoblasts have also been described.

When the liver is involved there may be jaundice,[108,117] but in other cases there is usually no icterus nor is there any indication of excessive blood destruction. In two cases of myelosclerosis the corpuscular fragility was increased,[116] and in several cases associated with benzene poisoning the hemolytic manifestations were quite marked.[105]

Diagnosis.—Since splenomegaly

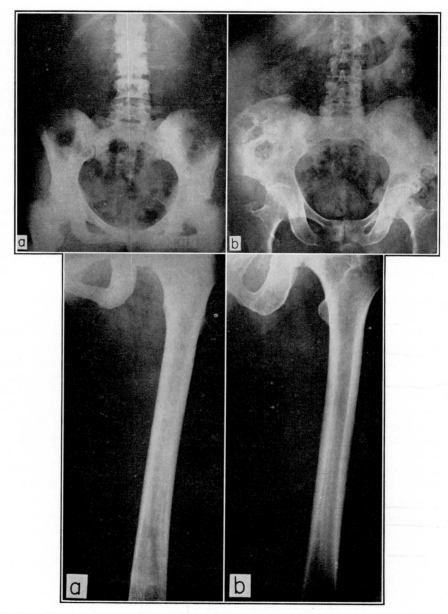

Fig. 11–11.—Roentgenograms of the spine, hip bones and femur of a woman with myelosclerosis (*a*), compared with those of a normal woman of the same age (*b*). Note especially the striking contrast between the density of the vertebrae and of the spongiosa of the long bones in the two subjects.

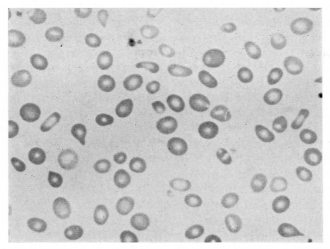

Fig. 11–12.—"Tear-drop" poikilocytes from a case of myelofibrosis. (Wright's stain × 720).

usually a prominent finding, leukemia and other conditions in which splenomegaly occurs are readily confused with myelofibrosis. Roentgenography may be helpful in differentiation but the characteristic picture, described above, is not observed in all cases. Myelofibrosis should not be confused with marble bone disease (p. 776).

Bone marrow examination is essential but puncture alone does not suffice. When the needle is introduced, the marrow may feel gritty and, in any event, little is obtained. That which is withdrawn usually is found to contain fewer nucleated cells than the blood. In the various cases which have been reported, aplastic, hypoplastic and normal marrow have been described. When some hyperplasia has been found, it has been relatively orderly in nature and the florid picture of leukemia has been lacking, thus providing an important means of differentiation. To confirm the diagnosis, surgical biopsy of marrow is necessary. Stained sections of bone marrow reveal diffuse fibrosis (Fig. 11–13).

Splenomegaly is due to myeloid metaplasia. This may cause enlargement of the liver and lymph nodes as well. The

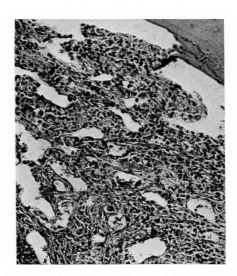

Fig. 11–13.—Diffuse fibrosis of the sternal marrow in a case of myelofibrosis. The nuclei are those of fibroblasts, not of blood cells.

myeloid hyperplasia in the spleen in myelofibrosis can be distinguished from the changes occurring in chronic myelocytic leukemia by *splenic puncture*:[111a] in the former the fundamental lymphatic structure of the spleen is retained and 50 to 60 per cent of the cells are found to be lymphocytes whereas in leukemia the proliferation is so extensive that the lymphoid structure is suppressed and only 50 to 30 per cent lymphocytes are found in the splenic puncture aspirate. The existence of extramedullary hemopoiesis in the spleen is indicated by the presence of immature cells of both the myeloid and erythroblastic series and a variable number of megakaryocytes.[112] Myeloid metaplasia may also be demonstrated by *lymph node puncture.*

Treatment.—Treatment should be conservative and designed to keep the patient in a reasonably satisfactory state of well-being and activity. Since the anemia is insidious in development, the patient has usually adjusted to the moderate impairment which this usually imposes. Artificial bolstering with blood transfusions is undesirable unless the anemia is severe. Various antianemic agents such as vitamin B_{12}, folic acid and iron are ineffective, as is also adrenocorticosteroid or cobalt therapy. On the ground that estrogenic substances administered in large amounts have been observed to cause endosteal thickening and fibrosis of the marrow in experimental animals which could be prevented by the administration of testosterone propionate, the latter hormone was given a therapeutic trial.[101,112] Results have been equivocal but the subject deserves further study.

In general *splenectomy* is not indicated.[97,100,102a] If the enlargement of the spleen is the result of an attempt to compensate for hypofunctioning bone marrow by extramedullary blood formation, splenectomy or *irradiation* of the spleen would not be expected to be helpful and might be harmful. Of Hickling's[104] series of 27 cases in which splenectomy had been performed, 24 died within a year, 12 within four days of splenectomy and seven more within several months. Nevertheless, the same writer subsequently observed good results from irradiation in patients with a high leukocytosis and a high proportion of immature cells in the circulating blood. In particular, abdominal discomfort due to the large spleen was decreased. Furthermore, a review of the results in 29 other splenectomized cases indicated that only three patients died within the first month of operation, 15 were known to have survived for periods in excess of two years and eight for four years.[102a] Comparison of blood values before and after splenectomy did not suggest that removal of the spleen resulted in lower blood values.

It appears, therefore, that with modern surgical technic splenectomy in myelofibrosis or "agnogenic myeloid metaplasia" is not followed by disastrous consequences. It is also clear, however, that the operation is not justified in most instances since no improvement occurs and the operative risk is not insignificant. However, when abnormal bleeding as the result of thrombocytopenia has been present, improved hemostasis has followed splenectomy. Again, in some cases of myelofibrosis a hemolytic component is associated and contributes greatly to the anemia. In such cases splenectomy may also be beneficial.[39d,102a] Erythrokinetic studies may be employed to determine whether, in cases in which erythrocyte life span is short, sequestration is occurring in the spleen.[111b]

A few patients have been treated with busulfan with the object of reducing the size of the spleen. This may occur but the drug must be used with great caution and in doses smaller than those employed in chronic myelocytic leukemia since these patients are sensitive to the drug and leukopenia is easily produced.[111c]

Prognosis.—This depends on the effectiveness of compensation for a hypofunctioning bone marrow and the wisdom exercised in supplementing rather than interfering with such compensatory changes as well as in managing the complications which may arise, such as hemorrhage and infections. Many patients have survived for several years and a few have lived a decade or longer.

Pathology. — Hepatosplenomegaly, occasionally generalized lymphadenopathy, and sclerotic or fibrotic marrow are usually found. The spleen may be huge. Microscopically, myeloid metaplasia is present in the spleen and often in the liver, renal capsules and lymph nodes as well. In the bones, an increase in the number of bony trabeculae and replacement of the marrow spaces with a loose, fairly cellular connective tissue are the principal microscopic findings. In cancellous bone there may be five or six times the normal number of trabeculae. In the connective tissue a few small islands of hemopoietic tissue often persist. In a study of the histopathologic changes in 30 cases, Wyatt and Sommers[118] concluded that the primary lesion in myelofibrosis is necrosis of partly matured, erythroid and myeloid bone marrow cells. Reactive overgrowth of the surviving, usually more immature cells follows and then extramedullary hematopoiesis develops. Repeated necrobiosis such as this is followed by overgrowth of marrow reticulum and, frequently, by ossification.

Pathogenesis.—The nature of this disorder is uncertain but many have considered it to be related in some manner to leukemia and the neoplastic reticuloses.[111d] It has been proposed that myelofibrosis, like myelocytic leukemia, "megakaryocytic myelosis" and polycythemia vera are very similar or related processes, all being "myeloproliferative disorders."[104a] In favor of this view is the fact that enormous enlargement of the spleen may occur at a time when the bone marrow is cellular and the myelofibrosis may be a late development;[96d] in reported cases of the disease the bone marrow has been variously hypoplastic, fibrotic and hyperplastic;[105] fibrosis of the bone marrow has been described in some cases of leukemia; some cases of

polycythemia vera have terminated with a clinical and hematological picture resembling the syndrome of myeloid metaplasia;[102a] and finally, as stated earlier (p. 586), removal of the spleen is not followed by the disastrous consequences which would be expected if this organ were compensating for bone marrow which has been destroyed.

This concept is not universally accepted,[106a] however, and the subject must be considered open. Pathological analogies between myelofibrosis and hepatic cirrhosis have been drawn and the suggestion was made that these are both morphologic entities without etiologic unity.[118] Thus it is possible that some stimulus causes activity of osteoblasts, fibroblasts, hemocytoblasts and megakaryocytes, cells which by their origin from the primitive mesenchyme reticulum cell are related, and that sclerosis is a secondary development.[116] It is also possible that, in certain instances at least, some toxic agent has caused destruction of the marrow and that the changes indicating hematopoiesis represent attempts at compensation.

MYELOPHTHISIC ANEMIA

(Leuko-erythroblastosis)

Definition and Synonyms.—This term is applied to the type of anemia associated with space-occupying disorders of the bone marrow. It does not refer to a specific entity but is encountered under a variety of circumstances. Because it is characterized by the presence in the circulating blood of immature leukocytes of the myeloid series as well as nucleated red cells in numbers sometimes quite out of proportion to the degree of anemia, this form of anemia has also been called **"leuko-erythroblastic" anemia.**[115] Since anemia may not be severe and since even polycythemia has been observed in certain cases, a better term is **leuko-erythroblastosis.** Other names are **myelopathic anemia** and **osteosclerotic anemia.**

Etiology.—Metastatic carcinoma in bone marrow is perhaps the commonest cause of this type of anemia. Malignancies of the breast, prostate, lungs, adrenals, or thyroid are especially apt to be accompanied by metastases to bones. The bones involved, unlike those invaded by other disorders, are usually those in which the bone marrow is normally active during life. Whether or not "leuko-erythroblastosis" develops in association with such metastases does not seem to depend on the nature of the primary site, the duration of the illness, the character of the bone changes (osteoclastic or osteoblastic), or the degree of skeletal involvement.

In **multiple myeloma** (p. 1068), perhaps in 5 per cent of cases,[115] the blood picture resembles that of myelophthisic anemia. Less frequently, myelophthisic anemia is encountered in other conditions which invade bone.[101] Bone involvement occurs in many cases of **Hodgkin's disease** and this may sometimes be associated with no demonstrable enlargement of lymph nodes (p. 1024). It is usually stated that in such cases thrombocytopenia does not occur even when there is severe anemia. We have observed at least one case, however, in which there was thrombocytopenia. In the **primary xanthomatoses,** Gaucher's disease, Niemann-Pick's disease, and Schüller-Christian's disease, myelophthisic anemia may also be encountered. The anemia of myelofibrosis (p. 583) and of marble bone disease (p. 776) is also of this type.

Symptomatology.—This will naturally vary with the underlying condition. The symptoms may be such as to suggest the true diagnosis but, in many instances, the signs and symptoms are non-specific.

Blood Changes.—Anemia is variable in degree. The most significant abnormality in the erythrocyte series is the presence of nucleated cells in the circulating blood in numbers quite out of proportion to the severity of the anemia. Most of the cells are normoblasts but some primitive forms may be found as well.[115] As many as 53 nucleated red cells per 100 leukocytes have been observed in cases in which there was little anemia. Reticulocytes may be increased, and polychromatophilia and stippling may be found.

The leukocyte count may be normal or reduced. Leukocytosis is unusual in the myelophthisic anemia associated with metastases.[111] Sometimes, however, a leukemoid picture may be observed (p. 265). As in myelofibrosis, the proportions of the different types of leukocytes are more or less the same as in normal blood, even when there is leukopenia. However, an occasional immature leukocyte, not normally seen in the blood, will be found.

The platelet count may be normal or moderately reduced. Thrombocytopenia may be present even when the leukocytes are normal in number. Bizarre forms of platelets may be noted.

Diagnosis. — Myelophthisic anemia should be suspected whenever nucleated red cells or myelocytes are observed in the circulating blood in cases in which there is little anemia. This type of anemia should also be considered whenever such cells as well as polychromatophilia, stippling, reticulocytosis and a decrease in lymphocytes rather than in myeloid forms are found in the face of quantitative evidence of impaired bone marrow function (anemia, leukopenia, thrombocytopenia). In fact, so subtle may the manifestations of myelophthisic anemia be that, when a bizarre blood picture is found which does not fit that characteristic of one of the commoner blood dyscrasias, the bones should be palpated systematically for tenderness or swelling, the urine should be examined for Bence-Jones protein, the blood for

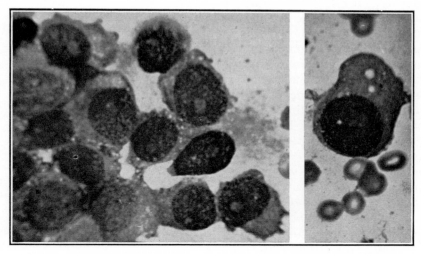

FIG. 11–14.—Tumor cells in the sternal marrow in a case of carcinoma of the prostate with myelophthisic anemia.

the total protein content, roentgenograms of the bones should be made, and a search for malignancy and for evidence of exposure to toxic agents instituted. Rectal examination may reveal unsuspected carcinoma of the prostate. If splenomegaly is present, as has been very occasionally observed in some cases of metastatic carcinoma,[115] myelophthisic anemia is easily confused with leukemia and with myelosclerosis. Bone marrow examination will be helpful in such cases. Even in the absence of splenomegaly, marrow examination may be helpful, since the tumor cells may be demonstrated thereby (Fig. 11–14). (See also Plate III, p. 70).

The primary xanthomatoses are associated with hemochromatosis and pigmentation of exposed skin. Schüller-Christian's disease is distinguished by a characteristic triad; exophthalmos, symptoms of diabetes insipidus and large bony defects, especially in the skull.[113] Gaucher's and Niemann-Pick's diseases are congenital and familial and the latter affects predominantly female Jewish infants. In Gaucher's disease a brownish wedge-shaped thickening of the cornea is found.

Biopsy of bone marrow reveals large "foam" cells containing lipoid. These disorders are discussed in Chapter 15.

Hodgkin's disease may be suspected if there is fever. In one of our cases of severe anemia, leukopenia, and thrombocytopenia in which there was neither lymphadenopathy nor splenomegaly the occurrence of a Pel-Ebstein type of fever as well as radiating pain, lesions in the skull, reticulocytosis, nucleated red cells and occasional myelocytes in the circulating blood suggested the diagnosis. This was subsequently confirmed at autopsy.

Treatment.—This depends on the nature of the underlying disorder. Transfusions have proved to be of only temporary benefit.

Prognosis.—The prognosis depends upon the nature of the causative disorder.

Pathology.—In cases of myelophthisic anemia associated with carcinomatous metastases, the metastatic areas may be surrounded by areas of active blood formation with large groups of primitive erythroblasts surrounded by normoblasts, many megakaryocytes and comparatively few leukocytes.[115] The marrow may appear red. In the primary xanthomatoses characteristic foam cells are present in the marrow.

Pathogenesis.—It is generally assumed that myelophthisic anemia associated with carcinomatous metastases or other focal lesions of the bone marrow is the result of mechanical limitation of hemopoietic tissue through invasion of the bone marrow. It has been pointed out,[115] however, that the total quantity of red marrow is often quite in excess of the amount normally present. Vaughan was not able to find adequate evidence of crowding out, and concluded that in cases of myelophthisic anemia hematopoiesis is in some way stimulated. She suggested that there may be a local nutritional deficiency as the result of consumption by the cells of the new growth of some necessary substance. Since then it has been shown that shortened survival of red corpuscles contributes to the anemia in many cases of neoplastic disease[71a,88a] and this in turn stimulates erythropoiesis. As pointed out elsewhere (p. 580) anemia develops because production does not increase sufficiently to compensate for the increased destruction.

BIBLIOGRAPHY

Acute Posthemorrhagic Anemia

1. Brøchner-Mortensen, K.: Iron Contents of the Serum in Patients with Hemorrhagic Anemia, Acta med. scandinav., *113*, 345, 1943.

1a. Chunn, C. F. and Harkins, H. N.: Alimentary Azotemia, Am. J. M. Sc., *201*, 745, 1941.

2. Coleman, D. H., Stevens, A. R., Jr., Dodge, H. T. and Finch, C. A.: Rate of Blood Regeneration after Blood Loss, Arch. Int. Med., *92*, 341, 1953.

2a. Ebert, R. V., Stead, E. A., Jr. and Gibson, J. G., II: Response of Normal Subjects to Acute Blood Loss, Arch. Int. Med., *68*, 578, 1941.

2b. Fowler, W. M. and Barer, A. P.: Rate of Hemoglobin Regeneration in Blood Donors, J.A.M.A., *118*, 421, 1942; Am. J. M. Sc., *205*, 9, 1943.

2c. Gordon, A. S.: Quantitative Nature of the Red Cell Response to a Single Bleeding, Proc. Soc. Exper. Biol. & Med., *31*, 563, 1934.

3. Jones, N. C. H.: Measurement of Red-Cell Loss from Gastro-Intestinal Tract, Using Radioactive Chromium, Brit. M. J., *1*, 493, 1958.

4. Lindebaum, I. S.: Das Knochenmark in den ersten Stunden und Tagen nach dem Aderlass, Folia hæmat., *39*, 501, 1930.

5. Meulengracht, E.: The Treatment of Hæmatemesis and Melæna With Food, Lancet, *2*, 1220, 1935.

6. Neumann, B.: Experimentelle Beiträge zum Studium des Blutverlustes, Arch. klin. Chir., *172*, 529, 1932.

6a. Pareira, M. D., Serkes, K. D. and Lang, S.: Early Response of Plasma Volume, Red Cell Mass and Plasma Proteins to Massive Hemorrhage, Proc. Soc. Exper. Biol. & Med., *103*, 9, 1960.

7. Schiødt, E.: Observations on Blood Regeneration in Man, Am. J. M. Sc., *193*, 313 and 327, 1937; *Ibid.*, *196*, 632, 1938.

9. Steele, B. F.: The Effects of Blood Loss and Blood Destruction Upon the Erythroid Cells in the Bone Marrow of Rabbits, J. Exper. Med., *57*, 881, 1933.

10. Warren, J. V., Brannon, E. S., Stead, E. A., Jr. and Merrill, A. J.: The Effect of Venesection and the Pooling of Blood in the Extremities on the Atrial Pressure and Cardiac Output in Normal Subjects, J. Clin. Invest., *24*, 337, 1945.

11. Wintrobe, M. M.: Anemia, Arch. Int. Med., *54*, 256, 1934.

Refractory Anemias

11a. Abels, J. C. and Rhoads, C. P.: Hemolysin in the Urine in Aplastic Anemia, Proc. Soc. Exper. Biol. & Med., *38*, 849, 1938.

12. Albahary, C. and Boiron, M.: Anémie primitive réfractaire avec hypersidérose sanguine médullaire et hépatique (cas féminin), Acta med. scandinav., *163*, 429, 1959.

12a. Anderson, J. P.: Coexistent Aplastic Anaemia and Coarctation of the Aorta, Arch. Dis. Childhood, *31*, 131, 1956.

12b. Arrau, C. M., Contreras, V., Nijamkin, A. and Cabezas, J.: Tres casos fatales de anemia aplastica por cloramfenicol, Rev. méd. de Chile, *85*, 606, 1957.

12c. Astaldi, G., Rondanelli, E. G., Gorini, P. and Zelaschi, C.: Recherches sur la prolifération des érythroblastes en culture dans un plasma irradié par les rayons roentgen, Rev. hémat., *8*, 477, 1953.

12d.AUB, J. C., EVANS, R. D., HEMPLEMANN, L. H. and MARTLAND, H. S.: The Effects of Internally Deposited Radioactive Materials in Man, Medicine, *31*, 221, 1952.

12e.BALDRIDGE, C. W.: Macrocytic Anemia With Aplastic Features Following the Application of Synthetic Organic Hair Dye, Am. J. M. Sc., *189*, 759, 1935.

12f. BAXTER, C. F., BELCHER, E. H., HARRISS, E. B. and LAMERTON, L. F.: Anæmia and Erythropoiesis in the Irradiated Rat, Brit. J. Hæmat., *1*, 86, 1955.

13. BERNARD, J. and ATTAL, C.: Les aplasies de la moelle et du sang provoquées par le chloramphénicol, Semaine d. hôp. Paris, *31*, 1150, 1955.

13a.BLOOM, M. A. and BLOOM, W.: The Radiosensitivity of Erythroblasts, J. Lab. & Clin. Med., *32*, 654, 1947.

13c. BOMFORD, R. R. and RHOADS, C. P.: Refractory Anæmia, Quart. J. Med., *10*, 175, 1941.

14. BOON, T. H.: Aplastic Anemia With Complete Recovery, Brit, M. J., *2*, 1041, 1938.

15. BOWDITCH, M., ELKINS, H. B., HUNTER, F. T., MALLORY, T. B., GALL, E. A. and BRICKLEY, W. J.: Chronic Exposure to Benzene (Benzol), J. Indust. Hyg. & Toxicol., *21*, 321, 1939 (Bibliography).

15a.BROD, R. C.: Blood Dyscrasias Associated with Tolbutamide Therapy, J. A. M. A., *171*, 296, 1959.

15b.BROWN, W. M. C. and ABBATT, J. D.: The Effect of a Single Dose of X-Rays on the Peripheral Blood Count of Man, Brit. J. Hæmat., *1*, 75, 1955.

15c. BURRELL, C. D.: Fatal Marrow Aplasia after Treatment with Carbimazole, Brit. M. J., *1*, 1456, 1956.

15d.CARLSON, G. W.: Aplastic Anemia Following Exposure to Products of the Sulfite Pulp Industry, Ann. Int. Med., *24*, 277, 1946.

15e. CAROLI, J. et al.: Hémochromatose avec anémie hypochrome et absence d'hémoglobine anormale, Presse méd., *65*, 1991, 1957.

15f. CASTLE, W. B., DRINKER, K. R. and DRINKER, C. K.: Necrosis of the Jaw in Workers Employed in Applying a Luminous Paint Containing Radium, J. Indust. Hyg. & Toxicol., *7*, 371, 1925.

15g.COOPER, W.: Pancytopenia Associated with Disseminated Tuberculosis, Ann. Int. Med., *50*, 1497, 1959.

16. CRAWFORD, M. A. D.: Aplastic Anæmia Due to Trinitrotoluene Intoxication, Brit. M. J., *2*, 430, 1954.

16a.CRONKITE, E. P.: Ionizing Radiation Injury. Its Diagnosis by Physical Examination and Clinical Laboratory Procedures, J. A. M. A., *139*, 366, 1949; Ann. Rev. Physiol., *18*, 483, 1956.

16b.CRONKITE, E. P., JACOBS, G. J., BRECHER, G. and DILLARD, G.: The Hemorrhagic Phase of the Acute Radiation Syndrome Due to Exposure of the Whole Body to Penetrating Ionizing Radiation, Am. J. Roentgenol., *67*, 796, 1952, J. Lab. & Clin. Med., *39*, 449, 1952.

16c. CUSTER, R. P.: Aplastic Anemia in Soldiers Treated with Atabrine, Am. J. M. Sc., *212*, 211, 1946.

16d.DACIE, J. V. and GILPIN, A.: Refractory Anæmia (Fanconi Type), Arch. Dis. Child., *19*, 155, 1944.

16e. DACIE, J. V., SMITH, MARY D., WHITE, J. C. and MOLLIN, D. L.: Refractory Normoblastic Anaemia, Brit. J. Haemat., *5*, 56, 1959.

17. DASSEN, R. and REY, J. C.: Acute Intoxication by Bismuth, Semana méd., *2*, 1152, 1930.

17a.DYKE, V. F. and WALLACE, J. B.: Development of Aplastic Anemia During the Use of Streptomycin, J.A.M.A., *136*, 1098, 1948.

17b.DICKIE, A. and HEMPLEMANN, L. H.: Morphologic Changes in the Lymphocytes of Persons Exposed to Ionizing Radiation, J. Lab. & Clin. Med., *32*, 1045, 1947.

18. DOBRINER, K., RHOADS, C. P., and HUMMEL, L. E.: The Excretion of Porphyrin in Refractory and Aplastic Anemia, J. Clin. Invest., *17*, 125, 1938.

18a.DOWDY, A. H., BENNETT, L. R. and CHASTAIN, S. M.: Protective Action of Anoxic Anoxia Against Total Body Roentgen Irradiation of Mammals, Radiol., *55*, 879, 1950.

18b.DUANE, G. W.: Aplastic Anemia Fourteen Years Following Administration of Thorotrast, Am. J. Med., *23*, 499, 1957.

19. DUNLAP, C. E.: Effects of Radiation on the Blood and the Hemopoietic Tissues, Including the Spleen, the Thymus and the Lymph Nodes, Arch. Path., *34*, 749, 1942.

20. EHRLICH, P.: Uber einen Fall von Anämie, mit Bermerkungen über regenerative Veränderungen des Knochenmarks, Charité-Ann., *13*, 300, 1888.

20a.EISEMANN, G. and DAMESHEK, W.: Splenectomy for "Pure Red Cell" Hypoplastic (Aregenerative) Anemia Associated with Autoimmune Hemolytic Disease, New England J. Med., *251*, 1044, 1954.

21. ERF, L. A. and RHOADS, C. P.: The Hematological Effects of Benzene (Benzol) Poisoning, J. Indust. Hyg. & Toxicol., *21*, 421, 1939.

22. FOUNTAIN, J. R. and DALES, M.: Pure Red-Cell Aplasia Successfully Treated with Cobalt, Lancet, 1, 541, 1955.

22a.FOY, H. and KONDI, A.: A Case of True Red-Cell Aplastic Anæmia Successfully Treated with Riboflavin, J. Path. & Bact., 65, 559, 1953.

22b.FREEMAN, H. E.: Aplastic Anemia With Thrombocytopenic Purpura and Agranulocytosis Complicating Mapharsen Therapy, Arch. Dermat. & Syph., 50, 320, 1944.

22c. FREEMAN, Z.: Pure Red-Cell Anaemia and Thymoma, Brit. M. J., 1, 1390, 1960.

22d.FRIBERG, L. and MARTENSSON, J.: Case of Panmyelophthisis after Exposure to Chlorophenothane and Benzene Hexachloride, Arch. Indus. Hyg. & Occupat. Med., 8, 166, 1953.

23. GARBY, L., SJÖLIN, S. and VAHLQUIST, B.: Chronic Refractory Hypochromic Anaemia with Disturbed Haem-Metabolism, Brit. J. Haemat., 3, 55, 1957.

23a.GARRIGA, S. and CROSBY, W. H.: The Incidence of Leukemia in Families of Patients with Hypoplasia of the Marrow, Blood, 14, 1008, 1959.

24. GASSER, C.: Pure Red Cell Anemia Due to Auto-Antibodies, Sang, 26, 6, 1955.

24a.GELPI, A. P. and ENDE, N.: An Hereditary Anemia with Hemochromatosis, Am. J. Med., 25, 303, 1958.

25. GOLDWATER, L. J.: Disturbances in the Blood Following Exposure to Benzol, J. Lab. & Clin. Med., 26, 957, 1941.

26. GLASSMIRE, C. R.: Fatal Pancytopenia Following Antihistamine Administration. Maine M. A. J., 42, 83, 1951.

27. GREENBURG, L., MAYERS, M. R., GOLDWATER, L. and SMITH, A. R.: Benzene (Benzol) Poisoning in the Rotogravure Printing Industry in New York City, J. Indust. Hyg. & Toxicol., 21, 395, 1939.

27a.GUNZ, F. W.: Culture of Human Leukaemic Blood Cells in Vitro; Some Effects of X-rays, Brit. J. Cancer, 3, 330, 1949.

27b.HALBERSTAEDTER, L. and ICKOWICZ, M.: The Effects of X-rays on the Lymphatic Organs of Normal and Adrenalectomized Rats, Radiol. Clin., 16, 240, 1947.

27c.HALE, G. S. and DE GRUCHY, G. C.: Aplastic Anaemia Following the Administration of Phenylbutazone, Med. J. Australia, 2, 449, 1960.

27d.HAVARD, C. W. H. and SCOTT, R. B.: Thymic Tumour and Erythroblastic Aplasia, Brit. J. Haemat., 6, 178, 1960.

28. HAYHURST, E. R. and NEISWANDER, B. E.: A Case of Chronic Benzene Poisoning, J. A. M. A., 96, 269, 1931.

29. HEATON, L. D., CROSBY, W. H. and COHEN, A.: Splenectomy in the Treatment of Hypoplasia of the Bone Marrow, Ann. Surg., 146, 637, 1957.

29a.HEILMEYER, L., KEIDERLING, W., BILGER, R. and BERNAUER, H.: Uber chronische refraktäre Anämien mit sideroblastischem Knochenmark (Anaemia refractoria sideroblastica), Folia haemat., 2, 49 and 61, 1958; Deutsche med. Wchnschr., 84, 1761, 1959; Schweiz. med. Wchnschr., 90, 934, 1960.

30. HERZOG, F. and ROSCHER, A.: Zur klinik und Pathogenese der Kollargolintoxikation beim Menschen, Virchows Arch. path. Anat., 236, 361, 1922.

31. HODGKINSON, R.: Blood Dyscrasias Associated with Chloramphenicol, Lancet, 1, 285, 1954.

31a.HOLSINGER, D. R., HANLON, D. G. and WELCH, J. S.: Fatal Aplastic Anemia Following Sulfamethoxypyridazine Therapy, Proc. Staff Meet., Mayo Clin., 33, 679, 1958.

31b.HORRIGAN, D. L., WHITTINGTON, R. M., WEISMAN, R., JR. and HARRIS, J. W.: Hypochromic Anemia with Hyperferricemia Responding to Oral Crude Liver Extract, Am. J. Med., 22, 99, 1957.

31c.HUNTER, D.: Industrial Toxicology, Quart. J. Med., 12, 185, 1943.

32. IMERMAN, S. W. and IMERMAN, C. P.: Dinitrophenol Poisoning, J.A.M.A., 106, 1085, 1936.

32a.INGRAM, M. and BARNES, S. W.: Experimental Confirmation of a Previously Reported Unusual Finding in the Blood of Cyclotron Workers, Science, 113, 32, 1951; Ibid. 116, 706, 1952.

33. ISAACS, R.: Effect of Arsenic on Maturation of Red Blood Cells, Folia hæmatol., 37, 389, 1928.

34. ISAACSON, S., GOLD, J. A. and GINSBERG, V.: Fatal Aplastic Anemia after Therapy with Nuvarone (3-Methyl-5-Phenylhydantoin), J. A. M. A., 160, 1311, 1956.

34a.JACOBSON, L. O., MARKS, E. K. and LORENZ, E.: The Hematological Effects of Ionizing Radiations, Radiol., 52, 371, 1949.

34b.JACOBSON, L. O., MARKS, E. K., ROBSON, M. J., GASTON, E. and ZIRKLE, R. E.: The Effects of Spleen Protection on Mortality Following X-Irradiation, J. Lab. & Clin. Med., 34, 1538, 1949; Ibid., 36, 40, 1950; Progress in Hematology, New York, Grune & Stratton, 1956, p. 311.

35. KADIN, M.: Aplastic Anemia Following Use of Neoarsphenamine, Arch. Dermat., 37, 787, 1938.

36. KAHN, J. B. and FURTH, J.: The Pathogenesis of Postirradiation Anemia, Blood, 7, 404, 1952; ibid, 8, 545, 1953.

36a. KOSZEWSKI, B. J. and HUBBARD, T. F.: Congenital Anemia in Hereditary Ectodermal Dysplasia, A. M. A. Arch. Dermat., 74, 159, 1956.

36b. KRAKOFF, I. H., KARNOFSKY, D. A. and BURCHENAL, J. H.: Effects of Large Doses of Chloramphenicol in Human Subjects, New England J. Med., 253, 7, 1955.

37. KRUMBHAAR, E. B.: Blood and Bone Marrow in Gas Poisoning, J.A.M.A., 72, 39, 1919.

37a. KURNICK, N. B., MASSEY, B. W. and SANDEEN, G.: The Effect of Radiation on Tissue Deoxyribonuclease, Radiation Res., 11, 101, 1959.

38. LATTA, J. S. and DAVIES, L. T.: Effects on the Blood and Hemopoietic Organs of the Albino Rat of Repeated Administration of Benzene, Arch. Path., 37, 55, 1941.

38a. LAWRENCE, J. S., DOWDY, A. H. and VALENTINE, W. N.: Effects of Radiation on Hemopoiesis, Radiol., 51, 400, 1948.

38b. LAWRENCE, J. S., VALENTINE, W. N. and DOWDY, A. H.: The Effect of Radiation on Hemopoiesis. Is There an Indirect Effect? Blood, 3, 593, 1948.

39. LAWSON, G. B., JACKSON, W. P. and CATTANACH, G. S.: Arsenic Poisoning, J.A.M. A., 85, 24, 1925.

39a. LEROY, G. V.: Hematology of Atomic Bomb Casualties, Arch. Int. Med., 86, 691, 1950.

39b. LEVINE, B. and ROSENBERG, D. V.: Aplastic Anemia During the Treatment of Hyperthyroidism with Tapazole, Ann. Int. Med., 41, 844, 1954.

39c. LIEBOW, A. A., WARREN, S. and DE COURSEY, E.: Pathology of Atomic Bomb Casualties, Am. J. Path., 25, 853, 1949.

39d. LOEB, V., JR., MOORE, C. V. and DUBACH, R.: The Physiologic Evaluation and Management of Chronic Bone Marrow Failure, Am. J. Med., 15, 499, 1953.

39e. LOONEY, W. B.: Late Clinical Changes Following the Internal Deposition of Radioactive Materials, Ann. Int. Med., 42, 378, 1955.

39f. LUKL, P., WIEDERMANN, B. and BARBOŘÍK, M.: Hereditäre Leptocyten-Anämie bei Männern mit Hämochromatose, Folia haemat., 3, 17, 1958.

39g. MAIER, C.: Anaemia refractoria sideroblastica, Schweiz. med. Wchnschr., 89, 1074, 1959.

39h. MALASSENET, R.: Les anémies hypochromes avec hypersidérémie, Sang, 29, 486, 1958.

40. MARTLAND, H. S.: Occupational Poisoning in Manufacture of Luminous Watch Dials, J.A.M.A., 92, 466, 522, 1929.

41. ———— The Occurrence of Malignancy in Radio-active Persons, Am. J. Cancer, 15, 2435, 1931.

41a. McDONALD, R. and GOLDSCHMIDT, B.: Pancytopenia with Congenital Defects (Fanconi's Anaemia), Arch. Dis. Childhood, 35, 367, 1960.

41b. MEYER, L. M., HEEVE, W. L. and BERTSCHER, R. W.: Aplastic Anemia after Meprobamate Therapy, New England J. Med., 256, 1232, 1957.

42. MINOT, G. R. and SPURLING, R. G.: Effect on Blood of Irradiation, Especially Short Wave Length Roentgen-Ray Therapy, Am. J. M. Sc., 168, 215, 1924.

42a. MITCHELL, J. S.: Metabolic Effects of Therapeutic Doses of X and Gamma Radiations, Brit. J. Radiol., 16, 339, 1943.

42b. MOESCHLIN, S., MARTI, H. R. and GERMANN, W.: Tödliche Panmyelopathie durch Thorotrast (Thoriumdioxyd), Schweiz. med. Wchnschr., 83, 1061, 1953.

42c. MOHLER, D. N. and LEAVELL, B. S.: Aplastic Anemia, Ann. Int. Med., 49, 326, 1958.

42d. MOLE, R. H.: Risks from Chronic Irradiation and their Hæmatological Control, J. Clin. Path., 7, 267, 1954.

43. MOORE, J. E. and KEIDEL, A.: Stomatitis and Aplastic Anemia Due to Neoarsphenamin, Arch. Dermat. 4, 169, 1921.

43a. MORGAN, A. D., JAYNE, W. H. W. and MARRACK, D.: Primary Liver Cell Carcinoma 24 Years after Intravenous Injection of Thorotrast, J. Clin. Path., 11, 7, 1958.

44. NAJEAN, Y. et al.: Exploration isotopique de l'érythrocinétique dans 31 cas de pancytopénie idiopathique chronique a moelle histologiquement normale ou riche, Sang, 30, 101, 1959.

44a. NILSSON, L. R.: Chronic Pancytopenia with Multiple Congenital Abnormalities, Acta paediat., 49, 518, 1960.

44b. PATON, M. D., RIDDELL, M. J. and STRONG, J. A.: Aplastic Anæmia Following Mepacrine Treatment of Lupus Erythematosus, Lancet, 1, 281, 1955.

44c. PETERS, J. T.: Equine Infectious Anemia Transmitted to Man, Ann. Int. Med., 23, 271, 1945.

44d. PROSSER, C. L.: The Clinical Sequence of Physiological Effects of Ionizing Radiation in Animals, Radiol., 49, 299, 1947.

45. PUCK, T. T.: The Action of Radiation on Mammalian Cells, Am. Naturalist, 94, 95, 1960.

46. RIGDON, R. H., CRASS, G. and MARTIN, N.: Anemia Produced by Chloramphenicol

38

(Chloromycetin) in the Duck, Arch. Path., *58*, 85, 1954.

47. ROSENTHAL, M. and GRACE, E. J.: Experimental Radium Poisoning, Am. J. M. Sc., *191*, 607, 1936.

47a. RUBIN, D., WEISBERGER, A. S., BOTTI, R. E. and STORAASLI, J. P.: Changes in Iron Metabolism in Early Chloramphenicol Toxicity, J. Clin. Invest., *37*, 1286, 1958; J. Lab. & Clin. Med., *56*, 453, 1960.

47b. SAIDI, P., WALLERSTEIN, R. O. and AGGELER, P. M.: Effect of Chloramphenicol on Erythropoiesis, J. Lab. & Clin. Med., *57*, 247, 1961.

48. SCOTT, J. L., CARTWRIGHT, G. E. and WINTROBE, M. M.: Acquired Aplastic Anemia: an Analysis of Thirty-Nine Cases and Review of the Pertinent Literature, Medicine, *38*, 119, 1959.

48a. SELLING, L.: Benzol as a Leucotoxin, The Johns Hopkins Hosp. Reports, *17*, 83, 1916.

48b. SHAHIDI, N. T. and DIAMOND, L. K.: Testosterone-Induced Remission in Aplastic Anemia, New England, J. Med., *264*, 953, 1961.

49. SÉZARY, A. and BOUCHER, G.: Agranulocytose Bismuthique, Bull. et mém. Soc. méd. hôp. de Paris, *47*, 1795, 1931.

49a. SHAW, R. G. and McLEAN, J. A.: Chloramphenicol and Aplastic Anaemia, Med. J. Australia, *1*, 352, 1957.

49b. SHELTON, J. G., KINGSTON, W. R. and McRAE, C.: Aplastic Anaemia and Agranulocytosis Following Chlorpromazine Therapy, Med. J. Australia, *1*, 130, 1960.

49c. SMILEY, R. K., CARTWRIGHT, G. E. and WINTROBE, M. M.: Fatal Aplastic Anemia Following Chloramphenicol (Chloromycetin) Administration, J. A. M. A., *149*, 914, 1952.

50. SNELL, F. M., NEEL, J. V. and ISHIBASHI, K.: Hematologic Studies in Hiroshima and a Control City Two Years after the Atomic Bombing, Arch. Int. Med., *84*, 569, 1949.

50a. SOUTTER, L. and EMERSON, C. P.: Elective Thymectomy in the Treatment of Aregenerative Anemia Associated with Monocytic Leukemia, Am. J. Med., *28*, 609, 1960.

50b. STOHLMAN, F., JR., BRECHER, G., SCHNEIDERMAN, M. and CRONKITE, E. P.: The Hemolytic Effect of Ionizing Radiations and Its Relationship to the Hemorrhagic Phase of Radiation Injury, Blood, *12*, 1061, 1957.

50c. STRAUS, B.: Aplastic Anemia Following Exposure to Carbon Tetrachloride, J. A. M. A., *155*, 737, 1954.

50d. STEINBERG, B.: Bone Marrow Regeneration in Experimental Benzene Intoxication, Blood, *4*, 550, 1949.

50e. THOMAS, E. D.: The Treatment of Refractory Anemia with Cobalt, Ann. Int. Med., *44*, 412, 1956.

51. THOMPSON, W. P., RICHTER, M. N. and EDSALL, K. S.: Analysis of So-called Aplastic Anemia, Am. J. M. Sc., *187*, 77, 1934.

51a. TROWELL, O. A.: The Sensitivity of Lymphocytes to Ionizing Radiation, J. Path. & Bact., *64*, 687, 1952.

51b. TSAI, S. Y. and LEVIN, W. C.: Chronic Erythrocytic Hypoplasia in Adults, Am. J. Med., *22*, 322, 1957.

51c. UNDERWOOD, L. C.: Fatal Bone Marrow Depression after Treatment with Acetazolamide (Diamox), J. A. M. A., *161*, 1477, 1956.

51d. UYEKI, E. M., LEUCHTENBERGER, CECILIE and SALERNO, P. R.: Effect of X-irradiation on the DNA Content of Individual Nuclei of Rabbit Bone Marrow, Exper. Cell Res., *17*, 405, 1959.

52. VALENTINE, W. N. and PEARCE, M. L.: Studies on the Radiosensitivity of Bone Marrow, Blood, 7, 1, 1952.

52a. VILTER, R. W. et al.: Refractory Anemia with Hyperplastic Bone Marrow, Blood, *15*, 1, 1960.

52b. WARREN, S. and BOWERS, J. Z.: The Acute Radiation Syndrome in Man, Ann. Int. Med., *32*, 207, 1950.

52c. WEICKER, H.: Die genetischen Grundlagen der Fanconi-Anämie, Schweiz. med. Wchnschr., *89*, 1081, 1959.

52d. WELCH, H., LEWIS, C. N. and KERLAN, I.: Blood Dyscrasias, Antibiotics & Chemother., *4*, 607, 1954.

53. WHEELIHAN, R. Y.: Granulocytic Aplasia of Bone Marrow Following Use of Arsenic, Am. J. Dis. Child., *35*, 1032, 1928.

56. WINTROBE, M. M., STOWELL, A. and ROLL, R. M.: Report of a Case of Aplastic Anemia Following Gold Injections in Which Recovery Occurred, Am. J. M. Sc., *197*, 698, 1939.

56a. WITKIND, E. and WAID, M. E.: Aplasia of the Bone Marrow During Mesantoin Therapy, J. A. M. A., *147*, 757, 1951.

Simple Chronic Anemia

57. ADAIR, F. L., DIECKMANN, W. J. and GRANT, K.: Anemia in Pregnancy, Am. J. Obst. & Gynec., *32*, 560, 1936.

57a. ADAMS, E. B.: Anæmia in Kwashiorkor, Brit. M. J., *1*, 537, 1954.

58. BAÉZ-VILLASEÑOR, J., RATH, C. E. and FINCH, C. A.: The Blood Picture in Addison's Disease, Blood, *3*, 769, 1948.

59. BALDERSTON, S. V.: Anemia Associated With Biliary Fistula, Arch. Int. Med., *50*, 223, 1932.

60. BERK, L., BURCHENAL, J. H. and CASTLE, W. B.: Erythropoietic Effect of Cobalt in Patients with or without Anemia, New England J. Med., 240, 754, 1949.

60a. BERLIN, N. I., GOETSCH, C., HYDE, G. M. and PARSONS, R. J.: The Blood Volume in Pregnancy as Determined by P³² Labeled Red Blood Cells, Surg., Gynec. & Obst., 97, 173, 1953.

60b. BETHELL, F. H., GARDINER, S. H. and MacKINNON, F.: The Influence of Iron and Diet on the Blood in Pregnancy, Ann. Int. Med., 13, 91, 1939; J. Am. Diet. A., 19, 165, 1943.

61. BEUTLER, E. and HOFSTRA, DIANA: Auto-cannibalism: the Etiology of Nerve-Resection Anemia, Blood, 15, 370, 1960.

61a. BLOOM, A. and BRYSON, C. C.: Aplastic Anæmia in Simmonds' Disease, Brit. M. J., 2, 75, 1948.

62. BOCK, H. E. and THEDERING, F.: Über Anämien bei Nierenkrankheiten, Deutsches Arch. klin. Med., 199, 130, 1952; Ztschr. ges. exper. Med., 118, 459, 1952.

63. BRAVERMAN, M. M.: The Anæmia of Pulmonary Tuberculosis, Am. Rev. Tuberc., 38, 466, 1938; Ibid., 46, 27, 1942.

65. BRUGSCH, H.: Hyperchrome Anämie bei chronischen Pankreaserkrankungen, Deutsch. Arch. klin. Med., 173, 199, 1932.

65a. BUSH, J. A., ASHENBRUCKER, H., CARTWRIGHT, G. E. and WINTROBE, M. M.: The Kinetics of Iron Metabolism in the Anemia Associated with Chronic Infection, J. Clin. Invest., 35, 89, 1956.

65b. CALLEN, I. R. and LIMARZI, L. R.: Blood and Bone Marrow Studies in Renal Disease, Am. J. Clin. Path., 20, 3, 1950.

66. CARTWRIGHT, G. E., LAURITSEN, M. A., JONES, P. J., MERRILL, I. M. and WINTROBE, M. M.: The Anemia of Infection, J. Clin. Invest., 25, 65 and 81, 1946; J. Biol. Chem., 184, 563, 575, and 579, 1950; J. Clin. Invest., 29, 1505, 1950; Ibid., 30, 161, 1951; Blood, 9, 183, 1954.

66a. CARTWRIGHT, G. E. and WINTROBE, M. M.: The Anemia of Infection XVII. A Review, Advances in Internal Medicine, 5, 165, 1952, Chicago, Year Book Publishers, Inc.

67. CHENEY, G.: The Megalocytic Hypochromic Anemia of Pancreatic Disease, Folia hæmat., 56, 28, 1936.

67a. DAUGHADAY, W. H., WILLIAMS, R. H. and DALAND, G. A.: The Effect of Endocrinopathies on the Blood, 3, 1342, 1948.

68. EVANS, T. S., DeLUCA, V. A. and WATERS, L. L.: The Association of Miliary Tuberculosis of the Bone Marrow and Pancytopenia, Ann. Int. Med., 37, 1044, 1952.

69. FAY, J., CARTWRIGHT, G. E. and WINTROBE, M. M.: Studies on Free Erythrocyte Protoporphyrin, Serum Iron, Serum Iron-Binding Capacity and Plasma Copper During Normal Pregnancy, J. Clin. Invest., 28, 487, 1949.

69a. FOUNTAIN, J. R.: Blood Changes Associated with Disseminated Tuberculosis, Brit. M. J., 2, 76, 1954.

69b. FREIREICH, E. J., MILLER, A., EMERSON, C. P. and ROSS, J. F.: The Effect of Inflammation on the Utilization of Erythrocyte and Transferrin Bound Radioiron for Red Cell Production, Blood, 12, 972, 1957.

69c. FREIREICH, E. J. et al.: Radioactive Iron Metabolism and Erythrocyte Survival Studies of the Mechanism of the Anemia Associated with Rheumatoid Arthritis, J. Clin. Invest., 36, 1043, 1957.

70. GARDNER, F. H.: The Use of Cobaltous Chloride in the Anemia Associated with Chronic Renal Disease, J. Lab. & Clin. Med. 41, 56, 1953.

70a. GERRITSEN, T. and WALKER, A. R. P.: The Effect of Habitually High Iron Intake on Certain Blood Values in Pregnant Bantu Women, J. Clin. Invest., 33, 23, 1954.

70b. GREEN, H. N., WAKEFIELD, JUNE and LITTLEWOOD, G.: The Nature of Cancer Anaemia and Its Bearing on the Immunological Theory of Cancer, Brit. M. J., 2, 779, 1957.

71. HUBBARD, J. P. and McKEE, M. H.: Anemia of Rheumatic Fever, J. Pediat., 14, 66, 1939.

71a. HYMAN, G. A.: Studies on Anemia of Disseminated Malignant Neoplastic Disease, Blood, 9, 911, 1954; Am. J. Med., 19, 350, 1955; Blood, 12, 1114, 1957; Am. J. Roentgenol., 79, 511, 1958; Cancer Res., 18, 959, 1958.

72. JAFFÉ, R. H.: Severe Anemia of Aplastic Type Associated With Sclerosis of Thyroid Gland, Arch. Int. Med., 61, 19, 1938.

72a. JONES, P. N., WEINSTEIN, I. M., ETTINGER, R. H. and CAPPS, R. B.: Decreased Red Cell Survival Associated with Liver Disease, Arch. Int. Med., 95, 93, 1955.

72b. KAYE, M.: The Anemia Associated with Renal Disease, J. Lab. & Clin. Med., 52, 83, 1958.

73. KEEFER, C. S., YANG, C. S. and HUANG, K. K.: Anemia Associated With Chronic Dysentery, Arch. Int. Med., 47, 436, 1931.

73a. KEIDERLING, W.: Uber die Ferrokinetik beim Infekt, Schweiz. med. Wchnschr., 88, 965, 1958.

73b. KHO LIEN-KENG: Erythroblastopenia with Giant Pro-Erythroblasts in Kwashiorkor, Blood, 12, 171, 1957.

74. KÜHNEL, P.: Untersuchungen über die physi-

ologische Schwangerschaftsanämie, Ztschr. Geburtsh. u. Gynäk., *90*, 511, 1926.

74a. LACHMANN, A., LUND, E. and VINTHER-PAULSEN, N.: Severe Refractory Anæmia in Pregnancy, Acta obst. et gynec. scandinav., *33*, 395, 1954.

74b. LEWIS, S. M. and PORTER, I. H.: Erythrocyte Survival in Rheumatoid Arthritis, Ann. Rheumat. Dis., *19*, 54, 1960.

75. LOGE, J. P., LANGE, R. D. and MOORE, C. V.: Characterization of the Anemia Associated with Chronic Renal Insufficiency, Am. J. Med., *24*, 4, 1958.

76. LUNDSTRÖM, P.: Studies on Erythroid Elements and Serum Iron in Normal Pregnancy, Upsala Läkaref ör. Förhandlingar, *55*, 1, 1949.

77. MAYER, C. F.: Epidemic Panmyelosis in the Russian Grain Belt, Mil. Surgeon, *113*, 173 and 295, 1953.

78. MIDDLETON, W. S. and BURKE, M.: Streptococcus Viridans Endocarditis Lenta, Am. J. M. Sc., *198*, 301, 1939.

78a. MILLER, A., CHODOS, R. B., EMERSON, C. P. and ROSS, J. F.: Studies of the Anemia and Iron Metabolism in Cancer, J. Clin. Invest., *35*, 1248, 1956.

79. MORGENSEN, E.: The Anemia of Gastric Cancer, Folia hæmat., *56*, 206, 1936.

79a. MUIRHEAD, E. E., JONES, F. and GROLLMAN, A.: The Anemia of Renal Insufficiency as Induced by Bilateral Nephrectomy of the Rabbit, J. Lab. & Clin. Med., *39*, 505, 1952; Ann. Int. Med., *40*, 307, 1954; J. Lab. & Clin. Med., *51*, 49, 1958.

79b. NAETS, J. P., BRAUMAN, H. and KRAYTMAN, M.: Etude de l'érythropoïèse au cours de l'insuffisance rénale aigue et chronique, Acta haemat., *24*, 169, 1960.

80. NORDENSON, N. G.: The Bone Marrow in the Anemia of Chronic Nephritis, Folia hæmat., *59*, 1, 1938.

80a. OPPENHEIM, A., ABELS, J. C., PACK, G. T. and RHOADS, C. P.: Metabolic Studies in Patients With Cancer of the Gastrointestinal Tract, J.A.M.A., *127*, 273, 1945.

81. OTTO, G. F.: Blood Studies on Trichuris-infested and Worm-free Children in Louisiana, Am. J. Trop. Med., *15*, 693, 1935.

82. PRICE, V. E. and GREENFIELD, R. E.: Anemia in Cancer *in Advances in Cancer Research*, New York, Academic Press Inc., 1958, p. 199; J. Nat. Cancer Inst., *21*, 641, and 1099, 1958.

82a. PRITCHARD, J. A. and ADAMS, R. H.: Erythrocyte Production and Destruction during Pregnancy, Am. J. Obst. & Gynec., *79*, 750, 1960.

83. ROBSCHEIT-ROBBINS, F. and WHIPPLE, G.:

Infection and Intoxication: Their Influence Upon Hemoglobin Production in Experimental Anemia, J. Exper. Med., *63*, 767, 1936.

84. RODRIGUEZ-MOLINA, R. and PONS, J. A.: Hematological Studies on Schistosomiasis Mansoni in Puerto Rico, Puerto Rico J. Pub. Health & Trop. Med., *11*, 369, 1936.

85. ROSAHN, P. D. and PEARCE, L.: Blood Cytology in Untreated and Treated Syphilis, Am. J. M. Sc., *187*, 88, 1934.

86. SAIFI, M. F. and VAUGHAN, J. M.: The Anæmia Associated With Infection, J. Path. & Bacteriol., *56*, 189, 1944; Brit. M. J., *1*, 35, 1948.

86a. SCHARFMAN, W. B. and PROPP, S.: Anemia Associated with Vitamin D Intoxication, New England J. Med., *255*, 1207, 1956.

87. SCHIAVONE, D. J. and RUBBO, S. D.: Anæmia Associated with Hæmophilus Influenzæ Meningitis, Lancet, *2*, 696, 1953.

88. SHARP, E. A. and MACK, H. C.: The Relationship of Hemopoietic Phenomena to Endocrine Disorders in Women, Endocrinology, *24*, 202, 1939.

88a. SHEETS, R. F., HAMILTON, H. E., DEGOWIN, E. L. and JANNEY, C. D.: Spontaneous and X-ray-Induced Hemolysis in Malignancy. J. Clin. Invest., *33*, 179, 1954.

88b. SHERMAN, J. D., RICKARD, CARMEN, CHRISTIAN, R. S. and FRIEDELL, G. H.: In Vitro Studies on the Anemia of Tumor-Bearing Hamsters, Blood, *15*, 130, 1960.

89. SNAPPER, I., GROEN, J., HUNTER, D. and WITTS, L. J.: Achlorhydria, Anemia and Subacute Combined Degeneration in Pituitary and Gonadal Insufficiency, Quart. J. Med., *6*, 195, 1937; Lancet, *2*, 307. 1942.

89a. SUMMERS, V. K.: The Anæmia of Hypopituitarism, Brit. M. J., *1*, 787, 1952.

90. TAUBER, E. G. and GOLDMAN, L.: Syphilitic Anemia With Diffuse Osteitis Superinfection, Am. J. Syph., *19*, 339, 1935.

91. TOWNSEND, S. R. and PIJOAN, J.: Action of Urea, Indican, and Phenol on Red Cell Hemolysis, Proc. Soc. Exper. Biol. & Med., *37*, 236, 1937.

92. VEREL, D., TURNBULL, A., TUDHOPE, G. R. and ROSS, J. H.: Anaemia in Bright's Disease, Quart. J. Med., *28*, 491, 1959.

93. VERLOOP, M. C., BLOKHUIS, E. W. M. and BOS, C. C.: Uber die Ursachen der (physiologischen) Schwangerschaftsanämie, Schweiz. med. Wchnschr., *88*, 1051, 1958; Acta haemat., *22*, 158, 1959.

94. WEINSTEIN, I. M.: A Correlative Study of the Erythrokinetics and Disturbances in Iron Metabolism Associated with the Anemia of Rheumatoid Arthritis, Blood, *14*, 950, 1959.

95. WINTROBE, M. M.: Erythrocyte in Man, Medicine, *9*, 195, 1930.

96. WINTROBE, M. M.: Relation of Disease of the Liver to Anemia, Arch. Int. Med., *57*, 289, 1936.

96a.WINTROBE, M. M., GREENBERG, G. R., HUMPHREYS, S. R., ASHENBRUGKER, H., WORTH, W. and KRAMER, R.: The Anemia of Infection, J. Clin. Invest., *26*, 103, 114, and 121, 1947; Blood, *2*, 323, 1947; J. Clin. Invest., *27*, 245, 1948; J. Lab. & Clin. Med., *33*, 532, 1948.

96b.WOLFF, J. R. and LIMARZI, L. R.: Anemia in Pregnancy, J.A.M.A., *128*, 482, 1945.

96c.ZIEVE, L.: Jaundice, Hyperlipemia and Hemolytic Anemia, Ann. Int. Med., *48*, 471, 1958.

Myelofibrosis and Myelophthisic Anemia (Leuko-erythroblastosis)

96d.BOWDLER, A. J. and PRANKERD, T. A. J.: Primary Myeloid Metaplasia, Brit. M. J., *1*, 1352, 1961.

97. CARPENTER, G. and FLORY, C. M.: Chronic Non-leukemic Myelosis, Arch. Int. Med., *67*, 489, 1941.

98. CHAPMAN, E. M.: Osteosclerotic Anemia, Am. J. M. Sc., *185*, 181, 1933.

98a.COOK, J. E., FRANKLIN, J. W., HAMILTON, H. E. and FOWLER, W. M.: Syndrome of Myelofibrosis, Arch. Int. Med., *91*, 704, 1953.

99. CRAIL, H. W., ALT, H. L. and NADLER, W. H.: Myelofibrosis Associated with Tuberculosis, Blood, *3*, 1426, 1948.

100. DOWNEY, H. and NORDLAND, M.: Hematologic and Histologic Study of a Case of Myeloid Megakaryocytic Hepato-Splenomegaly, Folia hæmat., *62*, 1, 1939.

101. ERF, L. A. and HERBUT, P. A.: Primary and Secondary Myelofibrosis, Ann. Int. Med., *21*, 863, 1944.

102. FAVRE, M., CROIZAT, P. and GUICHARD, A.: La myélose aleucémique mégacaryocytaire, Ann. de Méd., *35*, 5, 1934.

102a.GREEN, T. W., CONLEY, C. L., ASHBURN, L. L. and PETERS, H. R.: Splenectomy for Myeloid Metaplasia of the Spleen, New England J. Med., *248*, 211, 1953.

103. HEWER, T. F.: Megakaryocytic Myelosis With Osteosclerosis, J. Path. & Bact., *45*, 383, 1937.

104. HICKLING, R. A.: Chronic Non-leukemic Myelosis, Quart. J. Med., *6*, 253, 1937; Brit. M. J., *2*, 411, 1953.

104a.HUTT, M. S. R., PINNIGER, J. L. and WETHERLEY-MEIN, G.: The Myeloproliferative Disorders, Blood, *8*, 295, 1953.

105. JACKSON, H., JR., PARKER, F., JR. and LEMON, H. M.: Agnogenic Myeloid Metaplasia of the Spleen, New England J. Med., *222*, 985, 1940; Science, *93*, 541, 1941.

105a.KORST, D. R., CLATANOFF, D. V. and SCHILLING, R. F.: On Myelofibrosis, Arch. Int. Med., *97*, 169, 1956.

106. LEIGH, T. F. *et al.:* Myelofibrosis, Am. J. Roentgenol., *82*, 183, 1959.

106a.LEONARD, B. J., ISRAËLS, M. C. G. and WILKINSON, J. F.: Myelosclerosis, Quart. J. Med., *26*, 131, 1957.

107. LINDEBOOM, G. A.: Über die sogenannte aleukämische megakaryocytäre Myelose, Acta med. scandinav., *95*, 388, 1938.

108. LUCEY, H. C.: Leuco-erythroblastic Anæmia Resembling Acholuric Jaundice, Lancet, *2*, 76, 1939.

110. MENDELOFF, J. and ROSENTHAL, N.: Leukoerythroblastic Anemia With Diffuse Osteosclerosis, Ann. Int. Med., *19*, 518, 1943.

111. METTIER, S. R.: Hematologic Aspects of Space Consuming Lesions of the Bone Marrow (Myelophthisic Anemia), Ann. Int. Med., *14*, 436, 1940.

111a.MOESCHLIN, S.: Leucémies myéloides et pseudo-leucémies. Leur diagnostic différentiel par la ponction de la rate, Rév. méd., de la Suisse rom., *69*, 633, 1949.

111b.NATHAN, D. G. and BERLIN, N. I.: Studies of the Production and Life Span of Erythrocytes in Myeloid Metaplasia, Blood, *14*, 668, 1959.

111c.OISHI, N., SWISHER, S. N. and TROUP, S. B.: Busulfan Therapy in Myeloid Metaplasia, Blood, *15*, 863, 1960.

111d.ROHR, K.: Myelofibrose und Osteomyelosklerose, Acta haemat., *15*, 209, 1956; *ibid.*, *20*, 63, 1958.

112. ROSENTHAL, N. and ERF, L. A.: Clinical Observations on Osteopetrosis and Myelofibrosis, Arch. Int. Med., *71*, 793, 1943.

113. ROWLAND, R. S.: Schüller-Christian's Disease, Am. J. Roentgenol., *30*, 649, 1933.

114. STEPHENS, D. J. and BREDECK, J. F.: Aleukemic Myelosis With Osteosclerosis, Ann. Int. Med., *6*, 1087, 1933.

115. VAUGHAN, J. M.: Leuco-erythroblastic Anæmia, J. Path. & Bact., *42*, 541, 1936.

116. VAUGHAN, J. M. and HARRISON, C. V.: Leuco-erythroblastic Anæmia and Myelosclerosis, J. Path. & Bact., *48*, 339, 1939.

117. WAUGH, T. R.: Hemolytic Anemia in Carcinomatosis of the Bone Marrow, Am. J. M. Sc., *191*, 160, 1936.

118. WYATT, J. P. and SOMMERS, S. C.: Chronic Marrow Failure, Myelosclerosis and Extramedullary Hematopoiesis, Blood, *5*, 329, 1950.

Chapter 12

Normocytic Anemias—(*Continued*)
Hemolytic Anemias

HEMOLYTIC ANEMIAS

Definition and Classification.— Studies of erythrokinetics have shown that many forms of anemia are associated with shortened survival of the patient's erythrocytes. In many instances, however, this is not the primary fault responsible for the development of the anemia. Thus, for example, a shortened red cell life span has been observed in iron deficiency anemia. Here it is clear that such shortened survival as may be present is the consequence of impaired construction of erythrocytes resulting from lack of iron. No evidence of increased breakdown is found in studies of pigment metabolism; in fact, the serum bilirubin tends to be extremely low. The same can be said of the anemia associated with infection and of the anemia accompanying many forms of illness. These are not considered to be hemolytic anemias.

In another group of disorders, of which pernicious anemia is a prime example, clear signs of increased blood destruction are demonstrable. Measurements of erythrocyte life span are not needed to demonstrate the breakdown of red cells. In pernicious anemia breakdown of red corpuscles or a shunt in pigment metabolism takes place in the bone marrow (p. 483). In a sense these are hemolytic anemias. However, they are not usually classified as such. They are thought of, as a rule, as anemias associated with nutritional deficiency.

There remains a large variety of disorders in which signs of increased blood destruction are usually obvious. In contrast to the disorders mentioned above, the shortened survival of the red cells is more clearly associated with the clinical manifestations. The term "hemolytic anemia" is generally reserved for these conditions. This is admittedly an imperfect compromise since the magnitude of the increased blood destruction ranges from slight to extremely marked. Furthermore, in some instances no anemia is present because the increased breakdown is compensated by increased production. A distinction between hemolytic *disease* and hemolytic *anemia* could be made, if one wishes, but patients with hemolytic disease often develop decompensation at some time in their course. In general, it is

(598)

better to refer to each disease falling under this head by its specific name, if one is known.

The hemolytic anemias have been *classified* as acute and chronic, in accordance with their clinical manifestations but this has limited usefulness since fulminating symptoms may develop in the course of chronic disorders. On much firmer ground is their differentiation as congenital and acquired. This classification is based not only on a genetic foundation but also on the fact that the manifestations of the congenital forms are the consequence of an intrinsic abnormality of the erythrocytes whereas in the acquired forms, as a rule, the defect is extracorpuscular; that is, due to the action of external agents on normally constructed cells. Thus it has been shown that when normal corpuscles are transfused to patients in whom there is an extracorpuscular cause for hemolysis, the donated corpuscles are destroyed as rapidly as the patient's own cells. If, on the other hand, the patient's corpuscles are removed from their unfavorable environment and are transfused to a normal recipient, their survival time is normal.[20a] When the disorder is due to an intrinsic defect of the red corpuscles, the patient's corpuscles, when given to a normal recipient, are disposed of more rapidly than those of the recipient; the latter's corpuscles, if transfused into the patient, maintain a normal "life span". This is the basis for the classification presented in Table 12–1.

Even this classification has its limitations, however. Thus, paroxysmal nocturnal hemoglobinuria seems to be due to an intrinsic abnormality of the patient's red cells; yet there is no evidence of a genetic cause. Again, hemolytic disease of the newborn is congenital, yet not hereditary, and is acquired from the mother. Finally, in certain drug-induced hemolytic anemias, the susceptibility to hemolysis appears to be inherited.

Development of Knowledge Concerning the Hemolytic Anemias.— Hayem (1898), and later Widal, Abrami and Brule (1907–12) pointed out that, whereas the classical congenital hemolytic anemia of Minkowski and Chauffard often caused few symptoms, another type, which they regarded as acquired, often was associated with severe anemia and profound illness.[46,115] They included cases of excessive blood destruction associated with various infections or intoxications, as well as cases of unknown etiology. In the latter, autohemagglutination was frequently noted. Chauffard[43b] was able to demonstrate autohemolysins in the serum of a few cases of acute, acquired hemolytic anemia and spoke of "hemolysinic icterus." Nevertheless, doubt existed for many years that there is a true "acquired" form of hemolytic jaundice and little attention was paid to the possibility that an immune body reaction might play an important rôle. Lederer[63] called attention to an acute, idiopathic hemolytic anemia which was dramatically cured by a single blood transfusion. Subsequently similar cases attracted attention[51] and the fact that they were distinct from cases of congenital hemolytic jaundice in crisis came to be recognized. The existence of acquired hemolytic anemia in contrast to the congenital form was clearly established by Dameshek and Schwartz[46] who demonstrated abnormal hemolysins in patients suffering from acute hemolytic anemia and showed that spherocytosis and increased osmotic fragility can develop during the course of such anemia in man and in acute hemolytic anemia produced experimentally in animals.

The subsequent development of the field can be credited in large part to the application of serological technics to the study of hematological disorders. In particular, the discovery that erythrocytes sensitized by "incomplete" antibodies can be recognized by the use of

Table 12–1—Classification of Hemolytic Disorders

I. *Intracorpuscular Defects.*
  A. Hereditary spherocytosis (familial or congenital hemolytic jaundice)
  B. Hereditary elliptocytosis
  C. Congenital non-spherocytic hemolytic anemias
  D. Miscellaneous congenital hemolytic anemias ("Inclusion-body," "Heinz body," "Pappenheimer body")
  E. Hereditary leptocytosis (thalassemia, Mediterranean anemia)
  F. Sickle cell disease
  G. Other hereditary hemoglobinopathies (C, D, E, G, H, I, etc.)
  H. Combinations of thalassemia and sickle cell disease or other hemoglobinopathies
  I. Paroxysmal nocturnal hemoglobinuria

II. *Extracorpuscular Causes.*
  A. Infectious Agents
    1. Protozoal parasites: malaria
    2. Non-protozoal blood parasites: *Bartonella* (Oroya fever)
    3. Viruses: primary atypical pneumonia, infectious mononucleosis
    4. Bacteria: *Cl. welchii, V. comma,* rarely others

  B. Chemical Agents
    a. Those related to size of dose:

Phenylhydrazine	Phenacetin	Methyl chloride
Trinitrotoluene	Dinitrobenzene	Allyl-propyldisulfide
Toluene	Anilin	Arsine
Benzene	Saponin	Lead
Nitrobenzene	Lecithin	Colloidal silver
Acetanilid	Promin	Water

    b. Those depending on hypersensitivity:

Sulfonamides	Sulfones	Benzedrine
Primaquine	Nitrofurantoin	Neoarsphenamine
Pamaquin	Phenothiazine	p-aminosalicylic acid
Naphthalene	Paraphenylinediamine	"cryogénine"
Quinine	Vit. K substitutes	"myanesin"
Quinidine	Mesantoin	Probenecid

  C. Physical Agents (heat—severe thermal burns)

  D. Vegetable and animal poisons
    a. Vegetable poisons:
      (1) Fava bean (Favism)
      (2) Baghdad Spring Anemia
      (3) Castor bean
    b. Animal poisons:
      (1) Snake venoms
      (2) Endogenous agents

  E. Iso-agglutinins
    1. Mismatched transfusions (anti-A, anti-B)
    2. "Intra-group" transfusion reactions (anti-Rh, anti-Kell, etc.)
    3. Hemolytic disease of the newborn (anti-Rh [D,c,E], etc.), anti-A, anti-B, anti-Kell, etc.

  F. Paroxysmal cold hemoglobinuria

  G. Symptomatic hemolytic anemias
    a. Hemopoietic disorders
      (1) Chronic lymphocytic leukemia
      (2) Hodgkin's disease
      (3) Lymphosarcoma
      (4) Miscellaneous (sarcoidosis, myelofibrosis, etc.)
    b. Collagen disorders, especially disseminated lupus erythematosus
    c. Miscellaneous conditions (ovarian tumors, liver disease, etc.)
    d. Thrombotic thrombocytopenic purpura

  H. Idiopathic acquired hemolytic anemias

anti-human globulin sera prepared by immunizing rabbits against human serum proteins (Coombs' test, p. 622) proved to be of unique value in the study of acquired hemolytic anemias, as did also the observation that enzymes such as trypsin increase the susceptibility of human erythrocytes to certain types of antibodies. In another direction, the rediscovery of the usefulness of differential agglutination in the study of the survival of red corpuscles in the circulation and the introduction of other methods for this purpose (p. 163), made it possible to distinguish hemolytic anemias due to defects intrinsic in the red corpuscles from those produced by external factors.

In still another direction, progress came from recognition of the distinctive features of sickle cell hemoglobin and of the importance of molecular abnormalities in the causation of disease (p. 686) as well as from studies of the metabolism of the red corpuscle (p. 123). These developments led to the discovery of a variety of abnormal hemoglobins, each of which produces its characteristic marks in those who form them (p. 162), and also opened the door to a better understanding of the nature of intracorpuscular defects such as occur in hereditary spherocytosis. They may also give some insight into the means whereby toxic agents damage red corpuscles (p. 624).

Since there are a number of features common to all hemolytic anemias and since, from the clinical standpoint, it is necessary first to recognize that the case at hand represents a hemolytic disorder rather than some other type of anemia, it is proposed to consider first certain general aspects of the symptomatology, classification and etiology, diagnosis, treatment and pathogenesis of the hemolytic anemias. Subsequently, in this and the following chapter, certain well defined entities among the hemolytic diseases will be considered separately. The catabolism of hemoglobin has been considered already in Chapter 3 (p. 173).

General Symptomatology. — Hemolytic anemias may be acute, subacute or chronic, and the course of the latter may be interrupted by phases of more or less rapid destruction of cells. There may be only slight icterus of the skin and sclerae without anemia and no complaints: the description, "more yellow than sick" has been applied to some cases of chronic hereditary jaundice. Symptoms other than slight exertional dyspnea may be entirely absent. In patients with familial hemolytic jaundice and in sickle cell anemia, it is the interruptions of the chronic course of the disease, as by attacks of abdominal pain, which bring the disorder to attention. In other cases, complications which are the result of the chronic blood destruction and anemia, such as gall bladder disease and leg ulcers, are the outstanding complaints. In still other cases of hemolytic anemia the course may be acute and fulminating.

Onset.—The onset of hemolytic anemia may be fulminating, symptoms developing in the course of a few days; in other cases the history indicates the rapid progression of symptoms in the course of about a month, while in still others the development of the disorder appears to have been very gradual. In congenital and familial cases, an episode of weakness or yellowness may be recalled months or years before, which may have been repeated; or no symptoms whatever and no time of onset may have been recognized.

In acute forms of hemolytic anemia, and during the acute episodes which may punctuate the course of the chronic variety, the symptoms often suggest an acute febrile illness: sudden weakness, malaise, headache, restlessness, irritability, pain in the back and extremities, and anorexia. Nausea, vomiting, diarrhea and abdominal pain may be present.

Hemolysis may be so rapid that hemoglobinuria results. Hemorrhagic manifestations such as epistaxis, purpura, hematuria, and retinal hemorrhages are unusual but may appear in severe cases. Coma and paralysis may develop.

Symptoms of Rapid Destruction of Blood.—Rapid destruction of blood is associated with aching pain in the back, abdomen or limbs, headache, malaise and a severe shaking chill, followed by fever. The abdominal pain may be so severe and may be accompanied by such marked muscular rigidity and spasm as to simulate an acute surgical condition. Profound prostration and shock may occur. The cause of the shock is not clear but one of the important factors in its production may well be a reduction in total blood volume resulting from the rapid destruction of red cells and their removal from the circulation.[13] It appears that the greatest proportion of the products of red cell destruction is neither left in the circulation nor excreted by the kidneys but is rapidly removed by the body tissues.

Anuria or oliguria may develop, more because of circulatory collapse than as the result of obstruction of the renal tubules by precipitated hemoglobin (p. 362). When urine is passed, it is found to be very dark. Jaundice develops very rapidly. With the production of anemia, weakness, palpitation and other characteristic symptoms make their appearance.

Vascular Disturbances.—In transfusion reactions, particularly, urticaria is common and in paroxysmal cold hemoglobinuria vascular disturbances suggesting those of Raynaud's disease frequently appear. Such symptoms occur in other types of hemolytic anemia as well and they may be not only of a spastic and temporary character but signs of thrombosis and gangrene may develop.[101c] These complications suggest that hemolysis in many instances is preceded by agglutination of red corpuscles or may be accompanied by damage to the endothelial lining of blood vessels or accumulation in the blood vessels of the products of red cell destruction. Absence of the normal vasodilatation which occurs below 15° C. has been demonstrated in association with high-titer cold hemagglutination.[58] Red node-like spots on the hands, abdominal pain followed by hemorrhage from the bowel, infarction of the spleen, the lungs, and in the nervous system, and thrombosis in the arteries and veins of the extremities have been observed in cases of sickle cell anemia, acute hemolytic anemia and nocturnal hemoglobinuria.

Physical Findings.—In addition to the manifestations already mentioned, pallor of varying degree is found, as well as jaundice. The latter may be barely perceptible or very obvious. Pruritus is not associated with the icterus due to increased blood destruction. Splenomegaly, except in sickle cell anemia, is common in hemolytic anemias, whether acute or chronic, and enlargement of the liver may occur as well. Patients with sickle cell anemia often appear underdeveloped and they, as well as those who are the victims of familial hemolytic jaundice, may show skeletal abnormalities such as tower-shaped skull or excessive numbers of digits. In these conditions, as well as in thalassemia, characteristic changes in the bones are often demonstrable by roentgenoscopic examinations. These no doubt represent the effect of the continuously stimulated hematopoiesis on bone formation. Chronic leg ulcers are common in sickle cell anemia and may be seen in hereditary spherocytosis.

Findings in the Blood, Urine and Stool.—In an earlier chapter (p. 167), the manner of blood destruction was described and the appearance of the products of hemoglobin breakdown in the blood, urine and stools was discussed

(p. 173). The nature of the breakdown products depends on the rate of blood destruction and the extent to which breakdown is occurring intra- or extravascularly. *When destruction is rapid,* free hemoglobin reaches the blood stream and hemoglobinemia and methemalbuminemia develop. If the capacity of the haptoglobin and albumin to combine with hemoglobin and its breakdown products is exceeded the hemoglobin passes the kidney barrier and hemoglobinuria occurs as well. An interesting possibility which deserves investigation is that the amount or rate of haptoglobin production may be abnormal in certain disorders and this, rather than rapid utilization of haptoglobin because of continuing intravascular hemolysis, may be the cause of persisting hemoglobinemia and hemoglobinuria.[3b] When hemoglobinuria occurs, hemosiderin is likely to be found in the urine as well. In addition, the urine may contain protein and granular and red cell casts.

More often, blood destruction is less rapid. In such cases hemoglobinemia and hemoglobinuria are not found and there is only an increase in the icterus index, serum bilirubin, and urobilinogen excretion in the urine and stools. Even though there may be no demonstrable hemoglobinuria, hemosiderin may nevertheless be found in the urine. The urine does not contain bile (therefore the term acholuric). The stools assume a dark color and from 300 to 4000 mg. of urobilinogen may be found in the 24-hour stool, as compared with the normal of 40 to 280 mg. The 24-hour urine may contain 5 to 200 mg. of urobilinogen (normal, 0 to 3.5 mg.). It is noteworthy that the fecal urobilinogen may be increased when the urine urobilinogen and the bilirubin in the blood are not significantly greater than normal.

The intensity of bilirubinemia depends not only on the extent of blood destruction but also on the capacity of the liver to remove the pigment from the blood stream and excrete it in the bile. Only a small proportion passes through the kidneys. The normal liver has been found to excrete in twenty-four hours an amount of bilirubin derivable from the destruction of about $12\frac{1}{2}$ grams of hemoglobin but its reserve capacity is much greater than this.[13] In cases of hemolytic anemia, however, the added burden of work is met by a liver functionally impaired as the result of degenerative changes in the liver epithelial cells resulting from the anoxemia produced by the anemia.

When the hemolytic anemia is due to the presence of autoantibodies, agglutination of the red cells may be seen by allowing oxalated blood to flow in a thin layer along the side of a glass container. The agglutination may also be observed in the blood film, especially when the disorder is due to the presence of cold antibodies. It may, in fact, be difficult to make good blood smears in the latter case unless the coverslip or slide has first been warmed to 37° C.

The anemia may be of any degree, depending upon the severity of the hemolytic process and the rate of regeneration. As pointed out in an earlier chapter (p. 181), the bone marrow is capable of a seven- or eight-fold increase in productive capacity and thus it is possible for erythrocyte survival to be reduced even to fifteen days without anemia necessarily developing. To parallel the terminology of the cardiologist, this might be termed *"compensated hemolytic disease."* Anemia represents "decompensation."

The anemia may be normocytic or macrocytic. The *morphology of the blood* to some extent is correlated with the severity of the hemolytic process. The classical picture consists of marked variation in the size of the red corpuscles, usually relatively little poikilocytosis (except in sickle cell anemia), and signs of active red cell regeneration. **Reticulocytes** are greatly increased in number, it being common to find 10 to 25 per cent in chronic cases, and as many as 60 per cent or even more in acute cases. There is marked polychromatophilia and numerous normoblasts and macroblasts are present. The immature cells are usually larger than the mature corpuscles and, when immature forms are very numerous, the anemia is likely to be macrocytic.

At the same time that there is delivery of premature red cells (normoblasts and reticulocytes) from the bone marrow, there is marked stimulation of the **leukopoietic tissues.** There is leukocytosis, a "shift to the left" and myelocytes and even rare myeloblasts may be found. Leukocyte counts as high as 132,000 have been recorded. **Platelets** may be very numerous and are often unusually large or otherwise abnormal in appearance. It is noteworthy that these morphological and numerical abnormalites in the leukocytes and platelets, although most common in acute hemolytic anemias, may be encountered even in chronic forms of hemolytic anemia, such as sickle cell anemia, in the absence of an acute phase of blood destruction. In certain cases, however, leukopenia[46] and even slight thrombocytopenia are found (see p. 641).

Spherocytes, which stain bright red and show no central pallor are characteristic of hereditary spherocytosis and may be found in other forms of hemolytic anemia. Their appearance results from their excessive thickness, which is due to their relatively spherical shape. These cells are usually smaller in diameter than normal cells. All grades of spherocytosis are found. The unusual shape of the red corpuscles can be observed also by studying rouleau formation in fresh preparations of blood. Instead of the long rouleaux made up of erythrocytes of equal thickness which are characteristic of normal blood, the rouleaux are hardly ever straight, rarely lengthy and often decidedly bizarre in appearance. These changes are due to the spherical shape of some of the red corpuscles and the great diversity in their thickness.[6] The corpuscular hemoglobin concentration of spherocytes is greater than normal and this is reflected often in a greater mean corpuscular hemoglobin concentration (M.C.H.C.).[13c]

There are actually two types of spherocytes, namely, the hereditary form characteristic of hereditary spherocytosis and the type found in acquired hemolytic anemias. The former, although governed by a genetic factor, are not spherical at their origin; that is, their nucleated precursors in the bone marrow are not abnormal and even in the reticulocyte stage there is little or no evidence of the spherical shape. It is in the course of their life span that a progressive and striking increase in their thickness occurs. These cells undergo autohemolysis *in vitro* more rapidly than do normal cells.[5c] The "acquired" spherocyte is similar morphologically to the hereditary form but represents a normal corpuscle whose cell surface has been damaged. Spherocytes should be distinguished from *spherical forms* of red corpuscles which can be produced by suspending normal red cells in saline or sugar-containing media, a process which can be reversed by the addition of plasma or serum to the suspension.

Schistocytes, the products of red cell fragmentation, are seldom seen in normal blood but are common in hemolytic anemias. They may take a variety of forms: triangular cells, small elliptical cells, cells appearing to have been indented and irregularly crenated cells ("burr cells"). These fragmented corpuscles are found, in particular, in hemolytic anemias associated with burns or due to chemical poisons.

In cases of hemolytic anemia due to

auto-immune hemolytic disease, in paroxysmal cold hemoglobinuria, in hemolytic disease of the newborn and even in hemolytic disorders associated with septicemias,[25] protozoan infections and chemical poisoning, erythrocytes may be seen occasionally in blood films which have undergone phagocytosis by monocytes and, sometimes, neutrophils. Such **erythrophagocytosis** can be demonstrated more rapidly by incubating the heparinized blood at 37° C. or even at room temperature for an hour.[4e] Blood from patients with non-hematological disorders has not been found to behave in this manner. The same phenomenon has been produced artificially by incubating red and white blood cells with antisera containing specific iso-antibodies and with serum from cases of auto-immune hemolytic disease. It has been observed also that only those antibodies which are capable of causing hemolysis in the presence of complement regularly produce erythrophagocytosis.[5c] It is likely that phagocytes containing red corpuscles are rapidly removed from the circulation by the lungs and spleen. There is no clinical evidence that erythrophagocytosis contributes significantly to the degree of anemia.

Alterations in the osmotic and mechanical fragility of the erythrocytes may occur and, in certain types of hemolytic anemia, Heinz bodies (p. 624) may be demonstrable. These and other findings which assist in differentiating the various types of hemolytic anemia will be considered later in the section on Diagnosis (p. 617).

Bone Marrow. — As might be expected from the character of the blood findings, the bone marrow is very hyperplastic. As many as 60 per cent, or more, of the nucleated cells in smears of sternal marrow as obtained by puncture or biopsy may belong in the erythrocytic series, instead of about 20 per cent or less, which is the normal number. In other words, the myeloid: erythroid (M:E) ratio shifts from the normal of 4 or 5:1 to about 1:1 or even less.

These cells are of the normoblast or the macroblast type, and even when deeply basophilic, primitive forms are found, they do not show the peculiar, scroll-work type of nuclear chromatin which is characteristic of many of the nucleated red cells in the marrow of cases of pernicious anemia and related forms of macrocytic anemia. There may be numerous mitoses.

Because of the increased proportion of nucleated red corpuscles, the number of leukocytes is relatively reduced. The ratio of the various types of leukocytes to one another is about normal or there is a slight "shift to the left." The bizarre forms found in pernicious anemia (p. 480) are absent.

Etiology.—The underlying disturbance which is responsible for the changes which have been described varies in different types of hemolytic anemia. Many of the chronic forms of hemolytic anemia are the result of an inherited defect in the formation of the red corpuscles, whereas the more acute and subacute forms are more often the consequence of the action of hemolytic agents or hemolysins of one type or another. The findings in the blood and bone marrow represent the products of blood destruction and the effects of the stimulation of the marrow and of the tissues responsible for the removal of the residua of hemolysis. Splenomegaly and demonstrable abnormalities in bone structure may be regarded as the effects of long-continued overactivity of the spleen and bone marrow. It is less evident why leg ulcers and peculiar abnormalities in the heart should occur in sickle cell anemia.

I. Hemolytic Anemias Due to Intracorpuscular Defects.—These include hereditary spherocytosis, sickle cell anemia and a number of other well defined disease entitites listed in Table 12–1. Since these disorders, in addition to the manifestations common to all hemolytic diseases, are marked by features which are unique, each will be described separately in subsequent sections (p. 640 *et seq.*).

II. **Hemolytic Anemias Due to Extracorpuscular Factors.**—Because malaria, taking the world as a whole, is so common, hemolytic anemias due to infectious agents are the most frequent of the acquired hemolytic anemias. In ordinary practice in the Western world, however, such hemolytic anemias are rare. Even those attributable to chemical agents are less often encountered than "idiopathic" hemolytic anemias, with or without demonstrable autoantibodies, or hemolytic anemias associated with various disorders ("symptomatic hemolytic anemias"). Nevertheless, since the differentiation of the idiopathic varieties is in part based on the exclusion of recognized causes and requires a knowledge of them, the known factors concerned in the development of hemolytic anemias due to extracorpuscular causes will be discussed first.

(A) **Infectious Agents.**—1. **Protozoal Parasites.**—The anemia in **malaria** is due to the destruction of red corpuscles by the Plasmodia which develop within them and the severity of the anemia is in large measure directly correlated with the intensity and duration of the infection. Although the cause of this form of hemolytic anemia is originally extrinsic, the malarial organisms actually produce erythrocyte destruction through their presence in the corpuscles. The osmotic and mechanical fragility of parasitized corpuscles have been shown to be increased.[32h] As the parasites complete their cycle of development and invade and destroy new corpuscles, more anemia and deeper jaundice are produced. The anemia is usually normocytic although, when blood destruction

LEGEND FOR PLATE X.—*P. falciparum*

1. Very young ring form trophozoite.
2. Double infection of single cell with young trophozoites, one a "marginal form," the other "signet ring" form.
3, 4. Young trophozoites showing double chromatin dots.
5, 6, 7. Developing trophozoite forms.
8. Three medium trophozoites in one cell.
9. Trophozoite showing pigment, in a cell containing Maurer's spots.
10, 11. Two trophozoites in each of two cells, showing variation of forms which parasites may assume.
12. Almost mature trophozoite showing haze of pigment throughout cytoplasm. Maurer's spots in the cell.
13. Aestivo-autumnal "slender forms."
14. Mature trophozoite, showing clumped pigment.
15. Parasite in the process of initial chromatin division.
16, 17, 18, 19. Various phases of the development of the schizont ("presegmenting schizonts").
20. Mature schizont.
21, 22, 23, 24. Successive forms in the development of the gametocyte—usually not found in the peripheral circulation.
25. Immature macrogametocyte.
26. Mature macrogametocyte.
27. Immature microgametocyte.
28. Mature microgametocyte.

Reproduced with permission from the Manual for the Microscopical Diagnosis of Malaria in Man, National Institutes of Health Bulletin No. 180. (By Aimee Wilcox.)

PLATE X

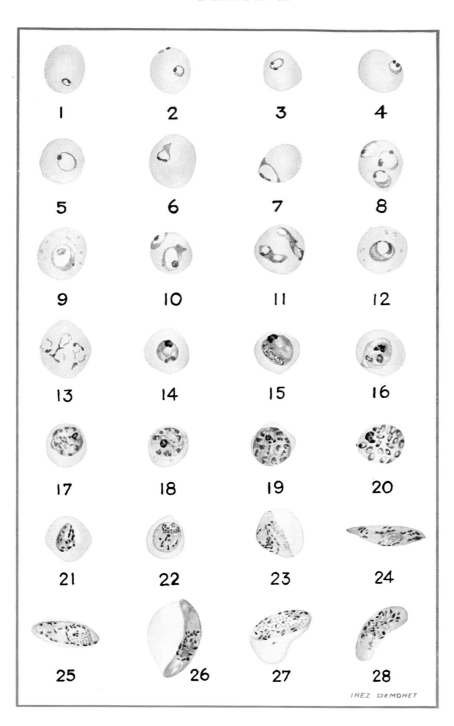

INEZ DEMONET

is very rapid, it may become slightly macrocytic.

Anemia in malaria may also be due in part to toxic inhibition of bone marrow activity, for the percentage of reticulocytes, which tends to be low during the period of infection, increases temporarily when the parasites are destroyed by effective treatment. An inhibitory effect on hematopoiesis is also suggested by the leukopenia which often accompanies malarial infection. *Plasmodium vivax* (tertian malaria) appears to have a particular affinity for reticulocytes.[36]

Blackwater fever (hemoglobinuric fever, hemorrhagic malarial fever, black jaundice, canebrake yellow fever) is a form of acute hemolytic anemia with hemoglobinuria which develops in connection with malarial infection. The clinical manifestations are fulminating, for there is intravascular hemolysis and this is associated with a rigor, general prostration, vomiting and pyrexia. Methemalbumin (p. 176) is constantly present in the plasma, as well as bilirubin. The osmotic fragility is usually normal but the red cells are sensitive to the hemolytic action of lysolecithin (p. 173). Although associated with infection by *P. falciparum*, the characteristic ring forms of the estivo-autumnal ("malignant tertian") parasite may not be detected during the attack. The condition is seen throughout the tropical and subtropical regions of Africa, in Southwest Asia, India and the Far East and sometimes in the Americas.

The pathogenesis of this serious disorder is not clear. Europeans who have had repeated attacks of malaria and have taken quinine irregularly are the chief victims of the disease.[2d] The attack often appears to be precipitated by the taking of quinine. This has been interpreted as suggesting that the pathogenesis of the disorder involves an auto-immune mechanism which depends, perhaps, on the combination of the drug in some manner with the red corpuscles to produce an antigen, thereby stimulating antibody formation. If this is the case, conventional methods have failed to demonstrate the antibodies. Sensitization to protein antigens of the malarial parasite which are released when anti-malarial drugs destroy them has also been postulated as the underlying mechanism.[12] It is noteworthy that red corpuscles from cases of blackwater fever are destroyed rapidly even in normal recipients.[13a] A possibility which deserves investigation is that an inherited defect in the red cells (p. 633) is the underlying cause. Whatever may be the underlying mechanism, it is important in the treatment of the disorder to control the shock and prostration, promote diuresis and maintain the acid-base equilibrium. Blood transfusions must be avoided during the paroxysm since normal cells undergo rapid hemolysis in the patient's circulation. Caution must guide the use of anti-malarial drugs following the attack.

2. **Non-protozoal Blood Parasites.** —A severe, acute hemolytic anemia is produced by *Bartonella*, an organism which was originally thought to be a protozoön but is now classified as a flagellated bacillus.[38] The disease is encountered in Peru under the name of **Oroya fever,** a condition marked by malaise, headache, muscle pains, remittent fever and chills, and very rapidly developing anemia. The blood picture is that characteristic of acute blood destruction and there is very marked leukocytosis.[28a, 32a] The mortality is high (30 to 98 per cent). The causative organism, *Bartonella bacilliformis*, is transmitted by the sand fly, Phlebotomus, and probably by other arthropods. *Verruca peruana*, a benign condition characterized by a wart-like eruption on the skin, is caused by the same organism. With Oroya fever it is classified as *Carrion's disease*, named after the student

who lost his life while investigating the infection.[32a]

Bartonella muris is found in rats (Fig. 20–21, p. 1057). Anemia due to related organisms has been described in the dog and other animals as well as in rats. An interesting feature of the infection in animals is that anemia rarely occurs in the normal animal whereas it develops in splenectomized rats[26] (p. 1051) or in dogs[31] receiving a deficient diet or deprived of plasma substances by plasmapheresis.[23] It has been clearly demonstrated in the animal studies that the anemia is due to blood destruction.[38]

The organism is rounded or rod-shaped, 1 to 2 μ in length by 0.2 to 0.5 μ in width, or 0.3 to 1 μ in diameter when round. In smears stained with Wright's stain it appears to be on the red corpuscles. It may be within or merely adherent to them. The organisms appear singly, in pairs, or in end to end chains which may assume a V or Y form.

3. **Viruses.**—Although cold antibodies (p. 169) frequently develop in high concentration in *primary atypical pneumonia*, associated hemolytic anemia is rare.[12d,24e] When it has occurred, hemolysis usually has developed suddenly towards the end of the second week.[5c] Hemoglobinuria has been observed and, in rare instances, gangrene has developed. In one case the hemolysis was followed ten days later by severe granulocytopenia and thrombocytopenia which were probably also due to the action of the incomplete antibodies of the cold agglutinin type.[104a]

A small number of instances of acute hemolytic anemia occurring during the course of infectious mononucleosis has been described (p. 1114). This complication has also been reported in association with acute viral hepatitis[27c] and with herpes simplex infection.[35e] The reported isolation of Newcastle disease virus from the blood stream in several

---

Legend for plate XI.—*P. vivax*

1. Normal sized red cell with marginal ring form trophozoite.
2. Young signet ring form trophozoite in a macrocyte.
3. Slightly older ring form trophozoite in red cell showing basophilic stippling.
4. Polychromatophilic red cell containing young tertian parasite with pseudopodia.
5. Ring form trophozite showing pigment in cytoplasm, in an enlarged cell containing Schüffner's stippling.*
6, 7. Very tenuous medium trophozoite forms.
8. Three ameboid trophozoites with fused cytoplasm.
9, 11, 12, 13. Older ameboid trophozoites in process of development.
10. Two ameboid trophozoites in one cell.
14. Mature trophozoite.
15. Mature trophozoite with chromatin apparently in process of division.
16, 17, 18, 19. Schizonts showing progressive steps in division ("presegmenting schizonts").
20. Mature schizont.
21, 22. Developing gametocytes.
23. Mature microgametocyte.
24. Mature macrogametocyte.

* Schüffner's stippling does not appear in all cells containing the growing and older forms of *P. vivax* as would be indicated by these pictures, but it can be found with any stage from the fairly young ring form onward.

Reproduced with permission from the Manual for the Microscopical Diagnosis of Malaria in Man, National Institutes of Health Bulletin No. 180. (By Aimee Wilcox.)

PLATE XI

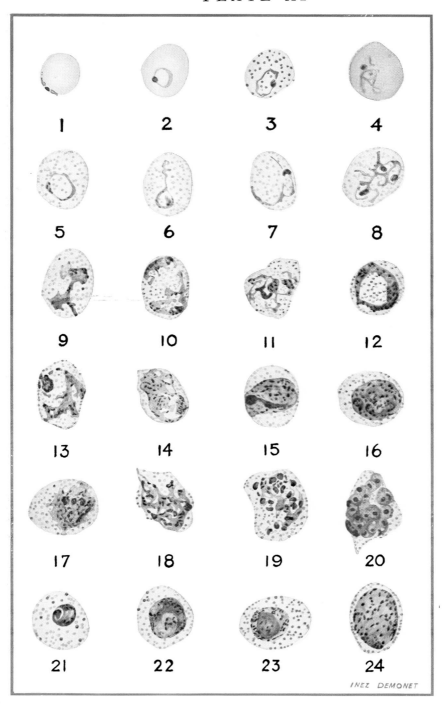

INEZ DEMONET

cases of acquired hemolytic anemia[24a] could not be confirmed.[24b]

4. Bacterial Infections.—*Cl. welchii* septicemia, usually following abortion, quite regularly produces a profound hemolytic anemia.[19g] *Vibrio comma* is another bacterial agent which is presumably responsible for severe hemolytic anemia and hemoglobinuria occurring in some cases of cholera.[8d] These manifestations may also rarely complicate *typhoid* fever[22e] and *salmonella* infection.[86a] Hemolytic anemia has been reported in children suffering from endocarditis due to *streptococcus pyogenes* (nonhemolytic), anaerobic enterococci and anaerobic staphylococci, in a child with pyemia due to the pneumococcus[14] and could be produced by the intradermal injection of living pneumococci in rabbits.[33a] It has been described also in hilar, acute areactive, miliary[5e] and pulmonary[24a] *tuberculosis*, as well as in association with tuberculosis of the spleen,[5e] and in streptococcal septicemia,[24a] scarlet fever and *H. influenzae* meningitis.[5e]

(B) Chemical Agents.—Hemolytic anemia associated with exposure to chemical agents can be considered under several categories. Some chemical agents cause anemia which is related in its severity to the quantity of the chemical absorbed. Other chemicals, such as benzene and trinitrotoluene, may have an earlier hemolytic effect which is followed by a toxic, inhibitory action on the bone marrow with aplastic anemia as the ultimate result. Another group are the derivatives of anilin and the nitro compounds, which more regularly cause methemoglobinemia (p. 194) but may also cause blood destruction. Plumbism represents still another category.

It has long been recognized that, in addition to these, cases are encountered in which the hemolytic reaction seems to have been one of unusual sensitivity on the part of the host. These have involved exposure to a variety of chemical agents and the subject has been the object of intense investigation. The various groups will be considered separately.

(a) *Chemical agents which are likely to produce hemolytic anemia in any person more or less regularly if a sufficiently large dose is given* include phenylhydrazine, trinitrotoluene, benzene, nitrobenzene, acetanilid, phenacetin, saponin,[4] lecithin,[35f] promin, methyl chloride, allyl-propyl disulfide (oil of onions),[39] arsine, lead and colloidal silver.[33] The hemolytic effects of phenylhydrazine (pyrodin) will be discussed later (p. 804) since this agent is sometimes used in the treatment of polycythemia vera. *Trinitrotoluene*[23a] and *toluene* produce methemoglobinemia and hepatic damage as well as hemolytic anemia[24] and T.N.T. has been known to produce aplastic anemia (p. 554). Early signs of industrial exposure to toluene are enlargement of the liver, macrocytosis with only moderate anemia, and absolute lymphocytosis.[16b] That inhibition of bone marrow activity takes place at the same time that increased blood destruction occurs, is suggested by the observation that a higher level of reticulocytes, resembling a reticulocyte crisis, developed in the ten-day period following removal of the subjects from exposure.[17a] In *benzene* (benzol) poisoning the usual signs of increased blood destruction may be associated with a normal leukocyte count or leukopenia rather than leukocytosis,[10a] recalling the fact that this agent often produces aplastic anemia (p. 553). *Nitrobenzene* produces methemoglobinemia and cyanosis as well as acute hemolytic anemia.[17c] This is also true of chronic acetanilid[33b] and phenacetin[23b,23c] intoxication. The dark urine observed in cases of nitrobenzene, acetanilid and phenacetin intoxication has been attributed to the excretion of para-amidophenol as well as hemoglobin derivatives. Similar effects are produced by other amino and nitro compounds of phenol, toluol and benzol, including *dinitrobenzol* and *anilin*.[16f]

39

The sulfone derivative *promin*, used in the treatment of leprosy and tuberculosis, causes the blood to change to a chocolate brown color as the result of the formation of methemoglobin, sulfhemoglobin and perhaps still another pigment,[17b] and produces hemolytic anemia of various degrees of severity. *Methyl chloride*, once widely used as a refrigerant in domestic refrigerators, is another potential cause of hemolytic anemia.[19]

Arsine (arseniuretted hydrogen), used in the manufacture of bleaching powder, tin refining, fertilizers[39a] and in other industries,[17c] especially those in which acids and alloys or ores containing arsenic are used, has produced fatalities through the development of acute hemolytic anemia. This gas was also found to produce the typical picture of acute hemolytic anemia with, however, a normal leukocyte count or leukopenia, in submarine crews who inhaled it.[9] Methemoglobin and other hemoglobin derivatives are produced as well.

Hemoglobinuria and even death from renal failure have been observed in association with transurethral resection of the prostate, apparently as the result of penetration of the irrigating fluid, **distilled water,** into the blood stream *via* lymphatic and venous channels opened by the operation.[19c] It has been shown

that the entry of 600 or more ml. of water into the circulation will produce hemoglobinemia and hemoglobinuria. This is probably the cause of the hemolysis seen in survivors of drowning in fresh water.[28] In such situations the normal protective mechanisms (p. 170) are overwhelmed.

The acute effects of **lead** on the blood have been observed in patients treated for cancer.[16] In these, progressive anemia developed in several weeks, reticulocytes increased and normoblasts appeared, and many of the latter, as well as a number of non-nucleated corpuscles showed basophilic stippling. Cabot rings and Howell-Jolly bodies were noted in some instances, and leukocytosis, usually marked, was found in the majority of the cases. In chronic poisoning,[40a] anemia is usually not severe and frank hemolytic anemia with bilirubinemia is rare.[8] However, a continuously increased breakdown of moderate degree takes place. The direct Coombs' test has been found to be positive.[35a] Lead has been shown to inhibit heme synthesis *in vitro*[15] and may have a toxic effect on porphyrin-forming organs.[10b] Consistent with these observations is the fact that the urinary excretion of coproporphyrin III is greatly increased in plumbism and is one of the most reliable early signs of lead intoxication.[22a]

LEGEND FOR PLATE XII.—*P. malariae*

1. Young ring form trophozoite of quartan malaria.
2, 3, 4. Young trophozoite forms of the parasite showing gradual increase of chromatin and cytoplasm.
5. Developing ring form trophozoite showing pigment granule.
6. Early band form trophozoite—elongated chromatin, some pigment apparent.
7, 8, 9, 10, 11, 12. Some forms which the developing trophozoite of quartan may take.
13, 14. Mature trophozoites—one a band form.
15, 16, 17, 18, 19. Phases in the development of the schizont ("presegmenting schizonts").
20. Mature schizont.
21. Immature microgametocyte.
22. Immature macrogametocyte.
23. Mature microgametocyte.
24. Mature macrogametocyte.

Reproduced with permission from the Manual for the Microscopical Diagnosis of Malaria in Man, National Institutes of Health Bulletin No. 180. (By Aimee Wilcox.)

PLATE XII

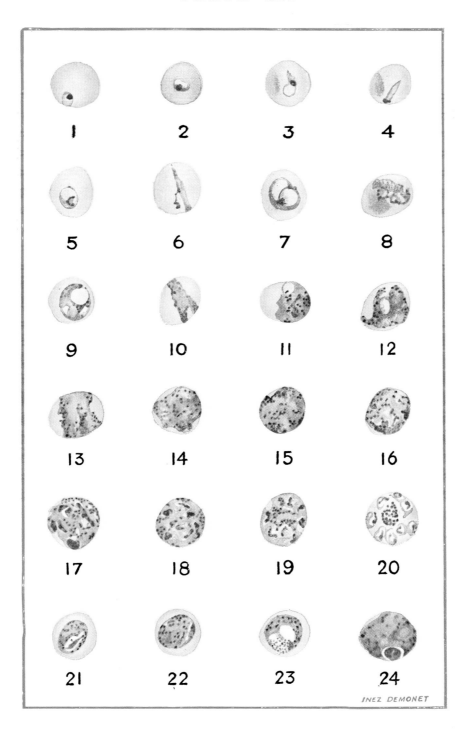

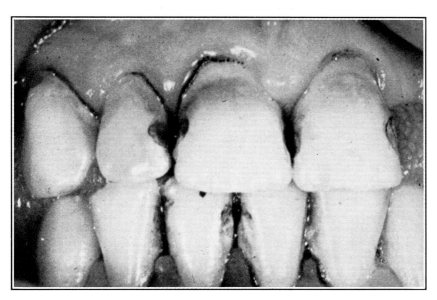

FIG. 12–1.—Lead "line" in a case of plumbism. Under a hand lens the lead line of blue-black lead sulfide, actually deposited in the gums immediately opposite to the teeth, appears as a clear row of dots or vertical streaks. (Belknap and Sanger, courtesy of J.A.M.A.)

The excretion of δ-aminolevulinic acid is also increased.[16c] These compounds, it should be noted, are also excreted in large amounts in porphyria (p. 188). Erythrocyte portoporphyrin and copper are also increased.[32b]

Coproporphyrinuria is often found in plumbism before *basophilic stippling* is demonstrable in the red corpuscles. These granules have been found to contain ribonucleic acid and their formation has been attributed to vital aggregation of RNA around mitochondria in the cytoplasm of the cells.[32c] When viewed with the electron microscope numerous granules of iron can also be seen in the cytoplasm of red cells, thus providing further evidence of arrested or impaired heme synthesis.[2] However, only a proportion of the cells are siderocytes (p. 100). Since stippled cells are found in greater proportion in the bone marrow than in the blood, and since splenectomy results in a very considerable increase in the number of stippled cells in the blood as well as amelioration of anemia,[22f] it

seems likely that lead intoxication results in the production of defective erythrocytes which are removed from the circulation by the spleen and other parts of the reticuloendothelial system. This appears to be a better explanation of the hematologic manifestations of plumbism than the original view that lead alters the surface of the red corpuscle, thus causing it to be more susceptible to trauma in the circulation.[1b]

(b) *Hypersensitivity to Chemical Agents.*— Because only a small proportion of those exposed developed hemolytic anemia, hypersensitivity was considered to be the underlying fault in cases of such anemia following exposure to sulfonamide drugs, *quinine,*[20] *quinidine,*[13b] *sulfones* used in the treatment of leprosy[8f,34] *nitrofurantoin,*[19a] *pamaquin* (plasmochin)[8g] *primaquine,*[8e] *paraaminosalicylic acid* (P.A.S.) (given with a sodium salt of ascorbic acid),[20d] *cryogénine* (phenylsemicarbazide), an anti-pyretic drug,[24f] *phenothiazine,* a urinary tract antiseptic,[18a] *neoarsphenamine,*[40d] *benzedrine,*[8a] *mesantoin,*[34a] *paraphenylinediamine* (used in hair dyes),[8b] "*myanesin*,"[27a] *pro-benecid*,[19a] and certain other drugs (p. 631). Also possibly belonging in this group is *naphthalene* which, in the form of moth balls and toilet-bowl deodorant, has been ingested by children who then developed acute hemolytic anemia.[8c,32d,40f] Hemolytic anemia has also been observed occasionally in premature infants whose only medication was prophylactic daily injections of the *vitamin-K substitute*, Synkayvite.®[1,32e] The pathogenesis of these and other forms of acquired hemolytic anemia will be discussed later (p. 633).

(C) **Physical Agents.**—Anemia of varying severity may be present in patients with full-thickness burns.[24c] It is very great in third degree burns of more than 20 per cent and has been attributed to an early hemolytic process, followed by a period of dyshemopoiesis.[17d] The hemolysis may be due to many factors but the actual heating of the blood, with consequent alterations in the osmotic and mechanical fragility of the red corpuscles[16d] is no doubt very important. It was shown that the intravenous injection into dogs of dog red blood cells rendered spheroid and osmotically and mechanically fragile by previous heating resulted in prompt hemoglobinemia and hemoglobinuria with selective removal of the abnormal cells within a few hours. Heated plasma, on the other hand, produced no such effects. It was postulated that red blood corpuscles, even though insufficiently altered in osmotic fragility to be hemolyzed by isotonic plasma, may nevertheless be broken down as a result of trauma resulting from the motion of the circulation as well as because of intravascular stagnation in certain tissues.[16d]

Whether or not ionizing radiation has a hemolytic action, in addition to the effects already described elsewhere (p. 557), is uncertain.[47] Maier[22] has listed still other physical agents which may produce hemolytic anemia.

(D) **Vegetable and Animal Poisons.** — Inhalation from bean plants when in blossom or ingestion of fava beans (*Vicia faba*), particularly when fresh, causes in sensitive persons an acute hemolytic anemia with all the characteristics which have been described. When due to inhalation, the attack may commence within a matter of minutes; when the broad beans are ingested there is usually a time lag of five to twenty-four hours. Blood destruction may be so severe and rapid as to cause death. The attack is followed by a period of immunity of about six weeks duration. *Favism* occurs mainly in Sardinia, Sicily and Calabria but was once widespread throughout the Mediterranean basin.[20c] A few cases have been reported in the United States and Great Britain but, with one exception the victims have been of Italian or Greek ancestry.[22d] Not only has this racial predisposition been observed but it was noted that more than one member of a family was likely to be affected. In cross transfusion experiments, erythrocytes from susceptible persons showed increased destruction when injected in victims of favism but normal cells survived normally.[36a] This would suggest an intrinsic defect in the red cells of the victims of favism, a possibility which was borne out by studies of glutathione instability and glucose-6-phosphate dehydrogenase deficiency[19d] which will be described below (p. 632). It has not been explained, however, why parents and relatives of affected persons who show similar enzymatic defects may be exposed to the bean with impunity.[19d] The possible rôle of serum[71a] or other [52a] factors is being studied.

It is very likely that the same enzyme deficiency is responsible for "Bagdad spring anemia."[19f]

The castor bean contains a powerful hemolytic agent (*ricin*[19b]) as do some *snake venoms*. The latter contain a lecithinase which converts lecithin to *lysolecithin*, which may act by causing swelling of the red cells.[38a]

The possibility that, under certain conditions, endogenous poisons of various types may produce hemolytic anemia is suggested by experiments in which it was found that canine black tongue-producing diets made dogs susceptible to the action of indol, a toxin formed in the intestinal tract, which became hemolytic in amounts not toxic when normal diets were given.[29] These studies also suggested a mechanism whereby drugs not usually toxic may have detrimental effects on the blood. Thus, amidopyrine caused anemia in dogs fed a deficient diet whereas this did not occur when the diet was supplemented with yeast.[30] Hemolytic anemia resulting from the action of endogenous substances has been described.[10c]

(E) The role of **isoagglutinins** in the production of hemolysis was discussed in an earlier chapter (p. 338). The relative importance of the various isoantibodies as causes of hemolytic transfusion reactions is indicated in Table 7–5 (p. 365). Hemolytic disease of the newborn will be discussed in a later chapter (p. 756).

(F) **Paroxysmal cold hemoglobinuria,** a well-defined clinical syndrome produced by a hemolysin activated by cold, will be considered separately (p. 637).

(G) **Symptomatic Hemolytic Anemias.**—In the preceding chapter it was pointed out that in many instances of simple chronic anemia accompanying a variety of diseases, shortened survival of transfused red corpuscles can be demonstrated (p. 577). In such cases, bilirubinemia and the various other signs of overt increased blood destruction are lacking, although a moderate degree of reticulocytosis may be demonstrable in some cases. The same is true of the anemia usually encountered in leukemia, Hodgkin's disease and many other dis-

orders involving the hemopoietic system. Occasionally, however, obvious hemolytic anemia is found in association with certain diseases and sometimes the first manifestations of illness are those of a hemolytic process rather than those of the underlying condition. It is these cases of overt hemolytic anemia which are referred to as "symptomatic hemolytic anemias." The clinical features may represent a combination of symptoms and signs of the primary disorder together with those of hemolytic anemia or may consist only of those of the hemolytic process.

The conditions in which overt hemolytic anemia has been observed, other than the infectious processes which have been discussed already (p. 606), may be considered in three categories; namely, (1) hemopoietic disorders, among which chronic lymphocytic leukemia and Hodgkin's disease stand out prominently; (2) the so-called collagen group, notably disseminated lupus erythematosus; and (3) a number of miscellaneous conditions, of which tumors of the ovary may be mentioned especially.

Frank hemolytic anemia in *chronic lymphocytic leukemia* is by no means rare[108] (approximately 15 per cent of cases[118]), whereas few examples of such anemia in chronic myelocytic leukemia[60a] or in acute leukemia[93b] have been reported (p. 925). In *Hodgkin's disease* symptomatic hemolytic anemia was observed in eight of 104 consecutive cases in one series[118] and has been reported from time to time by others.[85,86a,119] (p. 1024). In lymphosarcoma such anemia has been observed frequently[108,110] and it has been described also in giant follicular lymphoblastoma,[118] reticulum cell sarcoma,[109c] reticuloendotheliosis,[86] sarcoidosis[122a] and infectious mononucleosis[95b](p. 1114). The occasional occurrence of hemolytic anemia in association with myelosclerosis has been mentioned already (p. 586).

It is becoming recognized that hemolytic anemia may be the first evidence of *disseminated lupus erythematosus*.[108c] The incidence of frank hemolytic anemia in this disease was 10 per cent in one series.[118] This type of anemia has been reported also in periarteritis nodosa[6a] and even in scleroderma[93d] and in dermatomyositis.[116a]

Among the *miscellaneous disorders* in which hemolytic anemia has been described, those associated with ovarian tumors[68a] form a unique group since most of the tumors were dermoids[68b,110] or teratomas.[78] Hemoglobinemia, hemoglobinuria, thrombocytopenia and clotting defects have been reported in eclamptogenic toxemia of pregnancy[106a] and non-megaloblastic hemolytic anemia has been seen also in uncomplicated pregnancy and appeared to be related to it.[81a] Hemolytic anemia has been encountered in association with carcinoma of the tail of the pancreas,[86a] in the gastrointestinal tract (especially the stomach[100]) and at various other sites.[118] In cirrhosis of the liver[85,119] and, less often, in other forms of liver disease, including serum hepatitis,[118] increased blood destruction has been described. This has also been observed in a variety of other disorders, including generalized Kaposi's sarcoma,[100,103a] primary hemochromatosis,[109b] amyloidosis[60] and Gaucher's disease.[118]

The course of the anemia in these cases varied from that of a rapidly developing and fulminating process[46] to that of a chronic disorder with remissions and relapses. The anemia has frequently been macrocytic[85] but was nonmegaloblastic. Spherocytosis and increased osmotic fragility have been demonstrated in many instances[68b,110] but this was often not as pronounced as in hereditary spherocytosis or was absent entirely.

Many of these observations were made before the Coombs' test was devised. Studies carried out since that time indicate that the mechanism of hemolysis

in symptomatic hemolytic anemia is like that in "idiopathic" auto-immune hemolytic anemias in that the direct Coombs' test has usually been positive.[68b,81a] This was the case, for example, in 20 cases of chronic lymphocytic leukemia and lymphosarcoma and in several of them the positive test antedated the development of any other evidence of a hemolytic process by several months or a year.[108] Circulating hemagglutinins were demonstrated in 11 to 19 cases so tested. Positive direct antiglobulin tests have been found in almost all patients with disseminated lupus erythematosus and hemolytic anemia[5c,118] and have often antedated demonstrable increased blood destruction.

The etiologic relationship of the underlying disorder and the observed hemolytic anemia is suggested by the disappearance of all signs of increased blood destruction following successful treatment of the associated disease; as for example, by the treatment of Hodgkin's disease with nitrogen mustard,[109c] or by the removal of a dermoid cyst[68b,110] or other type of ovarian tumor.[78] In certain cases splenectomy seemed necessary in addition to treatment of the underlying disorder[60a,110] but in a few splenectomy alone was effective,[86] even when treatment of the underlying condition was of no value.[118] In one case of dermoid cyst and endometriosis, neither steroid therapy or splenectomy was helpful but removal of the tumor was immediately effective.[68b]

In *"thrombotic thrombocytopenic purpura"* severe hemolytic anemia is characteristic. This disorder will be discussed elsewhere (p. 831).

(H) Idiopathic Acquired Hemolytic Anemias.—Although the number of possible causes of hemolytic anemia is large, as the preceding pages indicate, in a very significant number of cases of acquired hemolytic anemia no cause is found and no associated disease is recognized. Some indication of the relative numbers of cases of various types is given by a review of pertinent literature from 1940 to 1951; there were 35 associated with primary atypical pneumonia, 5 cases of infectious mononucleosis, 27 "lymphomas" (chronic lymphocytic leukemia, Hodgkin's disease, lymphosarcoma), 5 collagen diseases and 13 miscellaneous symptomatic hemolytic anemias, as compared with 147 cases of the idiopathic variety.[108b] Cases attributable to chemical or physical agents or other causes listed in Table 12–1 were not mentioned. Thus it is evident that, even when allowance is made for the fact that some of the symptomatic hemolytic anemias make their first appearance in the guise of the idiopathic disorder, the underlying condition not being recognized at first, there remains a large proportion of cases in which present methods fail to reveal an etiologic factor.

The idiopathic cases range in the extreme insofar as their course and outcome are concerned. They may be acute, severe and fulminating or they may be insidious in onset and chronic in course. The latter may sometimes be punctuated by repeated attacks of hemolysis, followed by spontaneous remissions.[125] By and large, however, the manifestations are rarely as mild as they may be in hereditary spherocytosis, where the patient may be "more yellow than sick."

Idiopathic cases have been observed at all ages, from five months to seventy-eight years,[5c] but females are more often affected than males (2:1).[5c,108b] The hematological features are similar to those of other hemolytic anemias, varying according to the severity of the condition, but certain phenomena related to the immunological character of these anemias distinguish them from the hereditary hemolytic diseases.

Autoimmune mechanisms appear to be the basis of all, or at least almost all, cases of idiopathic acquired hemolytic anemia. Admittedly, the older literature contains reports of many cases which did not seem to be related to agglutinins or hemolysins[34c] but these cases were examined before the complexity of the antibodies and the need for improved technics to demonstrate them was appreciated.

In a statistical study of 128 cases of autoimmune hemolytic anemia 73 per cent were idiopathic, the remainder being associated with malignant conditions of the lymphocytic or reticuloendothelial systems, disseminated lupus or a virus infection.[84] Both the idiopathic and the symptomatic groups could be subdivided according to the presence of a "warm" or a "cold" antibody. The ratio of the "warm" to the "cold" type among the idiopathic cases was 8:1, among the symptomatic ones 2:1. Except for the features characteristic of the underlying disease, the idiopathic and the symptomatic cases were similar. Others have observed a somewhat higher proportion of cases with "cold" antibodies.[5e,105b]

Warm autoantibodies react well at 37° C. and are not potentiated at lower temperatures. The most common ones are "incomplete" (p. 352); that is, they sensitize normal erythrocytes to antiglobulin serum but do not cause agglutination in a saline medium. It is rare for saline dilutions of these antibodies to cause direct agglutination at 37° C.; that is, they are rarely "complete." The sensitization is not inhibited by previous heat-inactivation of the patient's serum at 56° C. and it is increased only slightly by acidification of the serum to pH 7.0 or 6.5. Typically these antibodies cause agglutination and not hemolysis. They almost invariably cause the agglutination of trypsinized red corpuscles and this, in fact, may occur in the absence of a positive antiglobulin test. These sensitizing antibodies usually are gamma globulins.[5d]

"Cold" antibodies are markedly potentiated by reducing the temperature below 37° C. These antibodies act as "incom-

plete" antibodies but they may also act as "complete" agglutinating antibodies and under certain circumstances may also bring about hemolysis.[5b] Warm antibodies only rarely do this. Two main forms of "cold" antibodies have been demonstrated in acquired hemolytic anemias. The common typical type is a powerful agglutinin; the rare variety is similar to the Donath-Landsteiner antibody of paroxysmal cold hemoglobinuria (p. 638). Cold antibodies are usually detectable by the direct antiglobulin test. The indirect test may not be positive at 37° C. unless the serum is acidified, but it is usually positive at 20° C.

From the standpoint of clinical manifestations, prognosis and treatment, there are striking differences between the hemolytic anemias associated with warm antibodies and those with cold antibodies. The course of the latter is often chronic and the manifestations may be mild, except for signs which develop in the cold, such as cyanosis or a blotchy appearance of the skin, Raynaud's phenomena or hemoglobinuria. Splenomegaly is uncommon. This type most frequently occurs in elderly subjects.[5e] Spherocytes are not conspicuous and osmotic fragility may be normal.

Clinical manifestations in the "warm" variety are likely to be more pronounced and may be severe. This type is seen at all ages. Icterus, moderate splenomegaly and macrocytic anemia are present. When leukopenia and thrombocytopenic purpura[11] are associated, the prognosis is likely to be more grave. In the series of 128 cases mentioned above, 46 per cent of the idiopathic cases with warm antibodies were fatal.[84] The persistence of a positive *indirect* Coombs' test tended to be associated with an unfavorable outcome. In these cases, however, in contrast to the "cold" variety, corticosteroid therapy was likely to be efficacious.

The antibody pattern from one case to another has not always been the same, however. Thus, it has been observed that the antibodies of one patient may differ considerably from those of another in temperature requirements, specificity and chemical nature and in their reactions *in vitro*.[67d] Furthermore, a single sample of serum may contain several autoantibody components, as well as isoantibodies formed as the result of past transfusions.[5d] Again, a few cases have been described in which the patients' serum contained a potent agglutinin for enzyme-treated cells but this was not associated with a positive direct Coombs' test.[105a]

In addition to the warm and cold autoantibodies, it is not uncommon to find other manifestations of abnormal protein formation in patients with acquired hemolytic anemia. Thus, antibodies against lipoid antigens may be present and may give rise to false-positive Wassermann and Kahn reactions. This is frequently the case in disseminated lupus erythematosus; this false-positive serological reaction may anticipate the appearance of frank hemolytic anemia. Again, serum complement may be reduced and hypergammaglobulinemia and cryoglobulins may develop. In several instances cryoglobulinemia has been observed in association with cold antibodies and hemolytic anemia.[4f]

It was assumed at first that the autoantibodies found in acquired hemolytic anemia are nonspecific; that is, that they react with all types of human red cells without relation to any known blood group antigens. It is now recognized that the autoantibodies may be specific.[121] In the main those encountered have been directed against various Rh antigens (e, D, E, c, C)[52, 61d, 102b, 121] but anti-K,[93a] anti-Fy[a], anti-Jk[a], anti-B and anti-O have also been reported.[102b] At the same time, autoantibodies without apparent specificity were often present. This led to the suggestion that the warm autoantibodies of acquired hemolytic anemias are usually directed against the nucleus of the Rh substance.[122] Since cold autoantibodies parallel in their behavior the natural isoagglutinins, it is possible that they are directed against the nucleus of the ABO substance.

It was at first thought that the type-specific antibodies were always of the "warm" variety. However, several cases have now been reported in which "cold" antibodies were present. The antigen on the reacting cells has been designated I.[121,122]

Chronic hemolytic anemia accompanied by leukopenia and thrombocytopenia in association with polyagglutinability of the red cells due to an antigen (Tn) which differed from the type encountered in aging red cells (p. 170) has also been described.[84a]

"Thrombotic thrombocytopenic purpura" may well belong with the autoimmune hemolytic anemias, but will be discussed elsewhere (p. 831).

Diagnosis.—Three steps are necessary in the diagnosis of the hemolytic anemias. It must first be suspected that one is dealing with a hemolytic disorder. The clinical pictures of the different hemolytic anemias are so varied that confusion with many other disorders is easily possible. The abdominal pain of the acute form may suggest some primary intraabdominal disease. Oliguria and edema suggest renal disease. An enlarged spleen may arouse suspicion of acute leukemia, a view which may find temporary support in the leukemoid blood picture which may be encountered. The more chronic forms of hemolytic anemia, on the other hand, may suggest a great variety of conditions characterized by anemia and splenomegaly; it would be impossible to list them all. Finally, it may be added that in the symptomatic hemolytic anemias the primary disorder may be apparent but the complication of hemolytic anemia may not be at once discerned; or, as has been mentioned before,

the manifestations of the hemolytic anemia may be obvious but the underlying condition may be obscure.

Once suspicion has been aroused, it is then necessary to prove that the case is one of hemolytic disease. The third step is the differentiation of the various types of hemolytic anemia. These last two aspects of the diagnosis of hemolytic disease will be considered here.

Recognition of Hemolytic Anemia. —Increased blood destruction may be suspected from the presence of the symptoms and signs which have been described already. Its existence in a given case is demonstrated by the appropriate examination of the blood, urine and stools. The evidence which such examinations may reveal was discussed in an earlier chapter (p. 178). Certain clinical aspects, however, may be considered here.

The *sudden destruction of blood* is indicated by the presence of free hemoglobin in the plasma and this may soon be reflected by the appearance of hemoglobin in the urine. It is obvious, however, that neither red plasma nor red urine necessarily means that this color is due to the presence of hemoglobin. Hemoglobinemia was discussed in detail earlier (p. 176). The significance of red urine may be considered briefly here.

The *urine may be red* because of the presence of red corpuscles (hematuria) or because of some drug (pyridium, antipyrine) or food (beets) taken by the patient. This color may also be produced by hemoglobinuria, porphyrinuria and myoglobinuria. Porphyrinuria was discussed fully elsewhere (p. 155). Hemoglobinuria must be distinguished from **myoglobinuria.** Muscle hemoglobin is found in the urine as the result of crushing injuries to the extremities ("crush syndrome"). In association with this a characteristic renal lesion has been described.[4a] Thrombosis of an artery which supplies a large muscle-mass, such as the femoral artery, may likewise cause myoglobinuria.[4b] High-voltage electric shock and other types of trauma in which a considerable mass of muscle is suddenly damaged will do the same. In man a condition known as **Haff disease** was described in inhabitants of Königsberg, Germany, and its environs.[35] The condition was characterized by severe pain, stiffness and limitation of movement, occurring in paroxysms. Degeneration of the voluntary muscles occurred. This was thought to be due to the action of poisonous resinous acids, by-products of the cellulose factories in this region, which found their way into a nearby inlet ("haff") and were ingested by the fish and eels, which were in turn eaten by the villagers. A characteristic symptom was the passage of dark urine. This contained myoglobin from the damaged muscles rather than hemoglobin and could be distinguished only by spectroscopic examination of the urine.[18] A similar disorder was described in Sweden where there was no recognized exposure to a poisonous agent.[1c]

There is, in addition, a rare spontaneous disorder, **idiopathic myoglobinuria**[77a] which is characterized by the acute onset of severe muscle pain and spasm followed by pseudo-paralysis of the involved muscles and the appearance of myoglobin in the urine. The attacks tend to recur and appear to be precipitated by exercise. In several instances a familial occurrence was observed. Muscle biopsy showed severe degenerative changes.[70a] A similar disorder in horses (equine myoglobinuria) has been attributed to the damage of muscles by lactic acid, suddenly released by activity from the excessive amounts of glycogen accumulating in the muscles during rest. Evidence of a disturbance in carbohydrate metabolism has been found in a chronic form of myoglobinuria.[74a]

Myoglobin is a heme pigment of small molecular weight (17,500) and is readily excreted by the kidneys. It gives a positive benzidine test but does not fluoresce under ultra-violet illumination. Spectroscopic examination is necessary to differentiate it from hemoglobin and this is facilitated by treatment with carbon monoxide since there is greater divergence between the bands of carboxy-hemoglobin and carboxy-myoglobin than between the oxy-forms. In contrast to hemoglobin, myoglobin remains in solution after 80 per cent saturation of the urine with ammonium sulfate.[41b]

The detection of hemoglobinuria, therefore, requires specific identification. In addition to hemoglobin in the urine, and even in its absence, *hemosiderinuria* (p. 176) will be demonstrable whenever the plasma hemoglobin level has exceeded 20 mg. per cent.

More gradual breakdown of red corpuscles is associated with the development of bilirubinemia and the appearance of increased quantities of urobilinogen in the urine and stools (p.178). The van den Bergh reaction is indirect and there is no bilirubin in the urine. The fecal urobilinogen (F.U.) ranges from 300 to 4000 mg. per day, the urinary urobilinogen (U.U.) from 1 to 200 mg. The quantity of these breakdown products in plasma, urine and stools, however, depends on many factors in addition to the degree of blood destruction. These include the adequacy of blood regeneration and the functional capacity of the liver. The amount of urobilinogen in the feces is affected by a great number of factors (p. 175) and, therefore, this must be looked upon as but a crude measure of blood destruction. Nevertheless, it has proved to be a useful clinical tool, especially when allowance is made for the quantity of hemoglobin available for destruction, as is done in the hemolytic index (p. 180).

In addition to circumstances in which there is exaggerated blood destruction, bilirubinemia of the indirect type is found also in association with chronic passive congestion, in pneumonia and various other infections and in the convalescent or later stages of any type of hepatitis. The urinary urobilinogen is also increased in such cases of pre-hepatic jaundice; F.U. however, is often only moderately increased (100 to 500 mg.).[36c] A type of retention jaundice which is more readily confused with chronic hemolytic icterus than are these conditions is **"familial non-hemolytic jaundice"** or **"constitutional hepatic dysfunction."** These terms refer to a rare form of constitutional hepatocellular inferiority in bilirubin excretion which results in accumulation of bilirubin.[79] Anemia, micro- and spherocytosis, reticulocytosis, increased red cell fragility and splenomegaly are absent and the excretion of urobilinogen in the urine and stools is normal. The plasma bilirubin, which may attain high levels, is of the "indirect" variety. In some instances[81] measurement of red cell survival may be required to differentiate this condition from congenital non-spherocytic hemolytic disease (p. 651). Other forms of nonhemolytic acholuric jaundice which must be distinguished from hemolytic jaundice are the syndromes described by Crigler and Najjar[78c] and by Israels et al.[101]

In contrast, in post-hepatic or regurgitation jaundice the van den Bergh reaction is mainly "direct" and bilirubin is found in the urine. In the mechanical type, as in cancer of the biliary tract, the F.U. is less than 5 mg., the U.U. less than 0.5 mg. per day; if the obstruction is varying or incomplete (calculi, stricture), a greater range of values for F.U. and U.U. is found.[36c] The same is true in cases of the parenchymal type of regurgitation jaundice (diffuse liver damage). In all of these conditions, even if anemia is present, the signs of greatly increased blood regeneration which characterize the hemolytic anemias, are lacking.

The *presence of hemolytic anemia, therefore,* *is indicated by* demonstration of the products of red cell destruction in the blood, urine and stools. The nature of the products which will be found will depend on the rate and, to some extent, the site of blood destruction as well as on the efficiency of the liver and kidneys in excreting them. It should not be overlooked that evidence of the response of the hemopoietic system to the need for blood replacement will also be present. This will be found in the blood and in the bone marrow. In particular, it should be stressed that the examination of the blood smear will be helpful in supporting the diagnosis of hemolytic anemia. Polychromatophilia, nucleated red cells and other signs of exaggerated erythropoiesis will be found and the accelerated activity may also be reflected in the leukocytes and platelets. Reticulocytes will be greatly increased in number. In addition, spherocytes will be found in many types of hemolytic anemia.

Differentiation of Various Types of Hemolytic Anemia.—Having established the fact that one is dealing with hemolytic anemia, differentiation of the various types is necessary. The history alone may suffice to reveal an etiologic agent or may suggest that one is dealing with one of the familial or hereditary disorders. In regard to the latter, it is important to *examine* other members of the family for, in congenital hemolytic disorders particularly, the existence of the condition in other members may have been overlooked or mistaken for some other ailment. A history of splenectomy in some relative may be an important clue. Again, physical examination may reveal one of the conditions of which hemolytic anemia can be symptomatic. In addition, certain *special tests* have been devised which give some clue to the nature of the disorder. Some of these will be only mentioned here since they have been described and discussed already. Considered in the order of their utility and yet simplicity and availability in various laboratories they may be classified in several groups:

(*a*) Examination of the blood smear for spherocytes; osmotic fragility; presumptive test for agglutinins and hemolysins (below); direct Coombs' test; test for sickle cells (p. 680); examination of the urine for hemosiderin (p. 641); examination of the urine formed overnight.

(*b*) Antibody tests with enzyme-treated cells;[84a] indirect Coombs' test; paper electrophoresis of hemoglobin (p. 717); mechanical fragility.

(*c*) Spectroscopic examination of the plasma for hemoglobin and methemalbumin (p. 399) and chemical measurement by the benzidine method;[16g] examination of the blood for Heinz bodies, for siderocytes (p. 101) and for erythrophagocytosis (p. 605).

(*d*) Survival of normal cells in patient's circulation and of patient's cells in normal subject (p. 163); ferrokinetics (p. 182).

Some of the more striking differences which are encountered in the hemolytic anemias are presented in Table 12–2.

Osmotic (hypotonic saline) fragility. (p. 171) is almost invariably increased in hereditary spherocytosis. This may be because many of the corpuscles, by their spherical shape, need to absorb very little fluid to bring them to the form in which their membrane is stretched to the bursting point (Fig. 12–9) but other factors may be more important (p. 635). Osmotic fragility is likely to be increased also in autoimmune hemolytic anemia, in hemolytic disease of the newborn due to anti-A (less commonly in sensitization due to anti-Rh), in hemolytic anemia due to chemical poisoning and in severe burning. Sometimes, however, the deviations from the normal are slight. In most cases of symptomatic hemolytic anemia, osmotic fragility is normal or essentially so and this is true also in paroxysmal nocturnal hemoglobinuria.

When samples of defibrinated blood from patients with hereditary spherocytosis are incubated *in vitro* under sterile conditions at 37° C. for exactly 24 hours, a symmetric increase in fragility occurs (Fig. 12–2), in contrast to other anemias in which the increase is asymmetric if it occurs at all. The osmotic fragility of unincubated blood may, in fact, be normal in some cases of congenital nonspherocytic hemolytic anemia and incubation of the red corpuscles may be necessary to demonstrate their abnormality.

Increased *resistance* to breakdown in hypotonic saline solutions is observed in thalassemia, sickle cell anemia and other disorders in which many thin red corpuscles are found (especially "target" cells) although sometimes a small proportion of unusually fragile cells may also be detectable.

Increased sensitivity to lysolecithin (p. 173) may be observed in blackwater fever even though saline osmotic fragility is normal.

The **test for autohemolysis**[4c] depends on the incubation of sterile defibrinated blood at 37° C. for 24 and 48 hours and measurement of the amount of spontaneous hemolysis which occurs. Normally 0 to 0.5 per cent hemolysis takes place in 24 hours, 0.4 to 3.5 per cent in 48 hours. In general, autohemolysis is increased when osmotic fragility is increased and when there is hemolysis *in vivo*.[117] The procedure may have some value in differentiating certain forms of nonspherocytic hemolytic anemia from hereditary spherocytosis (p. 651).

Increased mechanical fragility (p. 173) has been observed in some cases of acquired hemolytic anemia, even when osmotic fragility was normal. Spherical, agglutinated and sickled cells are especially sensitive to this type of trauma.

In seeking to demonstrate the presence of hemolysins, a **simple presumptive test**[40b] consists in placing fresh defibrin-

Table 12-2—Comparison of Findings in Five Types of Hemolytic Disease

	Hereditary Spherocytosis	Hemolytic Disease		Paroxysmal Hemoglobinuria	
		Auto-immune	Iso-immune	Cold*	Nocturnal
Inheritance	Mendelian dominant	Occurs	None	None	Common
Thrombophlebitis	Uncommon	In cold type	Shock	Common	None
Vasomotor disturbances	None				
Response to:					
Splenectomy	Excellent	Irregular	None	None	None
Adrenocorticosteroids	None	Good	?	?	Contraindicated
Spherocytosis	Characteristic	During crisis chiefly	In anti-A & B; not in anti-Rh	Unusual	None
Fragility:					
Osmotic	Inc., esp. after incubation	Normal or inc. (in active phase)	Normal in anti-Rh. Inc. in anti-A & B	Normal	Normal
Mechanical	Increased	Inc. in crises	Normal	Normal	Normal
RBC survival:					
Normal cells in pt.	Normal	Decreased (curve exponential)	Normal	Same as pts.' cells	Normal
Pt. cells in normal	Decreased	Normal or sl. dec.	Normal	Normal	Decreased
Hemoglobinemia	None	May occur	May occur	In attacks	In active phase
Methemoglobinemia	None	May occur	None	In attacks	In active phase
Coombs': Direct	Usually neg.	Positive	Positive (neg. in ABO)	Positive (after sensitization in the cold)	Neg.
Indirect	Negative	Positive	Positive	Neg.	Neg.
Auto-agglutinins:					
Warm Complete	None	Rare	None	None	None
Incomplete	None	Frequently present	Present (in anti-Rh)	None	None
Cold	None	May be present	None	Minimal or none	None
Auto-hemolysins	None	Rare	None	Characteristic	None
Acid hemolysis	None	Sometimes	None	None	Characteristic
Hemosiderinuria	None	Moderate	May occur	Following attacks	Characteristic

* Type associated with syphilis

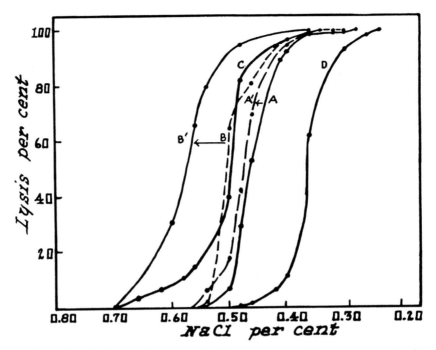

FIG. 12–2.—Normal and abnormal osmotic fragility curves. *A*, Normal curve; *A*[1], the moderate increase in osmotic fragility on incubation. *B*, Hereditary spherocytosis; *B*[1], greatly increased osmotic fragility following incubation. *C*, "Acquired" hemolytic anemia. *D*, Increased resistance of red corpuscles from a case of thalassemia minor.

ated blood into each of three test tubes. The first is incubated for one or two hours at body temperature and then centrifuged. If hemoglobin is present in the supernatant fluid, the presence of a warm hemolysin is suggested. The second tube is chilled for 20 minutes in cracked ice, then incubated for one hour and centrifuged. If the supernatant shows hemolysis, the presence of a cold hemolysin is indicated. The test tube should be examined before it has been warmed. If only cold agglutinins are present and no hemolysins, it will be seen that the red corpuscles agglutinate in the cold but fail to hemolyze when the tube is warmed, the clumps disappearing instead. When cold agglutinins are present, the cells must not be shaken too much while they are agglutinated in the cold, since they may hemolyze for mechanical reasons and give a false cold

hemolysin test. The blood placed in the third tube is acidified with carbon dioxide. If hemolysis is apparent after incubation for one hour and subsequent centrifugation, increased acid hemolysis is suggested.

When positive results are obtained in any one of these tubes, the test should be repeated with adequate controls.[4e] If a cold hemolysin appears to be present, the Donath-Landsteiner test (p. 639) should be carried out. A positive carbon dioxide test requires the performance of an acid-serum test with appropriate controls (p. 644).

The *Coombs' antiglobulin test* (p. 353) is used to demonstrate the presence of isoimmune mechanisms in a case of hemolytic anemia. The "direct" test, which is carried out by mixing the patient's washed red cells with serum from rabbits immunized to human gam-

Table 12-3—Antiglobulin (Coombs') Test

	Direct Test	Indirect Test	
Antihuman globulin serum is mixed with	Patient's RBC's	Normal RBC's Rh+ (after incubation in patient's serum)	Rh—
Hemolytic Disorders:			
Hereditary spherocytosis*	—	—	—
Acquired hemolytic anemia			
Auto-immune (symptomatic and idiopathic)			
Without circulating serum antibodies	+	—	—
With circulating serum antibodies	+	+	+
Iso-immune (Erythroblastosis fetalis due to			
Rh antibodies in Rh+ infant)	+	+	—
Due to physical or chemical agents	±	—	—
Sickle cell anemia	—	—	—
Paroxysmal nocturnal hemoglobinuria	—	—	—
Paroxysmal cold hemoglobinuria	+	—	—
(type associated with syphilis)			

* The occasional finding of a positive direct Coombs' test in hereditary spherocytosis and in other hemolytic disorders in which the test is usually negative, when not due to faulty technic, is assumed to be due to autosensitization superimposed on the primary disorder as the result of repeated transfusions or for other causes.

ma globulin, serves to demonstrate "incomplete" antibodies on the red corpuscles. The "indirect" test detects antibodies in the patient's serum: normal group O, Rh-positive and Rh-negative red corpuscles are first incubated in the patient's serum and they are then tested with the rabbit serum to determine whether they have become coated with "incomplete" antibodies.

The most constant immunologic finding in acquired hemolytic anemias is a positive direct antihuman globulin (Coombs') test. This is true of the "symptomatic" variety[108] as well as the idiopathic and has been observed in hemolytic anemia associated with primary atypical pneumonia[5c] and in favism,[22b] and even in bacterial[22e] and drug[24d, 34a] induced hemolytic anemia, provided the blood was examined at the time of the hemolytic episode. The regularity with which positive results have been obtained differs from one laboratory to another, probably because

the test possesses many technical hazards.[40c] In one series[84b] the antiglobulin test was positive in 97 per cent of 33 cases of the idiopathic variety and in 50 per cent of 28 cases of the symptomatic type, whereas only 21 per cent were positive among 14 cases of hereditary spherocytosis. Others have encountered even fewer positives in the hereditary disorder[5c] but experience has not borne out the original hope that the antiglobulin test would be negative in all cases of the hereditary hemolytic diseases and thus would always differentiate them from the acquired forms.

Some typical results are presented in Table 12-3.

It is important to bear in mind the different responses of warm and cold antibodies to the Coombs' test.[105b] Warm antibodies on red cells may be demonstrated with high dilutions of antiglobulin serum whereas warm antibodies in the patient's serum are found in much lower titers and may not be demonstrable at all unless trypsinized cells are used. Physiological saline is practically useless as a diluent. Cold hemagglutinins, on the other hand, are demonstrable in the serum by dilution in physiological saline solution. The reaction may be enhanced by the use of trypsin or bovine albumin as adjuvants. The antiglobulin test, although positive in most instances of cold hemagglutination, is of far weaker titer than that observed in warm agglutination. Hemolysins are demonstrated relatively infrequently and are most consistently associated with cold agglutinins. Hemolysins require complement to bring out their activity.

Hemosiderinuria is characteristic of paroxysmal nocturnal hemoglobinuria but it may be found whenever the plasma continuously contains abnormal amounts of hemoglobin.[44a] Only very small amounts have been found when the plasma hemoglobin levels were less than 20 mg. per 100 ml. but with plasma hemoglobin levels greater than 40 mg., hemosiderin is readily detected by the Prussian blue reaction (p. 641).

The measurement of the haptoglobin content of serum is a sensitive method for detecting hemolysis. When hemolysis, as measured by the hemoglobin turnover per day, exceeded twice the normal rate, haptoglobins were absent.[3b]

A search for **Heinz bodies**[12b] is helpful in recognizing hemolytic anemia due to certain drugs and in detecting red cells of the "primaquine-sensitive" type (p. 631). Heinz bodies are intracorpuscular structures which result from the oxidative injury of hemoglobin and loss of its normal configuration because of the oxidation of the thiol groups.[17f] This can occur spontaneously but is accelerated by such electron-carrying compounds as phenylhydrazine. In this process, reduced glutathione (GSH) is oxidized to GSSG and a portion of the GSH becomes bound to hemoglobin by forming mixed disulfides with the globin sulfhydryl groups; at the same time, hemoglobin is converted to methemoglobin. The Heinz bodies are the result of polymerization of the denatured hemoglobin molecules and their precipitation to form coccoid bodies. The presence of GSH appears to slow the precipitation of hemoglobin so that fewer, larger Heinz bodies are formed. It is well known that reticulocytes resist the development of Heinz bodies.[5a]

Heinz bodies appear as refractile, irregularly shaped bodies often lying at or close to the periphery of the red cells, sometimes attached to the outer surface of the cell. They range in size from minute particles to bodies up to 3 μ in size. Several bodies may be present in the same cell but the largest ones usually appear singly. They are not visible in blood films fixed in methanol and stained with Romanowsky dyes since the bodies and the surrounding hemoglobin stain the same pink color but can be stained supravitally by mixing a drop of blood with 4 drops of 0.5 per cent methyl violet in saline or by using a saline solution of brilliant cresyl blue (p. 90) and examining the preparation, after ringing it with petroleum jelly, under the oil immersion lens of the microscope. In methyl violet Heinz bodies stain deep purple; Howell-Jolly bodies, which are always round, and Pappenheimer bodies (p. 626) stain darkly, almost black with a bluish tinge. The reticulo-filamentous material of reticulocytes stains a pale blue. In brilliant cresyl blue Heinz bodies stain a distinctly lighter shade of blue than the reticulocyte substance. The spleen appears to be able to filter off red cells containing Heinz bodies from the circulation or perhaps removes the Heinz bodies from the red corpuscles.[32f]

In a test[8e] for the detection of "primaquine-sensitive" cells 0.1 ml. blood, collected in heparin, is mixed with 2 ml. of acetylphenylhydrazine (100 mg. per cent in a buffer solution). The suspension is mixed well, aerated and allowed to stand

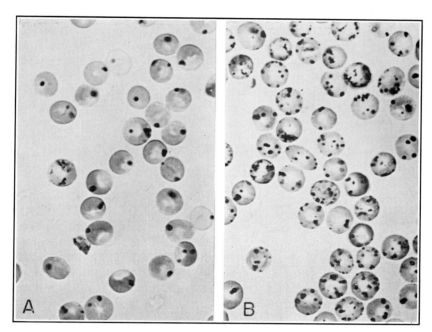

Fig. 12–3.—Heinz body formation in blood of persons sensitive to primaquine (*B*) compared with that in nonsensitive individuals (*A*). The red corpuscles were incubated with 100 mg. per cent acetylphenylhydrazine solution for four hours. Wet preparations stained with crystal violet. Magnification, 1300 ×. (Beutler *et al.*,[8e] courtesy of J. Lab. & Clin. Med.)

for two hours in a water bath at 37° C. When a small drop of such a suspension is placed on a coverslip and inverted over a larger drop of 2 per cent crystal violet solution on a microscope slide, red corpuscles containing Heinz bodies can be seen on oil immersion magnification (Fig. 12–3). In preparations containing sensitive erythrocytes 45 to 92 per cent of the red corpuscles were found to contain numerous small Heinz bodies whereas, in the blood of normal persons, the percentage of cells developing five or more Heinz bodies ranged from 0 to 28 per cent, with only two "false-positive" exceptions.

A wide range of aromatic nitrogen compounds of the nitrobenzene series and those related to aniline, as well as aliphatic nitro-compounds, hydroxylamine, sodium nitrate, sodium chlorate and naphthalene are capable of producing Heinz bodies.[12b] It will be noted that many of the same agents also produce methemoglobinemia (p. 194). In man chronic consumption of acetanilid or acetophenetidine (phenacetin)[23c] has resulted in the appearance of a few Heinz bodies in the blood. Although Heinz bodies may be found in the absence of anemia, and though Heinz body production is not the sole determinant of the instability of erythrocytes exposed to various drugs,[16h] large doses of the drugs producing them will cause hemolytic anemia. Heinz body formation has also been observed in hemolytic anemia associated with the taking of erythrol tetranitrate,[12a] salicylazosulfapyridine[34b] and diaminodiphenyl sulphone.[34] When patients with polycythemia vera are treated with phenylhydrazine or acetylphenylhydrazine (p. 804) Heinz bodies are produced.

More reliable than the Heinz body test is the glutathione stability test which depends on the measurement of reduced glutathione (GSH) levels before and after incubation of blood samples with acetylphenylhydrazine.[2a] A rapid screening test for glucose-6-phosphate dehydrogenase (G6PD) activity is also available,[104c] as well as methemoglobin reduction tests[3a] and a simple colorimetric method for determination of erythrocyte GSH.[110b]

Heinz Bodies in Absence of Drug Exposure. —Gasser[14a] reported 14 premature infants who developed hemolytic anemia and Heinz bodies. The condition was self-limited, providing the child survived the original severe hemolytic episode, but kernicterus developed in several. In retrospect it appears that ten of these cases may have been drug induced since hemorrhagic manifestations preceding the onset of anemia led to intensive Synkayvite® therapy. In four instances, however, and in other reported cases in a full term infant,[76a] and a child of 18 months,[1] no drug therapy was involved. In the last case other congenital abnormalities were present and the disease was fatal. An inborn error of erythrocyte metabolism may have been responsible.

These last cases may belong in one or more different categories of **inclusion body anemia**. One of these categories is associated with the passage of an abnormal pigment in the urine and possibly with the presence of an abnormal hemoglobin. Thus, in one patient, a 14 year old girl who was known to have had hemolytic anemia since the age of 30 months, dark urine had been passed since infancy. This contained a dark brown pigment thought to be a dipyrolmethene, mesobilifuscin. Inclusion bodies resembling Heinz bodies but not entirely identical with them were observed.[62a] A similar disorder was described in a father and his only son.[74] The inclusion bodies were indistinguishable from Heinz bodies. In addition, many erythrocytes containing basophilic stippling, siderotic granules and rod-like structures were present. A

possible elevation of the normal A_2 hemoglobin component was reported. Transfusion of the patient's erythrocytes into a normal recipient resulted in rapid removal of the heterologous cells from the circulation and the excretion of dark pigments in the urine. In a similar case studied in our laboratory (Fig. 12–4) an abnormal hemoglobin component of reduced anodal mobility at pH 8.6 was found which, on starch electrophoresis, migrated between the normal A_1 and A_2 fractions.[74b] The intracorpuscular defect was associated with an increased rate of erythrocyte autohemolysis *in vitro*. It could not be determined with certainty that the inclusion bodies were true Heinz bodies. They were thought to contain ribose nucleic acid.

Differing from these are cases with iron-staining erythrocytic inclusions (**"Pappenheimer bodies"**) or siderocytes (p. 100).[22e,25] In these cases of hemolytic anemia of obscure etiology, following splenectomy the erythrocytes were found to contain one to 20 or more iron-containing, coccoid or bacillary inclusions which also stained with Romanowsky dyes, methylene blue and pyronin but not with nuclear stains such as hematoxylin. The Pappenheimer bodies were numerous in the sternal marrow but were plentiful in the blood only after splenectomy. "Sideroblastic" refractory anemias were discussed in the preceding chapter.

Erythrokinetic studies (p. 185) will show whether the increased blood destruction is due to intracorpuscular or extracorpuscular causes and whether the breakdown of cells is taking place mainly in the spleen or elsewhere.[108d] These techniques also provide the means whereby erythrocyte production and destruction can be quantitated. As a rule, however, such measurements are not required to arrive at a diagnosis.

Prognosis, Treatment and Complications.—The outlook in hemolytic

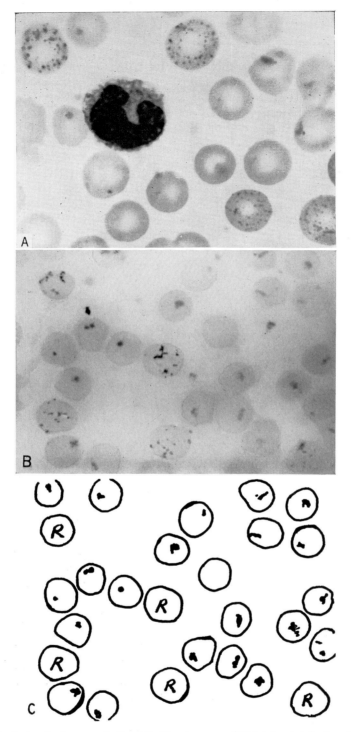

Fig. 12–4.—"Inclusion-body anemia." (A) Blood smear (Wright's stain) showing four red cells containing fine densely basophilic material as well as other red cells which contain larger and less dense, irregular basophilic bodies, probably corresponding to refractile inclusions demonstrable under phase microscopy and staining supravitally with aqueous stains. The latter are shown in (B) which is a wet blood film stained supravitally with aqueous methyl violet and allowed to dry. The cells in (C) marked R are reticulocytes, while the other structures appearing in red cells are inclusion bodies. (Scott, Haut, Cartwright and Wintrobe, courtesy of Blood).

anemias varies greatly, depending on their nature and cause. Where a specific etiologic agent is involved, the outlook is good if the cause can be removed, provided death does not occur during the acute hemolytic episode. Of the idiopathic variety, prognosis is generally better in the "cold" type, many such cases running a benign course. In hemolytic anemia associated with "warm" antibodies, prognosis is much less favorable but the introduction of steroid therapy has changed the outlook from grave to good.

An acute attack of hemolysis is treated by the use of appropriate measures to relieve shock, if present, maintain fluid balance and allow renal repair, if the kidneys have been damaged, as fully outlined elsewhere (p. 369). If the anemia is due to a bacterial agent, the organism must be eliminated or, if due to some chemical, exposure to the latter should be prevented.

Blood Transfusion.—Blood transfusions, so useful in acute anemia of other types, must be employed with caution in hemolytic anemias for, even when great care is taken in matching the blood, hemolysis with an increase in the burden on the excretory organs and sometimes with ensuing thromboses, may occur. Nevertheless, when blood destruction is rapid, the dangerous consequences of shock can only be met by intravenous administration of adequate amounts of blood. The presence of autoantibodies makes matching of blood difficult. Whenever possible the patient's blood should be genotyped before the first transfusion and the specificity of his antibodies determined. Blood homologous as to ABO and Rh blood groups should be matched with that of the patient and the best match used. It should be ascertained that the recipient's serum does not contain hemolysins against a prospective donor's cells by incubating them in a test tube at 37° C. for one hour. In spite of all such precautions, transfusion may nevertheless accelerate hemolysis. In such a case exchange transfusion has been used successfully.[3]

With the availability of hormone therapy, the necessity for blood transfusion, even at the initiation of treatment, is greatly reduced. In many instances, blood transfusion can be avoided entirely.

Steroid Hormones.—These are the agents of choice in acquired hemolytic anemias. In the idiopathic disorder with "warm" antibodies, complete relief from anemia can be expected in 70 to 90 per cent of cases.[7,53,84] In the symptomatic form results are somewhat less good. When "cold" antibodies are present, the beneficial effect is less dependable[84] but avoidance of exposure to cold is very helpful. Failures with steroid therapy are, in part at least, attributable to the use of inadequate doses. The therapeutic dose is the amount necessary to produce the desired results. Thus, in the case illustrated in Figure 12–5, as much as 200 mg. cortisone per day had little effect. When this dose was doubled a prompt response occurred. It is often found that a smaller amount than that necessary to relieve the anemia will suffice to maintain the patient in good condition. In some cases hormone may not be required to maintain the remission;[125] in others, anemia, increasing reticulocytosis, a greater proportion of nucleated red cells and even deep (bone ?) pain indicate that hormone therapy must be continued.

The oral administration of prednisone or a similar compound is preferable to parenteral therapy. It has been suggested that ACTH may be helpful when steroid hormones fail[5c] but we have not been impressed with the need for ACTH. The steroid dose should be spaced at six hourly intervals. Dietary salt restriction and, rarely, the administration of potassium salts (potassium chloride 8 to 16 Gm. daily) may be needed to minimize

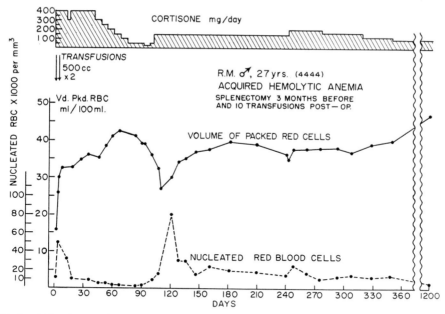

FIG. 12–5.—Effectiveness of large doses of cortisone in a patient with acquired hemolytic anemia (Coombs' positive) in whom splenectomy, ten blood transfusions and smaller amounts of cortisone (up to 200 mg. daily) had been of little value. The patient still requires steroid hormone therapy (prednisone, 12.5 mg. daily) 9 years after splenectomy.

salt retention. Once anemia has been relieved the dose of steroid should be reduced gradually over a period of weeks, sometimes longer. In many patients treatment with steroids must be continued a long time, sometimes permanently. The continued use of hormone in cases in which this is essential raises serious problems. Not only are the effects of the large doses which are sometimes necessary disfiguring, but other serious ill effects develop, especially osteoporosis. The administration of testosterone once every three weeks may possibly reduce this serious hazard. Muscular weakness may also develop. In our experience other untoward effects, such as the development of hypertension or diabetes, are less common.

The mode of action of the steroids or ACTH is uncertain. In most patients the production of autoantibodies persists, although usually at a lower level. The direct Coombs' test seldom becomes negative.[5e]

Splenectomy.—In contrast to the remarkable benefit from splenectomy in hereditary spherocytosis, this operation is much less valuable in the treatment of the acquired forms of hemolytic anemia. Although, before the discovery of the steroids, splenectomy was found helpful in approximately 50 per cent of cases,[120] now this operation should only be considered if steroid therapy fails. Even then there is no assurance that splenectomy will be useful. In some patients who could be maintained only on large doses of steroids, splenectomy made it possible to maintain the patient on smaller doses. However, this has by no means always been true. Splenectomy is even less likely to be helpful when cold antibodies are present than in the warm variety.[84] There are no well defined criteria on which to base the decision for operation.

The decision for operation cannot be made lightly for there is not only the surgical risk but complications such as postoperative atelectasis, thromboses and infections may plague the patient and his physicians. Because there are so many uncertainties, attempts have been made to devise objective criteria whereby a decision concerning the advisability of splenectomy could be made. These have been based on observations of body-surface scanning after the injection of radioactive chromate. Thus 25 to 50 ml. venous blood may be withdrawn and mixed with ACD solution and 50 to 150 microcuries of radioactive chromate. The mixture is incubated at room temperature for 30 to 60 minutes, as in the procedure for measuring erythrocyte life span with Cr^{51} (p. 164). Following reinjection of the tagged red cells, the anterolateral projection of the spleen is monitored with a unidirectional scintillation counter.[103b] After equilibrium over the spleen has been attained, the anterior projections of the liver and the heart, as well as the spleen are counted. From these counts ratios may be constructed between spleen and precordium (S/P) and the liver and precordium (L/P). This procedure can be repeated daily or twice a week until a definite trend in the ratios becomes evident. A "splenic localization index" (SLI) has been devised, as follows:

$$\frac{\frac{\triangle S/P}{S/P_o} \times 10}{d_{max}} = SLI,$$

where $\triangle S/P$ is the maximum change in the ratio, S/P_o is the initial ratio and d_{max} is the day on which the maximum ratio is found. Others have studied the ratio of radioactivity over the spleen as compared with that over the liver.[108d]

It was noted that a maximum S/P ratio of 1.5 or more and an SLI of 1.0, or more, correlated well with other information regarding the major site of increased blood destruction. When the clinical picture together with data from scintillation counts focused major blame on the spleen, splenectomy was found to be successful.[103b,108d] Further investigation of technics of this kind may well provide a useful guide for decisions involving splenectomy in the treatment of hemolytic anemias.

Iron and Other Antianemic Agents.—It has been shown in experimental acetylphenylhydrazine anemia in bile fistula dogs that iron from destroyed red cells is utilized readily and nearly quantitatively for the regeneration of hemoglobin.[5a] From clinical experience it is also evident that the materials required for blood formation are largely conserved when hemolysis occurs. Treatment with iron, vitamin B_{12}, folic acid or liver extracts is unnecessary but the diet should be adequate in proteins, vitamins and minerals.

In cases in which other therapy failed, the administration of radioactive colloidal gold[115a] or of heparin[103c] was said to be beneficial. If cold agglutinin disease is troublesome, mercaptanes deserve a trial.[70b]

As in hereditary spherocytosis (p. 646), episodes of marrow hypoplasia, accompanied by reticulocytopenia and continued hemolysis may occur, especially in association with infections.[79c] It has been postulated that the antibody involved in the pathogenesis of the hemolytic anemia in such cases causes destruction of red cell precursors in the marrow.[105b,108a]

Folic acid deficiency with megaloblastic marrow hyperplasia may develop in acquired hemolytic anemia of the autoantibody type or in the symptomatic variety, as well as in other forms of hemolytic anemia (hereditary spherocytosis, paroxysmal noctural hemoglobinuria, sickle cell anemia, thalassemia).[80b] This has been attributed to the great demands of an active erythroid marrow but other factors, such as impaired intestinal absorption, may be important as well.

Pathology.—The *spleen* is usually enlarged, one and a half to many times the normal size. Histologically, extreme congestion of the pulp, histiocytic proliferation with giant cell formation and erythrophagocytosis and myeloid metaplasia are often found.[46] Multiple areas of thrombosis and infarction may be observed. Congested sinuses with few red blood cells in the cords were seen in patients without spherocytosis whereas congestion of the splenic cords was associated with selective retention of morphologically abnormal red cells.[106c] Hemosiderosis in the spleen and liver is common and the bone marrow shows pronounced normoblastic hyperplasia. Renal lesions may be present, such as those which follow the administration of mismatched blood (p. 362). In hereditary spherocytosis (p. 653) and in sickle cell anemia (p. 685), as well as in nocturnal hemoglobinuria (p. 643) certain other changes have been described.

Pathogenesis.—In a discussion of the pathogenesis of the hemolytic anemias a number of factors must be considered. These include inherited or congenital abnormalities of the red corpuscles, exogenous factors injuring them and endogenous influences affecting them. Among these influences the spleen must be included. The agents acting upon the red corpuscles may do so directly, as is the case with a simple hemolysin such as saponin, or the mediation of some accessory factor or factors may be necessary. The latter is, by far, the more common occurrence in the hemolytic disorders encountered in man.

The pathogenesis of the various types of hemolytic disease due to intracorpuscular defects will be discussed separately in the sections dealing with each of these disorders. The *pathogenesis of the acquired hemolytic conditions* may be considered here.

In the section on Etiology (p. 605), a great number and variety of factors were listed as being associated with increased blood destruction. In regard to chemical factors, it was pointed out that the effect of some is closely correlated with the dose received; the action of others depends upon the *sensitivity of the host*. Thus hemolytic anemia was observed only in approximately 2 to 4 per cent of patients treated with sulfanilamide,[40] in 0.6 per cent of those receiving sulfapyridine[10] and only in a few instances of individuals treated with sulfathiazole,[27b] sulfadiazine,[19d] sulfadimidine[16b] and salicylazosulfapyridine.[34b] It was observed that only a small dose precipitated the hemolytic crisis and readministration had a similar effect.[40] Although increased urinary excretion of coproporphyrin III was demonstrated[12c] there was no other evidence of interference with hemoglobin production[37] or of the formation of unusual oxidation products of the sulfonamide drugs.[13] Investigations of the mechanism whereby sulfonamides produce hemolytic anemia led to the production of anemia in rats[21a] and mice[32] by the administration of these agents but it was difficult to relate these observations with the evidence of individual susceptibility which marked the problem in human subjects.

An important advance in the understanding of the pathogenesis of many forms of acquired hemolytic anemia arose from studies of the antimalarial compounds, *pamaquin*[9a] and *primaquine.*[8e] It was found that Negroes were more likely to develop acute hemolytic anemia from these agents than white persons and that about 10 per cent of American Negroes were susceptible.[8e] That this susceptibility resides in the subjects' erythrocytes was shown by the fact that the erythrocytes of such a subject, tagged with radiochromium and transferred into a nonsensitive subject, were hemolysed when primaquine was given to the recipient. On the other hand, non-sensitive red corpuscles were not hemolysed when transfused to a sensitive subject to whom primaquine had been given. Furthermore, the hemolysis was observed to be self-limited. Thus, the administration of primaquine to drug-sensitive recipients resulted in acute hemolysis followed by complete recovery even though drug administration was continued. This was shown to be due to a change in the reactivity of the red cell population. The sensitive cells were found to be the older ones and formed Heinz bodies (p. 624) more readily than do nonsensitive red cells. This led to the hypothesis that primaquine sensitivity is related to a deficiency in some enzyme system which decreases in activity as the red cell ages, making it more vulnerable to the action of noxious agents. Such an enzyme deficiency might well be undetected unless the red cells were challenged in some way.

It was found that glucose-6-phosphate dehydrogenase (G6PD) activity is reduced in the red blood cells of primaquine-sensitive subjects.[8e] As discussed elsewhere (p. 126) this enzyme is concerned with regeneration of TPNH and this, in turn, is required in the reduction of oxidized glutathione. Reduced glutathione (GSH) was found to be related to sensitivity to primaquine and other 8-aminoquinoline compounds, as well as to certain other compounds.[2b] Thus, it was observed that the GSH level of sensitive cells was consistently lower than that of nonsensitive cells, a rapid fall in red cell GSH occurred *in vivo* when primaquine was administered to sensitive individuals but not to nonsensitive ones, and the same was found *in vitro* when sensitive cells were incubated with acetyl phenylhydrazine. It could not be determined whether GSH depletion plays a primary role in the ultimate break-up of sensitive red cells when they are exposed to certain noxious agents or whether this is only a convenient indicator of other important changes. It was observed that glutathione reductase, aldolase and TPN are increased in the cells of sensitive persons and the rate of incorporation of glycine, *in vitro*, into GSH is decreased.[27d]

The GSH stability of red cells can be determined by incubating blood samples with acetylphenylhydrazine and measuring the GSH level before and after incubation.[2a] This procedure, as well as the Heinz body test described above (p. 624) showed that GSH instability can be demonstrated in the blood of subjects sensitive to sulfanilamide, sulfoxone, thiazolsulfone, sulfamethoxypyridazine (Kynex), N₂-acetylsulfanilamide, sulfacetamide, paraminosalicylic acid, probenecid acetanilid, acetophenetidine (phenacetin),[2b] acetylsalicylic acid,[35d] nitrofurantoin,[19a] α-naphthol and α-naphthoquinone,[8c,40f] naphthalene,[32d] certain vitamin K derivatives[32e] and perhaps other drugs,[2b,8e,35d] as well as the fava bean. It was shown, furthermore, that G6PD deficiency is relatively common not only among American Negroes[2a,4d] (7.2 per cent)[22c] but also in Caucasians of Italian and Greek extraction[22c] as well as in Sephardic (Oriental) Jews, Arabs, desert Bedouins and Druses.[35d] The incidence of the deficiency is low among Ashkenazy Jews[35d] and in subjects of Chinese and Javanese descent.[22c] Thus the ethnographic distribution of favism and of drug-induced hemolytic anemias of the "primaquine-sensitivity" type was found to be the same.[35b]

It has now been shown that the abnormality of erythrocyte metabolism which the primaquine studies disclosed is an inherited trait which appears to be transmitted as a sex-linked, incompletely dominant gene of intermediate penetrance.[4d,35d] The abnormality is not limited to the red cells. Although normal levels were present in leukocytes,[22c] a significantly reduced level of G6PD was found in the platelets and saliva of deficient subjects.[27d] That more remains to be learned, however, is suggested by the report that there is a quantitative difference in G6PD deficiency in affected Caucasians and Negroes.[22c] This has led to the suggestion that different genetic mechanisms account for the deficiency in these two races. Other studies have revealed morphologic differences in the erythrocyte membranes of G6PD deficient subjects, when examined by electron microscopy, as compared with those of normal individuals.[7a]

A special situation has been found in the *newborn*. The GSH concentration of cord blood is somewhat elevated but at the age of 30 to 75 hours the level becomes unstable in spite of the fact that the concentration of G6PD is not reduced. This, however, can be corrected with glucose or inosine in normal but not in sensitive infants.[35c] Thus, there is in newborns a non-genetic type of GSH instability. Whether such infants are unusually susceptible to the hemolytic effects of certain drugs or chemicals has not been settled.[40e]

To what extent inherited metabolic abnormalities of red cells can explain the hemolytic effects of various agents is not known. GSH instability and deficiency of G6PD apparently characterize the abnormality which permits the hemolytic action of a large number of drugs and chemical agents. Possibly some of those included in the list of agents which will cause hemolytic anemia in all persons exposed may be shown to belong in the "hypersensitivity" group. It seems very likely that in the case of certain agents an intrinsic red cell abnormality is responsible for the development of anemia from a dose which in many individuals has little or no effect, even though a large dose will be injurious to everyone. Phenylhydrazine may belong in this category.

It is also possible that some instances of hemolytic anemia occasionally occurring in the course of certain infections may be due to the existence of an intrinsic defect in the red corpuscles which had not been recognized. Blackwater fever (p. 607) is a case in point. However, there is some evidence to suggest that, as in the case of the sickling phenomenon (p. 670), G6PD deficiency may offer some protection against *P. falciparum* malaria.[40g]

The fact that Heinz bodies can be demonstrated in the red cells of patients who develop hemolytic anemia following exposure to many drugs and chemical agents indicates that the cells are actually damaged. It is now known that susceptibility to such damage not only varies, but in many instances can be attributed to an abnormality of the red cells themselves. However, red cells are probably subject to injury in other ways. Thus it was pointed out that, in the case of malaria and in the hemolysis associated with severe burns (p. 612), the osmotic and mechanical fragility of parasitized or heated red cells is increased. Again, sensitivity to fuadin[17] and to quinidine[13b] was shown to have an immunologic basis. Thus, in the latter case, it appeared that union of the chemical with the patient's serum caused agglutination of the red cells. In the presence of complement, hemolysis occurred. Still other pathogenetic mechanisms are involved when lead (p. 610), distilled water (p. 610) or other substances (p. 606) are the injurious agents.

Immunologic Mechanisms.— It has been postulated that some drugs and perhaps viruses, bacteria and other agents damage the surface of red corpuscles, rendering them more vulnerable to the action of endogenous factors or perhaps even altering them in such a way that they become antigenic and thereby set up antibody formation and an autoimmune reaction. In most cases of acquired hemolytic anemia, however, obvious sensitization is not present. Yet it has been found that erythrocytes from cases of acquired hemolytic anemia survive normally when transfused into normal persons whereas normal red corpuscles transfused into these patients are rapidly eliminated.[20a] Differential cell survival studies have shown that such normal cells become sensitized and give a positive direct Coombs' test before being eliminated from the patient's circulation.[32g] These and other observations which have been cited already have led to the conclusion that antibodies are involved in the pathogenesis of many instances of acquired hemolytic anemia.

In explanation of the mode of development of such autosensitization, it has been suggested that some endogenous process which is a normal one is set in motion in an exaggerated form under certain circumstances. Thus, autoagglutinins are found in normal individuals but they are weak and are active only in the cold; normally the tissue cells are sufficient to absorb them and thus protect the body from any harmful effects. Under exceptional circumstances, as in certain infections, autoagglutinins may be formed in such great excess that the means for coping with them are insufficient. When this occurs, time alone usually suffices to permit a diminution or disappearance of these hemolytic factors, provided the patient can survive the crisis. In other instances recovery occurs only after the organ in which certain changes take place, namely, the spleen, has been removed.

Immunologic changes in the "symptomatic" hemolytic anemias have usually been identical with those found in the idiopathic forms. Their frequent occurrence in diseases associated with abnormal proliferation of the reticuloendothelial system and lymphatic tissues has suggested to many investigators that the autoantibodies may be derived from these hyperplastic tissues.[108,118] Such antibodies have been extracted in high concentration from lymphosarcoma tissue[78c] and the demonstration of large amounts of intracellular periodic acid-Schiff positive protein in the neoplastic tissue of patients with malignant lymphomas, hemolytic anemia and positive antiglobulin tests has been interpreted as evidence that these tissues are capable of synthesizing abnormal proteins.[107] In the "collagen diseases" it has been suggested that the autoantibodies represent another manifestation of the disordered protein formation or the sensitivity to antigenic stimulation which is so characteristic of these conditions. Still other mechanisms have been postulated,[118] such as the development of autoimmune antibodies through the phenomenon of cross reactivity and the influence of repeated transfusions in altering the specificity of antibodies.

A substance coating erythrocytes in idiopathic and in symptomatic cases of autoimmune hemolytic disease of the "warm" variety, has been eluted from them and was found to be either a gamma globulin or a substance cross reacting with this protein.[93c] The life span of the erythrocytes was inversely proportional to the concentration of the erythrocyte-coating substance. A decrease in its concentration was associated with corticosteroid therapy. This substance failed to react with "cold" antibody, suggesting thereby that the erythrocytes in "cold" hemolytic anemias are coated by an adsorbed protein lacking antibody characteristics.

There is considerable evidence to support the hypothesis of autoimmunization, which is now so popular. Yet it should be remembered that an antigen has not been demonstrated[21b] and that a different explanation may ultimately be found.

Mechanism of Destruction of Red Cells.—The mechanism of erythrocyte destruction initiated by antibodies has been the subject of intensive study and it is clear that a number of different processes may be involved. Direct physicochemical injury of the erythrocyte has been mentioned already as a means whereby red corpuscles may be injured by chemical and other agents. As the result of studies of the metabolism of the erythrocyte it has become clear that important processes are normally at work to maintain the integrity of this corpuscle and that these processes may diminish in activity as the cell ages (p. 126) or may be defective as the result of genetic influences (p. 632). Even in the absence of such factors, exogenous influences may so alter the red corpuscles as to render them more vulnerable than normally to the stresses of the circulation[40c]

Agglutination is a fundamental factor in the mechanism of destruction of red cells by antibodies. Agglutination has been observed to take place intravascularly in experimental animals and in human subjects.[117a] Injected sensitized red cells agglutinate, probably as a consequence of the action of rouleaux-producing concentrations of plasma globulins.[17e] This is probably an intermediate step in the mechanism of sequestration. Sequestration occurs in the spleen and in tissue capillaries elsewhere, and this in turn may lead to arrest of the circulation, tissue ischemia and release of substances from the autolysing tissues. Such substances may have a local damaging effect on the impacted erythrocytes.[80a]

In many instances of autoimmune hemolytic anemia, agglutination occurs but the presence of a hemolysin cannot be demonstrated *in vitro*. However, in cases in which marked hemoglobinemia is found it may be assumed that intravascular *hemolysis* has taken place. Whereas, in the case of hemolytic agents of chemical or physical nature, their action both *in vitro* and *in vivo* is similar and consists of the production of gradual changes in the red corpuscles which become manifest in increased mechanical and osmotic fragility, the action of immune hemolysins *in vivo* is not the same as that *in vitro*. In paroxysmal nocturnal hemoglobinuria and paroxysmal cold hemoglobinuria lytic factors exists in the plasma. In the first instance a fall in pH (p. 643) and in the second a fall in temperature (p. 637) are required for maximum activity of the hemolytic system. In other examples of acquired hemolytic anemia, however, no such lytic factor has been demonstrated in the plasma. In some instances complement is required and this may explain why the level of serum complement is reduced in certain cases of acquired hemolytic anemia. In other cases there is nothing to suggest the participation of complement.

It was pointed out earlier that *erythrophagocytosis* can be demonstrated in some cases of acquired hemolytic anemia and that this phenomenon can be produced artificially by incubating red and white blood cells with the serum of patients with this disorder (p. 605). The quantitative importance of this mechanism as a means of red cell destruction is difficult to evaluate but it seems likely that when the action of tissue macrophages is added to that of the blood leukocytes, this mechanism may play a significant role in certain instances.[127]

The significance of *spherocytosis* is a central point in any consideration of hemolytic disorders. The spherocytosis which is so characteristic of hereditary spherocytosis is probably the consequence of an inherited metabolic defect in these corpuscles (p. 654). Their increased osmotic fragility has been attributed to the fact that in the spheroid form the red corpuscle is closer to the bursting point than is the normal biconcave corpuscle, but evidence has been presented that intracellular protein osmotic pressure is the important factor.[109a] The spherocytosis of acquired hemolytic anemias is probably the result of the action of factors acting after the cells have been released from the bone marrow and their breakdown may be due to changes in the tensile strength of their membranes.[109a] Osmotic lysis does not occur *in vivo* except under very unusual circumstances (p. 610).

There is increasing evidence that red cells may be subjected to *erythrostasis* in the spleen or in other sites by such processes as intravascular agglutination or sequestration of spheroidal cells.[16e] Erythrostasis may lead to a variety of changes in the red cells, such as increase in spheroidicity and in osmotic and mechanical fragility. It is possible that erythrostasis in the spleen permits accumulation of metabolites with resulting swelling of the cells. Erythrostasis may not be important in corpuscular breakdown under normal circumstances but, when it is of unusual degree or when abnormal cells, such as those damaged by various means are presented to the spleen, erythrostasis may play a very important role. Thus, it was shown that normal erythrocytes, perfused through spleens removed for nonhemolytic disorders, passed through the splenic sinusoids whereas uncoated spherocytes were retained.[9b, 40b]

The *spleen* appears to be a site for selective removal and sequestration of abnormal erythrocytes, it may permit further injury to the cells and, in certain instances, it may supply antibodies which coat the red corpuscles. Thus, it was found that incubation of normal red cells of compatible blood groups with the splenic pulp of patients with acquired hemolytic anemia caused these cells to become agglutinable by Coombs' serum.[36b] In contrast, this could not be accomplished by incubation of normal cells with spleens from patients with hereditary spherocytosis, thrombocytopenic purpura, congestive splenomegaly or Gaucher's disease. Furthermore, washed red cells removed from the splenic pulp of patients with acquired hemolytic anemia were more strongly agglutinated by Coombs' serum than those derived from normal blood.

Experience with the effects of splenectomy fits well with these concepts of the role of the spleen in the hemolytic anemias. In hereditary spherocytosis splenectomy is almost always successful. This can be attributed to the fact that erythrostasis in the spleen adds just enough damage to the congenitally abnormal spherocytes to cause their breakdown. When the spleen is removed the corpuscles which are produced are the same as before the operation but the hazard of passage through the spleen has been removed. In acquired hemolytic anemias, if the formation and release of damaging immune bodies is chiefly localized in the spleen, splenectomy will be successful. In such cases spherocytes disappear.[99a] In other cases extrasplenic tissues participate actively in the production of the abnormal antibodies or serve as sites for sequestration. In such cases splenectomy fails to eliminate the hemolytic processes.[36b] In still other conditions in which splenectomy is of no value, such as sickle cell anemia, paroxysmal nocturnal hemoglobinuria and thalassemia, processes unrelated to the spleen are involved in the pathogenesis of the disorder.

There is good evidence that the *liver* can be an important site for sequestration[16e] and also for hemolysis of red cells. By techniques of surface counting it was possible to show that cells which are removed very rapidly are destroyed in the liver.[82a] These were cells which had bound complement. Destruction in the spleen was slower and tended to be more concerned with cells whose surface properties were so slightly changed that they passed through the liver intact. In other experiments in which antibody/antigen proportions could be altered it was observed that a spectrum of effects could be produced, ranging from a slow partial trapping by the spleen with small doses to a brisk hepatic trapping with large doses, while still larger amounts caused intravascular hemolysis.[17e]

The *leukopenia* and possibly also the *thrombocytopenia* accompanying acute immune hemolysis may well be the result of the injurious action of antigen-antibody complexes released from the hemolyzing red cells.[17e] This may cause leukocytes to adhere to endothelial surfaces and may damage the platelets. Other systemic effects of immune hemolysis, such as chills and fever, urticaria and even renal injury may be due to the release of constituents of injured cells, such as pyrogen, histamine and serotonin.

PAROXYSMAL (COLD) HEMOGLOBINURIA

Definition. — Paroxysmal hemoglobinuria *e frigore* is a condition characterized by the sudden passage of hemoglobin in the urine following local or general exposure to cold.

History, Etiology, and Pathogenesis.—Pavy, in 1866, first clearly differentiated this disorder from the hemoglobinuria encountered in cases of malaria. In the same year Gull recognized the effect of chilling. Various writers defined the clinical features in the last quarter of the nineteenth century. In 1904, Donath and Landsteiner[67] showed that the hemoglobinuria is due to the sudden hemolysis of blood, probably intravascularly, as the result of the action of an autohemolysin contained in the patient's own blood. The hemolysin unites with the red corpuscles only at a low temperature but destruction of the cells occurs only after the blood is again warmed.

Complement is necessary for the hemolysis, which occurs in the warm phase. It is also more or less essential for the effective fixation of the antibody in the cold phase,[75a] perhaps in order to prevent the antibody from being rapidly eluted on subsequent warming.[5c] The C'4 component of complement may be required for this fixation.[61a]

Other factors than cold influence the hemolytic system, notably carbon dioxide.[75a] The latter probably affects hemolysis by decreasing pH and may be related to a second hemolysin.[69b] For the cold phase to be effective, at least thirty minutes are necessary and temperatures below 10° or 15° C. are usually needed.[5c] However, many variations have been observed insofar as thermostability, optimal period of the cold phase and the need for complement are concerned.[65]

Strongly positive direct antiglobulin (Coombs') reactions have been observed at the time of hemolytic attacks produced by chilling but these become negative after the attacks.[61a] Positive indirect reactions have also been reported.[5c,61a] The positive Coombs' test is probably due to interaction between the antiglobulin serum and the complement adsorbed on the test cells, this adsorption being promoted by the cold antibodies.[69d]

The disorder is quite rare.[41a] The typical condition is a manifestation of syphilis, the congenital form particularly, but also the acquired infection.[41a,67] The hemolysin has also been demonstrated in the sera of some patients with late syphilis who had had no symptoms of the disease.[62] It has been suggested, on experimental grounds, that during syphilitic infection antigens are liberated either from the spirochete or from the organs of their host and that the antibodies of the Wassermann reaction (reagin) and of the Donath-Landsteiner reaction are formed as a result.[69]

Burmeister[43] noted that, although the Wassermann reaction was positive in almost all cases of the disorder, indications of syphilis were present in less than half. It is now recognized that paroxysmal (cold) hemoglobinuria may be *unrelated to syphilis*. In such cases, not only are the serological reactions for syphilis negative and clinical or historical evidence of the disease lacking[14,48,72,76] but, in contrast to the luetic disorder, the titer of cold hemagglutinins is high, the Donath-Landsteiner test (p. 639) is negative and hemolysis can take place without first warming the blood. The cold agglutinin titer may be greater than 1:3000 and may cause difficulty in performing routine red cell counts (p. 386). The red corpuscles show increased susceptibility to trauma and complement is not required for hemolysis to occur.

In contrast to other anti-erythrocyte antibodies, the Donath-Landsteiner antibody readily causes lysis of normal human red corpuscles instead of predominantly causing agglutination. However, some agglutinating effect has been demonstrated.[5c]

Symptomatology. — Aching and pain in the back, legs or abdomen, cramps, headache, malaise, and even vomiting or diarrhea develop suddenly and are followed by a severe, shaking chill and fever (102° to 104° F.; 38.9° to 40° C.), usually of short duration. Dark brownish or almost black urine is passed, but this may be noticeable only in the first two or three specimens. It is usually possible to obtain a history of preceding exposure to cold, but the exposure may be very slight and may be limited to only one part of the body. Symptoms appear at any time from a few minutes to seven or eight hours following exposure.

The patient is weak, pale, and may be slightly icteric. The spleen is often somewhat enlarged, and the liver may be palpable. Vasomotor disturbances, such as urticarial wheals or symptoms of Raynaud's syndrome, are common.[57] Thus, the fingers, toes, tip of the nose, lips or ears may become blanched or deeply cyanotic. In addition to these signs, evidence of syphilis may be discovered.

In other cases, or at other times in the same case, the symptoms are milder, hemoglobinemia may occur without hemoglobinuria, and only moderate fever and icterus may develop. Recovery from the attack is usually rapid, and between attacks the patient may be entirely symptom-free.

Laboratory Findings.—Morphology of the Blood.—The blood findings are the same as those which have been described as characteristic of acute hemolytic anemia (p. 603). The red cell count and the color of the plasma depend on the severity of the attack. Sharp decreases in hemoglobin level may occur and, in persons subjected to continuous cold weather and repeated attacks, chronic anemia may develop. Marked decreases in leukocyte count take place after exposure to cold and erythrophagocytosis may be observed. Complement is required for the phagocytosis.[61b] It has been suggested that the trapping of phagocytic leukocytes in organ capillaries is responsible, at least in part, for the leukopenia. Leukocytosis follows later. This is of the myeloid type and is accompanied by the appearance of immature forms.[41]

Urine.—Spectroscopic examination reveals that the urine contains oxyhemoglobin and methemoglobin and these give it the dark red, brown, or almost black appearance. Few if any red corpuscles are found but in the urinary sediment "ghosts" of red cells may be seen, as well as red cell casts. Albuminuria will be noted. As already stated, these abnormalities may be found only in the first one or two specimens after an attack.

Tests for Demonstrating Hemolysins.—An attack may be reproduced by immersing the hands or feet in ice water for ten to twenty minutes. This is known as the *Rosenbach test*. Very occasionally all four extremities must be immersed to cause hemoglobinuria.[59b] This should not be attempted, however, unless it is known that less exposure will not produce an attack, as otherwise serious symptoms may ensue.

In the *Ehrlich test*, a ligature is tied around a finger, this is immersed in ice water, and local hemoglobinemia is then demonstrated after the finger has been warmed.

In the *Donath-Lansteiner test*, hemolysis following chilling of the blood is demonstrated *in vitro*. A *rough test* (Mackenzie)[67] is carried out as follows: 2 or 3 ml. of blood are taken from the patient and the same amount from a normal individual. Each sample is placed in a separate test tube and allowed to clot. Both tubes are then immersed in ice water for ten minutes and are subsequently warmed in a water bath for thirty minutes at 37° C. In a positive test hemolysis will be found in the blood taken from the patient whereas the serum in the control tube will be clear.

A more satisfactory test (modified from Mackenzie) is as follows: All syringes, tubes and salt solution used in carrying out the test are warmed. About 10 ml. of blood is taken from the arm vein of the patient. Half is placed in a dry, clean centrifuge tube, allowed to clot and centrifuged for serum. The remainder is placed in a bottle containing ammonium and potassium oxalate (p. 378). Some of these red cells are next washed three times in warm 0.85 per cent sodium chloride solution and then a 5 per cent suspension of cells is made. About 2 ml. of the suspension will be required.

Blood is obtained from a normal individual of the same blood group and prepared in the same way.

Complement is prepared by making a 1 to 10 dilution of fresh guinea pig serum. A total of 5 ml. should be prepared.

Six test tubes are prepared in a rack. Into each is measured 0.2 ml. of complement. Into tubes 1, 2, 3 and 4 is measured 0.1 ml. normal saline and into tubes 5 and 6, 0.6 ml. normal saline is placed. Patient's serum, 0.5 ml., is placed in tubes 1 and 3. Suspension of the patient's red cells, 0.2 ml., is placed in tubes 1, 4 and 5. Control serum, 0.5 ml., is placed in tubes 2 and 4. Suspension of control red cells, 0.2 ml., is placed in tubes 2, 3 and 6. The set of 6 tubes is next immersed in ice water for ten to thirty minutes and then warmed in a water bath for thirty minutes at 37° C.

When the test is positive hemolysis will be found in tubes 1 and 3 whereas the other tubes will be clear.

Diagnosis.—Appropriate tests for the study of cases of hemolytic anemia have been discussed already (p. 617). Where the preliminary tests suggest the presence of a cold hemolysin, the procedures described above should be carried out. When these are positive, the diagnosis is clear. There will also be serological and often clinical evidence of syphilis. As already stated (p. 637), *paroxysmal hemoglobinuria unrelated to syphilis* should be differentiated.

March Hemoglobinuria.[50a]—A rare type of hemoglobinuria has been observed to occur following prolonged walking or running, as in soldiers or marathon runners. Equal or more strenuous exercise of other types in man does not cause it, nor does chilling. The symptoms are trivial. There may be vague pains in the abdomen, back or thighs. However, the passage of dark urine may cause alarm. In one instance the spleen and liver were enlarged. The amount of blood which is hemolysed is probably slight, for jaundice is unusual and anemia does not develop. There may be a slight leukocytosis. Spectroscopic examination reveals that the pigmentation of the urine and blood is due to hemoglobin. After a few hours the hemoglobin is replaced by bilirubin or urobilinogen in the blood and urine respectively. About 83 cases have been described to date,[43a, 50a,58a,70,73,75b,77,77b] almost all in males, and particularly in the second decade of life. Spontaneous recovery occurs usually after a few months. A case has also been described in which a similar picture followed a blow in the region of the kidneys which led the patient to maintain a lordotic position.[75c] Contrary to typical cases, in five instances the hemoglobinuria followed excessive, strenuous exercise carried out within a short period of time[75b] and in one case the syndrome developed after exercise in the horizontal position.[43a]

The cause of the hemoglobinuria is not altogether clear. Although the condition is not unlike "march albuminuria" and orthostatic albuminuria, a relationship to circulatory disturbances in the kidneys or to lordosis, though postulated, is unproved. It has been shown[50b] that hemoglobinemia occurs frequently in marathon runners and in a few of these hemoglobinuria developed. This disappeared within a few hours after the end of the run. No alteration in erythrocyte fragility could be detected. Hemoglobinuria of this type is of no serious significance because hemoglobin from less than 10 ml. of normal blood is sufficient when released into the plasma to yield approximately 50 mg. per 100 ml. of plasma as measured by the benzidine method (p. 176). As little as 15 mg. is sufficient to produce red discoloration detectable by the eye. The destruction of so small an amount of blood following strenuous exertion may be regarded as within physiologic limits but why this should follow exercise of a special type and occur only in certain individuals, are questions which remain to be answered.

Idiopathic myoglobinuria and Haff disease have been described already (p. 618). These conditions, like march hemoglobinuria, are not accompanied by anemia. Furthermore, these disorders, as well as the various types of acute hemolytic anemia in which hemoglobinuria may occur, can be distinguished from hemoglobinuria *e frigore* by the history of the case and the negative

reactions to cold. On similar grounds a chronic type of hemolytic anemia, in which hemoglobinuria often occurs (paroxysmal nocturnal hemoglobinuria), which will be described shortly, can be differentiated.

Treatment.—Without treatment, attacks of paroxysmal hemoglobinuria were said to continue for years. Death following renal tubular necrosis has been described.[75d] Thorough and prolonged antisyphilitic treatment was found to end the clinical manifestations in at least the majority of the cases although the autohemolysin, as demonstrated by the Donath-Landsteiner test, may persist.[62,67] Transfusions with *fresh* whole blood could be harmful since this would supply complement.[65]

CHRONIC HEMOLYTIC ANEMIA WITH PAROXYSMAL NOCTURNAL HEMOGLOBINURIA

Definition, Synonyms and History.—This is an uncommon disorder of insidious onset and chronic course characterized by signs of hemolytic anemia and marked by attacks of hemoglobinuria which occur chiefly at night. It has been generally believed that the condition was first recorded by Marchiafava and Nazari in 1911, and was fully described by Micheli in 1931.[75] Consequently it is known as the *Marchiafava-Micheli syndrome*. The name *"haemoglobinuria recurrens vel nocturna cum anaemia haemolytica"* is also sometimes used. It appears,[43c] however, that the disease was known in the nineteenth century and that an excellent account was given by Strübing in 1882. By 1945 some 46 cases had been recorded.[42,42a,44d,45,52b,53,55,59a,61,67a,69b, 71,75,77b] Crosby[43d] in 1953 cited 162 cases. Undoubtedly there are a number of others, some overlooked.[76b]

Symptomatology.—Both sexes are affected, most commonly in adult life, usually in the third or fourth decade.

However, a few cases have been described in childhood[69c] and in elderly subjects. Weakness and yellowish discoloration of the skin and mucous membranes may be the first and only symptoms for many years or abdominal, lumbar or substernal pain together with a drowsy and ill sensation and fever may usher in an attack of hemoglobinuria early in the course of the ailment. Examination reveals jaundice, sometimes a bronzing of the skin, pallor, functional cardiac murmurs, usually moderate splenomegaly, and sometimes a degree of hepatic enlargement. The tongue is normal and so is the nervous system. The attacks of hemoglobinuria are unrelated to cold but it may have been noted that urine passed during the night or on arising is dark whereas the day urine may be quite normal in appearance. Exacerbations may occur at irregular intervals and attacks of hemoglobinuria may be precipitated by infections (even quite minor ones[53,67a]), menstruation,[5c] transfusions,[44b,53,55] operations, including splenectomy, the taking of iron salts[5c] and injections of liver extract or vaccine.[75]

The Blood.—There is usually well-marked anemia, the red cell count often being less than 2,000,000 cells. The anemia is usually macrocytic and there may be considerable variation in the size of the red corpuscles.[71] No spherocytes or evidence of erythrophagocytosis or abnormal leukocytes is usually seen. Reticulocytosis is well marked (10 to 20 per cent), there is polychromatophilia, and normoblasts and macroblasts may be found in the blood smear. The fragility of the red corpuscles to hypotonic saline solutions is normal. Mechanical fragility is also normal.[44b] The icterus index is raised and the plasma may actually be brownish in color. The van den Bergh reaction is positive, indirect. Spectroscopic examination reveals free hemoglobin in the plasma. This may be found even when there is no hemoglobinuria.[52b] Methemalbumin will also be found.

Leukopenia is usual and may be very marked (2500 per c.mm.). There may or may not be neutropenia and relative lymphocytosis.[57a] Thrombocytopenia of moderate degree is common but hemorrhagic manifestations are unusual.[55] Iron deficiency develops occasionally.[57a]

Urine.—The urine contains increased amounts of urobilinogen. Hemoglobinuria may be marked, or scarcely noticeable. Spectroscopic examination of the urine demonstrates the presence of varying amounts of free hemoglobin. The urinary sediment is tobacco-yellow in color and gives a positive iron reaction. Brown granules of altered blood pigment may be seen in the leukocytes or epithelial cells or outside the cells. The pigment has been identified as hemosiderin and is a very common, if not a constant finding.

The *hemosiderin can be demonstrated* as follows: A fresh sample of urine is centrifuged, the supernatant fluid is poured off and the residue is suspended in a fresh mixture of 2 per cent potassium ferrocyanide (5 ml.) plus 2 per cent hydrochloric acid (5 ml.). The preparation is allowed to stand ten minutes and is then centrifuged. The sediment is examined microscopically. When positive, blue granules of hemosiderin will be seen, especially within the cells. A permanent preparation can be made by smearing the urinary deposit on a glass slide, allowing this to dry in air and then fixing it by dipping the slide in methyl alcohol for ten to twenty minutes. It is then stained in freshly prepared acid-potassium ferrocyanide solution for ten minutes in a water-bath at 56° C. The slide is then washed in running water for twenty minutes, rinsed in distilled water and finally counterstained with 0.1 per cent safranin or eosin.

Relatively large amounts of iron are continuously lost in the urine. As much as 3.6 mg. in twenty-four hours has been demonstrated even in the absence of hemoglobinuria[42] and average daily ex-

41

cretions up to 15.9 mg. have been observed.[5c] It is noteworthy that, despite the continuous presence of hemoglobinuria, *renal function* is not seriously affected unless there is some unrelated complicating factor. Albumin has been detected immediately before and after an episode of hemoglobinuria[43d] but usually no protein can be demonstrated between attacks.

Bone Marrow.—Normoblastic hyperplasia is the characteristic finding on bone marrow examination. As many as 50 per cent of the nucleated cells may be normoblasts or macroblasts, but the megaloblasts of pernicious anemia are absent.[75] Sometimes the number of megakaryocytes may be decreased, or hypoplastic marrow may be found (*see* below).

Diagnosis.—This chronic hemolytic anemia has been confused with hereditary spherocytosis, but can be distinguished by the negative family history and the absence of increased fragility of the red corpuscles to hypotonic saline solutions. Cases which have been reported as "hemoglobinuria occurring in congenital hemolytic jaundice"[50] probably were examples of the condition under discussion. The same may be true of some cases heretofore described as "atypical" or "acquired" hemolytic jaundice.[75] Pernicious anemia can be excluded because glossitis and neural symptoms are absent, and achlorhydria is not found. Furthermore, the reticulocyte percentage is high even before any attempts at treatment have been made.

A sudden attack of hemoglobinuria may call to mind one of the acute hemolytic anemias, but in the latter leukocytosis is found rather than leukopenia and the clinical history reveals an illness of brief duration rather than a chronic one. Sickle cell anemia is recognized by the finding of sickle cells in wet films. Lack of a history indicating that cold activates the hemolysis helps to distinguish nocturnal hemoglobinuria from paroxysmal hemoglobinuria *e frigore*. Many of the other types of hemoglobinuria, it will be recalled, are not associated with severe anemia. In blackwater fever severe anemia is found but the history and the finding of malarial parasites will aid differentiation.

Atypical forms may present greater difficulty in differential diagnosis. In some cases hemoglobinuria occurs exceedingly infrequently[64] and, unless special tests are used the condition may be overlooked. In addition, several instances have been reported in which there was temporary[43e] or chronic pancytopenia[64, 69a] with hypoplastic bone marrow. Such cases can be mistaken for primary refractory or aplastic anemia.

Tests for the investigation of hemolytic anemias were discussed earlier (p. 619). Special procedures for the recognition of nocturnal hemoglobinuria will be described below.

Prognosis and Treatment. — No satisfactory form of treatment has been described. It is well known that blood transfusion may be followed by untoward reactions but this is due to hemolytic factors in the plasma. The transfusion of saline-washed red cells is not harmful.[44b] Normal cells survive well in these patients and consequently the raising of the hemoglobin level to the normal range by transfusions of washed red cells has been recommended and has been observed to produce temporary remissions.[44b, 57a] It has been suggested that the relief of anoxia produced in this way leads to a reduced production of the patient's abnormal cells, with a consequent decrease in hemolysis.

Splenectomy has produced no permanent benefit and has been followed by death in some instances.[75] A few patients have been reported to have had less frequent episodes of hemoglobinuria after splenectomy[53] but it is impossible to know that this was not coincidental.

ACTH or corticosteroids have not been of therapeutic value.[61c]

Infection, thromboses and aregenerative crises are the more serious complications of paroxysmal nocturnal hemoglobinuria. In almost fifty per cent of cases death was due to thrombosis in the brain or the portal system[43d] and thrombosis in the extremities or elsewhere is common.[75,77b] During crisis, transfusions of red cells washed in saline, the administration of penicillin or other antibiotics and moderate dicoumarolization are recommended.[43e] Dicoumarol, if used, should be given when recovery begins since this is the time of greatest danger from thrombosis. Prothrombin levels of 15 per cent of normal should be maintained. Dicoumarol has also been recommended in severely anemic patients who are not in crisis, on grounds which will be mentioned below, and was found not only to prevent thrombosis but also to bring about disappearance of abdominal pain and headaches and some relief of anemia.[43d,61c] Heparin, however, is contraindicated.[69a] Dextran (mean molecular weight 75,000, 6 per cent) infusions have been found to temporarily control hemolysis associated with infection, trauma and transfusion reactions, perhaps by binding properdin.[49] Long-term administration, however, is not recommended since hemorrhagic complications are likely to develop.

This is a chronic disorder and, if such serious threats as thrombosis[42a,52b] can be avoided, patients may live for many years. One patient was known to have lived for thirty-three years and another underwent four pregnancies and other stressful events and is known to have survived 32 years from the time of diagnosis.[55,76b] Some patients show a tendency to improve as time passes[43d] and even spontaneous cure with serological tests becoming negative has been described.[5c]

Pathology.—Venous thromboses may be found in the systemic or portal circulation.[75] There is hepatomegaly with central zone necrosis; moderate splenomegaly with little deviation from the normal; and marked erythropoietic hyperplasia of the bone marrow. The kidneys may be enlarged and snuff-brown in color. Hemosiderosis is found but it is peculiar in distribution. Free iron pigment is present in large amounts in the kidneys (convoluted tubules and ascending loops of Henle), but only traces are found in other organs.

Pathogenesis.—It has been observed that increased blood destruction occurs during sleep, whether it be in the day or night and is not related to posture or to fluid or food intake.[53] This led to the hypothesis, as yet unproved,[43d] that destruction of cells is promoted by accumulation of carbon dioxide and the consequent lowering of the pH of the blood. Hemolysis is increased by the administration of ammonium chloride and decreases when the patient is given alkalies or hyperventilates. These procedures are not recommended therapeutically, however, because blood destruction has been found to become more marked than ever when the administration of alkalies is discontinued. This, perhaps, is due to the accumulation of very sensitive cells in the circulation while hemolysis is depressed.[5c]

The fault appears to reside in the red corpuscles[44c,54,61] but certain serum factors are concerned as well. Normal erythrocytes survive for a normal length of time after transfusion into patients suffering from nocturnal hemoglobinuria but when patients' red corpuscles are transfused to a normal recipient, a proportion is rapidly destroyed.[44c] Not all the erythrocytes of the patient are very sensitive to hemolysis, however, and a wide range in sensitivity has been noted.[5c] Reticulocytes and fully mature red corpuscles do not seem to differ in their sensitivity to lysis. The nature of the abnormality is unknown. Abnormalities in the lipoproteins in the stroma of the red cells have been reported[56,68c] but the problem requires further investigation.[41] Also requiring further study are the reports of changes in the erythrocytic surface as viewed by electron microscopy.[67b] The significance of a reported marked reduction in erythrocyte acetylcholinesterase activity is uncertain.[57a] Such a reduction appears to be a regular finding in severe and moderately severe cases.[67e] The demonstration of thromboplastic activity by the nonhemolyzed red cells of this disease may explain the common occurrence of thrombosis.[67c]

A proportion of the red corpuscles of patients with paroxysmal nocturnal hemoglobinuria will hemolyze *in vitro* after incubation at 37° C. for one hour in autogenous fresh serum or in that of normal human subjects of the same blood group. The hemolytic system in the serum is thermolabile; hemolysis of the cells is influenced by change in pH and to demonstrate a significant amount of hemolysis it is necessary to add acid or carbon dioxide to the serum to compensate for the alkalinity which follows loss of carbon dioxide when serum is exposed to air.[53] Hemolysis is increased by the addition of fresh guinea pig serum but does not occur with guinea pig serum in the absence of thermolabile components of human serum. Normal red cells are not lysed by the patient's serum.

It has been shown that the hemolysis of PNH (paroxysmal nocturnal hemoglobinuria) red cells *in vitro* requires complement, the Mg^{++} ion[56a] and an optimum acid pH (6.7 to 7.1). In addition it appears that properdin, a normal constituent of serum which is distinct from complement and the components of the clotting system, is required although properdin is not itself hemolytic for PNH cells.[56a] It is obvious that the hemolytic process is a complex one. It has been postulated that *four* distinct factors are involved, all probably proteins.[43d] Two of these factors are hemolytic against PNH red cells, but not against normal red cells. Two others inhibit PNH hemolysis. One of the hemolytic factors is heat labile and is destroyed slowly by thrombin. It is inactive unless the other hemolytic factor, which is heat labile, is present. One of the inhibitors is heat labile and the other is heat stable. The latter is destroyed rapidly by thrombin. Both calcium and magnesium are necessary for hemolysis but in excess both cause inhibition. Thrombin acts as an activator of hemolysis because of its more rapid action on the inhibitor than on the hemolytic factor. The therapeutic value of Dicoumarol is explained by its inhibition of thrombin formation. Heparin and protamine in appropriate amounts increase hemolysis because of action on the inhibitors. The intensity of PNH hemolytic activity, according to these observations, depends on a delicately poised equilibrium of activators whose balance is easily disturbed.

It has been reported that the leukocytes and platelets in this disorder are prone to undergo autolysis *in vitro* more readily than normal cells and thus the PNH abnormality may be shared by all the formed elements of the blood.[43d] The susceptibility to infections has been attributed to a defect in the leukocytes and the thrombocytopenia and tendency to thrombosis to the proneness of the platelets to agglutinate.

Two **diagnostic procedures** for the recognition of paroxysmal nocturnal hemoglobinuria depend on the described abnormalities of the red corpuscles. In the *acid-serum* (Ham) *test*,[53] as originally described, 5 per cent by volume of 0.85 normal lactic acid or N/3 HCl was used. It has been pointed out that the effects of the acid will vary with the buffering power of the serum proteins and other factors.[44c] A recommended procedure, therefore, consists in defibrinating blood in an open flask and, to serum so obtained, adding 10 per cent by volume N/5 HCl and 10 per cent by volume of a 50 per cent suspension of washed patient's red corpuscles. A positive result is revealed by frank hemolysis.

It has not been generally appreciated that this test is not specific for nocturnal hemoglobinuria. In congenital or acquired hemolytic anemia the red corpuscles, if sufficiently spherocytic, will undergo hemolysis at a pH at which normal cells do not hemolyze. Positive tests have also been observed when certain "warm" and "cold" hemolysins were present.[44c] Two control tests are, therefore, regarded as essential: (1) patient's corpuscles suspended in acidified normal serum inactivated by heating; and (2) normal corpuscles suspended in the patient's acidified serum. These will both be negative in cases of nocturnal hemoglobinuria. A third control test may be made by adding the patient's corpuscles to normal serum. A trace or no hemolysis will take place if the case is one of nocturnal hemoglobinuria whereas hemolysis may occur if immune hemolysins are concerned. In the latter case, contrary to the finding in nocturnal hemoglobinuria, the Coombs' test will be positive. It may be added that heat inactivation does not prevent hemolysis of cells that are spherocytic.

Another test, which is simpler and is claimed to be specific for paroxysmal nocturnal hemoglobinuria, depends on the increase in hemolysis which occurs when *thrombin* is added to an acidified cell-serum suspension.[44] Another confirmatory test depends on the greatly increased sensitivity of PNH corpusclse to hemolysis by high-titer cold antibodies.[5c,45a]

HEREDITARY SPHEROCYTOSIS

Definition, History and Synonyms. —This is a form of jaundice characterized by spherocytosis, diminished resistance of the red corpuscles to hemolysis by hypotonic saline solutions, a variable degree of anemia of hemolytic type, and splenomegaly. The disorder is chronic, congenital and often familial, but the manifestations may be so mild that the disease may not be recognized even until late adult life. The first accurate description is said to have been published by Minkowski in 1900, and Chauffard first discovered the increased fragility[90a] of the erythrocytes in 1907.[43b,115] The condition is therefore also known by the names of these investigators, or by the terms *congenital hemolytic* or *chronic familial jaundice (icterus)*, *chronic acholuric jaundice*, and *spherocytic* or *globe-cell anemia*. A very significant report by Vanlair and Masius in 1871, who recognized the spherocytes and suspected their signifiicance, was overlooked.[43c]

Etiology.—Congenital hemolytic icterus is perhaps the least rare of the familial hemolytic anemias but its incidence in various localities varies, probably on account of its hereditary character. Thus Gänsslen,[95] in southern Germany, was able to study about 120 cases. The condition is rare in Negroes but 44 cases have been reported, including two in African Bantu.[101a,104]

Many family trees extending through three and even four generations have been published.[88,95,124] The trait appears to be a Mendelian dominant, transmissible through either parent.[106b] This implies that one parent of every patient should be affected and that signs of the disorder should be found in one-half of the siblings and offspring; the offspring of those who escape should also be free. A number of investigators[88,106b,124] have observed patients, however, neither of whose parents appeared to be affected. An analysis of reported families has shown a shortage of affected siblings but no shortage of affected offspring.[124] These observations could be explained either by assuming that the abnormal gene was formed in the patient by mutation or that the inherited gene was so poorly expressed in some of the siblings or in the parents that present methods fail to detect it.

The sexes are equally affected. Hereditary spherocytosis has been recognized at all ages, from infants soon after birth (36 hours)[79b,110a] to old age (seventy-seven years[106b]). These extremes are unusual, however. In a series of 28 cases,[124] anemia or jaundice was first detected at age five or younger in 14 cases and between ten and forty-five years of age in 8 cases.

Symptomatology.—The symptoms vary greatly, both in regard to their time of onset and their severity. As stated above, they are frequently noticed in childhood or adolescence. At this age the disease is likely to be more severe than in cases in which symptoms first appear late in life. In other instances, the manifestations may be so slight as to pass unnoticed, and may be forgotten. Thus, one of our patients, a woman of fifty-seven years, who presented the complete clinical and hematological picture of this disease, was considered to be an example of "acquired" hemolytic jaundice until careful questioning revealed spells of jaundice and anemia in her childhood, a similar illness in her brother and possibly also in her sister, and gall bladder disease in her mother. Because the signs of this disorder may be so insignificant, a family history not accompanied by examination of the relatives of a patient cannot be regarded as negative.

The icterus is usually not intense, but varies considerably and is said to increase with fatigue, cold, emotion, or pregnancy. There may be no detectable jaundice despite other signs of active hemolysis,[95,115] or there is a constant sallow complexion, and even when icterus is well marked the patients are generally "more yellow than sick." The jaundice, no matter how intense, is not accompanied by itching

of the skin, bradycardia, or xanthomata. Once severe jaundice and anemia have developed, complete spontaneous remission is unusual.[113]

From time to time jaundice may deepen and the anemia increase. These minor hemolytic episodes may be accompanied by vomiting, pyrexia, tachycardia and abdominal pain[88] and often follow intercurrent infections. In addition, at any time, even for the first time in late adult life, there may be a sudden, acutely developing illness, the **"crise de déglobulization."** This is accompanied by fever, lassitude, palpitation and shortness of breath, or there may be violent abdominal pain, as well as vomiting and anorexia. Such episodes had been regarded as due to a sudden acceleration of blood destruction. This view was challenged, however, by Owren[104d] who studied 4 cases occurring in members of the same family. He was impressed by the disappearance of reticulocytes from the blood, and the presence of leukopenia, thrombocytopenia and acute aplasia of the erythropoietic tissue in the bone marrow. Jaundice, serum bilirubin and urobilinuria decreased to normal values. These features not only suggested bone marrow arrest but a paradoxical cessation of blood destruction.

That "acute erythroblastopenia"[95a] or aplasia occurs and that this may develop at the same time in several affected members of a family has been confirmed a number of times.[83b,95c,103d] The crisis may last six to 12 days. Environmental factors, such as infections have been thought to precipitate the crisis in some cases.[95c,123] The persistence of spherocytosis in association with the crisis[83b] may simply be the consequence of diminished production of young cells which are less spherocytic than older ones and does not necessarily imply that increased blood destruction is the primary factor in the crisis; neither does the fact that crises have not been observed in

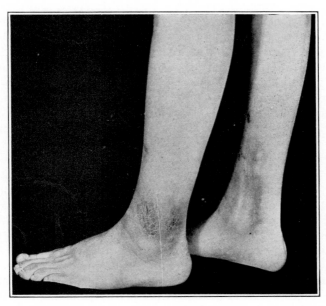

Fig. 12–6.—Marked pigmentation of the skin about the ankles in a case of hereditary spherocytosis.

splenectomized patients necessarily mean that the spleen is essential for their development.[88b] Its presence may merely favor the destruction of spherocytes which would otherwise remain in the circulation and, as a consequence, temporarily arrested production of red corpuscles would be less noticeable.[95c]

Symptoms of biliary tract disease may first bring the patient to the physician. **Cholelithiasis** has been found in 43[78d] to 85[124] per cent of cases and has been described even at the age of three years.[94] An uncommon complication, which may nevertheless be the chief complaint, is **chronic leg ulcer.**[92,111] This occurs over the internal or external malleoli and may persist for years unless splenectomy is performed. This can be the primary complaint if the disease has been unrecognized until late adult life or a chronic dermatosis[79] and pigmentation (Fig. 12–6) may be the only signs.

An indication of the differences in the severity of the disease which may be encountered is given by a study of 68 members of a family comprising 161 persons in three generations, of whom 10 were completely healthy, 11 showed all the manifestations of the disease, 34 had the disease but were compensated (no anemia) and in 13 the condition was in mild form.[95]

The **spleen** is almost always enlarged in active cases and may be huge. In latent cases, however, and especially in brothers or sisters of the patient, the spleen may not be felt or may be just at the costal border. Such individuals may, nevertheless, show other characteristics of this disorder. It has been stated that the spleen may not be palpable in as many as 30 per cent of cases.[95] This number must include a very large proportion of "formes frustes." In another series the spleen was readily palpable in 23 of 28 patients.[124] The spleen may be discovered accidentally, it may attract attention by producing a sense of oppression or weight, due to its size, or it may be the site of a sudden attack of pain.

The **liver** may not be enlarged at all,

or it may extend 1 to 3 cm. below the costal margin. In 10 of our cases the liver was not felt while in 6 it was slightly enlarged. Only in 1 case was the liver very big (7 cm. below the costal margin). The finding of an exceptionally large liver should arouse suspicion of a complication, or an error in diagnosis.

Nosebleeds are common in childhood in these patients but hemorrhage from other parts of the body, as in Banti's syndrome or in cirrhosis of the liver, does not occur. Sometimes the lymph nodes may be enlarged.[88] Neural symptoms have been reported,[82] but they must be exceedingly rare.

Abnormalities in the skeleton or other **developmental anomalies** may be found but their number has varied greatly in different series of cases.[124] The tower skull ("Turmschädel") is perhaps the most common but more than two dozen other anomalies have been described.[95,97] These include prominent eyes,[88] epicanthus, persistent pupillary membrane, abnormally wide root of the nose, persistence of deciduous teeth in adults, misplacement of permanent teeth, palatal deformities, polydactylia, and brachydactylia. If symptoms commence in childhood, growth may be impaired.[89,95] Infantilism may occur[79a] and other endocrine disorders have been observed.[93]

Changes in the bones demonstrable by **roentgen examination** are similar though less marked than those observed in sickle cell anemia and erythroblastic anemia. Thickening and striation of the frontal and parietal bones are the most frequent findings.[80]

The Blood.—The anemia is usually only moderate in degree, red cell counts between 3,000,000 and 4,000,000 per c.mm. being most common. There may be no anemia at all, however, or it may be quite severe. A rapid fall to as few as 1,000,000 cells may occur during a crisis, and even in its absence a count in the neighborhood of 2,000,000 cells

may be observed and may be found to be maintained for a long time. The reduction in hemoglobin and volume of packed red cells may or may not be proportional. Most frequently the *mean corpuscular volume* is somewhat below normal, but it may be normal, increased, or greatly decreased. In our cases values between 77 and 87 c.μ have been most frequent but in 1 patient the mean corpuscular volume was as low as 62 c.μ while in 2 cases the anemia was macrocytic (M.C.V. 102 to 125 c.μ). Macrocytic anemia is more likely to occur in cases with very severe anemia. Variations in mean corpuscular hemoglobin usually correspond to changes in volume but not infrequently the *mean corpuscular hemoglobin concentration* is high (37 to 39 per cent) (p. 604).

There may be the widest variation in the **size of the red corpuscles,** and the presence of macrocytes has led to confusion with pernicious anemia in some instances. Characteristically, the *mean diameter* is reduced, owing to the presence of round, bright corpuscles of small size (Fig. 12–7). These cells show no central pallor because of their spherical rather than biconcave shape. In the majority of our cases the mean diameter in stained smears was 6.2 to 7.0 μ and ranged from 5.4 to 7.6 μ. In wet films of blood the diameter is 0.5 to 1.0 μ greater, which is also below the normal value. The spherocytes, themselves, are often much smaller than the average and may measure even 4 μ in diameter.

The unusual *thickness* of these corpuscles accounts for the low mean cell diameter despite normal or only slightly reduced mean corpuscular volume. Calculations give values of 2.2 to 3.4 μ instead of 2.0 μ or less as is found in normal blood.[116b] The disproportionate thickness of the red corpuscles in hereditary spherocytosis (Fig. 12–8) has been confirmed by direct observation.[96,113] The

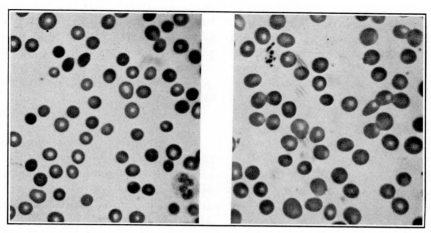

Fig. 12–7.—Blood smears from two cases of hereditary spherocytosis. There were many more sphero-cytes (the small, round, dark cells) in the case on the left than in that on the right. Note the lack of poikilocytosis. Wright's stain, × 900.

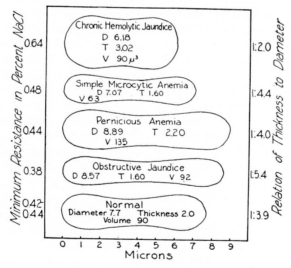

Fig. 12–8.—Diagram representing cross-section of erythrocytes in different clinical conditions. D re-fers to mean diameter, T means thickness, and V means corpuscular volume. (Haden, Am. J. M. Sc.)

degree of spherocytosis varies from case to case.

Reticulocytes are characteristically increased in number. Values between 5 and 20 per cent are common but they may be as high as 50 and even 92 per cent,[78e] or as low as 2 per cent. Poly-chromatophilia will often be observed in variable degree, as well as occasional normoblasts and microblasts. After a

crisis such signs of active erythropoiesis are prominent. Poikilocytosis is rarely very marked, although structures sug-gestive of fragmented red corpuscles may be seen.

The **fragility** of the red corpuscles in hypotonic saline solutions is increased in typical cases. The point of beginning hemolysis varies from about 0.51 to 0.72 per cent, and may be as high as 0.87

per cent. Hemolysis may be complete at the point where it normally commences. If the amount of hemolysis in various strengths of saline solution is measured and the results are plotted as a curve (Fig. 12–2, p. 622), it may be found that the curve of hemolysis is normal in shape but shifted to the left; it may be "tailed" with only a small proportion of the red corpuscles hemolysing in saline concentrations greater than 0.45 per cent;[83] or increased osmotic fragility may not be demonstrable until after 24 hour incubation of the cells.[40b]

Mechanical fragility is greater than normal[124] but acid fragility is normal. Spontaneous autohemolysis of sterile blood at 37° C. occurs sooner and in greater degree than is found in normal blood[108e] or in autoimmune hemolytic disease except at times of very active blood destruction.[124] There is no correlation between the degree of anemia and the fragility of the corpuscles.

The **Coombs' test** is usually negative.[124] Reported positive results (p. 623), when not attributable to the use of inadequately absorbed rabbit serum or inadequate characterization of the tested cases, may be explained, at least in some cases, by antibody development superimposed upon the original congenital disease.[83b]

The **leukocytes** are usually normal in number or only slightly increased but after a crisis there is marked leukocytosis and a "shift to the left." During the chronic stage of anemia, lymphocytes, plasma cells and basophils may be increased.[95]

Usually the **platelet** count is normal. It may be somewhat increased. In several of our cases it was moderately reduced (130,000 per c.mm.).

The **icterus index** may be as high as 100 but values of 15 to 30 are more common. The indirect van den Bergh reaction is positive.

The **urine** may or may not contain increased amounts of urobilinogen and coproporphyrin, but bile pigments and bile salts are absent. Hemoglobinuria is very unusual. The **stools** contain bile pigment as well as excessive quantities of urobilinogen. The increased urobilinogen excretion may be five to twenty times the normal.[99,105]

The plasma or **serum iron** may be increased or normal.

In the **bone marrow,** erythropoietic hyperplasia of the normoblastic type is found. Such cells may make up 25 to 60 per cent of all the nucleated cells, and many mitotic forms are evident.[103] Megaloblasts of the type seen in pernicious anemia are absent and the giant, abnormal leukocytes are also lacking.[116]

Diagnosis.—The presenting clinical picture may suggest a great variety of disorders: the various causes of jaundice, fever, abdominal pain, splenomegaly, or anemia. Complete examination, however, should make the diagnosis clear because the combination of hemolytic anemia, reticulocytosis, spherocytosis, markedly increased osmotic fragility, splenomegaly, and jaundice is found in no other condition. It is unsafe to assume that one is not dealing with hereditary spherocytosis if the symptoms make their appearance for the first time late in life. In some cases symptoms may be so mild that they are overlooked for many years or mistaken for those of other disorders. The manifestations of acquired forms of hemolytic anemia are usually more severe than those of the congenital condition. The findings in several different forms of hemolytic anemia are compared in Table 12–2 (p. 621). When there is a definite familial history of jaundice, sickle cell disease, thalassemia and various hemoglobinopathies (p. 668), as well as a rare familial disorder, "constitutional hepatic insufficiency" (p. 619) must be considered.

When the anemia is severe, macrocytosis may be marked and there may be confusion with pernicious anemia. Usuually the patients are younger than those found to have the latter disease, achlorhydria does not occur, and neural involvement is absent. In pernicious anemia, furthermore, reticulocytes are normal in number as a rule except during the response to therapy.

Confusion may occur if the fragility of the red corpuscles is not found to be increased. The value of incubation of the cells under these circumstances has been mentioned. Unless the diagnosis is clear-cut, the patient should be studied in the manner already described (p. 619) in order to rule out various other causes of hemolytic anemia (Table 12–1).

The ellipitical appearance of the cells in hereditary elliptocytic anemia (p. 103), a very rare disorder, should make it easy to differentiate that condition from hereditary spherocytosis. It is especially important to distinguish cases of **congenital non-spherocytic hemolytic anemia** because these usually have not been benefited by splenectomy. A number of cases have been described.[81,95e,110c] They do not appear to constitute a single entity. Although many of the reported cases have been characterized by a brisk hemolytic state, others may have manifested only a moderate rate of hemolysis and, in some, it was mild.[81] Cases of moderate or mild severity may be confused with "constitutional hepatic dysfunction" (p. 619) and it has been proposed that normal erythrocyte survival must be demonstrated before the latter diagnosis can be considered established.[81]

The congenital non-spherocytic hemolytic anemias may be defined as familial hemolytic disorders characterized by the presence of an intracorpuscular defect of the erythrocytes. They are distinquished from hereditary spherocytosis and hereditary elliptocytosis by the absence of definitive morphologic abnormalities. The mode of inheritance may be similar to that of hereditary spherocytosis. The anemia may date back to infancy and even hemolytic disease of the newborn has been simulated. In other cases clinical onset was noted only in adult life.[95e] The anemia may be macrocytic or normocytic. There may be a moderate degree of ovalocytosis, or mild hypochromia. Spherocytes are not found and osmotic fragility has been normal[81c,96a] or decreased, even after incubation; or incubation may increase osmotic fragility.[95e] Sometimes there has been conspicuous basophilia. The spleen has usually although not invariably, been palpable.

Studies of autohemolysis revealed at least two forms of the nonspherocytic disorder.[108e] In type I, which was characterized by the presence of oval macrocytes, the changes occurring on incubation were similar to those of normal cells but, when glucose was added, the rate of autohemolysis was diminished less than occurs with normal cells. In type II, characterized by rounded macrocytes, autohemolysis and potassium losses were much greater than normal and these were unaffected by glucose. In both types the cells seemed to be unable to utilize glucose at the normal rate. Thus, as in hereditary spherocytosis (p. 654) a defect in glycolysis seemed to be present. The abnormality in type II may be the result of pyruvate kinase deficiency with consequent deficient regeneration of ATP.[116e] Another investigator[128] distinguished three groups; namely (1) cases in which red cell glutathione was unstable in the presence of phenylhydrazine and G6PD activity was absent, a finding which has also been noted by others;[108f] (2) cases in which these abnormalities were lacking; (3) a patient in whom G6PD activity was increased. This patient had been reported previously[62a] as a possible case of inclusion body anemia (p. 626). The last observation as well as the descriptions of other reported cases, in which crenated and irregularly contracted corpuscles were described, or Pappenheimer bodies were abundant, or extreme variations in

red cell size and shape[83a] or some suggestion of porphyrin abnormality[81c,115b]
was noted, indicate that the nonspherocytic hemolytic anemias, as reported in
the literature, represent a heterogenous
group which only further study will
clarify.

Differentiation of hereditary spherocytosis from the various causes of splenomegaly (p. 1055) is usually easy if a
complete examination is carried out.

Complications.—The frequency of
biliary tract disease has been mentioned
already. So also has the occurrence of
chronic leg ulcers and various developmental anomalies. Gout has been observed in several instances.[115]

The discovery of gall stones in a young
person should cause one to suspect the
existence of hereditary spherocytosis.
If the latter is found, splenectomy must
be done before cholecystectomy, since
the bilirubinemia requires correction if
the deposition of bilirubin salts is to be
avoided. *Megaloblastic anemia* occurring
during successive pregnancies, and even
in their absence,[88a] until splenectomy
relieved the chronic anemia has been
reported several times.[101b] Primary carcinoma of the gall bladder was encountered at the early age of 36 years in a
patient with hereditary spherocytosis.[96b]

Treatment.—This is the one disorder in which splenectomy is followed
by almost uniformly beneficial and lasting results. The red cell count rises
500,000 to 1,000,000 cells immediately.[90]
This effect may last only a few hours but
it is nevertheless followed in a few days
by fading of the jaundice and a gradual
rise in the red cell count, hemoglobin
and volume of packed red cells to normal
limits, which are reached in several
weeks.[109] The reticulocytes decrease and
other signs of exaggerated erythropoiesis
disappear. Microcytosis often persists,
however, and spherocytes may continue
to be found in the blood smear. Mean
corpuscular volume and thickness may

or may not change, but in most instances
they are modified in the direction of
normal.[116b] The corpuscular fragility is
usually unaltered[115] although it may
decrease or even return to normal.
Rarely it is increased.[114] The platelet
count usually rises following splenectomy.
Leukocytosis, even to 48,000, follows
splenectomy immediately and persists
in moderate degree for a long time[87]
after operation. It has been observed
that similar changes in the red and white
corpuscles usually did not follow splenectomy in cases of atypical hemolytic
anemia nor did they follow cholecystectomy in splenectomized cases of hereditary spherocytosis.[109]

Splenectomy should be advised in any
patient who has typical hereditary spherocytosis if he has been continuously
anemic or gives a history of hemolytic
or aplastic crises. The presence of
cholelithiasis would indicate the need
for splenectomy. Chronic leg ulcers may
clear up only after splenectomy.[111] It is
difficult to see what is gained by delaying
operation unless the patient is completely
compensated and has been always symptom free. Even in such cases there is no
conclusive evidence that this good fortune
will persist. In the present day, the
operative mortality in good hands is extremely low. Only in infancy should the
operation be delayed since the risk of
infection is greater in the first year of
life than later.[79b] However, splenectomy
in childhood does not carry the high
risk which has been claimed (p. 1051)
and operation at four to five years of
age has the advantage that impairment
of growth and risks from crises or other
complications are avoided.

Some advise the use of anticoagulants
post-operatively to prevent thrombosis
but the writer has observed many patients
whose post-operative course was uneventful without anticoagulants, in spite of
marked post-operative thrombocytosis.
Cases have been reported in which the

dramatic improvement which usually follows splenectomy did not occur. Some of these were not true examples of hereditary spherocytosis, while in other cases complications were present. Failure to relieve the jaundice and anemia also raises the possibility that accessory spleens were overlooked, but there is but one well documented case of such a situation.[102a]

Other measures are of little value in this condition. Blood transfusions are usually unnecessary except in a crisis. There is no indication for corticosteroid therapy. Some surgeons recommend the injection of epinephrine, 1 ml. subcutaneously, just before the splenic pedicle is tied, in order to force blood out of the spleen.

The administration of iron, vitamin B_{12}, folic acid or arsenic is of no value.

Prognosis.—The illness is usually more serious if symptoms appear in childhood.[89] Death may occur during a crisis. Repeated attacks are associated with impairment of bodily and sometimes mental development, cardiac decompensation may occur and biliary tract disease may ensue.[89] Many patients, however, have attained an advanced age in spite of chronic anemia.[113] The histories of some patients[80c] suggest that there may be prolonged spontaneous improvement without recurrence of jaundice until late adult life,[103e] but usually, once jaundice has set in, it does not clear up completely until splenectomy has been performed.

Pathology.—The **spleen** is enlarged, weighing 1000 to 1500 Gm., and is usually easily removed at operation. Adhesions are uncommon. The cut surface is relatively dry, dark purplish-red in color, homogeneous in texture and bulges slightly above the capsule. The Malpighian bodies cannot be distinguished. Microscopically they are found to be small and widely separated. The pulp is a mass of closely packed red cells which distend, distort, and dilate it. The sinusoids, on the other hand, are conspicuous and empty. There may or may not be increased iron pigment[122b] and phagocytosis of red cells is slight in amount. Unlike the finding in the spleen of Banti's syndrome, there is no thickening of the trabeculae.

The **liver** is not enlarged in most cases, nor is it usually cirrhotic, but the quantity of iron pigment may be increased in the hepatic and the Küpffer cells, while bilirubin stones may be found in the gall bladder. The **kidneys** often show well-marked hemosiderosis and the **lymph glands** may also contain pigment.

The **bone marrow** is strikingly hyperplastic, dark red in color and free from fat. The microscopic picture, already described, shows marked erythropoietic hyperplasia of the normoblastic type. In this disease **heterotopia of the bone marrow** may occur. Such masses have been observed alongside the vertebral column in the thorax[96c, 98] and may also be found in the kidney pelvis.[87] They may also be encountered in other forms of chronic hemolytic anemia.[5]

Pathogenesis.—It is generally recognized that the fundamental abnormality is an inherited trait whereby red corpuscles of unusual thickness, closely approaching spheres in shape, are produced.[95] Such cells are similar in form to that which red corpuscles assume when they are about to burst in hypotonic solutions of sodium chloride[96] (Fig. 12–9). As the erythrocytes mature they become more and more spherocytic. Even the reticulocytes in this disorder have smaller diameters and are less disc-like than normal cells. It has been pointed out that the survival of the cells of hereditary spherocytosis is greatly reduced, even when they are transfused to normal individuals, whereas normal cells survive normally in the circulation of the victims of this disease. It has been demonstrated

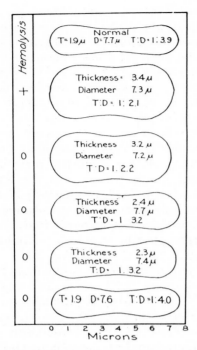

Fig. 12–9.—Changes in the shape and measurements of the mean erythrocytes of normal blood on the addition of varying amounts of distilled water to the plasma. (Haden, Am. J. M. Sc.)

by several groups of investigators[9b,126] that the spheroid cells are readily trapped in the splenic pulp because their abnormal thickness does not permit them to escape easily. Furthermore, the cells stagnating in the pulp are removed from the protective factors present in actively circulating blood. The spleen thus acts as a filter and a trap and there, in addition, a significant proportion of the red cells are made more vulnerable to the hazards of the circulation.[95d] Yet it would seem that the shape of the red cell is not of itself responsible for its destruction. Thus, when two non-anemic patients with hereditary spherocytosis were phlebotomized until their cells became hypochromic and thin, their life span in the circulation was not improved.[81d] Later splenectomy corrected the hemolytic disease. Splenectomy does not abolish the disease process. The abnormal cells continue to be manufactured. However, by splenectomy the major hazard in the circulation is removed.

The point of chief interest is the nature of the corpuscular defect. The observations on the rapid spontaneous hemolysis of spherocytes,[9b,108e] already alluded to, gave the first clues. An extension of these investigations[108e] showed that the continued presence of glucose during incubation markedly retarded the potassium loss and the increase in osmotic fragility which accompany the increased rate of autohemolysis of hereditary spherocytes, as compared with normal cells. Other studies[106] showed that intracellular glycolysis is abnormal. Using radioactive phosphorus as a tracer, it was found that in cells from patients with hereditary spherocytosis there is a smaller flux of P^{32} into adenosine triphosphate and 2,3-diphosphoglyceric acid than in normal cells and a concurrent increase in the flux into orthophosphate. These observations have been confirmed.[104b] They may indicate that a basic intracellular defect in phosphorylation is present in the red cells which, as a consequence, are less well able to maintain their integrity than normal ones. Such a metabolic abnormality might be a genetically controlled enzymatic deficiency, perhaps of enolase.[106] In other studies a significantly higher proportion of lysophosphatidyl ethanolamine and a significantly lower proportion of phosphatidyl ethanolamine were demonstrated in spherocytes as compared with normal cells.[78a] These observations led to the suggestion that the primary genetically controlled abnormality in hereditary spherocytosis is a partial block in the enzyme system for conversion of lysophosphatidyl ethanolamine to phosphatidyl ethanolamine. Other metabolic differences in the erythrocytes of hereditary spherocytosis, it is postulated, are secondary to the defect in the phospholipid component of the red cell membrane.

It may be expected that additional metabolic studies of hereditary spherocytosis and of congenital nonspherocytic anemias (p. 651) as well as of other atypical hemolytic anemias (p. 614) will demonstrate fundamental differences among disorders which in the past were only vaguely recognized as being "atypical." Possibly the discovery of counterparts of some of these disorders in animals[78b] will also be helpful.

The pathogenesis of the "crise de déglobulization" was discussed earlier (p. 646).

BIBLIOGRAPHY

Hemolytic Anemias in General—Miscellaneous Causes

1. ALLISON, A. C.: Acute Haemolytic Anaemia with Distortion and Fragmentation of Erythrocytes in Children, Brit. J. Haemat., *3*, 1, 1957.

1a. ALLISON, A. C., MOORE, T. and SHARMAN, I. M.: Haemolysis and Haemoglobinuria in Vitamin-E Deficient Rats after Injections of Vitamin-K Substitutes, Brit. J. Haemat., *2*, 197, 1956.

1b. AUB, J. C., FAIRHALL, L. T., MINOT, A. S. and REZNIKOFF, P.: Lead Poisoning, Medicine, *4*, 1, 1925 (Bibliography).

1c. BERLIN, R.: Haff Disease in Sweden, Acta med. scandinav., *129*, 560, 1948.

2. BESSIS, M. and BRETON-GORIUS, JANINE: Étude au microscope électronique du sang et des organes hémopoiétiques dans le saturnisme expérimental, Path. biol. (Semaine hôp. Paris), No. 4, 441, 1956.

2a. BEUTLER, E.: The Glutathione Instability of Drug-sensitive Red Cells, J. Lab. & Clin. Med., *49*, 84, 1957.

2b. BEUTLER, E.: The Hemolytic Effect of Primaquine and Related Compounds, Blood, *14*, 103, 1959.

2d. BLACKIE, W. K.: Blackwater Fever, Clin. Proc., Cape Town, *3*, 272, 1944.

3. BOWMAN, J. M.: Acquired Hemolytic Anemia, Am. J. Dis. Child., *89*, 226, 1955.

3a. BREWER, G. J., TARLOV, A. R. and ALVING, A. S.: Methaemoglobin Reduction Test, World Health Org., *22*, 633, 1960.

3b. BRUS, I. and LEWIS, S. M.: The Haptoglobin Content of Serum in Haemolytic Anaemia, Brit. J. Haemat., *5*, 348, 1959.

4. BUNTING, C. H.: Experimental Anæmias in the Rabbit, J. Exper. Med., *8*, 625, 1906.

4a. BYWATERS, E. G. L. and DIBLE, J. H.: Renal Lesions in Traumatic Anuria, J. Path. & Bact., *54*, 111, 1942.

4b. BYWATERS, E. G. L. and STEAD, J. K.: Thrombosis of the Femoral Artery with Myohaemoglobinuria and Low Serum Potassium Concentration, Clin. Sc., *5*, 195, 1945.

4c. CARTWRIGHT, G. E.: *Diagnostic Laboratory Hematology*, 2nd edition, New York, Grune & Stratton, 1958.

4d. CHILDS, B. *et al.*: A Genetic Study of a Defect in Glutathione Metabolism of the Erythrocyte, Bull. Johns Hopkins Hosp., *102*, 21, 1958.

4e. CONWAY, H.: The Production of Erythrophagocytosis in Peripheral Blood, J. Clin. Path., *6*, 208, 1953.

4f. CONN, H. O.: Acute Hemolytic Anemia, Cryoglobulinemia and Cold Agglutination, New England J. Med., *253*, 1011, 1955.

5. COVENTRY, W. D. and LaBREE, R. H.: Heterotopia of Bone Marrow Simulating Mediastinal Tumor, Ann. Int. Med., *53*, 1042, 1960.

5a. CRUZ, W. O., HAWKINS, W. B. and WHIPPLE, G. H.: Acetylphenylhydrazine Anemia, Am. J. M. Sc., *203*, 848, 1942.

5b. DACIE, J. V.: The Presence of Cold Hæmolysins in Sera Containing Cold Hæmagglutinins, J. Path. & Bact., *62*, 241, 1950.

5c. DACIE, J. V.: *The Hæmolytic Anæmias*, New York, Grune & Stratton, 1954 and 1960.

5d. ———— Acquired Hemolytic Anemia with Special Reference to the Antiglobulin (Coombs') Reaction, Blood, *8*, 813, 1953; Sang, *25*, 675, 1954.

5e. DACIE, J.V.: Acquired Haemolytic Anaemias, Brit. M. Bull., *15*, 67, 1959.

6. DAMESHEK, W.: Rouleaux Formation in Fresh, Unmodified Blood as a Diagnostic Test for Hemolytic Anemia, New England J. Med., *221*, 1009, 1939.

7. DAMESHEK, W. and KOMNINOS, Z. D.: The Present Status of Treatment of Autoimmune Hemolytic Anemia with ACTH and Cortisone, Blood, *11*, 648, 1956.

7a. DANON, D., SHEBA, CH. and RAMOT, B.: The Morphology of Glucose 6 Phosphate Dehydrogenase Deficient Erythrocytes: Electron-microscopic Studies, Blood, *17*, 229, 1961.

8. DAVIDSON, L. S. P.: Macrocytic Hæmolytic Anæmia, Quart. J. Med., *1*, 543, 1932.

8a. DAVIES, I. J.: Benzedrine: A Review of Its Toxic Effects, Brit. M. J., *2*, 615, 1937.

8b. DAVIS, J. E.: Hemolytic Anemia as a Manifestation of Paraphenylene-Diamine Toxicity, J. Pharmacol. & Exper. Therap., 88, 133, 1946.

8c.DAWSON, JEAN P., THAYER, W. W. and DESFORGES, JANE F.: Acute Hemolytic Anemia in the Newborn Infant Due to Naphthalene Poisoning, Blood, 13, 1113, 1958.

8d.DE, S. N., SINGUPTA, K. P. and CHANDA, N. N.: Intravascular Hæmolysis in Cholera, Lancet, 1, 807, 1954.

8e.DERN, R. J., WEINSTEIN, I. M., LEROY, G. V., TALMAGE, D. W. and ALVING, A. S.: The Hemolytic Effect of Primaquine, J. Lab. & Clin. Med., 43, 303, 1954; ibid., 44, 171 and 439, 1954; ibid., 45, 30 and 40, 1955; Science, 124, 484, 1956; Ann. Int. Med., 49, 240, 1958.

8f.DESFORGES, JANE F., THAYER, W. W. and DAWSON, JEAN P.: Hemolytic Anemia Induced by Sulfoxone Therapy, with Investigations into the Mechanisms of Its Production, Am. J. Med., 27, 132, 1959.

8g.DIMSON, S. B. and McMARTIN, R. B.: Pamaquin Haemoglobinuria, Quart. J., Med., 15, 25, 1946.

9. DUDLEY, S. F.: Toxemic Anemia From Arseniuretted Hydrogen Gas in Submarines, J. Indust. Hyg. & Toxicol., 1, 215, 1919.

9a.EARLE, D. P., JR., BIGELOW, F. S., ZUBROD, C. G. and KANE, C. A.: Effect of Pamaquine on the Blood Cells of Man, J. Clin. Invest., 27, 121, 1948.

9b.EMERSON, C. P., SHEN, S. C. and CASTLE, W. B.: The Osmotic Fragility of the Red Cells of the Peripheral and Splenic Blood in Patients with Congenital Hemolytic Jaundice Transfused with Normal Red Cells, J. Clin. Invest., 25, 922, 1946; ibid., 26, 1180, 1947; A.M.A. Arch. Int. Med., 97, 1, 1956.

10. ERF, L. A. and MacLEOD, C. M.: Increased Urobilinogen Excretion and Acute Hemolytic Anemia in Patients Treated With Sulfapyridine, J. Clin. Invest., 19, 451, 1940.

10a.ERF, L. A. and RHOADS, C. P.: The Hematological Effects of Benzene (Benzol) Poisoning, J. Indust. Hyg. & Toxicol., 21, 421, 1939.

10b.ERIKSEN, L.: The Effect of Lead on the in Vitro Biosynthesis of Heme and Free Erythrocyte Porphyrins, Scandinav. J. Clin. & Lab. Invest., 7, 80, 1955.

10c.EVANS, A. S., ENZER, N., EDER, H. A. and FINCH, C. A.: Hemolytic Anemia with Paroxysmal Methemoglobinemia and Sulfhemoglobinemia, Arch. Int. Med., 86, 23, 1950.

11. EVANS, R. S. and DUANE, R. T.: Acquired Hemolytic Anemia, Blood, 4, 1196, 1949; Arch. Int. Med., 87, 48, 1951; A. M. A. Arch. Int. Med., 100, 371, 1957.

12. FERNÁN-NUÑEZ, M.: Hemoglobinuric Fever, Am. J. Trop. Med., 16, 563, 1936.

12a.FERTMAN, M. H. and DOAN, C. A.: Irreversible Toxic "Inclusion Body" Anemia, Blood, 3, 349, 1948.

12b.FERTMAN, M. H. and FERTMAN, M. B.: Toxic Anemias and Heinz Bodies, Medicine, 34, 131, 1955.

12c.FIGGE, F. H. J., CAREY, T. N. and WEILAND, G. S.: Porphyrin Excretion by a Patient Treated with Sulfadiazine and Later with Sulfanilamide, J. Lab. & Clin. Med., 31, 752, 1946.

12d.FINLAND, M., PETERSON, O. L., ALLEN, H. E., SAMPER, B. A. and BARNES, M. W.: Cold Agglutinins: Occurrence of Cold Isohemagglutinins in Various Conditions, J. Clin. Invest., 24, 451, 1945.

13. FOX, C. L., JR. and OTTENBERG, R.: Acute Hemolytic Anemia from the Sulfonamides J. Clin. Invest., 20, 593, 1941.

13a.FOY, H., KONDI, A., REBELO, A. and SOEIRO, A.: Survival of Transfused Red Cells in Blackwater Fever Circulation and of Blackwater Red Cells in Normal Circulation, Trans. Roy. Soc. Trop. Med. & Hyg., 38, 271, 1945.

13b.FREEDMAN, A. L., BARR, P. S. and BRODY, E. A.: Hemolytic Anemia Due to Quinidine, Am. J. Med., 20, 806, 1956.

13c.GAFFNEY, FAY M.: Experimental Haemolytic Anaemia with Particular Reference to the Corpuscular Haemoglobin Concentrations of the Erythrocytes, Brit. J. Haemat., 3, 311, 1957.

14. GASSER, C.: Die Hämolytischen Syndrome im Kindesalter, Stuttgart, Georg Thieme 1951.

14a.——— Die hämolytische Frühgeburtenanämie mit spontaner Innenkörperbildung, Ein neues Syndrom, beobachtet an 14 Fällen, Helvet. pædiat. acta, 8, 491, 1953.

15. GOLDBERG, A., ASHENBRUCKER, HELEN E., CARTWRIGHT, G. E. and WINTROBE, M. M.: Studies on the Biosynthesis of Heme in vitro by Avian Erythrocytes, Blood, 11, 821, 1956.

16. GOULD, S. E., KULLMAN, H. J. and SHECKET, H. A.: Effect of Lead Therapy on Blood Cells of Cancer Patients, Am. J. M. Sc., 194, 304, 1937.

16a.GRECH, J. L. and CACHIA, E. A.: Acute Haemolytic Anaemia Associated with

Sulphadimidine Therapy, Brit. M. J., *2*, 1309, 1959.

16*b*.GREENBURG, L., MAYERS, M. R., HEIMANN, H. and MOSKOWITZ, S.: The Effects of Exposure to Toluene in Industry, J.A.M.A. *118*, 573, 1942.

16*c*.HAEGER-ARONSEN, BIRGITTA: Studies on Urinary Excretion of δ-aminolaevulic Acid and Other Haem Precursors in Lead Workers and Lead-intoxicated Rabbits, Scandinav. J. Clin. & Lab. Invest. (Suppl. 47), *12*, 9, 1960.

16*d*.HAM, T. H., SHEN, S. C., FLEMING, E. M. and CASTLE, W. B.: Studies on the Destruction of Red Blood Cells. IV. Thermal Injury, Blood, *3*, 373, 1948.

16*e*.HAM, T. H., WEISMAN, R., JR. and HINZ, C. F., JR.: Mechanisms of Destruction of Red Cells in Certain Hemolytic Conditions, A. M. A. Arch. Int. Med., *96*, 574, 1956.

16*f*.HAMILTON, A.: *Industrial Poisons in the United States*, New York, The Macmillan Company, 1925.

16*g*.HANKS, G. E. *et al.*: Further Modification of the Benzidine Method for Measurement of Hemoglobin in Plasma, J. Lab. & Clin. Med., *56*, 486, 1960.

16*h*.HARLEY, J. D. and MAUER, A. M.: Studies on the Formation of Heinz Bodies, Blood, *16*, 1722, 1960, *ibid.*, *17*, 418, 1961.

17. HARRIS, J. W.: Studies on the Mechanism of a Drug-induced Hemolytic Anemia, J. Lab. & Clin. Med., *47*, 760, 1956.

17*a*.HIGGINS, G., O'BRIEN, J. R. P., STEWART, A. and WITTS, L. J.: Some Early Effects of Exposure to T.N.T., British Ministry of Supply, London, 17 pp., 1944.

17*b*.HIGGINS, G. M.: Toxic Effects of Promin on the Erythrocytes of Guinea Pigs, Am. J. M. Sc., *205*, 834, 1943; Am. J. Clin. Path., *13*, 28, 1943.

17*c*.HUNTER, D.: Industrial Toxicology, Quart. J. Med., *12*, 185, 1943.

17*d*.JAMES, G. W., III, PURNELL, O. J. and EVANS, E. I.: The Anemia of Thermal Injury, J. Clin. Invest., *30*, 181, 1951; J. Clin. Invest., *33*, 150, 1954.

17*e*.JANDL, J. H., JONES, A. R. and CASTLE, W. B.: The Destruction of Red Cells by Antibodies in Man, J. Clin. Invest., *36*, 1428, 1957; *ibid.*, *37*, 1202, 1958; *ibid.*, *39*, 1145, 1960.

17*f*.JANDL, J. H., ENGLE, LOUISE K. and ALLEN, D. W.: Oxidative Hemolysis and Precipitation of Hemoglobin, J. Clin. Invest., *39*, 1818, 1960, *ibid.*, *40*, 454, 1961.

18. ZU JEDDELOH, B.: Haffkrankheit, Ergebn inn. Med. u. Kinderh., *57*, 138, 1939.

18*a*.JOHNSTONE, R. D. C.: Acute Hæmolytic Anæmia Following Phenothiazine Therapy, Brit. M. J., *1*, 259, 1942.

19. KEGEL, A. H., McNALLY, W. D. and POPE, A. S.: Methyl Chloride Poisoning From Domestic Refrigerators, J.A.M.A., *93*, 353, 1929.

19*a*.KIMBRO, E. L., JR., SACHS, MARIE V. and TORBERT, J. V.: Mechanism of the Hemolytic Anemia Induced by Nitrofurantoin (Furandantin[R]), Bull. Johns Hopkins Hosp., *101*, 245, 1957.

19*b*.KUNITZ, M. and McDONALD, M. R.: Isolation of Crystalline Ricin, J. Gen. Physiol., *32*, 25, 1948.

19*c*.LANDSTEINER, E. K. and FINCH, C. A.: Hemoglobinemia Accompanying Transurethral Resection of the Prostate, New England J. Med., *237*, 310, 1947.

19*d*.LARIZZA, P., BRUNETTI, P., GRIGNANI, F. and VENTURA, S.: L'individualità bio-enzimatica dell'eritrocito "Fabico," Haematologica, *43*, 205, 1958.

19*e*.LAYNE, J. A. and SCHEMM, F. R.: Acute Macrocytic Hemolytic Anemia Occurring Following Administration of Sulfadiazine, J. Lab. & Clin. Med., *29*, 347, 1944.

19*f*.LEDERER, R.: New Forms of Acute Hemolytic Anemia "Baghdad Spring Anemia," Trans. Roy. Soc. Trop. Med. & Hyg., *34*, 387, 1941.

19*g*.LENHARTZ, H.: Das Blutbild bei den septischen Erkrankungen, Deutsch. Arch. klin. Med., *146*, 257, 1925.

20. LICCIARDELLO, A. T. and STANBURY, J. B.: Acute Hemolytic Anemia from Quinine Used as an Abortifacient, New England J. Med., *238*, 120, 1948.

20*a*.LOUTIT, J. F. and MOLLISON, P. L.: Hæmolytic Icterus (Acholuric Jaundice), Congenital and Acquired, J. Path. & Bact., *58*, 711, 1946; J. Clin. Path., *2*, 109, 1949.

20*c*.LUISADA, A.: Favism, Medicine, *20*, 229, 1941 (Bibliography).

20*d*.LUST, M.: Severe Acute Hemolytic Anemia Following Ingestion of Sodium Ascorbate-Para-Aminosalicylic Acid Solution, Scalpel, Brussels, *106*, 287, 1953.

21. LUNDSTEEN, E., MEULENGRACHT, E. and RISCHEL, A.: Chronic Acetanilid Poisoning, Acta med. scandinav., *96*, 462, 1938; Folia hæmat., *63*, 89, 1939.

21*a*.MACHELLA, T. E. and HIGGINS, G. M.: Anemia Induced in Rats by Means of Sulphanilamide, Am. J. M. Sc., *198*, 804, 1939.

21*b*.MACKAY, I. R., LARKIN, LOIS and BURNET, F. M.: Failure of "Autoimmune" Antibody to React with Antigen Prepared

42

from the Individual's Own Tissues, Lancet, 2, 122, 1957.

22. MAIER, C.: *Hämolyse und hämolytische Krankheiten*, verlag Hans Huber, Bern, 1950.

22a.MALOOF, C. C.: Rôle of Porphyrins in Occupational Diseases, Arch. Indust. Hyg. & Occup. Med., 7, 296, 1950.

22b.MARCOLONGO, F.: Anemia emolitiche acquisato, Recenti Prog. Med., 15, 137, 1953.

22c.MARKS, P. A. and GROSS, RUTH T.: Erythrocyte Glucose-6-phosphate Dehydrogenase Deficiency: Evidence of Differences between Negroes and Caucasians with Respect to this Genetically Determined Trait, J. Clin. Invest., 38, 2253, 1959; Nature, 183, 1266, 1959; J. Biol. Chem., 236, 10, 1961.

22d.McCARTHY, O.: A Case of Favism, Lancet, 1, 748, 1955.

22e.McFADZEAN, A. J. S. and CHOA, G. H.: Hæmolytic Anæmia in Typhoid Fever, Brit. M. J., 2, 360, 1953.

22f.McFADZEAN, A. J. S. and DAVIS, L. J.: Iron-Staining Erythrocytic Inclusions with especial Reference to Acquired Hæmolytic Anæmia, Glasgow M. J., 28, 237, 1947; Quart. J. Med., 18, 57, 1949.

23. McNAUGHT, J. B., WOODS, F. M. and SCOTT, V.: Bartonella Bodies in the Blood of a Non-splenectomized Dog, J. Exper. Med., 62, 353, 1935.

23a.MINOT, G. R.: Blood Examination of Trinitrotoluene Workers, J. Indust. Hyg. & Toxicol., 1, 301, 1919.

23b.MIESCHER, P. and PLETSCHER, A.: Zur Pathogenese der Anämie bei Patienten mit Abusus phenacetinhaltiger Analgetica, Schweiz. med. Wchnschr., 88, 1056, 1958.

23c.MOESCHLIN, S.: Phenacetinsucht und-schäden, Schweiz. med. Wchnschr., 87, 123, 1957.

24. MOLLISON, P. L.: The Survival of Transfused Erythrocytes, with Special Reference to Cases of Acquired Hæmolytic Anæmia, Clin. Sc., 6, 137, 1947.

24a.MOOLTEN, S. E., CLARK, E., GLASSER, B. F., KATZ, E. and MILLER, B. S.: Blood Stream Invasion by Newcastle Disease Virus Associated with Hemolytic Anemia and Encephalopathy, Am. J. Med., 14, 294, 1953.

24b.MORGAN, H. R.: Acquired Hemolytic Anemia and Viremia, J. Lab. & Clin. Med., 46, 580, 1955.

24c.MOORE, F. D., PEACOCK, W. C., BLAKELY, E. and COPE, O.: The Anemia of Thermal Burns, Ann. Surg., 124, 811, 1946.

24d.MUIRHEAD, E. E., GROVES, M. and BRYAN, S.: Positive Direct Coombs' Test Induced by Phenylhydrazine. J. Clin. Invest.,

33, 1700, 1954; A.M.A. Arch. Int. Med., 101, 87, 1958.

24e.NEELY, F. L., BARIA, W. H., SMITH, C. and STONE, C. F., JR.: Primary Atypical Pneumonia With High Titer of Cold Hemagglutinins, Hemolytic Anemia, and False Positive Donath-Landsteiner Test, J. Lab. & Clin. Med., 37, 382, 1951.

24f.OLTRAMARE, M.: Anémie hémolytique aiguë chez une malade traitée par la Cryogènine et l'Irgafène, J. Suisse Méd., 83, 156, 1953.

25. PAPPENHEIMER, A. M., THOMPSON, W. P., PARKER, D. D. and SMITH, K. E.: Anæmia Associated With Unidentified Erythrocytic Inclusions After Splenectomy, Quart. J. Med., 14, 75, 1945.

26. PERLA, D. and MARMORSTON–GOTTESMAN, J.: Studies on Bartonella Muris Anemia, J. Exper. Med., 56, 777 and 783, 1932.

27a.PUGH, J. I. and ENDERBY, G. E. H.: Hæmoglobinuria after Intravenous Myanesin, Lancet, 2, 387, 1947.

27b.QUICK, E. D. and LORD, F. D.: Acute Hemolytic Anemia Following Sulfathiazole Administration, J.A.M.A., 117, 1704, 1941.

27c.RAFFENSPERGER, E. C.: Acute Acquired Hemolytic Anemia in Association with Acute Viral Hepatitis, Ann. Int. Med., 48, 1243, 1958.

27d.RAMOT, BRACHA et al.: A Study of Subjects with Erythrocyte Glucose-6-phosphate Dehydrogenase Deficiency: Investigation of Platelet Enzymes, J. Clin. Invest., 38, 1659, 1959; Nature, 185, 931, 1960.

28. RATH, C. E.: Drowning Hemoglobinuria, Blood, 8, 1099, 1953.

28a.REYNAFARJE, C. and RAMOS, J.: Estudios fisiopatologicos en la anemia de la enfermedad de Carrion, Rev. méd. peruana, 29, 74, 80 and 84, 1958; An. Fac. med., Lima, 42, 9, 1959.

29. RHOADS, C. P., BARKER, W. H. and MILLER, D. K.: The Increased Susceptibility to Hemolysis by Indol in Dogs Fed Deficient Diets, J. Exper. Med., 67, 299, 1938.

30. RHOADS, C. P. and MILLER, D. K.: Effect of Diet on Susceptibility of Canine Hematopoietic System to Damage by Amidopyrine, Proc. Soc. Exper. Biol. & Med., 36, 654, 1930.

31. ———— The Association of Bartonella Bodies With Induced Anemia in the Dog, J. Exper. Med., 61, 139, 1935.

32. RICHARDSON, A. P.: The Production of Anemia in White Mice by Sulfanilamide, Sulfapyridine and Diaminodiphenylsulfone, J. Pharmacol. & Exper. Therap., 67, 429, 1939; *Ibid.*, 72, 99, 1941.

32a.RICKETTS, W. E.: Bartonella Bacilliformis

Anemia (Oroya Fever), Blood, *3*, 1025, 1948; Arch. Int. Med., *84*, 751, 1949.

32*b*.RUBINO, G. F., PAGLIARDI, E., PRATO, V. and GIANGRANDI, E.: Erythrocyte Copper and Porphyrins in Lead Poisoning, Brit. J. Haemat., *4*, 103, 1958.

32*c*.SANO, S.: Studies on the Nature of the Basophilic Stippled Cells in Lead Poisoning, Acta Scholae med. Univ. Kioto, *35*, 149 and 158, 1958.

32*d*.SANSONE, G.: L'anemia emolitica acuta da ingestione accidentale di naftalina nel bambino, Haemat. latina, *1*, 45, 1958.

32*e*.SANSONE, G. and LEVI, A. T.: Sui rapporti fra vitamina K idrosolubile ed anemia dell'immaturo a corpi inclusl, Minerva pediat., *9*, 985, 1957.

32*f*.SELWYN, J. G.: Heinz Bodies in Red Cells After Splenectomy and after Phenacetin Administration, Brit. J. Hæmat., *1*, 173, 1955.

32*g*.SELWYN, J. G. and HACKETT, W. E. R.: Acquired Hæmolytic Anæmia: Survival of Transfused Erythrocytes in Patients and Normal Recipients, J. Clin. Path., *2*, 114, 1949.

32*h*.SHEN, S. C., FLEMING, E. M. and CASTLE, W. B.: Osmotic and Mechanical Fragilities of Erythrocytes of Monkeys Infected with *P. knowlesi* Malaria, Proc. Soc. Exper. Biol. & Med., *63*, 419, 1946.

33. SHOUSE, S. S. and WHIPPLE, G. H.: Effects of the Intravenous Injection of Colloidal Silver Upon the Hematopoietic System in Dogs, J. Exper. Med., *53*, 413, 1931.

33*a*.SHUMWAY, C. N., JR.: Spherocytic Hemolytic Anemia Associated with Acute Pneumococcal Infection in Rabbits, J. Lab. & Clin. Med., *51*, 240, 1958.

33*b*.SMITH, P. K.: Prolonged Administration of Large Doses of Acetanilid in Monkeys With Special Reference to Blood Changes, J. Pharmacol. & Exper. Therap., *68*, 1, 1940; *Ibid.*, *70*, 171, 1940.

34. SMITH, R. S. and ALEXANDER, SUZANNE: Heinz-body Anaemia Due to Dapsone, Brit. M. J., *1*, 625, 1959.

34*a*.SNAPPER, I., MARKS, D., SCHWARTZ, L. and HOLLANDER, L.: Hemolytic Anemia Secondary to Mesantoin, Ann. Int. Med., *39*, 619, 1953.

34*b*.SPRIGGS, A. I., SMITH, R. S., GRIFFITH, H. and TRUELOVE, S. C.: Heinz-body Anaemia Due to Salicylazosulphapyridine, Lancet, *1*, 1039, 1958.

34*c*.STICKNEY, J. M. and HECK, F. J.: Primary Nonfamilial Hemolytic Anemia, Blood, *3*, 431, 1948.

35. STOELTZNER, W.: Untersuchungen über die Haffkrankheit, Deutsch. med. Wchnschr., *58*, 1929, 1932.

35*a*.SUTHERLAND, D. A. and EISENTRAUT, ANNA M.: The Direct Coombs Test in Lead Poisoning, Blood, *11*, 1024, 1956.

35*b*.SZEINBERG, A., ASHER, Y.and SHEBA, Ch.: Studies on Glutathione Stability in Erythrocytes of Cases with Past History of Favism or Sulfa-drug-induced Hemolysis, Blood, *13*, 348, 1958.

35*c*.SZEINBERG, A. *et al.*: Glutathione Metabolism in Cord and Newborn Infant Blood, J. Clin. Invest., *37*, 1436, 1958.

35*d*.SZEINBERG, A., SHEBA, CH. and ADAM, A.: Selective Occurrence of Glutathione Instability in Red Blood Corpuscles of the Various Jewish Tribes, Blood, *13*, 1043, 1958; Acta Genet. Med. (Suppl. 2), *8*, 151, 1959; Acta haemat., *23*, 58, 1960.

35*e*.TODD, R. McL. and O'DONOHOE, N. V.: Acute Acquired Haemolytic Anaemia Associated with Herpex Simplex Infection, Arch. Dis. Childhood, *33*, 524, 1958.

35*f*.TOMPKINS, E. H.: Effects of Repeated Intravenous Injections of Lecithin in Rabbits, Arch. Path., *35*, 695, 1943.

36. VRYONIS, G.: Observations on the Parasitization of Erythrocytes by *Plasmodium Vivax*, With Special Reference to Reticulocytes, Am. J. Hyg., *30*, 41, 1939.

36*a*.VULLO, C. and PANIZON, F.: The Mechanism of Haemolysis in Favism, Acta haemat., *22*, 146, 1959.

36*b*.WAGLEY, P. F., SHEN, S. C., GARDNER, F. H., CASTLE, W. B.: The Spleen as a Source of a Substance Causing Agglutination of the Red Blood Cells of Certain Patients with Acquired Hemolytic Jaundice by an Anti-human Serum Rabbit Serum (Coombs' Serum), J. Lab. & Clin. Med., *33*, 1197, 1948; Proc. Soc. Exper. Biol. & Med., *72*, 411, 1949.

36*c*.WATSON, C. J.: The Bile Pigments, New England J. Med., *227*, 665 and 705, 1942.

37. WATSON, C. J. and SPINK, W. W.: Effect of Sulfanilamide and Sulfapyridine on Hemoglobin Metabolism and Hepatic Function, Arch. Int. Med., *65*, 825, 1940.

38. WEINMAN, D.: Infectious Anemias Due to Bartonella and Related Red Cell Parasites, Trans. Am. Phil. Soc., *33*, pt. 3, Philadelphia, 1944; Bull. N. Y. Acad. Med., *22*, 647, 1946.

38*a*.WILBUR, K. M. and COLLIER, H. B.: A Comparison of the Hemolytic Actions of Lysolecithin and Saponin, J. Cell. & Comp. Physiol., *22*, 233, 1943.

39. WILLIAMS, H. H., ERICKSON, B. N., BEACH, E. F. and MACY, I. G.: Biochemical

Studies of the Blood of Dogs With N-propyl Disulfide Anemia, J. Lab. & Clin. Med., *26*, 996, 1941.

39a.WILSON, R., JR. and MANGUN, G. H.: Acute Hemolytic Anemia in Fertilizer Workers, South. M. J., *36*, 212, 1943.

40. WOOD, W. B., JR.: Anemia During Sulfanilamide Therapy, J.A.M.A., *111*, 1916, 1938.

40a.WORMSER, F. E. and others: Conference on Lead Poisoning, Occup. Med., *3*, 13, 77 and 135, 1947.

40b.YOUNG, L. E.: Hemolytic Disorders, New York State J. Med., *47*, 1875, 1947.

40c.YOUNG, L. E., MILLER, G. and CHRISTIAN, R. M.: Clinical and Laboratory Observations on Autoimmune Hemolytic Disease, Ann. Int. Med., *35*, 507, 1951; Tr. A. Am. Physicians, *67*, 124, 1954.

40d.YOUNG, L. E., VALENTINE, W. N. and HOWLAND, J. W.: Acute Hemolytic Anemia Due to Neoarsphenamine, Ann. Int. Med., *24*, 104, 1946.

40e.ZINKHAM, W. H.: An in-vitro Abnormality of Glutathione Metabolism in Erythrocytes from Normal Newborns, Pediatrics, *23*, 18, 1959.

40f.ZINKHAM, W. H. and CHILDS, B.: A Defect of Glutathione Metabolism in Erythrocytes from Patients with a Naphthalene-induced Hemolytic Anemia, Pediatrics, *22*, 461, 1958.

Paroxysmal, Nocturnal, March and Paralytic Hemoglobinurias and Miscellaneous Hemolytic Anemias

40g.ALLISON, A. C. and CLYDE, D. F.: Malaria in African Children with Deficient Erythrocyte Glucose-6-Phosphate Dehydrogenase, Brit. M. J., *1*, 1346, 1961.

41. BARRY, R. M.: The Phospholipid Distribution in the Erythrocyte in Paroxysmal Nocturnal Haemoglobinuria, Brit. J. Haemat., *5*, 212, 1959.

41a.BECKER, R. M.: Paroxysmal Cold Hemoglobinurias, Arch. Int. Med., *81*, 630, 1948.

41b.BLONDHEIM, S. H., MARGOLIASH, E. and SHAFRIR, E.: A Simple Test for Myohemoglobinuria (Myoglobinuria), J. A. M. A., *167*, 453, 1958.

42. BRULE, M., HILLEMAND, P. and GAUBE, R.: Un nouveau Cas d'Anémie hémolytique avec Hémoglobinurie et Hémosidérinurie, Presse méd., *46*, 1329, 1938.

42a.BUELL, A. and METTIER, S. R.: Paroxysmal Nocturnal Hemoglobinuria with Hemolytic Anemia, J. Lab. & Clin. Med., *26*, 1434, 1941.

43. BURMEISTER, J.: Über paroxysmale Hämoglobinurie und Syphilis, Ztschr. klin. Med., *92*, 19, 1921.

43a.CHAIKEN, B. H., WHALEN, E. J., LEARNER, N. and SMITH, N. J.: Variants of "March Hemoglobinuria," Am. J. M. Sc., *225*, 514, 1953.

43b.CHAUFFARD, M. A. and TROISIER, J.: Anémie grave avec hémolysine dans la sérum, etc., Sem. méd., 28, 904, 1908; *Ibid.*, 29, 601, 1909; Bull. et mém. Soc. méd. hop. de Paris, 26, 94, 1908; *Ibid.*, 32, 726, 1912.

43c.CROSBY, W. H.: Paroxysmal Nocturnal Hemoglobinuria. A Classical Description by Paul Strübing in 1882, and a Bibliography of the Disease, Blood, *6*, 270, 1951.

43d.CROSBY, W. H.: Paroxysmal Nocturnal Hemoglobinuria: Plasma Factors of the Hemolytic System, Blood, *8*, 444 and 769, 1953.

43e.CROSBY, W. H.: Paroxysmal Nocturnal Hemoglobinuria: A Case Complicated by an Aregenerative (Aplastic) Crisis, Ann. Int. Med., *39*, 1107, 1953.

44. CROSBY, W. H. and DAMESHEK, W.: Paroxysmal Nocturnal Hemoglobinuria, Blood, *5*, 822 and 843, 1950; Blood, *13*, 684, 1958; *ibid.*, *15*, 505, 1960.

44a.CROSBY, W. H. and DAMESHEK, W.: The Significance of Hemoglobinuria and Associated Hemosiderinuria, with Particular Reference to Various Types of Hemolytic Anemia, J. Lab. & Clin. Med., *38*, 829, 1951.

44b.DACIE, J. V.: Transfusion of Saline-Washed Red Cells in Nocturnal Hæmoglobinuria, Clin. Sci., *7*, 65, 1948.

44c.————Diagnosis and Mechanism of Hemolysis in Chronic Hemolytic Anemia with Nocturnal Hemoglobinuria, Blood, *4*, 1183, 1949.

44d.DACIE, J. V. and FIRTH, D.: Blood Transfusion in Nocturnal Hæmoglobinuria, Brit. M. J., *1*, 626, 1943.

45. DACIE, J. V., ISRAËLS, M. C. G. and WILKINSON, J. F.: Paroxysmal Nocturnal Hæmoglobinuria of the Marchiafava Type, Lancet, *1*, 479, 1938.

45a.DACIE, J. V., LEWIS, S. M. and TILLS, D.: Comparative Sensitivity of the Erythrocytes in Paroxysmal Nocturnal Hæmoglobinuria to Hæmolysis by Acidified Normal Serum and by High-Titre Cold Antibody, Brit. J. Haemat., *6*, 362, 1960.

46. DAMESHEK, W. and SCHWARTZ, S. O.: Acute Hemolytic Anemia, Medicine, *19*, 231, 1940 (Bibliography).

47. DAVIS, R. W., DOLES, H., IZZO, M. J. and YOUNG, L. E.: Hemolytic Effect of Radiation, J. Lab. & Clin. Med., *35*, 528, 1950.

48. ERNSTENE, A. C. and GARDNER, W. J.: The

Effect of Splanchnic Nerve Resection and Sympathetic Ganglionectomy in a Case of Paroxysmal Hemoglobinuria, J. Clin. Invest., *14*, 799, 1935.

49. GARDNER, F. H. and LAFORET, MITSUKO T.: The Use of Clinical Dextran in Patients with Paroxysmal Nocturnal Hemoglobinuria, J. Lab. & Clin. Med., *55*, 946, 1960.

50. GIFFIN, H. Z.: Hemoglobinuria in Hemolytic Jaundice, Arch. Int. Med., *31*, 573, 1923.

50a.GILLIGAN, D. R. and BLUMGART, H. L.: March Hemoglobinuria, Medicine, *20*, 341, 1941; New England J. Med., *243*, 944, 1950.

50b.GILLIGAN, D. R., ALTSCHULE, M. D. and KATERSKY, E. M.: Physiological Intravascular Hemolysis of Exercise. Hemoglobinemia and Hemoglobinuria Following ing Cross-Country Runs, J. Clin. Invest., *22*, 859, 1943.

51. GIORDANO, A. S. and BLUM, L. L.: Acute Hemolytic Anemia (Lederer Type), Am. J. M. Sc., *194*, 311, 1937.

52. GOLD, E. R., IKIN, ELIZABETH W. and MOURANT, A. E.: Serum Containing Three Rh Autohaemagglutinins, Brit. M. J., *2*, 1273, 1958.

52a.GREENBERG, M. S. and WONG, HELENA: Studies on the Destruction of Glutathione-Unstable Red Blood Cells. The Influence of Fava Beans and Primaquine Upon Such Cells *in Vivo*, J. Lab. & Clin. Med., *57*, 733, 1961.

52b.HAM, G. C. and HORACK, H. M.: Chronic Hemolytic Anemia with Paroxysmal Nocturnal Hemoglobinemia, Arch. Int. Med., *67*, 735, 1941.

53. HAM, T. H.: Chronic Hemolytic Anemia With Paroxysmal Nocturnal Hemoglobinuria, Arch. Int. Med., *64*, 1271, 1939.

54. HAM, T. H. and DINGLE, J. H.: Chronic Hemolytic Anemia With Paroxysmal Nocturnal Hemoglobinuria: Certain Immunological Aspects of the Hemolytic Mechanism With Special Reference to Serum Complement, J. Clin. Invest., *18*, 657, 1939.

55. HAMBURGER, L. and BERNSTEIN, A.: Chronic Hemolytic Anemia With Paroxysmal Nocturnal Hemoglobinuria, Am. J. M., Sc., *192*, 301, 1936.

56. HARRIS, I. M., PRANKERD, T. A. J. and WESTERMAN, M. P.: Abnormality of Phospholipids in Red Cells of Patients with Paroxysmal Nocturnal Haemoglobinuria, Brit. M. J., *2*, 1276, 1957.

56a.HARRIS, J. W., JORDAN, W. S., PILLEMER, L. and DESFORGES, J. F.: The Enzymatic Nature of the Factor in Normal Serum which Hemolyzes the Erythrocytes in Paroxysmal Nocturnal Hemoglobinuria, J. Clin. Invest., *30*, 646, 1951; J. Lab. & Clin. Med., *44*, 811, 1954; Science, *120*, 279, 1954.

57. HARRIS, K. E., LEWIS, T. and VAUGHAN, J. M.: Hæmoglobinuria and Urticaria From Cold Occurring Singly or in Combination, Heart, *14*, 305, 1929.

57a.HARTMANN, R. C. and AUDITORE, J. V.: Paroxysmal Nocturnal Hemoglobinuria, Am. J. Med., *27*, 389, 1959; J. Clin. Invest., *38*, 702, 1959; J. Applied Physiol., *14*, 589, 1959.

58. HILLESTAD, L. K.: The Peripheral Circulation during Exposure to Cold in Normals and in Patients with the Syndrome of High-titre Cold Haemagglutination, Acta med. scandinav., *164*, 203 and 211, 1959.

58a.HOBBS, R. E.: March Hemoglobinuria, Am. J. Clin. Path., *14*, 485, 1944.

59. HOFFMANN, W.: Paroxysmal Hemoglobinuria Elicited by Marching, Med. Welt, *11*, 1640, 1937.

59a.HOFFMAN, B. J. and KRACKE, R. R.: Chronic Hemolytic Anemia With Paroxysmal Nocturnal Hemoglobinuria, J. Lab. & Clin. Med., *28*, 817, 1943.

59b.HOWARD, C. P., MILES, E. S. and TOWNSEND, S. R.: Paroxysmal Hemoglobinuria, Am. J. M. Sc., *196*, 792, 1938.

60. JAMRA, M. *et al.*: Amiloidose primária, Rev. Hosp. clin., *14*, 76, 1959.

60a.JONSSON, U., HANSEN-PRUSS, O. C. and RUNDLES, R. W.: Hemolytic Anemia in Myelogenous Leukemia With Splenectomy, Blood, *5*, 920, 1950.

61. JORDAN, F. L. J.: Etudes sur l'hémoglobinurie, Acta med. scandinav., *95*, 319, 1938.

61a.JORDAN, W. S., JR., PILLEMER, L. and DINGLE, J. H.: The Mechanism of Hemolysis in Paroxysmal Cold Hemoglobinuria, J. Clin. Invest., *30*, 11 and 22, 1951.

61b.JORDAN, W. S., JR., PROUTY, R. L., HEINLE, R. W. and DINGLE, J. H.: The Mechanism of Hemolysis in Paroxysmal Cold Hemoglobinuria, Blood, *7*, 387, 1952.

61c.KALANT, N. and CYR, D. P.: Treatment of Paroxysmal Nocturnal Hemoglobinuria with ACTH, Blood, *7*, 607, 1952.

61d.KISSMEYER-NIELSEN, F., BICHEL, J. and HANSEN, P. B.: Specific Auto-Antibodies in Immunohaemolytic Anaemia, Acta hæmat., *15*, 189, 1956.

62. KUMAGAI, T. and NAMBA, M.: Weitere Beiträge zur Kenntnis der paroxysmalen Hämoglobinurie, Deutsch. Arch. klin. Med., *156*, 257, 1927.

62a.LANGE, R. D. and AKEROYD, J. H.: Congenital Hemolytic Anemia with Abnormal Pigment Metabolism and Red Cell Inclusion Bodies: a New Clinical Syndrome, Blood, *13*, 950, 1958.

63. LEDERER, M.: Form of Acute Hemolytic Anemia Probably of Infectious Origin, Am. J. M. Sc., *170*, 500, 1925.

64. LETMAN, H.: Possible Paroxysmal Nocturnal Hemoglobinuria with Pronounced Pancytopenia, Reticulocytopenia, and without Hemoglobinuria Simulating Aplastic Anemia, Blood, *7*, 842, 1952.

65. VAN LOGHEM, JR., J. J., MENDES DE LEON, D. E., FRENKEL-TIETZ, H. and VAN DER HART, M.: Two Different Serologic Mechanisms of Paroxysmal Cold Hemoglobinuria, Blood, *7*, 1196, 1952.

67. MACKENZIE, G. M.: Paroxysmal Hemoglobinuria, A Review, Medicine, *8*, 159, 1929 (Bibliography).

67a. MANCHESTER, R. C.: Chronic Hemolytic Anemia With Paroxysmal Nocturnal Hemoglobinuria, Ann. Int. Med., *23*, 935, 1945.

67b. MARTIN, H., HUG, O. and LIPPERT, W.: Paroxysmale nächtliche Hämoglobinurie—Anämia Marchiafava-Micheli. Eine morphologische Studie, Folia haemat., *76*, 141, 1959.

67c. McKELLAR, M. and DACIE, J. V.: Thromboplastic Activity of the Plasma in Paroxysmal Nocturnal Haemoglobinuria, Brit. J. Haemat., *4*, 404, 1958.

67d. MEHROTRA, T. N.: Individual Specific Nature of the Cold Auto-Antibodies of Acquired Haemolytic Anaemia, Nature, *185*, 323, 1960.

67e. METZ, J., BRADLOW, B. A., LEWIS, S. M. and DACIE, J. V.: The Acetylcholinesterase Activity of the Erythrocytes in Paroxysmal Nocturnal Haemoglobinuria in Relation to the Severity of the Disease, Brit. J. Haemat. *6*, 372, 1960.

68. MEYER, E. and EMMERICH, E.: Über paroxysmale Hämoglobinuria, Deutsch. Arch. klin. Med., *96*, 287, 1909.

68a. MIESCHER, P., v. RECHENBERG, H. K., BERGER, J. and HOLLÄNDER: Hämolytische Anämie bei Ovarialtumor, Schweiz. med. Wchnschr., *88*, 498, 1958.

68b. MÜLLER, W. and SCHUBOTHE, H.: Symptomatische hämolytische Anämien bei Dermoidcysten, Folia haemat., *2*, 321, 1958.

68c. MUNN, J. I. and CROSBY, W. H.: Paroxysmal Nocturnal Hemoglobinuria. Evidence of Defect of Red Cell Stroma Manifested by Abnormalities of Lipids, Proc. Soc. Exper. Biol. & Med., *96*, 480, 1957.

69. NAMBA, M.: Uber die kunstliche Erzeugung

des Autohämolysins, Deutsch. med. Wchnschr., *51*, 594, 1925.

69a. NELSON, M. G. and BRUCE, J. H.: Paroxysmal Nocturnal Hemoglobinuria with the Development of Aplastic Anemia, Blood, *8*, 664, 1953.

69b. PETERSON, E. T. and WALFORD, R. L.: Serologic Properties of a Cold Hemolysin and an Acid Hemolysin Occurring in a Case of Syphilitic Paroxysmal Cold Hemoglobinuria, Blood, *7*, 1109, 1952.

69c. PIERCE, P. P. and ALDRICH, C. A.: Chronic Hemolytic Anemia With Paroxysmal Nocturnal Hemoglobinuria (Marchiafava-Micheli Syndrome), J. Pediat., *22*, 30, 1943.

69d. PARISH, D. J. and MITCHELL, J. R. A.: Syphilitic Paroxysmal Cold Haemoglobinuria, J. Clin. Path., *13*, 237, 1960.

70. PORGES, O. and STRISOWER, R.: Marschhämoglobinurie, Wien. klin. Wchnschr., *26*, 193, 1913.

70a. REINER, L. *et al.*: Idiopathic Paroxysmal Myoglobinuria, A.M.A. Arch. Int. Med., *97*, 537, 1956.

70b. RITZMANN, S. E. and LEVIN, W. C.: Effect of Mercaptanes in Cold Agglutinin Disease, J. Lab. & Clin. Med., *57*, 718, 1961.

71. ROSENTHAL, F.: Über eine neue Form von paroxysmaler Hämoglobinurie, Ztschr. klin. Med., *119*, 449, 1932.

71a. ROTH, K. L. and FRUMIN, A. M.: Studies on the Hemolytic Principle of the Fava Bean, J. Lab. & Clin. Med., *56*, 695, 1960.

72. SALÉN, E. B.: Thermostabiles, nicht komplexes (Auto-) Hämolysin bei transitorischer Kältehämoglobinurie, Acta med. scandinav., *86*, 570, 1935.

73. SCHELLONG, F.: Untersuchungen über Marschhämoglobinurie; ihre Beziehungen zur Kältehämoglobinurie und orthostatischen Albuminurie, Ztschr. ges. exper. Med., *34*, 82, 1923.

74. SCHMID, R., BRECHER, G. and CLEMENS, T.: Familial Hemolytic Anemia with Erythrocyte Inclusion Bodies and a Defect in Pigment Metabolism, Blood, *14*, 991, 1959.

74a. SCHMID, R. and MAHLER, R.: Chronic Progressive Myopathy with Myoglobinuria; Demonstration of a Glycogenolytic Defect in the Muscle, J. Clin. Invest., *38*, 2044, 1959.

74b. SCOTT, J. L., HAUT, A., CARTWRIGHT, G. E. and WINTROBE, M. M.: Congenital Hemolytic Disease Associated with Red Cell Inclusion Bodies, Abnormal Pigment Metabolism and an Electrophoretic Hemoglobin Abnormality, Blood, *16*, 1239, 1960.

75. SCOTT, R. B., ROBB-SMITH, A. H. T. and SCOWEN, E. F.: The Marchiafava-Micheli

Syndrome of Nocturnal Hæmoglobinuria With Hæmolytic Anæmia, Quart. J. Med., 7, 95, 1938.

75a. SIEBENS, A. A., ZINKHAM, W. H. and WAGLEY, P. F.: Observations on the Mechanism of Hemolysis in Paroxysmal (Cold) Hemoglobinuria, Blood, 3, 1367, 1948.

75b. STAHL, W. C.: March Hemoglobinuria, J. A. M. A., 164, 1458, 1957.

75c. STEINMETZ, I.: Ein Fall von Marschhämoglobinurie, Deutsch. Arch. klin. Med., 196, 314, 1949.

75d. SUSSMAN, R. M. and KAYDEN, H. J.: Renal Insufficiency Due to Paroxysmal Cold Hemoglobinuria, Arch. Int. Med., 82, 598, 1948.

76. SWEETNAM, W. P., MURPHY, E. F. and WOODCOCK, R. C.: Acute Idiopathic Paroxysmal Cold Hæmoglobinuria of Nonsyphilitic Type in a Child, Brit. M. J., 1, 465, 1952.

76a. VARADI, S. and HURWORTH, E.: Heinz-body Anaemia in the Newborn, Brit. M. J., 1, 315, 1957.

76b. WAGLEY, P. F. and RUMSFELD, J. A.: A Clinical Note on Marchiafava-Micheli Disease, A. M. A. Arch. Int. Med., 101, 300, 1958.

77. WATSON, E. M. and FISCHER, L. C.: Paroxysmal "March" Hemoglobinuria, Am. J. Clin. Path., 5, 151, 1935.

77a. WHISNANT, C. L., JR., OWINGS, R. H., CANTRELL, C. G. and COOPER, G. R.: Primary Idiopathic Myoglobinuria in a Negro Female, Ann. Int. Med., 51, 140, 1959.

77b. WITTS, L. J.: The Paroxysmal Hæmoglobinurias, Lancet, 2, 115, 1936.

Hemolytic Jaundice, Congenital and "Acquired"

78. ALLIBONE, E. C. and COLLINS, D. H.: Symptomatic Hæmolytic Anæmia Associated with Ovarian Teratoma in a Child, J. Clin. Path., 4, 412, 1951.

78a. ALLISON, A. C., KATES, M. and JAMES, A. T.: An Abnormality of Blood Lipids in Hereditary Spherocytosis, Brit. M. J., 2, 1766, 1960.

78b. ANDERSON, R., HUESTIS, R. R. and MOTULSKY, A. G.: Hereditary Spherocytosis in the Deer Mouse, Blood, 15, 491, 1960.

78c. ARIAS, I. M.: Gilbert's Disease, Bull. New York Acad. Med., 35, 450, 1959.

78d. BATES, G. C. and BROWN, C. H.: Incidence of Gallbladder Disease in Chronic Hemolytic Anemia (Spherocytosis), Gastroenterology, 21, 104, 1952.

78e. BATY, J. M.: A Case of Congenital Hemolytic Jaundice With an Unusually High Percentage of Reticulocytes, Am. J. M. Sc., 179, 546, 1930.

79. BEINHAUER, L. G. and GRUHN, J. G.: Dermatologic Aspects of Congenital Spherocytic Anemia, A. M. A. Arch. Dermat., 75, 642, 1957.

79a. BERNARD, J., BOIRON, M. and ESTAGER, J.: Une grande famille hémolytique, Semaine hôp., Paris, 28, 3741, 1952.

79b. BURMAN, D.: Congenital Spherocytosis in Infancy, Arch. Dis. Childhood, 33, 335, 1958.

79c. BURSTON, J., HUSAIN, O. A. N., HUTT, M. S. R. and TANNER, E. I.: Two Cases of Autoimmune Haemolysis and Aplasia, Brit. M. J., 1, 83, 1959.

80. CAFFEY, J.: Skeletal Changes in Chronic Hemolytic Anemias (Erythroblastic Anemia, Sickle Cell Anemia and Chronic Hemolytic Icterus), Am. J. Roentgenol., 37, 293, 1937.

80a. CASTLE, W. B., HAM, T. H. and SHEN, S. C.: Observations on the Mechanism of Hemolytic Transfusion Reactions Occurring without Demonstrable Hemolysin, Tr. A. Am. Physicians, 63, 161, 1950.

80b. CHANARIN, I., DACIE, J. V. and MOLLIN, D. L.: Folic-acid Deficiency in Haemolytic Anaemia, Brit. J. Haemat., 5, 245, 1959.

80c. CHENEY, W. F. and CHENEY, G.: Chronic Hereditary Hemolytic Jaundice, Am. J. M. Sc., 187, 191, 1934.

81. CONRAD, M. E., JR., CROSBY, W. H. and HOWIE, D. L.: Hereditary Non-Spherocytic Hemolytic Disease, Am. J. Med., 29, 811, 1960.

81a. CRAIG, G. A. and TURNER, R. L.: A Case of Symptomatic Hæmolytic Anæmia in Pregnancy, Brit. M. J., 1, 1003, 1955.

81c. CROSBY, W. H.: Hereditary Nonspherocytic Hemolytic Anemia, Blood, 5, 233, 1950.

81d. CROSBY, W. H. and CONRAD, M. E.: Hereditary Spherocytosis: Observations on Hemolytic Mechanisms and Iron Metabolism, Blood, 15, 662, 1960.

82. CURSCHMANN, H.: Funicular Myelosis in Hemolytic Icterus, Deutsch. Ztschr. Nervenh., 122, 119, 1931.

82a. CUTBUSH, MARIE and MOLLISON, P. L.: Relation between Characteristics of Blood-group Antibodies *in vitro* and Associated Patterns of Red-cell Destruction *in vivo*, Brit. J. Haemat., 4, 115, 1958.

83. DACIE, J. V.: Familial Hæmolytic Anæmia (Acholuric Jaundice), With Particular Reference to Changes in Fragility Produced by Splenectomy, Quart. J. Med., 12, 101, 1943.

83a. DACIE, J. V., MOLLISON, P. L., RICHARDSON,

N., SELWYN, J. G. and SHAPIRO, L.: Atypical Congenital Hæmolytic Anæmia, Quart. J. Med., 22, 79, 1953.

83b. DAMESHEK, W. and BLOOM, M. L.: The Events in the Hemolytic Crisis of Hereditary Spherocytosis, with Particular Reference to the Reticulocytopenia, Pancytopenia and an Abnormal Splenic Mechanism, Blood, 3, 1381, 1948.

84. DAUSSET, J. and COLOMBANI, J.: The Serology and the Prognosis of 128 Cases of Autoimmune Hemolytic Anemia, Blood, 14, 1280, 1959.

84a. DAUSSET, J., MOULLEC, J. and BERNARD, J.: Acquired Hemolytic Anemia with Polyagglutinability of Red Blood Cells Due to a New Factor Present in Normal Human Serum (Anti-Tn), Blood, 14, 1079, 1959.

84b. DAVIDSOHN, I. and OYAMADA, A.: Specificity of Auto-antibodies in Hemolytic Anemia, Am. J. Clin. Path., 23, 101, 1953.

85. DAVIDSON, L. S. P.: Macrocytic Hæmolytic Anæmia, Quart. J. Med., n.s., 1, 543, 1932.

86. DAVIDSON, L. S. P. and FULLERTON, H. W.: Some Rare Types of Macrocytic Anæmia, Quart. J. Med., 7, 43, 1938.

86a. DAVIS, L. J.: Symptomatic Hæmolytic Anæmia, Edinburgh M. J., 51, 70, 1944.

87. DAWSON, L.: Hume Lectures on Hemolytic Icterus, Brit. M. J., 1, 963, 1931.

88. DEBRÉ, R., LAMY, M., SÉE, G. and SCHRAMECK, G.: Congenital and Familial Hemolytic Disease in Children, Am. J. Dis. Child., 56, 1189, 1938.

88a. DELAMORE, I. W., RICHMOND, J. and DAVIES, S. H.: Megaloblastic Anaemia in Congenital Spherocytosis, Brit. M. J., 1, 543, 1961.

88b. DENNY, W. F., BIRD, R. M. and DuVAL, M. K.: Hereditary Spherocytosis, A. M. A. Arch. Int. Med., 101, 894, 1958.

89. DIAMOND, L. K.: Indications for Splenectomy in Childhood, Am. J. Surg., n.s., 39, 400, 1938.

90. DOAN, C. A., CURTIS, G. M. and WISEMAN, B. K.: The Hemolytopoietic Equilibrium and Emergency Splenectomy, J.A.M.A., 105, 1567, 1935.

90a. DREYFUS, C.: Chronic Hemolytic Jaundice, Bull. New England Med. Center, 4, 122, 1942.

92. EPPINGER, H.: Über schwer heilbare Füssgeschwüre bei hämolytischen Ikterus, Klin. Wchnschr., 9, 10, 1930.

93. FALCONER, E. H.: Familial Hemolytic Icterus Associated With Endocrine Dysfunction, Endocrinology, 20, 174, 1936.

93a. FLÜCKIGER, P., RICCI, C. and USTERI, C.: Zur Frage der Blutgruppenspezifität von Autoantikörpern, Acta haemat., 13, 53, 1955.

93b. FRUMIN, A. M. and KOHN, A.: Autoimmune Hemolytic Disease in Acute Leukemia, Arch. Int. Med., 95, 326, 1955.

93c. FUDENBERG, H. H. and KUNKEL, H. G.: Physical Properties of the Red Cell Agglutinins in Acquired Hemolytic Anemia, J. Exper. Med., 106, 689, 1957; Blood, 8, 201, 1958.

93d. FUDENBERG, H. and WINTROBE, M. M.: Symptomatic Hemolytic Anemia: Report of a Case with Scleroderma, Ann. Int. Med., 43, 201, 1955.

94. GAIRDNER, D.: Association of Gallstones With Acholuric Jaundice in Children, Arch. Dis. Child., 14, 109, 1939.

95. GÄNSSLEN, M., ZIPPERLEN, E. and SCHÜZ, E.: Die hämolytische Konstitution, Deutsch. Arch. klin. Med., 146, 1, 1925.

95a. GASSER, C.: Erythroblastopénie aiguë dans les anémies hémolytiques, Sang, 21, 237, 1950.

95b. GREEN, N. and GOLDENBERG, H.: Acute Hemolytic Anemia and Hemoglobinuria Complicating Infectious Mononucleosis, A. M. A. Arch. Int. Med., 105, 108, 1960.

95c. GREIG, H. B. W. et al.: The Familial Crisis in Hereditary Spherocytosis: Report of Five Cases, South African J. M. Sc., 23, 17, 1958.

95d. GRIGGS, R. C., WEISMAN, R., JR. and HARRIS, J. W.: Alterations in Osmotic and Mechanical Fragility Related to in vivo Erythrocyte Aging and Splenic Sequestration in Hereditary Spherocytosis, J. Clin. Invest., 39, 89, 1960.

95e. DE GRUCHY, G. C., SANTAMARIA, J. N., PARSONS, I. C. and CRAWFORD, H.: Nonspherocytic Congenital Hemolytic Anemia, Blood, 16, 1371, 1960.

96. HADEN, R. L.: The Mechanism of the Increased Fragility of the Erythrocytes in congenital Hemolytic Jaundice, Am. J. M. Sc., 188, 441, 1934.

96a. ———A New Type of Hereditary Hemolytic Jaundice without Spherocytosis, Am. J. M. Sc., 214, 255, 1947.

96b. HAGER, H. G., JR. and VAN CAMP, W.: Primary Carcinoma of the Gall Bladder in a Patient with Congenital Hemolytic Jaundice, Ann. Int. Med., 27, 823, 1947.

96c. HANFORD, R. B., SCHNEIDER, G. F. and MAC CARTHY, J. D.: Massive Thoracic Extramedullary Hemopoiesis, New England J. Med., 263, 120, 1960.

97. HANSEN, K. and KLEIN, E.: Symptomatology and Heredity of Hemolytic Jaundice, Deutsch. Arch. klin. Med., 176, 567, 1934

98. HARTFALL, S. J. and STEWART, M. J.: Massive Paravertebral Heterotopia of Bone Marrow in a Case of Acholuric Jaundice, J. Path. & Bact., 37, 455, 1933.

99. HEILMEYER, L.: Blutfarbstoffwechselstudien, Deutsch. Arch. klin. Med., 172, 628, 1932.

99a. HEILMEYER, L.: Hemolytic Hypersplenia: Acquired Hemolytic Icterus, Deutsch. Arch. klin. Med., 178, 89, 1935; Ibid., 179, 292, 1936.

100. HOGEMAN, O.: Hyperhemolysis of Nonsplenic Origin, Acta med. scandinav., 144, 247, 1953.

100a. HOLLIDAY, T. D. S.: Familial Non-spherocytic Hæmolytic Anæmia, J. Clin. Path., 6, 219, 1953.

101. ISRAËLS, L. G., SUDERMAN, H. J. and RITZMANN, S. E.: Hyperbilirubinemia Due to an Alternate Path of Bilirubin Production, Am. J. Med., 27, 693, 1959.

101a. KLINE, A. H. and HOLMAN, G. H.: Hereditary Spherocytosis in the Negro, A. M. A. J. Dis. Child., 94, 609, 1957.

101b. KOHLER, H. G., MEYNELL, M. J. and COOKE, W. T.: Spherocytic Anaemia, Complicated by Megaloblastic Anaemia of Pregnancy, Brit. M. J., 1, 779, 1960.

101c. KUMAR, S., SINGH, M. M., BHATIA, B. B. and MANGALIK, V. S.: Symmetrical Peripheral Gangrene in Acquired Hemolytic Anemia, Acta haemat., 19, 369, 1958.

102a. LOEB, V., JR., SEAMAN, W. B. and MOORE, C. V.: The Use of Thorium Dioxide Sol (Thorotrast) in the Roentgenologic Demonstration of Accessory Spleens, Blood, 7, 904, 1952.

102b. VAN LOGHEM, J. J. and VAN DER HART, M.: Varieties of Specific Auto Antibodies in Acquired Hæmolytic Anæmia (II), Vox sanguinis, 4, 129, 1954; in Proceedings of the Sixth International Congress of the International Society of Hematology, New York, Grune and Stratton, 1958, p. 858.

103. LÖWINGER, S.: Das Bild des Knochenmarkes bei der konstitutionellen hämolytischen Anämie (Ikterus Hæmolyticus), Folia hæmat., 54, 27, 1935.

103a. MÄRTENSSON, J. and HENRIKSON, H.: Immuno-Hemolytic Anemia in Kaposi's Sarcoma with Visceral Involvement Only, Acta med. scandinav., 150, 175, 1954.

103b. McCURDY, P. R. and RATH, C. E.: Splenectomy in Hemolytic Anemia, New England J. Med., 259, 459, 1958.

103c. McFARLAND, W., GALBRAITH, R. G. and MIALE, A., JR.: Heparin Therapy in Autoimmune Hemolytic Anemia, Blood, 15, 741, 1960.

103d. MARCHAL, G., BILSKI-PASQUIER, G. and VORIAS, N.: L'érythroblastopénie aiguë, Sang, 31, 209, 1960.

103e. MENDELBAUM, H.: Congenital Hemolytic Jaundice; Initial Hemolytic Crisis Occurring at the Age of 75, Ann. Int. Med., 13, 872, 1939.

104. METZ, J.: Hereditary Spherocytosis in the Bantu, South African M. J., 33, 1034, 1959.

104a. MOESCHLIN, S., SIEGENTHALER, W., GASSER, C. and HASSIG, A.: Immunopancytopenia Associated with Incomplete Cold Hemagglutinins in a Case of Primary Atypical Pneumonia, Blood, 9, 214, 1954.

104b. MOTULSKY, A. G., GIBLETT, E., COLEMAN, D., GABRIO, B. and FINCH, C. A.: Life Span, Glucose Metabolism and Osmotic Fragility of Erythrocytes in Hereditary Spherocytosis, J. Clin. Invest., 34, 911, 1955.

104c. MOTULSKY, A. et al.: Glucose-6-Phosphate Dehydrogenase Dye Test, Clin. Res., 7, 89, 1959.

104d. OWREN, P. A.: Congenital Hemolytic Jaundice. The Pathogenesis of the "Hemolytic Crisis," Blood, 3, 231, 1948.

105. PASCHKIS, K.: Beiträge zur Kenntnis und Wertung der Blutzerstörung beim hämolytischen Ikterus, Ztschr. klin. Med., 116, 680, 1931.

105a. PAYNE, R., SPAET, T. H. and AGGELER, P. M.: An Unusual Antibody Pattern in a Case of Idiopathic Acquired Hemolytic Anemia, J. Lab. & Clin. Med., 46, 245, 1955.

105b. PISCIOTTA, A. V. and HINZ, A. C. E.: Detection and Characterization of Autoantibodies in Acquired Auto-immune Hemolytic Anemia, Am. J. Clin. Path., 27, 619, 1957; A. M. A. Arch. Int. Med., 104, 264, 1959.

106. PRANKERD, T. A. J., ALTMAN, K. I. and YOUNG, L. E.: Abnormalities of Carbohydrate Metabolism of Red Cells in Hereditary Spherocytosis, J. Clin. Invest., 34, 1268, 1955; Am. J. Med., 22, 724, 1957; Quart. J. Med., 29, 199, 1960.

106a. PRITCHARD, J. A., WEISMAN, R., JR., RATNOFF, O. D. and VOSBURGH, G. J.: Intravascular Hemolysis, Thrombocytopenia and Other Hematologic Abnormalities Associated with Severe Toxemia of Pregnancy, New England J. Med., 250, 89, 1954.

106b. RACE, R. R.: On the Inheritance and Linkage Relations of Acholuric Jaundice, Ann. Eugen., 11, 365, 1942.

106c. RAPPAPORT, H. and CROSBY, W. H.: Autoimmune Hemolytic Anemia, Am. J. Path., 33, 429, 1957.

107. RAPPAPORT, H. and JOHNSON, F. B.: Intra-

cellular Protein Resembling Russell Bodies in Malignant Lymphomas Associated with Acquired Hemolytic Anemia, Blood, *10*, 132, 1955.

108. ROSENTHAL, M. C., PISCIOTTA, A. V., KOMNINOS, Z. D., GOLDENBERG, H. and DAMESHEK, W.: The Auto-Immune Hemolytic Anemia of Malignant Lymphocytic Disease, Blood, *10*, 197, 1955.

108a. SACCHETTI, C., ROSSI, V. and DIENA, F.: Behaviour of Erythroblasts *in vitro* in Sera from Cases of Acquired Haemolytic Anaenia, Brit. J. Haemat., *4*, 416, 1958.

108b. SACKS, M. S., WORKMAN, J. B. and JAHN, E. F.: Diagnosis and Treatment of Acquired Hemolytic Anemia, J. A. M. A., *150*, 1556, 1952.

108c. SARLES, H. E. and LEVIN, W. C.: The Role of Splenectomy in the Management of Acquired Autoimmune Hemolytic Anemia Complicating Systemic Lupus Erythematosus, Am. J. Med., *26*, 547, 1959.

108d. SCHLOESSER, L. L., KORST, D. R., CLATANOFF, D. V. and SCHILLING, R. F.: Radioactivity over the Spleen and Liver following the Transfusion of Chromium^{51}-labelled Erythrocytes in Hemolytic Anemia, J. Clin. Invest., *36*, 1470, 1957.

108e. SELWYN, J. G. and DACIE, J. V.: Autohemolysis and Other Changes Resulting from the Incubation *in Vitro* of Red Cells from Patients with Congenital Hemolytic Anemia, Blood, *9*, 414, 1954.

108f. SHAHIDI, N. T. and DIAMOND, K. K.: Enzyme Deficiency in Erythrocytes in Congenital Nonspherocytic Hemolytic Anemia, Pediatrics, *24*, 245, 1959.

109. SHARPE, J. C., McLAUGHLIN, C. W. and CUNNINGHAM, R.: Hemolytic Jaundice: Immediate and Delayed Changes in the Blood After Splenectomy, Arch. Int. Med., *64*, 268, 1939.

109a. SHARPSTEEN, J. R., JR.: Physico-chemical Mechanisms in the Pathogenesis of Certain Hemolytic Anemias, Am. J. M. Sc., *229*, 506, 1955.

109b. SIDDOO, J. K.: Acquired Hemolytic Anemia Associated with Hemochromatosis, Arch. Int. Med., *93*, 977, 1954.

109c. SIEVERS, K. und HARWERTH, H.-G.: Zur Therapie symptomatischer hämolytischer Anämien, Acta hæmat., *9*, 208, 1953.

110. SINGER, K. and DAMESHEK, W.: Symptomatic Hemolytic Anemia, Ann. Int. Med., *15*, 544, 1941.

110a. STAMEY, C. C. and DIAMOND, L. K.: Congenital Hemolytic Anemia in the Newborn, A. M. A. J. Dis. Child., *94*, 616, 1957.

110b. STEVENSON, T. D., McDONALD, BERDENIA L.

and ROSTON, S.: Colorimetric Method for Determination of Erythrocyte Glutathione, J. Lab. & Clin. Med., *56*, 157, 1960.

110c. SUNDERMANN, A. and KÄMMERER, J.: Die atypische hereditäre korpuskuläre nicht sphärocytäre hämolytische Anämie, Folia haemat., *76*, 562, 1959.

111. TAYLOR, E. S.: Chronic Ulcer of the Leg Associated With Congenital Hemolytic Jaundice, J.A.M.A., *112*, 1574, 1939.

113. ————Hemolytic Jaundice, Bull. New York Acad. Med. *15*, 174, 1939.

114. THOMSON, A. P.: Acholuric Jaundice With Increased Fragility of Red Blood Corpuscles Appearing After Splenectomy, Lancet, *2*, 1139, 1933.

115. TILESON, W.: Hemolytic Jaundice, Medicine, *1*, 355, 1922.

115a. TOCANTINS, L. M. and WANG, G. C.: Radioactive Colloidal Gold in the Treatment of Severe Acquired Hemolytic Anemia Refractory to Splenectomy, *in Progress in Hematology*, New York, Grune and Stratton, 1956, p. 138.

115b. TÖNZ, O., MEREU, T. and KÄSER, H.: Familiäre, nicht-sphärocytäre hämolytische Anämie mit Ausscheidung von Porphyrinpräkursoren (Typ Crosby), Schweiz. med. Wchnschr., *90*, 1214, 1960.

116. TÖTTERMAN, G.: Das Knochenmark bei hämolytischem Ikterus mit einem Beiträg zur Frage nach der Natur der Megaloblasten, Acta med. scandinav., *90*, 527, 1936.

116a. UNGER, L. J.: The Effect of ACTH in Acquired Hemolytic Anemia, Am. J. Clin. Path., *21*, 456, 1951.

116b. VAUGHAN, J. M.: Red Cell Characteristics in Acholuric Jaundice, J. Path. & Bact., *45*, 561, 1937.

116c. VALENTINE, W. N. *et al.:* Tr. A. Am. Physicians, 1961.

117. VERLOOP, M. C., BAKKER-V. AARDENNE, W. I. T. and RICCI, C.: In Vitro Autohaemolysis in Congenital and Acquired Haemolytic Disorders, Acta med. scandinav., *163*, 385, 1959.

117a. WASARTJERNA, C., PISCIOTTA, A. and DAMESHEK, W.: Direct Observations of Intravascular Agglutination of Red Blood Cells in the Cheek Pouch of Hamsters with Experimental Hetero-Immune Hemolytic Anemia, Acta med. scandinav., *148*, 173, 1954; J. Lab. & Clin. Med., *43*, 98, 1954.

118. WASSERMAN, L. R., STATS, D., SCHWARTZ, L. and FUDENBERG, H.: Symptomatic and Hemopathic Hemolytic Anemia, Am. J. Med., *18*, 961, 1955.

119. WATSON, C. J.: Hemolytic Jaundice and Macrocytic Hemolytic Anemia, Ann. Int. Med. *12*, 1782, 1939.

120. WELCH, C. S. and DAMESHEK, W.: Splenectomy in Blood Dyscrasias, New England J. Med., *242*, 601, 1950.

121. WEINER, W., BATTEY, D. A., CLEGHORN, T. E., MARSON, F. G. W. and MEYNELL, M. J.: Serological Findings in a Case of Hæmolytic Anæmia, Brit. M. J., *2*, 125, 1953; Brit. M. J., *1*, 73, 1956; J. Clin. Path., *13*, 232, 1960.

122. WIENER, A. S., GORDON, E. B. and GALLOP, C.: Studies on Autoantibodies in Human Sera, J. Immunol., *71*, 58, 1953; Ann. Int. Med., *44*, 221, 1956; *ibid., 47*, 1, 1957.

122*a*.WEST, W. O.: Acquired Hemolytic Anemia Secondary to Boeck's Sarcoid, New England J. Med., *261*, 688, 1959.

122*b*.WILAND, O. K. and SMITH, E. B.: The Morphology of the Spleen in Congenital Hemolytic Anemia (Hereditary Spherocytosis), Am. J. Clin. Path., *26*, 619, 1956.

123. WRIGHT, C-S. and GARDNER, E., JR.: A Study of the Role of Acute Infections in Precipitating Crises in Chronic Hemolytic States, Ann. Int. Med., *52*, 530, 1960.

124. YOUNG, L. E., IZZO, M. J. and PLATZER, R. F.: Hereditary Spherocytosis. I. Clinical, Hematologic and Genetic Features in 28 Cases, with Particular Reference to the Osmotic and Mechanical Fragility of Incubated Erythrocytes, Blood, *6*, 1073, 1951.

125. YOUNG, L. E. and MILLER, G.: Differentiation between Congenital and Acquired Forms of Hemolytic Anemia, Am. J. M. Sc., *226*, 664, 1953; Tr. A. Am. Physicians, *66*, 190, 1953; J. Chron. Dis., *6*, 307, 1957.

126. YOUNG, L. E., PLATZER, R. F., ERVIN, D. M. and IZZO, M. J.: Hereditary Spherocytosis. II. Observations on the Role of the Spleen, Blood, *6*, 1099, 1951.

127. ZINKHAM, W. H. and DIAMOND, L. K.: *In Vitro* Erythrophagocytosis in Acquired Hemolytic Anemia, Blood, *7*, 592, 1952.

128. ZINKHAM, W. H. and LENHARD, R. E., JR.: Metabolic Abnormalities of Erythrocytes from Patients with Congenital Nonspherocytic Hemolytic Anemia, J. Pediatrics, *55*, 319, 1959.

Chapter 13

Sickle Cell Disease, Thalassemia and the Abnormal Hemoglobin Syndromes

IN AN earlier chapter (p. 160) it was pointed out that, in addition to fetal and adult types of human hemoglobin, a number of other "abnormal" hemoglobins have been discovered. The most common of these is the type found in sickle cell anemia. The epoch-making discovery of Pauling, Itano and their associates[91] not only revealed the underlying molecular abnormality of that disease but initiated a series of studies in their own and in many other laboratories which have led to the recognition of new clinical syndromes and have clarified the nature of hitherto puzzling variants of recognized disorders.

Sickle cell anemia and the other conditions associated with the presence of abnormal hemoglobins are the consequence of the inheritance of a genetic trait which, when heterozygous, gives little clinical evidence of its presence but, when homozygous, results in disease, an outstanding manifestation of which is an increased rate of red cell destruction. These, therefore, can be classified, like hereditary spherocytosis, as hemolytic anemias due to intracorpuscular defects.

Another disorder, thalassemia, though not proved to be due to the presence of an abnormal hemoglobin, is closely related to the abnormal hemoglobinopathies. Not only are the clinical manifestations of all of these conditions similar, but the genes which govern the various conditions have been found to have been inherited in various combinations, resulting in a variety of clinical syndromes. Similar technics are used to distinguish these disorders from other hemolytic anemias, namely, electrophoresis and studies of the rate of denaturation, the solubility and other properties of the different hemoglobins.

It is proposed to discuss all of these conditions in the present chapter and to consider the methods which may be employed for their differentiation. Some of the physical and chemical properties of the different types of hemoglobin have been discussed already (p. 160).

A table which summarizes the usual findings in a number of the hemoglobinopathies and in thalassemia, as well as in various combinations of these disorders, will be found on page 716 (Table 13–2).

(668)

SICKLE CELL ANEMIA

Definition and Synonyms.—This is a hereditary and familial form of chronic hemolytic anemia essentially peculiar to Negroes, which is characterized clinically by symptoms of anemia, rheumatoid manifestations, leg ulcers and acute attacks of pain, and is distinguished morphologically by the presence of peculiar sickle-shaped and oatshaped red corpuscles, as well as signs of excessive blood destruction and active blood formation. It was at one time referred to as *drepanocytic anemia*[49] or *menisocytosis*.[40]

Inheritance, Incidence and Geographic Distribution.—The phenomenon of sickling of the red corpuscles is an hereditary abnormality which of itself usually produces no ill effects. Thus, in a large series[27] it was found that children harboring the trait were no more anemic than a control group of children without the trait. Sickle cell anemia, on the other hand, is a morbid state characterized by hemolytic anemia and other manifestations. It has been shown that the survival of the red corpuscles of persons harboring the trait, transfused to normal individuals or to patients with sickle cell anemia, is normal, whereas the survival of cells from cases of sickle cell anemia is abnormally short.[14,115] Although some exceptions have been noted,[85] the great body of evidence supports the theory that, when the gene for sickling is heterozygous, only the sickle cell trait is found, whereas the homozygous state produces sickle cell anemia.[7,84] A clinical picture closely resembling that of sickle cell anemia is produced by simultaneous heterozygosity for the sickle cell gene and the genes responsible for thalassemia, hemoglobin C or hemoglobin D (see pp. 715, 691 and 694).

Sickle cell anemia was first described in Negroes in North America.[54] The incidence of the sickle cell trait varies somewhat among Negroes in different parts of the United States. The average figure is 8.5 per cent[82] but values as high as 13.4 per cent (South Carolina[121]) have been recorded. Sickle cell anemia, the homozygous state (SS) has been observed in 0.3 to 1.3 per cent of various groups of Negroes examined[82] but also in this respect higher values have been found in certain parts of the country (Memphis, 2.5 per cent[27]). Among American Indians abnormal hemoglobins appear to be absent or rare.[92]

In Central and South America and in the West Indies the incidence of the sickling trait is similar to that in North America. Thus, among 2,089 inhabitants of Puerto Rico, abnormal hemoglobins were found in 42 persons, all but one of whom was Negro or Negroid.[119] The incidence of the sickle cell trait among Negroes was 5.6 per cent. In British West Indian Negroes, 9.6 per cent were found to have the trait.[124] Figures for South America include 10.7 per cent among Negroes in Caracas,[104] 10.4 per cent in Negroids in Brazil[80] and 15 per cent in Surinam.[75] On the Isthmus of Panama the incidence of the trait was 14.3 per cent among Negroes, 12.2 per cent in mulattos, 1.3 per cent in mestizos and none in white persons.[13] Sickling has been reported in some Mexicans[68] but none was found among 1,545 pure Brazilian Indians.[112] As many as 9 per cent of those harboring the trait in Central and South America were found to have sickle cell anemia.[124] Cases of sickle cell anemia have been described in the Argentine[107] and in Peru.[132]

Studies in Africa have revealed a broad belt of high incidence of the sickling trait extending roughly across the middle third of the continent, with the highest figures in Eastern and Central Africa. An incidence of 46 per cent was found among pigmoids in East Africa,[96] 27 per cent in certain Nilotic tribes and, on the Western seaboard, 28.3 per cent in Gambia and 18.75 per cent in Nigeria and the Cam-

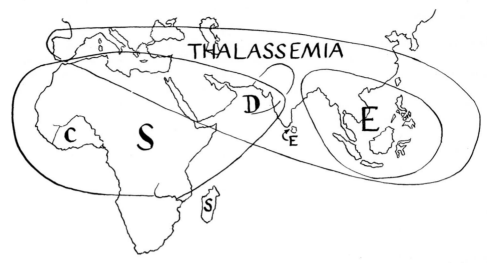

FIG. 13–1.—Distribution of the more common hemoglobinopathies, S, C, E and D, and thalassemia. (Courtesy of Dr. Hermann Lehmann.)

eroons[36] (Fig. 13–1). The incidence varies greatly from tribe to tribe.[75b] It is noteworthy that the trait was demonstrated among 19 per cent of Bantus but only in 2.9 per cent of the Hamitic peoples, who have Caucasian features. There is a rapid decrease in incidence as one proceeds either north or south. Sickling is relatively rare in South Africa. To explain this distribution of the sickling trait in Africa it was suggested that the trait may have been introduced there from the northeast via the former land bridge between Asia and Africa[73] (p. 671). The distribution of the sickle cell gene in Africa has been attributed to varying degrees of admixture of the Hamitic and Bantu races.

A remarkable phenomenon observed in Africa, in contrast to the United States, is the high incidence of the trait in certain regions of Africa and the comparative rarity of sickle cell anemia. The ratio of the trait to the anemia in Africa has been estimated as more than 1000:1. Since persons who are homozygous for this gene rarely reproduce, there must be a constant loss of sickle cell genes in each generation. If individuals who carry the sickle cell trait reproduced at a greater rate than did those without the trait, the loss of sickle cell genes through the early death of the homozygote might possibly be compensated (balanced polymorphism).[85] Another explanation might be found if the spontaneous mutation rate of the Hgb-S gene were very high. However, for these explanations no support has been found. The mutation rate is not sufficient to maintain the high frequencies of Hgb-S.[128]

These observations led to the suggestion that the heterozygote for Hgb-S must possess a selective advantage over the homozygote. In this connection it was proposed that the heterozygote for the sickle cell gene may possess a relative immunity to *falciparum* malaria because this organism may be able to metabolize sickle hemoglobin less well than normal hemoglobin.[2] Whether or not this is the correct explanation, considerable evidence now indicates that the distribution and high incidence of this gene in West Africa is the result of the interaction of both selection and gene flow and may well be related to the spread of malaria.[76] It has been shown that there the change from hunting to agriculture produced the conditions which favor the growth of the *Anopheles* mosquito. Thus, it would appear, the destruction of forests, the spread of agriculture and the growth of populations, made possible the spread of the selective advantage of the sickle cell gene.

Before the discovery of the various abnormal hemoglobins and the introduction of electrophoretic and other technics in the investigation of these disorders, certain exceptions to the exclusive occurrence of the sickling trait in Negroes had been noted. Although in some of the reported cases admixture with Negro blood was not ruled out satisfactorily,[5,111] or seemed possible[3] or very probable,[88] at least 12 instances of sickle cell anemia in white families seemed unchallengable.[20,21,22,42,43,44,48,77,102,131] Of these all but one were in persons of Greek or Italian (especially Sicilian) stock. Subsequently, admixture of the sickling and the thalassemia traits was recognized[94] and, since then, it has become clear that, in most instances at least, this is the explanation for the occurrence of "sickle cell anemia" in persons of Mediterranean stock (see p. 715). In one family[21] it was hemoglobin D which was later found to be associated with the sickling trait (p. 694).

Evidence is now accumulating which indicates that the sickling trait may not necessarily have originated in Africa. The finding of an incidence of 31.3 per cent among the primitive hill tribes of the negroid Veddoids of southern India[74] and southern Arabia (Figure 13–1) led to the suggestion that the sickle cell trait may have been introduced into Africa from the northeast via the former land bridge between Asia and Africa. It was noted that among the Veddoids the frequency of the cDe blood group chromosome, so common in African Negroes, is low. Among the Mahars around Nagpur in central India, an incidence of 22.2 per cent was found.[110a] Other "pockets" of

S hemoglobin were reported in several tribes in western India.[120] In Southern Turkey, among the Eti-Turks an incidence of the trait of 13.3 per cent was observed.[1] In individuals who were found to have sickle cell anemia, there was no suggestion of Negroid coloring or features. In certain cities and villages in Greece 17.7 to 32 per cent of the inhabitants have been found to exhibit the sickling phenomenon.[19,25] It was noted that the blood group frequencies among these subjects did not differ significantly from those of Greece as a whole and showed no excess of genes from Africa.

Contrary to earlier reports, there is no evidence for a linkage between the sickling gene and the MNS blood group genes.[86,129]

Age and Sex Incidence.—Though not sex linked, the trait may be somewhat commoner in females than in males.[96] The proportion of the red corpuscles which sickle is low at birth and increases in the next few months.[130] Thus, in one instance followed from birth, sickling was observed to increase progressively from 6 per cent at birth to 90 per cent at four and one-half months of age. It has been found that there is a corresponding progressive increase in the quantity of S hemoglobin.[105] The full complement of abnormal hemoglobin is reached, apparently, at about the same time as adult hemoglobin would normally replace fetal hemoglobin. These observations explain the rarity of sickle cell anemia in very young infants. In the American literature there is a record of but six cases of sickle cell anemia before three months of age and only a few more in the succeeding age period to one year.[7a,74a,130]

However, in those parts of Africa where the incidence of the sickle cell trait is known to be high, once a search among infants began to be made, many cases of sickle cell anemia were found among infants seven to 15 months of age.[127] The high mortality of sickle cell anemia at that age and in early child-hood, noted by investigators in the Congo,[71,127a] and elsewhere[127] probably accounts for the original, apparently erroneous, impression that sickle cell anemia is rare in Africa even though the incidence of the trait is high; it is in adults in Africa that sickle cell anemia is uncommon. In the western hemisphere it is not as uncommon.[134] Nevertheless, even in the United States not many patients with the homozygous condition are encountered over the age of 30 years. In individuals of middle and old age other forms of anemia, occurring in association with the sickling trait, may be mistaken for sickle cell anemia.

Symptomatology.—Individuals af-fected with sickle cell anemia show a remarkable adaptation to their state of chronic anemia and jaundice. They may have few or no complaints and examina-tion may unexpectedly reveal that the sclerae are greenish-yellow and the mu-cous membranes very pale. Others may fatigue more readily than do healthy persons. This state of adaptation is not a continuous one, however, for inquiry reveals that from time to time certain symptoms have appeared and have spon-taneously disappeared. Sometimes the clinical picture is so fulminating as to constitute a "crisis" (see below).

Extremities and Abdomen.—There may be a sudden increase of weakness and fatigability, or other symptoms of anemia; there may be episodes of aching pain in the joints or elsewhere in the extremities, which are often referred to as "rheuma-tism;" or there may be severe abdominal pain of sudden onset and associated with vomiting. The pain may be sharp and stabbing in character and it may be referred to the epigastrium or to the left or right in the abdomen. Prostration and abdominal tension may be associated and the picture may so closely simulate that of one of the abdominal emergencies that many patients have been operated on with the expectation of finding a ruptured peptic ulcer, intestinal obstruction or some other serious accident which re-quires surgical intervention.[15] The leu-kocytosis which is usually found in pa-tients with this disease contributes to the confusion. The problem is compounded by the fact that the incidence of chole-lithiasis in sickle cell anemia is high.[66]

Physical Signs. — Examination of such a patient may reveal the clinical picture of shock, there may be low grade fever or the temperature may be quite high (103° F.). There may be general-ized abdominal tenderness, or this may be confined to the right hypochondrium or to the splenic region where sometimes a friction rub may be heard. Attacks of pain in the extremities are rarely asso-ciated with tenderness, swelling or red-ness of joints, but there may be tenderness on pressure over the bones.

Further examination will reveal that the palms of the hands and the mucous membranes are pale and the sclerae greenish-yellow in color. There may be some general glandular enlargement but palpable **splenomegaly** occurs only in a small proportion of cases. In one series of 115 cases of sickle cell anemia,[130a] splenomegaly was found in 21 cases. It is noteworthy that two-thirds of these were in the first decade of life although only one-third of the entire series was in that age group. The liver may be en-larged.

In cases of severe sickle cell anemia of long standing, the physical appearance often presents a characteristic picture.[136] The patients are usually underweight, the trunk is short, the extremities long, and the habitus linear with comparatively narrow hips and shoulders (Fig. 13–4). The hands and feet may be long and narrow. There may be an increased upper dorsal kyphosis and lumbar lordo-sis and the chest may be increased in antero-posterior diameter, a finding often present even in children. In the latter a

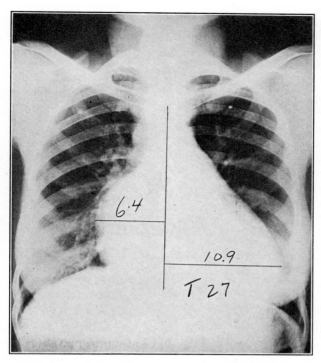

Fig. 13-2.—Teleoroentgenogram of the heart and great vessels in a case of sickle cell anemia. The heart is markedly enlarged with prominent left ventricle and right atrium. There is a slight prominence in the region of the pulmonary conus.

large abdomen and the small circumference of the legs may attract notice. The external genitalia may sometimes be atrophic and the facial hair may be somewhat scanty.

Heart.—The heart in sickle cell anemia offers some of the most interesting features of the disease.[70] Sinus arrhythmia is frequent. Pulsations may be prominent in the neck. The precordium is overactive. The tachycardia as well as the readily visible, diffuse wavy impulse are accentuated by the thin chest wall. Although the point of maximal impulse is not well localized, it is forceful and rolling in character. A diastolic tap may be felt in the pulmonic area and a systolic thrill may be perceptible over the precordium. The heart is enlarged both to the right and the left (Fig. 13–2) and frequently enlargement is made out in the

region of the pulmonary conus. Roentgenographically the heart may appear globular in shape. A systolic murmur of variable intensity is usually heard. It is maximal early in systole and may be loud enough to obscure the first sound, or a presystolic murmur may blend with the first sound. The second sound is accentuated. The murmurs have often been mistaken for those of mitral regurgitation or stenosis, or congenital heart disease. Electrocardiograms may show sinus arrhythmia, extrasystoles, or prolongation of the P–R interval. Unsaturation of the arterial blood is comparatively frequent. This appears to be due principally to intrapulmonary shunting of blood.[118] Cardiac output is usually high and blood volume may be increased. Although the hemodynamic pattern of cor pulmonale may be simulated, decreased pulmonary

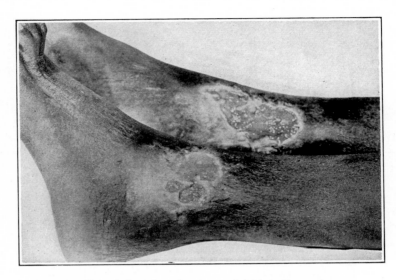

FIG. 13–3.—Chronic leg ulcers in a case of sickle cell anemia.
(Courtesy of Dr. A. F. Jonas, Jr.)

resistance has been found.[118] Thus, rather than cor pulmonale, the high cardiac output may be responsible for the cardiac findings.

Although the clinical findings frequently suggest those of rheumatic heart disease or sometimes simulate coronary occlusion, these conditions are extremely rare in patients with sickle cell anemia.[55]

Liver. — Moderate hepatic enlargement is not unusual, sometimes it is huge.[41] No relation to cardiac dysfunction has been noted. Jaundice is regularly found but is due chiefly to increased levels of indirect-reacting bilirubin and is accompanied by increased excretion of urobilinogen. There usually is no bile in the urine. Tests of hepatic function have revealed various degrees of dysfunction, especially after the second decade.

Genito-urinary System. — Spontaneous hematuria may occur in the absence of any of the usual causes.[72] This has also been described in persons harboring only the sickle trait.[23] In sickle cell anemia, and in many instances of sickle cell trait, the concentrating power of the kidneys after fluid deprivation is less than in normal subjects. In children this is not accompanied by a reduction in filtration rate or effective renal plasma flow but these functions may be decreased in adults, presumably in consequence of thrombus formation and loss of functioning tissue.[35] In infants the defect could be remedied temporarily if their erythrocytes were exchanged for normal cells and a normal hemoglobin was maintained for several weeks.[67] A specific tubular defect seems to be responsible.[52] Ultimately renal function may become seriously impaired.

Priapism has developed in a number of instances.[72]

Chronic Leg Ulcers.—Chronic leg ulcers (Fig.13–3) over the internal or external malleoli are common in adolescents and adults with sickle cell anemia, and not infrequently constitute the patient's main complaint. They are punched out in appearance, single or multiple, and unilateral or bilateral.

Bone Deformities. — Bone deformities, such as kyphosis, scoliosis, and saber shins, may be encountered, and the tower-shaped skull, like that seen in hereditary spherocytosis, has been observed in these patients (Fig. 13–4).[50] Abnormalities in the **roentgenographic appearance**[17] of the bones may be found, especially in the skull, vertebrae, tibiae, and fibulae. Such changes are more frequent in adolescents and adults than in children. However, bone lesions can appear in childhood and disappear.[78] The earliest change visible in the skull is the development of a ground glass appearance. In more advanced stages a peculiar radial striation is seen. This "hair-on-end" appearance in the skull (Fig. 13–5) is produced by trabecular striations which radiate outward, perpendicularly to the inner table. In later stages the diploë may be thickened, the outer table may be poorly defined, or there may be osteoporosis. The latter may be seen in the vertebral bodies, which may also appear flattened and may collapse.[53] In the long bones, osteosclerosis, with cortical thickening, new bone formation within the medullary cavity, and patchy irregularities in the density and pattern of the bone structure have been observed (Figs. 13–6, 13–7, 13–8). Pathologic fracture has occurred and bone infarcts have been described.[103] Although more common in sickle cell-hemoglobin C disease,[190] (p. 693), aseptic necrosis of the femoral capital epiphysis also has been observed in sickle cell anemia.[123] Permanent damage may take place in the joints, especially the hips, as the ultimate consequence of pathologic changes in small blood vessels and attendant focal hemorrhages.[110]

Osteomyelitis, due to *salmonella*, has been described in a number of cases of sickle cell anemia[56,101] and may be difficult to recognize since fever, pain and swelling in the extremities, and bone infarction may be seen in the absence of this complication.

Epistaxis.—This is a frequent complaint but purpura has not been observed.

Neurological Manifestations.—

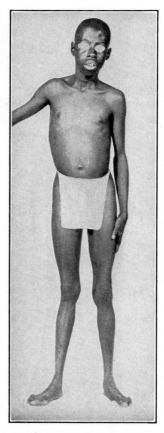

FIG. 13–4.—Negro, aged twenty-two years, with sickle cell anemia, showing tower-skull. He appeared younger than his stated age and was also found to have bilateral hypoplasia of the terminal phalanx of the fourth finger, a funnel chest, spina bifida, bilateral saber deformity of the tibiae, and hallux valgus. By the age of forty, severe renal junctional impairment was in progress.

Neurological manifestations are frequent.[58] The symptoms which have been observed include drowsiness, stupor or coma, hemiplegia, aphasia, headache, convulsions, stiffness of the neck, irritability, nystagmus, pupillary changes, blindness (temporary or permanent), cranial nerve palsies and paresthesias of the extremities. In one of our cases the initital complaints suggested poliomyelitis. The lesions in the central nervous system are most often due to thrombosis.[10] They are generally multiple and are vari-

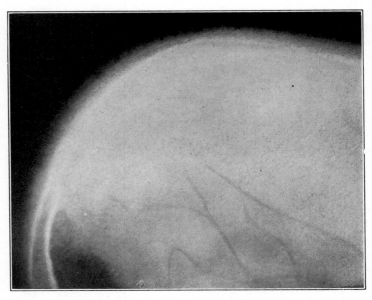

FIG. 13–5.—"Hair-on-end" appearance of skull produced by trabecular striations radiating outward from the inner table in a case of sickle cell anemia.

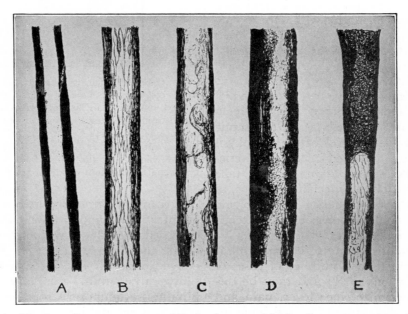

FIG. 13–6.—Tracings of roentgenograms of fibulae in cases of sickle cell anemia, to show the variation which may be observed: *A*, No change; *B*, osteoporosis with increase in trabecular markings; *C*, irregs ularities in thickness of the cortex and abnormal bone formation within the medullary cavity; *D*, cortical thickening, narrowing of the medullary cavity; *E*, complete obliteration of the marrow cavity. (Diggs, Pulliam and King, courtesy of South. M. J.)

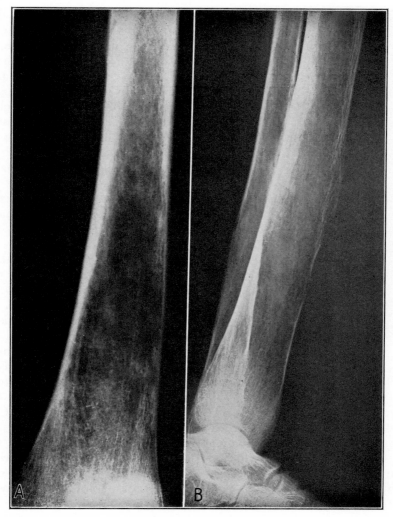

Fig. 13–7.—Sickle cell anemia. *A*, Femur. The cortex is thinned and the normal bony architecture is disturbed. Adjoining small areas of translucency there are areas of sclerosis. *B*, Tibia and fibula: marked thinning of the cortex of the bones as well as periosteal reaction and disarrangement of the trabeculae. The latter changes and the extensive coarseness of the cortical layers suggest that the bone is involved from within.

able in location. These symptoms may be the initial complaints or may develop as complications. The cerebrospinal fluid is often normal but there may be increased pressure, sickled erythrocytes, xanthochromia and an increase in protein and cells.

The veins of the retina may be dilated and tortuous to an extreme degree[50] (Fig. 13–9). Microaneurysms of the retinal vessels have been described.[34]

Crises.—The periodic episodes of severe pain, fever, extreme prostration and shock, which punctuate the course of patients with sickle cell anemia and may be fatal,[64] may develop without precipitating cause[130a] or may follow infections, or even blood transfusion.[90] As a rule,

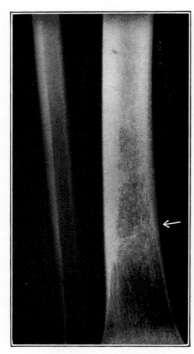

Fig. 13–8.—Sickle cell anemia. There is a striking disarrangement of the trabeculae in the lower third of the tibia. There is no cortical thickening or periosteal reaction.

they are self-limited (five to seven days) and without evidence of the development of a more severe anemia during or following the crisis.[26a] True "aplastic" crises, with hypocellularity of the bone marrow, absence of jaundice and a decrease in reticulocytes and nucleated red cells in the blood have been observed,[26a] but are extremely rare. Although it has often been stated that some crises are accompanied by increased blood destruction, there is doubt that true hemolytic crises occur.[26a]

Laboratory Findings. — Blood. — Anemia is usually well marked and may be severe (1,000,000 to 2,000,000 red corpuscles per c.mm.). The reduction in hemoglobin and in volume of packed red cells is often proportional so that normal values for mean corpuscular volume and hemoglobin content are found.[28] In some instances, especially if the anemia is very severe, the anemia may be macrocytic. In other cases the mean corpuscular volume has been as low as 75 or even 65 c.μ. Corresponding variations occur in mean corpuscular hemoglobin so that the hemoglobin concentration of the red corpuscles is found to be normal, whether the average cell size is normal, increased or decreased below normal.

It has been shown that variations in the size of the red corpuscles depend on their oxygen saturation, treatment of the blood with carbon dioxide producing a substantial increase in the volume of packed red cells.[135]

In *stained smears*, most of the cells are round or oval, although they vary in size and large macrocytes (13.5 μ) as well as tiny microcytes may be found. The mean diameter is often somewhat increased but may be normal or decreased. A few of the cells are elongated and narrow with rounded or pointed ends[28] (Fig. 13–10). Elongated structures of this type as long as 20 μ and even 50 μ, and 1 to 4 μ in width have been observed. Other irregularities in shape are unusual. Hypochromia is not common but target cells (p. 100), may be observed frequently.

Nucleated red corpuscles, chiefly normoblasts, are found, ordinarily 1 to 10 per 100 leukocytes, but sometimes as many as 40. In addition there are polychromatophilia, basophilic stippling, and sometimes Howell-Jolly bodies. Cabot's rings are rare. Nucleated sickle cells have been observed in a few instances.[122] Reticulocytes are characteristically increased in number (5 to 25 per cent, sometimes higher). The reticulocytes are usually round or oval and rarely assume the bizarre forms of the nonreticulated corpuscles.

In many instances the number and character of sickled cells in stained smears are too insignificant to warrant a diagnosis of sickle cell anemia being made.

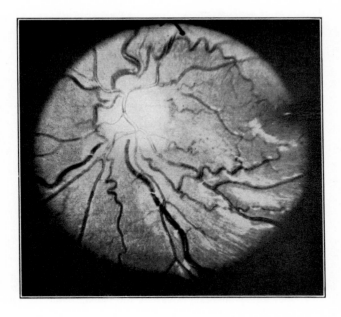

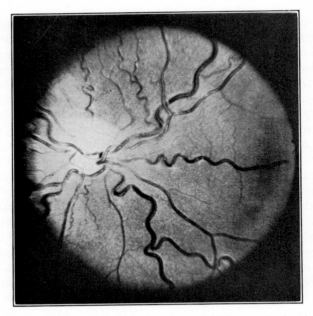

FIG. 13–9.—Photographs of fundus of each eye in a case of sickle anemia showing the extreme tortuosity of the blood vessels. (The white streaks are due to the reflection of light and are not exudates.) (Courtesy of Dr. James Bordley, III.)

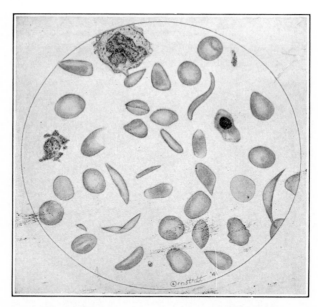

Fig. 13–10.—Drawing of blood smear from a case of sickle cell anemia. From a preparation dried and stained (Wright's, × 960) immediately on obtaining the blood. Note the bizarre shapes and the peculiar distribution of hemoglobin in some of the cells.

The characteristic phenomenon in this disorder is the change which can be observed to take place in the shape of the red corpuscles **when a drop of blood is sealed under a cover-slip on a slide** (p. 409) or in test tubes.[6,109] In such preparations a few bizarre, multipointed forms may be seen immediately, but changes occur at a maximal rate in from two to six hours after the blood is drawn. First there is thickening of the corpuscle on one side, with corresponding thinning on the opposite side. The diameter of the corpuscle then becomes greater and a series of transformations takes place (Fig. 13–11), which result in the formation of structures of which the most striking characteristics are a bizarre shape and the presence of elongated and pointed filaments. These modifications in structure in each cell take place in two to four minutes (*See* p. 687).

The changes in the shape of the red corpuscles can be observed in blood mixed with oxalate and other anticoag-ulant solutions and may be seen if diluted blood is left in the counting chamber for an hour or more. The process of sickling takes place more slowly, however, when the blood has been diluted.[109]

Leukocytosis is regularly found in sickle cell anemia. When there is active blood destruction it may be marked (10,000 to 30,000 or more leukocytes per c.mm.). The increase is due to the presence of cells of the myeloid series and there is often a "shift to the left" and a moderate number of myelocytes. Eosinophilia is not infrequent and the monocytes may be increased in number. Occasionally red corpuscles may be seen within some of the latter cells.[57]

Platelets are also increased in number (300,000 to 500,000 per c.mm.) and bizarre forms may be observed. Bleeding time and coagulation time are usually normal.

The **resistance of the red corpuscles** to hypotonic saline solutions is increased moderately, and sometimes extremely,

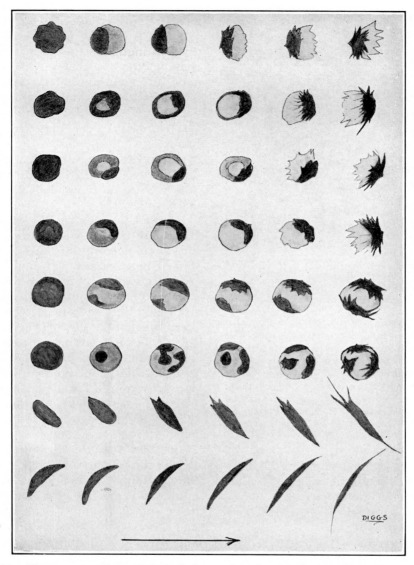

Fig. 13–11.—The sequence of morphological changes in red corpuscles in sealed moist preparations of the blood in sickle cell anemia. (Diggs and Bibb, courtesy of J.A.M.A.)

some of the red corpuscles failing to hemolyze even in distilled water.[28] The resistance to mechanical trauma is decreased.

The abnormal shape of sickled cells prevents rouleau formation. Probably as a result of this, the **sedimentation** of the corpuscles is slow, even though the anemia is severe.[11] This has been made

the basis of a test which has been found positive only in sickle cell anemia.[135] The rate of sedimentation of blood collected from a vein after venous stasis of six minutes' duration has been produced, is compared with that of the same sample after it has been thoroughly aërated. Within fifteen to sixty minutes the difference between the sedimentation rate of

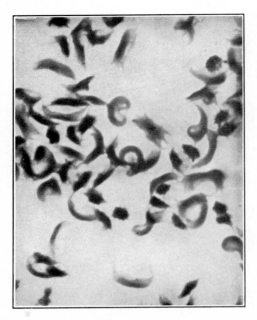

Fig. 13–12.—Sickled red corpuscles from a case of sickle cell anemia. The cells were washed several times with normal saline solution and the cell suspension was then allowed to remain under oil. After time had been allowed for sickling to occur, formalin was added in order to fix the cells in their abnormal shape. A smear was then made and stained with Wright's. × 1050. Prepared by Dr. Irving J. Sherman.

the sickled (venous) sample and that of the aërated, non-sickled cells, will be greater than 20 millimeters.

Gastric analysis reveals no characteristic abnormality.

Bone Marrow.—Nucleated red cells may constitute as many as 50 to 70 per cent of all the nucleated cells of the marrows. These are chiefly orthochromatic normoblasts. Some polychromatophilic normoblasts and a few, more immature forms are also found but the megaloblasts of pernicious anemia are absent. There may be a moderate "shift to the left" in the myeloid leukocytes and eosinophils may be relatively numerous. Megakaryocytes may be present in increased number, monocytes may be found to contain ingested red corpuscles, and nuclear fragments as well as pigment granules may be seen scattered about.

There is nothing in the bone marrow that distinguishes this from other forms of hemolytic anemia except the appearance of the non-nucleated red corpuscles. A few of the normoblasts may be abnormal in shape but this is unusual. Occasionally, very long, filamentous bands of what appears to be erythrocyte cytoplasm may be seen. These may extend across the whole oil-immersion field and may be no more than 2 μ in thickness.

Blood Changes in Persons Having Only the Sickle Cell Trait.—In persons who have only the *sickle cell trait* the stained blood smear will show no sickled cells. In sealed wet preparations changes similar to those found in patients with sickle cell anemia can be seen but they occur much more slowly (Fig. 13–13) and fewer cells are transformed to the bizarre forms which have been described. As long as twenty-four hours or even longer may be required for the changes to take place.[28] Furthermore, anemia of hemolytic type and signs of active red cell regeneration are absent.

In order *to hasten the formation of sickle cells* a rubber band may be placed around the proximal portion of the finger and allowed to remain five minutes.[106] The distal end of the finger is then punctured and a drop of the dark blood is removed and quickly sealed under a cover-slip. If it is available, it is still better to add a reducing agent to the blood: a drop of 2 per cent sodium metabisulfite ($Na_2S_2O_5$)[24] or a specially prepared reagent containing sodium dithionite ($Na_2S_2O_4$).[61]

If venous blood is collected by means of a Luer syringe in which the dead space has been filled with white oil, and about 1 ml. of the blood is injected into 2 or 3 ml. of isotonic saline-formalin (neutral formaldehyde [40 per cent] diluted to 4 per cent strength with 0.85 per cent sodium chloride) under oil, 30 to 60 per

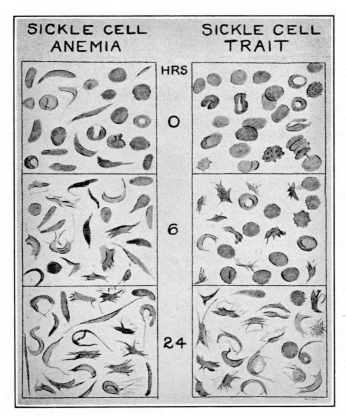

Fig. 13–13.—Drawing showing the morphology of sickled erythrocytes in sickle cell anemia and in the sickle cell trait as revealed in sealed moist preparations at the time of making the preparations, after six hours and after twenty-four hours. (Diggs, L. W., Ahmann, C. F., and Bibb, Juanita, courtesy of Ann. Int. Med.)

cent of the erythrocytes will be found sickled if the blood has been taken from a case of sickle cell anemia. The blood preparations should be made about five minutes after the mixture with formalin and must be examined shortly thereafter. When obtained in this way only a rare sickle cell has been found in the blood of persons who have only the sickle cell trait.[109] A modification of this method can be used to prepare permanent sickle cell preparations.[118a]

Diagnosis.—Unless the possibility of sickle cell anemia is kept in mind and an appropriate blood examination is made, an error in diagnosis may readily occur. As already described, the symptoms may suggest abdominal disease, rheumatic fever, osteomyelitis, or a neurological disorder. Even after the blood has been examined, the problem for the surgeon in a case in which there is severe abdominal pain, muscle spasm, and leukocytosis, as well as vomiting and constipation or diarrhea, is a very difficult one. He must be guided by the knowledge that all of these symptoms and signs may develop in cases of sickle cell anemia without anything having occurred which requires surgical intervention.[15] A conservative attitude in such cases, therefore, is advisable. The characteristic findings which allow a diagnosis of sickle cell anemia to be made are sickling of the red corpuscles in wet preparations, anemia with signs of active red cell regeneration, leukocytosis, and bilirubinemia. Sickling alone is not sufficient for it only indicates the presence of the sickle cell trait. In association with the trait alone, neither anemia nor the above symptoms are produced.

In cases with prominent cardiac signs and joint pains the differentiation of rheumatic fever may be very difficult. In sickle cell anemia it will be found that pain is not limited to the joints but is referred to the bones as well and the characteristic therapeutic response to salicylates fails to occur.

Sickle cells should not be confused with elliptical cells. The latter do not change in shape in wet preparations and are not usually related to anemia (p. 102). Hereditary spherocytosis has much in common with sickle cell anemia but, in addition to being very rare in Negroes, it is characterized by increased fragility rather than increased resistance of the red corpuscles in hypotonic saline solutions. Very rarely the two conditions may occur together.

It has been pointed out already that splenomegaly is not common in sickle cell anemia. The spleen was palpable in only 10 per cent of a series of 78 patients over the age of ten.[130a] Consequently the discovery of a palpable spleen should arouse suspicion of another diagnosis such as sickle cell-hemoglobin C disease (p. 691) or sickle cell-thalassemia (p. 715). If paper electrophoresis reveals the presence of normal hemoglobin in addition to S, instead of C or fetal hemoglobin, the likelihood is great that one is dealing with the sickle cell trait and a superimposed anemia of other etiology.

In association with sickle cell anemia, acute myeloblastic leukemia has been reported.[39]

As a rule, the *sickle cell trait* is asymptomatic. However, as already pointed out, hematuria and hyposthenuria may develop (p. 674) and even bone infarction and hemolytic anemia have been encountered,[191] although they must be rare. Ordinarily there is no anemia. Under conditions which produce severe anoxia, as in high altitude flights, massive splenic infarction may occur.[102a,116] Persons harboring the sickle cell trait may, of course, develop various forms of anemia and this must be differentiated from sickle cell anemia. Iron deficiency is not uncommon. The elliptical cell anomaly[37] (p. 102) and hereditary spherocytosis[65,79] have been reported in association with the sickle cell trait.

The demonstration of the sickling phenomenon in red corpuscles has been considered to be a specific indication of the presence of Hb S in such cells. A possible exception to this concept will be discussed shortly (p. 697).

Treatment.—Only palliative management is possible. Iron, vitamin B_{12} and folic acid are of no value. Multiple transfusions decrease both hemolysis and erythropoiesis, as manifested by a decrease in reticulocytes and in plasma bilirubin levels.[30] This is accompanied by a decrease in the number and concentration of sickle cells. These effects are so temporary that blood transfusion is rarely justified. Splenectomy does not influence the blood destruction as a rule but the operation has given symptomatic relief in patients whose spleens were huge as well as in rare instances in which an extracorpuscular factor in blood destruction could be demonstrated.[48,130a] Prolongation of erythrocyte survival time has been observed in patients with splenomegaly who were splenectomized.[117a] Corticotropin (ACTH) and adrenal steroids are of no value.

For the chronic leg ulcers, bed rest, maintenance of the blood at nearly normal levels by transfusion and local measures are helpful. Even under ambulatory conditions healing has been observed when proteolytic enzymes and antibiotics were used to debride, combat cellulitis, improve local circulation and promote epithelialization.[117]

The occurrence of a "crisis" calls for the liberal use of analgesics (aspirin 0.6 Gm.) and anodynes (codeine 30 mg.) but narcotics should be avoided, if possible, because of the danger of addiction. Rarely, muscle spasm is so great as to require general anesthesia. Blood transfusion may be helpful, and is essential in the rare aplastic crisis. Since infections may initiate a crisis, these should be looked for and treated appropriately. A variety of other measures has been recommended from time to time (steroids, intravenous alkalinization with bicarbonate, anticoagulants, carbonic anhydrase inhibitors and benzazoline) but none of these has stood the test of time.

Surgical procedures are rarely required for aseptic necrosis of the head of the femur. For hematuria nephrectomy should be considered only if conservative management fails, since the second kidney often becomes involved in the same process. If splenic infarction occurs, symptomatic treatment usually suffices. Splenic rupture naturally requires emergency splenectomy.

Course, Prognosis and Complications.—The degree of anemia and the depth of jaundice may wax and wane. Patients with sickle cell anemia show a remarkable adaptation to their chronic state of ill-health and often maintain hemoglobin levels of 7 or 8 Gm. per 100 ml. for long periods of time. With extremely rare exceptions,[190] remissions are never of such a degree that icterus and anemia disappear completely.

However, sickle cell anemia is a serious malady and the outcome is ultimately fatal. Most patients die in the first decade of life and very few survive the third.[190] Death may occur from intercurrent infections, especially tuberculosis, from cardiac or renal failure, or as the result of thrombosis or hemorrhage involving other vital tissues. Death may

occur following one of the abdominal crises, perhaps as a result of shock produced by the rapid removal of red cells from the circulation subsequent to their sickling.[125] The prognosis following central nervous system injury is poor, but it varies and is unpredictable.[58] Attacks of severe blood destruction are said to become less numerous as age advances.

Pregnancy is associated with greater than normal morbidity in women with sickle cell anemia but the high mortality once attributed to sickle cell anemia[72] has now been shown to belong to sickle cell-hemoglobin C disease rather than true sickle cell anemia[23a,190] (p. 693).

As in other forms of severe hemolytic anemia (p. 652), *megaloblastic erythropoiesis*, probably as the consequence of folic acid deficiency resulting from a high requirement in excess of the dietary intake, sometimes develops.[107a]

Pathology.—At autopsy,[29] evidence of chronic hemolytic anemia is found. The **bone marrow** of the flat and cancellous bones of the trunk, the calvarium, and the long bones of the extremities shows hyperplasia, but the smaller bones of the hands and feet may contain only fat. The marrow is soft and jelly-like, and uniformly dark red or purplish-black. Microscopically great cellularity and congestion are found, with islands of proliferating cells scattered among non-nucleated corpuscles. The details of the microscopic picture have been mentioned already (p. 682). Hemosiderosis has been observed in the liver, spleen, kidneys, lymph nodes and bone marrow.

Evidence of degenerative and reparative processes may also be observed: thrombosis, infarction, necrosis, and hemorrhage, as well as abnormal calcification and new bone formation such as would be expected from the roentgenoscopic appearance of the bones (Fig. 13–6). Although reference has been made frequently to the presence of thrombi, a critical analysis[69] revealed that these are relatively uncommon. Ischemic infarctions have been described more often in the absence of, than together with related thrombi.

Thickening of the walls of small and medium-sized arteries and end-arterial intimal proliferation in addition to or in the absence of thrombosis, have been found in various tissues. The lesions in the central nervous system are primarily intravascular.[58] In the brain dilatation of peripheral blood vessels and congestion with sickled erythrocytes have been described, as well as multiple thromboses of smaller blood vessels and even thrombosis of the larger dural sinuses. In addition there may be perivascular edema, cellular exudation, hemorrhage and necrosis.

The **spleen** in the earliest stages is enlarged and there is congestion of reticular spaces with sickled erythrocytes.[26] Tissues fixed in formalin may show more sickled cells than those preserved in Zenker's solution. The capillaries of the Malpighian bodies are often dilated and present the appearance of multiple varices. Infarction is common. Organization occurs and pigmentary changes with deposition of mineral salts follow. Eventually fibrosis and shrinkage in the size of the spleen occurs and in the last stages the spleen is reduced to a tiny wrinkled mass, weighing as little as 16 Gm. The spleen from cases of sickle cell anemia can be recognized by a characteristic malformation of the splenic sinuses immediately about the Malpighian follicles with collections of pools of blood in fibrosed and atrophic areas.[100] This malformation may be attributable to the clumps of sickled cells rather than to a congenital defect.[126]

The **liver** at autopsy gives evidence of anoxic necrosis, probably as the result of anemia, sickling of the red corpuscles in the sinusoids and obstruction by Kupffer cells engorged with phagocytized red cells.[116a] When cirrhosis develops, it is usually of the macronodular or postnecrotic type.

In **kidneys** removed from young patients because of hematuria, severe congestion, focal medullary or papillary hemorrhages, necrosis, repair and regeneration were observed.[29] In postmortem studies, the medullary pyramids showed edema, telangiectasia, fibrous scarring and obliteration of tubular elements.[7a] These sequelae of ischemic necrosis, by virtue of their predominant location in the papillae, offer a reasonable explanation for the inability of children with sickle cell anemia to concentrate urine during water deprivation. In older children, enlargement and increased vascularity of glomeruli, particularly those situated extraglomerularly, may explain the increased filtration rate seen sometimes. In still older subjects the glomerular congestion and enlargement appear to give way to progressive ischemia and fibrosis, leading to glomerular obliteration.[7a] In gross appearance and histologically, such kidneys show granularity of the surface, adherent capsule, ischemic and hemorrhagic infarcts, areas of cortical necrosis, interstitial fibrosis, abnormal calcification, papillary necrosis and submucosal hemorrhages in the pelvis.[35]

Pathogenesis.—Early studies of the sickling phenomenon showed that assumption of the crescentic shape occurs in an atmosphere deprived of oxygen and is favored by lowering of the pH and by increasing the temperature to that of the body, whereas exposure to oxygen or carbon monoxide restores sickle cells to a circular form.[49,109] Such evidence that the circular shape of the red corpuscles is assumed when they contain combined hemoglobin and that the crescentic shape develops when the hemoglobin is reduced, led to a study of the physical and chemical properties of sickle cell blood and resulted in the fundamental observations of Pauling and his associates.[91] They found that, in a buffer of suitable pH, the two components of a mixture of sickle cell and normal hemoglobins migrate electrophoretically in opposite directions. On the basis of the difference in their isoelectric points, it was concluded that the hemoglobin of sickle cell anemics has 2 to 4 more net positive charges per molecule than normal hemoglobin. Since the heme moiety is the same in sickle cell and in normal hemoglobin the electrophoretic differences were attributed to differences in the polypetide chains of globin. As discussed in an earlier chapter (p. 156), these investigations led to the discovery of other abnormal hemoglobins and brought about advances in our knowledge of human protein which are of far-reaching importance in relation to concepts of human disease and of human genetics. Ultimately it was shown that the fundamental difference between sickle cell and normal adult hemoglobin is the substitution of valine for glutamic acid in tryptic digest 4 of the β polypeptide chain.

In the blood of patients with sickle cell anemia 76 to almost 100 per cent is sickle cell hemoglobin, the remainder being fetal hemoglobin. In the blood of individuals with the sickle cell trait the amount ranges from 22 to 45 per cent, the remainder being normal hemoglobin.[133] Two modal values have been found, 34 to 36 per cent and 40 to 42 per cent. There are significant intrafamily correlations in this respect and it has been suggested that these are due to the action of segregating genetic modifiers.[87,133]

It should be borne in mind that electrophoretic observations such as have been described above are carried out on the whole red cell mass. Attempts to analyze the red cell population of cases of sickle cell anemia by transfusing sickle cell anemia red corpuscles into normal recipients, measuring their disappearance rates and quantitating the alkali-resistant component, have been interpreted as indicating that there are three main groups: (1) cells containing S hemoglobin and little or no F hemoglobin, (2) cells containing both pigments, and (3) cells containing F pigment and little or no S hemoglobin.[114] The corpuscles carrying mostly S hemoglobin were found to have the shortest life span whereas those containing mostly F hemoglobin survived the longest.[159d] The severity of the anemia in a given case would perhaps depend, then, on the size of that portion of the erythrocyte population which is most rapidly eliminated as well as on the ability of the bone marrow to replace these cells. Studies by various methods, including hemin N^{15} disappearance and fecal urobilin N^{15} appearance,[63] indicate that there is random destruction of the circulating red cells. However, the activity of this process varies from case to case.

It has been observed[108] that two types of sickled erythrocytes can be differentiated in the blood of patients with sicklemia. The first type, which exhibits filamentous processes, reverts to the discoidal form on exposure to oxygen. The second, which is sickle- or oat-shaped, does not revert under these conditions. When blood was incubated, it was found that non-reticulated cells largely lost their ability to resume the discoidal form while reticulocytes retained this ability. It has been suggested that sufficient intermittent or continuous stagnation of the red cells in various organs *in vivo* with consequent sickling may result in the production of irreversibly sickled forms. The fact that reticulocytes do not readily acquire the property of becoming irreversibly sickled after incubation *in vitro*, may explain the fact that sickled reticulocytes are rarely seen in stained blood films.

Sickling has not been observed in the circulating blood but much indirect evidence indicates that this phenomenon occurs *in vivo*. Thus, changes in partial oxygen pressure in a limb are associated with variations in the number of sickled cells in the blood collected therefrom.[106] In venous blood collected under oil, higher proportions of sickled cells are found as compared with similar specimens of arterial blood.[64a,109] Again, when patients with sickle cell anemia were allowed to breathe 70 to 100 per cent oxygen the percentage of abnormal forms was less in both arterial and venous blood than during pre- and post-oxygen periods.[99] It is of interest, however, that no consistent detectable change in rate of hemolysis occurred during eight- to twenty-day periods of oxygen administration. Both the percentage of reticulocytes and the number of red cells decreased during the periods of oxygen administration. After the latter was discontinued a striking reticulocytosis developed and the erythrocyte count rose to the pre-oxygen level.

It has been pointed out already that increased blood destruction is constantly present in sickle cell anemia. When such patients are transfused to a normal hemoglobin level, a prompt decline in the reticulocyte count occurs, which reaches normal values in five to seven days.[18,30,115] High-normal or super-normal levels of hemoglobin were associated with subnormal reticulocyte percentages whereas modest declines in hemoglobin were followed by a distinct reticulocyte response.[18]

The clinical and hematological manifestations and the pathologic changes found in sickle cell anemia can be explained by the peculiar physical properties of the sickle cell. Since sickle cell hemoglobin is relatively insoluble, some investigators suggested that sickling is due to incipient crystallization of the hemoglobin when reduced. This does not, however, appear to be the true explanation. It was observed many years ago, in the author's laboratory, that sickled cells are birefringent.[109] Pauling and his associates[91] later inferred that when sickle cell hemoglobin molecules lose oxygen they combine with one another to form highly anisomeric units which become partially aligned within the cell and have

enough rigidity to distort it into the sickle shape. Harris was able to show that, in the oxygen unsaturated state the sickle hemoglobin molecules undergo orderly orientation, forming, by specific linkage of the individual molecules, long chains of hemoglobin elements. Subsequent parallel alignment of these elements results in birefringement tactoids, the sickled cell being a "hemoglobin tactoid, thinly veiled and somewhat distorted by the cell membrane."[51]

These conclusions are supported by direct observation by phase microscopy and electron micrography.[8,98] That an oriented, birefringent gel is formed is also suggested by the fact that sickle cells do not give X-ray spacings.[93]

Much of the abnormal physiology of sickle cell anemia is attributable to the increased viscosity of the deoxygenated blood. The chronic hemolytic anemia is attributable to the increased mechanical fragility and diminished life span of the erythrocytes and the appearance of painful crises can be explained by the various circumstances which temporarily so alter the flow of blood in an organ that a vicious cycle is established. The intracellular molecular orientation described above produces the sickled form of the erythrocyte. At decreased oxygen tensions the viscosity of the whole blood and the mechanical fragility of the erythrocytes significantly increase, owing to the assumption of the sickled form.[51] With the increase in viscosity, a cycle is initiated in which the factors of stasis, lowered pH, and continuing oxygen uptake combine to augment the number of sickled cells and prolong the stasis. Plugs or masses of sickled erythrocytes become solid enough to occlude vessels and result in the "thrombotic" episodes associated with pain which are characteristic of the disease. Erythrostasis limits access to cell-maintaining energy as well as favoring the sickled state. When red cells after stasis are released into free circulation, a certain proportion, having been fixed in irreversibly sickled form, have also become more fragile in terms of mechanical trauma. Consequently they are more than normally susceptible to the trauma associated with circulation. These factors, as well perhaps as metabolic failure,[95] result in increased blood destruction. The development of these changes depends on the quantity of abnormal hemoglobin present. In the homozygous state the erythrocytes contain sufficient abnormal hemoglobin to result in sickling within the physiological range of oxygen tensions; in the heterozygous state the clinical course is essentially benign because sickling ordinarily fails to take place *in vivo*. It has been suggested that the increased cardiac output which accompanies the anemia in sickle cell disease provides lowered arteriovenous differences. This effectually maintains higher blood oxygen tensions and shortens the period of red cell deoxygenation, thereby decreasing the probability of massive *in vivo* sickling.[64a] A shift to the right in the oxygen dissociation curve also may prevent extremely low blood oxygen tensions.

The underlying mechanism responsible for many of the clinical manifestations of a crisis may be obstruction of vascular channels by tangles of sickled erythrocytes.[183a] The picture of shock which patients with the abdominal crisis of sickle cell anemia manifest may be due to the packing of sickled erythrocytes in small capillaries, thus removing them from a functional status and adding to the anemia already present.[125] The capillary anoxemia would result in plasma loss, hemoconcentration and further stagnation. Bone pain may be due to distention of the intramedullary cavity of the bones by the vascular engorgement. In some cases there may be focal infarction of bone marrow. It is possible that the irregular sclerosis visible in roentgenograms of the long bones is due to healing of such infarcted areas with scarring and subsequent osteoid deposition. Other changes in the bones may perhaps be the result of hyperplasia compensatory to the increased blood destruction. The degree of bone change seems to be related to the duration of the anemia rather than to its severity.[30]

HEMOGLOBIN C DISORDERS

The application of electrophoresis in the study of sickle cell anemia soon led to the discovery of another type of adult hemoglobin[164,169] in addition to normal hemoglobin A, and sickle cell hemoglobin, designated S. First called III and c, the third variety of hemoglobin is now known as C. This hemoglobin may be found in various combinations with normal and abnormal hemoglobins. In the following discussions, insofar as possible, combined disorders will be designated by listing the major pigment component first.

Hemoglobin C.—It was pointed out in an earlier chapter that the abnormality in Hb C resides in tryptic digest 4 of the β polypeptide chain (p. 161). Lysine replaces glutamic acid in residue no. 6 of the β chain (Table 3–5, p. 160). The resulting increase of two charges above that of normal hemoglobin may account for the distinctive electrophoretic mobility of Hb C (p. 718). Hb C is more stable in its reduced form than is normal hemoglobin and is more soluble than Hb A. However, under conditions which permit partial drying and partial hemolysis, crystallization of Hb C occurs *in vitro*, provided the concentration of Hb C is sufficiently great (more than 44 per cent).[154] Thus, tetragonal crystals of hemoglobin were demonstrable when suspensions of washed erythrocytes in 3 per cent sodium citrate solution were sealed under a cover slip, left at room temperature for hours, and allowed to dry slowly. Intraerythrocytic crystals of

44

Hb C have been observed in blood smears of individuals with Hb C disorders. Such red corpuscles may assume a rigid, rod-shaped form.[189] This phenomenon was thought to be unique for this abnormal hemoglobin but it has been reported to occur with a wide variety of other hemoglobins.[139]

The incidence of Hb C has been found to be highest in West Africa, especially in northern Ghana where 16.5 to 28 per cent of the Negroes were found to have this abnormal hemoglobin.[156] The river Niger seems to have acted as a barrier to its spread toward the east. It is rare in South Africa.[148] Surveys of randomly selected Negroes in the United States have yielded values of 2 to 3 per cent.[182,189] In Puerto Rican Negroes an incidence of 1.3 per cent was found.[119] Both of these are significantly lower than values for the incidence of Hb S and it is therefore curious that the incidence of Hb S and Hb C is the same in Lumbee Indians in the U.S.A., a people of uncertain origin.[92]

No extensive world-wide survey of the incidence of Hb C has been made but the trait does not appear to have spread widely. The African Gold Coast is thought to be its origin. However, sporadic cases among non-Negroes have been observed in individuals of Italian[154] and of Dutch ancestry.[189]

Unlike Hb S (p. 670), Hb C does not seem to offer protection against malaria.[155a] Yet the gene frequency in certain parts of Africa is high, as indicated above. This may, perhaps, be explained on the basis of balanced polymorphism in the case of an abnormality of lesser severity than sickle cell anemia which would consequently not require as much of an advantage in favor of heterozygosity than is necessary to maintain the high frequency of Hb S.[174]

Genetic data indicate that Hb C is transmitted as an autosomal dominant.

[164,178] Its clinical expression appears to be modified by the presence of other abnormalities of the erythrocyte. In the heterozygous state, the gene has incomplete expression. There is a greater degree of expression when some other abnormality of the red cell is present and presumably the gene has full expression in the homozygous state.

Hemoglobin C Trait (AC). —From 28 to 44 per cent of the hemoglobin of per ons harboring this trait is Hb C,[151] the remainder being normal adult hemoglobin. Target cells are found characteristically in association with Hb C trait but their number may range from 1 to 100 per cent and there appears to be no correlation between the amount of Hb C and the number of target cells.[189] Osmotic fragility is reduced, sometime markedly. There is no anemia and no evidence of increased blood destruction.[169] The survival of these cells when transfused into normal recipients was found to be normal.[199] Clinical manifestations are exceptional. Infarction of dental bones and unilateral renal hematuria have been noted but seem to be very rare.[189] No evidence of gene interaction was observed when Hb C trait was found in association with pernicious anemia, primaquine-sensitive erythrocytes or hereditary elliptocytosis[189].

Homozygous C Disease (CC). — Data are available for 36 Negroes,[166,179, 189] nine Algerian Mussulmans,[177] one subject of Sicilian origin,[154] two of Dutch extraction[162] and in one Anglo-Saxon family.[158b] Symptoms have been similar to but in general of much milder degree than in sickle cell anemia. These have included poorly localized, recurrent pain not associated with inflammatory joint change; abdominal pain, episodic but poorly localized, and in three instances severe enough to mimic intestinal obstruction; convulsive seizures; and hemorrhagic manifestations such as epistaxis, hemoptysis, hematuria and bilateral periorbital hemorrhage. The habitus of the patients has not been abnormal but jaundice was noticed frequently. Ocular, cardiac and pulmonary abnormalities have been lacking but splenomegaly, sometimes huge, has been observed in all but two persons. Skeletal abnormalities have not been observed.

Anemia is common, usually of moderate degree (volume of packed red cells 37 to 25 volumes per cent), normocytic or microcytic in type and accompanied by slight bilirubinemia (1.2 to 2.0 mg. per 100 ml.), increased urobilinogen excretion and normoblastic hyperplasia of the bone marrow. The blood smear shows many target cells (30 to 100 per cent) (Fig. 13–14) as well as some degree of anisocytosis, poikilocytosis and polychromatophilia, and occasional microspherocytes.[189] The microspherocytes appear as irregularly rounded dense cells with a diameter less than one third of that of a normal erythrocyte. Reticulocytes are increased (2 to 7 per cent) and nucleated red cells may be seen. Rodshaped erythrocytes with squared corners have been described and crystal formation can be produced by gradual drying of fresh blood smears.[199b] In the absence of the spleen these changes are much more marked.

The osmotic fragility of the erythrocytes is decreased but mechanical fragility may be increased slightly.[193] The serum iron has been found to be normal but the rate of iron turnover has been normal[193] or moderately accelerated.[166] Decreased survival time of the red corpuscles (30 to 55 days) when transfused into normal recipients has been demonstrated, whereas the life span of normal cells transfused into homozygous C patients was normal.[192] Electrophoresis has indicated that approximately all of the hemoglobin in the erythrocytes is Hb C.[185] One patient gave birth to a child who, at birth, had only fetal and some adult hemoglobin

but, after four months, the fetal hemoglobin had been replaced by Hb C.[193]

Thrombocytopenia has been observed in several cases. The specific gravity, protein content and microscopic sediment of the urine have not been abnormal.

Prognosis seems to be good. Many patients have lived a full life span. There is no evidence that pregnancy is tolerated poorly. Splenectomy has not been found to ameliorate the hemolytic process.[185] No characteristic pathological findings have been described.

Sickle Cell-Hemoglobin C Disease (SC).—It is very probable that most of the cases hitherto reported as representing forms of sickle cell anemia intermediate between the asymptomatic carrier state and the homozygous, classical disease, actually were cases simultaneously heterozygous for S and C hemoglobin.[187] This disorder is much milder in its manifestations than sickle cell anemia and, although virtually all of the manifestations of sickle cell anemia, with the exception of the cardiac signs, have been described in SC disease, they have been both less frequent and less severe.[161,196,197] Anemia in childhood has been observed in less than half the cases and normal hemoglobin values were found in the same patients later. Some have never been known to be anemic. However, transient hemolytic episodes do occur and even when there is no anemia, normoblastic hyperplasia of the bone marrow is present, suggesting that the absence of anemia is due to compensation rather than to a return to normal of the shortened red cell survival time. During hemolytic crises, reticulocytosis, extraordinary numbers of nucleated red cells and marked leukocytosis have been described.

Target cells are prominent in these cases, 20 to 85 per cent of the cells being in this form. Spherocytes are absent and sickling is not prominent in the stained smear, although it is demonstrable in wet preparations. Reticulocytes may not be

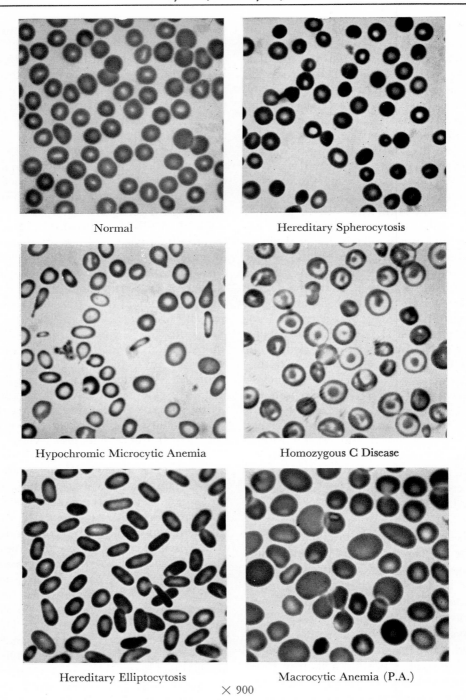

Normal   Hereditary Spherocytosis

Hypochromic Microcytic Anemia   Homozygous C Disease

Hereditary Elliptocytosis   Macrocytic Anemia (P.A.)

× 900

Fig. 13–14.—Photomicrographs of blood smears in various disorders. The dark microcytes of hereditary spherocytosis contrast with the hypochromic microcytes of iron deficiency anemia. The differences between the elliptical cells seen in hypochromic microcytic anemia and those found in hereditary elliptocytosis and in macrocytic anemia should be noted. The characteristic target cells of homozygous C disease are shown.

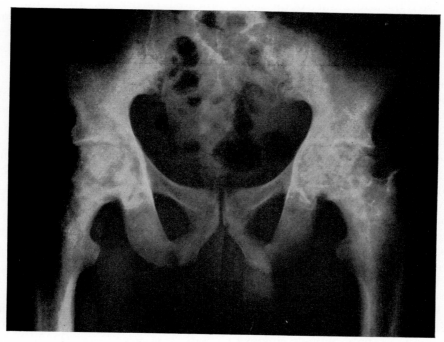

Fig. 13–15.—Aseptic necrosis of the femoral heads in a case of sickle-cell hemoglobin C disease. There is irregular erosion of the articular cartilage, erosion of the superior cortical margin of the femoral heads and a mixture of radiolucency and increased density throughout the femoral heads.

increased in number and the serum bilirubin may be normal. In contrast to sickle cell anemia, splenomegaly has been found in the majority of the cases and is progressive, and the body build characteristic of patients with sickle cell anemia has not been seen. Aseptic necrosis of the humoral or femoral heads (Fig. 13–15) has occurred in a high proportion of the cases and abnormalities of the retina have been described, especially intraocular hemorrhages and small aneurysmal dilatations of the retinal vessels.[187] Gross hematuria has been reported.[161]

Although, in general, prognosis is better in SC disease than in sickle cell anemia and some patients seem to live their full life span, the morbidity and mortality during **pregnancy** have been great; it appears that the poor prognosis during pregnancy, formerly attributed to sickle cell anemia, really should be charged

against SC disease.[190] In sickle cell-hemoglobin C disease anemia has been observed frequently to increase in severity as gestation progressed, in contrast to sickle cell anemia.[189] As in sickle cell anemia acute infarction of the bone marrow and fat embolization play an important role in the pathogenesis of many of the acute manifestations of this disorder.[175,183a,189]

Although a case of SC disease has been reported from Africa,[156] no data are available concerning the frequency of this association. It appears to be much less common than sickle cell anemia.

Hemoglobin C-Thalassemia. — Several cases representing simultaneous heterozygosity for Hb C and thalassemia have been described.[186,189] Those affected have been Negroes. Mild to severe bone pain may occur.[189] Splenomegaly is unusual. The most characteristic feature of the disease is the appearance of the blood smear. Large, thin target cells and small fragmentary erythrocytes predominate but target cells and microspherocytes similar to those present in Hb C disease are plentiful. Decreased osmotic fragility and moderate erythroid hyperplasia of the bone marrow are found. Sickling is absent. A noteworthy feature is that the amount of Hb C in the hemolysates has been 75 to 80 per cent. The remainder is Hb A and Hb F. This suggests that the thalassemia gene enhances the expressivity of the abnormal pigment, perhaps by suppressing the production of the β polypeptide chain of Hb A. However, this has not been the case in all instances,[286] presumably those cases of Hb C associated with α thalassemia (p. 703).

There is evidence that hemoglobins C, S and A are alleles and have a high order of penetrance.[178] The locus of the thalassemia gene is probably closely linked to that of the CSA gene.

OTHER DISORDERS ASSOCIATED WITH THE PRESENCE OF ABNORMAL HEMOGLOBINS

Hemoglobin D.—By paper electrophoresis the mobility of Hb D is the same as that of Hb S but it is more soluble than Hb S in the reduced state and its presence in erythrocytes does not cause sickling.[164] Agar gel electrophoresis at pH 6.2 permits the separation of Hb D from Hb S. By paper electrophoresis Hb SS, Hb SD and sickle-thalassemia cannot be distinguished.

The incidence of Hb D among American Negroes was found to be 0.4 per cent in North Carolina[151a] and 0.085 per cent in Baltimore.[172] Hb D has also been found among Algerian Moslems[150] and in India, and isolated cases have been encountered in Turkey,[1] in a Portuguese child[145] and among Caucasians elsewhere. This abnormal hemoglobin may well have originated in non-Negroes. As in-

dicated earlier (p. 162), a number of hemoglobins with the electrophoretic mobility of Hb D have been discovered,[158c] possibly as many as nine. The abnormal hemoglobin of the family of Irish, English and American Indian ancestry, originally reported as an example of sickle cell disease in Caucasians,[21] is now known as Hb D$_{Hollywood}$.[191] The abnormality in this hemoglobin resides in the β chain. Two different foci of Hb D have been found in India, one among the Sikhs (Hb D$_{Punjab}$, p. 160, formerly D$_\gamma$) and the other among the Gujerati.[146] Although the abnormality in Hb D$_{Punjab}$ also resides in the β chain, it probably differs from that of Hb D$_{Hollywood}$. There is some evidence that the abnormality in other D hemoglobins is present in the α chain.

No clinical or hematologic abnormality has been described in the heterozygous state, *hemoglobin D trait* (DA).[151a] Between 35 and 49 per cent of the hemoglobin has been of the abnormal type, the remainder being normal adult hemoglobin. The only instances of possible *homozygous-D disease* which have been reported[151a] have not been proved to be homozygous by family studies but, judging from these, it has been assumed that the homozygous state is virtually asymptomatic and is accompanied by an extremely mild hemolytic anemia. The red cells have been described as microcytic and normochromic and may have been of the target cell variety.

Sickle cell-hemoglobin D disease simulates sickle cell anemia but is less severe.[188,191] Pallor and splenomegaly have been observed to begin in infancy. Attacks of severe pain in the abdomen and extremities and recurrent jaundice are likely to occur but there are long periods of remission. A relatively large number of oat- and sickle-shaped red corpuscles, many hypochromic cells, a small number of target cells, conspicuous polychromatophilia and a few normoblasts may be seen in the blood smear. Sickling of the erythrocytes can be produced. The anemia, at times severe, may subside in great part or completely.

Genetic data indicate that Hb D is an autosomal mendelian dominant character which may be an allele of hemoglobins A, C and S.

A possible instance of *Hb D-thalassemia* has been reported in a Persian girl.[163] The manifestations resembled those of SD disease.

Hemoglobin E.—Distinctive electrophoretic mobility led to the recognition of this abnormal hemoglobin.[165] At pH 8.6 it moves close to Hb C but slightly faster and at pH 6.5 its position is close to Hb S, though just behind it. Its solubility is about the same as that of Hb A. The underlying amino acid abnormality was discusssed earlier (p. 160).

High incidences for Hb E have been found among Siamese (13.6 per cent),[152] Burmese (15.3 per cent)[153] and Cambodians (35 per cent)[149] and in some Indonesian, Ceylonese and Malaysian (1 per cent)[198a] populations. Thus, Hb E is characteristic of the peoples of southeast Asia.[143] Elsewhere only occasional cases have been encountered.[143,165]

The heterozygous abnormality, *Hb E trait* (EA) is asymptomatic. There is no sickling and minimal or no hypochromia, and no target cells or decreased osmotic fragility are found. In the carrier state 35 to 49 per cent of the hemoglobin is type E, the remainder being the normal adult form.[151]

Hemoglobin E disease, the homozygous state (EE), is characterized as a rule by mild microcytic, normochromic anemia with 25 to 60 per cent target cells, decreased osmotic fragility and minimal signs of hemolytic anemia. Splenomegaly is absent or slight. Approximately 92 to 100 per cent of the hemoglobin in the erythrocytes is E, and fetal hemoglobin values are normal or slightly increased.[152,171] Homozygous C disease closely resembles Hb E disease but, in addition to the racial difference, in the former more target cells are likely to be found and the spleen is large. In Hb E disease the anemia may be more definitely microcytic than is the case in Hb C disease. Polycythemia with microcytosis may be observed.

Hemoglobin E-thalassemia has been observed in southeast Asia,[152] as might be expected, and occasionally in the adjoining areas (Chinese,[198a] Bengalese [150b]). Approximately 60 to 80 per cent of the hemoglobin is E, the remainder being Hb F.[151] The clinical manifestations simulate those of thalassemia major (p. 705) in almost every respect and the blood is much the same. Differentiation therefore depends on the electrophoretic pattern.

One instance of *sickle cell-hemoglobin E disease* (SE) has been reported.[144] Slight anemia, mild reticulocytosis, hypochromia without microcytosis and a few target cells were noted.

Hemoglobin G. — A hemoglobin characterized by mobility between that of hemoglobin A and S in paper electrophoresis, veronal buffer, pH 8.6, was first described in a Negro West African family.[157] Since then several more hemoglobins have received this designation.[182b,183,184,198] That these are not identical is clear. This confusion has resulted from the use of electrophoresis as the sole means of differentiating one hemoglobin from another.[184] As indicated in Table 3–5 (p. 160), the nature of the abnormality in three G hemoglobins has been identified and these all differ from one another. In accordance with the proposed new nomenclature, the different G hemoglobins[158c] are designated according to the locality where each was first found. Thus, the following can be listed: $G_{San Jose}$ [160,183] and G_{Accra},[157,182b] both with β chain abnormalities; and $G_{Philadelphia}$,[145a] $G_{Honolulu}$, [159e] G_{Ibadan},[158c,184] and $G_{Bristol}$,[178b] all with α chain abnormalities. The G hemo-

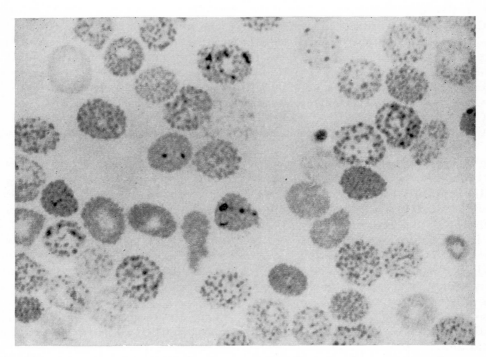

Fig. 13–16.—Erythrocyte inclusion bodies in blood of patient with Hb H-thalassemia.[155] The inclusion bodies appeared after incubation with brilliant cresyl blue for 20 minutes at 37° C. and may be seen in nearly every erythrocyte, in contradistinction to the reticulum of reticulocytes (dark black bodies in the photograph), which is present in only a few cells. ($\times$ 1000).

globins which have been found predominantly in Chinese[198] are probably the same as Hb $G_{Honolulu}$.[159e] Hb $G_{Azuakoli}$ is probably the same as Hb $G_{Philadelphia}$. A minor component of Hb G will be discussed shortly (p. 703).

No clinical or hematologic manifestations have been reported to be conferred by any of the G hemoglobins. When associated with Hb S or thalassemia, the presence of Hb G was not found to alter the expression of these genes.[183]

Hemoglobin H.—This is the first of a series of "fast" hemoglobins[180] which share the electrophoretic characteristic of a faster anodal mobility at pH 8.6 than that of normal adult hemoglobin. Other "fast" hemoglobins include I, J, K, N and three not yet identified by letters (see below). The anodal migration of Hb H on paper electrophoresis at pH 8.6 is dis-

tinct from all others except Hb I. At pH 6.5 the anodal migration of Hb H distinguishes it from Hb I. As discussed earlier (p. 162), Hb H is unique in that it is composed of four polypeptide chains which are all of one kind, the β chain of normal adult hemoglobin. Another special feature is that the spontaneous denaturation of Hb H within intact erythrocytes *in vitro* results in the formation of multiple inclusion bodies.[155] This process can be accelerated by the incubation of red cells at 37° C. with brilliant cresyl blue, or with the reducing agent, sodium dithionite. Thus, 3 or 4 drops of blood are mixed in a small tube with 0.5 ml. 1 per cent brilliant cresyl blue in citrate saline and left for some hours at room temperature. Films are then made and examined wet or dry for inclusion bodies.

This abnormal hemoglobin has been

described in Chinese,[167,180,198b] Greeks,[147] [159,176] Italians (Sardinian), Filipinos, Algerians, Thais, Malayans, Trans-Jordanians, Nepalese[155] and in an Oriental Jewess.[177a] However, Hb H has only been demonstrable when it was accompanied in the same individual by another genetic anomaly of hemoglobin formation, hitherto, in all but three instances,[176,177a,198b] the thalassemia trait or a closely related disorder. Differing from the finding in classical thalassemia trait (p. 702), is the fact that the Hb A₂ fraction has been low, less than 1 per cent.[155,159b] The amount of Hb H in the red cells has been found to be in the range of 15 to 20 per cent.[155] The possible significance of these facts will be discussed further, below (p. 703).

Clinical manifestations suggest thalassemia: chronic, iron-refractory, hypochromic microcytic anemia, reticulocytosis, slight bilirubinemia, decreased osmotic fragility of the erythrocytes, sometimes associated with splenomegaly. In the blood smear there are marked anisocytosis, tear drop cells, fragmented cells and target cells, occasional Howell-Jolly bodies, stippling and polychromatophilia. Heinz bodies have not been demonstrated but incubation of the red cells with cresyl blue reveals intraerythrocytic inclusion bodies (Fig. 13–16).

Hemoglobin I, very similar to Hb H, as indicated above, was identified in an asymptomatic American Negro male and in five members of his family.[181] No hematological abnormalities were detected. This hemoglobin was soon discovered also in Algiers.[150a]

As indicated earlier (p. 684), the demonstration of sickling in erythrocytes has been assumed to give evidence of the presence of Hb S in such cells. It appears that this assumption must be qualified. In a Negro woman whose hemoglobin disclosed the pattern of Hb I together with Hb A, with no Hb S component, sickling of the erythrocytes was usually produced when the blood was mixed with 2 per cent sodium metabisulfite,[145b] as in the test for sickling (p. 682). The phenomenon could be reproduced consistently if 4 per cent sodium metabisulfite was employed. However, unlike the findings when Hb S is present, the changes were not completely reversible, nor could they be observed in an untreated, sealed cover-glass preparation. In contrast to the finding in the original case of Hb I trait, where this pigment made up but 20 per cent of the total hemoglobin, in this case Hb I comprised 70 per cent of the total. Although a complete family study could not be carried out, it appeared that in this case the larger Hb I component was attributable to the simultaneous presence of a gene for thalassemia. It was postulated that the sickling differed from that seen in association with Hb S in that it was not attributable to gelation of the abnormal hemoglobin and the formation of paracrystalline tactoids but rather to a direct chemical action on a red cell stroma altered by the presence of the high concentration of Hb I.

Hemoglobin J was first discovered in an American Negress[194] but has since been reported in a few Algerians, Indonesians, Indians, Chinese and others.[168,198c,199a] Electrophoretic studies showed that this "fast" hemoglobin falls between Hb A and Hb I. The abnormality probably resides in the β chain (p. 160).[158c] Carriers were found to have 60 per cent Hb J.[194] Nevertheless, they showed no hematological abnormalities.[168] Most examples of this hemoglobin have been seen in association with Hb A. However, association with thalassemia minor, Hb D and Hb S has been observed.[199a] No evidence for a detrimental interaction between these genes has been found, the manifestations being those of the associated gene only.

Hemoglobin K was first reported in the Algerian Kabyles.[149a] It has since

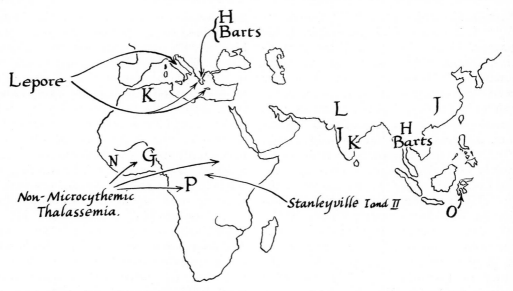

Fig. 13–17.—Distribution of the rare hemoglobinopathies: G (West Africa, Ghana, Nigeria); N (West Africa, Portuguese New Guinea, Liberia); P (Congo); Stanleyville I and II (Northern Congo); K (West and North Africa, India (Dravidians); L (Western India); J (India and China); H and Bart's (Greece, China, Thailand, Malaya and Indonesia); "Lepore trait" (Northern Italy, Greece, Cyprus); O (Celebes); "High F gene" ("non-microcythemic thalassemia") (Ghana, Nigeria, Congo, Uganda). (Courtesy of Dr. Hermann Lehmann.)

been observed in Liberia (and thus provisionally named *Liberian II*) and in Indians.[141] The relative electrophoretic mobilities at pH 8.6 of the four "fast" hemoglobins are $H = I > J > K > A$. No clinical or hematological abnormality has been described. The amino acid abnormality is thought to be in the α chain (p. 160).

Hemoglobin L was first discovered in a Punjabi Hindu.[140] It migrates on alkaline paper electrophoresis between hemoglobins A and S, slightly more slowly than Hb G. It has been differentiated from G and P (see below) by chromatography. So far Hb L has been seen only in Indians. No clinical abnormality has been noted.

The letter M has been used in reference to a form of hereditary methemoglobinemia (p. 196). Consequently, next in the alphabetical series of aberrant hemoglobins is **hemoglobin N,** provisionally designated *Liberian I*.[180a] This is another

"fast" hemoglobin.[141] Its mobility by paper electrophoresis at pH 8.6 is faster than that of Hb J but slower than that of H or I. At acid pH it separates from A towards the anode while J does not. It has also been reported from Portuguese Guinea.[195] The abnormality appears to be in the β chain (p. 160).

Hemoglobin O (*Buginese X*) was reported from Celebes.[171a] On alkaline electrophoresis its mobility lies between that of Hb S and Hb E and by chromatography it moves faster than L but more slowly than S. A somewhat similar compound was observed in a boy with congenital anemia associated with red cell inclusion bodies and abnormal pigment metabolism (p. 626). Hb O together with Hb S has been reported in an Arab family.[177b]

Hemoglobin P was first reported from Galveston, Texas.[182a] It was found in the blood of a Negro woman. In zone electrophoresis at pH 8.6 its mobility lies between that of G and S. In free electrophoresis it is identical with that of A. The same hemoglobin has been encountered in the Belgian Congo,[153a] in one instance in association with A and S,[169a] Hb P may not be allelic with A, S and C.

Hemoglobin Q, discovered in a Chinese male, in association with Hb H, moves more slowly at alkaline pH than Hb A but slightly faster than Hb G.[198b] The α chain differs from that of normal hemoglobin (p. 160).

No hematological abnormality was found to be associated with the inheritance of hemoglobins L, N, O, P or Q.

Few letters of the alphabet remain but a number of contenders have been described.[200b] Those moving on paper electrophoresis more slowly than Hb A include (1) the **"Lepore trait,"** which is characterized by altered red cell morphology resembling that of thalassemia minor.[159a] In a patient in whom the "Lepore trait" was associated with thalassemia minor, severe hemolytic anemia clinically indistinguishable from thalassemia major was observed (see p. 705). The abnormal hemoglobin which, in the heterozgyous condition, constituted 10 to 12 per cent of the total hemoglobin, migrated at pH 8.6 with a mobility indistinguishable from that of Hb S. Starch block electrophoresis was required to distinguish the Lepore pigment from other hemoglobins. There is good evidence that the Lepore hemoglobin is a variant of Hb A₂; that is, that the β chains of normal hemoglobin are replaced by delta (δ) chains (p. 160). It remains to be determined whether or not there is an abnormality in the δ chain of Lepore hemoglobin.

(2) **"Stanleyville I and II"** refers to two abnormal pigments encountered in the Belgian Congo which resemble Hb D.[153b] The first of these behaved like Hb L or P on paper electrophoresis at alkaline pH but on chromatography at pH 6 behaved like S or D. The second behaved like S or D on paper electrophoresis at pH

8.6 but on chromatography (amberlite resin) at pH 6 differed from both. The red cells did not sickle in either instance.

A number of "fast" hemoglobins, in addition to those described above (I, J, K, N) have been described. These include two abnormal hemoglobins found in Negroes with electrophoretic mobility at pH 8.6 greater than that of Hb A, the first of which had a mobility equal to that of Hb I **("Hopkins-1")** whereas the second **("Hopkins-2")** was comparable with Hb J.[190] "Hopkins-2" was inherited with Hb S in three matings, an observation which led to the suggestion, now confirmed,[147a] that its locus must be on a different chromosome than that of A, S and C.

Another "fast" hemoglobin **("Norfolk")** was discovered in a purely English family which resembles but is not identical with Hb J.[142]

Two abnormal hemoglobins have been observed in the cord blood of infants which were thought to be abnormal fetal hemoglobins. No abnormal hemoglobin was found in the blood of the parents. The first,[158a] originally designated according to the initials of its discovers, *"F and P,"* and then renamed **"Singapore-Bristol,"**[178a] differs from the second **("Bart's")**[141] in that the latter moved on paper electrophoresis at alkaline pH in front of Hb J whereas "F and P" did not, while Bart's was resistant to alkali denaturation whereas "F and P" was denatured as Hb A. The family of the infant with "F and P" hemoglobin had thalassemia. *Bart's,* which was so named because it was discovered at St. Bartholomew's Hospital, has been shown to possess only one type of polypeptide chain, which is similar to or identical with the γ polypeptide of fetal hemoglobin (p. 159). In the original observations Bart's was found to disappear as the child grew older, but another study showed this hemoglobin to persist, in association with thalassemia, to a later age.[152a] Other examples of these two hemoglobins have been encountered.[159c,195a] Hb Bart's has also been found to occur in association with Hb H.[161a]

Still another variant of fetal hemoglobin has been described **("Alexandra"),** in a newborn, which disappears progressively like Hb F but is distinct from this on paper and starch electrophoresis.[158]

As stated earlier, hemoglobins C, S and A are thought to be alleles. The locus of the thalassemia gene is thought to be closely lined to that of A, C and S but Hb P and "Hopkins-2" may not be allelomorphic with these hemoglobins. If the suggestion is correct that there are two genes responsible for hemoglobin structure, one controlling the amino acid sequence of the alpha chain peptides and the other controlling the beta chain (p. 703), mutations could occur in either or both of these genes and it would be possible to have from one to four different kinds of hemoglobin in one individual. In two families such variants of human hemoglobin with four distinct electrophoretic components have been reported.[145a,178b]

THALASSEMIA

Definition, Synonyms and History.—This disorder was first clearly separated by Cooley and Lee in 1925[211] from the complex of disorders in infancy and childhood which had been known as Von Jaksch's anemia or Jaksch-Hayem-Luzet anemia. The classical form is characterized by chronic progressive anemia commencing early in life, well-marked erythroblastosis in the peripheral blood, a characteristic facies, splenomegaly, and a familial and racial incidence. It is also known as *Cooley's anemia, erythroblastic anemia, Mediterranean disease or thalassemia*[280] and, because of the characteristic finding of flat, "target" cells, *"hereditary leptocytosis."*

A relatively mild anemia occurring in the United States in adolescents and adults of Mediterranean extraction which resembled thalassemia but was much less severe was described in 1940 by several investigators, independently.[217,273,283] It was suspected that this condition was related to Cooley's anemia and the writer, in the first edition of this book (1942), recorded findings in two families in which *both* parents of children with typical Cooley's anemia showed hematological changes like those he had observed in Italian adolescents and adults.[283] (Table 13–1). Thus evidence was presented which linked the disorder in adolescents and adults to Cooley's anemia of infancy and childhood and provided grounds for the hypothesis that Cooley's anemia represents the inheritance of an anomaly of the red corpuscle from both parents which, in an individual who is heterozygous for this factor, produces so few changes of clinical importance that symptoms are unusual and the abnormality may be discovered only accidentally. Until then, even though it had been recognized that two, three or even five siblings in a family might be affected,[280] Cooley's anemia had not been considered hereditary. However, examination of the early case reports in which it was claimed that adult members of affected families were normal, revealed that the examinations had not been sufficiently thorough to demonstrate the abnormality.

Subsequently, comprehensive reviews[210,250] brought to the attention of English-speaking readers the voluminous literature from the Mediterranean basin. At the same time that Cooley's anemia was attracting attention in the United States, Rietti described a syndrome which Italian writers ultimately called the *microelliptopoikilocytic anemia* of Rietti, Greppi and Micheli.[250] Other European investigators[201,207a] noted mild forms of "infantile erythroblastic anemia" and Caminopetros,[207a] in two families, found both

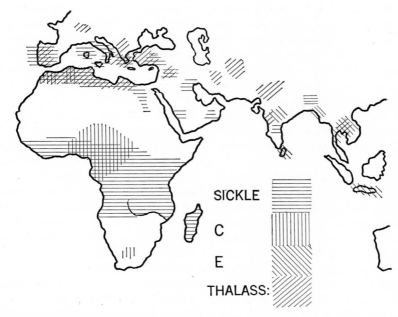

SICKLE

C

E

THALASS:

F‌ig. 13–18.—Geographic distribution of sickling trait, thalassemia and the hemoglobin anomalies, C and E. (Courtesy of Dr. Herman Lehmann.)

parents affected with the disorder. Later studies[278] further served to define the characteristic features of these disorders and to give additional evidence for the hereditary character of thalassemia.

Incidence and Racial Distribution. —Until attention was called to the milder forms of this condition and to additional characteristics by which the disorder might be identified, thalassemia had been regarded as quite rare. Until 1942 less than 100 cases of Cooley's anemia had been reported. Later, survey of persons of Italian descent in Rochester, New York,[253] revealed the severe form of the disease as occurring once in 2,368 births and the lesser anomaly once in each 25 persons. In another study of 16 families, 63 persons were examined and, in 54, abnormalities of the blood were revealed.[269] Twelve, all children, were severely anemic and 42, including parents and siblings, had the milder condition.

It is now clear that thalassemia affects many of the peoples of the eastern hemisphere.[209a] In Italy an incidence of the anomaly as high as 20 per cent has been observed in some communities near Ferrara in the delta of the Po River.[248] Sicily has proved to be almost as important a source of the disease and Sardinia also has many examples.[210,250,267] It is frequent in Greece,[208] Crete, Cyprus,[204] Syria, Turkey and adjacent geographical areas.[209a,262] Isolated case reports record the disorder in persons of northern European origin[209a,250a] and even in American Indians and Negroes.[209a] Larger numbers are being discovered in India,[279] Thailand,[252] China, the Philippines and elsewhere in the East. It has also been shown that thalassemia may be associated with the sickling trait (see below) and with a number of other abnormal hemoglobins, as already discussed. The trait has lately been encountered in various parts of Africa[209a,254] and in the West Indies.[279b]

One wonders how thalassemia achieved

so widespread a geographic distribution (Fig. 13–18). It is possible that mass migrations and commerce served to carry the defect eastward from a large pool in the Mediterranean basin.[265] Other theories propose that the trait arose in Indochina and moved westward or that it originated in Armenia and spread both to the east and west.[209a] Spontaneous mutation arising in a number of areas is another possibility.

No one has satisfactorily explained why a potentially lethal gene like thalassemia continues to be prevalent. It is assumed that this depends on a state of balanced polymorphism, as in the case of the sickling trait (p. 670), but there is less good reason than there is for the sickling trait to assume that the thalassemia trait offers partial resistance to malarial infection. There are interesting speculations that a fatal hemolytic process similar to thalassemia may have contributed to the disappearance of the Peruvian Incas and the pre-Columbian Mayan Indians.[209a]

Varieties of Thalassemia and Inheritance of the Trait.—It was at first assumed that thalassemia represents a single abnormality, *thalassemia minor* being the comparatively mild disorder observed in adolescents and adults who are *heterozygous* for the autosomal dominant trait whereas *thalassemia major*, or Cooley's anemia, is the severe, usually fatal disorder inherited from both parents which represents the *homozygous* condition.[278] However, the studies of the Italian investigators,[210] in particular, showed that the list of Mediterranean hemolytic syndromes is a long one. Even in the United States it was observed very early that thalassemia minor ranges in severity from a barely perceptible erythrocytic anomaly to a form in which there is moderate anemia, icterus and splenomegaly.[186,283] The Italian investigators referred to the completely benign form as *thalassemia minima*, or the *microcythemia* of Silvestroni and Bianco.[267]

Confusion with syndromes later recognized to be due to double heterozygosity for thalassemia and various abnormal hemoglobins no doubt accounts for some of the variations from the usual clinical picture which have been noted. In addition, the lack of more distinctive characteristics than those furnished by the classical clinical and hematologic picture made it necessary to differentiate thalassemia by a process of exclusion. Of great importance in this connection was the demonstration by starch block electrophoresis of a Hb E-like component (A_2[247]) of normal adult hemoglobin which moves more slowly than the major component. This is present in normal blood in small amounts ($2.54 \pm 0.35 \%$) but in thalassemia minor increased amounts were demonstrated (mean, $5.11 \pm 1.36 \%$). It has been observed that, within a given pedigree, the degree of elevation of Hb A_2 has been of the same order of magnitude. This finding has been so consistent[249b] that some have proposed that the minimum diagnostic criteria for the thalassemia trait should include increased Hb A_2 together with microcytosis.[231] In thalassemia major the quantity of A_2 is about normal. However, the suggestion that an elevated Hb A_2 level be regarded as the *sine qua non* for the diagnosis of thalassemia minor has not found universal acceptance,[210b] for several reasons which will be discussed shortly.

Two more features, both noted in cases of thalassemia major, should be considered here. These are the fact that the production of normal adult hemoglobin is suppressed, apparently completely, in some instances. The second is that fetal hemoglobin is found in increased amounts (10 to 90 per cent).[257, 268] In thalassemia minor, on the other hand, Hb F is normal or minimally elevated as a rule.[249b] In several instances of thalassemia minor, however, large amounts of fetal hemoglobin have been demonstrated.[200] It may be added that

Hb F not infrequently is increased in hemoglobinopathies due to simultaneous heterozygosity for the thalassemia gene and Hb S,[151] Hb C,[186] Hb E,[152] the Lepore trait[159a] and other hemoglobinopathies.[200c]

Significance of Hb A₂ and Genetic Control of Hemoglobin Production.—It was pointed out earlier (p. 160) that Hb A_2 is similar to Hb A in its α chain composition but that its second pair of chains differs sufficiently from the β chains to justify their special designation as δ chains. It has been found that the Hb A_2 from individuals with thalassemia minor is indistinguishable from that of normal people.[240] There is evidence, furthermore, that the δ chains are under genetic control which is separate from that of the β chains.[240] Abnormal minor components[238a] (B_2,[208b] A'_2[238b]) have been described which can replace some of the normal Hb A_2. Thus, in a person homozygous for the abnormal Hb G_{Ibadan}, which differs from Hb A in the α chain, no normal Hb A_2 was found; instead, there was a new minor component, G_2, which differed in electrophoretic mobility from Hb A_2 in the same way that Hb G differs from Hb A.[158c,184] It has therefore been inferred that the genetic control of the production of Hb A_2 is exercised by α and δ genes, whereas Hb A is controlled by α and β genes.[240] It appears, furthermore, that the β and δ genes are linked[208b] and that the hemoglobins of a normal individual are under the control of four genes, α, β, γ and δ. According to this view,[240] the α gene is concerned in the manufacture of all three types of hemoglobin; namely F as $\alpha_2^A \gamma_2^A$, A as $\alpha_2^A \beta_2^A$ and A_2 as $\alpha_2^A \delta_2^{A_2}$. The production of these various hemoglobins depends on whether or not the β, γ or δ genes are "active," which in turn may depend upon the stage of development of the individual. The study of an individual with the four hemoglobins A, G, C and G/C[184] provided evidence that the last step in

hemoglobin synthesis is the combination of the independently synthesized α_2 and β_2 units.[183b]

The studies on Hb A_2 are important in relation to thalassemia. One hypothesis[239] suggests that thalassemia is attributable to mutations that are similar to those which lead to the single amino acid substitutions in the recognized abnormal adult hemoglobins, such as Hb S, C and E. However, thalassemia is thought to differ from the abnormal hemoglobin diseases in that the hypothetical thalassemia mutations lead to amino acid substitutions which do not affect the electrophoretic mobility of the hemoglobin produced, but merely its rate of synthesis. According to this view there would be different thalassemias, according to whether the α or the β chain production of Hb A is decreased, so-called "α" and "β" thalassemias. The occurrence of high proportions of fetal hemoglobin, observed in some cases of thalassemia minor, could be explained as compensation for the decreased production of β chains in β thalassemia since fetal hemoglobin incorporates only α and γ chains, whose synthesis, according to this hypothesis, would be unimpaired. This would not happen in α thalassemia, since fetal hemoglobin uses α chains. The observed high levels of Hb A_2 in many cases of thalassemia minor could thus be ascribed to the presence of a β chain defect.

This concept is also consistent with descriptions of cases in which the usual clinical and morphological findings of thalassemia were present but no increased concentrations of Hb A_2 were found.[210b, 247] Among 15 Negroes with thalassemia, ten, representing four families, failed to show Hb A_2 elevation. It is also compatible with findings in individuals who appeared to be doubly heterozygous for thalassemia and Hb H,[155] or Hb J[260] or an unidentified abnormal hemoglobin,[208a] if in these subjects the production of α

chains was deficient. It is also consistent with the description of a clinical picture intermediate in severity between that of thalassemia major and minor in patients with the Lepore trait[159a] (p. 699), again in the absence of increased Hb A$_2$.

In families of thalassemia-H disease, it is the α type of thalassemia which would be expected to be present, according to the above hypothesis.[155,191a] It is plausible to assume that Hb H is completely recessive in the heterozygote but that, in association with α thalassemia, the defect in production of α chains, augmented perhaps by interference with production of α chain by the H gene, results in the production of four β chains. An alternative explanation is that Hb H disease results from the interaction of two genes for α thalassemia which markedly reduces the rate of synthesis of α polypeptide chains.[161a] However, on the basis of these hypotheses, it is difficult to classify the family with thalassemia-H disease in which a high level of Hb A$_2$ was found.[284]

The suggestion that the last step in hemoglobin synthesis is the pairing of fully formed subunits, mentioned above, serves to explain the formation of Hb H (β_4^A) and of Bart's (γ_4^F). In these instances the rate of synthesis of abnormal α_2 subunits or the reduced synthesis of α_2^A subunits permits the appearance of either Hb H or Bart's, or both.[183b] It is noteworthy that trace amounts of Bart's have been demonstrated in adult cases of Hb H disease.[161a] There is evidence to suggest that only one abnormal gene is needed for the production of Hb Bart's.[145b]

There are observations which suggest that elevated fetal hemoglobin concentrations may also be under independent control. In one family in Liberia, a disorder resembling thalassemia was described which appeared as if it might be attributable to the double inheritance of a **high F hemoglobin gene** and a **high Hb A$_2$ gene**.[254] In other

instances it was noted that a high level of F was inherited as a dominant trait in association with Hb A in persons who were hematologically normal.[159d,175a,279a] Several members of these families were found to have inherited the gene for Hb S in addition to that resulting in persistence of fetal hemoglobin. These persons appeared to be well and had none of the manifestations of sickle cell anemia, perhaps because the presence of high concentrations of Hb F in the red cells tended to prevent sickling. It has been suggested that in the conditions characterized by hereditary persistence of fetal hemoglobin, a factor allelic with the genes for hemoglobins A, S and C causes failure of production of hemoglobin A, with formation of fetal hemoglobin occurring as an indirect result.[159d] Combinations with other abnormal hemoglobins have been described.[172a]

It is apparent that the spectrum of disorders which has been included under the designation of thalassemia represents a great variety of heritable abnormalities, inherited in various combinations.[279b] The genetic mechanisms involved are highly complex and are not yet fully described by the terms of current genetic theory. According to one suggestion,[208b] there are three types of thalassemia, (1) those characterized by microcytosis and an increase in the Hb A$_2$ fraction above 3 per cent; (2) those with microcytosis and no increased A$_2$; and (3) those without microcytosis but with high A$_2$. This hypothesis, however, ignores the behavior of Hb F. Another proposal[287] is that the polypeptides of the γ and δ type represent primitive, incomplete or altered β chains. According to this view, certain types of thalassemia are the consequence of mutations of β genes affecting the synthesis of β chains and therefore represent multiple alleles at the β chain locus. The nature of the particular amino acid substitutions in the anomalous β chain would determine whether predominantly δ or γ chains, and

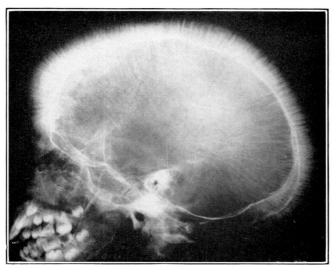

Fig. 13–19.—"Hair-on-end" appearance of skull produced by trabecular striations radiating outward from the inner table in a case of thalassemia major. (Courtesy of Dr. Robert A. Strong.)

consequently Hb A_2 or F, or still other fractions, are formed. The "high F gene" might be a mutant β gene which conveys the structure of β chains on the non-α polypeptide under its control or, if γ chains may be considered to be primitive β chains, is a "throwback" to an earlier evolutionary stage in which the β genes had not yet developed the structure necessary to make the step from γ to β chain synthesis possible.

Linkage studies have failed to show any relation of the thalassemia trait to the ABO or Rh blood group or to taste, eye color,[249] or the haptoglobin locus.[268a]

Symptomatology.—The following is a description of the classical picture of thalassemia major and minor.

Thalassemia Major. Cooley's Anemia.—The onset is insidious. Pallor is usually the first evidence of the disease and may be present from birth or soon thereafter. It is usually noticed in the first two years of life. An intercurrent infection may attract attention to the condition. It is not long before the abdomen becomes exceptionally prominent, due to the enlargement of the *spleen* and often of the *liver* as well. The spleen may reach the crest of the ilium. The symp-

toms are those of anemia, but there may be periodic attacks of fever as well.

When the condition is fully developed, the clinical picture is characteristic. The child is small for its age but the head is large. The skin is of a pale, muddy yellow color, the cheek bones are prominent, the cranial bones thickened ,the bridge of the nose may be sunken, the eye-lids may be puffy, and there may be an epicanthal fold; thus the designation, "mongoloid facies." Outright jaundice is unusual. The skin is pale and yellowish brown. There may be moderate lymphadenopathy but this is never striking. Cardiac dilatation is often found, and in advanced stages there is edema and effusion into serous cavities, and ecchymoses as well as free bleeding may develop. Chronic leg ulcers, like those seen in sickle cell anemia, are rare.[255,285]

Skeletal System.—Roentgenograms reveal striking changes in the skeletal system. There is thickening of the diploë of the skull to several times the normal depth. The outer and inner tables are thin, the former sometimes being invisible, and perpendicular striations appear between the tables. The result suggests hair standing erect on the scalp (**Fig.**

45

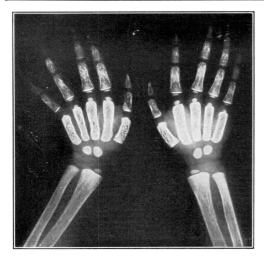

Fig. 13–20.—Mosaic pattern produced by trabeculation in the bones of the hand, in a case of thalassemia major. Note the rectangular contour of the metacarpals.

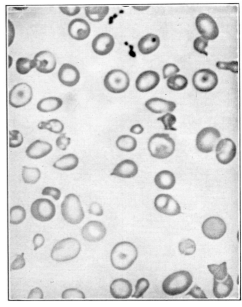

Fig. 13–21.—Blood smear in a case of thalassemia major. Note the hypochromia, target cells and poikilocytes. Photomicrograph. (× 1050.)

13–19). In the long bones, widening due to increase in the medullary portion, decreased density of the medulla and thinning of the compact bone of the cortex are found; and in the short bones, which are often rectangular in contour, trabeculation of the medulla which gives the bones a mosaic pattern, is the characteristic finding (Fig. 13–20).

Demonstrable abnormalities in the bone structure have been observed as early as four and a half months of age. The earliest lesions in the skull are in the frontal bones but the picture in the skull varies considerably even in cases of apparently equal severity. In the long bones the most striking findings have been in the distal ends of the femora. The lesions in the tubular bones of the extremities regress with age while the changes in the central segments of the skeleton, such as the skull, spine and pelvic bones, persist and increase.[207] Retarded pneumatization of cranial air sinuses is common. Spontaneous fractures are unusual.

The Blood.—The anemia is usually pronounced when it is first discovered. The red cell count is often between 2,000,000 and 3,000,000, but it may be as high as 4,000,000 or as low as 1,000,-

000. The reduction in hemoglobin and in volume of packed red cells is even greater, the anemia being hypochromic, microcytic in type.

The appearance of the *red corpuscles* in blood smears is very characteristic (Fig. 13–21). They vary greatly in size, ranging from 3 to 15 μ in diameter. Even more striking is the fact that they contain little pigment and may be so distorted in shape and unusual in appearance that it is easy to accept the view that they are composed almost exclusively of a thin, almost colorless membrane. The coloring matter which is present may outline only the periphery. It may also form a circular area in the center ("target corpuscles") or there may be a bridge joining the central and peripheral zones of pigment. Sometimes the red corpuscles appear to be ridged. Few fully colored cells are present.

In wet preparations the distortion of the red corpuscles is still more evident and there may be considerable fragmentation.[212] The edges of some corpuscles may be folded over and then the several layers may be seen to be remarkably transparent. Sickling is not found.

The presence of *nucleated red cells* is a charactertistic finding. There may be only 10 or 20 per 100 leukocytes, or the nucleated red cells may be several times as numerous as the white cells; in absolute terms, 200 to 125,000 per c.mm. may be found.[205] The majority are typical normoblasts and microblasts but a comparatively large minority of very immature normoblasts may be seen. The most primitive forms are round or oval in shape, about 15 μ in diameter, with deep blue cytoplasm, and granular nuclear chromatin.[246] Nucleoli are not often visible. These cells have been well illustrated and described by Kato and Downey.[246] They are unlike the megaloblasts found in pernicious anemia (Plate V, p. 94).

In addition to these signs of active red cell regeneration, many polychromatophilic cells, a moderate or large number of stippled erythrocytes, and occasional corpuscles with Howell-Jolly bodies are found. Reticulocytes are increased, often to 5 or even 15 per cent. Sometimes these immature forms of red corpuscles are found when nucleated cells are few or even absent.

As tested by hypotonic saline solutions, the *fragility of the red corpuscles* is not increased as a rule, although in some instances slight initial hemolysis has been noted in 0.54 per cent saline.[205] More often fragility is decreased. Hemolysis may not be complete in 0.2 per cent saline and sometimes not even in water: a pale, gelatinous layer remains in the bottom of the test tubes.[205,212]

A method has been described whereby red blood cells containing different types of hemoglobin can be distinguished.[261]

Differences in sensitivity of red corpuscles from thalassemia major and minor to Heinz body formation have been reported.[251]

The *leukocytes* are often increased in number, counts of 10,000 to 25,000 per c.mm. being common. Values as high as 50,000 and even 100,000 have been recorded. There may be well-marked myeloid stimulation with many immature forms, including myelocytes and myeloblasts.[246] As a rule, however, these forms are not numerous. Monocytes may be somewhat increased in number or, especially in infants, there may be lymphocytosis.

No significant abnormalities in the *platelet count* have been recorded.

The *icterus index* is slightly or moderately increased (8 to 30), the van den Bergh reaction is positive, indirect. The protoporphyrin content of the erythrocytes was reported as increased in 2 cases.[229] The plasma copper may be increased above normal.[208] The serum iron is high[208] and the serum possesses no unbound iron-binding capacity,[269] as is the case in other conditions characterized by increased blood destruction.

Urine. — The urine often contains slightly or moderately increased quantities of urobilinogen or urobilin. An occasional, iron-laden, kidney epithelial cell may be found in the urinary sediment. The output of amino acids in the urine was found to be markedly increased in children with thalassemia major.[210a] This was attributed to decreased kidney reabsorption.

Gastric analysis has revealed no abnormalities.

The **feces** and the gall bladder bile have been found to contain greatly increased amounts of coproporphyrin.[229]

Thalassemia Minor. — As stated earlier (p. 702) the manifestations of thalassemia minor vary but, in general, symptoms are lacking or at most there is some increased fatigability. The cases are usually discovered by chance, as in the first case described by the writer and his associates.[283] Admitted because of pneumonia, this son of Sicilian parents was discovered to have splenomegaly and iron-refractory, hypochromic microcytic anemia of moderate degree (hemoglobin

10.1 Gm.). The icterus index varied from 13 to 35. The reticulocytes were 3.6 per cent and the stained smear showed marked anisocytosis, poikilocytosis, hypochromia, "target" corpuscles, and numerous stippled red cells (Fig. 13–22). No nucleated red cells were found. Marked fragmentation of red corpuscles was evident in wet films of blood but there was no sickling. Few red corpuscles hemolyzed in hypotonic saline solutions in the normal range (Fig. 13–23) and a gelatinous layer of unbroken cells remained even in 0.03 per cent salt solution. There was marked erythroblastosis of the sternal marrow, as well as increased osteoporosis and thinning of the cortex of the long bones (Fig. 13–24). This boy's father and his brother, the latter aged thirty years, were found to have splenomegaly, icterus, and the same abnormalities of the red corpuscles. Other members of this family, as well as of another Italian

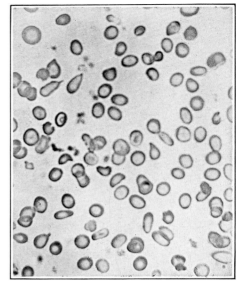

Fig. 13–22.—Stained smear showing the marked hypochromia, moderate poikilocytosis and microcytosis, as well as a few target cells, in a case of thalassemia minor in a boy aged eighteen years. Photomicrograph ($\times$ 800).

CONTROL

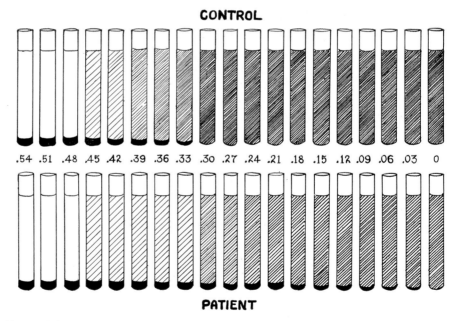

.54 .51 .48 .45 .42 .39 .36 .33 .30 .27 .24 .21 .18 .15 .12 .09 .06 .03 0

PATIENT

Fig. 13–23.—Diagrammatic representation of results of fragility tests in a case of thalassemia minor. The clear tubes indicate no hemolysis, light hatching indicates slight hemolysis, heavy hatching marked hemolysis. Note the early appearance of well-marked hemolysis and the disappearance of all cell residue in the sample of normal blood, and the slow development of hemolysis and persistence of corpuscular residue in the patient's blood.

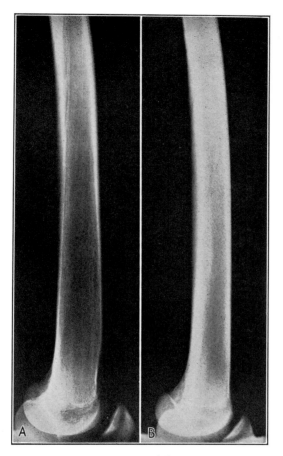

Fig. 13–24.—Femur of a boy, aged eighteen years (*A*) who had thalassemia minor, compared with that of a healthy boy of the same age (*B*). Note the thinness of the cortex and the general decreased density.

family and one Italian whose family could not be studied, were found to have similar abnormalities.

The red cell count in these individuals may actually be somewhat higher than normal (as high as 6,300,000 in 1 case) even though the hemoglobin and volume of packed red cells are reduced below normal.[278] There is microcytosis and hypochromia but there is no evidence of chronic blood loss, and iron therapy, even iron supplemented with copper or with vitamin B_6, is ineffective in relieving the anemia. Morphological changes in the red corpuscles are far out of proportion to

the degree of anemia. Stippling of the red corpuscles brought several of these cases to our attention. This was very marked but evidence of lead or other poisoning was not found. In addition to stippling, hypochromia, poikilocytosis, and the presence of "target" corpuscles were noteworthy findings in the blood smears. As already described, there was a striking increase in resistance to hemolysis by hypotonic saline solutions.

As in cases of thalassemia major, the plasma copper may be increased above normal, the free erythrocyte protoporphyrin may be raised[208] (although this

Table 13–1.—Blood Findings in Two Cases of Cooley's Anemia and in Their Respective Parents

	Family C.			Family S.		
	Cl. C., age 2 yrs.	Ca. C., father	B. C., mother	A. S., age 6 mos.	P. S., father	L. S., mother
R.B.C., 10^6/c.mm. . . .	3.30	5.53	4.27	3.58	6.11	6.11
Hemoglobin, Gm./100 ml. .	6.7	11.6	9.5	7.5	12.0	12.0
Vol. Packed R.B.C., ml./100 ml.	23.5	43.3	33.5	26.0	39.7	41.0
M.C.V., c.μ.	71	78	78	73	65	67
M.C.H., $\gamma\gamma$	20	21	23	21	20	20
M.C.H.C., per cent . . .	28	27	29	29	30	29
Retics., per cent	7.4	1.0	0.4	3.0	. .	. .
Icterus index	20	9	6	12	8	12
Fragility	0.45— 0.03	0.45— 0.21	0.45— 0.03	0.48— 0.15	0.51— 0.24	0.48— 0.24

(Control 0.45–0.33)

Marked poikilocytosis, hypochromia, microcytosis and slight to moderate stippling as well as some "target cells" were present in all instances. In Cl. C. there were 24 normoblasts per 100 leukocytes. The spleen was palapable in Cl. C. and in her mother, B. C., but was not made out in the parents of A. S. whose own spleen, however, was enlarged.

Cl. C. was the fifth child. Two children, ages thirteen and ten, were said to be well but could not be examined. Two had died in infancy. A. S. had a brother aged thirteen years who was said to be well and could not be examined. Another sibling had died in infancy.

is not always the case[233,275]) and none of the iron-binding capacity of the serum may be free.[271]

The blood findings in the symptomless parents of children with classical Cooley's anemia (Table 13–1) show the characteristics described in adolescents and adults with thalassemia minor.

Persons carrying the thalassemia trait are asymptomatic but, as mentioned above, splenomegaly and signs of moderately increased blood destruction may be found, and even extramedullary hematopoiesis may result in the production of tumors, as in other forms of chronic hemolytic anemia.[246a]

Diagnosis.—The clinical picture of the classical case is so striking that it can hardly be missed: mongoloid facies, splenomegaly, skeletal changes, severe anemia and thin pale corpuscles of various shapes and sizes, erythroblastosis, polychromatophilia, stippling, reticulocytosis, leukocytosis and slight icterus. It should

be remembered that erythroblastosis may be slight or even absent. Resistance to hemolysis by hypotonic saline solutions is increased and sickling is absent.

This combination of features distinguishes the condition from hereditary spherocytosis and from sickle cell anemia, two disorders with which thalassemia has much in common. The racial and familial incidence help to distinguish it from other "erythroblastic anemias" which may be found in infants and very young children in association with celiac disease or congenital syphilis. The skin, mucous membrane, and bone changes of syphilis are absent and the serological reaction is negative. The splenomegaly may suggest leukemia but it is to be noted that the cell immaturity in thalassemia major involves the red cells much more strikingly than the leukocytes. Furthermore, the platelets are unaffected. Blood and roentgen ray studies should make it possible to rule out Gaucher's disease, Niemann-

Pick's disease, the Schüller-Christian syndrome, rickets, and other conditions to which there is a superficial resemblance.

The carrier state (thalassemia minor) is recognized by hypochromia and microcytosis of the red cells, with or without slight anemia and sometimes associated with an abnormally high red cell count; the striking morphologic abnormalities in the red corpuscles, including stippled, "target" and oval cells, quite out of proportion to the degree of anemia, if any exists at all; the increased resistance of the cells to hemolysis in hypotonic saline solutions; the refractoriness of the blood to iron therapy; and, finally, in most cases the racial factor already described. Lead poisoning, hemolytic diseases and other conditions associated with splenomegaly must be ruled out. As pointed out already, occasional individuals with thalassemia minor, the heterozygous state, may show a rather severe degree of anemia.

A_2, as already stated, is present in amounts above 3 per cent in carriers of the most common variety of thalassemia, the so-called β type (p. 703). For the demonstration of Hb A_2, paper electrophoresis can be used if special buffers together with a stain for protein are employed (p. 718). Best of all is starch block electrophoresis. It is important also to look for abnormal hemoglobins which may be associated with the thalassemia trait. Such double heterozygosity accounts for some of the atypical and "intermediate" forms of thalassemia. The test for sickling will be positive in sickle cell-thalassemia (p. 715). The chief characteristics of the various hemoglobinopathies are summarized in Table 13–2 (p. 716).

Hypochromic microcytic anemia is most commonly due to iron deficiency. Next in frequency is one of the thalassemic disorders and very rare is pyridoxine-responsive anemia (p. 136) or the copper deficient syndrome occasionally seen in infants (p. 141). In iron deficiency anemia target cells and cells showing punctate basophilia are fewer than in thalassemia and the increase in osmotic resistance is less likely to be as severe. The serum iron is low and iron is not found in the bone marrow, in striking contrast to the increased amounts in thalassemia. Some evidences of increased blood destruction may be demonstrable in thalassemia (bilirubinemia, increased excretion of urobilinogen) and family studies may reveal additional cases of the disorder, whereas a therapeutic trial of iron will be ineffective.

An obscure form of hypochromic microcytic anemia defying classification was reported under the title, "hereditary (? sex-linked) anemia."[259] This was unassociated with skeletal abnormalities or signs of increased blood destruction but was accompanied by splenomegaly and the presence of strikingly deformed erythrocytes. The condition had affected the male members in several generations but appeared to be transmitted by females, many of whom had splenomegaly and minor red cell abnormalities without anemia. Cases similar to these were discussed elsewhere (p. 563).

The erythrocytosis found in some cases of thalassemia minor and minima should not cause confusion with polycythemia vera, in spite of the splenomegaly which may be present. Although the erythrocyte count is high, the hemoglobin level is normal or low, the red corpuscles are microcytic and hypochromic, and bizarre forms are likely to be found in thalassemia. In polycythemia vera the red corpuscles are normal in appearance. In hereditary elliptocytosis, the red cells are not hypochromic, nor do they show the great variations in size and shape which are so characteristic of thalassemia.

Course and Prognosis.—As an ever greater variety of syndromes comes to be included under the term thalassemia, it becomes more difficult to describe the syndrome. The classical form of Cooley's anemia was fatal and was noted to be more rapidly so the earlier it became manifest; if it was discovered in the first year of life, death often occurred within six months.[205] An intercurrent infection was the usual cause of death. When it appeared later, death might be delayed for several years. Cardiac failure, perhaps in relation to the heavy deposits of iron in the myocardium is not rare.[270]

With the recognition of less serious cases, it has become evident that prognosis is not always this bad and cases extending into adolescence[283] and even into adult life[241] have been recognized. In classical thalassemia minor the prognosis is comparatively good and ranges from that of a condition associated with moderately severe anemia and splenomegaly to that of a hematological stigma which only painstaking examination will disclose.

In classical Cooley's anemia crises and remissions are unusual but this is not true of the whole gamut of conditions which falls under this head. Intercurrent infections may be associated with "aplastic" crises and pregnancy sometimes is accompanied by aggravation of anemia.[209] In a few instances, "pernicious anemia" of pregnancy may have developed and responses to folic acid were observed; in others a dietary deficiency of folic acid may have been involved.[209] In another instance, Addisonian pernicious anemia which responded to vitamin B_{12} was described.[214] In one case episodes of hematologic decompensation due to bone marrow failure were observed which responded in a striking fashion to the administration of large doses of folic acid.[241] Since physiologic amounts of folic acid had no effect, it was postulated that increased red cell turnover associated with chronic hemolytic anemia may sometimes produce an acute "relative" deficiency of certain metabolites. It is of interest that the response to

therapy was associated with diffuse, intense bone pain and tenderness, especially in the lower extremities, possibly as the result of the rapid expansion of the intramedullary erythroid mass. The writer has observed the same phenomenon, accompanied by fever, in other instances of exceptionally active blood cell regeneration.

Treatment.—The anemia ordinarily is unaffected by any form of antianemic therapy (iron, copper, cobalt, pyridoxine, vitamin B_{12}) or by the great variety of organ extracts[280] and other substances which have been tried from time to time. The rare occurrence of "relative folic acid deficiency" was discussed in the preceding paragraph. Transfusion of blood has only temporary value and should be avoided whenever possible. These patients are able to adapt remarkably well to their state of chronic anemia. When transfusions are given it may be found that the requirement in time becomes greater and greater. When an extracorpuscular mechanism can be demonstrated as the cause of the increased transfusion requirement, splenectomy may be very helpful and greatly reduce the need for transfusions.[256,270] The operation also has sometimes been recommended to afford mechanical relief when the spleen is huge. It was claimed that splenectomized thalassemics may be abnormally susceptible to infection and their growth in height and sexual development may be retarded[270] but this has not been the universal experience.[284a]

The chronic leg ulcers should be treated in the same manner[213] as those seen in sickle cell anemia (p. 684).

Pathology.—In cases of Cooley's anemia the main findings at autopsy are the evidences of anemia and of active blood formation, both medullary and extramedullary, splenomegaly, striking changes in the bones, and pigmentation of various organs resembling that of hemochromatosis.

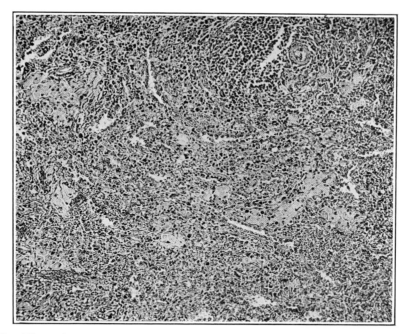

FIG. 13–25.—Photomicrograph of spleen from a case of Mediterranean anemia (thalassemia major), showing nests of foam cells in the pulp and thickened sinusoids. (× 200.) (Whipple and Bradford, courtesy of Am. J. Dis. Child.)

The **spleen** is much enlarged and may show infarcts and adhesions. It is firm and hard. There are foci of extramedullary blood formation, with nucleated red cells, myelocytes, and megakaryocytes.[205] In other areas an increase of stroma and accumulations of foam cells are seen (Fig. 13–25). The latter give at best a faint pink color with fat stains but they give an intense reaction with the periodic acid-Schiff (PAS) stain.[263] In some cases eosinophils have been very numerous. The malpighian corpuscles are approximately normal, or small.[280]

The gross changes in the **bones** have been mentioned. The bones may be greatly thickened and the long bones may tend to be rectangular in shape. There is atrophy of the bone shafts and trabeculae and, at the same time, proliferation of delicate new bone. In the skull this is arranged in a more or less parallel, centrifugal pattern (Fig. 13–26).

The **bone marrow** is hyperplastic and contains many parent stem cells, numerous nucleated red cells, and many myelocytes as well as megakaryocytes. There may be a number of phagocytes, some containing small amounts of hemosiderin. Foam cells may be present in small islands. These as well as stroma may sometimes dominate the picture in the marrow and spleen. Thus, confusion with Gaucher's disease may arise. A PAS positive substance has been demonstrated in the marrow normoblasts.[202,232]

Iron-containing pigment[280] is abundant in the liver, pancreas, lymph glands, gastric mucosa, thyroid, and adrenals and is usually demonstrable in Brunner's glands, the salivary and mucous glands, the parathyroids, hypophysis, heart muscle, and kidney tubules. In the spleen, however, there is a conspicuous lack of pigment. Iron-staining pigment in the skin has not been found.

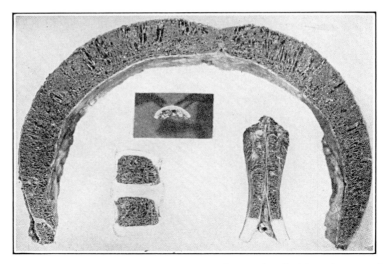

FIG. 13–26.—Coronal section of the calvarium, a rib and costochondral junction, vertebrae and cross-section of the shaft of the femur.   Case of Mediterranean anemia.   (Whipple and Bradford, courtesy of Am. J. Dis. Child.)

Pathogenesis.—In an earlier section observations on the nature of the hemoglobin found in the blood of thalassemics were discussed (p. 702).   It was pointed out that in the majority of cases of thalassemia minor the quantity of the slow normal hemoglobin component, A_2, is increased, whereas in thalassemia major the quantity of Hb F is increased and Hb A production is suppressed.[239]   No close correlation has been observed, however, between these differences in amounts and kinds of hemoglobin and the severity of the anemia.

Nevertheless, it would appear that the clinical manifestations of thalassemia are in some manner related to a genetically determined defect in red cell formation. The red corpuscles one sees in the blood seem to be formed with an adequate or excessive membrane but with little substance.   Their extreme thinness accounts for some of the bizarre forms which are observed, including the "target" cells and fragmented corpuscles; it also explains their increased resistance to hypotonic saline solutions.   They are able to absorb more fluid without bursting than can normal cells.   The mechanical fragility of these deformed corpuscles is increased[250] and this may be responsible in part for the manifestations of increased blood destruction which are found in thalassemia major.   The morphological abnormalities which characterize the disorder are more striking in thalassemia major than in thalassemia minor[249c] and, correspondingly, it has been found that the survival of the red corpuscles from subjects with thalassemia minor who had no icterus was normal[236,244] when transfused into normal individuals whereas the survival of cells from subjects with thalassemia major was shortened.[244]   It is noteworthy that between 25 and 50 per cent of the cells in thalassemia major blood disappeared from the recipient's circulation in twenty to thirty days, whereas the remainder followed the normal rate of elimination.   It has been observed by electron microscopy that the surface texture of red cell ghosts from thalassemia major blood is distinctly different from that of cells from thalassemia minor or from normal blood.[238]

The bone marrow hyperplasia probably represents an attempt to compensate for the red cell destruction and the immature forms of the erythroid series found in the circulation simply reflect this. It is plausible to assume that continuous marrow hyperplasia from early life can cause bone changes such as are found in children suffering from this disorder.

Patients with Cooley's anemia have been shown to have an increased turnover of hemoglobin constituents comparable to the maximal response seen in other hemolytic anemias.[274] However, there is a marked decrease in the maximal delivery of erythrocytes to the blood, thus indicating that the severity of the anemia is largely related to a production defect.[222] *In vitro* studies in which incorporation of glycine-2-C^{14} or Fe^{59} was measured suggested that there is a quantitative impairment of hemoglobin synthesis by immature red cells.[203] *In vivo* studies with similarly labelled heme and globin confirmed these findings and showed also that there is either an abnormal degree of premature destruction of red cells or hemoglobin within the bone marrow, or an anabolic pathway for the production of stercobilin since radioactivity appeared extremely rapidly in the fecal stercobilin.[233] The basic abnormality would therefore seem to be in the erythroblast.

The resemblance of the morphological characteristics of the abnormally formed red corpuscles to the red corpuscles of iron deficiency anemia, as well as the excessive amounts of iron which are found in the tissues, would lead one to suspect that the defect is associated in some manner with an inability to utilize iron in hemoglobin synthesis. In thalassemia large quantities of iron have been observed to have accumulated in the erythroblasts and have even been found in the erythrocytes as ferritin.[206] Of uncertain significance is the observation that the iron which is deposited so abundantly in the tissues of thalassemics is distributed more in the manner seen in hemochromatosis than like that encountered in hemolytic anemias (p. 631).

Combinations of Thalassemia and Various Abnormal Hemoglobins. — A number of such combinations were described in the preceding sections. Actually the first of these to be recognized was the association of thalassemia with the sickling trait, **sickle cell-thalassemia disease** or **microdrepanocytic disease.**[267a] In such individuals 60 to 80 per cent of the hemoglobin has been Hb S and up to 20 per cent Hb F, the remainder (0 to 20 per cent) being Hb A.[151] Thus the electrophoretic pattern may be indistinguishable from that of sickle cell anemia. In fact, such cases when first observed in the United States were reported as examples of sickle cell anemia occurring in white persons (p. 671). The condition has been recognized most often in white persons, especially in Italians,[267a] Greeks and Eti-Turks.[200a] Cases have also been reported from Tunisia[258] and India,[208b] as well as in the American Negro[264] and in persons of mixed Chinese and African ancestry.[249a] In the majority of reported cases one gene has been inherited from each parent but, exceptionally, both seem to have been derived from the same parent.[267a] Sickling of the red corpuscles, microcytosis, hypochromia, target cells, decreased osmotic fragility of the red corpuscles and the pigmentary manifestations of a rather severe hemolytic process, are the usual laboratory findings. Abdominal crises, leg ulcers and hepatosplenomegaly have been described. The manifestations, however, are not always severe and only mild anemia, and even no anemia whatever, have been observed. It should be noted, however, that in some families the proportion of Hb S has been comparatively low (27 per cent).[210b] Thus, as in the case of SC disease (p. 691), the abnormal hemoglobin may be associated with the α type of thalas-

Table 13–2.—Summary of Usual Findings in Abnormal Hemoglobinopathies And Thalassemia

Condition	Hb Types[1]	Sickling	Micro-cytosis	Hypo-chromia	Target Cells[2] Per Cent	Hemolytic Anemia[3]	Spleno-megaly
None-adult	AA	0	0	0	0	0	0
None-newborn	AF	0	0	0	0	0	0
Traits[11]							
Sickle cell trait[4]	AS	+	0	0	4	0	0
Hb C trait[4]	AC	0	0	+	1–100	0	0
Hb D trait	AD	0	0	0	0	0	0
Hb E trait	AE	0	0	0	0	0	0
Hb G trait[4]	AG	0	0	0	0	0	0
Hb I trait	AI	0	0	0	<2	0	0
Diseases							
Sickle cell anemia[4]	SS	++	0	0, +	5–30	++++	0
Homozygous Hb C[4,9] . . .	CC	0	±	+	30–100	++	++
Homozygous Hb E . . .	EE	0	++	0	25–60	+[7]	±
Homozygous Hb G[4] . . .	GG	0	0	0	0	0	0
Sickle cell-Hb C[4,5] . . .	SC	+	±	+	20–85	++	++
Sickle cell-Hb D[6]	SD	+	+	++	+	++	++
Sickle cell-Hb G	SG	+	0	0	0	0	0
Thalassemia minor . . .	AA₂[8]	0	+	+ *	+	+[7]	±
Thalassemia major . . .	AF	0	++	++ *	10–35	+++	++++
Sickle cell-thalassemia[6] . . .	SF	+	+	+ *	20–40	++	++
Hb C-thalassemia[4]	CA	0	+	± *	+++	+	0
Hb E-thalassemia	EF	0	++	++ *	10–40	++	+++
Hb G-thalassemia (?) . . .	GF	0	+	+	+	+	0
Hb H-thalassemia[10] . . .	AH	0	++	++	++	++	±
Sickle cell-hereditary spherocytosis	SA	+	+	0	+	++	++

[1] The major hemoglobin component is shown first. In sickle cell anemia especially, there may also be a substantial proportion of Hb F.

[2] Osmotic fragility is reduced more or less proportionately to the number of target cells.

[3] Mechanical fragility and RBC survival correspond *as a rule* to the presence and degree of hemolytic anemia.

[4] Chiefly in Negroes.

[5] Cases of sickle cell anemia intermediate in severity between sickle cell trait and sickle cell anemia.

[6] Sickle cell disease in Caucasians.

[7] Or polycythemia with microcytosis.

[8] In the majority of cases.

[9] Partial drying and partial hemolysis are associated with crystallization of hemoglobin. Rod shaped erythrocytes with squared corners are seen in blood smear.

[10] Inclusion bodies demonstrable in red corpuscles.

[11] No clearly defined hematological abnormalities have been reported to be associated with the inheritance of the following traits: J, K, L, N, O, P, Q. The manifestations of the Lepore trait are like those of thalassemia minor; when Lepore is associated with the thalassemia trait, the clinical picture is that of thalassemia major.

* Basophilic stippling of the red corpuscles.

semia rather than the more common β variety (p. 703).

DIFFERENTIATION OF THE ABNORMAL HEMOGLOBIN SYNDROMES AND THALASSEMIA

The most important clinical and hematological differences among the various hemoglobinopathies are summarized in Table 13–2 (p. 716). As described in Chapter 3 (p. 156), the important advances which have been made in our knowledge of the variations which occur in the structure of human hemoglobin have required the use of a number of highly specialized technics. Some of these were discussed in an earlier section (p. 156). It is significant, however, that the initial observations which led to such painstaking analysis often have been made by comparatively simple means. In this section only those procedures which can be carried out in a clinical laboratory will be discussed.

In addition to a thorough history and physical examination, as well as the usual blood examination (volume of packed red cells, hemoglobin, red cell count, calculation of red cell indices, leukocyte and platelet counts *and* careful examination of the blood smear) the following procedures should be carried out when a hemoglobinopathy is suspected:

(1) Test for sickle cells (pp. 680, 682);
(2) Test for osmotic fragility of the red corpuscles (p. 171);
(3) Serum bilirubin (p. 177) and urinary urobilinogen (p. 178);
(4) Reticulocyte count (p. 90);
(5) Test for inclusion bodies (p. 696) and for Heinz bodies (p. 624);
(6) Test for siderocytes (p. 101) and, if the bone marrow is examined, test for hemosiderin in the bone marrow sample (p. 60);
(7) Paper electrophoresis of hemoglobin; and

(8) Quantitation of alkali-resistant hemoglobin (p. 719).

These examinations will provide information concerning the nature of the anemia, if any is present, and will indicate whether it is associated with gross evidences of increased blood destruction, signs of active blood regeneration, altered osmotic fragility of the erythrocytes, disturbed iron metabolism and chemical abnormalities in the red corpuscles (sickle cells, inclusion bodies, Heinz bodies, siderocytes). The alkali-resistance test is a measure of Hgb F and electrophoresis may serve to identify the abnormal hemoglobin.

If these examinations confirm the possibility that one is dealing with one of the syndromes discussed in this chapter, as many members of the patient's family as possible should be examined in the same way. In particular, it is important to examine *both* parents, as well as the siblings. In addition, it may be necessary to measure the solubility of the hemoglobin[164a] and to carry out other procedures discussed earlier, such as starch block electrophoresis, moving boundary electrophoresis and ion exchange chromatography. In the identification of an abnormal hemoglobin suspected of being a new one, it is absolutely essential to test it side by side with well-authenticated specimens of the hemoglobins which it more superficially resembles. For such an investigation it is necessary to call for the assistance of one of the special laboratories concerned with investigation in this field.

Paper Electrophoresis.—A number of different types of apparatus have been devised which can be made up in one's own laboratory, provided a constant source of voltage is available.[151] They utilize sheets or strips of filter paper suspended between bars in appropriate relation to chambers containing buffer solutions. Such instruments are less elabor-

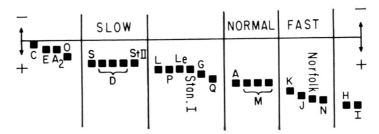

Fig. 13–27.—Relative mobilities of normal and abnormal adult hemoglobins on paper electrophoresis at pH 8.6.

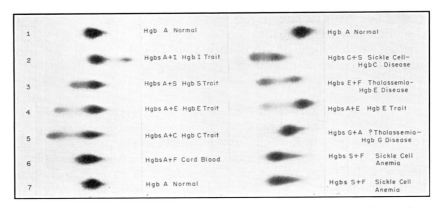

Fig. 13–28.—Paper electophoresis of human hemoglobins. On the left are shown the actual runs of specimens from persons with the heterozygous Hb C, E, I and S traits as well as that of cord blood, as compared with the electrophoretic pattern of normal hemoglobin (Hb A) alone. On the right are shown the electrophoretic patterns of sickle cell anemia, sickle cell-Hb C disease, thalassemia-Hb E disease and thalassemia-Hb G disease. (Courtesy of Dr. Amoz Chernoff[151] and New England J. Med.)

ate than the various types of commercially available apparatus but are quite satisfactory and are inexpensive.

Hanging-strip rather than horizontal paper electrophoresis has been recommended for comparison of hemoglobins which migrate at about the same rate[142a] and, as will be indicated below, electrophoresis at pH 6.5 is sometimes useful in addition to the customary alkaline pH (8.6). Electrophoresis in agar gel has also been found helpful.[180b] This technic has been especially useful in the electrophoretic separation of Hb F from other hemoglobins.[180b] The latter has been used for the rapid demonstration of Hb A₂.[277] Paper electrophoresis with a special (TRIS) buffer has been employed

successfully[213a] but probably the best procedure for measurement of Hb A₂ is the original starch grain block technic of Kunkel.[247]

The mobilities of various adult hemoglobins on paper electrophoresis at pH 8.6 are represented diagrammatically in Figure 13–27, patterned after Lehmann.[169b] There are two main groups, those moving more slowly and those moving faster than normal adult hemoglobin (A). Of the former, there are the *very slow* abnormal hemoglobins, such as C, E and O, as well as Hb A₂. Electrophoresis at pH 6.5 serves to distinguish between C and E. E and A₂ are indistinguishable by electrophoresis but A₂ never exceeds 15 per cent of the total hemoglobin even in thalassemia whereas Hb E, when present, amounts to 20 per cent or more.

The *slow* hemoglobins which move like Hb S include the several varieties of Hb D and Stanleyville II. Hb D can be distinguished from S by the solubility test.[164a,165]

The group of hemoglobins which move *more slowly than Hb A but more rapidly than S* are similar to fetal hemoglobin in this respect and include the G hemoglobins as well as L, P, Q, Lepore and Stanleyville I. To separate these, ion exchange chromatography is necessary.

Hemoglobins which move like Hb A are the M hemoglobins (p. 703). Hb F, if mixed with a sufficiently large proportion of A, will also simulate Hb A in mobility.

The *fast* hemoglobins can be divided into two groups, fast and very fast. The former include K, J, Norfolk and N. The *very fast* hemoglobins include H and I. Bart's hemoglobin is intermediate between fast and very fast. Electrophoresis at pH 6.5 facilitates differentiation of these hemoglobins. Bart's resembles Hb F in being alkali resistant.

Alkali Denaturation.[151,268]—A stock solution of standardized N/4 KOH is prepared and kept in a tightly stoppered paraffin bottle. One part of the stock solution is diluted with 2 parts distilled H_2O to produce N/12 KOH. Fifty per cent saturated $(NH_4)_2SO_4$ is prepared by adding 500 ml. saturated $(NH_4)_2SO_4$ to 500 ml. distilled water plus 2.5 ml. concentrated HCl (11 N).

The red cell hemolysate is prepared as described for paper electrophoresis but a concentration of 10 Gm. hemoglobin per 100 ml. is required. This is solution A. Of solution A 0.1 ml. is pipetted into 1.6 ml. N/12 KOH in a test tube. The 0.1 ml. blow-out pipette is rinsed five or six times with the KOH-hemoglobin mixture, which is then agitated gently 10 to 20 times. The reaction is permitted to proceed for *exactly one minute* and is stopped by the addition of 3.4 ml. of the 50 per cent saturated $(NH_4)_2SO_4$ solution. (In this time interval all the normal adult hemoglobin plus a small amount of Hb F is denatured.) The test tube is then inverted three or four times and the mixture is filtered into a clean test tube. This is solution B.

To calculate the percentage of hemoglobin F the optical density of solution B is determined in a colorimeter at 540 millimicrons and this reading is related to the hemoglobin concentration in the original solution (solution A). The latter may be obtained by diluting 0.02 ml. (Sahli pipetteful) of solution A with 4 ml. of distilled H_2O and reading at a wave length of 540 millimicrons in a Beckman spectrophotometer. This is solution C.

The percentage of hemoglobin F is obtained by the following ratio:

$$\frac{\frac{1}{4} \text{ optical density solution B}}{\text{optical density solution C}} \times 100 = \% \text{ Hb F}$$

The factor, 1/4, is used because the hemoglobin in solution B is diluted one part in 50 whereas the dilution factor in solution C is 1:200; that is, solution B is four times as concentrated as solution C. In some colorimeters it may be necessary to use larger volumes of filtrate which will alter the dilution factor employed in the calculation.

There is considerable evidence derived from immunologic, crystallographic, spectrophotometric and solubility studies which indicates that the alkali resistant hemoglobin is identical with the normal fetal hemoglobin of the newborn infant.[151] In the concentrations described above, over 2.0 per cent Hb F will impart a brownish to red color to solution B. Blood specimens from normal persons will appear colorless although spectrophotometric readings up to 1.8 per cent alkali resistant hemoglobin may be obtained on the colorless filtrate. It is not known whether this residual reading represents hemoglobin F or some other material as yet unidentified. Since the alkali denaturation procedure is insensitive to less than 2 per cent Hb F, all figures below that level are considered normal.

BIBLIOGRAPHY

Sickle Cell Anemia and the Sickling Trait

1. AKSOY, M.: Sickle-Cell Trait in South Turkey, Lancet, *1*, 589, 1955; Blood, *11*, 460, 1956; Brit. M. J., *2*, 937, 1958.
2. ALLISON, A. C.: Protection Afforded by Sickle-Cell Trait against Subtertian Malarial Infection, Brit. M. J., *1*, 290, 1954.
3. ALTMANN, A.: Sickle Cell Anæmia in a South African-Born European, Clin. Proc., Cape Town, *4*, 1, 1945.
5. ARCHIBALD, R. G.: Sickle Cell Anæmia in the Sudan, Trans. Roy. Soc. Trop. Med. & Hyg., *19*, 389, 1926.
6. BECK, J. S. and HERTZ, C. S.: Standardizing Sickle Cell Method and Evidence of Sickle Cell Trait, Am. J. Clin. Path., *5*, 325, 1935.
7. BEET, E. A.: The Genetics of the Sickle-Cell Trait in a Bantu Tribe, Ann. Eugenics, *14*, 279, 1949.
7a.BERNSTEIN, J. and WHITTEN, C. F.: A Histologic Appraisal of the Kidney in Sickle Cell Anemia, Arch. Path., *70*, 407, 1960.
8. BESSIS, M., BRICKA, M., BRETON-GORIUS, J. and TABUIS, J.: New Observations on Sickle Cells With Special Reference to Their Agglutinability, Blood, *9*, 39, 1954; Rev. hémat., *13*, 249, 1958.
10. BRIDGERS, W. H.: Cerebral Vascular Disease Accompanying Sickle Cell Anemia, Am. J. Path., *15*, 353, 1939.
11. BUNTING, H.: Sedimentation Rates of Sickled and Non-sickled Cells From Patients With Sickle Cell Anemia, Am. J. M. Sc., *198*, 191, 1939.
13. CALERO, C.: Drepanocitemia y Anemia Drepanocitica en el Istmo de Panamá, Arch. Hospital Santo Tomás, *1*, 27, 1946.
14. CALLENDER, S. T. E., NICKEL, J. F., MOORE, C. V. and POWELL, E. O.: Sickle Cell Disease: Studied by Measuring the Survival of Transfused Red Blood Cells, J. Lab. & Clin. Med., *34*, 90, 1949.
15. CAMPBELL, E. H.: Acute Abdominal Pain in Sickle Cell Anemia, Arch. Surg., *31*, 607, 1935.
17. CARROLL, D. S. and EVANS, J. W.: Roentgen Findings in Sickle-Cell Anemia, Radiology, *53*. 834, 1949; South. M. J., *50*, 1486, 1957.

18. CHAPLIN, H., JR., KEITEL, H. G. and PETERSON, R. E.: Hematologic Observations on Patient with Sickle Cell Anemia Sustained at Normal Hemoglobin Levels by Multiple Transfusions, Blood, *11*, 834, 1956.
19. CHOREMIS, C., IKIN, E. W., LEHMANN, H., MOURANT, A. E. and ZANNOS, L.: Sickle-Cell Trait and Blood-Groups in Greece, Lancet, *2*, 911, 1953; *Ibid.*, *2*, 1333, 1957.
20. CLARKE, F.: Sickle Cell Anemia in White Race, Nebraska Med. J., *18*, 376, 1933.
21. COOKE, J. V. and MACK, J. K.: Sickle Cell Anemia in a White American Family, J. Pediat., *5*, 601, 1934.
22. COOLEY, T. B. and LEE, P.: Sickle Cell Anemia in a Greek Family, Am. J. Dis. Child., *38*, 103, 1929.
23. CRONE, R. I., JEFFERSON, S. C., PILEGGI, V. J. and LOWRY, E. C.: Gross Hematuria in Sickle-Cell Trait, A. M. A. Arch. Int. Med., *100*, 597, 1957.
23a.CURTIS, E. M.: Pregnancy in Sickle Cell Anemia, Sickle Cell-Hemoglobin C Disease, and Variants Thereof, Am. J. Obst. & Gynec., *77*, 1312, 1959.
24. DALAND, G. A. and CASTLE, W. B.: A Simple and Rapid Method for Demonstrating Sickling of the Red Blood Cells: The Use of Reducing Agents, J. Lab. & Clin. Med., *33*, 1082, 1948.
25. DELIYANNIS, G. A. and TAVLARAKIS, N.: Sickling Phenomenon in Northern Greece, Brit. M. J., *2*, 299, 1955.
26. DIGGS, L. W.: Siderofibrosis of the Spleen in Sickle Cell Anemia, J.A.M.A., *104*, 538, 1935.
26a.DIGGS, L. W.: The Crisis in Sickle Cell Anemia, Am. J. Clin. Path., *26*, 1109, 1956.
27. DIGGS, L. W., AHMANN, C. F. and BIBB, J.: Incidence and Significance of Sickle Cell Trait, Ann. Int. Med., *7*, 769, 1933.
28. DIGGS, L. W. and BIBB, J.: The Erythrocyte in Sickle Cell Anemia, J.A.M.A., *112*, 695, 1939.
29. DIGGS, L. W. and CHING, R. E.: Pathology of Sickle Cell Anemia, South. M. J., *27*, 839, 1934; *ibid.*, *30*, 249, 1937; A. M. A. Arch. Path., *63*, 336, 1957.
30. DONEGAN, C. C., JR., MACILWAINE, W. A. and LEAVELL, B. S.: Hematologic Studies on Patients with Sickle Cell Anemia Following Multiple Transfusions, Am. J. Med., *17*, 29, 1954.
34. EDINGTON, G. M. and SARKIES, J. W. R.: Two Cases of Sickle-Cell Anæmia Associated with Retinal Microaneurysms, Tr. Roy. Soc. Trop. Med. & Hyg., *46*, 59, 1952.

35. ETTELDORF, J. N., TUTTLE, A. H. and CLAYTON, G. W.: Renal Hemodynamics in Children with Sickle Cell Anemia, Am. J. Dis. Child., 83, 185, 1952; Am. J. Med., 18, 243, 1955.

36. EVANS, R. W.: The Sickling Phenomenon in the Blood of West African Natives, Trans. Roy. Soc. Trop. Med. & Hyg., 37, 281, 1944.

37. FADEM, R. S.: Ovalocytosis Associated with Sickle Cell Trait, Blood, 4, 505, 1949.

39. GOLDIN, A. G., KELTY, K. C. and BEARD, M. F.: Sickle Cell Anemia Terminating in Acute Myeloblastic Leukemia, Ann. Int. Med., 39, 920, 1953.

40. GRAHAM, G. S. and McCARTY, S. H.: Sickle Cell (Meniscocytic) Anemia, South. M. J., 23, 598, 1930.

41. GREENBERG, M. S., KASS, E. H. and CASTLE, W. B.: Factors Influencing the Role of S Hemoglobin in the Pathologic Physiology of Sickle Cell Anemia and Related Disorders, J. Clin. Invest., 36, 833, 1957.

42. GREENWALD, L. and BURRETT, J. B.: Sickle-Cell Anemia in a White Family, Am. J. M. Sc., 199, 768, 1940.

43. GREENWALD, L., SPIELHOLZ, J. B. and LITWINS, J.: Sickling Trait in a White Adult Associated With Hemolytic Anemia, Endocarditis and Malignancy, Am. J. M. Sc., 206, 158, 1943.

44. GUYTON, R. A. and HEINLE, R. W.: Sickle Cell Anemia in the White Race, Am. J. M. Sc., 220, 272, 1950.

48. HADEN, R. L. and EVANS, F. D.: Sickle Cell Anemia in the White Race, Arch. Int. Med., 60, 133, 1937.

49. HAHN, E. V.: Sickle Cell (Drepanocytic) Anemia, Am. J. M. Sc., 175, 206, 1928.

50. HARDEN, A. S.: Sickle Cell Anemia, Changes in the Vessels and in the Bones, Am. Jour. Dis. Child., 54, 1045, 1937.

51. HARRIS, J. W.: Molecular Orientation in Sickle Cell Hemoglobin Solutions, Proc. Soc. Exper. Biol. & Med., 75, 197, 1950; Arch. Int. Med., 97, 145 and 315, 1956.

52. HEINEMANN, H. O. and CHEUNG, M. W.: Renal Concentrating Mechanism in Sickle-Cell Anemia, J. Lab. & Clin. Med., 49, 923, 1957.

53. HENKIN, W. A.: Collapse of the Vertebral Bodies in Sickle Cell Anemia, Am. J. Roentgenol., 62, 395, 1949.

54. HERRICK, J. B.: Peculiar Elongated and Sickle-shaped Red Corpuscles in a Case of Severe Anemia, Arch. Int. Med., 6, 517, 1910.

55. HIGGINS, W. H., JR.: The Heart in Sickle Cell Anemia, South. M. J., 42, 39, 1949.

56. HOOK, E. W., CAMPBELL, C. G., WEENS, H. S. and COOPER, G. R.: Salmonella Osteomyelitis in Patients with Sickle-Cell Anemia, New England J. Med., 257, 403, 1957.

57. HUCK, J. B.: Sickle Cell Anemia, Bull. Johns Hopkins Hosp., 34, 335, 1923.

58. HUGHES, J. G., DIGGS, L. W. and GILLESPIE, C. E.: The Involvement of the Nervous System in Sickle-Cell Anemia, J. Pediat., 17, 166, 1940.

61. ITANO, H. A. and PAULING, L.: A Rapid Diagnostic Test for Sickle Cell Anemia, Blood, 4, 66, 1949.

63. JAMES, G. W., III, and ABBOTT, L. D., JR.: Erythrocyte Destruction in Sickle-Cell Anemia: Simultaneous N^{15}-Hemin and N^{15}-Stercobilin Studies, Proc. Soc. Exper. Biol. & Med., 88, 398, 1955.

64. JENKINS, M. E., SCOTT, R. B. and BAIRD, R. L.: Sudden Death during Sickle Cell Anemia Crises in Young Children, J. Pediat., 56, 30, 1960.

64a. JENSEN, W. N., RUCKNAGEL, D. L. and TAYLOR, W. J.: In Vivo Study of the Sickle Cell Phenomenon, J. Lab. & Clin. Med., 56, 854, 1960.

65. JONES, BARBARA and KLINGBERG, W. G.: Hemoglobin S-Hereditary Spherocytosis, J. Pediat., 54, 375, 1959.

66. JORDAN, R. A.: Cholelithiasis in Sickle Cell Disease, Gastroenterology, 33, 952, 1957.

67. KEITEL, H. G., THOMPSON, D. and ITANO, H. A.: Hyposthenuria in Sickle Cell Anemia, J. Clin. Invest., 35, 998, 1956.

68. KILLINGSWORTH, W. P. and WALLACE, S. A.: Sicklemia in the Soutwest, J.A.M.A., 107, 1508, 1936.

69. KIMMELSTIEL, P.: Vascular Occlusion and Ischemic Infarction in Sickle Cell Disease, Am. J. M. Sc., 216, 11, 1948.

70. KLINEFELTER, H.: The Heart in Sickle Cell Anemia, Am. J. M. Sc., 203, 34, 1942.

71. LAMBOTTE-LEGRAND, J. and LAMBOTTE-LEGRAND, C.: L'anémie à hématies falciformes en Afrique Noire, Sang, 23, 560, 1952; Ann. Soc. belge de méd. trop., 35, 47, 1955.

72. LEAVELL, B. S. and MacILWAINE. W. A.: Sickle Cell Anemia, Monographs in Medicine, Ed. by W. B. Bean, Baltimore, Williams & Wilkins Co., 1952.

73. LEHMANN, H.: Distribution of the Sickle Cell Gene, Eugenics Rev., 46, 3, 1954.

74. LEHMANN, H. and CUTBUSH, M.: Sickle-Cell Trait in Southern India, Brit. M. J., 1, 404, 1952.

74a. LEIKIN, S. L. and McCOO, J. W., JR.: Sickle-

Cell Anemia in Infancy, A. M. A. J. Dis. Child., *96*, 51, 1958.

75. LIACHOWITZ, CLAIRE, ELDERKIN, JANET, GUICHIRIT, I., BROWN, H. W. and RANNEY, HELEN M.: Abnormal Hemoglobins in the Negroes of Surinam, Am. J. Med., *24*, 19, 1958.

76. LIVINGSTONE, F. B.: Anthropological Implications of Sickle Cell Gene Distribution in West Africa, Am. Anthropol., *60*, 533, 1958.

77. MAKRYCOSTAS, K.: Über die Sichelzellänamie, Wien, Arch. inn. Med., *33*, 330 and 390, 1940.

78. MARGOLIES, M. P.: Sickle Cell Anemia: A Composite Study and Survey, Medicine, *30*, 357, 1951.

79. MARTIN, W. W., JR., KOUGH, R. H. and BRANCHE, G. C., JR.: Hereditary Spherocytosis-Sicklemia in the Negro, Blood, *14*, 688, 1959.

80. MARTINS DA SILVA, E.: Estudos sôbre indice de siclemia, Mem. Inst. Oswaldo Cruz, Brasil, *42*, 315, 1945.

82. MYERSON, R. M., HARRISON, ESTHER and LOHMULLER, H. W.: Incidence and Significance of Abnormal Hemoglobins, Am. J. Med., *26*, 543, 1959.

84. NEEL, J. V.: The Inheritance of Sickle Cell Anemia, Science, *110*, 64, 1949; Cold Spring Harbor Symp. on Quant. Biol., *15*, 141, 1951.

85. NEEL, J. V.: Data Pertaining to the Population Dynamics of Sickle Cell Disease, Am. J. Human Genet., *5*, 154, 1953; *ibid.*, *6*, 208, 1954.

86. NEEL, J. V., SCHULL, W. J. and SHAPIRO, H. S.: Absence of Linkage between the Genes Responsible for the Sickling Phenomenon, the MN Blood Types, and the S-agglutinogen, Am. J. Human Genet., *4*, 204, 1952.

87. NEEL, J. V., WELLS, I. C. and ITANO, H. A.: Familial Differences in the Proportions of Abnormal Hemoglobin Present in the Sickle Cell Trait, J. Clin. Invest., *30*, 1120, 1951.

88. OGDEN, M. A.: Sickle Cell Anemia in the White Race, Arch. Int. Med., *71*, 164, 1943.

90. PATERSON, J. C. S. and SPRAGUE, C. C.: Observation on the Genesis of Crises in Sickle Cell Anemia, Ann. Int. Med., *50*, 1502, 1959.

91. PAULING, L., ITANO, H. A., SINGER, S. J. and WELLS, I. C.: Sickle Cell Anemia, a Molecular Disease, Science, *110*, 543, 1949; J. Biol. Chem., *187*, 221, 1950.

92. POLLITZER, W. S., CHERNOFF, A. I., HORTON,

L. L. and FROEHLICH, M.: Hemoglobin Patterns in American Indians, Science, *129*, 216, 1959.

93. PONDER, E.: The Specific Heat and the Heat of Compression of Human Red Cells, Sickled Red Cells, and Paracrystalline Rat Red Cells, J. Gen. Physiol., *38*, 575, 1955.

94. POWELL, W. N., RODARTE, J. G. and NEEL, J. V.: The Occurrence in a Family of Sicilian Ancestry of the Traits for Both Sickling and Thalassemia, Blood, *5*, 887, 1950.

95. PRANKERD, T. A. J.: The Uptake of Radioactive Phosphate and Its Distribution amongst Esters in Sickled Cells, Clin. Sc., *14*, 381, 1955.

96. RAPER, A. B.: Sickle-Cell Disease in Africa and America—A Comparison, J. Trop. Med. & Hyg., *53*, 49, 1950; Nature, *164*, 494, 1949.

98. REBUCK, J. W., STURROCK, R. M. and MONTO, R. W.: Sequential Electron Micrography of Sickling, Lab. Investigation, *4*, 175, 1955.

99. REINHARD, E. H., MOORE, C. V., DUBACH, R. and WADE, L. J.: Depressant Effects of High Concentrations of Inspired Oxygen on Erythrocytogenesis, J. Clin. Invest., *23*, 682, 1944.

100. RICH, A. R.: Splenic Lesion in Sickle Cell Anemia, Bull. Johns Hopkins Hosp., *43*, 398, 1928.

101. ROBERTS, A. R. and HILLBURG, L. E.: Sickle Cell Disease with Salmonella Osteomyelitis, J. Pediat., *52*, 170, 1958.

102. ROSENFELD, S. and PINCUS, J. B.: Occurrence of Sicklemia in White Race, Am. J. M. Sc., *184*, 674, 1932.

102a.ROTTER, R. *et al.*: Splenic Infarction in Sicklemia during Airplane Flight, Ann. Int. Med., *44*, 257, 1956.

103. ROWE, CAROLINE W. and HAGGARD, MARY E.: Bone Infarcts in Sickle-Cell Anemia, Radiology, *68*, 661, 1957.

104. VAN DER SAR, A.: Sickle Cell Disease, Nederl. Tijdsch. v. Geneesk., *93*, 1833, 1949.

105. SCHNEIDER, R. G. and HAGGARD, M. E.: Sickling, a Quantitatively Delayed Genetic Character, Proc. Soc. Exper. Biol. & Med., *89*, 196, 1955.

106. SCRIVER, J. B. and WAUGH, T. R.: Studies on a Case of Sickle Cell Anemia, Canad. M.A.J., *23*, 375, 1930.

107. SEGURA, G., RADICE, J. C., DONIN, L. and GIUSTI, C. Z.: Estudio Anatoma-Patologico del Primer Caso Argentino de Anemia

Falciforme, Rev. Asociacion Med. Argent., *58*, 731, 1944.

107a. SHALDON, S.: Megaloblastic Erythropoiesis Associated with Sickle-Cell Anaemia, Brit. M. J., *7*, 640, 1961.

108. SHEN, S. C., FLEMING, E. M. and CASTLE, W. B.: Irreversibly Sickled Erythrocytes: Their Experimental Production *in Vitro*, Blood, *4*, 498, 1949.

109. SHERMAN, I. J.: The Sickling Phenomenon, With Special Reference to the Differentiation of Sickle Cell Anemia From the Sickle Cell Trait, Bull. Johns Hopkins Hosp., *67*, 309, 1940.

110. SHERMAN, MARY: Pathogenesis of Disintegration of the Hip in Sickle Cell Anemia, South. M. J., *52*, 632, 1959.

110a. SHUKLA, R. N. and SOLANKI, B. R.: Sickle-Cell Trait in Central India, Lancet, *7*, 297, 1958.

111. SIGHTS, W. P. and SIMON, S. D.: Marked Erythrocytic Sickling in White Adult Associated With Anemia, Syphilis and Malaria, J. Med., *12*, 177, 1931.

112. DA SILVA, E. M.: Absence of Sickling Phenomenon of the Red Blood Corpuscle Among Brazilian Indians, Science, *107*, 221, 1948.

114. SINGER, K. and FISHER, B.: Studies on Abnormal Hemoglobins, Blood, *7*, 1216, 1952; *ibid.*, *8*, 270, 1953; J. Lab. & Clin. Med., *42*, 193, 1953.

115. SINGER, K., ROBIN, S., KING, J. C. and JEFFERSON, R. N.: The Life Span of the Sickle Cell and the Pathogenesis of Sickle Cell Anemia, J. Lab. & Clin. Med., *33*, 975, 1948.

116. SMITH, E. W. and CONLEY, C. L.: Sicklemia and Infarction of the Spleen during Aerial Flight, Bull. Johns Hopkins Hosp., *96*, 35, 1955.

116a. SONG, Y. S.: Hepatic Lesions in Sickle Cell Anemia, Am. J. Path., *33*, 331, 1957.

117. SPIER, I. R. and CLIFFTON, E. E.: Local Ambulatory Treatment of Chronic Leg Ulcers with Hyaluronidase, Plasminogen, and Antibiotics, Surg., Gynec. & Obst., *98*, 667, 1954.

117a. SPRAGUE, C. C. and PATERSON, J. C. S.: Role of the Spleen and Effect of Splenectomy in Sickle Cell Disease, Blood, *13*, 569, 1958.

118. SPROULE, B. J., HALDEN, E. R. and MILLER, W. F.: A Study of Cardiopulmonary Alterations in Patients with Sickle Cell Disease and Its Variants, J. Clin. Invest., *37*, 486, 1958.

118a. STENTON, P.: Permanent Sickle Cell Preparations, J. Clin. Path., *12*, 484, 1959.

119. SUAREZ, R. M., BUSO, R., MEYER, L. M. and

OLAVARRIETA, S. T.: Distribution of Abnormal Hemoglobins in Puerto Rico and Survival Studies of Red Blood Cells Using Cr^{51}, Blood, *14*, 255, 1959.

120. SUKUMARAN, P. K., SANGHVI, L. D. and VYAS, G. N.: Sickle-Cell Trait in Some Tribes of Western India, Current Sc., *25*, 290, 1956.

121. SWITZER, P. K.: The Incidence of the Sickle Cell Trait in Negroes from the Sea Island Area of South Carolina, South. M. J., *43*, 48, 1950.

122. SYDENSTRICKER, V. P.: Further Observations on Sickle Cell Anemia, J.A.M.A., *83*, 12, 1924.

123. TANAKA, K. R., CLIFFORD, G. O. and AXELROD, A. R.: Sickle Cell Anemia (Homozygous S) with Aseptic Necrosis of Femoral Head, Blood, *11*, 998, 1956.

124. TOMLINSON, W. J.: The Incidence of Sicklemia and Sickle Cell Anemia in 3000 Canal Zone Examinations Upon Natives of Central America, Am. J. M. Sc., *209*, 181, 1945.

125. ——————Abdominal Crises in Uncomplicated Sickle Cell Anemia, Am. J. M. Sc., *209*, 722, 1945.

126. ——————A Study of the Circulation of the Spleen in Sicklemia and Sickle Cell Anemia, Am. J. Path., *21*, 877, 1945.

127. TROWELL, H. C., RAPER, A. B. and WELBOURN, H. F.: The Natural History of Homozygous Sickle-Cell Anaemia in Central Africa, Quart. J. Med., *26*, 401, 1957.

127a. VANDEPITTE, J. M.: Aspects quantitatifs et génétiques de la sicklémie à Léopoldville, Ann. Soc. belge de méd. trop., *34*, 501, 1954.

128. VANDEPITTE, J. M., ZUELZER, W. W., NEEL, J. V. and COLAERT, J.: Evidence Concerning the Inadequacy of Mutation as an Explanation of the Frequency of the Sickle Cell Gene in the Belgian Congo, Blood, *10*, 341, 1955.

129. WALLER, M., WALLER, R. K. and HUGHES, R. D.: Linkage Studies of Genes for Sickling and MNS Blood Groups, Proc. Soc. Exper. Biol. & Med., *80*, 479, 1952.

130. WATSON, J.: The Significance of the Paucity of Sickle Cells in Newborn Negro Infants, Am. J. M. Sc., *215*, 419, 1948.

130a. WATSON, R. J., LICHTMAN, H. C. and SHAPIRO, H. D.: Splenomegaly in Sickle Cell Anemia, Am. J. Med., *20*, 196, 1956.

131. WEINER, S. B.: Sickle Cell Anemia in Italian Child, J. Mt. Sinai Hospital, *4*, 88, 1937.

132. WEISS, P., ALTUNA, M. T. and DIAZ, H. C.: Sobre dos casos de anemias con erytrocitos en forma de hoz encontrados en Lima, Actualidad Médica Peruana, *7*, 2, 1935.

133. WELLS, I. C. and ITANO, H. A.: Ratio of Sickle Cell Anemia Hemoglobin to Normal Hemoglobin in Sicklemics, J. Biol. Chem., *188*, 65, 1951.

134. WENT, L. N. and MacIVER, J. E.: Sickle-Cell Anaemia in Adults and Its Differentiation from Sickle-Cell Thalassaemia, Lancet, *2*, 824, 1958.

135. WINSOR, T. and BURCH, G. E.: Diagnostic Physicochemical Blood Tests in Sickle Cell Anemia, Am. J. M. Sc., *207*, 152, 1944; J.A.M.A., *129*, 793, 1945.

136. ————Habitus of Patients With Active Sickle Cell Anemia of Long Duration, Arch. Int. Med., *76*, 47, 1945.

Abnormal Hemoglobinopathies Other than Sickle Cell Anemia

139. AGER, J. A. M. and LEHMANN, H.: Intra-Erythrocytic Haemoglobin Crystals, J. Clin. Path., *10*, 336, 1957.

140. AGER, J. A. M. and LEHMANN, H.: Haemoglobin L, Brit. M. J., *2*, 142, 1957; Acta genet. statist. med., *9*, 202, 1959.

141. AGER, J. A. M. and LEHMANN, H.: Observations on Some "Fast" Haemoglobins: K, J, N, and "Bart's", Brit. M. J., *1*, 929, 1958; Nature, *187*, 158, 1960.

142. AGER, J. A. M. and LEHMANN, H.: Haemoglobin "Norfolk", Brit. M. J., *2*, 539, 1958.

142a.AGER, J. A. M., LEHMANN, H. and VANDE-PITTE, J. M.: Role of Paper Electrophoresis in the Identification of Human Hemoglobin, Lancet, *1*, 318, 1958.

143. AKSOY, M., BIRD, G. W. G., LEHMANN, H., MOURANT, A. E., THEIN, H. and WICKRE-MASINGHE, R. L.: Haemoglobin E in Asia, J. Physiol., *130*, 56, 1955.

144. AKSOY, M. and LEHMANN, H.: The First Observation of Sickle-Cell Haemoglobin E Disease, Nature, *179*, 1248, 1957.

145. ARENDS, T., LAYRISSE, M. and RINCON, A. R.: Sickle Cell-Haemoglobin D Disease in a Portuguese Child, Acta haemat., *22*, 118, 1959.

145a.ATWATER, JEAN, SCHWARTZ, I. R. and TOCANTINS, L. M.: A Variety of Human Hemoglobin with 4 Distinct Electrophoretic Components, Blood, *15*, 901, 1960.

145b.ATWATER, JEAN *et al.:* Sickling of Erythrocytes in a Patient with Thalassemia-Hemoglobin-I Disease, New England J. Med., *263*, 1215, 1960.

146. BENZER S., INGRAM, V. M. and LEHMANN, H.: Three Varieties of Human Haemoglobin D, Nature, *182*, 852, 1958.

147. BINGLE, J. P., HUEHNS, E. R. and PRANKERD, T. A. J.: Haemoglobin-H Disease, Brit. M. J., *2*, 1389, 1958.

147a.BRADLEY, T. B., JR., BOYER, S. H. and ALLEN, F. H., JR.: Hopkins-2-Hemoglobin, Bull. Johns Hopkins Hosp., *108*, 75, 1961.

148. BRAIN, P.: Incidence of Haemoglobin C in the 'Coloured' Population of Cape Town, Nature, *175*, 262, 1955.

149. BRUMPT, L., BRUMPT, V., COQUELET, M. L. and DE TRAVERSE, P. M.: La détection de l'hémoglobine E, Rev. hémat., *13*, 21, 1958.

149a.CABANNES, R. and BUHR, L.: Une nouvelle fraction hémoglobinique humaine à migration electrophorique plus rapide que l'hemoglobine A et moins rapide que l'hemoglobine H, Pédiatrie, *10*, 838, 1955.

150. CABANNES, R., SENDRA, L., et DALAUT: Hémoglobinose D, Algérie-méd., *59*, 387, 1955.

150a.————: Nouvelle hémoglobine humaine héréditaire à migration plus rapide que l'hémoglobine normale, Compt. rend. Soc. de biol., *149*, 914, 1955.

150b.CHATTERJEA, J. B., SAHA, A. K., RAY, R. N. and GHOSH, S. K.: Hemoglobin E-Thalassemia Disease, Indian J. Med. Sc., *11*, 553, 1957.

151. CHERNOFF, A. I.: The Human Hemoglobins in Health and Disease, New England J. Med., *253*, 322, 365 and 416, 1955; Am. J. Human Genet., *13*, 151, 1961.

151a.CHERNOFF, A. I.: The Hemoglobin D Syndromes, Blood, *8*, 116, 1958.

152. CHERNOFF, A. I. and MINNICH, V.: Hemoglobin E, a Hereditary Abnormality of Human Hemoglobin, Science, *120*, 605, 1954; J. Lab. & Clin. Med., *47*, 455 and 490, 1956; Blood, *12*, 529, 1957.

152a.CHOREMIS, C., ZANNOS-MARIOLEA, L., AGER, J. A. M. and LEHMANN, H.: Persistence of Haemoglobin "Bart's" beyond Infancy in a Child with Thalassaemia, Brit. M. J., *2*, 348, 1959.

153. COLBOURNE, M. J. *et al.:* Haemoglobin E and the Diego Blood Group Antigen in Sarawak and Burma, Nature, *181*, 119, 1958.

153a.DHERTE, PAULETTE, LEHMANN, H. and VANDEPITTE, J.: Haemoglobin P in a Family in the Belgian Congo, Nature, *184*, 1133, 1959.

153b.DHERTE, PAULETTE, VANDEPITTE, J., AGER, J. A. M. and LEHMANN, H.: Stanleyville I and II, Brit. M. J., *2*, 282, 1959.

154. DIGGS, L. W., KRAUS, A. P., MORRISON, D. B. and RUDNICKI, R. P. T.: Intra-erythrocytic Crystals in a White Patient with Hemoglobin C in the Absence of Other Types of Hemoglobin, Blood, *9*, 1172, 1954; J. Lab. & Clin. Med., *47*, 700, 1956.

155. DITTMAN, W. A., HAUT, A., WINTROBE, M. M. and CARTWRIGHT, G. E.: Hemoglobin H Associated with an Uncommon Variant of Thalassemia Trait, Blood, *15*, 975, 1960.

155a. EDINGTON, G. M. and LAING, W. M.: Relationship between Hemoglobins C and S and Malaria in Ghana, Brit. M. J., *1*, 143, 1957.

156. EDINGTON, G. M. and LEHMANN, H.: A Case of Sickle Cell-Hæmoglobin C Disease and a Survey of Hæmoglobin C Incidence in West Africa, Tr. Roy. Soc. Trop. Med. & Hyg., *48*, 332, 1954; Man, *56*, 34, 1956; Nature, *183*, 1587, 1959.

157. ———Hæmoglobin G. A New Hæmoglobin Found in a West African, Lancet, *2*, 173, 1954; Nature, *175*, 850, 1955.

158. FESSAS, P., MASTROKALOS, N. and FOSTIROPOULOS, G.: New Variant of Human Foetal Haemoglobin, Nature, *183*, 30, 1959.

158a. FESSAS, P. and PAPASPYROU, ATHENA: New "Fast" Hemoglobin Associated with Thalassemia, Science, *126*, 1119, 1957.

158b. GALBRAITH, P. A. and GREEN, P. T.: Hemoglobin C Disease in an Anglo-Saxon Family, Am. J. Med., *28*, 969, 1960.

158c. GAMMACK, D. B., HUEHNS, E. R. and SHOOTER, E. M.: Identification of the Abnormal Polypeptide Chain of Haemoglobin G_{Ib}, J. Mol. Biol., *2*, 372, 1960; Acta genet., *11*, 1, 1961.

158d. GÖKSEL, V. and TARTAROGLU, N.: Hämoglobin D, Blut, *6*, 213, 1960.

159. GOUTTAS, A., FESSAS, P., TSEVRENIS, H. and XEFTERI, E.: Déscription d'une nouvelle varieté d'anémie hémolytique congénitale, Sang, *26*, 911, 1955.

159a. GERALD, P. S. and DIAMOND, L. K.: A New Hereditary Hemoglobinopathy (the Lepore Trait) and Its Interaction with Thalassemia Trait, Blood, *13*, 835, 1958; A. M. A. J. Dis. Child., *97*, 464, 1959.

159b. HEDENBERG, F., MÜLLER-EBERHARD, U., SJÖLIN, S. and WRANNE, L.: Haemoglobin H and Inclusion-Body Anaemia in a Swedish Family, Acta paediat., *47*, 652, 1958.

159c. HENDRICKSE, R. G., BOYO, A. E., FITZGERALD, P. A. and KUTI, S. R.: Studies on the Haemoglobin of Newborn Nigerians, Brit. M. J., *1*, 611, 1960.

159d. HERMAN, E. C., JR. and CONLEY, C. L.: Hereditary Persistence of Fetal Hemoglobin, Am. J. Med., *29*, 9, 1960; Bull. Johns Hopkins Hosp., *108*, 242, 1961.

159e. HILL, R. L.: Personal Communication.

160. HILL, R. L., SWENSON, R. T. and SCHWARTZ, H. C.: Characterization of a Chemical Abnormality in Hemoglobin G, J. Biol. Chem., *235*, 3182, 1960.

161. HOOK, E. W. and COOPER, G. R.: The Clinical Manifestations of Sickle Cell-Hemoglobin C Disease and Sickle Cell Anemia, South. M. J., *51*, 610, 1958.

161a. HUEHNS, E. R., FLYNN, F. V., BUTLER, ELIZABETH A. and SHOOTER, E. M.: The Occurrence of Haemoglobin 'Bart's' in Conjunction with Haemoglobin H, Brit. J. Haemat., *6*, 388, 1960.

162. HUISMAN, T. H. J., VAN DER SCHAAF, P. C. and VAN DER SAR, A.: Some Characteristic Properties of Hemoglobin C, Blood, *10*, 1079, 1955.

163. HYNES, M. and LEHMANN, H.: Haemoglobin D in a Persian Girl: Presumably the First Case of Haemoglobin-D-Thalassaemia, Brit. M. J., *2*, 923, 1956.

164. ITANO, H. A.: A Third Abnormal Hemoglobin Associated with Hereditary Hemolytic Anemia, Proc. Nat. Acad. Sc., *37*, 775, 1951.

164a. ITANO, H. A.: Solubility of Naturally Occurring Mixtures of Human Hemoglobins, Arch. Biochem., *47*, 148, 1953; Advances in Protein Chemistry, *12*, 213, 1957.

165. ITANO, H. A., BERGREN, W. R. and STURGEON, P.: Identification of a Fourth Abnormal Human Hemoglobin, J. Am. Chem. Soc., *76*, 2278, 1954.

166. JENSEN, W. N., SCHOEFIELD, R. A. and AGNER, R.: Clinical and Necropsy Findings in Hemoglobin C Disease, Blood, *12*, 74, 1957.

167. JIM, R. T. S.: Hemoglobin H Disease, A. M. A. Arch. Int. Med., *102*, 400, 1958.

168. JIM, R. T. S.: Hemoglobin J in a Healthy Hawaiian-Chinese-Caucasian Male, Blood, *15*, 285, 1960.

169. KAPLAN, E., ZUELZER, W. W. and NEEL, J. V.: A New Inherited Abnormality of Hemoglobin and Its Interaction with Sickle Cell Hemoglobin, Blood, *6*, 1240, 1951.

169a. LAMBOTTE-LEGRAND, J., LAMBOTTE-LEGRAND, C., AGER, J. A. M. and LEHMANN, H.: L'hémoglobinose P. A propos d'un cas d'association des hémoglobines P et S, Rev. hémat., *15*, 10, 1960.

169b. LEHMANN, H.: Classification and Identification of Human Haemoglobins, Proc. Roy. Soc. Med., *52*, 959, 1959.

170. LEHMANN, H., STORY, P. and THEIN, H.: Haemoglobin E in Burmese. Two Cases of Haemoglobin E Disease, Brit. M. J., *1*, 544, 1956.

171. LIE-INJO LUAN ENG and OEY HOEY GIOK: Homozygous Haemoglobin-E Disease in Indonesia, Lancet, *1*, 20, 1957.

171a.Lie-Injo Luan Eng and Sadono: Haemoglobin O (Buginese X) in Sulawesi, Brit. M. J., 7, 1461, 1958.

172. Marder, V. J. and Conley, C. L.: Frequency of Hemoglobin D in a Negro Population, Bull. Johns Hopkins Hosp., 105, 77, 1959.

172a.McCormick, W. F. and Humphreys, Eleanor W.: High Fetal-Hemoglobin C Disease, Blood, 16, 1736, 1960.

173. Neel, J. V.: Human Hemoglobin Types. Their Epidemiologic Implications, New England J. Med., 256, 161, 1957.

174. Neel, J. V. et al.: Data on the Occurrence of Hemoglobin C and Other Abnormal Hemoglobins in Some African Populations, Am. J. Human Genet., 8, 138, 1956.

175. Ober, W. B., Bruno, M. S., Simon, R. M. and Weiner, L.: Hemoglobin S-C Disease with Fat Embolism, Am. J. Med., 27, 647, 1959.

175a.Olivia, J. and Myerson, R. M.: Hereditary Persistence of Fetal Hemoglobin, Am. J. M. Sc., 241, 215, 1961.

176. Perosa, L., Ramunni, M., Bini, L. and Manganelli, G.: Su quattro casi di una sindrome emopatica osservata in complessi familiari greci, caratterizzata da una Hb elettroforeticamente più veloce dell'Hb A (cosiddetta Hb H ?) e da una spiccata ovalocitosi, Haematologica, 43, 1, 1958.

177. Portier, A., Cabannes, R., Massonnat, J. and Duzer, A.: L'hémoglobinose C, Semaine hôp. Paris (Arch. biol. med.), 32, 1, 1956.

177a.Ramot, B., Sheba, Ch., Fisher, S., Ager, J. A. M. and Lehmann, H.: Haemoglobin H Disease with Persistent Haemoglobin "Bart's" in an Oriental Jewess and Her Daughter, Brit. M. J., 2, 1228, 1959.

177b.Ramot, B. et al.: Haemoglobin O in an Arab Family, Brit. M. J., 2, 1262, 1960.

178. Ranney, H. M.: Observations on the Inheritance of Sickle-Cell Hemoglobin and Hemoglobin C, J. Clin. Invest., 33, 1634, 1954.

178a.Raper, A. B., Ager, J. A. M. and Lehmann, H.: Haemoglobin "Singapore-Bristol", Brit. M. J., 1, 1537, 1960.

178b.Raper, A. B., Gammack, D. B., Huehns, E. R. and Shooter, E. M.: Four Haemoglobins in One Individual, Brit. M. J., 2, 1257, 1960.

179. Rice, H. M.: Haemoglobin C Disease and Trait, Brit. M. J., 1, 25, 1957.

180. Rigas, D. A., Koler, R. D. and Osgood, E. E.: New Hemoglobin Possessing a Higher Electrophoretic Mobility than Normal Adult Hemoglobin, Science, 121, 372, 1955; J. Lab. & Clin. Med., 47, 51, 1956.

180a.Robinson, A. R. et al.: Two "Fast" Hemoglobin Components in Liberian Blood Samples, Blood, 11, 902, 1956.

180b.Robinson, A. R., Robson, M., Harrison, A. P. and Zuelzer, W. W.: A New Technique for the Differentiation of Hemoglobin, J. Lab. & Clin. Med., 50, 745, 1957.

181. Rucknagel, D. L., Page, E. B. and Jensen, W. N.: Hemoglobin I: An Inherited Hemoglobin Anomaly, Blood, 10, 999, 1955.

182. Schneider, R. G.: Incidence of Hemoglobin C Trait in 505 Normal Negroes: A Family with Homozygous Hemoglobin C and Sickle-Cell Trait Union, J. Lab. & Clin. Med., 44, 133, 1954.

182a.Schneider, Rose G. and Haggard, Mary Ellen: Haemoglobin P (the 'Galveston' Type), Nature, 182, 322, 1958.

182b.Schneider, Rose G. and Haggard, Mary Ellen: A Family with Hemoglobin G, J. Lab. & Clin. Med., 55, 60, 1960.

183. Schwartz, H. C. and Spaet, T. H.: Hemoglobin G: Clinical and Genetic Observations on the Occurrence of a Fifth Abnormal Hemoglobin, Clin. Res. Proc., 3, 51, 1955; Blood, 12, 238, 1957.

183a.Shelley, W. M. and Curtis, E. M.: Bone Marrow and Fat Embolism in Sickle Cell Anemia and Sickle Cell-Hemoglobin C Disease, Bull. Johns Hopkins Hosp., 103, 8, 1958.

183b.Shooter, E. M.: Personal Communication.

184. Shooter, E. M., Skinner, E. R., Garlick, J. P. and Barnicot, N. A.: The Electrophoretic Characterization of Haemoglobin G and a New Minor Haemoglobin, G₂, Brit. J. Haemat., 6, 140, 1960.

185. Singer, K., Chapman, A. Z., Goldberg, S. R., Rubinstein, H. M. and Rosenblum, S. A.: Pure (Homozygous) Hemoglobin C Disease, Blood, 9, 1023, 1954.

186. Singer, K., Kraus, A. P., Singer, L., Rubinstein, H. M. and Goldberg, S. R.: A New Syndrome: Hemoglobin C-Thalassemia Disease, Blood, 9, 1032, 1954; ibid., 12, 593, 1957.

187. Smith, E. W. and Conley, C. L.: Clinical Features of the Genetic Variants of Sickle Cell Disease, Bull. Johns Hopkins Hosp., 94, 289, 1954.

188. Smith, E. W. and Conley, C. L.: Sickle Cell-Hemoglobin D Disease, Ann. Int. Med., 50, 94, 1959.

189. Smith, E. W. and Krevans, J. R.: Clinical Manifestations of Hemoglobin C Disorders, Bull. Johns Hopkins Hosp., 104, 17, 1959.

190. Smith, E. W. and Torbert, J. V.: Study of Two Abnormal Hemoglobins with Evi-

dence of a New Genetic Locus for Hemoglobin Formation, Bull. Johns Hopkins
Hosp., *101*, 38, 1958.

191. STURGEON, P., ITANO, H. A. and BERGREN,
W. R.: The Interaction of Hemoglobin-S
with Hemoglobin-D, Blood, *10*, 389, 1955.

191a. STURGEON, P., JONES, R. T., BERGREN, W.
R. and SCHROEDER, W. A.: Observations
on "Bart's" and the "Fast" Hemoglobins of
Thalassemia H Disease, (to be published).

192. TERRY, D. W., MOTULSKY, A. G. and RATH,
C. E.: Homozygous Hemoglobin C, New
England J. Med., *251*, 365, 1954.

193. THOMAS, E. D., MOTULSKY, A. G. and
WALTERS, D. H.: Homozygous Hemoglobin C Disease, Am. J. Med., *18*, 832,
1955.

194. THORUP, O. A., ITANO, H. A., WHEBY, M.
and LEAVELL, B. S.: Hemoglobin J,
Science, *123*, 889, 1956.

195. TRINCÂO, C., DE ALMEIDA FRANCO, L. T. and
NOGUEIRA, A. R.: Haemoglobin N in
Portuguese Guinea, Nature, *183*, 193, 1959.

195a. TUCHINDA, S., VAREENIL, C., BHANCHIT, P.
and MINNICH, VIRGINIA: "Fast" Hemoglobin Component Found in Umbilical-
Cord Blood of Thai Babies, Pediatrics, *24*,
43, 1959.

196. TUTTLE, A. H. and KOCH, B.: Clinical and
Hematological Manifestations of Hemoglobin CS Disease in Children, J. Pediat.,
56, 331, 1960.

197. VEGAS, F. and ORTIZ RIVAS, E.: Estudio sobre
las hemoglobinas, Med. latina, *15*, 183,
1956.

198. VELLA, F., AGER, J. A. M. and LEHMANN, H.:
An Abnormal Haemoglobin in a Chinese:
Haemoglobin G, Nature, *182*, 460, 1958.

198a. VELLA, F. and YEOH, O. S.: Haemoglobin
E-Thalassaemia in Two Unrelated Chinese
Patients, Proc. Alumni A., Malaya, *11*,
159, 1958; *ibid.*, *12*, 97, 1959.

198b. VELLA, F., WELLS, R. H. C., AGER, J. A. M.
and LEHMANN, H.: A Haemoglobinopathy
Involving Haemoglobin H and a New (Q)
Haemoglobin, Brit. M. J., *1*, 752, 1958.

198c. WASI, P., GITHENS, J. and HAHTAWAY, W.:
Hemoglobin J in an American Caucasian
Family of Swedish Ancestry, Blood, *16*,
1795, 1960.

199. WEINSTEIN, I. M., SPURLING, C. L., KLEIN,
H. and NECHELES, T. F.: Radioactive
Sodium Chromate for the Study of Survival
of Red Blood Cells, Blood, *9*, 1155, 1954.

199a. WENT, L. N. and MACIVER, J. E.: Sickle-
Cell/Haemoglobin-J Disease, Brit. M. J., *2*,
138, 1959.

199b. WHEBY, M. S., THORUP, O. A. and LEAVELL,
B. S.: Homozygous Hemoglobin C Disease

in Siblings: Further Comment on Intra-
erythrocytic Crystals, Blood, *11*, 266, 1956.

Thalassemia

200. AKSOY, M.: Thalassaemia Minor with Large
Amount of Fetal Haemoglobin, Acta
haemat., *22*, 188, 1959; *ibid.*, *25*, 136 and
200, 1961.

200a. AKSOY, M. and LEHMANN, H.: Sickle-Cell-
Thalassaemia Disease in South Turkey,
Brit. M. J., *1*, 734, 1957.

200b. ALBAHARY, C. *et al.*: Hémoglobines anormales
au Sud-Vietnam, Rev. hémat., *13*, 163,
1958.

200c. ANDRÉ, R. *et al.*: Association d'un syndrome
thalassémique et d'une hémoglobine anormale à l'électrophorése, non encore identi-
fiée, chez un français d'origine picarde,
Rev. hémat., *13*, 31, 1958.

201. ANGELINI, V.: Primi resultati di richerche
ematologiche nei familiari di ammalati di
anemia di Cooley, Minerva med., *28*, (II),
331, 1937.

202. ASTALDI, G. and TOLENTINO, P.: Studies on
the Pathogenesis of Thalassaemia, J. Clin.
Path., *5*, 140, 1952; Acta haemat., *12*,
145, 1954.

203. BANNERMAN, R. M., GRINSTEIN, M. and
MOORE, C. V.: Haemoglobin Synthesis in
Thalassaemia; *in vitro* Studies, Brit. J
Haemat., *5*, 102, 1959.

204. BANTON, A. H.: A Genetic Study of Mediterranean Anæmia in Cyprus, Am. J. Human
Genet., *3*, 47, 1951.

205. BATY, J. M., BLACKFAN, K. D. and DIAMOND,
L. K.: Blood Studies in Infants and in
Children; Erythroblastic Anemia, Am.
J. Dis. Child., *43*, 667, 1932.

206. BESSIS, M., ALAGILLE, D. and BRETON-GORIUS,
J.: Particularités des érythrocytes dans la
maladie de Cooley, Rev. hémat., *13*, 538,
1958; Blood, *14*, 423, 1959.

207. CAFFEY, J.: Cooley's Anemia: A Review of the
Roentgenographic Findings in the Skeleton, Am. J. Roentgenol., *78*, 381, 1957.

207a. CAMINOPETROS, J.: Researches on Infantile
Erythroblastic Anemia in People of Eastern
Mediterranean, Ann. de méd., *43*, Jan.,
27–61, Feb., 104–125, 1938.

208. CARTWRIGHT, G. E., HUGULEY, C. M., JR.,
ASHENBRUCKER, H., FAY, J. and WINTROBE,
M. M.: Studies on Free Erythrocyte Proto-
porphyrin, Plasma Iron and Plasma Cop-
per in Normal and Anemic Subjects,
Blood, *3*, 501, 1948.

208a. CAROLI, J. *et al.*: Hémochromatose avec
anémie hypochrome et absence d'hémoglobine normale. Étude au microscope
électronique, Presse méd., *65*, 1991, 1957.

208b. CEPPELINI, R.: L'emoglobina normale lenta A₂, Acta Genet. med., Suppl. 2, p. 47, 1959.

208c. CHATTERJEA, J. B., SWARUP, SUSHIELA, GHOSH, S. K. and RAY, R. N.: Hb. S-Thalassaemia Disease in India, J. Indian M. A., 30, 4, 1958.

209. CHANARIN, I., DACIE, J. V. and MOLLIN, D. L.: Folic Acid Deficiency in Hemolytic Anemia, Brit. J. Haemat., 5, 245, 1959.

209a. CHERNOFF, A. I.: The Distribution of the Thalassemia Gene: A Historical Review, Blood, 14, 899, 1959.

210. CHINI, V. and VALERI, C. M.: Mediterranean Hemopathic Syndromes, Blood, 4, 989, 1949.

210a. CHOREMIS, C., KIOSSOGLOU, K., MAOUNIS, F. and BASTI, B.: Amino-Acid Tolerance Curves and Amino-Aciduria in Cooley's and Sickle-Cell Anaemias, J. Clin. Path., 12, 245, 1959.

210b. COHEN, FLOSSIE, ZUELZER, W. W., NEEL, J. V. and ROBINSON, A. R.: Multiple Inherited Erythrocyte Abnormalities in an American Negro Family: Hereditary Spherocytosis, Sickling and Thalassemia, Blood, 14, 816, 1959.

211. COOLEY, T. B. and LEE, P.: Series of Cases of Splenomegaly in Children With Anemia and Peculiar Bone Change, Trans. Am. Pediat. Soc., 37, 29, 1925.

212. ———Erythroblastic Anemia, Am. J. Dis. Child., 43, 705, 1932.

213. COOPER, C. D. and WACKER, W. E. C.: The Successful Therapy with Streptokinase-Streptodornase of Ankle Ulcers Associated with Mediterranean Anemia, Blood, 9, 241, 1954.

213a. CRADOCK-WATSON, J. E., FENTON, J. C. B. and LEHMANN, H.: TRIS Buffer for the Demonstration of Haemoglobin A₂ by Paper Electrophoresis, J. Clin. Path., 12, 372, 1959.

214. CROSBY, W. H. and SACKS, H. J.: The Co-incidence of Mediterranean Anemia and Pernicious Anemia in a Young Sicilian, Blood, 4, 1267, 1949.

217. DAMESHEK, W.: "Target Cell" Anemia: Anerythroblastic Type of Cooley's Erythroblastic Anemia, Am. J. M. Sc., 200, 445, 1940; Ibid., 205, 643, 1943.

222. ERLANDSON, M. E., SCHULMAN, I., STERN, GERTRUDE and SMITH, C. H.: Rates of Destruction and Production of Erythrocytes in Thalassemia, Pediatrics, 22, 910, 1958.

229. FREUDENBERG, E. and ESSER, M.: Pathogenesis of Cooley's Anemia, Ann. pædiat., 158, 128, 1942.

231. GERALD, P. S. and DIAMOND, L. K.: The Di-agnosis of Thalassemia Trait by Starch Block Electrophoresis of the Hemoglobin, Blood, 13, 61, 1958.

232. GREIG, H. B. W. and METZ, J.: The Periodic-Acid-Schiff Reaction as a Diagnostic Aid in Thalassaemia, South African J. M. Sc., 22, 7, 1957.

233. GRINSTEIN, M., BANNERMAN, R. M., VAVRA, J. D. and MOORE, C. V.: Hemoglobin Metabolism in Thalassemia, Am. J. Med., 29, 18, 1960.

236. HAMILTON, H. E., SHEETS, R. F. and DE-GOWIN, E. L.: Analysis of Mechanism of Cooley's Anemia, J. Clin. Invest., 29, 693, 1950.

238. HOFFMAN, J. F., WOLMAN, I. J., HILLIER, J. and PARPART, A. K.: Ultrastructure of Erythrocyte Membranes in Thalassemia Major and Minor, Blood, 11, 946, 1956.

238a. HUEHNS, E. R. and SHOOTER, E. M.: The Polypeptide Chains of Haemoglobin A₂, Nature, 1961 (to be published).

238b. HUISMAN, T. H. J. and MEYERING, C. A.: Studies on the Heterogeneity of Hemoglobin I. The Heterogeneity of Different Human Hemoglobin Types in Carboxymethyl Cellulose and in Amberlite IRC-50 Chromatography: Qualitative Aspects, Clin. Chim. Acta, 5, 103, 1960; Nature, 190, 357, 1961.

239. INGRAM, V. M. and STRETTON, A. O. W.: Genetic Basis of the Thalassaemia Diseases, Nature, 184, 1903, 1959.

240. INGRAM, V. M. and STRETTON, A. O. W.: Human Haemoglobin A₂: Chemistry, Genetics and Evolution, Nature, 1961 (to be published).

241. JANDL, J. H. and GREENBERG, M. S.: Bone-Marrow Failure Due to Relative Nutritional Deficiency in Cooley's Hemolytic Anemia, New England J. Med., 260, 461, 1959.

244. KAPLAN, E. and ZUELZER, W. W.: Erythrocyte Survival Studies in Childhood, J. Lab. & Clin. Med., 36, 517, 1950.

246. KATO, K. and DOWNEY, H.: Hematology of Erythroblastic Anemia, Folia hæmat., 50, 55, 1933.

246a. KNOBLICH, R.: Extramedullary Hematopoiesis Presenting as Intrathoracic Tumors, Cancer, 13, 462, 1960.

247. KUNKEL, H. G., CEPPELLINI, R., MÜLLER-EBERHARD, U. and WOLF, J.: Observations on the Minor Basic Hemoglobin Component in the Blood of Normal Individuals and Patients with Thalassemia, J. Clin. Invest., 36, 1615, 1957.

248. LOVISETTO, P., LUCCI, R., CASTELLANO, M. and VALLISNERI, E.: A Study of the Haemo-

globin Types Found in the Thalassaemic Population of the Delta of the Po, Acta haemat., *22*, 38, 1959.

249. LUDWIN, I., LIMENTANI, D. and DAMESHEK, W.: Linkage Tests of Mediterranean Anemia with Blood Groups, Blood Types, Rh Factors and Eye Color, Am. J. Human Genet., *4*, 182, 1952.

249a. MacIVER, J. E., WENT, L. N. and CRUICKSHANK, E. K.: Sickle Cell-Thalassemia Dissease in Jamaica, Blood, *13*, 359, 1958.

249b. MARINONE, G. and BERNASCONI, C.: Das Verhalten des langsamen Hämoglobins des Erwachsenen (HbA$_\beta$) bei Normalen und bei Thalassämie. Quantitative elektrophoretische Studie, Folia haemat., *2*, 28, 1958.

249c. MARINONE, G., BERNASCONI, C., GAUTIER, A. and MARCOVICI, I.: Studi di citologia elettronica nella talassemia, Haematologica, *43*, 1123, 1958.

250. MARMONT, A. and BIANCHI, V.: Mediterranean Anemia, Acta hæmat., *1*, 4, 1948.

250a. MARTI, H. R. and BETKE, K.: Das Vorkommen der Thalassämie in der deutschen Schweiz, Schweiz. med. Wchnschr., *89*, 1079, 1959.

251. MATIOLI, G. and DEL PIANO, E.: Emazie talassemiche e corpi di Heinz, Haematologica, *44*, 739, 1959.

252. MINNICH, V., NA-NAKORN, S., CHONGCHAREONSUK, S. and KOCHASENI, S.: Mediterranean Anemia. A Study of Thirty-two Cases in Thailand, Blood, *9*, 1, 1954.

253. NEEL, J. V. and VALENTINE, W. N.: The Frequency of Thalassemia, Am. J. M. Sc., *209*, 568, 1945; Genetics, *32*, 38, 1947.

254. OLESEN, E. B. *et al.*: Thalassaemia in Liberia, Brit. M. J., *1*, 1385, 1959.

255. PASCHER, FRANCES and KEEN, R.: Ulcers of the Leg in Cooley's Anemia, New England J. Med., *256*, 1220, 1957.

256. REEMTSMA, K. and ELLIOTT, R. H. E., JR.: Splenectomy in Mediterranean Anemia: An Evaluation of Long-Term Results, Ann. Surg., *144*, 999, 1956.

257. RICH, A.: Studies on the Hemoglobin of Cooley's Anemia and Cooley's Trait, Proc. Nat. Acad. Sc., *38*, 187, 1952.

258. ROCHE, R. *et al.*: Coexistence des tares sicklémique et thalassémique dans une famille tunisienne, Rev. hémat., *11*, 26, 1956.

259. RUNDLES, R. W. and FALLS, H. F.: Hereditary (?Sex-Linked) Anemia, Am. J. M. Sc., *211*, 641, 1946.

260. SANGHVI, L. D., SUKUMARAN, P. K. and LEHMANN, H.: Haemoglobin J Trait in Two Indian Women Associated with Thalassaemia in One, Brit. M. J., *2*, 828, 1958.

261. SANSONE, G. and MASSIMO, L.: Riconoscimento dei globuli rossi a diverso tipo emoglobinico su strisci di sangue fissati. Importanza del metodo nello studio delle talassemia, Minerva pediat., *11*, 245, 1959.

262. SCHIEBER, C. L.: Target Cell Anemia, Lancet, *2*, 851, 1945.

263. SEN GUPTA, P. C., CHATTEREA, J. B., MUKHERJEE, A. M. and CHATTERJI, ANJALI: Histochemical Study of the Foam Cell in Thalassaemia, Bull. Calcutta S. T. M., *7*, 145, 1959.

264. SHIELDS, G. S., WETHERS, DORIS, GAVIS, G. and WATSON, R. JANET: Hemoglobin-S-Thalassemia Disease, A. M. A. Am. J. Dis. Child., *91*, 485, 1956.

265. SIDDOO, J. K., SIDDOO, S. K., CHASE, W. H., MORGAN-DEAN, L. and PERRY, W. H.: Thalassemia in Sikhs, Blood, *11*, 197, 1956.

267. SILVESTRONI, E. and BIANCO, I.: Rare Constitutional Abnormality of Blood in Relation to Hereditary Microcytic Anemia, Policlinico, *52*, 137, 1945; Am. J. Human Genet., *1*, 83, 1949.

267a. SILVESTRONI, E. and BIANCO, I.: Genetic Aspects of Sickle Cell Anemia and Microdrepanocytic Disease, Blood, *7*, 429, 1952; *ibid.*, *8*, 1061, 1953.

268. SINGER, K., CHERNOFF, A. I. and SINGER, L.: Studies on Abnormal Hemoglobins. I. Alkali Denaturation, Blood, *6*, 413, 1951.

268a. SINISCALCO, M. *et al.*: Indagini sulla genetica delle aptoglobine del siero umano in una popolazione talassemica, Haematologica, *43*, 1157, 1958.

269. SMITH, C. H.: Familial Blood Studies in Cases of Mediterranean (Cooley's) Anemia, Am. J. Dis. Child., *65*, 681, 1943; *Ibid.*, *75*, 505, 1948.

270. SMITH, C. H., ERLANDSON, M. E., STERN, GERTRUDE and SCHULMAN, I.: The Role of Splenectomy in the Management of Thalassemia, Blood, *15*, 197, 1960.

271. SMITH, C. H., SISSON, T. R. C., FLOYD, W. H., JR. and SIEGAL, S.: Serum Iron and Iron-Binding Capacity of the Serum in Children With Severe Mediterranean (Cooley's) Anemia, Pediatrics, *5*, 799, 1950; Proc. Soc. Exper. Biol. & Med., *74*, 258, 1950.

273. STRAUSS, M. B., DALAND, G. A. and FOX, H. J.: Familial Microcytic Anemia, Am. J. M. Sc., *201*, 30, 1941; Blood, *3*, 438, 1948.

274. STURGEON, P. and FINCH, C. A.: Erythroki-

netics in Cooley's Anemia, Blood, *12*, 64, 1957.

275. STURGEON, P., ITANO, H. A. and BERGREN, W. R.: Genetic and Biochemical Studies of 'Intermediate' Types of Colley's Anæmia, Brit. J. Hæmat., *1*, 264, 1955.

277. VAKULIS, V. J., *et al.*: Rapid Demonstration of A₂ Hemoglobin by Means of Agar Gel Electrophoresis, Am. J. Clin. Path., *34*, 28, 1960.

278. VALENTINE, W. N. and NEEL, J. V.: Hematologic and Genetic Study of the Transmission of Thalassemia, Arch. Int. Med., *74*, 185, 1944; Am. J. M. Sc., *215*, 456, 1948.

279. WEATHERALL, D. J. and VELLA, F.: Thalassaemia in a Gurkha Family, Brit. M. J., *1*, 1711, 1960.

279a. WENT, L. N. and MacIVER, J. E.: An Unusual Type of Hemoglobinopathy Resembling Sickle Cell-Thalassemia Disease in a Jamaican Family, Blood, *13*, 559, 1958.

279b. WENT, L. N. and MacIVER, J. E.: Thalassemia in the West Indies, Blood, *17*, 166, 1961.

280. WHIPPLE, G. H. and BRADFORD, W. L.:

Mediterranean Disease — Thalassemia, J. Pediat., *9*, 279, 1936.

283. WINTROBE, M. M., MATTHEWS, E., POLLACK, R. and DOBYNS, B. M.: A Familial Hemopoietic Disorder in Italian Adolescents and Adults, J.A.M.A., *114*, 1530, 1940.

284. WOLFF, J. A., MICHAELS, R. H. and VON HOFE, F. H.: Hemoglobin H-thalassemia Disease, Blood, *13*, 492, 1958.

284a. WOLFF, J. A., SITARZ, ANNELIESE L. and VON HOFE, F. H.: Effect of Splenectomy on Thalassemia, Pediatrics, *26*, 674, 1960.

285. ZELICKSON, A. S.: Leg Ulcers Associated with Mediterranean Anemia (Thalassemia Major and Minor), A. M. A. Arch. Dermat., *76*, 351, 1957.

286. ZUELZER, W. W. and KAPLAN, E.: Thalassemia-Hemoglobin C Disease, Blood, *9*, 1047, 1954.

287. ZUELZER, W. W., ROBINSON, A. R. and BOOKER, C. R.: Reciprocal Relationship of Hemoglobins A₂ and F in Beta Chain Thalassemias, a Key to the Genetic Control of Hemoglobin F, Blood, *17*, 393, 1961; Nature, *190*, 237, 1961.

Chapter 14

Hypochromic Microcytic (Iron Deficiency) Anemia

Definition.—In this type of anemia the hemoglobin, and to a lesser degree the volume of packed red cells, are reduced much more than is the red cell count. This is due to the fact that the majority of the red corpuscles making up the blood are smaller than normal and are poorly filled with hemoglobin. These changes are expressed quantitatively in the reduced mean corpuscular volume, low mean corpuscular hemoglobin, and —what is most significant—reduced mean corpuscular hemoglobin concentration (below 30 per cent). Only in this type of anemia is the mean corpuscular hemoglobin concentration significantly lower than normal.

It should be pointed out that the term "hypochromic" refers to the hemoglobin concentration of the red corpuscles. The same term is used less specifically by some writers in referring to a variety of "secondary" anemias which may include all those which are not macrocytic and "hyperchromic." Such usage is confusing. This subject has been discussed more fully elsewhere (p. 428).

Synonyms and Sub-groups.—These will be enumerated fully in the succeeding pages, but the following may be mentioned here: *nutritional hypochromic anemia*, chronic or "idiopathic" hypochromic anemia, chloranemia, chlorosis, chlorotic anemia, asiderotic anemia, hypochromic anemia of pregnancy, of prematurity, and of infancy and childhood.

Etiology and Pathogenesis.—By far the most common cause of hypochromic microcytic anemia is a deficiency of iron of such a degree that hemoglobin production is impaired. Next in frequency, but much less common, is thalassemia or an associated disorder, as discussed in the preceding chapter (p. 700). The hypocupremic syndrome occasionally seen in infants (141) is accompanied by hypochromic microcytic anemia only when associated with iron deficiency. Pyridoxine-responsive anemia (p. 136), which is also hypochromic and microcytic, and refractory sideroblastic microcytic hypochromic anemias (p. 562), are extremely rare.

Factors concerned with the absorption of iron, the relative value of different foods, iron transport and storage and the requirements for iron were discussed in an earlier chapter (p. 143). On theoretical grounds the circumstances under which iron deficiency might occur can be enumerated as follows: inadequate intake, defective absorption, increased requirements, imperfect utilization, and excessive loss (Fig. 14–1). In many instances, more than one of these factors is involved. Time is an additional factor. Until the body stores of iron have been

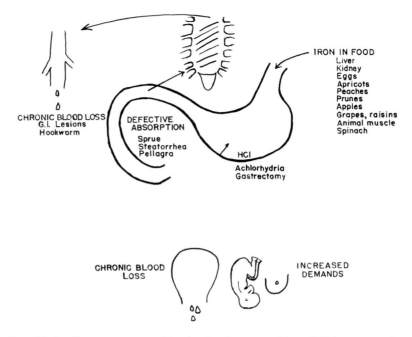

Fig. 14–1.—Factors concerned in the development of iron deficiency anemia. (Wintrobe, Internat. Clinics, courtesy of J. B. Lippincott Company.)

drained, hypochromic microcytic anemia will not develop.

Diet.—It is rare in ordinary practice to find cases of hypochromic anemia in which the consumption of a diet lacking meat, liver, vegetables, fruit and other foods containing iron, is the only discoverable etiological factor.[33] It is true, however, that food idiosyncrasies, bad dentition, gastrointestinal disturbances, or well-intentioned but misguided treatment of such disorders, as well as poverty,[18] the exigencies of war,[176] the cultivation of "money crops" to the exclusion of farm products necessary for home consumption,[59] or religious tenets and caste practices[71] result in the use of a diet which can furnish little hemoglobin-building material. In cases of chronic hypochromic anemia in women it was possible to elicit a history indicating a diet poor in iron in 32 to 70 per cent of the cases.[28, 33, 50] The average diet of a group of women of the poorer classes in Scotland

was found to supply only 2.5 mg. of iron per day. As economic conditions improve, such grades of deficiency become less and less common but in many parts of the world they are still prevalent.

Hypochromic anemia was found to be common in regions where the soil was deficient in iron and the vegetables grown were low in iron content.[1]

Impaired Absorption.—The role of gastric secretion in the absorption of iron was discussed in an earlier chapter (p. 145) where it was pointed out that hydrochloric acid is only of minor importance except perhaps where iron requirements are high and therefore even minor factors may be significant. Although it is true that many normal individuals can be found who have achlorhydria and yet show no anemia[58] and in spite of the fact that iron deficiency is uncommon in pernicious anemia (p. 487) where achlorhydria is characteristic, it is noteworthy that chronic hypochromic anemia is not

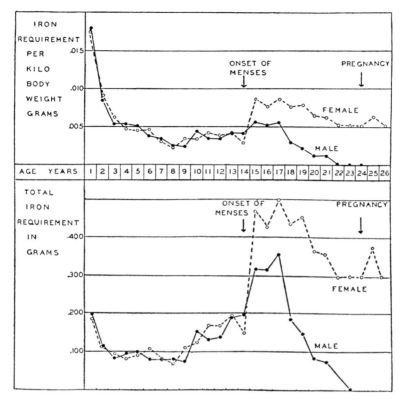

Fig. 14–2.—Annual iron requirements of males and females at various age periods.
(Heath and Patek, courtesy of Medicine.)

unusual in men following gastrectomy even though this type of anemia is rare in the male sex otherwise. Hypochromic microcytic anemia is more common following this operation than macrocytic anemia both in man[8a,49] and in experimental animals.[45,57] Such animals were found to be particularly prone to develop anemia during pregnancy.[36] It was observed that large quantities of mucus in the gastric juice such as are found in cases of chronic hypochromic anemia, decreased absorption of iron[32] and that utilization of iron by achlorhydric patients was as low as 3.1 per cent, whereas in patients with normal gastric secretion and similar anemia, 11.8 per cent of the iron given was used.[33] It would seem that achlorhydria alone will rarely cause iron deficiency but, when other factors

are contributing to the development of iron deficiency and, in consequence, iron requirements are high, the handicap of achlorhydria may be of some importance.

In addition to gastrectomy other defects in the gastrointestinal tract may contribute to the development of iron deficiency. Thus, this type of anemia is often associated with sprue, idiopathic steatorrhea[30a] (p. 501) and celiac disease[31] and sometimes is seen in other disorders characterized by chronic diarrhea and impaired absorption.[38]

Increased Requirements.—In the absence of disease, requirements for iron in a male adult vary little. In infancy, childhood and adolescence, on the other hand, because of the increased needs for the rapidly growing tissues, and in the female sex from the menarche to the menopause, the requirements for iron are great (Fig. 14-2).

In *infants* from four to six months until three years of age, hypochromic anemia is common.[61b] In surveys made in Great Britain among the poorer classes, such anemia was found in 20 per cent or more[27] of children under three years of age. The anemia is particularly common in premature infants[18] and in twins, and is more frequent in artificially as compared with breast-fed infants.[44] A similar type of anemia is observed in older children with abnormal eating habits.

The development of hypochromic anemia in infancy (p. 765) is not a matter for surprise when it is recalled that during the first year of life the total blood volume must be tripled and the quantity of hemoglobin doubled. It has been aptly stated that "the infant bleeds into his own increasing blood volume."[33] The view that defective antenatal storage is the cause of the hypochromic anemia of infancy has been rather generally accepted. It is based on the observation that anemia was more frequent in a series of infants born of anemic mothers than in those whose mothers were in good health.[61,65] Other factors have been mentioned as contributing to the iron deficiency of infancy; for example, early clamping of the umbilical cord, which may deprive the infant of iron for storage.[71a] Again, the heavier the child at birth, the greater the amount of blood available for destruction and storage. It has been estimated that as much as 250 to 300 mg. of iron may be stored as the result of the blood destroyed during the first few days of life.[62a] The development of iron deficiency anemia in infants and twins can be attributed to their small size at birth and, in premature infants, to the more rapid rate of growth which places additional burdens on the iron stores.[37]

Notwithstanding all these factors, abnormal diet is probably the most important factor in the development of iron deficiency in infants. In many instances excessive milk consumption and the exclusion of other foods is the underlying fault.[74] A high caloric intake is supplied thereby but the iron content of milk is low, more so in cows' milk than in breast milk.[27] Contributory factors may be infectious, which impair food consumption[37] and disturb iron metabolism; gastrointestinal disorders, such as colitis or celiac disease; and, perhaps, achlorhydria.[27a,31,63] Blood loss from the gastrointestinal tract may be another factor. In studies in which Fe^{59} was given intravenously to 13 iron deficient infants and its appearance in the feces was noted and measured, it was calculated that as much as 71 to 107 ml. of blood was lost in the stools of three infants in a period of three to four weeks and 24 to 39 ml. in eight more.[35b]

The greater demands for iron in the female (p. 149) readily account for the prevalence of iron deficiency anemia in the *female sex*. After the age of puberty, such anemia is much more common in the female than in the male. The female requirement for iron during the reproductive period is four times that of the male.[33] The average iron loss of normal women is 30 mg. per period and in anemic women it may be 120 mg. or more.

Severe anemia *in pregnancy* (hemoglobin less than 10 Gm.) is usually hypochromic and is amenable to iron therapy. Symptoms appear about mid-pregnancy. The women affected are more often those who have borne several children already and it is often found that symptoms suggestive of anemia were present before pregnancy.[53b,66]

Iron deficiency is common in pregnancy and in lactating women. This is to be expected if consideration is given to the fetal requirement, the quantity of blood in the placenta and uterus and the ultimate loss at parturition, especially if these drains involve a person whose stores may already have been taxed by a number of years of menstrual losses and perhaps several preceding pregnancies. As pointed out elsewhere (p. 149), child-bearing represents a drain of approximately 725 mg., which is by no means made up by the saving of losses through menstruation.

So common is iron deficiency anemia in the female that two clinical syndromes have been described which have occurred almost exclusively in females.

Chlorosis.—Chlorosis is the name given to a disorder which was common until the first part of the twentieth century. It was observed in girls at puberty or somewhat later, but was rare after the age of 25 years. Lange separated it as a clinical entity in 1520 under the title "De morbo virgineo."[24] It was depicted in many paintings, especially by the Dutch school. The name chlorosis arose from the greenish-yellow color of affected girls, a color which perhaps required "the eye of faith" to discern. In the 1830's the affection was classified as a disease of the blood by Ashwell,[7] the deficiency of iron was recognized by Foedisch and the value of iron therapy was demonstrated by Blaud. Yet the cause of the anemia remained obscure. Love-sickness was popularly considered to be an etiological factor, and homesickness, worry, constipation and "autointoxication," ovarian insufficiency, and the wearing of corsets with resulting splanchnoptosis and displacement of the spleen were all given serious attention as causative factors.[60] In time nutritional insufficiency was suggested, and it was noted that the condition was often found in girls whose idiosyncrasies as to diet included the avoidance of meats and subsistence on an almost exclusively carbohydrate diet.[64]

The present rarity of chlorosis makes the study of this condition by modern methods impossible. However, from earlier observations it would appear that inadequate intake of iron and menstrual

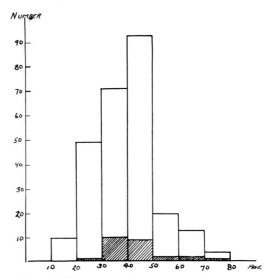

Fig. 14–3.—Age incidence of chronic hypochromic anemia. (Wintrobe and Beebe, courtesy of Medicine.) The shaded portion represents the authors' own cases while the remainder were derived from the literature.

loss at a time of rapid growth and exceptional needs were the chief factors concerned. A diet poor in iron may also have been aggravated in many instances by a decreased intake and possibly lowered absorption during illness from infections. It has been estimated that the iron requirement in the female in adolescence is as great as or even greater than in pregnancy[33] (Fig. 14–2). It is difficult to understand how the wearing of tight corsets could have played an important role.

The disappearance of "chlorosis" has perhaps been exaggerated. Whatever "chlorosis" may be, it should be noted that hypochromic anemia of moderate degree is by no means rare in girls and young women[3, 35a, 56] and in many cases of such anemia in older women one can obtain a history of symptoms extending back to early adult life. This was true of 25 per cent of our cases.[72]

A disorder in *males* similar to chlorosis is extremely rare, but has been observed.[9,21] This is most commonly seen

Table 14–1.—*Pernicious Anemia and Chronic Hypochromic Anemia Compared*

	Pernicious anemia	Chronic hypochromic anemia	
		Similarity to P. A.	Points of difference
Etiologic features:			
Age, years	Especially 45 to 60		Especially 35 to 50
Sex incidence	Approximately equal		Females 96 per cent
Constitutional type	Often characteristic	Often similar to P.A. type	
Familial incidence	Common	Described, even in P. A. families	
Symptomatology:			
Onset of symptoms	Insidious	Insidious	
Duration	Years	Years	
Character: Symptoms of anemia	Characteristic	Characteristic	
Gastro-intestinal	Common	Common	
Tongue sore or atrophic	Characteristic	Common, but perhaps less than in P.A.	
Sore mouth	Uncommon		Not unusual
Dysphagia	Rare		Fairly common
Neurological symptoms	Common and characteristic	Paresthesias in 18 per cent	
P. E. neurological signs	Characteristic		Very rare
Nutrition	Often good	Good or poor	
Color	Characteristically yellowish pallor		White or waxy pallor (but may be yellowish)
Spleen palpable	30 per cent	33 per cent	
Koilonychia	None		30 per cent
Gastric analysis:			
Free hydrochloric acid	Absent in 99 per cent	Absent in 84 per cent	
Mucus	Absent		Greatly increased
Pepsin	Absent	Absent in 25 per cent, decreased in majority	
Influence of histamine	None		Slight increase in volume, HCl and pepsin
Blood findings:			
R. B. C., Number	Characteristically under 3.5 million		Usually 3.5 to 5.0 million
Hemoglobin	Not proportionately reduced		Very markedly reduced
Size of red cells	Increased (95 to 160 c.μ)		Decreased (50 to 80 c.μ)
Hemoglobin concentration of red cells	Normal (32 to 34 per cent)		Decreased (22 to 29 per cent)
Nucleated red cells and polychromatophilia	Common in severe cases		Less common
Plasma iron	Increased or normal usually		Reduced (50 μgm. per cent or less)
Serum copper	Normal		High
Erythrocyte protoporphyrin	Low normal (15–30 μgm.)		Increased (50–600 μgm. per 100 ml. red cells)

Table 14–1—Pernicious Anemia and Chronic Hypochromic Anemia Compared
(Continued)

	Pernicious anemia	Chronic hypochromic anemia	
		Similarity to P. A.	Points of difference
W. B. C.	Leukopenia		Normal or slight leukopenia
Platelets	May be decreased		Normal usually
Bilirubin in blood plasma	Increased		Normal or decreased
Bone marrow	Megaloblastic		Normoblastic
Course	Remissions and relapses		Remissions rare without treatment
Prognosis	Fatal without treatment		Only 1 death reported
Treatment:			
Liver, liver extract or B₁₂	Excellent		No or little value
Follic acid	Often good at first		Valueless
Iron	No value		Very effective
Effect of stopping treatment	Relapse	Relapse in some cases	

at a time when adolescent growth is being completed and may be associated with inefficient food iron absorption, in addition to the requirements for growth.[12a]

Under the name of **chronic hypochromic anemia,** or a variety of other terms (simple achlorhydric anemia, achylic chloroanemia, late chlorosis, essential, primary or idiopathic hypochromic anemia) a syndrome akin to chlorosis but occurring in women in the third to fifth decades of life (Fig. 14–3), received wide attention.[72] Again, like chlorosis, this clinical picture was infrequent (4 per cent) among men.[13]

It was observed that the anemia was more common and certainly more pronounced in the poorer classes of society. In a survey among the poorest classes in Scotland, this type of anemia was found in 45 per cent of the adult women examined.[18] It was common to obtain a history of inadequate convalescence following illnesses; and particularly following pregnancy. In many instances it was possible to obtain a history of several pregnancies, repeated at frequent inter-

47

vals or terminating in abortions with excessive loss of blood. The diet often had been deficient, especially in foods known for their hemoglobin-building value. Menstrual disturbances were common.

One of the most striking characteristics of chronic hypochromic anemia was the frequency with which *achlorhydria* was found (p. 746). It was this association of achylia with "simple anemia" that caused Faber to suggest that it might be a nosological entity.[20] It is interesting that a number of the patients possessed the constitutional features[72] described as characteristic of pernicious anemia (Table 14–1); namely, light-colored eyes set widely apart, prematurely gray hair, and wide costal angle. It was not unusual to find a family history of anemia in these patients and in a few instances one or more male members of the family had had pernicious anemia while hypochromic anemia occurred in some of the women (Fig. 14–4). Although many such cases were reported from Europe and North America, unlike pernicious anemia the

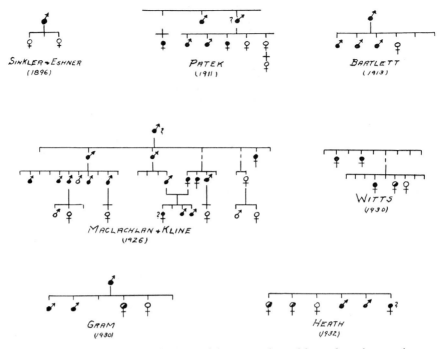

Fig. 14–4.—Seven families in which both pernicious anemia and hypochromic anemia were encountered. Black circles, pernicious anemia; open circles, hypochromic anemia; circles half open, half black, cases in which hypochromic anemia was followed by pernicious anemia. Members of these families who had no anemia are indicated only by short strokes. (Wintrobe and Beebe, courtesy of Medicine.)

condition was also common in Italy[2] and in Asia.

"Idiopathic" hypochromic anemia attracted considerable attention in the first three decades of the twentieth century and was the subject of much study and some bewilderment. This preoccupation can be appreciated if it is recalled that iron metabolism was not well understood at that time. Furthermore, considerable confusion existed concerning the differentiation of various types of anemia and in regard to the relative merits of organic, as compared with inorganic, iron in the treatment of anemia (p. 457).

Blood Loss.—Hypochromic microcytic anemia is encountered most often when blood loss, open or concealed, has occurred over a long period of time. This may be only as an exaggeration of physiological blood loss, as by menstruation, or

because of disease. Thus, common causes are menorrhagia and metrorrhagia from uterine fibroids, or peptic ulcer, hernia at the esophageal hiatus, non-specific ulcerative colitis, carcinoma of the stomach or colon, cirrhosis of the liver with bleeding varices or bleeding hemorrhoids. Sometimes such anemia may result from recurrent severe epistaxes, as in multiple hereditary telangiectasia. It is possible to a certain extent to make up for loss of blood by consuming an adequate diet, as the absence of anemia in many men with chronically bleeding hemorrhoids indicates. Nevertheless, if sufficiently great and when continued for a long enough time, the chronic loss of blood will result in iron deficiency even where other demands for iron, as in men, are small. Since the chronic loss of blood in the male, if detected, would usually lead to his seeking attention, the discovery of iron deficiency anemia in a male patient almost always signifies the presence of an occult source of chronic blood loss, such as peptic ulcer or carcinoma of the ascending colon or stomach.

Hookworm.—Of the variety of intestinal parasites which infest man, hookworm is the one which characteristically is associated with hypochromic microcytic anemia.[59] At one time the view was widely held that hookworm anemia is due to the elaboration of a toxin. No such mysterious concept is necessary. The blood picture and the clinical state are similar to that observed in iron deficiency anemia in the absence of the hookworm, a noteworthy difference being, however, that no predilection for the female sex has been described. The anemia possesses all the characteristics of iron deficiency and can be relieved by the administration of iron, whether the worms are removed or not.[16a] Studies in infected individuals whose erythrocytes had been tagged with Cr^{51} showed intestinal blood losses ranging from 2 to 251 ml. per day, the loss being roughly in proportion to the severity of the infection.[59a] The same investigators found that a wide range of iron was reabsorbed (13 to 76 per cent, average 44 per cent) but the net loss was substantial nevertheless. The loss from *Necator americanus* infestation was greater than that attributable to *Ancylostoma duodenale*. These observations are consistent with those of others[26] and with the results of experimental studies in animals.[22,54,70]

There is no doubt, however, that in cases of hookworm infestation, blood loss caused by the worm is only one of the factors involved. Deficient diet, other drains on iron stores, as for example from repeated pregnancies, and achlorhydria have been found to be contributory factors in studies of hookworm anemia in Puerto Rico[59] and in Brazil.[16,56a] It is significant that in hookworm carriers in Argentina, those who consumed much

meat were not anemic. Marked decreases of serum vitamin B_{12} levels and impaired intestinal absorption of folic acid in persons with heavy hookworm infestation[42] give further evidence of their impaired state of nutrition.

A theoretically possible additional factor, not hitherto mentioned, is the role of faulty *utilization of iron*. It is known that iron balance is disturbed when there is an infection (p. 577). There is no evidence that infections are ever a primary cause of iron deficiency; in fact, the iron which is unused remains in the body stores. Nevertheless, impaired utilization of iron as the result of infection might possibly serve as a contributory factor in the development of anemia.

From the above considerations, it should be apparent that a multiplicity of factors may be involved in the production of iron deficiency. Often, in a given case, more than one factor has played a role. Whichever of the above single or multiple factors is involved in a given case, the ultimate result is the same; namely a negative iron balance with ultimate depletion of the iron stores of the body.

Attention has so far been focused on the ultimate development of hypochromic microcytic anemia. Iron plays an important role in other tissues, in addition to the hemopoietic system. The changes in the nails so characteristic of iron deficiency (p. 743) give evidence of the place of iron in epithelial tissues,[68] as do also the angular stomatitis and glossitis which may accompany chronic hypochromic anemia. These can be corrected by iron therapy, even in the face of a deficient diet.[17a] The dysphagia of the Plummer-Vinson syndrome (p. 740) has been attributed to lack of iron.[69]

As a component of heme, iron forms a part of myoglobin, as well as hemoglobin. It is found in the cytochromes, cytochrome oxidase, catalase and peroxidase. It is also involved in several other important enzymic reactions.[10] Contrary to earlier conclusions, there is evidence that varying degrees of depletion in several iron enzymes occur in the iron deficiency state.[10,28a] The differences observed, however, have been small and have not been shown to be of biologic significance.

Attention has been called to the fact that the severity of symptoms of patients with iron deficiency anemia is often not proportional to the degree of anemia. This can be admitted readily and could well be expected in persons who have developed anemia over a long period of time and under a great variety of social and economic circumstances. The attempt to relate the symptomatology of iron deficient patients or of chronically fatigued, non-anemic women to deficiency of iron enzymes has, so far, been unconvincing.[10a]

Symptomatology.—Certain features are common to all the forms of hypochromic microcytic anemia which have been mentioned. Their *onset* is insidious and their progress is gradual. In our cases of chronic hypochromic anemia in *adult women* the duration of symptoms varied from two to 22 years and averaged eight years. Symptoms common to all anemias may be found, such as weakness, fatigability and pallor. Nervous irritability, deficient mental application, headache, and disturbances of sleep are common. An ever-present feeling of "dead-tiredness" is a frequent symptom. Nevertheless, in some cases the onset is so slow that the patient becomes adjusted to the chronic state of ill-health and severe grades of anemia may be maintained with remarkably few complaints.

In *infants* with hypochromic anemia, edema of the extremities, as well as enlargement of the liver, spleen and lymph nodes, may develop when the anemia is marked.

Gastro-intestinal Disturbances.—Gastro-intestinal disturbances of the type which have been attributed to gastro-intestinal "neuroses" are often encoun-

tered. Just as anemia may contribute to the development of such symptoms, it is to be noted that a poor appetite and an inadequate diet favor the development of iron deficiency. In chlorosis capricious appetite and sometimes marked abnormalities associated with craving for unusual or even disgusting articles, together with flatulence, heartburn, vague and often shifting and irregular epigastric distress after meals, and hunger pain were described as prominent features. Constipation was regarded as a troublesome and relatively constant symptom.

Similar complaints are present in the chronic hypochromic anemia of later life but in this condition there may be diarrhea. Since achlorhydria is frequently present, the bowel movements may be of the type often associated with defective gastric secretion; namely, the passage of one stool immediately on arising and another semi-soft one after breakfast or later. As already stated, hypochromic anemia, instead of macrocytic anemia, may be found in cases of sprue, idiopathic steatorrhea, and celiac disease. In such cases the symptoms characteristic of these disorders (p. 496) are prominent.

Sore tongue or *sore mouth* has been found in approximately 28 per cent of cases, but it is noteworthy that the glossitis rarely approaches the intensity observed in pernicious anemia. There may be pain or "spasm" in the throat or actual *dysphagia*. Difficulty in swallowing may be the presenting symptom and as such has been described as the **Plummer-Vinson syndrome.**[35c,72,75]

Waldenström[69] found *sideropenic dysphagia* (a name he proposed in preference to Plummer-Vinson syndrome) to be the most common disease of the esophagus in Sweden, more than twice as common as carcinoma. Pain and burning sensations when solid food passed behind the larynx, or a sensation as if food remained there, were the commonest complaints. The dysphagia was usually of long standing and was sometimes so severe as to interfere with nutrition. Anemia was not present in all of his cases but low plasma iron (sideropenia) was consistently found and symptomatic relief followed iron therapy even though the roentgenographic appearance of the esophagus was not altered. Changes in the latter were regarded as characteristic. In order to distend the esophagus adequately a large quantity of thick barium was swallowed and fluoroscopic as well as repeated antero-posterior and lateral plates were taken, using as short exposures as possible. The most frequent finding, usually seen in the upper part of the esophagus just below the cricoid cartilage and never as low as the crossing of the aorta, was a thin defect in the opacity produced by the barium. This pointed into the lumen of the esophagus approximately at right angles to the wall and resembled a thin membrane. Rarely several of these were seen and in advanced cases a circular fold of the esophageal wall was described or even a broader, cuff-like stricture below the membrane, was found. As a rule the wall of the esophagus was smooth and its lumen above and below the stricture was the same.

A relatively rare symptom is hematemesis,[72] which, when it is associated with anemia and splenomegaly, suggests the diagnosis of Banti's syndrome.

Cardio-respiratory Disturbances.— Cardio-respiratory complaints include palpitation, a common symptom which may be more or less persistent or most troublesomely recurrent; arrhythmias of the simpler variety; dyspnea on exertion, and choking sensations. Edema about the ankles and, less frequently, puffiness of the face may produce a clinical picture which suggests congestive cardiac failure or chronic nephritis. In severe cases, heart failure may actually supervene.[62]

Genito-urinary System.—Disturbances of menstruation are frequent. In chlorosis the periods may appear late,

they may be very profuse, or there may be dysmenorrhea or irregularity of flow. In 35 per cent of our cases of chronic hypochromic anemia there was unexplained menorrhagia.[28] In 13 per cent endometrial hyperplasia was found and in 20 per cent there were myomata uteri. In 30 per cent the history revealed that there had been repeated pregnancies, postpartum hemorrhages, or abortions. In only 23 per cent was the history or pelvic examination entirely negative. In other series of cases pelvic abnormalities have been less prominent.[29,50] It is noteworthy that in some cases menorrhagia ceased as the anemia was relieved.[72]

Pruritis vulvae occurs but is uncommon.[72] Urinary complaints are rare unless there is complicating cystitis.

Endocrine Features. — In addition to the disturbances of menstrual function already mentioned, there may be signs of mild hypothyroidism[50] which do not disappear as the anemia is relieved but require specific treatment.

Neuromuscular System. — There may be neuralgic pains, vasomotor disturbances, or numbness and tingling. The last-mentioned complaints have been observed in 15 to 30 per cent of cases of chronic hypochromic anemia but, like glossitis, they rarely attain the prominence found in pernicious anemia. More serious symptoms, such as disturbances of gait and objective neurological findings are very unusual.[67]

In addition to the symptoms described above, in patients in whom the anemia is primarily due to blood loss, there may be complaints referable to the system where the blood loss is occurring. Thus there may be signs and symptoms indicative of **peptic ulcer.** It is essential to bear in mind, however, that the symptoms of anemia may completely obscure those of the underlying condition. Thus in one of our patients, a young man with severe hypochromic microcytic anemia, the discovery of the anemia led to a

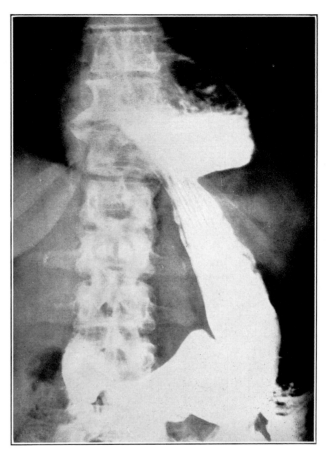

FIG. 14–5.—Roentgenogram showing hernia at the esophageal hiatus. This was associated with marked hypochromic microcytic anemia.

thorough search which revealed a "silent," chronically bleeding, duodenal ulcer.

Murphy and Hay[53a] observed severe hypochromic anemia in 26.6 per cent of their cases of **hernia at the esophageal hiatus** (Fig. 14–5). They pointed out that hypochromic anemia for which no cause is readily demonstrated should lead one to suspect the presence of a hiatal hernia, particularly if such symptoms as substernal distress or pain, postprandial discomfort aggravated by reclining, and regurgitation or vomiting with relief, are present. Hiatal hernia is much more commonly seen in women than in men, free hydrochloric acid is more often present in the gastric juice than absent, and not infrequently the feces give a positive guaiac test for blood.

In *infants*, of course, the majority of the symptoms outlined are absent but disturbances of appetite and of bowel function, irritability, and fretfulness are uncommon.

In *hookworm anemia* the symptoms, in general, are similar to those already outlined. Epigastric pain, abdominal cramps, vomiting, diarrhea, or constipation, are common. Often no history of "ground-itch" is obtained. Long-infested children show retarded development, both physical and mental.

Physical Examination.—The appearance of these patients is often quite characteristic. They do not look acutely ill but appear tired and lifeless. In chlorosis, pallor is the most striking outward symptom. Although in some cases the pallor was associated with a greenish-yellow tint, in the larger proportion of cases this feature was absent. In some patients, the "rosy chlorotics," there was said to be a rosy color in the cheeks and a vivid red in the lips but we have never seen this in cases of chronic hypochromic anemia. In some instances of the latter condition a peculiar brownish hue may be observed in the skin and, as in pernicious anemia, vitiligo may be found. The yellowish pallor of pernicious anemia is rare. Depigmentation of the skin is a prominent symptom of *Kasai*, a syndrome seen in the Belgian Congo[57a] which is characterized, in addition, by anemia, edema and digestive disturbances and is attributed to iron deficiency.

The mucous membranes of the gums and pharynx are pale, as are the nailbeds and the ocular conjunctivae. The last-mentioned are blue or pearly white instead of icteric as in pernicious anemia. The skin, especially in adult patients, is inelastic and may be wrinkled and dry. The hair usually feels dry and dead and is often scanty. There may be no evidence of weight loss and some patients are actually obese.

In at least 39 per cent of cases of chronic hypochromic anemia, some degree of **papillary atrophy of the tongue** (Fig. 14–6) has been observed. This, however, is rarely if ever as striking as is found in pernicious anemia. There may be swelling, a blotchy, irregular denudation of the papillae or dusky red irregular spots on the tongue.[17a] Fissures may be present at the angles of the mouth. On the mucous membranes of

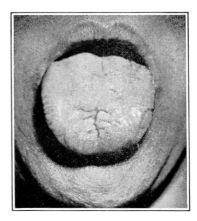

Fig. 14–6.—Tongue of patient with chronic hypochromic anemia, showing moderate papillary atrophy.

the mouth there may also be small, blister-like lesions surrounded by areas of erythema.

Slight cardiac enlargement may be found. Functional systolic murmurs are very common. The presence of edema has been mentioned. The abdominal wall is often atonic and inelastic. The "pot-belly" of hookworm disease is a classical feature of advanced cases of that condition. The liver is often palpable and in some patients with marked anemia it has been quite large. In about 10 per cent of chlorotics and in at least a third of the cases of hypochromic anemia in later life, the spleen has been palpable.[72] Excessive enlargement, however, is unusual.

A remarkable finding, which can be observed in a third of the patients with chronic hypochromic anemia, is longitudinal ridging and flattening of the finger nails, which appear dull and lusterless. They are unusually brittle, break easily, may be "sore," and sometimes are actually concave instead of convex[5] (Fig. 14–7). We have observed severe grades of **koilonychia** only in patients who had subjected their hands to much water and caustic cleansing agents. Waldenström[69a] described cases of koilonychia in which

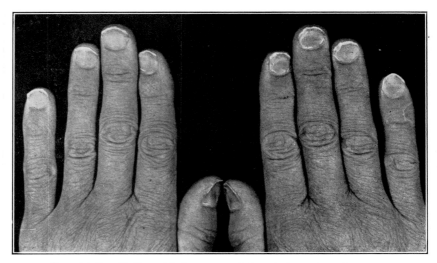

FIG. 14–7.—Koilonychia in a case of chronic hypochromic anemia.

anemia was absent but improvement followed treatment with iron nevertheless.

Fever is unusual except in severely anemic patients, in whom a low-grade elevation of temperature may be found.[58a]

Laboratory Findings.—The Blood. —The changes in the blood necessarily vary with the severity of the anemia. The chief characteristic is the poverty of hemoglobin in the **individual red corpuscles.** This is indicated by an exaggeration of their central pallor. The more severe the anemia, the greater the degree of this change and the more numerous the corpuscles affected. In extreme grades of hypochromic anemia, most of the red corpuscles are mere rings (Fig. 14–8). Tiny microcytes and a moderate number of poikilocytes, particularly elongated, ellipitical forms are also found.

In almost all instances, however, a variable number of well-filled red corpuscles are present and some macrocytes, often polychromatophilic, can be distinguished. These probably represent the feeble effort to form hemoglobin-containing corpuscles. The number of these cells is increased as iron is made available.

Reticulocytes are normal in number or reduced, unless a recent hemorrhage has occurred. A large hemorrhage may induce temporary reticulocytosis. Stippling is not common but occasional normoblasts and microblasts are found in the more severe cases.

The morphological changes are reflected in the quantitative data. The hemoglobin is reduced out of proportion to the red cell count and volume of packed red cells. The red cell count may be normal or even somewhat above normal when the hemoglobin is as low as 8 Gm. Extreme reductions in the red cell count, such as are seen in pernicious anemia, are not found. It is the hemoglobin and volume of packed red cells which reach extremely low levels. We have seen cases in which the hemoglobin was as low as 2.5 Gm. per 100 ml. and the volume of packed red cells 10 ml. In 90 per cent of our cases of chronic hypochromic anemia the red cells numbered between 3,000,000 and 5,150,000 per c.mm.; in 74 per cent the hemoglobin was 6 to 10 Gm., and in 80 per cent the volume of packed red cells was 23 to 35 ml. per 100 ml.

In 75 per cent of the same series the

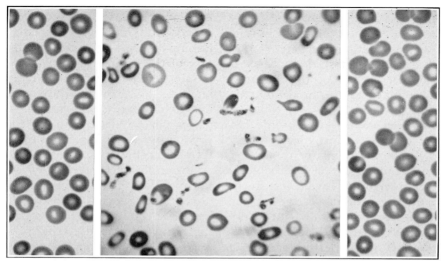

Fig. 14–8.—Blood smear from a case of hypochromic microcytic anemia due to iron deficiency. Red corpuscles from normal blood are shown, for comparison, on each side. Wright's stain, ×900.

mean corpuscular volume ranged between 55 and 74 c.μ while the mean corpuscular hemoglobin was 15 to 21 $\gamma\gamma$ in 70 per cent. In 83 per cent the mean corpuscular hemoglobin concentration was 25 to 30 per cent. In extremely severe cases the mean corpuscular volume may be as low as 50 c.μ, the mean corpuscular hemoglobin 12 $\gamma\gamma$ and the mean corpuscular hemoglobin concentration 22 per cent.

Measurements of the diameters of the red corpuscles show that the mean diameter is reduced (6.2 to 6.7 μ) and the distribution ("Price-Jones") curve has a broadened base and is swung to the left of normal. The corpuscles are also extremely thin, indirect measurements giving mean values even as low as 1 μ.

The **fragility** of the red corpuscles may be normal but often there is some increased resistance to destruction in hypotonic salt solutions, a pale layer of unbroken cells remaining in tubes of salt concentration as low as 0.21 per cent.[17] Extreme grades of corpuscular resistance, however, such as are found in Mediterranean anemia are unusual. The abnor-

mal osmotic fragility returns to normal following adequate therapy.[58b]

The **blood plasma** is very pale and no evidence of increased blood destruction is found in the urine or stools. The plasma protein content is often reduced. The content of *iron* in the plasma is very low, usually below 35 μgm. per cent. The serum *copper* content, on the other hand is raised and the *erythrocyte protoporphyrin* (p. 155) is increased above normal,[55a] reaching values even as high as 500 μgm. per 100 ml. of red cells.

The **leukocytes** may be normal in number or slightly reduced. A few multisegmented neutrophils may be found, and there may be slight absolute granulocytopenia as well as relative lymphocytosis in long-standing cases. A fresh hemorrhage of large size, however, may cause slight leukocytosis of the neutrophilic type, even with the appearance of an occasional myelocyte. In hookworm anemia, eosinophilia is common.[59]

The **platelets** are usually normal in number and small. In chlorosis their number was said to be increased in some cases.[55] In long-standing cases of chronic hypochromic anemia in adults the number of platelets rarely may be slightly reduced. Significant changes in the bleeding or coagulation time, clot retraction and tourniquet test do not occur unless the case is one of hypochromic anemia secondary to thrombocytopenic purpura.

Gastric Secretion.—In chronic hypochromic anemia, achlorhydria is a very common finding. As many as 83 per cent of cases fail to secrete hydrochloric acid in response to the Ewald test meal; in 50 to 60 per cent of cases even the injection of histamine failed to cause secretion of hydrochloric acid.[72] Frequently there is an excessive secretion of mucus and decreased formation of pepsin.[19] The volume of the gastric contents is generally less than normal. The intrinsic factor of Castle is present, although often in diminished quantity.[15,30] Some writers considered achlorhydria a fundamental feature of this anemia and consequently designated it as "simple achlorhydric anemia."[73]

Regarding the gastric secretion in chlorosis, conflicting views have been expressed. The most convincing report is that of Arneth,[6] who found normal or high values for free hydrochloric acid in 23 patients, low values in none.

In the hypochromic anemia of infancy and childhood, the acidity is normal or decreased or there may be achlorhydria.[27a,31] In the hypochromic anemia of pregnancy normal gastric acidity was found only in 2 patients in a series of 29 cases whereas achlorhydria, which persisted after delivery, was present in 17 cases.[66] Even in cases of hookworm anemia, achlorhydria is common. In a series of 54 cases in Puerto Rico,[59] the alcohol test revealed achlorhydria in 24.

Other laboratory findings are not noteworthy except those which may reveal occult bleeding, as for example from the gastro-intestinal tract. The urine shows no significant changes.

Bone Marrow.—The bone marrow is hyperplastic and shows a relative as well as absolute increase of normoblasts, a finding contrasting sharply with the poverty of the peripheral blood and calling to mind the similar situation in pernicious anemia. Unlike the latter condition, megaloblasts are not found, although young normoblasts are in evidence. The predominant cell is a small polychromatophilic normoblast. Large and atypical neutrophilic metamyelocytes suggesting the peculiar cells found in pernicious anemia have been described in a few instances, but in general granulopoiesis shows no significant deviation from the normal.

The increase in normoblasts is roughly proportional to the degree of anemia. The percentage of these cells increases after the administration of iron but as the blood is restored to normal the cellularity of the marrow likewise becomes normal.

Roentgenographic Changes. — In the skull, widening of the diploic spaces and a "hair-on-end" appearance like that seen in congenital hemolytic anemias (p. 705) have been observed in iron deficiency anemia in infants, especially in premature infants and in twins, in whom iron depletion may have an early onset.[12,61a]

Diagnosis.—If the blood is not examined carefully there may be much confusion. The history of many cases of chronic hypochromic anemia, in adults particularly, reveals that these patients have been subjected to fruitless and expensive investigations and ineffective methods of treatment, or that they have been labeled "psychoneurotic" without further investigation. The long duration of the symptoms, their persistence and the frequent nervous instability of the patients lend credence to such a hasty conclusion. Other patients, whose chief symptom may be local, as in the genito-urinary system, may be treated without regard to their general condition. We have known patients subjected to curettage, hysterectomy, exploratory laparotomy, or splenectomy who were unrelieved by these measures. Improvement took place only after iron therapy. Occult tuberculosis, heart disease, infective endocarditis, myxedema, rheumatism, pyelitis, pernicious anemia, aplastic anemia, leukemia, Banti's syndrome, and colitis are some of the incorrect diagnoses which had been made in our patients.

Examination of the blood should include not only inspection of the blood smear but also calculation of the size and hemoglobin content of the red corpuscles. The smear may contain some macrocytes and this has sometimes led to the erroneous conclusion that the case is one of pernicious anemia. Measurement of the mean cell diameter by one of the halometer methods is often misleading because the cell size may seem to be normal or only slightly reduced, and the most significant feature, the low mean corpuscular hemoglobin concentration, is not demonstrated by this means.

Other methods for the recognition of iron deficiency which may be used are usually impractical or unnecessary. It is generally accepted that lack of stainable iron in the bone marrow (p. 60) is a reliable sign of iron deficiency, but the discomfort involved in such an examination is usually not justified. The same can be said of the enumeration of bone marrow sideroblasts (p. 101). The measurement of serum iron and iron-binding capacity can be helpful if correctly interpreted (p. 146) but these procedures are not always available, nor always dependable. Iron tolerance curves are of no value.[11]

The degree of hypochromia and microcytosis is correlated with the severity of the anemia. When the deficiency of iron is only moderate in degree, little anemia and consequently few morphologic changes in the red cells can be expected. In such cases, the recognition of iron deficiency anemia may be difficult.

Sometimes a therapeutic trial with iron is necessary.

Whenever iron deficiency is found or suspected, careful inquiry concerning possible causes is important. This is especially true if a cause is not obvious, since the development of iron deficiency may be the first sign of an occult malignancy. As already stated, if the patient is a man, except when there has been a gastric resection, occult blood loss is almost always due to an ulcerative lesion in the gastrointestinal tract. Rarely steatorrhea is a factor.[30a] If the patient is a woman, a careful review of menstrual losses is necessary since deviations from the normal are not always appreciated by the patient. In infants and young children especially, the dietary history is important and in all cases the stool should be examined for occult blood and parasites.

A smooth tongue, numbness and tingling, achlorhydria, the general appearance of the patient and sometimes even the family history may make a strong case for pernicious anemia. (See Table 14–1.) Blood examination should make the differentiation simple. Although a few macrocytes may be present, the majority of the red cells are small and poor in hemoglobin content. Furthermore, there is no evidence of increased blood destruction.

Easy bruising and a palpable spleen may suggest thrombocytopenic purpura. In chronic hypochromic anemia, thrombocytopenia, if present, is slight and anemia is relatively great, whereas the reverse is true in purpura hemorrhagica unless there has been a great deal of bleeding. It should be kept in mind that excessive menstrual bleeding may be the only symptom of both of these conditions.

Some cases which have been classed as examples of Banti's syndrome probably belong with chronic hypochromic anemia, because iron therapy has brought complete relief.[72] The extreme degree of splenomegaly which may be seen in the Banti disorder is not observed in chronic hypochromic anemia.

Little need be said regarding the recognition of chlorosis for this condition is rare, at least in the classical form. In mild form, however, hypochromic anemia is not uncommon in girls and young women.[35a]

Thalassemia major (Cooley's anemia) is characterized by microcytosis and hypochromia, and target cells are found in a number of syndromes associated with the presence of certain abnormal hemoglobins. These have been described already (p. 668). There should be no confusion with these disorders. The presence of strikingly deformed erythrocytes, the existence of some evidence of increased blood destruction together with signs of active red cell regeneration such as stippling, polychromatophilia and nucleated red cells, and the presence of well marked splenomegaly are some of the distinguishing features. These conditions do not respond to iron therapy.

Complications and Sequelae.—The most frequent complication is the recurrence of anemia if iron therapy is stopped. Recurrence is less common after the menopause.[28] In chlorosis, thrombosis was common especially in the leg veins but sometimes it occurred in the cerebral sinuses with serious consequences.[7]

Associated diseases include arthritis, rheumatic heart disease, chronic cholecystitis, syphilis, uveitis, and focal infections.[72]

Pernicious anemia has developed in several cases of chronic hypochromic anemia[50a,72] (Fig. 14–4). The occasional coexistence of these two types of anemia has been discussed already (p. 487). One type of anemia may overshadow the other and the latter may be discovered only after treatment for the former has been instituted. In other cases the mixture of macrocytes and microcytes is such that the mean corpuscular volume is normal (Fig. 10–8, p. 488).

Treatment.—The administration of adequate amounts of inorganic iron salts is so regularly followed by a well-marked therapeutic response that such treatment can be regarded as specific. The dosage, preparations to be employed, and methods of administration, were discussed in detail in Chapter 9. In addition to iron, the general measures previously outlined for the treatment of anemia should be carried out and a diet containing adequate amounts of vitamins as well as of foods known for their hemoglobin-building value is desirable. This is sometimes difficult to enforce but it is advisable for the complete restoration of the patient's health, even though the blood itself may return to normal and the changes in the nails, tongue[17a] and other epithelial tissues[68] disappear on iron therapy alone.

The earliest evidence of response to treatment with iron is an increase in the percentage of reticulocytes. The magnitude of this increase is inversely proportional to the degree of anemia as measured by the quantity of hemoglobin. The maximum percentage of reticulocytes is attained about the fifth to eighth day following the institution of treatment.[52] When only moderate or slight degrees of anemia are present a well pronounced reticulocyte response cannot be expected.

When effective treatment is given, hemoglobin regeneration occurs at the rate of 0.2 to 0.3 Gm. per day (Fig. 14–9) during the first few weeks, after which time the rate of increase may be less rapid. The red cell count and volume of packed red cells rise at the same time, the former sometimes increasing temporarily to values above normal (Fig. 9–5, p. 461). Usually the hemoglobin per 100 ml. blood is restored more rapidly than the hemoglobin concentration of the cells. The plasma iron level is restored to normal more slowly than the hemoglobin level.

In the writer's experience, cases of iron deficiency anemia which are refractory

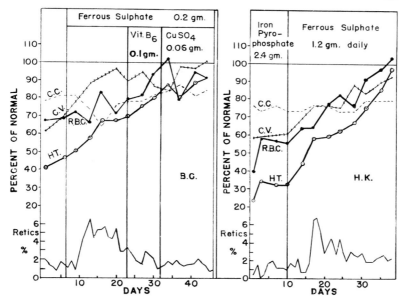

Fig. 14–9.—Results of treatment in 2 cases of chronic hypochromic anemia. All data except the percentage of reticulocytes are recorded in relation to the average normal values. Note the relative efficiency but submaximal response to a small dose of ferrous sulphate (0.2 Gm.) in patient B. C. and the failure of vitamin B_6 or copper sulphate therapy to speed up the response. In patient H. K. a relatively large dose of iron pyrophosphate (2.4 Gm.) had little effect, whereas the recommended dose of ferrous sulphate (1.2 Gm. daily) caused rapid blood regeneration. The average increase in hemoglobin was 0.3 Gm. per day.

to oral iron therapy are extremely rare. Most of those that have been reported have been associated with a fat-absorption defect.[30a] Even in sprue, however, oral iron therapy is usually effective. Frequently lack of adequate instruction of the patient concerning the best way to take iron orally (p. 458) or lack of co-operation by the patient is the cause of iron refractoriness unless, of course, the anemia is not really due to iron deficiency.

A most unusual explanation of relative refractoriness to iron therapy is concurrent increased red cell destruction. This was described in two women in whom extracorpuscular factors were thought to be the cause of the increased hemolysis.[67a] Theoretically, at least, another possible cause of refractoriness to iron therapy would be absence of transferrin.

Administration of iron is recommended as a prophylactic measure in pregnancy, and in premature infants or in those whose birth weight is less than 7 pounds.[27] Hypochromic anemia is likely to develop in artificially fed infants and in those who have had infective illnesses. In such children particularly, the blood should be examined at three or four months of age in order to determine the need for iron. A dietary source of iron is desirable for all infants before six months of age.[62a] Where hookworm infestation is widely prevalent and its persistence is based on deeply rooted habits, the development of anemia is more readily prevented by incorporating 0.2 Gm. ferrous sulfate in the diet than by attempts to eradicate the infestation.[16]

As was pointed out earlier (p. 140), there is little evidence to support the view that copper must be added as a supplement to iron therapy. Nothing is to be gained from the use of liver extracts,[25] folic acid or vitamin B_{12}. Whole liver, however, should be included in the diet because it is a source of valuable vitamins and proteins. It has been shown quite clearly that, when true iron deficiency anemia exists, satisfactory hemoglobin regeneration occurs in response to the administration of iron without the addition of the B vitamins, even in cases in which signs of niacin deficiency, ariboflavinosis or multiple neuritis may be present.[52a]

Transfusion is rarely, if ever, needed, even in severely anemic cases. Such patients, unless a recent severe hemorrhage has occurred, are already adjusted to the anemia and require no sudden bolstering by transfusion.

The administration of free hydrochloric acid is unnecessary as an aid in antianemic therapy but it is of value when there are gastro-intestinal symptoms resulting from achlorhydria. In such cases, 4 ml. of dilute hydrochloric acid (U.S.P.), in water or fruit juices with meals may be useful.

It is advisable to delay treatment of complications such as menorrhagia until the anemia has been at least partly relieved. In many instances the menstrual flow becomes more normal as the anemia disappears. When it does not, the patient's improved condition will at least allow other measures to be used more successfully.

Prognosis and Course.—Unlike pernicious anemia, temporary remissions are uncommon. Under the influence of iron therapy, however, the blood returns to normal and many of the symptoms disappear. This is particularly true of the glossitis and acroparesthesias of chronic hypochromic anemia. The writer has observed the return of the tongue papillae and restoration of the nails to normal. The cardiac murmurs may persist for a long time although dyspnea disappears. Menorrhagia may cease but in other cases it becomes worse and requires attention. Failure to attain normal blood values

has been described,[73] but in our experience this has occurred only in cases in which menorrhagia persisted or increased in severity. Failure to respond to iron given orally and a need for parenteral iron therapy[18a] is very rare and, as already mentioned, is usually associated with a defect in fat absorption.[30a] In some patients a certain degree of fatigability or other complaints may persist for a long time. Since many of these patients have been ill for many years and have acquired faulty habits of various kinds, it sometimes requires all the art of the physician to bring about complete restoration of health.

In many cases relapse occurs unless iron therapy, at least in small doses, is continued. This is true particularly in women before the climacteric in whom great demands for iron continue.[28]

Pathology.—Little is known about the pathology of chlorosis or of chronic hypochromic anemia because the anemia itself has not been known to cause death. The few autopsies available have revealed no characteristic findings other than those common to anemias which are not associated with increased blood destruction. In cases of the Plummer-Vinson syndrome lesions in Auerbach's plexus have been described[46] but this requires confirmation. Others have noted hyperkeratinization of the epithelium or chronic esophagitis. On esophagoscopy a thin semilunar membrane on the anterior wall has been observed.[69]

Gastroscopy has revealed a pale, gray atrophic mucosa.[53] The histological appearance of the mucosa, as obtained by biopsy, has ranged from normal to that of atrophic gastritis and gastric atrophy.[8] In a few cases severe atrophy like that seen in pernicious anemia has been observed. The etiology of these changes in the gastric mucosa is uncertain. Although it has been thought for years that the achlorhydria so commonly associated with chronic iron deficiency anemia precedes the development of the anemia[30] and persists in spite of relief of the anemia, there are differences of opinion as to whether the lack of iron produces the observed gastric changes[8] or is in part the consequence of these histologic alterations.[43]

BIBLIOGRAPHY

Hypochromic Microcytic (Iron Deficiency) Anemia

1. ABBOTT, O. D.: Nutritional Anemia in Florida, distributed by U. S. Dept. Agr. Extension Service, 1078–40.
2. ALLODI, A., PENATI, F. and QUAGLIA, F.: Sulle anemie ipocromiche essenziali, Minerva med., *1*, 489, 1934.
3. ALSTED, G.: Chlorosis: Essential Juvenile Iron Deficiency Anemia, Am. J. M. Sc., *201*, 1, 1941.
5. ANDERSON, N. P.: Syndrome of Spoon Nails, Anemia, Cheilitis and Dysphagia, Arch. Dermat. and Syph., *37*, 816, 1938.
6. ARNETH, J.: Parallel laufende Magensaft- und Blutuntersuchungen bei der Chlorose, Deutsch. med. Wchnschr., *32*, 66, 1906.
7. ASHWELL, S.: Observations on Chlorosis and Its Complications, Guy's Hosp. Rep., *1*, 529, 1836.
8. BADENOCH, J., EVANS, J. R. and RICHARDS, W. C. D.: The Stomach in Hypochromic Anaemia, Brit. J. Haemat., *3*, 175, 1957.
8a. BAIRD, I. McL., BLACKBURN, E. K. and WILSON, G. M.: The Pathogenesis of Anaemia after Partial Gastrectomy, Quart. J. Med., *28*, 21, 1959.
9. BECKERT, W.: Occurrence of Chlorosis in Male Subjects, München. med. Wchnschr., *85*, 823, 1938.
10. BEUTLER, E.: Iron Enzymes in Iron Deficiency, Acta haemat., *21*, 371, 1959; J. Clin. Invest., *38*, 1605, 1959.
10a. BEUTLER, E., LARSH, S. E. and GURNEY, C. W.: Iron Therapy in Chronically Fatigued, Nonanemic Women: A Double-Blind Study, Ann. Int. Med., *52*, 378, 1960.
11. BEUTLER, E., ROBSON, M. J. and BUTTENWIESER, E.: A Comparison of the Plasma Iron, Iron-Binding Capacity, Sternal Marrow Iron and Other Methods in the Clinical Evaluation of Iron Stores, Ann. Int. Med., *48*, 60, 1958; *ibid.*, *50*, 313, 1959.
12. BRITTON, H. A., CANBY, J. P. and KOHLER, COLETTE M.: Iron Deficiency Anemia Producing Evidence of Marrow Hyperplasia in the Calvarium, Pediatrics, *25*, 621, 1960.
12a. BRUMFITT, W.: Primary Iron-Deficiency Anae-

13. BURGER, G. N. and WITTS, L. J.: Hypochromic Anemia in Men, Guy's Hosp. Rep., *84*, 14, 1934.
14. CAMPBELL, J. M. H.: Chlorosis, Guy's Hosp. Rep., *73*, 247, 1923.
15. CASTLE, W. B., HEATH, C. W. and STRAUSS, M. B.: Observations on Etiologic Relationship of Achylia Gastrica to Pernicious Anemia. Am. J. M. Sc., *182*, 741, 1931.
16. CRUZ, W. O.: Pathogenesis of Anæmia in Hookworm Disease, Memorias do Instituto Oswaldo Cruz, Rio de Janeiro, Brazil, *27*, 423, 1933; *ibid.*, *28*, 391, 1934; *ibid.*, *29*, 263, 1934; *ibid.*, *34*, 261, 1939; *ibid.*, *42*, 401, 1945; Blood, *3*, 457, 1948.
17. DALAND, G. A. and WORTHLEY, K.: The Resistance of the Red Blood Cells to Hemolysis in Hypotonic Solutions of Sodium Chloride, J. Lab. & Clin. Med., *20*, 1122, 1935.
17a. DARBY, W. J.: The Oral Manifestations of Iron Deficiency, J.A.M.A., *130*, 830, 1946.
17b. DAVIDSON, L. S. P., DONALDSON, G. M. M., LINDSAY, S. T. and McSORLEY, J. G.: Nutritional Iron Deficiency Anæmia in Wartime, Brit. M. J., *2*, 95, 1943.
18. DAVIDSON, L. S. P. and FULLERTON, H. W.: Chronic Nutritional Hypochromic Anæmia, Edinburgh M. J., n.s., *45*, 1, 1938.
18a. DAVIDSON, L. S. P. and GIRDWOOD, R. H.: Refractory Iron-Deficiency Anæmia Treated With Intravenous Saccharated Oxide of Iron, Brit. M. J., *1*, 733, 1948.
19. DAVIES, D. T.: Studies on Achlorhydria and Anæmia, Quart. J. Med., *24*, 447, 1931.
19a. DAWSON, JEAN P. and DESFORGES, JANE F.: Dietary and Storage Factors in Iron-Deficiency Anemia of Infancy, A. M. A. J. Dis. Child., *96*, 169, 1958.
20. FABER, K.: Anämische Zustände bei der chronischen Achylia gastrica, Berl. klin. Wchnschr., *50*, 958, 1913.
21. FORSHAW, J. W. B.: Idiopathic Hypochromic Anæmia in Males, Brit. M. J., *2*, 908, 1954.
22. FOSTER, A. O. and LANDSBERG, J. W.: Nature and Cause of Hookworm Anemia, Am. J. Hyg., *20*, 259, 1934.
24. FOWLER, W. M.: Chlorosis—An Obituary, Ann. Med. Hist., *8*, 168, 1936.
25. FOWLER, W. M. and BARER, A. P.: The Etiology and Treatment of Idiopathic Hypochromic Anemia, Am. J. M. Sc., *194*, 625, 1937.
26. FOY, H., KONDI, ATHENA, and AUSTIN, W. H.: Hookworms as a Cause of Tropical Iron Deficiency Anaemia. Radio-active Studied East African M. J., *35*, 607, 1958.
27. FULLERTON, H. W.: Iron Deficiency Anemia

of Late Infancy, Arch. Dis. Childhood, *12*, 71, 1937.

27a.GASSER, C.: Achylische Chloranämie im Kindesalter, Helv. pæd. acta, *3*, 167, 1948.

28. GRAY, L. A. and WINTROBE, M. M.: Chronic Hypochromic Anemia in Women, Am. J. Obst. & Gynec., *31*, 3, 1936.

28a.GUBLER, C. J., CARTWRIGHT, G. E. and WINTROBE, M. M.: Enzyme Activities and Iron Metabolism in Copper and Iron Deficiencies, J. Biol. Chem., *224*, 533, 1957.

29. HADEN, R. L. and SINGLETON, J. M.: Disturbances of Menstruation Due to Simple Achlorhydric Anemia, Am. J. Obst. & Gynec., *26*, 330, 1933.

30. HARTFALL, S. J. and WITTS, L. J.: Intrinsic Factor of Castle in Simple Achlorhydric Anæmia, Guy's Hosp. Rep., *83*, 24, 1933.

30a.HAWKINS, C. F., PEENEY, A. L. P. and COOKE, W. T.: Refractory Hypochromic Anæmia and Steatorrhœa, Lancet, *2*, 387, 1950.

31. HAWKSLEY, J. C., LIGHTWOOD, R. and BAILEY, U. M.: Iron-deficiency Anæmia in Children, Arch. Dis. Childhood, *9*, 359, 1934.

32. HEATH, C. W., MINOT, G. R., POHLE, F. J. and ALSTED, G.: The Influence of Mucin Upon the Absorption of Iron in Hypochromic Anemia, Am. J. M. Sc., *195*, 281, 1938.

33. HEATH, C. W. and PATEK, A. J., JR.: The Anemia of Iron Deficiency, Medicine, *16*, 267, 1937 (Bibliography).

35. VON HOESSLIN, H.: Zur Abnahme der Chloroes, München. med. Wchnschr., *73*, 853, 1926.

35a.HERVEY, G. W., McINTIRE, R. T. and WATSON, V.: Low Hemoglobin Levels in Women as Reavealed by Blood Donor Records, J.A.M.A., *149*, 1127, 1952.

35b.HOAG, M. SILVIJA, WALLERSTEIN, R. O. and POLLYCOVE, M.: Occult Blood Loss in Iron Deficiency Anemia of Infancy, Pediatrics, *27*, 199, 1961.

35c.HOWELL, J. T. and MONTO, R. W.: Syndrome of Anemia, Dysphagia and Glossitis (Plummer-Vinson Syndrome), New England J. Med., *249*, 1009, 1953.

36. IVY, A. C., MORGAN, J. E. and FARRELL, J. I.: Effects of Total Gastrectomy, Surg., Gynec. & Obst., *53*, 611, 1931.

37. JOSEPHS, H. W.: Anemia of Infancy and Early Childhood, Medicine, *15*, 307, 1936.

38. KEEFER, C. S., YANG, C. S. and HUANG, K. K.: Anemia Associated With Chronic Dysentery, Arch. Int. Med., *47*, 436, 1931.

42. LAYRISSE, M., BLUMENFELD, NORMA, DUGARTE, IRIS and ROCHE, M.: Vitamin B_{12} and Folic Acid Metabolism in Hookworm-Infected Patients, Blood, *14*, 1269, 1959.

43. LEES, F. and ROSENTHAL, F. D.: Gastric Mucosal Lesions before and after Treatment in Iron Deficiency Anaemia, Quart. J. Med., *27*, 19, 1958.

44. MacKAY, H. M. M.: Nutritional Anemia in Infancy, Spec. Rep. Ser. Med. Res. Coun., London, No. 157, 1931.

45. MAISON, G. L. and IVY, A. C.: Gastrectomy and Subsequent Hematologic Studies in the Hog, Proc. Soc. Experl Biol. & Med., *31*, 554, 1934.

46. McGEE, L. C. and GOODWIN, T. M.: The Syndrome of Dysphagia and Anemia, Ann. Int. Med., *11*, 1498, 1938.

49. MEULENGRACHT, E.: Simple Achylic Anemia After Gastro-enterostomy and Partial Gastrectomy, Acta med. scandinav., *81*, 87, 1934.

50. MEYERS, S. G., PRICE, A. H., MACK, H. C., FOSTER, L. J. and SHARP, E. A.: Chronic Hypochromic Anemia in Women, Ann. Int. Med., *11*, 1590, 1938.

50a.MILLER, E. B. and DAMESHEK, W.: "Primary" Hypochromic Anemia Terminating in Pernicious Anemia, Arch. Int. Med., *68*, 375, 1941.

52. MINOT, G. R. and HEATH, C. W.: The Response of the Reticulocytes to Iron, Am. J. M. Sc., *183*, 110, 1932.

52a.MOORE, C. V., MINNICH, V., VILTER, R. W. and SPIES, T. D.: Hypochromic Anemia in Patients With Deficiency of the Vitamin B Complex, J.A.M.A., *121*, 245, 1943.

53. MORRISON, L. M., SWALM, W. A. and JACKSON, C. L.: Syndrome of Hypochromic Anemia, Achlorhydria and Atrophic Gastritis, J.A.M.A., *109*, 108, 1937.

53a.MURPHY, W. P. and HAY, W. E.: Symptoms and Incidence of Anemia in Hernia at the Esophageal Hiatus, Arch. Int. Med., *72*, 58, 1943.

53b.NAPIER, L. E. and EDWARDS, M. I. N.: *Anæmia in Pregnancy in Calcutta*, Indian Med. Res. Mem., No. 33, Thacker, Spink and Co., Ltd., Calcutta, 1941.

54. NISHI, M.: Experimental Observations on the Blood-sucking Activities of Ancylostomidæ, Especially Ancylostoma Caninum, J. M. A. Formosa, *32*, 61, 1933.

55. OLEF, I.: Chlorosis, Ann. Int. Med., *10*, 1654, 1937.

55a.PAGLIARDI, E., PRATO, V., GIANGRANDI, E. and FIORINA, L.: Behaviour of the Free Erythrocyte Protoporphyrins and of the Erythrocyte Copper in Iron Deficiency Anaemias, Brit. J. Haemat., *5*, 217, 1959.

56. PATEK, A. and HEATH, C.: Chlorosis, J.A.M.A., *106*, 1463, 1936.

56a.PESSÔA, S. B.: Considerações sobre as verminoses no nordeste brasileiro, Rev. Inst. Med. trop. São Paulo, 1, 57, 1959.

57. PETRI, S., NORGAARD, F. and BING, J.: Pathological Changes Produced by Gastrectomy in Young Swine, Am. J. M. Sc., 195, 717, 1938.

57a. PIERAERTS, G.: Étude sur le syndrome depigmentation-œdème au Kasai, Rec. Travaux Sci. Méd. Congo Belge, 1, 104, 1942.

58. POLLAND, W. S.: The Blood in Cases of Unexplained Gastric Anacidity, J. Clin. Invest., 12, 599, 1933.

58a. REIMANN, F.: Das Eisenmangelfieber, Acta haemat., 2, 247, 1949.

58b. REIMANN, F. and ARKUN, N. S.: Die Einwirkung der Eisenbehandlung auf das Verhalten der osmotischen Resistenz der Erythrocyten bei den eisenempfindlichen chronischen Chloranämien (Asiderosen), Ztschr. klin. Med., 153, 589, 1956.

59. RHOADS, C. P., CASTLE, W. B., PAYNE, G. C. and LAWSON, H. A.: Observations on Etiology and Treatment of Anemia Associated With Hookworm Infection in Puerto Rico, Medicine, 13, 317, 1934.

59a. ROCHE, M., PEREZ-GIMENEZ, MARIA ENRIQUETA, LAYRISSE, M. and DI PRISCO, ESTELA: Gastrointestinal Bleeding in Hookworm Infection, Am. J. Digest. Dis., 2, 265, 1957; J. Clin. Invest., 36, 1183, 1957; J. Lab. & Clin. Med., 54, 49, 1959; Rev. hémat., 15, 19, 1960.

60. SCHWARZ, E.: Chlorosis, Supp. Acta medica belgica, 1951.

61. SISSON, T. R. C. and LUND, C. J.: The Influence of Maternal Iron Deficiency on the Newborn, Am. J. Clin. Nutrition, 6, 376, 1958.

61a. SHAHIDI, N. T. and DIAMOND, L. K.: Skull Changes in Infants with Chronic Iron-Deficiency Anemia, New England J. Med., 262, 137, 1960.

61b. SMITH, N. J. and ROSELLO, S.: Iron Deficiency in Infancy and Childhood, J. Clin. Nutrition, 1, 275, 1953.

62. SOMERS, K.: Acute Reversible Heart Failure in Severe Iron-Deficiency Anemia Associated with Hookworm Infestation in Uganda Africans, Circulation, 19, 672, 1959.

62a. STEARNS, G. and McKINLEY, J. B.: The Conservation of Blood Iron During the Period of Physiological Hemoglobin Destruction in Early Infancy, J. Nutrition, 13, 143, 1937.

63. STEWART, A.: Gastric Acidity in Infants and Young Children Under Normal and Pathologic Conditions, With Especial Reference to Nutritional Anemia, Brit. J. Child. Dis., 34, 1, 1937.

64. STOCKMAN, R.: On the Amount of Iron in Ordinary Dietaries and in Some Articles of Food, J. Physiol., 18, 848, 1895.

65. STRAUSS, M. B.: Anemia of Infancy From Maternal Iron Deficiency in Pregnancy, J. Clin. Invest., 12, 345, 1933.

66. STRAUSS, M. B. and CASTLE, W. B.: Studies on Anemia in Pregnancy, Am. J. M. Sc., 184, 655, 663, 1932; ibid., 185, 539, 1933.

67. SUH, T. H. and MERRITT, H. H.: Combined System Disease Without Obvious Evidence of Pernicious (Macrocytic) Anemia, Am. J. M. Sc., 196, 57, 1938.

67a. VERLOOP, M. C., VAN DER WOLK, M. and HEIER, A. J.: Radioactive Iron Studies in Patients with Iron Deficiency Anemia with Concurrent Abnormal Hemolysis, Blood, 15, 791, 1960.

68. WALDENSTRÖM, J.: Iron and Epithelium. Some Clinical Observations. I. Regeneration of the Epithelium, Acta med. scandinav., Supp., 90, 380, 1937.

69. WALDENSTRÖM, J. and KJELLBERG, S. R.: The Roentgenological Diagnosis of Sideropenic Dysphagia (Plummer-Vinson's Syndrome), Acta radiol., 20, 618, 1939.

70. WELLS, H. S.: Observations on Blood Sucking Activites of Hookworm, Ancylostoma Caninum, J. Parasitol., 17, 167, 1931.

71. WILLS, L., MEHTA, M. M., TALPADE, S. N. and BILIMORIA, H. S.: Studies in Pernicious Anemia of Pregnancy, Indian J. Med. Res., 17, 777, 1930; ibid., 18, 283, 1930; ibid., 20, 391, 1932; ibid., 21, 669, 1934.

71a. WILSON, E. E., WINDLE, W. F. and ALT, H. L.: Deprivation of Placental Blood as a Cause of Iron Deficiency in Infants, Am. J. Dis. Child., 62, 320, 1941.

72. WINTROBE, M. M. and BEEBE, R. T.: Idiopathic Hypochromic Anemia, Medicine, 12, 187, 1933 (Bibliography).

73. WITTS, L. J.: Simple Achlorhydric Anemia, Guy's Hosp. Rep. 80, 253, 1930; ibid., 81, 205, 1931.

74. WOODRUFF, C. W.: Multiple Causes of Iron Deficiency in Infants, J. A. M. A., 167, 715, 1958; Am. J. Clin. Nutrition, 7, 634, 1959.

75. WYNDER, E. L. and FRYER, J. H.: Etiologic Considerations of Plummer-Vinson Syndrome, Ann. Int. Med., 49, 1106, 1958.

Chapter 15

Anemia and Other Disorders in Infancy and Childhood

General Considerations.—Anemia and other disorders occurring in infancy and childhood require special consideration for several reasons. Thus, the fetus and infant are exposed to certain hazards not encountered in later life. Again, the demands for growth increase the requirements for blood building factors. Finally, many congenital and hereditary disorders make their appearance early in life.[37a] At the same time the responsiveness of the hemopoietic system of the infant is not the same as that of adults.

The first important hazard is the possibility of maternal isoimmunization by fetal blood factors, with grave consequences for the fetus. Another is hemorrhage into the placenta or from umbilical vessels. Next comes the tying of the cord and this, if tied too early, may deprive the infant of blood which, aside from any immediate value, furnishes materials such as iron that can be used even after the red corpuscles have served their life span. If the infant has been born prematurely, an additional hazard arises and anemia in some way associated with this may develop. In the newborn, as at other times, hemorrhage may occur, thrombocytopenic purpura may appear and even leukemia may develop and in rare instances an obscure congenital aregenerative anemia has been observed. Fortunately hemorrhagic disease of the newborn is now unusual.

Genetically controlled hemopoietic disorders may appear early in life but one in particular, sickle cell anemia, does not develop before six months of age, the presence of fetal hemoglobin offering some protection (p. 671). Other abnormal hemoglobin syndromes may appear early, even so early as to cause confusion with hemolytic disease of the newborn (p. 710). Hereditary spherocytosis usually does not cause trouble in the first year of life but this is not invariable.

Dietary restrictions, deliberate or as the consequence of unwise infant care, when combined with the increased requirements which *growth* demands, result in anemia which is most often due to iron deficiency, but the megaloblastic anemia of infancy is due to lack of other factors. Growth requirements make special demands and thus may leave their mark in the way of anemia even throughout adolescence. Playing an equally important rôle are *infections*. Rarely these are congenital, as in the case of syphilis, and often they are acquired. These are important not only because they influence the diet but also because they may have a more profound effect on hematopoiesis in early life than in adults.[7]

The hemopoietic equilibrium is less well established in the infant than in the adult; as a result, the effect of any given stimulus may differ, not only quantitatively, but also qualitatively. Leukocytosis may be more striking, anemia more profound, nucleated red cells may appear where only polychromatophilia and reticulocytosis would develop in an adult, and myelocytes and even myeloblasts are found instead of the usual slight or moderate "shift to the left" of adults. Lymphocytosis develops frequently and to a more striking degree, and the spleen, lymph nodes, and liver become enlarged more readily than in adults.

If these differences are not recognized, new and unusual clinical entities will be suspected when only the same factors which also produce anemia in adults are present. An example is the **"anemia pseudoleukemica infantum"** described by Rudolf von Jaksch in 1890.[6] This anemia was characterized by him as a deficiency in hemoglobin and erythrocytes with marked anisocytosis and poikilocytosis, numerous erythroblasts and macroblasts, extreme leukocytosis with relative lymphocytosis, splenomegaly, and enlargement of the liver and lymphatic glands. The patients were all under three years of age. The onset of the illness was insidious and the manifestations included listlessness, weakness, gastrointestinal disturbances, marked pallor, and often irregular fever. In some instances there was evidence of increased blood destruction. A majority of the patients recovered completely.

It is now recognized that the syndrome described by Von Jaksch is not a disease entity, but represents a symptom-complex which may be associated with a large variety of factors, among which malnutrition, gastrointestinal disturbances, syphilis, tuberculosis, and a number of other infections, iron deficiency and thalassemia may be included.

The normal blood values and their physiological variations in the newborn, in infancy, and in childhood have been discussed in Chapters 2, 4 and 5. Conclusions regarding anemia, leukocytosis, macrocytosis or microcytosis in any given instance should only be drawn in relation to these normal standards. Because the normal values are not the same as for adults and because immature red cells appear more readily, classification of anemias on morphological grounds is somewhat less useful in infancy than in later life. Anemia in the first six weeks to three months of age is predominantly macrocytic, but this is only rarely accompanied by megaloblastic bone marrow and is rarely responsive to the administration of folic acid and related substances (p. 768). Hypochromic microcytic anemia in a child, on the other hand, is as significant as in adults; it usually represents nutritional iron deficiency.

Of the anemias encountered in infants and children that due to infection is by far the most common. The pathogenesis of such anemia has been discussed already (p. 576). It has been reported that in the course of various diseases in children the erythroblasts may suddenly disappear from the bone marrow for a short period of time (**"acute erythroblastopenia"**).[4a] Such an "aplastic crisis," if of short duration and if the "life" of the circulating red corpuscles is normal, would have no noteworthy influence on the blood. If the aplasia is prolonged, anemia or other changes may develop. Observations concerning the occurrence of this phenomenon in hereditary spherocytosis have been discussed already (p. 646).

ANEMIAS OF THE NEWBORN BABY

HEMOLYTIC DISEASE OF THE NEWBORN

(ERYTHROBLASTOSIS FETALIS)

Definition.—This is a disorder occurring in the fetus *in utero* or manifest in the first few days of life, which is produced by excessive destruction of the erythrocytes. The bone marrow, liver and spleen engage actively in erythropoiesis and the peripheral blood often reflects this by the presence of numerous nucleated red cells (erythroblastosis). Edema, jaundice, pallor, and enlargement of the spleen and liver are the outstanding manifestations and may be observed either singly or in combination. According to the symptoms which predominate, this condition has been referred to as **hydrops fetalis, icterus gravis neonatorum,** and **congenital anemia of the newborn**. It was shown by Levine[9] and others that the condition is caused by iso-immunization of the pregnant mother with consequent destruction of the red cells of the fetus.

Etiology.—Characteristically, in cases due to Rh incompatibility, the first-born child is very rarely affected, sometimes the first two or three offspring have been normal; once the disorder has appeared, however, succeeding pregnancies have usually, though not always,[13b] resulted in the birth of affected infants or a macerated and dead fetus, or in abortion. The condition has been observed in identical twins,[1, 6a] and only in one of double ovum twins where one twin was Rh-positive and the other Rh-negative.[10b] In hemolytic disease due to incompatibility within the ABO groups, infants born of first pregnancies are not infrequently affected. This is perhaps due to the fact that many heterogenic factors such as injections of tetanus toxoid may stimulate the formation of anti-A in group O subjects. Unlike Rh incompatibility, the disease does not become more severe in subsequent infants than in the first affected infant in the family.

The mother may appear perfectly normal or excessive uterine enlargement may be noted.[6a] Toxemias of pregnancy may be somewhat more common in this group of pregnant women. It was observed[6a] that the average duration of gestation was shorter (36.3 weeks) when the fetus showed the picture of hydrops than when icterus was the outstanding symptom (thirty-nine weeks).

Although earlier figures indicated an incidence of hydrops only about once in 1400 to 3800 births and icterus gravis once in 900 to 1500 births, more recent data indicated an incidence of hemolytic disease of the newborn of once in 200 pregnancies.[9h] This is, in part at least, due to more accurate diagnosis but may be caused also by the greater readiness with which transfusions have been used therapeutically, thereby immunizing the mother even before pregnancy. Rh-positive women rarely bear children with hemolytic disease (p. 763). In Rh-negative women, it has been calculated, the incidence of the disorder increases from 1:42 deliveries in the second to 1:12 deliveries by the fifth pregnancy.[10d]

There is good correlation between the incidence of the disease and the proportion of Rh-negative individuals in different races.[12a] Thus, it is rare among Negroes.[12e] When erythroblastosis fetalis occurs in the Negro, ABO incompatibility is the more common cause. The incidence of hemolytic disease due to ABO incompatibility is about 0.6 to 1.0 per cent of all deliveries.[12k]

Symptomatology. — The **hydropic** child is heavier than average, shows marked and extensive pitting edema, the neck appears short and there may be a suggestion of the mongoloid facies. There often is pronounced thoracic and abdominal distention due in part to effusions in the pleural, pericardial and peritoneal cavities and in part caused by hepatic enlargement. The arms and legs may seem shorter than normal and the skin is macerated if the child is stillborn, as is usually the case. The child with the **icterus gravis** form is usually born alive. The amniotic fluid and vernix caseosa are likely to be discolored. Icterus, although rarely present at birth,[13] appears within 24 to 48 hours and increases rapidly in intensity to produce a picture simulating that of an obstructive jaundice. It is likely to be detected earlier if care is taken to look at the infant several times during the first two days of life and if proper light is available. Inspection of the skin can be aided by blanching it with a piece of polished leucite which can be kept sterile and through which the yellowish color can be detected. The spleen as well as the liver is greatly enlarged. When anemia exists in the absence of marked hydrops or icterus it is sometimes referred to as **congenital anemia of the newborn** (see p. 765). The last group and the icteric form comprise approximately 70 per cent of all cases of hemolytic disease of the newborn.[10a]

There is little to be gained by differentiating icterus gravis from congenital anemia, however. These terms simply emphasize two important features of hemolytic disease. Pallor may not be apparent at birth because of the reddening and irritation of the skin consequent to delivery. Jaundice is present in all cases but is more pronounced in some. In the more fulminating cases jaundice increases rapidly and reaches a maximum after three to five days if death does not take place sooner. In the milder types, the jaundice may regress rapidly after the first few days and anemia may become the dominating feature. A general lethargy, dyspnea, cardiac enlargement and systolic cardiac murmurs are prominent features in infants with the most severe

degrees of anemia. The majority of infants who die, do not die from anemia. They become increasingly jaundiced, remain drowsy and feed poorly and die with terminal convulsions or cyanotic attacks during the first few days of life.

In the more severe cases hemorrhagic manifestations may appear with purpura as a prominent feature.[8a] Very occasionally hemorrhage, such as melena, is the predominating evidence of disease.[6a] In such cases hepato- and splenomegaly are also present and other features of hemolytic disease of the newborn are usually discernible if they are looked for.

Cerebral signs may appear in some cases. In somewhat less than 16 per cent of the severely icteric cases[3] these may consist of convulsions, twitchings, opisthotonos and respiratory difficulties, with death resulting in the first week of life; or, if the infant survives, there may be choreo-athetosis, extrapyramidal spasticity or mental retardation. These changes have been shown to be due to damage to the nuclei of the brain (*"Kernicterus"*)[4c]. In other cases cerebral symptoms may be due to spontaneous intracerebral hemorrhages.

When the hemolytic disease is due to ABO incompatibility, the infant as a rule is not seriously affected.[13e] Anemia at birth is absent or minimal and there may be little fall in hemoglobin subsequently. Jaundice occurs, however and, unlike "physiologic" icterus, is manifest within the first 24 hours of life. Sometimes it is pronounced and kernicterus has been described.[9a]

The Blood.—The great increase in the number of nucleated red cells is the most striking change in the blood. There may be from 10,000 to 100,000 nucleated red cells per c.mm. of blood, as compared with 200 to 2000 in the blood of normal premature or full-term infants in the first two days of life.[1b] The nucleated red cells are often very large and are found in every stage of maturation. Certain writers[1b,11a] have referred to some of these cells as megaloblasts but their illustrations do not show cells like those found in the bone marrow in pernicious anemia. They resemble immature cells of the normoblastic series. Marked polychromatophilia, red cells with nuclear fragments and other evidences of immaturity, and large numbers of reticulocytes (10 to even 60 per cent) are also found. The erythrocytes are macrocytic and well filled with hemoglobin; thus the mean corpuscular volume and mean corpuscular hemoglobin are increased above the normal for the newborn and the mean corpuscular hemoglobin concentration is normal. Red cell diameter measurements show a biphasic curve with a macrocytic and a normocytic peak or two macrocytic peaks.[11a] There is little variation in the shape of the red corpuscles. Spherocytosis is not usually obvious when the immunization is caused by Rh antigens. On the other hand, when due to ABO incompatibility, spherocytosis may be a marked feature of the blood smear. This is accompanied by a marked increase in osmotic fragility which is seldom found in anti-Rh incompatibility. There is no increase in mechanical fragility.[4g]

The red cell count varies considerably, ranging from 0.5 to 6 million with corresponding values for hemoglobin.[11a] Only in the severe forms is there more than a slight degree of anemia. Generally much lower counts have been found in the hydrops form than in icterus gravis. Blood from the umbilical cord[6a] shows all the changes which have been described above.

The concentration of fetal hemoglobin at birth is usually lower than normal while the concentration of adult hemoglobin is increased.[12d] This has been attributed to effective synthesis of adult hemoglobin rather than preferential destruction of fetal hemoglobin.

As the disease progresses, the erythrocytes decrease rapidly in number, sometimes by as much as a million per c.mm.

per day.[1b] Thus a profound anemia may be found in the third or fourth day where little was present at birth. The nucleated red cells tend to diminish and may disappear by this time but the macrocytosis persists.

The leukocyte count is often 15,000 to 30,000 per c.mm. Much higher counts have been recorded but in many instances nucleated red cells, which do not disappear on the addition of acetic acid, have been included in the counts. Immature forms of the granulocytes are generally present and immature lymphocytes have been described.[1b]

Platelets may be normal in number or, in the severe cases, may be greatly reduced in number. In the latter instances prolonged bleeding time and poor clot retraction, as well as purpura are found. Prothrombin[1b,8a] and even fibrinogen[11b] deficiency may be present to augment the bleeding tendency. After the first week the platelets return to normal levels.

Other Laboratory Findings.—The icterus index is generally high immediately after birth and may rise to 100 or more.[8a] Whereas the *serum bilirubin* level of blood samples from the umbilical cord of normal mature infants is usually below 3 mg. per 100 ml., in the erythroblastotic child the initial level will usually be higher and then will rise much more rapidly.[5a] In erythroblastosis, by the end of the third day levels of 30 mg. are found, on the average, in untreated infants whereas 7 mg. is the average and 13 mg. is the maximum in the normal infant. In the premature normal infant the initial level is usually lower than in the mature child; however, it rises to higher levels than in the mature infant (even 27 mg.[1a]). A rapid rise to high levels is characteristic in erythroblastosis and is not seen even in babies with biliary atresia. The elevation is due to the indirect fraction of the bilirubin. When the bile ducts become obstructed by inspissated bile, or if liver damage occurs, the direct bilirubin rises.[10] Corresponding to these changes, the excretion of urobilinogen in the feces and urine increases greatly.[2] Without treatment, by the sixth to the twelfth day the feces is likely to become clay colored and the urine bile tinged.[1b]

When the condition is due to the Rh antibodies, cord blood erythrocytes give a strongly positive *direct antiglobulin (Coombs') test*. This test also detects antibodies of the Kell, Kidd and Duffy blood group systems. In contrast, this reaction is usually weak when the erythroblastosis is due to anti-A and it may even be negative.[1f] The positive direct test in Rh sensitization often remains positive for weeks in untreated infants but usually becomes negative within a few days if they have been effectively treated by means of exchange transfusion.

The indirect reaction is usually positive in an affected infant at birth but the titer of free antibody does not seem to be correlated with the severity of the hemolysis.[12i]

Diagnosis.—This condition should be suspected in a pregnant woman who has had a stillbirth or miscarriage after one or two normal deliveries; and in one who has had abortions after the fifth month. If her red cells are Rh-negative and her husband is Rh-positive this suspicion gains support. Roentgenography may reveal a "halo" about the fetal head due to edema of the scalp or the fetus may be seen to be occupying a Budda or frog-like position on account of the great abdominal enlargement.[6a] The roentgenogram may show the placenta to be very large. The placenta in cases of hydrops is pale on the maternal surface and deeply fissured and it closely resembles the placenta seen in syphilis.

As will be discussed below (p. 763), the likelihood of Rh sensitization is at least twice as great when the husband's blood is compatible with that of his wife in the ABO group than when this is not the case.

The *possibility* of the presence of hemolytic disease is increased when Rh antibodies are detectable in such an expectant mother and the *probability* is increased if her husband is homozygous Rh-positive.[13e] Although the presence of antibodies in the maternal serum is not diagnostic, since they may have been formed by a previous pregnancy or transfusion, a rise in the antibody titer during the pregnancy is strong evidence for the Rh-positivity of the fetus. The indirect antiglobulin (Coombs') technic for titrating the antibodies in the maternal serum is generally preferred. In conjunction with this, a "partial absorption" test has been found useful in discriminating between mild and severe cases of hemolytic disease of the newborn.[7b] Regular titrations should be carried out at least from the 24th week of pregnancy. It has been claimed that, with some exceptions, the severity of the disease in the newborn can be expected to be directly proportional to the mathematical product of the height of the antibody titer multiplied by the length of intrauterine exposure of the fetus to the antibodies.[12f]

In cases of ABO sensitization, however, prenatal tests have little diagnostic or predictive value. Furthermore, since a woman may give birth to infants who are entirely free of hemolytic disease even though she had previously had an affected child, the past history is of little value.

Early recognition of the likelihood and of the possible severity of hemolytic disease in the prospective newborn is important in management, as will be discussed below. In the newborn, the appearance of jaundice in the first 24 hours of life should suggest the diagnosis and this is confirmed, for practical purposes, if the serum bilirubin level is above 10 mg. per 100 ml. in the first twenty-four hours and above 15 mg. on the second day.[1a] Other signs of hemolytic anemia, including marked erythroblastosis, further support the diagnosis.

It must be kept in mind, however, that an increased number of nucleated red cells may be found in cases of congenital syphilis, in other instances of ante-natal or early post-natal infection, in cases of anoxia due to atelectasis of the lungs, in infants of diabetic mothers and in those with congenital anomalies of the gastro-intestinal tract, in traumatic or spontaneous hemorrhage due to any cause, in thalassemia, and in extreme prematurity. Congenital syphilis may be distinguished by the blood serology and by roentgeno-grams of the bones. Severe anemia is not found in congenital heart disease but otherwise the latter may present many features suggesting hemolytic disease of the newborn. Congenital hemolytic ane-mias such as hereditary spherocytosis should be kept in mind.

Simple *icterus neonatorum*, in contrast to icterus gravis, usually has its onset about the third day after birth and is not asso-ciated with severe anemia or enlargement of the liver and spleen. The number of nucleated red cells in the circulating blood is rarely greater than 5000 per c.mm. and even these disappear within two or three days.

Severe anemia is not found in congen-ital obliteration of the bile ducts where the jaundice, furthermore, becomes ac-centuated in the second or third week rather than earlier.

The infant's, or cord blood should be examined at the time of birth. The most significant finding there is a positive di-rect Coombs' test, which indicates that the infant's corpuscles have been sensi-tized. If both the mother and the infant are Rh-negative or Rh-positive, when other evidence is compatible with the diagnosis, sensitization against antigens other than D, such as c, E or Kell, and ABO incompatibility must be considered. In ABO incompatibility, the Coombs' test may be negative. In such cases,

isoagglutinins anti-A or anti-B which have traversed the placenta and are capable of reacting with the red cells of the infant, have been demonstrated.[12f]

Course, Prognosis and Sequelae.— The mortality in the past was 70 to 80 per cent.[8] With modern therapy the number of stillbirths has not been altered significantly but, of those infants born alive, the complete recovery rate has in-creased to greater than 84 per cent.[1a] In the series cited, of the 16 per cent who died, 9 per cent were due to hydrops and 7 per cent to other causes. Others have reported even better results.[9g,13b] The incidence of kernicterus has been reduced to zero in well-treated cases.[1a]

The prognosis is worse the earlier the manifestations appear. The fetus is prone to die *in utero* in the seventh or eighth month of gestation. Those born alive may die within twenty-four to forty-eight hours. If edema is absent and jaundice and anemia develop more gradually, the infant may survive. The degree of sensi-tization and the amount of free antibody in the serum by themselves do not in-dicate the severity of the disease but must be considered in conjunction with the hematological findings.[10a] Another im-portant factor is the capacity of the liver to deal with the products of hemolysis. The outlook is poorer in premature in-fants, partly because of the functional inefficiency of their livers. At one time one of the chief causes of death was hemorrhage associated with hepatic dam-age and prothrombin deficiency. Hemo-lytic disease of the newborn is self-limited and if death does not occur or can be prevented by appropriate treatment, re-covery can be complete provided no serious complication develops. Kernic-terus is the only important cause of death and crippling after the first day of life.[1a] It is possible that some cases of idiopathic juvenile cirrhosis may have their begin-ning in hemolytic disease of the new-born.[4h] In those that survive there may be a deep green staining of the deciduous teeth, produced by pigment deposition in the growing enamel.[3,4] This does not affect the permanent teeth.

Treatment. — The management of hemolytic disease of the newborn includes the problem of recognition of impending difficulties and preparation for these, and the treatment of the newborn infant itself. All pregnant women should be typed for Rh to determine whether they are positive or negative. This is particularly important if a primipara has received one or more transfusions or injections of blood; or if a multipara is found to have given birth to an infant with jaundice or unexplained anemia, or has had a stillbirth. If a woman is Rh-negative and her husband is Rh-positive, it is helpful whenever possible to determine whether the prospective father is homozygous or heterozygous[12i] by the use of appropriate antisera. A test for antibodies should be carried out at the first prenatal visit and this should be repeated at intervals. The diagnostic and prognostic value of examinations made during the pregnancy has been discussed already (p. 759).

There is no convincing evidence of the value of any form of antenatal treatment of the mother, such as the use of Rh hapten,[1e] adrenocorticosteroids,[5c] progesterone or vitamin K.[4f] What is most important is to ensure, if possible, the delivery of a viable infant and to be prepared for its prompt treatment if that is necessary. Earlier views opposing the premature induction of labor because of the increased hazards which prematurity adds and the greater likelihood of kernicterus,[13] have been modified, on the basis of later experience, to recommend this step where an Rh-immunized mother has already had a stillbirth due to Rh incompatibility and an expert team is available for early exchange transfusion.[1a,5b,7c] It has been recommended that the pregnancy be terminated at the 36th week if the indirect antiglobulin titer at that time is 1/512 or higher.[7c]

The value of exchange transfusion is well established.[1a,13f] *Exchange transfusion is recommended* (1) whenever there is clinical evidence of disease at the time of birth as manifested by enlargement of the spleen and liver or by anemia (hemoglobin of cord blood less than 15 Gm. per 100 ml.); (2) when there is a history of severe disease or of kernicterus in a previous baby; (3) in all premature erythroblastotic infants (because of their marked tendency to become severely jaundiced); (4) when the maternal titer of anti-Rh is 1 : 64 or higher (since there is a marked tendency for severe jaundice to occur in such cases); (5) if exchange transfusion is not done at birth, (*a*) it should be carried out if jaundice becomes apparent before the infant is six hours of age, (*b*) if the serum bilirubin level reaches 10 mg. per 100 ml. or more in the first twelve hours even though the hemoglobin is above 15 Gm. but is less than 17.5 Gm. Exchange transfusion should be repeated within the first twelve to twenty-four hours if the serum bilirubin still rises; it should not be permitted to exceed 20 mg. per 100 ml. A third exchange transfusion is rarely necessary if the first two are done early.[1a]

Mature infants whose cord hemoglobin exceeds 17.5 Gm., in whom jaundice is absent and the Coombs' test is negative will probably not require active therapy. If the Coombs' test is positive and clinical signs (icterus, anemia, rising erythroblast count) do not appear in the first twenty-four hours, exchange transfusion will probably not be needed.

The results of repeated simple transfusions[10a] are less good than those claimed for exchange transfusions but it is important that the latter be done only by trained persons with sufficient experience to avoid the potential dangers. Various technics for "exsanguination" transfusion have been described,[13b,13f] a very satisfactory one being that of Diamond in which the umbilical cord, cannulated by a plastic catheter, is used.[1a] The objection has been raised that the latter is a "blind" procedure. Some prefer to withdraw blood from the radial artery at the wrist, the exchange blood being given via the saphenous vein at the ankle.[13f] For an Rh-positive infant Rh-negative blood is used, since Rh-negative blood will not induce isoimmunization and the red cells will not become coated by the circulating antibodies. Simultaneously the antibody-coated infant cells which are destined to be destroyed are removed. In this way the harmful effects of the products of blood destruction are avoided and a certain amount of anti-Rh antibody is also removed. At one time it was the practice to give more blood than was removed but this has been found to be dangerous since overloading of the infant's circulatory system can cause cardiac failure and death. A useful guide is the estimation of venous pressure, measured by holding the plastic catheter in the umbilical vein in a vertical position above the abdomen. The pressure should be maintained at 60 mm. or less.

Blood for transfusion is selected from an Rh-negative donor. The baby's father obviously would not be a suitable donor and his relatives would less likely be suitable than those of the mother. In an emergency the mother's blood may be used,[13d] preferably after replacing her plasma with plasma from a person of group AB. Some prefer to use blood of female donors[1a] but others have not found this to be advantageous.[12b] For *cross matching* the mother's serum is preferable to that of the infant since antibody that could be present in the serum of the baby is also present in the serum of the mother and usually in much greater concentration. The blood that is to be used for the baby must be blood that could be given to the mother; that is, the blood given the baby must lack the factor which the maternal antibody could attack. The donor should of course be of a blood group that is compatible with the baby also. Group O blood to which A and B substances have been added is recommended.[1a] Cross matching should be done by the indirect Coombs' test since the maternal antibody is often the type that does not agglutinate, but nevertheless coats the donor cells. If mother and baby are both Rh-positive donors should be tested.

Other than transfusion, the child should receive the usual care required for its age and state of maturity. There is no good evidence that ACTH or cortisone is of value.[4b] Although the mother's breast milk and particularly the colostrum, contains Rh antibodies,[14] there is no definite proof that antibodies are absorbed from the gastrointestinal tract of the infant and, thus, there appears to be no danger from breast feeding.

The disease process dies out after three to six weeks as the antibodies derived from the mother are eliminated. Occasionally an infant who has received one or more exchange transfusions is found to have a fairly severe anemia by the third or fourth week after birth. Specific supportive therapy is usually not necessary. Although the anemia is attributed to physiologic inactivity of the bone marrow, reticulocyte counts of 3 to 10 per cent are usually found. Only when the anemia becomes severe (hemoglobin 6 Gm. or less) and anorexia, sleeplessness, increasing irritability and other signs of impending anoxia develop, is it necessary to give a blood transfusion. A small transfusion of packed red cells (10 ml. per pound of body weight) will usually suffice.

Pathology.[4e]—Besides icterus, edema, pallor, effusions in the serous cavities and sometimes petechiae, the most striking finding is extensive extramedullary hematopoiesis. This is to be seen not only in the liver and spleen but also in the kidneys, adrenals, and other organs. In the macerated fetus the finding of erythroblasts in the pulmonary capillaries is the most important single diagnostic sign.[10c] The great enlargement of the liver and spleen has been mentioned. In the liver there may be necrosis and atrophy of some of the parenchymal cells, as well as distention of the bile capillaries with bile thrombi. The bone marrow shows pronounced hyperplasia. The brain[4c] may show a diffuse icteric staining or a localization of pigment in the region of the basal nuclei. Deposits of hemosiderin are found in other tissues as well.

Pathogenesis.—Before the outstanding discovery of Levine and his co-workers was made, such theories had been proposed as failure of the hematopoietic system to develop beyond the fourth or fifth month,[7] deficient supply of substances derived from the mother which are necessary for hematopoiesis,[31] and the inheritance of a dominant mutation. Darrow[2a] attributed the symptoms to an antigen-antibody reaction with passive sensitization to the hemoglobin of the red cells of the fetus and transmission of the antibody through the placenta.

The demonstration by Levine, Katzin and Burnham,[9] in 1941, of an abnormal hemagglutinin in the serum of mothers of infants with erythroblastosis fetalis which agglutinated the red cells of the infants as well as of the fathers, set in motion a series of investigations which have elucidated the pathogenesis of this disorder. It was shown that the blood factor in the fathers and infants was closely related to the Rh agglutinogen (p. 340). It was also found that, whereas random sampling of the white population in the United States revealed 85 per cent of persons to be Rh-positive, only 10 per cent of mothers of affected infants were Rh-positive and 100 per cent of the husbands and affected infants of Rh-negative mothers were Rh-positive.[8c] It has now been shown that in most instances of hemolytic disease of the newborn, the Rh-negative mother is immunized by the Rh-positive cells of the fetus; the anti-Rh agglutinin so produced in the mother passes into the circulation of the infant and destroys its red corpuscles. A severe hemolytic anemia with all its associated manifestations, such as jaundice, edema, pigment deposition and profound hemopoietic stimulation is the result. Chown[40] and others[5,7d] have demonstrated fetal red cells in the maternal circulation.

Unless a woman has been sensitized by blood transfusion or by the intramuscular injection of blood, at least one pregnancy is required to initiate sensitization to the Rh agglutinogen. Sometimes the first child to be affected develops relatively mild symptoms of jaundice and anemia and recovers spontaneously, subsequent offspring being injured more seriously. When a woman has been sensitized by transfusion the disease may appear in the first pregnancy and then the combined action of pregnancy and transfusion may produce the severest form of hemolytic disease of the newborn.[9b] It has been shown that a single transfusion of Rh-positive blood in an Rh-negative female, even if given in childhood, may immunize her forever.

It has been observed that an affected infant is not produced in all instances even though several pregnancies have occurred in the Rh-negative wife of an Rh-positive husband. It has been calculated that the incidence of hemolytic disease is no higher than one in ten in pregnancies which provide the necessary Rh conditions,[10e] even after allowing for the fact that 57 per cent of Rh-positive men are heterozygous and would therefore have offspring half of whom would be Rh-negative.[12j] The mechanism whereby such protection against immunization occurs is obscure. One theory postulates that the placental barrier differs in the extent to which fetal Rh-positive cells enter the mother's circulation.[9f] Of special interest is the curious observation that compatible matings in the ABO system are significantly more frequent in families in which hemolytic disease has occurred than in non-affected families.[8c] Various explanations have been offered; for example, it has been suggested that competition with a stronger antigen may prevent sensitization to the Rh antigen.[10a] It was found that volunteers could be more successfully immunized to Rh by injection of blood if the blood was ABO compatible.[12f] It is possible that fetal cells entering the maternal circulation, if ABO incompatible with the mother, may be eliminated before they have time to act as Rh antigen. It is also possible that ABO incompatible fetuses are eliminated early in pregnancy.[10e]

Although D is by far the most important of the Rh antigens which can cause hemolytic disease of the newborn, occasionally the infants are children of Rh-positive (D) mothers. This was observed in approximately 1 per cent of the cases in one large series[9e] and was due to antibodies against c, E and C.[w] Others have reported hemolytic disease due to sensitization to C^x,[12h] D^u,[9d] f[9c] (?) and other rare Rh antigens.[12c] Anti-K (Kell) has been the cause of severe hemolytic disease on many occasions[8b,10e] but hemolytic disease has been encountered only rarely in response to the M,[12g] S,[8d] s,[4d] Fy^a[1d] or Jk^a[1c] antigens (see also p. 344). In most of these cases the antibodies have been of the "incomplete" variety.

Hemolytic disease of the newborn due to ABO incompatibility is next in frequency to that caused by anti-D. Anti-A (A_1)[15a] has been a more common cause than anti-B. The interesting observation has been made that in hemolytic disease due to this form of incompatibility the mother has been almost invariably group O.[12] This has been explained on the hypothesis that the active antibody is the cross-reacting anti-"C" which only group O subjects can form.[13d] Wiener distinguished two patterns of ABO hemolytic

disease; namely, one in which the maternal isoantibodies are chiefly of hetero-immune origin (so-called "natural" antibodies) and the first-born incompatible infant is generally affected but the manifestations tend to be mild (*icterus praecox*); and another, more serious form in which one or more normal babies of an incompatible blood group may first be born. These babies are secretors and sensitize the mother so that subsequent babies of incompatible blood group develop typical erythroblastosis.[13d]

The development of *kernicterus* is closely correlated with the levels of serum bilirubin. Kernicterus may develop whenever the serum bilirubin is very high (20 to 25 mg./100 ml.), whatever the cause.[4c,13a,16] This is especially true in premature infants. The excess of "indirect" reacting, unconjugated bilirubin, which is regularly found in the human newborn, is probably due to the inadequate development of the glucuronide conjugating mechanism.[16] Another factor may be imperfect protein binding of bilirubin.[9i] It has been reported that bilirubin interferes with oxidative phosphorylation, thereby, perhaps, causing brain damage.[3a]

Hemolytic disease can be produced experimentally in newborn dogs following immunization of the dam by transfusion,[15] in rabbits,[7a] and in other species.[10e]

POSTHEMORRHAGIC ANEMIA

Although the hazards of maternal hemorrhage during labor and delivery are well recognized, the possibility that the fetus and newborn might develop anemia from hemorrhage into the placenta,[40] or from umbilical vessels, received little attention until recently. Nevertheless, this type of anemia is probably the second most common cause of anemia in the newborn, after hemolytic disease.[44] This type of anemia may be severe and all the symptoms of hypovolemia may be present.[47a] Death may ensue if the cause of the symptoms is not recognized and blood transfusion not given. In other cases, the anemia may be more moderate in degree and may not be immediately evident. It is normocytic or macrocytic in type and the striking erythroblastosis of hemolytic disease is lacking, as are signs of increased blood destruction. Whether severe or mild, the anemia is not accompanied be hepatosplenomegaly.

A curious phenomenon which has been attributed to the existence of direct communications between the two fetal circulations, such as arteriovenous shunts, or because of other abnormalities in the circulation, is the occurrence of anemia in one of a pair of monozygotic twins and polycythemia in the other.[43]

CONGENITAL HYPOPLASTIC ANEMIA

In an earlier chapter (p. 551) various hypoplastic and aplastic anemias occurring in childhood were mentioned, including congenital pancytopenia and acute erythroblastopenia. Acute erythroblastopenia has been discussed already in the present chapter (p. 755). Congenital pancytopenia or Fanconi's anemia, which is a rare, fatal disorder characterized by pancytopenia, bone marrow hypoplasia and congenital anomalies, is not usually detected until the age of four or later, although it has been observed as early as thirteen months of age (p. 561).

Aplastic anemia with acellular bone marrow and pancytopenia due to drug exposure is very rare in the newborn or in early infancy and the "idiopathic" form, like Fanconi's anemia is most unusual this early.[47] Congenital hypoplastic anemia[41] (**chronic congenital aregenerative anemia,**[46] erythrogenesis imperfecta,[39] anemia of Blackfan and Diamond[1b]), however, is encountered in the newborn.[7] The anemia develops insidiously within the latter part of the neonatal period or some time later in the first year of life, is progressive and of a non-regenerative type. There is no erythroblastosis or evidence of increased blood destruction and hepatosplenomegaly does not develop until many transfusions have been given. The term **"pure red cell anemia"** has also been applied because the leukocyte and platelet counts are normal or only very slightly reduced and hemorrhagic manifestations do not occur. The bone marrow is deficient in normoblasts. The condition may be of long duration and the ultimate prognosis is uncertain. Blood transfusion has been the only therapeutic measure which sustained life. Splenectomy has been effective occasionally in arresting the anemia and spontaneous recovery has occurred.[47] There are some reports of benefit from ACTH and cortisone therapy[42,45] but failures have also been recorded.[47] The cause of the disorder is unknown. In two instances an abnormality of tryptophane metabolism, as manifested by the finding of anthranilic acid in the urine, was reported.[37,45] In what was probably a different disorder, acquired hemolytic anemia may have produced the pseudo-aplastic picture.[38]

NUTRITIONAL ANEMIAS

"IRON DEFICIENCY" ANEMIA

Hypochromic anemia in infancy and childhood responding to the administration of iron has been discussed in the preceding chapter (p. 734). A number of factors are concerned in the development of iron deficiency at this age. It is now thought that it is important from the point of view of conservation of iron in the infant to delay tying the cord until it has stopped pulsating.[24] Iron derived from the mother apparently plays a very important rôle in the infant. Studies in which the importance of transplacental iron could be determined by tracing the

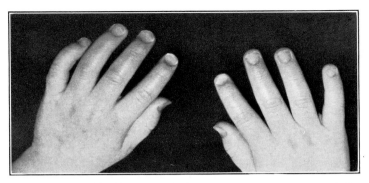

Fig. 15–1.—Koilonychia ("spoon-nails") in a child, aged one and a half years, with iron deficiency anemia.

Fe[55]-tagged iron of the mother showed that there is very little or no utilization of dietary iron for hemoglobin synthesis until three or four months after birth and even at one year iron of transplacental origin constituted approximately 70 per cent of the full-term infant's total hemoglobin iron.[34a]

Iron deficiency anemia is uncommon before the age of six months and is rather frequent at 18 months or later. It is during this period and later, that diet and growth become important factors in the development of iron deficiency. The so-called "physiologic anemia" of infancy is attributable in part, at least, to iron deficiency. Thus, when 5 mg. iron was supplied daily in the formula of infants three to six months of age, and 10 mg. daily thereafter, no "physiologic anemia" developed.[29a]

Infections of various types are often associated with hypochromic anemia in infants and children. These not only adversely affect the dietary intake of iron but also interfere with iron metabolism (p. 577). Chronic gastrointestinal disturbances may lead to the development of iron deficiency anemia both by influencing the quality of the diet and through impairment of absorption. In celiac disease[31] and in cases of chronic dysentery, hypochromic anemia is often found. Idiopathic steatorrhea often begins in childhood and may be associated with hypochromic anemia[18] (p. 501). Although achlorhydria has been demonstrated in many anemic infants, this probably is not an important factor in the development of iron deficiency since hypochlorhydria is common in early age groups.[7] Finally it may be pointed out that chronic hemorrhage may be a cause of hypochromic anemia in childhood, as it is in adults (p. 734). Hookworm anemia is not common in the first few months of life, but is notoriously frequent in young children. The potbellied, barefooted pale child represents the classic picture of the disease.

The *clinical manifestations* of hypochromic anemia in infancy and childhood are similar to those in adults and need no additional description. Except for pallor, the children usually look well nourished. There is no icterus. The writer has seen koilonychia ("spoon-nails") as striking in a child of one and a half years (Fig. 15–1) as in women of middle age. In the blood there may be found a number of erythroblasts, as well as the small, ring-like red corpuscles characteristic of this type of anemia.

The *treatment* of iron deficiency anemia has been discussed already (pp. 457, 748). There is no need to supplement iron with copper, in spite of the fact that copper is concerned in iron metabolism (p. 140).

The quantity of copper required by man is so small that the amount needed is easily acquired in drinking water, vegetables and other foods. However, in infants fed cows' milk, a poor source of both iron and copper, a syndrome of hypoferremia and hypoproteinemia has been observed which was accompanied by *hypocupremia* (p. 141). In such infants the administration of iron together with a liberal diet sufficed to relieve the anemia.

VITAMIN DEFICIENCY, GOAT'S MILK ANEMIA, MACROCYTIC ANEMIAS

The rôle of the various vitamins in hematopoiesis was discussed in an earlier chapter (p. 130). There is no convincing evidence that deficiency of vitamins A or D, *per se* is ever a cause of anemia. It is clear, however, that pyridoxine, pteroylglutamic ("folic") acid and vitamin B_{12} are actively concerned in hematopoiesis, and riboflavin and niacin probably play a rôle as well. The place of ascorbic acid is obscure. Anemia in scorbutic infants is less common than in scorbutic adults[32] and frequently when both scurvy and anemia are present, orange juice does not produce a specific hematologic response.[7] Evaluation of such cases is often difficult because other substances such as iron may be lacking as well, and infection may be present also. It has been shown, however, that ascorbic acid is involved in the metabolism of folic acid and vitamin B_{12}.

Macrocytic anemia is a characteristic finding in certain nutritional anemias in adults (see Chapter 10) but in infants and young children this has proved to be a less reliable sign. This is due in part to the fact that macrocytosis seems to develop more readily at a very early age than later and also because multiple deficiencies are more likely to occur in infants. The microcytosis of iron deficiency may neutralize the macrocytosis of another type of deficiency and normal

mean corpuscular volume may be the result.

It is theoretically possible for the factors leading to deficiency of vitamin B_{12} and folic acid and the production of macrocytic, megaloblastic anemia in adults to have the same effect in infants and children. True "intrinsic factor" deficiency, however, which is the fundamental disorder in pernicious anemia, is rare below 20 years of age (p. 469). Macrocytic anemia may be seen in association with celiac disease[25] (p. 501) although it is rare in comparison with the incidence of hypochromic microcytic anemia. Various other types of gastro-intestinal abnormalities, such as those produced by congenital defects or post-operative shunts could have this effect as well. In particular, however, macrocytic anemia from dietary deficiency of "extrinsic factor" would be expected to occur in infancy and childhood. This may have been a factor in the cases described by Cooley and Lee[20] and in those of Blackfan and Diamond.[16] The latter observed 15 infants between the ages of four and sixteen months in whom a severe macrocytic anemia developed which was corrected by the parenteral administration of liver extract. This anemia was attributed to acute infection and a temporary complete achlorhydria. It is significant that in only one patient was more than one course of liver therapy needed; the remaining children recovered completely after a single course of treatment. The usual symptoms of anemia, together with anorexia, loss of weight, vomiting and diarrhea were observed in these patients, together with some enlargement of both the liver and the spleen. In contrast to the finding in pernicious anemia, the leukocytes were often elevated in number.

Goat's milk anemia, a type of anemia observed particularly in Germany and in Italy in infants fed goat's milk exclusively, has frequently been described as macrocytic, and megaloblasts, thrombocytopenia and often leukopenia have been reported. Bilirubinemia and high plasma iron[22] complete the resemblance to pernicious anemia. These infants are often poorly nourished and may have chronic diarrhea. The anemia has been cured by increasing the amount of goat's milk,[17] by feeding liver or yeast extract,[23] by injections of liver extract[32a] or by giving folic acid.[22] European workers[33] reported the production of anemia in rats by feeding goat's milk which was cured by giving liver but not by giving ascorbic acid or iron. American investigators[30] were unable to confirm these results.

It seems likely that the cases of goat's milk anemia, and the other cases of macrocytic anemia mentioned above[1b, 20] are related to those reported more recently by Zuelzer and Ogden[35] in Detroit and by Amato and Gerbasi[19] in Italy which have been designated as **megaloblastic anemia of infancy.** The condition has been described in infants three to eighteen months of age, most frequently between nine and twelve months old. With the exception of twins, none of the patients' siblings have been affected. Pallor, irritability, loss of appetite and intermittent fever are usually noticed following an upper respiratory infection or gastro-enteric disorder from which the patient has failed to recover. Cough, coryza, earache, or vomiting and diarrhea are often present. In severe cases bleeding manifestations may be noted. The infant usually appears acutely ill. In addition to the marked pallor, an icteric tint can be discerned. The nutritional state is below par, petechiae may be found in the skin and mucous membranes and other signs suggesting scurvy may be present. Cardiac enlargement, hemic murmurs, hepatic enlargement and, less consistently, splenomegaly may be found. There may be evidence of infection in the ears, nose and throat or lungs and osteoporosis or frank signs of scurvy may be seen roentgenologically.

The blood findings are identical with those of pernicious anemia, except that infection may be present and leukocytosis may be found. Macrocytosis may not be so pronounced that the mean corpuscular volume is necessarily increased above normal but the blood smear is characteristic and the bone marrow contains typical megaloblasts as well as many forms intermediate between normoblasts and megaloblasts. Curiously, the erythropoietic activity of the bone marrow was found reduced when the anemia was most severe,[35] unlike the findings in nutritional anemias in adults. Hyperbilirubinemia, increased output of urobilinogen in the urine and stools, high serum iron and hypoproteinemia have been found. Free hydrochloric acid has been absent from the gastric juice in most cases during the height of the disorder, even after injection of histamine.

A reticulocyte increase and rapid regeneration of blood similar to those seen in pernicious anemia have been observed following the administration of liver extract,[35] folic acid or vitamin B_{12}[34, 34b] but the most consistent responses have followed folic acid. Partial or complete failure to respond to B_{12} has been described.[26] Only a short course of therapy is required and relapse does not occur. Even without specific therapy remissions have been observed but, as a rule, left to itself the anemia progresses rapidly and death eventually ensues.

The demands of growth, the impairment of hemopoiesis by infection[27] and the possibility of dietary deficiency have been considered as etiologic agents. The last is probably the most important.[27a] It was noted that a large proportion of the patients in this country had been fed a proprietary powdered milk of relatively low protein content[35] without added ascorbic acid.[26, 27] It is of great interest that of the two breast fed infants of Zuelzer's series, the mother of one had pernicious anemia and the mother of the second had hypochromic anemia with glossitis and achlorhydria. Two patients had received goat's milk. In South African Bantus, megaloblastic anemia of infancy was most commonly associated with kwashiorkor.[34c]

Further clinical[26] and experimental[27] studies have brought evidence of the importance of ascorbic acid deficiency in this syndrome. What seems to be an identical disorder has been produced in monkeys[27] by feeding a diet similar to the proprietary milk powder regime described above. Only when this was not supplemented with ascorbic acid did the disorder develop but the administration of folic acid, without ascorbic acid, produced a prompt hemopoietic response. Thus it would seem that this form of megaloblastic anemia results from folic acid deficiency which is somehow induced by a chronic deficiency of ascorbic acid.

It may be emphasized once more that not all instances of macrocytic anemia are the result of nutritional deficiencies. Thus, the anemia in hemolytic disease of the newborn (p. 757) is macrocytic but this is due to the presence of a great number of immature cells and is not influenced by the administration of folic acid or vitamin B_{12}.

ANEMIA OF PREMATURITY AND OF TWINS

The customary post-natal fall in hemoglobin level tends to be exaggerated in the premature infant even though the initial cord hemoglobin may be the same as in full-term babies. The lower the birth weight, the greater the decrease.[7,31] The same is true of twins or other full-term infants of low birth weight. The fall in mean corpuscular volume and in mean corpuscular hemoglobin is essentially parallel so that the mean corpuscular hemoglobin concentration remains normal although the mean cell size is

reduced from values in the range of 105 $c\mu$ to approximately 70 $c\mu$.[23a] The lowest levels are reached at approximately six to nine weeks of age. Usually slow improvement occurs about the fourth month, only to be followed by a second phase of anemia.[28] In the second phase hypochromia develops and a response to iron therapy is observed.[29,31] It is the first phase of the anemia of prematurity which has been the subject of much speculation for many years and the literature is filled with many conflicting statements.

Several quantitative studies are now available which permit a reasonably adequate picture to be drawn.[20a,21,33] Two major changes take place in the first two months of life. There is, first of all, a striking depression of hemopoietic activity soon after birth, as reflected by a fall in the reticulocyte count to very low levels during the first week of postnatal life, where it remains for the next five to seven weeks; at the same time growth takes place, usually at a rate which is more rapid than in the full-term infant. As a result the hemoglobin concentration decreases. Some evidence has been presented that red cell survival is somewhat shorter than in the normal (seventy-seven to ninety-eight days, as compared with one hundred to one hundred and twenty days).[33] Although the products of erythrocyte breakdown are utilized for new blood formation, the early sluggishness of erythropoiesis fails to make full use of the materials which are available. This concept explains the observations of many investigators that iron therapy does not significantly affect the early phase of the anemia of prematurity.

During the second month of life, a spontaneous resumption of erythropoiesis occurs, as indicated by a reticulocytosis and subsequent marked rise in *total* body hemoglobin.[33] At this time, even fetal hemoglobin synthesis has been found to be temporarily resumed. About sixteen

49

weeks are required before the hemoglobin mass present at birth is regained. It has been observed that the basic hematologic changes which occur in the full-term and in the premature infant are almost identical and the morphology of the cells in the bone marrow of the premature and the mature infant is the same.[21] It is noteworthy, however, that studies of the mother's tagged iron indicate that the premature infant has little stored iron to draw upon for hemoglobin formation and depends on dietary iron more than does the full-term infant.[34a]

Stated differently, the early anemia of premature infants is due mainly to the "physiological" postnatal depression of erythropoiesis, the effects of which are exaggerated by the rapidity of their growth.[21] The later anemia is due to iron deficiency.

These studies are significant from the standpoint of *therapy*. Blood transfusion for uncomplicated anemia of prematurity does not serve any useful purpose and may even retard the spontaneous process of recovery by reducing the erythropoietic stimulus which anemia induces. Iron given in the early phase can be stored for use in the second phase[23b,29] when continued rapid growth and an active bone marrow make demands which the original supply of blood-forming materials in an infant born with less than the normal stores is unable to meet. Thereby the severity of the second phase of the anemia is minimized.

It has been found that erythropoiesis can be stimulated in premature infants at a time when it is otherwise at a low ebb by the administration of cobalt.[21] It is doubtful, however, that this is advantageous to the infant and the possibility of toxic effects (p. 142) makes such treatment unwise.

HEMOLYTIC ANEMIAS

General Considerations.—Anemias which are predominantly hemolytic in character, similar to those described in Chapters 12 and 13 occur in infants and children as well as in adults. These include hereditary spherocytosis, sickle cell anemia, thalassemia, and the other hemoglobinopathies, the various types of hemoglobinuria, favism and the different forms of hemolytic anemia due to chemical agents or caused by immune bodies. For a discussion of these disorders the reader is referred to the preceding chapters (pp. 598 and 668). Acute hemolytic anemia has been described in infants and children after vaccination,[51] following gas poisoning,[49] and after eating "cranberries."[48] Hemolytic disease of the newborn has been discussed in this chapter already (p. 756).

The manifestations of hemolytic anemia are likely to be more acute in children. Anemia may be more severe, jaundice more marked, and erythroblastosis and reticulocytosis more striking. The last-mentioned changes may be so pronounced that the indications of increased blood destruction may appear insignificant in comparison. In all the forms of hemolytic anemia in infants and young children, leukocytosis may be very marked (50,000 to 100,000). This may be due to the presence of myeloid forms, including myelocytes, or there may be lymphocytosis.

DISEASES WITH OUTSTANDING SPLENOMEGALY

A number of diseases which may be referred to as conditions with outstanding splenomegaly are encountered at all ages. Some will be discussed in other chapters. These include "Banti's disease," thrombosis of the portal vein, kala-azar, leukemia, Hodgkin's disease, and tumors of the spleen. Certain other disorders, however, appear particularly or even exclusively in infancy or childhood and will be considered here.

GAUCHER'S DISEASE

Definition and History.—This is a rare, chronic, familial disorder characterized clinically by splenomegaly, skin pigmentation, pingueculae of the sclera, and bone lesions. Histologically, large kerasin-containing cells are found, particularly in the spleen. The condition was described by Gaucher in 1882[59] and the lipid in the cells was identified by Epstein[58] and Lieb[63] in 1924.

Etiology.—The condition may make its appearance early in infancy, in childhood or early or late in adult life[54,64a] but it is most often discovered in childhood. In one series of 71 cases,[61] the disease was recognized before the eighth year of age in 56 per cent. The diagnosis has been made at one week of life and as many as 17 per cent of cases have been in infants under one year of age. A considerable proportion of those affected have been Jews but the condition has been described in natives of Greece,[55c] India and Japan and has been seen in Negroes.[60a] It is common to find several cases in one family[55b] although it is very unusual for more than one generation to be affected. There is no preference for either sex. The mode of inheritance is still uncertain. It has been suggested that the condition is due to a mutation which is then transmitted as a simple dominant[54] but other evidence has been presented that Gaucher's disease is due to the action of an autosomal recessive gene which, in the homozygous state, causes an intracellular metabolic defect.[60] In the latter study the frequency of multiple cousin marriages was stressed.

Symptomatology.—There is considerable variation not only in the age of onset, as indicated above, but also in the rate of progression. As a rule, however, the earlier the onset the more rapid the course. Splenomegaly is usually the outstanding sign of the disease and may be discovered accidentally. Rarely the weight of the organ produces a dragging sensation, or infarction with sharp pain may develop. Much less frequently splenomegaly is inconspicuous or absent and anemia is the outstanding feature.[53,67,69a] Ascites is rare.[61a]

Hemorrhage, especially from the nose and gums, is relatively common. Occasionally, petechial or purpuric spots are found but other types of bleeding are rare. Pain in the limbs, due to bone involvement, may develop in long-standing cases.[64a]

In infants the onset is more acute and neurological symptoms (rigidity of the neck, convergent strabismus, opisthotonos) as well as retardation of development may be noted. A few similar cases have been observed in older children.

Skin pigmentation is found in 45 to 75 per cent of cases. This is ochre to brown in color with a yellow or leaden hue. The head, neck and hands are frequently affected and symmetrical pigmentation of the legs from just below the knees to the instep, has been described.[54]

Except in infants, or in terminal stages, cachexia is slight or absent. The splenomegaly may be extreme. The liver may be enlarged, sometimes markedly. There is little enlargement of the superficial lymph nodes. Wedge-shaped pingueculæ, light yellowish-brown discolorations of the conjunctiva on either side of the cornea may be found (Fig. 15–2), especially in those who survive to a late age. These contain the typical Gaucher cells.[57b] The fundi show no characteristic changes. Myopia is frequent.[54]

The accumulation of Gaucher cells in the bones may be associated with macroscopic areas of destruction. These may be found in the head, neck or lower end of the femur, sometimes to produce a swelling in the lower femur which resembles the shape of an Erlenmeyer flask; the hip bones, vertebræ, humerus or tibia may be involved.[59a] Collapse of vertebral bodies with gibbus and patho-

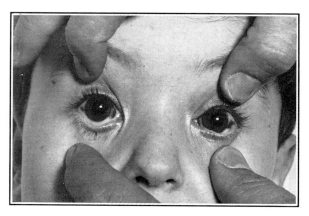

Fig. 15–2.—Pinguecula in a case of Gaucher's disease.

logical fractures may occur.[64a, 69a] The bone may be increased in diameter and the cortical layer thinned,[54] or there may be areas of rarefaction and condensation, giving a mottled appearance.

The Blood.—The anemia is usually moderate in degree and normocytic in type. There is little or no evidence of active blood regeneration such as polychromatophilia or nucleated red cells. Leukopenia with relative lymphocytosis is common and slight thrombocytopenia may be present as well. Thrombocytopenia without anemia or leukopenia but accompanied by a clinical picture of thrombocytopenic purpura and responding to splenectomy has been reported[56] and occurred in one of our cases, a child of eight years. Monocytosis may occur. In infants anemia is more severe than in cases encountered at a later age.[7] Gaucher cells were reported in the blood in one case.[53]

There is no evidence of increased blood destruction. The total fats, cholesterol, and lecithin of the blood have been found to vary within normal limits but in several cases the lipoid nitrogen has been observed to be elevated whereas the lipoid phosphorus was normal.[54] This contrasts with the findings in nephrosis and xanthomatosis, where the lipoid phosphorus as well as the lipoid nitrogen is increased. The serum acid phosphatase level may be elevated above normal[73b] and the cytoplasm of Gaucher cells shows strong acid phosphatase activity.[55a]

Diagnosis. — The classical findings which accompany this form of splenomegaly, namely, pinguecula, skin pigmentation, and generally good state of physical preservation suggest Gaucher's disease. When these signs are absent diagnosis is less easy. Niemann-Pick's disease must be considered in infants. The typical Gaucher cells can often be demonstrated by splenic or sternal puncture or biopsy[71] (Fig. 15-3 and Plate II, p. 64). In marrow smears the cells should be looked for at the end of the smear and with a low power lens.

Treatment. — Treatment is purely symptomatic. Splenectomy should be considered if the weight of the spleen is oppressive. This operation has also been performed successfully when secondary thrombocytopenic purpura was present, as indicated above. It has been claimed that bone lesions appear earlier after splenectomy.[77]

Prognosis.—Patients have lived as long as forty years after the diagnosis was first made. In a number of instances, patients with this disease have undergone

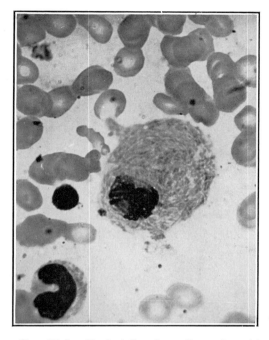

FIG. 15–3.—Typical Gaucher cell together with a lymphocyte and a juvenile neutrophil from the sternal bone marrow in a case of Gaucher's disease.

pregnancy, without difficulty, on purely conservative management.[60b] In infants the prognosis is less good.[62] If neurological involvement is present, death occurs early.

Pathology.[68]—Distinctive large cells, 20 to 80 μ in diameter, are found packed within the organs, especially in the spleen, bone marrow, liver, and lymph nodes ("Gaucher cells"). They are round, oval, or spindle-shaped and usually possess one or many, small, eccentrically placed nuclei. The cytoplasm stains faintly with eosin and not at all with fat stains, but with Mallory's aniline blue numerous wavy fibrillae can be demonstrated. Their arrangement suggests a spider's web. A pale, blue-staining material is seen between the fibrils.

The *spleen* on the average is increased tenfold in size (average normal weight 250 Gm.) and has been known to weigh 8100 Gm. The splenic pulp is almost entirely replaced by the Gaucher cells which are found not only in the sinusoids but also in the pulp and the Malpighian corpuscles. Pigment, chiefly hemosiderin, is also present.[68]

The *liver* is often twice normal in size. Small, pale areas suggest leukemic infiltration. Gaucher cells are found in the portal spaces and in the sinusoids of the lobules. In the *bone marrow* nests of these cells are found. Here they may be spindle-shaped. The deep *lymph nodes* are more likely to be enlarged than the superficial ones and these also contain large accumulations of the "foam" cells. The Gaucher substances may be stored in the cells of the *nervous system* as well.[61d, 67]

Pathogenesis.—The racial and familial characteristics of Gaucher's disease suggest a constitutional basis. The Gaucher cells have been thought[64] to be reticulum cells or histiocytes. In bone lesions,[53] the osteoblasts, osteoclasts, osteocytes and fibroblast-like spindle cells lining the bone spicules may be the source of the Gaucher cells. The lipid found in Gaucher cells was recognized as a cerebroside by Lieb[63] and was thought to contain galactose in its carbohydrate moiety. It was assumed that the total molecule is identical with brain kerasin. Later, others found that *d*-glucose is present rather than galactose and that behinic acid is the major fatty acid constituent.[69c] The identification of behenyl glucocerebroside was taken to imply that in Gaucher's disease there is a deviation in hexose metabolism which favors the utilization of glucose rather than galactose in the production of the spleen lipids. However, the conclusion that the cerebrosides from Gaucher's tissue contain exclusively glucose has not been confirmed by other investigators, who found significant quantities of galactose-cerebrosides as well as glucose-cerebrosides in the spleen lipids.[73a]

Gaucher's disease has been viewed as a generalized disturbance of lipid metabolism which results in abnormal lipid storage. Many of the symptoms can be attributed to abnormal accumulation of the cerebroside in certain cells, causing enlargement of organs and encroachment on blood-forming tissue and on bone structure. The cerebroside may constitute 6 to 10 per cent of the weight of the dried spleen.[74] It has been assumed that the condition represents an overproduction of the cerebroside or trapping of the compound, or its precursors, as it circulates in trace amounts.[57a] As viewed by electron microscopy, the cytoplasm of Gaucher cells was found to be filled with a number of dense elongate or crescent-shaped bodies. Each of these fibrils was bounded by a single dense limiting membrane and contained a homogeneous appearing matrix. Tubular-appearing subunits visible within this matrix were thought to represent the abnormal cerebroside.

It is also possible that the biochemical defect is catabolic rather than anabolic, since no greater *de novo* synthesis of cerebrosides could be demonstrated in Gaucher cells than in control tissue.[73a] The demonstration of marked amounts of intracellular iron within Gaucher cells led another investigator to postulate that some metabolic abnormality involving iron may be present in Gaucher's disease,[63b] in addition to the alterations already noted.

NIEMANN-PICK'S DISEASE

History and Symptomatology.— Niemann-Pick's disease, a condition similar to Gaucher's disease, was described by the authors[66, 68a] after whom it is named in 1914 and 1922. Originally thought to appear only in infancy, it has since been found that manifestations may be discovered for the first time in the second year of life and even later (6 years).[55] There is a marked predilection for the Jewish race; 30 per cent of one

series of 18 patients were of Jewish ancestry,[55] 50 per cent in another.[75]

Persistent early jaundice, enlarging abdomen or poor general nutritional and developmental progress are the commonest initial complaints. The enlargement of the liver occurs early in contrast to the late appearance of hepatomegaly in Gaucher's disease. Bile has been found in the urine and the alkaline phosphatase has been elevated in some cases. The jaundice may subside in a few months. The spleen is also enlarged. Severe constipation, difficult feeding and repeated bronchitis and bronchopneumonia mark the course of the disease. The skin may take on a pale, waxy, brown hue and skin xanthomas are common. There may be moderate or considerable lymph node enlargement. Cherry-red spots in the macular area of the fundus oculi, similar to those seen in amaurotic familial idiocy, have been found in perhaps a fourth, or more, of the cases. Mental retardation is very common, but not invariably present.

Roentgenography frequently reveals diffuse and intense miliary mottling of the lungs and coarse trabeculation of the long bones, widening and prominence of the medullary cavities and undermineralization.

The Blood.—Anemia is not conspicuous and, when present, is only moderate in degree. Leukopenia may be found and in some instances leukocytosis was present, in the absence of infection.[68a] The most interesting abnormality is the presence of vacuoles in the cytoplasm of circulating lymphocytes and monocytes (Fig. 15–4, A). These are discrete, unstained, round, 1/2 to 1 micron in diameter and are often present in groups of 2 to 15 or 20 per cell. Rarely they may seem to distend the cell membrane and displace the nucleus. The nature of the vacuoles is unknown. There may be moderate thrombocytopenia.

Serum lipids are usually normal but in

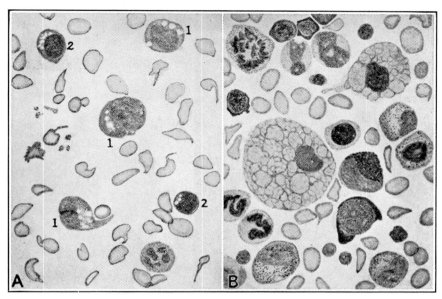

Fig. 15–4.—Drawings of representative cells in smears made from (*A*) peripheral blood and (*B*) sternal bone marrow in a case of Niemann-Pick's disease showing numerous vacuoles in the cytoplasm of monocytes (*A1*) and lymphocytes (*A2*) in the blood, and foam cells in the marrow. (Kato, courtesy of Am. J. Dis. Child.)

some cases elevations of cholesterol and phospholipids have been observed.[55]

The **diagnosis** is readily made on the basis of the characteristic clinical picture and the demonstration of the characteristic cells filled with lipid (Fig. 15–4, *B*) which are found by puncture of the bone marrow or spleen.

Prognosis and Treatment.—The disease is much more rapid in its course than Gaucher's disease and most patients die within a few months, invariably following a period of severe general deterioration. It is not true, however, that all patients die very early, for some have lived to 20 years of age.[55,58a] Whether three cases described in adults represent the same disorder as that seen in infants is uncertain.[73]

Treatment, in the absence of an understanding of the inherent defect, is necessarily symptomatic and supportive. Infections are treated as they arise. Splenectomy has had little value except

to relieve respiratory and gastrointestinal distress when the size of the spleen became a problem.

Pathology.—The cells of Niemann-Pick's disease are round, oval, or polyhedral and are filled with small round hyaline droplets in clusters which give the appearance of foam or a honeycomb (Fig. 15–4).[69] This contrasts with the wrinkled cytoplasm of the Gaucher cell. Furthermore, unlike the latter, the cells of Niemann-Pick's disease have only one or two, rarely many nuclei. The cells give positive reactions for sudan III and other fat stains. Their average diameter is 40 μ.

There is much more widespread involvement than in Gaucher's disease. All the organs are yellow and fatty. The bone marrow may appear strikingly yellow. The liver and spleen are enormously enlarged. The lymph nodes, suprarenals, thymus, thyroid, and lungs are extensively involved as are also the brain and

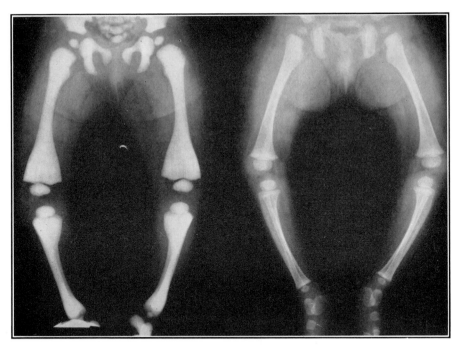

Fig. 15–5.—Roentgenogram of lower extremities and portion of pelvis of a nine-month-old infant (G.A.B.) with osteopetrosis (left) compared with those of a normal infant of the same age (right). Note the loss of differentiation between cortex and spongiosa, thus producing a homogeneous density.

spinal cord. In the central nervous system the histological picture resembles that of Tay-Sach's disease (amaurotic family idiocy).

Pathogenesis.—This, like Gaucher's disease, is thought to be a disorder of lipid metabolism. The involved organs show an increase in total lipids, usually total phospholipids, invariably cholesterol and, absolutely and relatively, sphingomyelin.[55] In many instances more than one sibling in a family has been affected.[75] The condition appears to be the result of a constitutional anomaly which is probably inherited as a recessive trait.

HURLER'S DISEASE

Commonly known as *gargoylism* and lipochondrodystrophy, this disorder of childhood which is characterized by physical and mental retardation, enlargement of the skull, corneal opacities,

thickness of the tongue, short stubby fingers and umbilical hernia, is also associated with hepatosplenomegaly and with certain changes in the hemopoietic tissues.[61b] These consist of the presence of lilac-colored granulations in the leukocytes of the blood and in the reticulum cells, the osteoblasts and the histiocytes of the bone marrow. The inclusions in the leukocytes closely resemble those seen in Alder's hereditary anomaly of leukocytes (p. 224). Especially when viewed by supravital staining of marrow fragments, phagocytic clasmatocytes containing inclusions are found.

MARBLE BONE DISEASE

Definition and Synonyms.—This is a rare congenital and probably hereditary disorder,[76] described by Albers-Schönberg in 1904, which is also known as osteopetrosis or Marmorknochenkrank-

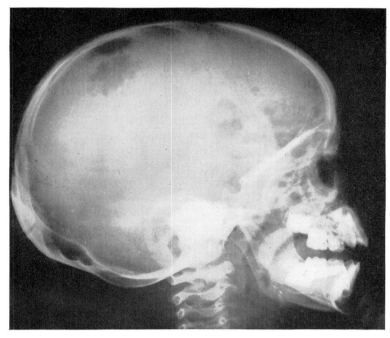

FIG. 15–6.—Osteolytic lesions in the skull in a case (D.E.J.) of Letterer-Siwe disease.

heit,[61c] chalky bones and osteopetrosis fragilis generalisata.[69] It occurs in infancy and childhood and is marked by splenomegaly, spontaneous fractures and a characteristic appearance of the bones.

Symptomatology.—An outstanding feature of this disease is the high incidence of fractures following trivial injury. The infant or child often appears older than its actual age, is frail and underdeveloped and the skin is dry and wrinkled. Loss of sight, and deafness or paralysis of muscles supplied by cranial nerves, have been observed, the result of narrowing of the cranial foramens with consequent nerve atrophy. Hydrocephalus is relatively common. The condition may cause death *in utero.* Hepatosplenomegaly and generalized lymphadenopathy are frequently associated with anemia but anemia is not necessarily found.[74a] In about a fourth of the cases[74b] the blood picture has been that of myelophthisic anemia (p. 588). Roentgenographically, the bones of the entire skeleton are homogeneously opaque (Fig. 15–5).

Diagnosis.—The characteristic clinical picture should suggest examination of the bones. On marrow puncture the bone is found to be stony hard and the needle will not penetrate through the cortex.

Treatment and Prognosis.—Treatment is supportive. Patients with osteopetrosis have been observed to live a few weeks to a few years, the duration depending on the severity and extent of the process, the adequacy of compensation and the successful management of intercurrent infections and hematological complications, such as hemorrhage or severe anemia. Splenectomy has been reported to be effective in relieving thrombocytopenia but did not influence the anemia.[71a] A benign form[54a,69] which permits the achievement of even a normal life span may or may not be related to the relatively malignant disorder of infancy and childhood.

Pathology.—The endosteum of most of the bones reveals a marked increase in the number and thickness of the trabeculae, which may encroach on the marrow to its exclusion. The periosteum may also be involved. The changes are present in the epiphysis, metaphysis, diaphysis and cortex. The fragility of the bones is attributed to the uncontrolled variability in the size and shape of the bone trabeculae and their purposeless architectural arrangement.[69] The fundamental abnormality would seem to consist of retardation or partial or total failure to resorb mineralized tissue and to form new bone.[57c]

HISTIOCYTOSIS X (EOSINOPHILIC GRANULOMA OF BONE, LETTERER-SIWE DISEASE, SCHULLER-CHRISTIAN DISEASE)

There is increasing evidence[62a] that a form of skeletal lesion of particular histologic type (eosinophilic granuloma of bone), a symptom complex consisting of exophthalmos, diabetes insipidus and bone lesions (Hand-Schüller-Christian disease) and a relatively acute, systemic disorder occurring particularly in young children (Letterer-Siwe disease) have a pathologic common denominator; namely, a distinctive and perhaps specific inflammatory histiocytosis. It appears that all three syndromes, with a number of variations between, represent a single entity probably due to the same underlying, and unknown, etiologic agent. Many names have been applied to such a disorder, especially *reticuloendotheliosis* (systemic, aleukemic, non-lipid) but the proliferating cells which characterize the condition, though admittedly derived largely from the reticulo-endothelium, appear to be already clearly differentiated histiocytes.[62a] There is even less good

evidence for use of the term xanthomatosis than for the name reticuloendotheliosis.

This disorder may be considered as occurring as a localized lesion or in disseminated form. The localized disorder, **eosinophilic granuloma of bone,**[65] is seen in infants, children and young adults, and occasionally in older adults,[52] and is marked by the presence of a single or several discrete, osteolytic lesions in bone which on biopsy reveal a characteristic histologic picture. The only complaints, if any exist, are referable to the local lesion. The lesions may occur in any bone and there may be local pain, swelling, tenderness, and occasionally heat. The pathologic picture is usually that of histiocytic proliferation and eosinophilic infiltration in what appears to be a granuloma. Giant cells and foam cells may be present and fat stains may be positive. There is no discernible visceral involvement and no constitutional symptoms are present and, with curettement or x-ray therapy, cure has been reported,[52,62a] although later additional skeletal lesions may sometimes appear.

The disseminated condition may be marked by an acute or subacute course, or the latter may be more or less chronic. The acute disorder **(Letterer-Siwe syndrome)**[65] is seen most often in infants and young children, particularly below the age of three years, but may be encountered occasionally even in young adults. There is evidence of a wasting disorder, with enlargement of the spleen and liver, generalized lymphadenopathy, a hemorrhagic diathesis, especially petechiae and purpura, skeletal lesions (Fig. 15–6), progressive anemia and cutaneous manifestations which are more or less characteristic.[70a] These consist of discrete, yellowish-brown maculo-papular lesions, or papules with a red border and yellow center. They are scattered over the face and trunk particularly, but may be found in the scalp and elsewhere. There may be whitish macules over the palate and the tongue. Weeping erosions may appear in the axillary, genital and perianal regions and tender tumefactions may develop in these areas. Slight or moderate fever may be present and there is often a predisposition to secondary infections. The course is very variable in duration, ranging from a few weeks to even several years. Though very serious, the disease may not always be fatal and occasionally the condition may become chronic or a remission may develop.

The **Schüller-Christian syndrome**,[65,70] which is usually chronic in course, is seen in children and young adults, occasionally in older adults and, in the classical form, is ushered in by increasing irritability, polydypsia, polyuria, swelling of the gums, loosening of the teeth, exophthalmos and persistent discharge from the ears. *Defects in membraneous bones* are manifested chiefly by sharply defined lesions in the skull, which may present a "geographic" pattern. The face may become deformed by the involvement of the bones of the orbit, the mastoid or maxilla. *Exophthalmos* develops as a consequence of the skull tumors. Symptoms of *diabetes insipidus* are presumably due to involvement of the pituitary stalk or hypothalamus. Associated destruction of the sella turcica is infrequent.[52] Other signs of pituitary insufficiency may develop.

Actually, this classic triad is not often found.[52] More often, one or more of these signs is accompanied by other manifestations. Erosions of the mandible are relatively common, usually in the tooth-bearing portions, and ultimately displacement of the teeth by the tumor causes them to appear to be suspended in space. Other bones may be involved, especially the pelvis, femur, ribs, humerus and spine.[52] In the long bones the lesions usually appear towards the ends of the shafts or epiphyses. There may be pain and tenderness in the limbs.

Chronic otitis media is a common presenting complaint. *Skin lesions* and mucous membrane ulcerations may be found which resemble those seen in Letterer-Siwe syndrome. Involvement of the *lungs* may produce dyspnea and cyanosis and diffuse, bilateral pleural and interstitial pulmonary infiltration, leading eventually to fibrosis,[69b] honeycombing of the lungs and episodes of spontaneous pneumothorax, may be found on roentgenography of the chest. Cor pulmonale and right heart failure may develop. Moderate enlargement of the liver, spleen and lymph nodes may occur. Involvement of the nervous system is rare.[57]

The ultimate prognosis is better than has been considered in the past.[72] It is true that the outlook may be less good when the condition begins very early in life and that progression may occur and death result from pulmonary fibrosis, pituitary involvment or other causes. However, spontaneous remissions have been observed or at least modest improvement takes place. Thus, in one series of 29 cases,[52] one-third recovered and one-half still had signs of active disease. The mortality was 13 per cent.

As these syndromes have attracted more attention and as more cases have been studied carefully, it has become apparent that a child with "eosinophilic granuloma of bone" may develop signs suggesting systemic disease; similar lesions may be found in extra-skeletal sites such as the lymph nodes, the skin, the oral cavity, the anogenital region or the lungs; the acute picture of the Letterer-Siwe syndrome may become chronic; in a typical instance of the Schüller-Christian syndrome an acute exacerbation may develop; the Schüller-Christian triad may be encountered in an otherwise typical example of the Letterer-Siwe syndrome; the skeletal defects in the Schüller-Christian form may not be situated in the calvarium or they may not appear until after lesions in extra-skeletal sites are already well established.

The Blood.—Anemia does not occur in eosinophilic granuloma and may or may not be present in the Schüller-Christian syndrome. In the latter, when it develops, it is of the non-regenerative type and leukopenia and slight thrombocytopenia may be found or, rarely, a pronounced picture of myelophthisic anemia may be seen.[7] In the Letterer-Siwe syndrome anemia is common, thrombocytopenia is frequent, leukopenia may occur and pancytopenia and even hemolytic anemia have been reported.[63a] Hemohistiocytes have been seen in the blood[67a] and a leukemic picture has been observed.[58b]

Diagnosis.—It is evident that, unless a characteristic combination of signs is present, a great variety of disorders may be simulated. Outstanding features are the presence of skeletal lesions, cutaneous, oral and anogenital manifestations, hepato-splenomegaly, adenopathy, exophthalmos and diabetes insipidus in various combinations and with or without signs of wasting disease. A focus of eosinophilic granuloma of bone may develop so rapidly and break through the cortex of the affected bone so readily that prior to biopsy it may be mistaken for a primary malignant tumor such as Ewing's sarcoma. Multiple foci may suggest a diagnosis of metastatic neuroblastoma. Chronic otitis media failing to respond to antibiotic therapy may be the first manifestation of the disease. Skin involvement may simulate intractable eczema from other causes. The miliary pulmonary infiltrations are usually asymptomatic but productive cough, loss of weight and other signs have led to the incorrect diagnosis of tuberculosis. Failure of growth and delayed puberty in association with diabetes insipidus should suggest Schüller-Christian disease. The diagnosis ultimately rests on histologic examination of involved tissue.

Course, Prognosis and Treatment.—Reference has been made already to the great variations in course and prognosis. The favorable response to curettement or x-ray therapy in many instances in which the lesions are localized has also been mentioned. When lesions are purely localized, it is probably better to avoid roentgen therapy since surgical management is satisfactory.[65] Although roentgen therapy is often quickly effective in the treatment of local lesions in the Schüller-Christian syndrome,[60a] some would avoid its use in a chronic disorder in children.[65] Adrenocorticosteroids[52] and folic acid antagonists have been used with some success.[65] The injection or insufflation of β-hypophamine (pitressin) has ameliorated the signs of diabetes insipidus when it has developed. Roentgen therapy may cause the pulmonary changes to disappear but in other cases the ultimate progress of the disease may not be stopped by any therapeutic agent.[72]

Therapeutic results are often quite unsatisfactory in the Letterer-Siwe syndrome. Nitrogen mustard (p. 1037) may produce diminution in the size of local tumefactions without over-all improvement.[65] Other chemotherapeutic agents and adrenocorticosteroids have been used, with uncertain results.[64a]

Pathology.[62a]—Grossly lesions such as those in the skull are found to consist of defects of various shapes and size which are filled with a light yellow or brownish, tough substance. Similar granulation tissue is found in the spleen, liver, lymph nodes and other tissues. The initial microscopic picture is essentially that of an inflammatory histiocytosis or granulomatosis which may or may not be accompanied by intense eosinophilic reaction. This character may be maintained for many months but eventually there is a tendency toward fibrosis, diminution in the number of eosinophilic leukocytes present, and conversion of histiocytes to lipophages, thus presenting a picture of "lipid granuloma." This, however, is a late phase of the evolution of the histiocytic lesion. The fibrosis which is seen at this stage is probably an expression of healing. In fatal cases of the acute disseminated disorder the rapidly proliferating histiocytes in fresh skeletal lesions may appear to become "foamy" as fast as they are formed. Charcot-Leyden crystals have been demonstrated in sections of eosinophilic granuloma of bone.[52a]

Pathogenesis.—Most students of this disorder regard it to be an inflammatory granuloma, possibly of infectious origin rather than a form of xanthomatosis, as was once assumed. Others, however, point out that the classical Letterer-Siwe syndrome resembles much more a generalized reticulum cell sarcoma or monocytic leukemia than a granulomatous disease.[65] Such discussions recall the disagreement concerning the nature of Hodgkin's disease and the relation of "Hodgkin's sarcoma" to the more common forms of that condition (p. 1007).

BIBLIOGRAPHY

Hemolytic Disease of the Newborn

1. AABERG, M. E. and ROLY, C.: Erythroblastosis Fetalis in Twin Pregnancy, Am. J. Obst. & Gynec., 50, 548, 1945.
1a. ALLEN, F. N., JR., DIAMOND, L. K. and WATROUS, J. B., JR.: Erythroblastosis Fetalis, New England J. Med., 241, 799, 1949; Ibid., 244, 39, 1951; Am. J. Dis. Child., 80, 779, 1950; J.A.M.A., 155, 1209, 1954; New England J. Med., 250, 283 and 324, 1954; ibid., 251, 453, 1954.
1b. BLACKFAN, K. D., DIAMOND, L. K. and LEISTER, C. M.: Atlas of the Blood in Children, New York, The Commonwealth Fund, 1944.
1c. BAILEY, J. P., HUTCHINSON-SMITH, B. H., BARBER, M. and DUNSFORD, I.: Immunization during Pregnancy to the Kidd (Jkª) Red-Cell Antigen, Brit. M. J., 1, 1329, 1959.
1d. BEVAN, B.: Haemolytic Disease of the Newborn Caused by Anti-Duffy (Fyª), Lancet, 1, 914, 1959.
1e. CARTER, B. B.: The Treatment of Erythroblastosis Fœtalis with Rh Hapten, Lancet, 1, 1267, 1954.
1f. CRAWFORD, H., CUTBUSH, M. and MOLLISON, P. L.: Hemolytic Diseases of the Newborn

Due to Anti-A, Blood, 8, 620, 1953; Am. J. Obst. & Gynec., 76, 1285, 1958.
2. DAMESHEK, W., GREENWALT, T. J. and TAT, R. J.: Erythroblastosis Fetalis (Acute Hemolytic Anemia of the Newborn), Am. J. Dis. Child., 65, 571, 1943.
2a. DARROW, R. R.: Icterus Gravis (Erythroblastosis) Neonatorum, an Examination of Etiologic Considerations, Arch. Path., 25, 378, 1938.
2b. DAY, R. and PERRY, E.: Intravascular Hemagglutination, Blood, 5, 1114, 1950.
3. DIAMOND, L. K.: The Clinical Importance of the Rh Blood Type, New England J. Med., 232, 447 and 475, 1945; Proc. Roy. Soc. Med., 40, 546, 1947.
3a. ERNSTER, L., HERLIN, L. and ZETTERSTRÖM, R.: Experimental Studies on the Pathogenesis of Kernicterus, Pediatrics, 20, 647, 1957.
4. FORRESTER, R. M. and MILLER, J.: The Dental Changes Associated with Kernicterus, Arch. Dis. Childhood, 30, 224, 1955.
4a. GASSER, C.: Acute Erythroblastopenie, Helv. pædiat. acta, 4, 107, 1949.
4b. GEPPERT, L. J., AKEROYD, J. H. and SIMPSON, J. W.: ACTH in the Treatment of Erythroblastosis, Pediatrics, 12, 72, 1953.
4c. GERRARD, J.: Kernicterus, Brain, 75, 526, 1952.
4d. GIBLETT, ELOISE, CHASE, JEANNE and CREALOCK, F. W.: Hemolytic Disease of the Newborn Resulting from Anti-s Antibody, Am. J. Clin. Path., 29, 254, 1958.
4e. GILMOUR, J. R.: Erythroblastosis Fetalis, Arch. Dis. Child., 19, 1, 1944.
4f. GLISSON, C. S., JR., TEATE, H. L. and SMITH, A. A.: Progesterone and Vitamin K for the Prevention of Erythroblastosis Fetalis, Am. J. Obst. & Gynec., 64, 498, 1952.
4g. GREENWALT, T. J., TRIANTAPHYLLOPOULOS, D. C. and MOORMAN, M.: In Vitro Studies of Red Cell Fragility in Anti-D Hemolytic Disease of the Newborn, J. Lab. & Clin. Med., 45, 135, 1955.
4h. HENDERSON, J. L.: Fourth Type of Erythroblastosis Fetalis Showing Hepatic Cirrhosis in Macerated Fetus, Arch. Dis. Child., 17, 49, 1942.
5. HOSOI, T.: Serological Identification of Fetal Blood in the Maternal Circulation, Yokohama M. Bull., 9, 61, 1958.
5a. HSIA, D. Y., ALLEN, F. H., JR., GELLIS, S. S. and DIAMOND, L. K.: Studies of Serum Bilirubin in Relation to Kernicterus, New England J. Med., 247, 668, 1952.
5b. HUBINONT, P. O. and MASSART-GUIOT, T.: Considérations sur le traitement de la maladie hémolytique du nouveau-né,

Bruxelles-méd., *35*, 1, 1955; Bull. Soc. roy. belge de gynéc. et d'obst., *28*, 30, 1958.

5c.Hunter, O. B., Jr. and Ross, J. B.: Cortisone in Rh Incompatibilities, South. M. J., *45*, 732, 1952; J. A. M. A., *154*, 905, 1954.

6. von Jaksch, R.: Über Leukämie und Leukocytose im Kindesalter, Wien. klin. Wchnschr., *2*, 435, 456, 1889.

6a.Javert, C. T.: Erythroblastosis Neonatorum, Surg. Gynec. & Obst., *74*, 1, 1942.

7. Josephs, H. W.: Anemia of Infancy and Early Childhood, Medicine, *15*, 307, 1936 (Bibliography).

7a.Kellner, A. and Hedal, E. F.: Experimental Erythroblastosis Fetalis in Rabbits, J. Exper. Med., *97*, 33 and 51, 1953.

7b.Kelsall, G. A., Vos, G. H., Kirk, R. L. and Shield, J. W.: The Evaluation of Cord-Blood Hemoglobin, Reticulocyte Percentage and Maternal Antiglobulin Titer in the Prognosis of Hemolytic Disease of the Newborn (Erythroblastosis Fetalis), Pediatrics, *20*, 221, 1957; Australasian Ann. Med., *7*, 346, 1958.

7c.Kelsall, G. A., Vos, G. H. and Kirk, R. L.: Case for Induction of Labour in Treatment of Haemolytic Disease of the Newborn, Brit. M. J., *2*, 468, 1958.

7d.Krivit, W., Goodlin, R., Ziegler, N. and Lienke, R.: Foetomaternal Transfusion as a Cause of Neonatal Anaemia, Arch. Dis. Childhood, *34*, 471, 1959.

8. Lehndorff, H.: Anæmia Neonatorum, Ergeben. inn. Med. u. Kinderh., *52*, 611, 1937 (Bibliography).

8a.Leonard, M. F.: Hemolytic Disease of the Newborn, J. Pediat., *27*, 249, 1945.

8b.Leventhal, M. L. and Wolf, A. M.: Erythroblastosis (Hydrops) Fetalis from Kell Sensitization, Am. J. Obst. & Gynec., *71*, 452, 1956.

8c. Levine, P.: Serological Factors as Possible Causes in Spontaneous Abortions, J. Hered., *34*, 71, 1943.

8d.Levine, P., Ferraro, L. R. and Koch, E.: Hemolytic Disease of the Newborn Due to Anti-S, Blood, *7*, 1030, 1952.

9. Levine, P., Katzin, E. M. and Burnham, L.: Isoimmunization in Pregnancy, J.A.M.A., *116*, 825, 1941; Blood, *3*, Supp. 2, 3, 1948; *Ibid.*, *3*, 404, 1948; Human Biol., *30*, 14, 1958.

9a.Levine, P., Vogel, P. and Rosenfield, R. E.: *Hemolytic Disease of the Newborn*, in *Advances in Pediatrics*, vol. VI, Chicago, Year Book Publishers, Inc., 1953, p. 97.

9b.Levine, P. and Waller, R. K.: Erythroblastosis Fetalis in the First-Born, Blood, *1*, 143, 1946.

9c.Levine, P. *et al.*: Haemolytic Disease of the Newborn Probably Due to Anti-f, Nature, *185*, 188, 1960.

9d.Lewi, S., Mayer, M. and Clarke, T. K.: Maladie hémolytique chez un enfant D^u, Rev. hémat., *15*, 183, 1960.

9e. van Loghem, J. J. and Hart, M. v. d.: Iso-Immunization by Rare Rh-Antigens as a Cause of Haemolytic Disease of the Newborn and Transfusion Reactions, J. Clin. Path., *2*, 284, 1949.

9f. Mengert, W. F., Rights, C. S., Bates, C. R., Jr., Reid, A. F., Wolf, G. R. and Nabors, G. C.: Placental Transmission of Erythrocytes, Am. J. Obst. & Gynec., *69*, 678, 1955.

9g.Mollison, P. L. and Cutbush, M.: A Method of Measuring the Severity of a Series of Cases of Hemolytic Disease of the Newborn, Blood, *6*, 777, 1951.

9h.Mollison, P. L., Mourant, A. E. and Race, R. R.: *The Rh Blood Groups and Their Clinical Effects*, Medical Research Council Memorandum No. 19, His Majesty's Stationery Office, London, 1948; Brit. M. J., *1*, 123, 1949.

9i. Odell, G. B.: Studies in Kernicterus. I. The Protein Binding of Bilirubin, J. Clin. Invest., *38*, 823, 1959.

10. Oppé, T. E. and Valaes, T.: Obstructive Jaundice and Haemolytic Disease of the Newborn, Lancet, *1*, 536, 1959.

10a.Pickles, M. M.: *Haemolytic Disease of the Newborn*, Springfield, Ill., Charles C Thomas, 1949.

10b.Potter, E. L.: A Double Ova Pregnancy in Which the Rh + Twin Developed Erythroblastosis, J. Pediat., *24*, 449, 1944.

10c.————: Diagnosis of Erythroblastosis Fetalis in the Macerated Fetus, Arch. Path., *41*, 223, 1946.

10d.———— *Rh, Its Relation to Congenital Hemolytic Disease and to Intragroup Transfusion Reactions*, The Year Book Publishers, Chicago, Ill., 1947.

10e.Race, R. R. and Sanger, Ruth: *Blood Groups in Man*, ed. 3, Oxford, Blackwell Scientific Publications, 1958.

11a.Reisner, E. H., Jr.: Morphology of Erythrocytes in Erythroblastosis Fetalis, Arch. Int. Med., *71*, 230, 1943.

11b.Rice, W. G. and Sister Mary Eloise: Deficient Prothrombin and Fibrinogen in Fatal Erythroblastosis Fetalis, J. Pediat., *42*, 231, 1953.

12. Rosenfield, R. E. and Eisinger, F.: AB Hemolytic Disease of the Newborn, Blood, *10*, 17, 1955.

12a.Sacks, M. S., Guilbeau, J. A., Jr., Bradford, G. T. and Jahn, E. F.: Rh Isosensitization in the American Negro, Blood, *4*, 1245, 1949.

12*b*.SACKS, M. S., KUHNS, W. J. and JAHN, E. F.: Studies in Rh-Isoimmunization in Pregnancy, Am. J. Obst. & Gynec., *54*, 400, 1947; Pediatrics, *6*, 772, 1950.

12*c*.SACKS, M. S. *et al.*: Isosensitization to a New Blood Factor, Rh^D, with Special Reference to its Clinical Importance, Ann. Int. Med., *51*, 740, 1959.

12*d*.SCHULMAN, I. and SMITH, C. H.: Fetal and Adult Hemoglobins in Hemolytic Disease of the Newborn, Am. J. Dis. Child., *87*, 167, 1954.

12*e*. SCOTT, R. B., JENKINS, M. E. and KESSLER, A. D.: Erythroblastosis Fetalis in the Negro Infant, J. Pediat., *39*, 680, 1951.

12*f*.STERN, K., DAVIDSOHN, I. and MASAITIS, LILLIAN: Experimental Studies on Rh Immunization, Am. J. Clin. Path., *26*, 833, 1956; Am. J. Obst. & Gynec., *75*, 369, 1958.

12*g*.STONE, B. and MARSH, W. L.: Haemolytic Disease of the Newborn Caused by Anti-M: Brit. J. Haemat., *5*, 344, 1959.

12*h*.STRATTON, F. and RENTON, P. H.: Hæmolytic Disease of the Newborn Caused by a New Rh Antibody, Anti-C^x, Brit. M. J., *1*, 962, 1954.

12*i*. STURGEON, P.: Immunohematologic Observations of Erythroblastotic Infants, Am. J. Clin. Path., *24*, 115, 1954.

12*j*. TAYLOR, G. L. and RACE, R. R.: Hæmolytic Disease of the Newborn, The Preponderance of Homozygous Rh-Positive Fathers, Brit. M. J., *1*, 288, 1944.

12*k*.TURMAN, C. M., VAUGHAN, V. C., III and SHELLY, R. M.: Incidence of Hemolytic Disease of the Newborn Due to A or B Incompatibility, Am. J. Obst. & Gynec., *71*, 885, 1956.

13. VAUGHAN, V. C., III, ALLEN, F. H., JR. and DIAMOND, L. K.: Erythroblastosis Fetalis, Pediatrics *6*, 173, 441, 630 and 706, 1950.

13*a*.VEST, M.: Austauschtransfuzionen zur Verhütung von Kernicterus bei der Hyperbilirubinämie der Frühgeburten und Neugeborenen, Schweiz. med. Wchnschr., *88*, 208, 1958.

13*b*.WALKER, W. and MURRAY, S.: The Management of Hæmolytic Disease of the Newborn, Brit. M. J., *2*, 126, 1954; *ibid.*, *1*, 681, 1955; *ibid.*, *1*, 187, 1956.

13*c*.WIENER, A. S.: Pathogenesis of Congenital Hemolytic Disease, J. Lab. & Clin. Med., *30*, 957, 1945; Am. J. Dis. Child., *71*, 14, 1946; Am. J. Obst. & Gynec., *59*, 178, 1950; Postgraduate Medicine, *7*, 1, 1950.

13*d*.WIENER, A. S., SAMWICK, A. A., MORRISON, H. and COHEN, L.: Studies on Immunization in

Man. II. The Blood Factor C, Exper. Med. & Surg., *11*, 276, 1953; J. Lab. & Clin. Med., *46*, 757, 1955; Am. J. Obst. & Gynec., *79*, 567, 1960.

13*e*.WIENER, A. S., WEXLER, I. B. and HURST, J. G.: The Use of Exchange Transfusion for the Treatment of Severe Erythroblastosis Due to A–B Sensitization, With Observations on the Pathogenesis of the Disease, Blood, *4*, 1014, 1949.

13*f*.WIENER, A. S., WEXLER, I. B. and BRANCATO, G. J.: Treatment of Erythroblastosis Fetalis by Exchange Transfusion, J. Pediat., *45*, 546, 1954; *ibid.*, *49*, 381, 1956; Lancet, *2*, 244, 1957.

14. WITEBSKY, E. and HEIDE, A.: Further Investigations on Presence of Rh Antibodies in Breast Milk, Proc. Soc. Exper. Biol. & Med., *52*, 280, 1943.

15. YOUNG, L. E., ERVIN, D. M., CHRISTIAN, R. M. and DAVIS, R. W.: Hemolytic Disease in Newborn Dogs Following Isoimmunization of the Dam by Transfusions, Science, *109*, 630, 1949; Blood, *6*, 291, 1951.

15*a*.ZUELZER, W. W. and KAPLAN, E.: ABO Heterospecific Pregnancy and Hemolytic Disease, Am. J. Dis. Child., *88*, 158, 179, 307 and 319, 1954; Blood, *12*, 883, 1957.

16. ZUELZER, W. W. and MUDGETT, R. T.: Kernicterus, Pediatrics, *6*, 452, 1950; J. Clin. Invest., *37*, 332, 1958.

Nutritional Anemia

17. BAAR, H.: Pathogenese und Therapie alimentären Kleinkinderanämien, Abdhand. a. d. Kinderh., Berlin, S. Karger, No. 16, 1927.

18. BENNETT, T. I., HUNTER, D. and VAUGHAN, J. M.: Idiopathic Steatorrhœa (Gee's Disease), Quart. J. Med., *1*, 603, 1932.

19. BURGIO, G. R.: Anémie pseudo-pernicieuse et autres anémies mégaloblastiques du nourrisson, Acta hæmat., *11*, 355, 1954; Archiv. Kinderheilk., *152*, 110, 1956.

20. COOLEY, T. B. and LEE, P.: Pernicious Blood Pictures in Infancy, J. Pediat., *1*, 184, 1932. 1932.

20*a*.DANCIS, J., DANOFF, S., ZABRISKIE, J. and BALIS, M. E.: Hemoglobin Metabolism in the Premature Infant, J. Pediat., *54*, 748, 1959.

21. GAIRDNER, D., MARKS, J. and ROSCOE, J. D.: The Early Anæmia of Prematurity, Arch. Dis. Childhood, *30*, 203, 1955.

22. GASSER, C.: Folsäure bei perniciosiformer Ziegenmilch-Anämie, Helv. pædiat. acta, *3*, 301, 1948.

23. GYÖRGY, P.: Pathogenesis of Goat's Milk Anemia, Ztschr. Kinderh., Berlin, *56*, 1, 1934.

23a.HADLEY, G. G. and CHINNOCK, R. F.: A Study of Hemograms in Premature Infants, J. Pediat., 45, 413, 1954.

23b.HAMMOND, D. and MURPHY, ARLENE: The Influence of Exogenous Iron on Formation of Hemoglobin in the Premature Infant, Pediatrics, 25, 362, 1960.

24. JOSEPHS, H. W.: Iron Metabolism and the Hypochromic Anemia of Infancy, Medicine, 32, 125, 1953; Pediatrics, 18, 959, 1956.

25. LEVY, W. and WIDROW, S. A.: A Case of Megaloblastic Anemia Associated with Steatorrhea and the Celiac Syndrome, J. Pediat., 47, 100, 1955.

26. LUHBY, A. L. and WHEELER, W. E.: Megaloblastic Anemia of Infancy: II. Failure of Response to Vitamin B₁₂ and the Metabolic Role of Folic Acid and Vitamin C, Health Center J., Ohio State Univ., 3, 1, 1949.

27. MAY, C. D., NELSON, E. N. and SALMON, R. J.: Experimental Production of Megaloblastic Anemia; An Interrelationship Between Ascorbic Acid and Pteroylglutamic Acid, J. Lab. & Clin. Med., 34, 1724, 1949; Am. J. Dis. Child., 80, 191, 1950; J. Lab. & Clin. Med., 36, 591, 1950; Am. J. Dis. Child., 84, 718, 1952.

27a.MacIVER, J. E. and BACK, E. H.: Megaloblastic Anaemia of Infancy in Jamaica, Arch. Dis. Childhood, 35, 134, 1960.

28. MACKAY, H. M. M.: Early Anemia of Premature Infants, Arch. Dis. Childhood, 10, 195, 1935.

29. MERRITT, K. K. and DAVIDSON, L. T.: The Blood During the First Year of Life: II. The Anemia of Prematurity, Am. J. Dis. Child., 47, 261, 1934.

29a.NICCUM, W. L., JACKSON, R. L. and STEARNS, G.: Use of Ferric and Ferrous Iron in the Prevention of Hypochromic Anemia in Infants, Am. J. Dis. Child., 86, 553, 1953.

30. ORTEN, J. and SMITH, A.: Goat's Milk Anemia, Yale J. Biol. & Med., 8, 637, 1936.

31. PARSONS, L. G. and HAWKSLEY, J. C.: The Anhæmatopoietic Anæmias (Deficiency Diseases of the Erythron): Nutritional Anæmia, and the Anæmias of Prematurity, Scurvy and Cœliac Disease, Arch. Dis. Child., 8, 117, 1933.

32. PARSONS, L. G. and SMALLWOOD, W. C.: The Anæmia of Infantile Scurvy, Arch. Dis. Childhood, 10, 327, 1935.

32a.PERKINS, E. M.: Goats' Milk Anemia, J. Pediat., 25, 439, 1944.

33. ROMINGER, E. and BOMSKOV, C.: Studies on Hyperchromic Anemias in Experimentally Produced Sprue-like Disturbances, Klin. Wchnschr., 14, 148, 1935.

34. SHNIER, M. H. and METZ, J.: Megaloblastic Anaemia in Infancy with Special Reference to Treatment with Vitamin B₁₂, South African M. J., 33, 1009, 1959.

34a.SMITH, C. A., CHERRY, R. B., MALETSKOS, C. J., GIBSON, J. G., 2ND, ROBY, C. C., CATON, W. L. and REID, D. E.: Persistence and Utilization of Maternal Iron for Blood Formation during Infancy, J. Clin. Invest., 34, 1391, 1955.

34b.STURGEON, P. and CARPENTER, G.: Megaloblastic Anemia of Infancy. Response to Vitamin B₁₂, Blood, 5, 458, 1950.

34c.WALT, F., HOLMAN, S. and NAIDOO, P.: Megaloblastic Anaemia of Infancy Treated with Folic Acid, Brit. M. J., 2, 1464, 1957.

35. ZUELZER, W. W. and OGDEN, F. N.: Folic Acid Therapy in Macrocytic Anemias of Infancy, Proc. Soc. Exper. Biol. & Med., 61, 176, 1946; Am. J. Dis. Child., 71, 211, 1946; J. Lab. & Clin. Med., 32, 1217, 1947; Nutritional Anemia, Cincinnati, Ohio, The Robert Gould Research Foundation, p. 79, 1948.

Congenital Hypoplastic and Miscellaneous Anemias

37. ALTMAN, K. I. and MILLER, G.: A Disturbance of Tryptophan Metabolism in Congenital Hypoplastic Anæmia, Nature, 172, 868, 1953.

37a.BJURE, J., FICHTELIUS, K. -E. and RANSTRÖM, S.: On the Problem of Congenital Hemopathies, Acta paediat., 49, 358, 1960.

38. BONHAM-CARTER, R. E., CATHIE, I. A. B. und GASSER, C.: Aplastiche Anämie (chronische Erythroblastophthise) bedingt durch Autoimmunisierung, Schweiz. med. Wchnschr., 84, 1114, 1954.

39. CATHIE, I. A. B.: Erythrogenesis Imperfecta, Arch. Dis. Childhood, 25, 313, 1950.

40. CHOWN, B.: Anæmia from Bleeding of the Fetus into the Mother's Circulation, Lancet, 1, 1213, 1954; Am. J. Obst. & Gynec., 70, 1298, 1955.

41. DIAMOND, L. K. and BLACKFAN, K. D.: Hypoplastic Anemia, Am. J. Dis. Child., 56, 464, 1938.

42. KÅSS, A. and SUNDAL, A.: Anæmia Hypoplastica Congenita (Anæmia Typus Josephs-Diamond-Blackfan), Acta pædiat., 42, 265, 1953.

43. KERR, MARGARET, M.: Anæmia and Polycythaemia in Uniovular Twins, Brit. M. J., 1, 902, 1959.

44. KIRKMAN, H. N. and RILEY, H. D., JR.: Posthemorrhagic Anemia and Shock in the Newborn Due to Hemorrhage during Delivery, Pediatrics, 24, 92, 1959.

45. PEARSON, H. A. and CONE, T. E., JR.: Con-

genital Hypoplastic Anemia, Pediatrics, *19*, 192, 1957.

46. SMITH, C. H.: Chronic Congenital Aregenerative Anemia (Pure Red Cell Anemia) Associated with Isoimmunization by the Blood Group Factor "A", Blood, *4*, 697, 1949.

47. SMITH, C. H.: Hypoplastic and Aplastic Anemias of Infancy and Childhood, J. Pediat., *43*, 457, 1953.

47a. WEISERT, O. and MARSTRANDER, J.: Severe Anemia in a Newborn Caused by Protracted Feto-Maternal "Transfusion," Acta pædiat., *49*, 426, 1960.

Hemolytic Anemia

48. FRENKIEL, H.: Ein Fall von Hämoglobinurie bei einem Kinde nach Genuss von Rauschbeeren, Ztschr. Kinderh., *52*, 608, 1932.

49. SYLVAN, H.: Two Cases of Disease of the Blood Forming Organs after Gas Poisoning, Acta pædiat., *14*, 197, 1933.

51. WILLIAMS, T. P.: "Pernicious" Blood Picture in an Infant, with Recovery, Proc. Roy. Soc. Med., *26*, 1367, 1933.

Diseases with Outstanding Splenomegaly

52. AVERY, MARY ELLEN, MCAFEE, J. G. and GUILD, HARRIET G.: The Course and Prognosis of Reticuloendotheliosis (Eosinophilic Granuloma, Schüller-Christian Disease and and Letterer-Siwe Disease), Am. J. Med., *22*, 636, 1957.

52a. AYRES, W. W. and SILLIPHANT, W. M.: Charcot-Leyden Crystals in Eosinophilic Granuloma of Bone, Am. J. Clin. Path., *30*, 323, 1958.

53. BLOCK, M. and JACOBSON, L. O.: The Histogenesis and Diagnosis of the Osseous Type of Gaucher's Disease, Acta hæmat., *1*, 165, 1948.

54. BLOEM, T. F., GROEN, J. and POSTMA, C.: Gaucher's Disease, Quart. J. Med., *20*, 517, 1936; Blood, *3*, 1221 and 1238, 1948.

54a. CASSIDY, W. J., ALLMAN, F. C. and KEEFE, G. J.: Osteopetrosis, Arch. Int. Med., *82*, 140, 1948.

55. CROCKER, A. C. and FARBER, S.: Niemann-Pick Disease, Medicine, *37*, 1, 1958; Am. J. Clin. Nutrition, *9*, 63, 1961.

55a. CROCKER, A. C. and LANDING, B. H.: Phosphatase Studies in Gaucher's Disease, Metabolism, *9*, 341, 1960.

55b. CRONE, R. I. and BERGIN, J. J.: Gaucher's Disease in Identical Twins, Ann. Int. Med., *49*, 941, 1958.

55c. DANOPOULOS, E. and LOGOTHETOPOULOS, J.: Klinische und hæmatologische Beobach-

tungen an zwei familiären Fällen der Gaucherschen Krankheit, Arch. klin. Med., *201*, 79, 1954.

56. DAVIS, F. W., GENECIN, A. and SMITH, E. W.: Gaucher's Disease with Thrombocytopenia, an Instance of Selective Hypersplenism, Bull. Johns Hopkins Hosp., *83*, 176, 1949.

57. DAVISON, C.: Xanthomatosis and the Central Nervous System, Arch. Neurol. & Psychiat., *30*, 75, 1933.

57a. DEMARSH, Q. B. and KAUTZ, JEAN: The Submicroscopic Morphology of Gaucher Cells, Blood, *12*, 324, 1957.

57b. EAST, T. and SAVIN, L. H.: A Case of Gaucher's Disease with Biopsy of the Typical Pingueculae, Brit. J. Ophth., *24*, 613, 1940.

57c. ENGFELDT, B., FAJERS, C. -M., LODIN, H. and PEHRSON, M.: Studies on Osteopetrosis. III., Acta pædiat., *49*, 391, 1960.

58. EPSTEIN, E.: Beitrag zur Chemie der Gaucherschen Krankheit, Biochem. Ztschr., *145*, 398, 1924.

58a. FORSYTHE, W. I., MCKEOWN, E. F. and NEILL, D. W.: Three Cases of Niemann Pick's Disease in Children, Arch. Dis. Childhood, *34*, 406, 1959.

58b. FREUD, P., PLACHTA, A., SPEER, F. D. and LUHBY, A. L.: Leukemic Xanthomatosis, Am. J. Dis. Child., *88*, 43, 1954.

59. GAUCHER, P. C.: De l'Epitheliome primitif de la Rate sans Leucémie. Thèse de Paris, 1882.

59a. GORDON, G. L.: Osseous Gaucher's Disease, Am. J. Med., *8*, 332, 1950.

60. HERNDON, C. N. and BENDER, J. R.: Gaucher's Disease: Cases in Five Related Negro Sibships, Am. J. Human Genet., *2*, 49, 1950.

60a. HODGSON, J. R., KENNEDY, R. L. J. and CAMP, J. D.: Reticulo-Endotheliosis, Radiology, *57*, 642 and 653, 1951.

60b. HOJA, W. A.: Gaucher's Disease in Pregnancy, Am. J. Obst. & Gynec., *79*, 286, 1960.

61. HORSLEY, J. S., BAKER, J. P. and APPERLY, F. L.: Gaucher's Disease of Late Onset with Kidney Involvement and Huge Spleen, Am. J. M. Sc., *190*, 511, 1935.

61a. IMPARATO, A. M.: Gaucher's Disease with Ascites, Ann. Surg., *151*, 431, 1960.

61b. JERMAIN, L. F., ROHN, R. J. and BOND, W. H.: Studies on the Role of the Reticuloendothelial System in Hurler's Disease, Am. J. M. Sc., *239*, 612, 1960.

61c. LAMB, F. H. and JACKSON, R. L.: Osteopetrosis (Marble Bone Disease), Am. J. Clin. Path., *8*, 255, 1938.

61d. LANDING, B. H. and FREIMAN, D. G.: Histochemical Studies on the Cerebral Lipidoses and Other Cellular Metabolic Disorders, Am. J. Path., *33*, 1, 1957.

50

62. LANGE, C. DE: Malignant Form of Gaucher's Disease, Acta pædiat., *27*, 34, 1939.

62a.LICHTENSTEIN, L.: Histiocytosis X, Arch. Path., *56*, 84, 1953.

63. LIEB, H.: Cerebrosidspeicherung bei Spleno-megaly, Typus Gaucher, Ztschr. physiol. Chem., *140*, 305, 1924.

63a.LIPTON, E. L.: Hemolytic and Pancytopenic Syndrome Associated with Letterer-Siwe Disease, Pediatrics, *14*, 533, 1954.

63b.LORBER, M.: The Occurrence of Intracellular Iron in Gaucher's Disease, Ann. Int. Med., *53*, 293, 1960.

64. MANDELBAUM, F. S. and DOWNEY, H.: The Histopathology and Biology of Gaucher's Disease, Folia hæmat., *20*, 139, 1916.

64a.MEDOFF, A. S. and BAYRD, E. D.: Gaucher's Disease in 29 Cases: Hematologic Compli-cations and Effect of Splenectomy, Ann. Int. Med., *40*, 481, 1954.

65. MERMANN, A. C. and DARGEON, H. W.: The Management of Certain Nonlipid Reticulo-Endothelioses, Cancer, *8*, 112, 1955.

66. NIEMANN, A.: Ein unbekanntes Krankheits-bild, Jahrb. Kinderh., *79*, 1, 1914.

67. NORMAN, R. M., URICH, H. and LLOYD, O. C.: The Neuropathology of Infantile Gaucher's Disease, J. Path. & Bact., *72*, 121, 1956.

67a.ORCHARD, N. P.: Letterer-Siwe's Syndrome, Arch. Dis. Childhood, *25*, 151, 1950.

67b.PETIT, J. V. and SCHLEICHER, E. M.: "Atypi-cal" Gaucher's Disease, Am. J. Clin. Path., *13*, 260, 1943.

68. PICK, L.: A Classification of the Diseases of Lipoid Metabolism and Gaucher's Disease, Am. J. M. Sc., *185*, 453, 1933.

68a.————— Niemann-Pick's Disease and Other Forms of So-called Xanthomatosis, Am. J. M. Sc., *185*, 601, 1933.

69. PINES, B. and LEDERER, M.: Osteopetrosis: Albers Schönberg Disease (Marble Bones), Am. J. Path., *23*, 755, 1947.

69a.REICH, C., SEIFE, M. and KESSLER, B. J.: Gaucher's Disease, Medicine, *30*, 1, 1951.

69b.RENZETTI, A. D., JR., EASTMAN, G. and AUCHINCLOSS, J. H., JR.: Chronic Dissemi-nated Histiocytosis X (Schüller-Christian Disease) with Pulmonary Involvement and Impairment of Alveolar-Capillary Diffu-sion, Am. J. Med., *22*, 834, 1957.

69c.ROSENBERG, A. and CHARGAFF, E.: A Rein-vestigation of the Cerebroside Deposited in Gaucher's Disease, J. Biol. Chem., *233*, 1323, 1958.

70. ROWLAND, R. S.: Xanthomatosis and the Reticulo-endothelial System, Arch. Int. Med., *42*, 611, 1928.

70a.RUCH, D. M.: Cutaneous Manifestations of Letterer-Siwe's Disease, A. M. A. Arch. Dermat., *75*, 88, 1957.

71. SCHARTUM-HANSEN, H.: Sternalpunktion bei Morbus Gaucher, Folia hæmat., *61*, 180, 1938.

71a.SJÖLIN, S.: Studies on Osteopetrosis, Acta paediat., *48*, 529, 1959.

72. SOSMAN, M. C.: Xanthomatosis (Schüller-Christian's Disease, Lipoid Histiocytosis), J.A.M.A., *98*, 110, 1932.

73. TERRY, R. D., SPERRY, W. M. and BRODOFF, B.: Adult Lipidosis Resembling Niemann-Pick's Disease, Am. J. Path., *30*, 263, 1954.

73a.TRAMS, E. G. and BRADY, R. O.: Cerebroside Synthesis in Gaucher's Disease, J. Clin. Invest., *39*, 1546, 1960.

73b.TUCHMAN, L. R. and SWICK, M.: High Acid Phosphatase Level Indicating Gaucher's Disease in Patient with Prostatism, J. A. M. A., *164*, 2034, 1957.

74. UZMAN, L. L.: The Lipoprotein of Gaucher's Disease, Arch. Path., *51*, 329, 1951; *ibid.*, *55*, 181, 1953.

74a.VAN CREVELD, S. and HEYBROEK, N. K.: Albers-Schönberg's Disease (Marble Bones), Acta paediat., *27*, 462, 1940.

74b.VAUGHAN, J. M.: Leuco-erythroblastic Anae-mia, J. Path. & Bact., *42*, 541, 1936.

75. VIEDEBAEK, A.: Niemann-Pick's Disease, Acta pædiat., *37*, 95, 1949.

76. WEICKER, H.: Zum Erbgang der Marmor-knochenkrankheit, Schweiz. med. Wchn-schr., *88*, 1019, 1958.

77. WELT, S., ROSENTHAL, N. and OPPENHEIMER, B. S.: Gaucher's Splenomegaly, J.A.M.A., *92*, 637, 1929.

Chapter 16

Polycythemia

THE term polycythemia is generally considered to signify an increase above the normal in the number of red corpuscles in the circulating blood. The increase in the number of red corpuscles is usually accompanied by a corresponding increase in the quantity of hemoglobin and volume of packed red cells, although this is not always the case.

Relative, Transient and Absolute Polycythemia.—The term polycythemia, as ordinarily used, is applied to all increases, whether they are only relative and transient or absolute and even permanent. *Relative polycythemia* occurs when, through loss of blood plasma, the concentration of the red corpuscles becomes greater than normal in the circulating blood. On the other hand, when, in response to some stimulus, red corpuscles are shunted into the circulation from some storehouse such as the spleen, *transient polycythemia* occurs. By *absolute polycythemia* is meant an increase in the total red cell mass.

The terms erythrocytosis and erythremia are used to refer to two forms of absolute polycythemia. **Erythrocytosis** denotes polycythemia which occurs in response to some known stimulus; **erythremia** refers to a disease of unknown etiology. Thus, these terms are employed in the same way as leukocytosis and leukemia.

Relative Polycythemia. — Relative polycythemia may result from abnormally lowered fluid intake or marked loss of body fluids, as occurs in persistent vomiting, severe diarrhea, copious sweating, or diabetic acidosis. Loss of electrolyte from the extracellular compartment, when not accompanied by corresponding loss of water, leads to a decline of osmolar concentration in the extracellular fluid. The resulting shift of water into the tissue cells may produce relative polycythemia, sometimes of high grade. In certain types of peripheral circulatory failure there is a loss of plasma into the interstitial fluid. Such a shift takes place largely in the periphery, with the result that the polycythemia may be more marked in capillary blood than in that from central blood vessels.[6]

Whether polycythemia is accompanied by an augmentation in total blood volume depends on the changes which take place in the fluid portion of the blood as well as in the corpuscular mass. In "relative polycythemia" the total blood volume is actually reduced owing to the decrease in plasma volume. Even in cases of absolute polycythemia the total blood volume may not be raised or may increase relatively little if a compensatory decrease in total plasma volume occurs.

The rôle of the spleen as a storehouse for red corpuscles has been discussed (p. 113). In the dog, cat and horse, exercise, anoxemia, drugs such as epinephrin, and emotional conditions produce temporary polycythemia, perhaps in part by splenic contraction and expulsion of cells. Undoubtedly an important additional factor is the redistribution of blood cells within the vascular system. In man the rôle of the spleen is not as great as in the dog. A rise in relative volume of packed red cells (hematocrit) occurs following administration of epinephrin in splenectomized but otherwise normal persons, as well as in normal individuals and in cases of polycythemia vera.[10b] In normal persons, injection of the drug was followed by a decrease in plasma volume and a slight increase in cell volume. Similar changes were observed in cases of polycythemia vera, but in splenectomized subjects both plasma and cell volumes decreased. The effect of exercise was similar to that of epinephrin.

ERYTHROCYTOSIS

In the Newly Born.—As indicated in an earlier chapter (p. 109), because of the large size and correspondingly higher hemoglobin content of the red corpuscles at birth, the hemoglobin and the volume of packed red cells are greater than normal even when the red cell count is little increased. This is an absolute polycythemia but it is transient.

Congenital Heart Disease.—Red cell counts of 7,000,000 to 8,500,000 are commonly found in cases of congenital heart disease and there are reports of counts as high as 10,000,000 and even 13,900,000.[20] The volume of packed red cells was as high as 86 ml. per 100 ml. blood in one of the writer's cases. Polycythemia occurs in cases in which there is a partial shunt of the blood from the pulmonary circuit. The most common defects producing such polycythemia are pulmonary stenosis, usually with defective ventricular or auricular septum, patent foramen ovale or patent ductus arteriosus; persistent truncus arteriosus; complete transposition of arterial trunks;

and cases with the tetralogy of Fallot (pulmonary stenosis, defective ventricular septum, dextroposition of the aorta, right ventricular hypertrophy). Such individuals exhibit evidence of disturbed cardio-respiratory function, marked cyanosis, clubbing of the fingers and toes, and sometimes stunted growth. It has been reported that an enlarged spleen is not uncommon but this has not been the writer's experience.

The cytological changes in erythrocytosis, as contrasted with those in erythremia will be discussed later (p. 799). The total plasma volume may be reduced below normal but the increase in the size of the red cell mass is so great that the total blood volume is higher than normal.[5,15b] Such pathological evidence as is available indicates that fat tissue in the bone marrow is replaced by hemopoietic marrow.[20,24,25]

In a series of 41 cases[15b] the serum bilirubin and the serum iron were found to be increased above normal but no more than would be expected from the total increase in hemoglobin metabolism as represented by the polycythemia.

It is generally assumed that the underlying stimulus to the hematopoietic system is low oxygen tension resulting from diminished blood flow to the lungs with consequent unsaturation of the arterial blood. The arterial oxygen saturation is often as low as 30 to 35 per cent. With successful operative intervention this may rise to 75 and even 88 per cent and, with this, the polycythemia disappears. The effect of the anoxia, however, is not a direct one on the bone marrow. Thus, in a case of patent ductus arteriosus occurring distal to the origin of the subclavian artery it was shown that the sternal marrow manifested the same pronounced normoblastic hyperplasia as the iliac marrow even though the oxygen saturation of the latter was markedly decreased as compared to the normal saturation of the sternal marrow.[17b] Such

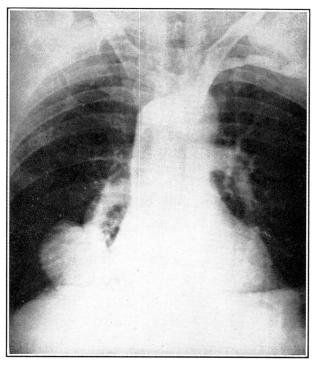

Fig. 16–1.—Pulmonary arteriovenous fistula associated with polycythemia.

observations give additional support for the view that humoral factors are concerned in the regulation of bone marrow activity (p. 49).

In *acquired heart disease* such polycythemia as may develop is of minor degree and is correlated to some extent with the degree of decompensation. The polycythemia has been reported as being accompanied by evidence of intensified erythropoiesis in the bone marrow, an increase in red cell mass and some macrocytosis.[9]

Pulmonary Disease. — If deficient oxygenation develops, pulmonary disease may lead to polycythemia. Emphysema is the most common of the chronic pulmonary conditions producing cyanosis and polycythemia, although this change in the blood is not always found. Silicosis with extensive pulmonary fibrosis may produce polycythemia, sometimes of marked degree. In the Peruvian Andes miners have been observed with extreme grades of erythrocytosis. Cavernous hemangiomata of the lung may be associated with polycythemia.[16] Pulmonary arteriovenous fistula should be suspected when a peculiar murmur in a lung field together with abnormal roentgenographic shadows is associated with polycythemia, cyanosis and other symptoms suggesting pulmonary disorder such as hemoptysis and clubbing of the fingers.[11b,25a] (Fig. 16–1). In a case of severe polycythemia associated with long-standing bronchopulmonary disease, increased intracranial pressure, choked disks and amblyopia developed together with increased internal jugular venous pressure in the absence of increased general venous pressure.[11c]

Ayerza's Syndrome.—Ayerza's syndrome, a condition characterized clinically by slowly developing asthma, bronchitis, dyspnea, and cyanosis and associated with polycythemia, was described by Ayerza in 1901. These patients are known as "*cardiacos negros*" (black cardiacs).[11a,15a] Cardiac complications may be present and there is usually evidence of dilatation and hypertrophy of the right auricle and ventricle. The essential pathological change, however, is primary disease of the pulmonary artery or its branches.[23] This has been attributed to syphilis[17] but more often there is pulmonary arterial and arteriolar sclerosis. In some cases, congenital narrowing or hypoplasia of the pulmonary artery may play a rôle, and changes in the lungs such as emphysema and pulmonary fibrosis may be contributory factors.[14] The spleen is sometimes enlarged, clubbing of the fingers is present and passive congestion of the liver and chronic heart failure eventually occur.

Chronic Cor Pulmonale.—The clinical picture of this syndrome is varied but oxygen deficiency with arterial desaturation is of central significance.[7] The role of polycythemia and of the associated increased viscosity of the blood in the production of the symptoms of decompensation which are found, is obscure. There is no clear evidence that venesection is helpful in relieving these manifestations. It has been observed that the mean corpuscular volume of the red cells tends to be increased above normal[1b] whereas the mean corpuscular hemoglobin concentration is generally lower than normal.[4a]

Obesity. The Pickwickian Syndrome.—Another form of hypoventilation associated with the development of polycythemia is a syndrome characterized by massive exogenous obesity, somnolence and cyanosis, together with hypercapnia, periodic respiration and ultimately right ventricular failure. The clinical picture is that of the fat boy described in Dickens' Pickwick Papers.[2]

Obesity does not necessarily produce alveolar hypoventilation[1a] but it seems likely that there is a critical degree of obesity at which ventilatory insufficiency appears.

At High Altitudes.—It was shown by Viault[21] in 1890 that polycythemia follows sojourn at high altitudes. He found erythrocyte counts of 7,500,000 and 8,000,000 cells, not only in natives living in the Peruvian Andes and working in a mine at an altitude of 4,392 meters above sea level, but in himself and in a fellow traveller as well, although his blood count at Lima (160 meters) had been normal. The change in the blood can be observed in animals as well as man.[26] They have already been described fully elsewhere (p. 106).

The ascent to high altitudes is accompanied in some persons by symptoms of fatigue, dizziness, headache at the vertex, nausea, ringing in the ears, and even vomiting, chills, and prostration. After a few days adaptation occurs. In individuals so acclimatized, as well as in others who may never have suffered any symptoms at the high altitude, a disorder may develop insidiously a few years later or even as long as twenty years after continued residence in these regions. This is known as **chronic mountain sickness** or seroche (Monge's disease).

Monge[13] described an "erythremic type" and an "emphysematous type." In the latter the dominant symptom is dyspnea and there is a long history of frequent bronchitis and laryngitis. Cyanosis is present. The thorax is globular and the vital capacity is diminished. The condition resembles Ayerza's disease, being distinguished chiefly by the symptomatic improvement which residence at sea level provides.

The erythremic type may be mild, when it is characterized by some diminution in mental and physical fitness, fatigue, an erythremic color which turns to cyanosis on the least exertion, occipital headache, anorexia which increases as the day goes on, nausea, vomiting, diminution of visual acuity, and paresthesias. In other instances headache, dizziness, tinnitus, vague pains in the extremities, cough and hemoptysis occur. When the disorder is more severe there is incessant dyspnea, aphonia is common, and there is profound lethargy and even coma. Crises of mental confusion have been observed. Frigidity is common. There are not only paresthesias but excruciating pain may be felt in the lower extremities. The face is bluish-violet, the eyelids are edematous and bluish, the scleræ are intensely colored by distended capillaries, the tongue is thick, the hands are enlarged and turgid, and the fingers are clubbed. Hypotension is often present. The liver and spleen have been found to be enlarged only in about 10 per cent of cases.

Polycythemia is characteristic and is more marked than in other residents at the same altitude who have no symptoms. Counts of 7,000,000 are common and 9,060,000 cells were found in one of Monge's cases.[13] There is a corresponding, sometimes a slightly greater, rise in hemoglobin and volume of packed red cells.[19] The mean corpuscular volume is normal or slightly increased and the mean corpuscular hemoglobin concentration is normal.[10,19] Reticulocytes may be increased,[10,13] although in most cases they are normal. The leukocyte count is often normal,[10] although Monge described slight leukocytosis together with monocytosis. Bilirubinemia may be pronounced, the van den Bergh reaction being positive, indirect. There is greater blood destruction, as measured by fecal urobilinogen, than in normal residents of high altitudes.[12] Remarkable increases in blood volume have been recorded, as high as 212 ml. per kg. body weight for total blood volume with 173 ml. for cell volume and 28 to 43 ml. per kg. body

weight for plasma volume.[10] More recent, and probably more accurate determinations have indicated a less striking although still greatly increased cell volume (88 and 95 ml. per kg. body weight).[12] Although platelet counts have been found to be normal or high, clot retraction is poor. Epistaxis is common and hemoptysis, bleeding of the gums, and purpura may occur.

Those affected are usually in the fourth to sixth decade of life. Remissions and relapses are described. Ascent to still higher altitudes results in aggravation of the symptoms whereas descent to sea level relieves them. Cardiac disorder does not appear until late and death occurs more often from hemorrhage, pulmonary tuberculosis, and bronchopneumonia than from cardiac insufficiency.

As already stated, there is considerable clinical similarity between Ayerza's disease and chronic mountain sickness. A person afflicted with the former disease, however, could probably not live at altitudes of 10,000 feet (3300 meters) or higher. Furthermore, the carbon dioxide content of the blood is increased,[19] whereas in patients with chronic mountain sickness it is decreased. Cases of congenital heart disease can be distinguished by the cardiac findings. In acquired heart disease cyanosis is associated with signs of failure whereas these are lacking when cyanosis is present in Monge's disease. The chief distinction from erythremia (polycythemia vera) is the failure of the latter to be affected by increased oxygen pressure. In Monge's disease descent to sea level brings about complete relief of symptoms, together with a pronounced reduction in the blood volume and restoration of normal blood counts.[10]

There is decreased oxygen saturation of the arterial blood in individuals residing in high altitudes but this is not correlated with the development of symptoms of chronic mountain sickness, nor is there any relationship to the O_2 and CO_2 tension of the alveolar air.[1] The pathogenesis of this disease is unknown. It is plausible to assume that intrinsic pulmonary disease, too mild to cause signs or symptoms at sea level, is the cause in many instances. This was the finding in a case observed in the Rocky Mountains.[8] Another possibility is the development of an abnormality in the normal regulatory mechanism which adjusts the degree of erythropoiesis to the state of anoxemia.[10]

Chemical and Physical Agents.— The excessive use of **coal-tar derivatives**, and other forms of chronic poisoning, by producing abnormal hemoglobin pigments such as sulfhemoglobin and methemoglobin (p. 193) may cause erythrocytosis. Polycythemia has been reported in cases of poisoning by **anilin and its derivatives**, such as toluyldiamine, atoxyl and nitrobenzol (shoe dye poisoning). **Gum shellac** appears to be a powerful agent in the experimental production of polycythemia, normoblastosis, and erythrocytic hyperplasia of the bone marrow.[14a] In **phosphorus poisoning**, especially in the match industry, polycythemia was found.[18] This may have been merely relative polycythemia and the result of acute liver damage.

A variety of agents have been mentioned from time to time as producing polycythemia but the evidence is unimpressive. These include digitalis, caffeine, nicotine, a number of minerals (manganese, mercury, iron, bismuth, arsenic, germanium), ultraviolet light, roentgen rays and radium salts. The claim that ephedrine sulfate produces polycythemia could not be confirmed.[17a] *Cobalt*, however, does affect erythropoiesis. This has been discussed fully elsewhere (p. 142).

Tumors and Miscellaneous Disorders.—Polycythemia has been described in association with a variety of disorders, as follows.

(1) *Infratentorial Vascular Tumors.*[18b]— Out of a series of 106 patients with this type of tumor, hemoglobin values greater than 18 Gm. were found in 11. Both cystic and solid tumors were found. Previously, 26 similar cases had been reported. However, few studies of blood volume have been carried out. In only two instances is it known that there was an absolute increase in red cell mass. In the remaining cases either relative polycythemia was found or no information was given. It is noteworthy that in 21 of the total of 37 cases in which polycythemia was reported, a return to normal hemoglobin followed operative intervention. It was noted that papilledema was usually associated with the polycythemia.[18b] Clearly, such a combination of findings should lead one to search for a vascular tumor in the posterior fossa of the skull.

Other neurologic conditions have also been described as being associated with polycythemia. In many instances anatomic evidence has been inadequate but a lesion affecting the mesodiencephalic region may be a common feature of all the cases. The pathogenesis of this form of polycythemia is obscure. Possibly an influence on a center affecting water balance or on centers associated with respiration is involved.

(2) *Hypernephroma and Other Renal Disorders.*—Polycythemia has been described in association with renal tumors in more than 40 patients.[2a,3,11,44a] When nephrectomy was possible, long remissions of the polycythemia were observed in many cases. Polycythemia has also been encountered in other forms of renal disease, such as polycystic kidneys[15] and hydronephrosis[3,3a,10a] and, as with the renal tumors, disappeared after removal of the renal lesions.[10a] In a number of instances there appeared to be a true increase in red cell mass. The plasma iron disappearance rate was similar to that found in polycythemia vera in two instances but not in another.[3a,10a] The

frequency of the association of poly-cythemia with the abovementioned renal disorders is uncertain and figures ranging from 2.6 per cent [2a] to 0.3 per cent [23a] have been reported. Because of the possibility that erythropoietin may be produced in the kidney (p. 51), the association of renal tumors with poly-cythemia has aroused considerable interest. Plasma erythropoietin levels, measured in two cases, were raised before operation and fell to normal after neph-rectomy.[10a] Curiously, in one of these cases the venous blood draining from the hydronephrotic kidney had a lower eryth-ropoietin level than blood from an arm vein. In none of these cases were the leukocyte or platelet counts significantly abnormal. The erythropoietin level, measured by Gurney (Chicago), was also above normal in an unreported case of our own.

Of special interest is the report that simple excision of the cysts, in two cases of cystic disease of the kidney associated with polycythemia, produced remission of the polycythemia.[15] In one of these cases, high levels of erythropoietin activity were demonstrated in the cyst fluid and cyst wall, an observation which suggests that the abnormal secretion may have arisen from the cyst itself, rather than from the kidney as a whole.

(3) *Other Tumors.*—Polycythemia was observed in about 10 per cent of cases of hepatocarcinoma[11d] and has been described in a few cases of uterine myoma[18a,44a] and, in mice, when mas-culinizing tumors (luteomas, adrenal rest tumors) were produced.[4]

(4) In *Cushing's syndrome* polycythemia is a frequent finding. Some degree of polycythemia can be produced by the administration of adrenocorticosteroids in large doses. This effect is probably attributable to the profound myeloid stimulation caused by these agents (p. 49).

Stress erythrocytosis (p. 106, 802) is the term applied to a form of relative poly-cythemia[84b] occasionally observed in very active, hard driving persons in whom a state of anxiety is regarded as the underlying cause.

In summary, it may be stated that erythrocytosis develops as the result of:

(1) *Defective saturation* of the arterial blood with oxygen either from (*a*) decreased atmospheric pressure, or (*b*) impaired pulmonary ventilation.

(2) *Circulatory failure*, because of (*a*) shunting (congenital heart disease, pulmonary A-V aneurysm), or (*b*) chronic acquired heart disease.

(3) *Inefficiency of the red corpuscles* due to the formation of an abnormal pigment (methemoglobin, sulfhemoglobin).

(4) In *miscellaneous* circumstances (brain tumors, hypernephroma, poly-cystic kidney) and in Cushing's syndrome.

ERYTHREMIA

Definition.—This is a disease of insidious onset and chronic course and of unknown etiology, which is characterized by a striking absolute increase in the number of red blood corpuscles and in the total blood volume and frequently by signs of increased bone marrow activity. Clinically there is a peculiar reddish-purple color of the skin, a variety of vasomotor and neurological manifestations and, usually, splenic enlargement.

Synonyms. — Polycythemia vera, splenomegalic polycythemia, Vaquez's disease, Osler's disease, polycythemia rubra, polycythemia with chronic cyanosis, myelopathic polycythemia (Weber), erythrocytosis megalosplenica (Senator), cryptogenic polycythemia (R. C. Cabot).

History. — Persistent polycythemia, as distinguished from relative and transient forms, was described in 1892 by Vaquez[134a] in a man whom he took to have a congenital cardiac lesion even though there were no auscultatory signs. At autopsy one year later, the heart was found to be normal. Türk,[134] in 1902

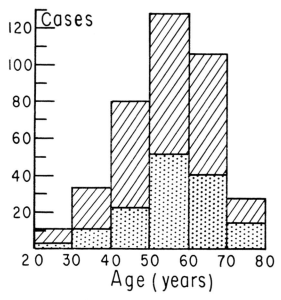

Fig. 16–2.—Age and sex of 386 cases of polycythemia vera [40a,44a,132a]. Males are represented by hatched columns, females by dotted columns.

called attention to the occurrence of leukocytosis in this disease, as well as immature forms of cells of the red and white series, thus suggesting a hyperplastic disorder of blood formation. The writings of Osler (1903, 1904)[103,104] crystallized the picture of the disease, which he considered a new clinical entity.[138a] Excellent reviews of the literature have been published[6,53,67,84b,139] but little of fundamental importance has been added since the earliest publications.

Etiology.—Polycythemia vera is rare among Negroes and comparatively common in Jews. Thus, to quote the largest reported series,[44a] there were only seven Negroes among 197 cases in a hospital where Negroes represent approximately 16 to 25 per cent of the patients. The high incidence among Jews was first noted by Türk and is supported by the data in several series of cases.[44a,87,114] The ratio as compared to other persons, chiefly of European stock, is 2:1 or higher. There is little to support the claim[67,139] that those affected tend to be of slender body build.[44a]

Males are somewhat more commonly affected than females. On the basis of a number of reports,[52,87,117a,134] some of which diverge a good deal from one another, one would estimate the ratio as somewhat less than 2:1. The sex incidence and age at time of diagnosis in 386 cases reported in three large series of cases[40a,44a,132a] is shown in Figure 16–2. The predominant age of onset of symptoms in classical cases is in middle or later life. Cases have been described as appearing early in life, even congenitally, but proof that these have not been examples of "secondary" polycythemia, has often been lacking. A more convincing report is that of Halbertsma regarding a boy of six years.[66] Another is a nine year old boy included in the series of 197 cases reported by Damon and Holub[44a] but not included in Figure 16–2. We have a similar patient, a girl of nine years in whom no etiological factor for the polycythemia has been demonstrated. A case in an eleven year old girl has also been reported.[92a] Such cases are extremely rare and may represent an entity different from the erythremia of later life.

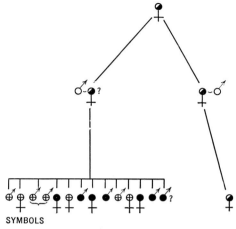

SYMBOLS

○ Well
⊕ Dead and therefore not examined
◑ Polycythemic (history only)
● Polycythemic (blood examined)

FIG. 16–3.—Tree of Engelking's polycythemic family. (Harrop and Wintrobe, Polycythemia, *in* Downey's Handbook of Hematology, courtesy of Paul B. Hoeber, Inc.)

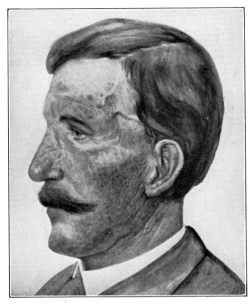

FIG. 16–4.—Photograph of a drawing (original in color) of one of Osler's cases of erythremia.

Erythremia as a *familial* anomaly, has been the subject of reports since 1907.[6] Most remarkable is the family described by Engelking[49] and Wieland[136] in which as many as 11 members in 3 generations may have been involved (Fig. 16–3). In several individuals the abnormality was noted in early childhood. It remains to be seen, however, whether cases of this type are the same in etiology as the sporadic cases which occur in persons of middle age. The familial condition is often symptomless and there is no leukocytosis or "shift to the left" in the myeloid series of leukocytes.[128] Cessation of body growth with signs of infantilism is common in the heredofamilial cases.[136] However, it is noteworthy that an increase above normal in total blood volume, like that found in sporadic cases, has been demonstrated.[28a, 98]

Symptomatology. — Onset. — It is evident from the history in most cases that the disorder probably has been present a long time. The presenting complaint may be headache, dizziness, ringing in the ears or visual disturbances, or there may be dyspnea, lassitude or weakness. Although the color of the skin is often admitted as having been unusual a long time, this alone rarely brings the patient to the physician. Skin and mucous membrane hemorrhages are not uncommon and these, or a sense of weight or swelling in the abdomen due to enlargement of the spleen, may be the initial symptoms. There may be so great a multiplicity of symptoms that neurasthenia is suspected. On the other hand there may be no complaints whatever and the polycythemia is then discovered only accidentally.

Skin and Mucous Membranes.— The color of the face is not like that of ordinary cyanosis but resembles more that of a chronic alcoholic patient or that produced by blushing or exposure to a warm fire. This "rubor" may be very intense so as to produce a startling appearance. The face, particularly the lips, cheeks, tip of the nose, the ears and the neck show this color (Fig. 16–4) but the skin of the trunk is not usually so strikingly affected. The distal portions of the extremities exhibit these changes more than the proximal portions and may be more truly cyanotic. The degree of red or blue depends upon the state of dilatation of the peripheral vascular network and upon the speed of circulation through these areas, since these factors determine the quantity of reduced hemoglobin present.[89] The delayed, sluggish peripheral circulation no doubt accounts for the sensitiveness to cold of which these patients may complain.

Ecchymoses of various sizes are common. Following the application of a mustard plaster, Zadek[139] observed in one case an extensive hemorrhage which soon included almost the entire skin surface. The writer has seen ecchymosis almost as extensive following a breast operation. Red or dark violet spots, or brownish pigmentation of the skin may be found and a great variety of skin lesions[36,110] has been observed (dry skin, eczema, acneform or urticarial changes, acne rosacea, acne urticata,[30a] urticaria pigmentosa[37] and even a nodular eruption similar to the specific infiltration found in leukemia).[54] Purpura was observed in 8 per cent of one series of 163 cases.[133]

The eyes may appear bloodshot. The mucous membranes possess a deep raspberry red color. Epistaxis and bleeding of the gums are common.

A curious but common complaint is intense itching after a bath. This may be so troublesome that bathing with hot or even warm water is avoided. Less frequently, a similar reaction occurs following the use of cold water. This complaint tends to disappear as the polycythemia is treated and returns with relapse. We have not observed this symptom in secondary polycythemia.

Reddening, swelling and pain (erythromelalgia) may occur,[39] especially in the extremities. Club-like thickening of the terminal phalanges is uncommon.

Cardiovascular System. — Cardiac symptoms are not particularly prominent and cardiac hypertrophy is more frequently absent than present. Vascular disease,[100] on the other hand, is extremely common, and vascular accidents are frequent and in many instances are the cause of death. Venous thromboses occur in many cases and varicosities and phlebitis are often observed. Moderate or marked thickening of the peripheral arteries is found, and coronary thrombosis, claudication without occlusion, arterial occlusion with gangrene, acroparesthesia, the Raynaud syndrome and thromboangiitis obliterans have been described.[39] The occurrence of erythromelalgia has been mentioned already.

Gaisböck's syndrome,[53] or *polycythemia hypertonica*, refers to cases in which there is polycythemia and hypertension but no splenomegaly. There is moderate or marked arteriosclerosis, the heart is enlarged, especially to the left, and the history may indicate that there have been a number of apoplectic strokes.

It has been stated that hypertension is so unusual in true erythremia that its presence indicates that the polycythemia is secondary in type.[24] This view seems extreme, for one might expect hypertension in a proportion of cases whenever a chronic disease of middle and late life is involved. It is doubtful whether Gaisböck's syndrome should be distinguished as a separate entity, for one may encounter cases with the symptoms and signs of erythremia but without splenomegaly or hypertension,[28] as well as other cases in which all of these changes are present.[61] In the course of time splenomegaly has been observed to develop in cases otherwise typical of Gaisböck's syndrome.[6] All grades and all possible combinations of symptoms have been observed. In one series of cases[44] systolic blood pressures greater than 140 mm. mercury were found in 11 out of 20 cases (55 per cent). The writer's experience is similar (42 per cent). In another series,[84a] in one-third of the 33 per cent of cases in which elevated blood pressures were present, there was a return to normal following successful treatment of the polycythemia.

Gastro-intestinal System.—Besides feelings of fulness, thirst, gas pains, belching and constipation, in a number of cases peptic ulcer, hemorrhage or thrombosis may occur. Duodenal *ulcer* has been found in as many as 8 per cent of cases of erythremia, almost four times the number in a control series.[137] In another series of 125 cases, duodenal ulcer was found in 16 per cent and gastric ulcer in 7 per cent.[135] It has been suggested that these follow thrombosis in the vessels of the first part of the duodenum and are produced by the action of the digestive juices upon the area of local necrosis.[38] *Hemorrhage* from varices in the esophagus, stomach or bowel may be massive.[28b] Bleeding from hemorrhoids is common and hemorrhage into the peritoneal cavity and into the spleen has been reported several times.[73] *Thrombosis* in the mesenteric veins and arteries may be mistaken for peritonitis or the perforation of an ulcer.[78] *Portal thrombosis* has been considered a cause of polycythemia by some authors.[84]

Enlargement of the liver is frequent (40 or more per cent of cases;[127] 50 per cent in our series). Cirrhosis of the liver has been reported in a number of instances and some writers have distinguished, without much justification, a separate group of cases of erythremia with liver cirrhosis (**Mosse syndrome**).[97] Occlusion of the hepatic veins (Budd-Chiari syndrome) has been observed.[49b,105a]

Splenomegaly. — Splenomegaly occurs in at least three-fourths of cases[40a,132a] (90 per cent of our cases). The size of the spleen varies greatly in individual patients and occasionally it may even extend to the pelvic brim.[44] It is usually quite hard and smooth. There may be pain in the splenic region and following infarction a friction rub can be heard in this area. It is usually supposed that polycythemia antedates the enlargement of the spleen and that engorgement of this organ with blood is the chief cause of the swelling.

Respiratory System. — Dyspnea on much exertion is common and hoarseness is not unusual. Respiratory infections are easily acquired by these patients. Massive hemoptysis or hemothorax may occur. Roentgenograms usually reveal prominent vascular markings in the thorax. Although some pulmonary function studies have been interpreted as indicating deficiencies in ventilation and gas exchange,[99] other investigators[111a] have reported essentially normal arterial oxygen saturation and pulmonary function. A slight reduction in arterial oxygen saturation may be encountered even in healthy persons in the age group usually affected by polycythemia vera. In rare instances inability to ventilate involuntarily sufficiently to arterialize the blood has been observed.[99,111a] This has been attributed to depression of the medullary respiratory center.

Genito-urinary System.—Vesical, vaginal, or uterine bleeding has been recorded, as well as a non-traumatic perirenal hematoma.[91] When there is hypertension, albuminuria and signs of nephritis may be found.

Neuromuscular System. — Headache is the most common neurological symptom but lassitude, vertigo and giddiness, transitory syncope, insomnia, weakness, a sensation of fulness in the head and numbness and tingling in the fingers, less often in the feet, are very common. As Osler remarked, these symptoms are like those of mountain sickness.

Visual disturbances are common and

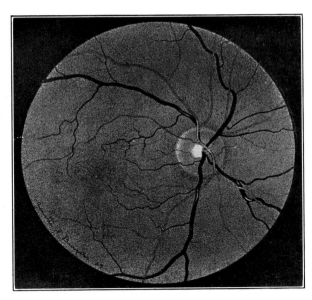

FIG. 16–5.—Drawing of fundus oculi in a case of erythremia. The retina was deeply colored and the veins very greatly engorged and extremely dark in color. The arteries were slightly tortuous and there was moderate compression of the veins at the arteriovenous crossings. The disk was of normal color and outline with physiological cupping. The macula and peripheral fundus were clear. (Courtesy of Dr. Alan C. Woods.)

include transitory dimness of vision, or even temporary blindness, scotomata, specks and bright points in front of the field of vision, diplopia and temporary paralysis of one of the eye muscles. On examination of the *eyegrounds* the vessels are observed to be engorged, tortuous and irregular in diameter; the veins are dark purple, the retina deeply colored (Fig. 16–5). Papilledema has been observed and embolism of the central retinal artery has been reported.[48] Ringing and roaring in the ears is exceedingly common. Ménière's syndrome has been reported.

Vascular lesions of the brain constitute the most serious complication. Various resulting paralyses may be the first symptoms of the disease. Myoclonia, chorea,[83a] grand mal attacks, and symptoms suggesting brain tumor, general paresis and tabes have been associated with erythremia, as well as narcolepsy, attacks of catalepsy and psychic disturbances of various types (loss of memory, mental depression, confusion, hallucinations, slurring of speech).

Pains in the limbs may be very troublesome and severe. These have been attributed to the pressure on the bone by swollen, hyperplastic bone marrow. Curious paresthesias may be encountered and pruritis may be very distressing. Anatomic evidence of spinal cord changes has not, however, been found at autopsy.

Blood.—The blood is characteristically dark in color. It may be so thick that it is drawn up in a pipet with difficulty and spreads slowly between cover-glasses. **Red cell counts** of 7,000,000 to 10,000,000 per c.mm. are common when patients are first seen with this disease and values as high as 12,000,000 and even 15,000,000 have been recorded.[6] It is difficult to accept some of the values reported. When red corpuscles are normal in volume (87 c.μ) there is "standing room" only for about

11,500,000 cells and it is inconceivable that anyone could live with the blood consisting of all cells and no plasma. The writer found the volume of packed red cells as high as 86 ml. per 100 ml. blood in a case of congenital heart disease and 80.8 ml. in a case of erythremia. The highest recorded is 92 ml. in a patient with polycythemia vera whose red cell count was 10,370,000.[139]

It is not unusual to find that, in cases with marked polycythemia, the mean corpuscular volume is reduced below normal. The average size in 22 of our cases was 80 c.μ. In one case the mean volume was as low as 61 c.μ. Somewhat more than 16,000,000 cells as small as these could be packed in 1 c.mm.

Hemoglobin values as high as 240 per cent (40 Gm.) have been recorded but the accuracy of such determinations must also be questioned. Values of 18 to 24 Gm. per 100 ml. blood are more usual. The hemoglobin may not be increased in proportion to the increase in red cell count, this being the case when the mean corpuscular volume and the mean corpuscular hemoglobin are reduced. Sometimes the hemoglobin content of the red cells is reduced even more than their size (low mean corpuscular hemoglobin concentration), which indicates hypochromia in association with polycythemia. This is found particularly after large and repeated hemorrhages.

The **individual red corpuscles** usually appear quite normal. There may be slight anisocytosis but poikilocytosis is unusual. Polychromatophilia and occasionally basophilic stippling may be found. An occasional normoblast may be observed in the blood smear and such a finding, in the presence of a relatively normal or definitely increased red cell count, should arouse suspicion of erythremia. The reticulocyte count, in per cent, is not significantly increased. Following a hemorrhage, however, the reticulocytes may be increased and a number of other immature forms of the red cell series may be encountered. If the hemorrhages are repeated the morphology of the red corpuscles may be like that in hypochromic microcytic anemia.

It is curious that neither Vaquez nor Osler appreciated the significance of the moderate or even marked **leukocytosis,** together with a "shift to the left" in the myeloid series of leukocytes which is often present in the disease named after them. Türk in 1902 called attention to this significant finding which suggests that the whole bone marrow is hyperactive rather than the erythropoietic tissue alone. The leukocyte counts were greater than 10,000 in half of Osler's patients. In another series of 96 cases, the white cell count was elevated in 67.7 per cent of the cases.[87] In 12 of our cases the leukocyte count was 12,850 to 58,000 whereas in 10 it was 6300 to 11,550.

Leukocyte counts of 25,000 per c.mm. are not uncommon[84b] and values above 50,000 have been recorded.[43,117] The myeloid leukocytes are relatively as well as absolutely increased, the metamyelocytes are increased in number and 1 or 2 per cent of myelocytes, sometimes more, are found. Myeloblasts are not usually observed. The basophilic as well as eosinophilic cells may be more numerous than normally. Monocytes may be absolutely increased. As discussed in an earlier chapter (p. 235), the test for *leukocyte alkaline phosphatase* is useful in helping to differentiate erythremia from chronic myelocytic leukemia.

The **blood platelets** are frequently increased, even five- to ten-fold. Counts as high as 3,000,000 and even 6,000,000 platelets per c.mm. have been recorded.[44] Rarely megakaryocytes may be found in the circulating blood. Bleeding time and coagulation time are normal but the clot may retract poorly, perhaps because the red cell mass is so great. The presence of a fibrinolytic factor in the plasma has been reported.[31c]

It should be noted, however, that the leukocyte and platelet counts are not always increased above normal in otherwise typical cases of erythremia. Such normal values were found in 20 per cent of the cases in one series.[132a]

Studies of the **fragility of the red corpuscles**[76,95] in solutions of hypotonic saline indicate a lengthened resistance span, with initial hemolysis appearing in more concentrated solutions and complete hemolysis occurring in more dilute solutions than is normal. The plasma of patients with erythremia has been found to exert a hemolytic effect on normal red corpuscles.[95]

There may be some evidence of increased **blood destruction** in cases of erythremia, although this is not common. Icterus index and van den Bergh tests may show bilirubinemia greater than normal,[95,139] and there may be an increase in urobilinogen and urobilin in the urine, as well as increased urobilin in the stools.[107]

The **viscosity** of the blood may be five to eight times greater than normal.[84b,139] The **specific gravity** is 1.075 to 1.080, as compared with 1.055 to 1.065 normally. The degree of abnormality varies with the relative quantity of red corpuscles. The viscosity and specific gravity of the serum have been found to be actually less than is normal.[102] The **sedimentation rate** of polycythemic blood is greatly delayed.

In most cases of polycythemia vera the **arterial oxygen saturation** has been found to be normal, even when the hemoglobin levels were high, indicating that the high viscosity of the blood does not prevent the normal saturation of the blood with oxygen.[49a] Breathing oxygen raises the oxygen of the arterial blood to a degree comparable to that observed normally, and the oxygen dissociation curve

is normal. The carbon dioxide combining power of the whole blood has been found to be less than normal but other acid-base properties usually are normal.

Total Blood Volume.—This is characteristically increased. The enormous increase in blood which distends even the smaller vessels of the whole body accounts, no doubt, for many of the symptoms of this disease. In a group of 30 patients whose volume of packed red cells was 55 ml. per 100 ml. or greater, the total red cell volume, measured by the P^{32}-labelled red cell method, was 38.8 to 93.9 ml. per Kg. body weight as compared with the normal average of 29.9 ml.[31a] In two-thirds of these cases the plasma volumes (29 ml. per Kg.) were below the lower limits of normal and in none was the plasma volume above normal. Similar observations have been made by the Cr^{51} method.[132a] Because of variations in plasma volume, the volume of packed red cells gives only a rough indication of the size of the red cell mass.

Bone Marrow.—The marrow is dark red in color and very cellular. The hyperplasia involves all the marrow elements, however, so that the ratio of the different types of cells to one another is not strikingly different from the normal. The percentage of nucleated red cells may be moderately elevated.[135d] These cells may be either orthochromic normoblasts or of less mature type, but megaloblasts are not found. There may be more myelocytes and myeloblasts than is normal and an unusual number of eosinophilic and basophilic leukocytes may be found. Megakaryocytes are sometimes more numerous than is normal.

Other Findings.—The **urine** may be normal, but not infrequently albuminuria, and less often casts are found.[84b] The increased urobilinogenuria found in some cases has been mentioned already. Studies of renal hemodynamics in three cases suggested that glomerular filtration is kept at almost normal values, in spite of the decreased fraction of plasma in the blood, by an increase in renal blood flow and in the proportion of plasma filtered.[135b] The **gastric acidity** may be normal or increased or there may be anacidity. A variety of **chemical analyses of the blood** have been reported but the conflicting results give the impression that no characteristic abnormality has yet been demonstrated. We have never found significant changes in serum albumin, total serum proteins, albumin-globulin ratio, blood cholesterol, fats, non-protein nitrogen constituents, serum calcium, magnesium, phosphorus or total serum base.[6] Hyperkaliemia has been noted when the platelets were greatly increased in number.[97a] The *uric acid* is usually normal. In a series of 47 patients, values from 2.8 to 11.7 mg. per cent were found (average 6.6 mg.)[84b] However, persistently increased endogenous uric acid excretion has been observed[125] and **gout** occurs in about 5 per cent of cases,[44a,132a] or more.[132b,135] It has been demonstrated by the cumulative labelling of urinary uric acid with glycine-N[15] that the occurrence of hyperuricemia in erythremia is attributable to overproduction of uric acid.[138c] A sharp contrast was noted between the rapid peak of isotope incorporation into uric acid in primary gout and the slow incorporation in secondary gout, such as that which may be seen in erythremia.

A moderate increase in **basal metabolic rate** is frequently found,[32] although this is not invariably the case. It was +35 or higher in 3 of our patients. The **circulatory minute volume** is reduced and the **velocity of blood flow** is greatly lowered,[34] but the cardiac output and work are normal.[27] The skin capillaries are distended and the capillary loops are enlarged.

An increased **cerebrospinal fluid** pressure has been reported.[36]

Diagnosis.—The classical triad is a

51

"ruddy cyanosis," splenomegaly and polycythemia. To this should be added the morphological signs of increased erythrogenesis such as occasional nucleated red cells and polychromatophilia, which are very often found if looked for, as well as the frequent association of leukocytosis, with moderate shift to the left, and thrombocytosis. These findings, in fact, are helpful in distinguishing erythremia from erythrocytosis for in the latter normoblastosis, leukocytosis and thrombocytosis are not found as a rule. Thus, in a series of cases of congenital heart disease, slight leukopenia with a slight absolute decrease in the number of eosinophils, monocytes and lymphocytes was found.[15b] However, it has been pointed out that normoblasts may be found in the peripheral blood in congestive heart failure.[60] This finding alone, therefore, cannot be taken as evidence of polycythemia vera. Even the co-existence of gout does not indicate that one is dealing with polycythemia vera since gout has been observed in polycythemia secondary to congenital heart disease.[25b]

It is noteworthy that the characteristic color is not invariably present and the spleen is not always enlarged. Furthermore, the symptoms are so varied that a great number of diseases, particularly those of the cardiovascular and nervous systems may be simulated. The first manifestations of the disorder[44] may suggest peripheral vascular disease (thromboangiitis obliterans, erythromelalgia), gastro-intestinal disease (appendicitis, ulcer, gall bladder disease), arthritis or nephritis; or the symptoms may be so numerous and unrelated that neurasthenia may be considered.

Blood examination, which includes enumeration of the three corpuscular constituents of the blood and careful examination of the blood smear, should make the diagnosis of polycythemia evident. It is necessary, however, to rule out the various conditions which lead to the production of "secondary" polycythemia (p. 788). Measurement of total blood volume is of value chiefly in ruling out relative polycythemia. In "stress erythrocytosis" (p. 106), which is actually a form of relative polycythemia, the total red cell volume is normal but the plasma volume is greatly reduced.[84b] As a consequence the high volume of packed red cells gives a misleading impression. In true erythrocytosis, that is, in secondary forms of absolute polycythemia, the total blood volume may be as much increased as in erythremia.[84b] To distinguish the secondary forms of polycythemia, it is useful to determine arterial oxygen saturation for this is normal in polycythemia vera and substantially reduced in the secondary form (p. 807).

The recognition of erythremia in the early stages is naturally difficult. The finding of splenomegaly and polycythemia, even when the latter is not striking, suggests erythremia but a similar picture may be associated with obliterative thrombophlebitis of the splenic and portal veins,[85] tuberculosis, syphilis and hydatid disease of the spleen. If the patient appears for the first time when a complication has developed, there may be considerable difficulty in diagnosis. A severe hemorrhage, for example, may reduce the red cell count even to normal and, as occurred in one of our cases, the splenomegaly and leukocytosis may then suggest leukemia. In one series of 163 cases, as many as 10 per cent of the patients presented a leukemoid reaction with marked leukocytosis and even myeloblasts in the blood which was of such a degree that, together with the marked splenomegaly, the picture of chronic myelocytic leukemia was closely simulated.[133] Furthermore, rare cases of chronic myelocytic leukemia have been described[95] which in their early stages were characterized by slight polycythemia rather than anemia. Sometimes

one must watch the progress of the disease before a final diagnosis can be made.

Course, Complications and Duration.—The course is chronic and of long duration (ten to fifteen years or longer) if serious complications do not develop. Many years may go by without progression of the symptoms. In other instances the intensity of the complaints waxes and wanes without any apparent relation to the blood findings. The "acute erythremia" of di Guglielmo is quite different from the disorder under discussion here. Its course is acute and it is characterized by anemia and marked erythroblastosis (p. 941).

Intercurrent infections are frequent, especially those of the respiratory tract. Bronchitis and emphysema may develop. Vascular complications, as already mentioned, are so common that they may be considered a part of the disease. It is noteworthy, however, that thromboses were found to occur much less frequently (4.2 per cent) in patients treated successfully with radioactive phosphorus[84a] than prior to the introduction of this form of therapy (approximately 25 per cent of cases). The association of duodenal ulcer, cirrhosis of the liver (Mosse syndrome), hypertension (Gaisböck's syndrome) and gout has been mentioned. Albuminuria is common and is possibly the result of blood stasis in the kidneys. Orthostatic albuminuria has been described.[70] In cases with hypertension particularly, chronic renal disease and arteriosclerosis are common.[24]

In view of the frequent finding of an increased basal metabolic rate, it is of interest that hyperthyroidism has been reported in only one well-studied case.[139] Paroxysmal hemoglobinuria has been described in one case[108] and "agranulocytosis" in another.[123] Termination of erythremia in leukemia or anemia has been reported and will be discussed shortly. Hemoblastic sarcoma[109] and osteosclerosis[117] have also been observed.

Treatment.—General Remarks.— As long as the cause of erythremia is unknown, its treatment must be symptomatic. A great number of methods has been recommended to relieve the symptoms of this disorder. Relief of most of the symptoms is accomplished by lowering the total blood volume. This can be done by removing blood (venesection), by destroying it (phenylhydrazine), or by affecting blood production (irradiation, chemotherapeutic agents, or a diet poor in blood building substances). In choosing a method of treatment the object should be to produce a reduction in the blood volume by a means which gives the least trouble to the patient and carries the smallest chance of causing harm.

The choice of a method is relatively simple if the above objectives are kept clear. In criticism of venesection, it has been stated that the method is somewhat troublesome and that hematopoiesis is stimulated by the blood loss. The latter objection is theoretical and has not been substantiated.[130] In any event, it is unimportant. Venesection has the advantage that the blood taken off is actually removed from the body and is not available for new blood formation.

When the red corpuscles are destroyed by phenylhydrazine, the products of destruction remain in large part with the body and may be used again.[93] This drug, furthermore, is a potent one with a delayed action which may produce severe anemia and deep jaundice. On the other hand, it is administered easily and, if only small doses are given for the purpose of maintaining a reduced blood volume, already lowered by other means, there is no danger from its use.

Irradiation by means of x-rays is relatively slow in action, requires special apparatus as well as skill and the effect produced, if greater than expected, may be irreparable. On the other hand, the remission produced with successful irradiation may be relatively prolonged. More satisfactory is radioactive phosphorus which has a similar effect, causes no nausea or vomiting and can be administered easily.

The employment of an iron-free **diet**[116] or of other dietary regimens (high fat diet,[119] low purine diet) has not only been unsuccessful but imposes an unnecessary hardship on patients with so chronic a disease as erythremia. It is also worth noting that rigorous use of some of the diets recommended might bring about serious nutritional deficiency disorders.

The feeding of *spleen* or splenic extracts, with the purpose of administering some hypothetical splenic hormone with a hemolytic effect, has not been followed by convincingly beneficial results.[6,80] The administration of *ascorbic acid*,[81] or *choline*[41] unlike their reputed effect in cobalt polycythemia, has not influenced the blood in cases of erythremia.

General measures in the management of this disease include avoidance of physical or mental strain, and of alcohol or stimulants, but rigorous dietary regulation, as already suggested, seems an unnecessary hardship. Too sedentary a life is to be avoided as further lagging of the circulation, with the possibility of thrombosis, is thereby favored. Because of the tendency to hemorrhage, surgical measures should be avoided as far as possible.

Venesection.—This is a valuable therapeutic agent which is useful primarily for its immediate effects in relieving symptoms, especially the vertigo, fulness in the head, headache, tinnitus, mental torpor, weakness and pain in the muscles, bones or joints. If 500 ml. is removed repeatedly (usually six to eight times) at intervals of one to three days, it is possible to reduce the blood volume to normal and to produce a remission which may last several, even fifteen months.[130] Blood viscosity is reduced, blood volume is lowered and circulatory efficiency improved. It is of interest that venesections have not been followed, in many instances, by reticulocytosis and other signs of stimulated blood formation.

Venesection can be used as the sole therapeutic measure for erythremia. Some patients can be controlled by one or two 500 ml. phlebotomies every three or four months. Generally patients are comfortable if the volume of packed red cells is brought to the upper limit of normal rather than to still lower levels. When venesections have to be performed more frequently than once in two months, it is generally found preferable to resort to other forms of therapy. Of those that will be described below, the agent most generally preferred is radioactive phosphorus (p. 805).

In India, patients with polycythemia vera have been treated successfully by deliberately producing hookworm infestation.[39a]

Phenylhydrazine.—This drug is a base related to antipyrine and is prepared on a large scale from the anilin used commercially to produce antipyrine. It was introduced for the treatment of erythremia by Eppinger and Kloss in 1918. The liquid phenylhydrazine is unstable but the crystalline hydrochloride is less easily decomposed except when it is exposed to air. It is best given in capsules. Its mode of action is not entirely clear, but a direct action on red corpuscles must be postulated. It has been suggested that by oxidation the benzene nucleus is liberated and permitted to act upon the blood.

As employed originally,[59] phenylhydrazine was given in amounts of 0.1 to 0.3 Gm. daily up to a total of 1.5 to 3.5 Gm. This was followed by a period of observation without medication for a week or ten days, more being given if necessary. The earliest noticeable effect is leukocytosis,[86] due to an increase in granulocytes. An increase in plasma bilirubin follows and a drop in erythrocyte count occurs.[57,58] The red cell count continues to fall and the signs of blood destruction persist for seven to ten days after the drug has been stopped. The red corpuscles preserve their normal size unless the blood destruction is great, when macrocytosis may develop.[90] At the same time there is an increase in the reticulocyte count, and nucleated red corpuscles, polychromatophilia, anisocytosis and poikilocytosis may appear.[90] Heinz bodies (p. 624) are formed. Erythrocyte fragility in solutions of hypotonic saline, instead of increasing, may decrease.[39] The total blood volume decreases.

Large doses given to bile fistula dogs have been shown to destroy almost all of the mature cells in the circulation.[43a] This is accompanied by an output of bile pigment which corresponds closely to the calculated amount which could be derived from the destroyed hemoglobin. At the same time there is almost maximal production of new hemoglobin and red cells, the iron and perhaps the globin from the destroyed hemoglobin being re-utilized.

Overdosage results in anorexia, vomiting, diarrhea, deep jaundice, pruritus, vertigo, lumbar pain and general weakness. Tenderness over the spleen may develop and hematuria as well as hematemesis has been reported. The urine may become dark in color, almost black. Reducing substances (phenol) may appear but these are distinguished from those found in glycosuria by a negative fermentation reaction.

Liver damage has been produced in dogs by phenylhydrazine[35] but the amounts necessary to produce this effect are far in excess of what is ever used in man.[57] The chief danger in man is from the production of severe anemia as the result of the use of excessive doses and from failure to appreciate the cumulative action of phenylhydrazine.[82]

It has been stated that the tendency

to thrombosis is increased by the action of this drug on the platelets. This complication is so common in untreated erythremia that one cannot be certain that phenylhydrazine is responsible if thrombosis occurs during its use. Nevertheless, it is undoubtedly wise to avoid using the drug in elderly patients, in anyone who is confined to bed or in any patient who has had thrombosis.[59]

The toxic effects of phenylhydrazine hydrochloride which have been described may be attributed to the large doses which have been used. The writer has found this drug to be a useful agent and has not observed toxic effects, probably because it has been used as an adjunct to therapy, not as the primary agent for reducing the red cell mass to lower levels. Venesection is the safest and most efficient means to achieve the latter. When phenylhydrazine is given in amounts of 0.1 Gm. at such intervals (daily, every other day, twice a week) as may be necessary to maintain the blood at a satisfactory level, no untoward effects are observed. There is only slight bilirubinemia and there may be no leukocytosis. Phenylhydrazine is useful, particularly, in cases in which thrombocytopenia has developed following treatment with radioactive phosphorus. We have not observed "tolerance" to the drug.[67] One of our patients took the drug regularly for nine years.

Irradiation. — Irradiation, in one form or another, has been used as a method of treatment for erythremia for many years. The radiations were first directed to the spleen, without benefit. Radiation of the bones was first successfully applied in 1916[88] and entails mapping out the entire skeleton and treating systematically one or more areas at a sitting.[105] Deep roentgen-therapy has been given, "grenzstrahlen" have been employed,[40] radium as well as thorium-X has been used,[115] and irradiation of the whole body ("spray therapy," "total radiation") has been recommended.[124]

A disadvantage of irradiation therapy is that it is not immediate in its effect. Thus the patient not only fails to be relieved symptomatically at once but it is also impossible to be certain that too much or too little irradiation has been given. In the latter case it can be repeated, but in the former irreparable damage has been done. In cases in which the leukocyte count is normal and falls quickly after irradiation, it may be difficult to give effective dosage with safety. On the other hand, if successfully carried out, the result is more lasting than can be achieved by many other forms of treatment of this disease. If immediate relief is desired, it can be secured by venesection. In patients who are bedridden or in those who have had thromboses, irradiation is preferable to phenylhydrazin.

Of particular value is treatment by means of **radioactive phosphorus.**[112] This substance (P^{32}) is obtained by bombardment of red phosphorus (P^{31}) with 12 million volt deuterons. The phosphorus is then synthesized into its dibasic sodium salt. The salt is soluble in water and, while it is effective when given by mouth,[138b] it has been used more successfully when given by vein.

The radioactive phosphorus passes to tissues which have a high phosphorus content and which metabolize phosphorus rapidly. Its uptake by rapidly dividing cells is greater than that of normal cells. Since its half-life is 14.3 days, steady irradiation of tissue takes place for several weeks.[51a] Its concentration in bone makes radioactive phosphorus particularly valuable in the management of hemopoietic disorders. Among these its value seems to be greatest in connection with the management of erythremia.

Radioactive phosphorus has been found to induce satisfactory clinical and hematologic remissions in this disease which have lasted as long as one to two or more years.[84a,112] As with roentgen therapy, the fall in the red cell count does not usually begin before thirty to sixty days after it has been given. Care must be taken to avoid producing anemia, leukopenia or thrombocytopenia. Unlike the effects of roentgen therapy, irradiation sickness does not occur.

A recommended method of treatment is as follows: The volume of packed red cells is brought down to 55 ml. per cent, or less, by phlebotomies. The patient is then given between 4 and 5 millicuries (mc.) of P^{32}, intravenously. No additional P^{32} is given for three months, in order to avoid cumulative effects. If the polycythemia increases above 55 ml. in the interval, venesection can be performed. If, after three months, the volume of packed red cells is above 55 ml., a second injection of 1 to 4 millicuries is given. Examinations are repeated at three-month intervals. Some patients do not require a second injection or further phlebotomies for six to 18 months or longer. Perhaps 10 per cent of patients will need a third injection. After this, it has been recommended that no further injections be given for at least a year, preferably 18 months.[112]

An analysis of 300 courses given to 139 patients showed that an average of 6.7 millicuries had been given in a "course," as represented by a six-month period.[84b] The majority of the patients were retreated within intervals of six to ten months. In another series of 241 cases[132] the average dose required to produce remissions was 5.7 millicuries in cases without leukocytosis or myeloid immaturity and as much as 8.3 millicuries in other cases. The range of doses required was 3 to 21 millicuries. Complications of the P^{32} therapy were acute leukemia in 3.3 per cent of the cases, "anemia with leukemoid reactions" (possibly myelofibrosis with myeloid metaplasia or myelocytic leukemia) in 10 per cent and hypoplastic anemia in only one case. Since approximately 80 per cent

of the patients were still alive at the time of the report, the ultimate incidence of such complications may prove to be much higher. As yet, however, it is difficult to establish the thesis that the incidence of leukemia in patients treated with P^{32} is greater than in untreated cases or in cases of erythremia treated by other means.

Various **chemotherapeutic agents** used in the treatment of leukemia, Hodgkin's disease and related disorders have been employed in the management of polycythemia vera. Benzene was once used in the treatment of erythremia[83] but the toxic effects of this drug led to its abandonment. Fowler's solution (potassium arsenite), administered in the same manner as in the treatment of chronic myelocytic leukemia (p. 962), was found effective in lowering the blood count in some cases,[50] but better agents are now available. When a total dose of 0.4 mg. of *nitrogen mustard* (methyl-bis, β-chloroethylamine hydrochloride) per Kg. of body weight was given intravenously, a 25 per cent fall in the quantity of red corpuscles occurred in an average of 4.4 weeks in 10 cases.[128a] Remissions averaged 6.4 months in duration. *Triethylene melamine*, in oral doses of 2.5 to 5 mg. every one to three days until a total of 15 to 40 mg. was given in a course, has also been reported favorably.[117a] In 20 out of 30 cases a satisfactory symptomatic and hematologic response was observed, with remissions lasting eight to nine months. Thrombocytopenia was a frequent complication, however, and purpura developed in one case. The experience of others[47a] has been similar. This agent has advantages over nitrogen mustard in that it can be given by mouth and gastro-intestinal discomfort does not occur or is minimal. *Busulfan* has been given in initial doses of 2 to 10 mg. per day, followed by maintenance therapy in amounts of 2 to 8 mg. per week.[86a,135a] The antimalarial, *pyrimethane*, has also been shown to have an effect in erythremia.[51b] All of these agents carry the disadvantage that much closer supervision of the patient is necessary than when P[32] is used and various untoward effects may develop.

Splenectomy has been performed in a number of cases. It is not only valueless but it may be harmful, for death has followed in a number of instances.

Pathology.—The extreme plethora, the engorgement of all the organs with blood which flows, when the heart is removed, as if "from an inexhaustible spring;" the enlarged and thrombosed veins "resembling bunches of thick worms;"[38] as well as the unusual color of the skin and the large and small hemorrhages in the skin, mucous membranes, brain, meninges, serous cavities and the various organs, make up a striking and characteristic picture.

The *spleen* is enlarged, smooth, moderately hard, dark bluish-red in color and may contain infarcts, thromboses and cysts produced by hemorrhage. The follicles are atrophied and the pulp hypertrophied and hyperemic. The spleen is crowded with adult red corpuscles but a few foci of extra-medullary hematopoiesis with nucleated red corpuscles in them are often seen. Tuberculosis has been found in the spleen in a number of cases,[121] including 2 of our own.

The liver is often enlarged and is strikingly hyperemic. Myeloid metaplasia may be found.[95] Cirrhosis may be discovered.[97] Renal changes are not found, unless chronic nephritis is associated, and there may be no cardiac hypertrophy. No remarkable changes are seen in the lymph nodes as a rule, although there may be deposits of hemosiderin and hematopoietic foci have been observed.

The bone marrow has been described (p. 800). It is red in the long bones as well as in the short and flat bones but in the former it is engorged chiefly with adult erythrocytes whereas in the short bones there is evidence of active hematopoiesis.[139]

Pathogenesis.—The symptoms and signs of erythremia can be attributed in large part to the slowing of the blood flow as the result of the increased viscosity of the blood.[27] The blood viscosity increases sharply as the concentration of red corpuscles rises to abnormal levels.[93a] The additional vascular space in the skin associated with the general distension of all the blood vessels may lead to a loss or impairment of the physiological heat mechanism and many of the sensory symptoms may be attributable to this.

The cause of the disorder is unknown. The fact that polycythemia is known to develop as a result of **oxygen want,** has led to the view that some defect which results in lack of oxygen is the fundamental cause. It has been suggested that the disease is the consequence of a lessened power of the red corpuscles to absorb oxygen; or that there is such a state of capillary dilatation that the corpuscles cannot unload their oxygen, this in turn stimulating increased erythropoiesis. For these hypotheses there is no proof. The oxygen combining power of the hemoglobin is not decreased, and tissue respiration is not increased.[67] In contrast to the findings in cases of secondary polycythemia, where the oxygen saturation may be as low as 75 per cent, the findings in polycythemia vera are essentially the same as in normal individuals (91 to 97 per cent) even at very high hematocrit levels.[42,135c] However, a significantly increased oxygen unsaturation after exercise has been observed, a finding which was attributed to changes in the rate of pulmonary gas diffusion.[68]

The capillaries of the lungs have been found to contain an unusually large number of megakaryocytes.[75] It has been suggested that these cells, produced in excess as the result of some unknown stimulus, plug the lung capillaries and produce oxygen want. One might, of course, view the question from another angle; namely, that the increased number of megakaryocytes is only a manifestation of a disorder in which megakaryocytes and leukocytes also, as well as erythrocytes, are produced in excess.

A suggestion that erythremia is the compensatory result of anoxemia of the bone marrow[114] was based on the observation of capillary thickening and subintimal and adventitial fibrosis of the subarteriolar capillaries, arterioles and arteries in bone marrow specimens from cases of polycythemia vera which were not found in control specimens. However, in the population group studied, thromboangiitis obliterans was common and it seems likely that the vascular changes in the bone marrow were coincidental rather than etiologically related to the polycythemia. Direct measurements of bone marrow oxygen saturation have failed to reveal significant differences between normal individuals and patients with polycythemia vera.[31,69] In another study[123a] the percentage saturation of bone marrow blood was greater and the arterial-bone marrow blood oxygen difference was smaller in patients with this disease than in controls.

It has been pointed out that polycythemia might be the result of increased activity of the blood-forming organs, decreased blood destruction or prolonged "life" of the red corpuscles. No evidence of abnormal red cell life span has been found.[85a] Fecal urobilinogen values are lower than would be anticipated on the basis of the increased amounts of hemoglobin that are degraded although they may be greater than is found in normal individuals. As to **functional hyperactivity of the hematopoietic organs,** this is suggested by the findings in the blood and bone marrow. Not only are the red corpuscles produced in excess and immature forms thrown into the cir-

culation, but signs of increased production are found in the myeloid leukocytes and platelets as well. Furthermore, studies of heme synthesis by the N^{15}-glycine method have shown a rate of hemoglobin production about $2\frac{1}{2}$ times the normal[85a] while measurement of plasma iron turnover also showed a marked increase.[75a] It cannot be easily assumed that this stimulus to overproduction of cells is anoxemia, for in such conditions as Monge's disease (p. 790), the exaggerated hemopoiesis is confined to the red cell series and, even of red cells, nucleated forms are not found in the blood. It is noteworthy that oxygen administration does not affect plasma iron turnover in polycythemia vera, whereas a marked decrease occurs in secondary forms.[75a]

It has been suggested that erythremia is the **antithesis of pernicious anemia,** the overproduction of cells being due to excessive formation of gastric hematopoietic factor. Attempts to demonstrate an excess of this factor did not yield convincing results.[30] An extract of the liver of a case of erythremia was reported as being more potent in the treatment of pernicious anemia than normal human liver.[138] There also have been reports of marked, though temporary decreases in the erythrocyte counts in cases of erythremia treated by gastric lavage.[74,101] Irradiation of the stomach in one case[74] and gastrectomy in another,[126] were reported as beneficial but failure of irradiation has also been recorded.[129] Thus the evidence is not at all convincing. It may be pointed out in regard to this hypothesis that the administration of excessive amounts of liver extract or vitamin B_{12} to patients with pernicious anemia or to normal individuals, does not produce polycythemia.

It is of interest that erythremia may occasionally terminate in a form which suggests the clinical picture of pernicious[29] or of aplastic anemia[46,51,92] and even the blood picture in such cases may be very much like that seen in these types of anemia. These cases do not include those in which roentgen therapy[47,122] was the possible cause of the anemia. Leuko-erythroblastic anemia has also been observed.[131]

The morphological picture, as well as the course of occasional cases of erythremia, suggest a **relationship to chronic myelocytic leukemia.**[93b] The leukocytosis in erythremia is sometimes so marked as to suggest a diagnosis of chronic myelocytic leukemia.[43,95,106,113] In some cases, in spite of a clinical and hematologic picture of erythremia, at autopsy the amount of leukoblastic tissue greatly exceeded the quantity of erythroblastic tissue and the pathological findings resembled those characteristic of chronic myelocytic leukemia.[33,140] In still other cases, anemia developed following a period of polycythemia whereas leukocytosis persisted, producing a picture very suggestive of leukemia.[45,95,118] Even acute myeloblastic leukemia has been known to develop as a terminal event in cases of erythremia.[71,79] In none of the cases cited above could the changes which occurred be attributed to irradiation therapy. Following roentgen therapy acute myeloblastic leukemia has been reported in one case[38a] and the writer observed another. As mentioned earlier (p. 806) acute leukemia has been observed to develop following treatment with radioactive phosphorus. In an even larger series (453 cases) than that cited earlier, acute leukemia was observed in 2.7 per cent of the P[32]-treated cases.[138b]

In several instances polycythemia has been observed to develop in cases of typical leukemia.[55] The writer has observed a patient who, after receiving roentgen therapy for what appeared to be classical chronic myelocytic leukemia, developed a typical picture of erythremia with a red cell count of 9,450,000, 19.5 Gm. hemoglobin, 66 ml. volume packed red cells and a leukocyte count of only 29,600, of which but 4 per cent were myelocytes. Venesections produced symptomatic improvement. Eight months later the spleen became huge, the leukocytes rose to 212,000 and anemia developed. Such cases are sometimes referred to under the designation, *"erythroleukemia"* (see p. 941). In a few cases erythremia and leukemia have been encountered in the same family.[63,64] It is difficult to believe that such uncommon conditions as erythremia and leukemia, especially acute leukemia, would occur merely by chance in the same individual. It is noteworthy that the cases of leukemia, whenever identified, have been myeloblastic or myelocytic rather than lymphoid. Only once has the association of chronic lymphocytic leukemia been recorded.[31b] Some fundamental relationship or, in certain cases, the effect of irradiation must be suspected.

Much has been written regarding the possible *relation* of erythremia to **abnormalities of endocrine secretion.** It has been suggested that erythremia is the result of a lack of balance in the hormonal control of the hematopoietic system.[6,49] With the renewed interest in "erythropoietin" (p. 49), attempts have been made to relate erythremia to overproduction of this humoral factor. However, to date, no consistent findings have been recorded. Elsewhere (p. 48) the influence of the various hormones on erythropoiesis was discussed. There is no evidence that any of the recognized endocrine or humoral factors is concerned in the development of erythremia.

The **role of the spleen** has been the subject of discussion not only because of its relationship to the hematopoietic system but because tuberculosis located primarily or chiefly in this organ has been discovered in a number of instances of polycythemia. The relationship of such tuberculosis to the polycythemia is quite

obscure.[121]   It has been suggested that
there may be (1) suppression of the
hemolytic role of the spleen; (2) increased
activity of the bone marrow due to suppression of the regulatory action of the
spleen; and (3) replacement of lymphoid
by myeloid tissue in the spleen as the
consequence of the presence of tubercle
bacilli or their toxins.   These suggestions
are purely conjectural.

BIBLIOGRAPHY

Erythrocytosis

1. BARRON, E. S. G., DILL, D. B., EDWARDS, H.
   T. and HURTADO, A.: Acute Mountain
   Sickness; the Effect of Ammonium Chloride, J. Clin. Invest., 16, 541, 1937.
1a. BEDELL, G. N., WILSON, W. R. and SEE-
    BOHM, P. M.: Pulmonary Function in
    Obese Persons, J. Clin. Invest., 37, 1049,
    1958.
1b. BERNDT, H.: Einfluss von Herz- und Lungen-
    erkrankungen auf das Volumen und die
    Farbstoffkonzentration der Erythrocyten,
    Acta med. scandinav., 165, 41, 1959.
2. BURWELL, C. S., ROBIN, E. D., WHALEY, R.
   D. and BICKELMANN, A. G.: Extreme
   Obesity Associated with Alveolar Hypoventilation—a Pickwickian Syndrome, Am.
   J. Med., 21, 811, 1956.
2a. DAMON, A., HOLUB, D. A., MELICOW, M. M.
    and USON, A. C.: Polycythemia and Renal
    Carcinoma, Am. J. Med., 25, 182, 1958.
3. FORSSELL, J.: Polycythemia and Hypernephroma, Acta med. scandinav., 150, 155,
   1954; *ibid.*, 161, 169, 1958.
3a. GARDNER, F. H. and FREYMANN, J. G.:
    Erythrocythemia (Polycythemia) and Hy-
    dronephrosis, New England J. Med., 259,
    323, 1958.
4. GOTTSCHALK, R. G. and FURTH, J.: Polycythemia With Features of Cushing's Syndrome   Produced   by   Luteomas,   Acta
   hæmat., 5, 100, 1951.
4a. GRANT, J. L. *et al.:* Red Cell Changes in
    Chronic Pulmonary Insufficiency, J. Clin.
    Invest., 37, 1166, 1958.
5. HALLOCK, P.: Polycythemia of Morbus
   Cæruleus (Cyanotic Type of Congenital
   Heart Disease), Proc. Soc. Exper. Biol. &
   Med., 44, 11, 1940.
6. HARROP, G. A., JR. and WINTROBE, M. M.:
   Polycythemia, *in Handbook of Hematology*,
   H. Downey, Ed., New York, Paul B.
   Hoeber, Inc., 4, 2366, 1938 (Bibliography).

7. HECHT, H. H.: Heart Failure and Lung Disease, Circulation, 14, 265, 1956.
8. HECHT, H. H. and McCLEMENT, J. H.: A
   Case of "Chronic Mountain Sickness" in
   the United States, Am. J. Med., 25, 470,
   1958.
9. HEDLUND, S.: Studies on Erythropoiesis and
   Total Red Cell Volume in Congestive
   Heart Failure, Acta med. scandinav.,
   146, 1, 1953, Suppl. 284.
10. HURTADO, A.: Chronic Mountain Sickness,
    J.A.M.A., 120, 1278, 1942; Ann. Int. Med.,
    53, 247, 1960.
10a. JONES, N. F., PAYNE, R. W., HYDE, R. D.
     and PRICE, T. M. L.: Renal Polycythae-
     mia, Lancet, 1, 299, 1960; Nature, 185,
     459, 1960.
10b. KALTREIDER, N. L., MENEELEY, G. R. and
     ALLEN, J. R.: The Effect of Epinephrine on
     the Volume of the Blood, J. Clin. Invest.,
     21, 339, 1942.
11. LAWRENCE, J. H. and DONALD, W. G., JR.:
    Polycythemia   and   Hydronephrosis   or
    Renal Tumors, Ann. Int. Med., 50, 959,
    1959.
11a. LEOPOLD, S. S.: The Etiology of Pulmonary
     Arteriosclerosis, Am. J. M. Sc., 219, 152,
     1950.
11b. LINDSKOG, G. E., LIEBOW, A., KAUSEL, H.
     and JANZEN, A.: Pulmonary Arteriovenous
     Aneurysm, Ann. Surg., 132, 591, 1950.
11c. LOMAN, J. and DAMESHEK, W.: Plethora of the
     Intracranial Venous Circulation in a Case
     of Polycythemia, New England J. Med.,
     232, 394, 1945.
11d. McFADZEAN, A. J. S., TODD, D. and TSANG,
     K. C.: Polycythemia in Primary Carci-
     noma of the Liver, Blood, 13, 427, 1958.
12. MERINO, C.: Studies on Blood Formation and
    Destruction in the Polycythemia of High
    Altitude, Blood, 5, 1, 1950.
13. MONGE, C.: High Altitude Disease, Arch.
    Int. Med., 59, 32, 1937; Physiol. Rev.,
    23, 166, 1943.
14. MORSE, P. F.: Symptomatic Polycythemia
    With Cyanosis and Dyspnœa, Arch. Int.
    Med., 33, 459, 1924.
14a. MULLER, G. L.: Experimental Bone Marrow
     Reactions, J. Exper. Med., 45, 399, 1927.
15. NIXON, R. K., O'ROURKE, W., RUPE, C. E.
    and KORST, D. R.: Nephrogenic Poly-
    cythemia, Arch. Int. Med., 106, 797, 1960.
15a. PORTO, J.: Analyse pathogénique de la
     cardiopathie noire, J. Suisse Méd., 78,
     913, 1948.
15b. PRADER, A., ROSSI, E. and WODENEGG, M.:
     Blutuntersuchungen beim Morbus coe-
     ruleus, Helv. pædiat. acta, 4, 267, 1949;
     Ibid., 5, 159, 172 and 185, 1950.

16. Rodes, C. B.: Cavernous Hemangiomas of the Lung With Secondary Polycythemia, J.A.M.A., *110*, 1914, 1938.

17. Rogers, L.: Extensive Atheroma and Dilatation of the Pulmonary Arteries, Quart. J. Med., *2*, 1, 1908.

17a.Schilling, R. F.: Failure to Produce Polycythemia in Man, Dog and Rabbit by Daily Administration of Ephedrine Sulfate, Am. J. Physiol., *167*, 59, 1951.

17b.Schmid, R. and Gilbertsen, A. S.: Fundamental Observations on the Production of Compensatory Polycythemia in a Case of Patent Ductus Arteriosus with Reversed Blood Flow, Blood, *10*, 247, 1955.

18. Silberman, R.: Ein Beitrag zur Polyzythämie bei Phosphorvergiftung, Prager med. Wchnschr., *32*, 167, 1907.

18a.Singmaster, L.: Uterine Fibroids Associated with Polycythemia, J. A. M. A., *163*, 36, 1957.

18b.Starr, G. F., Stroebel, C. F., Jr. and Kearns, T. P.: Polycythemia with Papilledema and Infratentorial Vascular Tumors, Ann. Int. Med., *48*, 978, 1958.

19. Talbott, J. H. and Dill, D. B.: Clinical Observations at High Altitude, Am. J. M. Sc., *192*, 626, 1936.

20. Todtenhaupt, W.: Kongenitaler Herzfehler und Erythrocytose, Deutsch. Arch. klin. Med., *154*, 79, 1927.

21. Viault, F.: Sur l'âugmentation considérable du nombre des globules rouges dans le sang chez les habitants des hautes plateaux de l'Amerique du Sud, Compt. rend. Acad. sc., *111*, 917, 1890.

23. Warthin, A. S.: A Case of Ayerza's Disease, Osler Memorial, *2*, 1042, 1919.

23a.Ways, P., et al.: Polycythemia and Histologically Proven Renal Disease, Arch. Int. Med., *107*, 154, 1961.

24. Weber, F. P.: *Polycythæmia, Erythrocytosis and Erythræmia (Vaquez-Osler Disease)*, London, Lewis, 1921.

25. Weil, E.: Note sur les organes hématopoiétiques et l'hématopoièse dans la cyanose congénitale, Compt. rend. Soc. biol., *53*, 713, 1901.

25a.Yater, W. M., Finnegan, J. and Giffin, H. M.: Pulmonary Arteriovenous Fistula (Varix), J.A.M.A., *141*, 581, 1949.

25b.Yü, T. F., Wasserman, L. R., Benedict, J. D., Bien, E. J., Gutman, A. B. and Stetten, D., Jr., A Simultaneous Study of Glycine-N[15] Incorporation into Uric Acid and Heme, and of Fe[59] Utilization, in a Case of Gout Associated with Polycythemia Secondary to Congenital Heart Disease, Am. J. Med., *15*, 845, 1953.

26. Zuntz, N., Loewy, A., Mueller, F. and

Casperi, W.: Hökenklima und Bergswanderungen, Berlin, 1906.

Erythremia

27. Altschule, M. D., Volk, M. C. and Henstell, H.: Cardiac and Respiratory Function at Rest in Patients With Uncomplicated Polycythemia Vera, Am. J. M. Sc., *200*, 478, 1940.

28. Arnstein, A.: Ein Fall von Polycythaemie ohne Blutdruckerhöhung und ohne Milztumor, Mitt. Gesellsch. inn. Med. u. Kinderh., *11*, 209, 1912.

28a.Auerback, M. L., Wolff, J. A. and Mettier, S. R.: Benign Familial Polycythemia in Childhood, Pediatrics, *21*, 54, 1958.

28b.Aufses, A. H., Jr.: Bleeding Varices Associated with Hematologic Disorders, A.M. A. Arch. Surg., *80*, 655, 1960.

29. Avery, H.: A Pernicious Type of Anemia Following Erythremia, Lancet, *1*, 342, 1930.

30. Baráth, E. and Fülöp, J.: Investigations on Pathogenic Connection of Pernicious Anemia and Splenomegalic Polycythemia, Ztschr. klin. Med., *129*, 172, 1935.

30a.Baxter, D. L. and Lockwood, J. H.: Acne Urticata Polycythemia, A. M. A. Arch. Dermat., *78*, 325, 1958.

31. Berk, L., Burchenal, J. H., Wood, T. and Castle, W. B.: Oxygen Saturation of Sternal Marrow Blood with Special Reference to Pathogenesis of Polycythemia Vera, Proc. Soc. Exper. Biol. & Med., *69*, 316, 1948.

31a.Berlin, N. I., Lawrence, J. H. and Gartland, J.: Blood Volume in Polycythemia as Determined by P[32] Labeled Red Blood Cells, Am. J. Med., *9*, 747, 1950.

31b.Bethard, W. F., Block, M. H. and Robson, M.: Coexistent Chronic Lymphatic Leukemia and Polycythemia Vera, Blood, *8*, 934, 1953.

31c.Björkman, S. E., Laurell, C. B. and Nilsson, I.-M.: Serum Proteins and Fibrinolysis in Polycythemia Vera, Scandinav. J. Clin. & Lab. Invest., *8*, 304, 1956.

32. Bliss, T. L.: Basal Metabolism in Polycythemia Vera, Ann. Int. Med., *2*, 1155, 1929.

33. Blumenthal, R.: Un cas de polycythémie myélognèe, Bull. Acad. roy. méd. belg., s. 4, *19*, 775, 1905.

34. Blumgart, H. L., Gargill, S. L. and Gilligan, D. R.: Studies on the Velocity of Blood Flow: XV. The Velocity of Blood Flow and Other Aspects of the Circulation in Patients With "Primary" and Secondary Anemia and in Two Patients With Polycythemia Vera, J. Clin. Invest., *9*, 679, 1930.

35. BODANSKY, M., MARR, W. L. and BRINDLEY, P.: An Experimental Study of the Action of Phenylhydrazine Hydrochloride and Acetylphenylhydrazine (Pyrodin), With Reference to Their Use in the Treatment of Polycythemia Vera, Am. J. Clin. Path., 2, 391, 1932.

36. BÖTTNER, A.: Zur Spinaldruckerhöhung und zur Einteilung der echten Polycythämie-formen mit Berücksichtigung ihrer Augenhintergrundsveränderungen, Deutsch. Arch. klin. Med., 132, 1, 1920.

37. BOWDLER, A. J. and TULLETT, G. L.: Urticaria Pigmentosa and Polycythaemia Vera, Brit. M. J., 1, 396, 1960.

38. BOYD, W.: The Relationship of Polycythemia to Duodenal Ulcer, Am. J. M. Sc., 187, 589, 1934.

38a. BRIEGER, H. and FORSCHBACH, J.: Zur Pathologie der Erythrämie, Klin. Wchnschr., 1, 845, 1922.

39. BROWN, G. E. and GIFFIN, H. Z.: Peripheral Arterial Disease in Polycythemia Vera, Arch. Int. Med., 46, 705, 1930.

39a. BRUMPT, L. C. and GUJAR, B. J.: Treatment of Polycythemia by Artificial Infection with Ancylostoma Duodenale, Indian Med. Gazette (Calcutta), 83, 166, 1948.

40. BUCKY, G. and FREUND, E.: Die Beeinflussung der Polycythaemia rubra durch Grenzstrahlen, München. med. Wchnschr., 75, 1405, 1928.

40a. CALABRESI, P. and MEYER, O. O.: Polycythemia Vera, Ann. Int. Med., 50, 1182, 1959.

41. CARPENTER, G.: Failure to Control Polycythemia Rubra Vera With Lipocaic and Choline, Am. J. M. Sc., 200, 462, 1940.

42. CASSELS, D. E. and MORSE, M.: The Arterial Blood Gases, the Oxygen Dissociation Curve, and the Acid-Base Balance in Polycythemia Vera, J. Clin. Invest., 32, 52, 1953.

43. CAUTLEY, E.: Chronic Polycythemia, Lancet, 1, 1204, 1908.

43a. CRUZ, W. O.: Acetylphenylhydrazine Anemia, Am. J. M. Sc., 202, 781, 1941; Ibid., 203, 848, 1942.

44. DAMESHEK, W. and HENSTELL, H. H.: The Diagnosis of Polycythemia, Ann. Int. Med., 13, 1360, 1940.

44a. DAMON, A. and HOLUB, D. A.: Host Factors in Polycythemia Vera, Ann. Int. Med., 49, 43, 1958.

45. DANIELS, L. P. and v. BUCHEM, F. S. P.: Uber einen Fall von Polycythaemia vera welche in eine myeloische Leukämie überging, Klin. Wchnschr., 7, 121, 1928.

46. DELHOUGNE, F., GOTSCHLICH, E. and FRO-

BOESE: Über Polyzythämie mit Ausgang in Anämie, Deutsch. Arch. klin. Med., 160, 257, 1928.

47. DETRE, L.: Ein in Panmyelophthisis übergegangener Fall von Polycythämie rubra, Med. Klin., 22, 1297, 1926.

47a. ELLISON, R. R., GINSBERG, V. and WATSON, J.: Triethylene Melamine in Polycythemia Vera, Cancer, 6, 327, 1953.

48. ELSCHNIG, A. and NONNENBRUCH, W.: Polycythämie und Embolie der Arteria centralis retinae, Klin. Monatsbl. f. Augenh., 88, 433, 1932.

49. ENGELKING, E.: Über familiäre Polyzythämie und die dabei beobachteten Augenveränderungen, Klin. Monatsbl. f. Augenh., 64, 645, 1920.

49a. FISHER, JUNE M., BEDELL, G. N. and SEEBOHM, P. M.: Differentiation of Polycythemia Vera and Secondary Polycythemia by Arterial Oxygen Saturation and Pulmonary Function Tests, J. Lab. & Clin. Med., 50, 455, 1957.

49b. FITZGERALD, O., FITZGERALD, P., CANTWELL, D. and MEHIGAN, J. A.: Diagnosis and Treatment of the Budd-Chiari Syndrome in Polycythaemia Vera, Brit. M. J., 2, 1343, 1956.

50. FORKNER, C. E., SCOTT, I. F. McN. and WU, S. C.: Treatment of Polycythemia Vera (Erythremia) With Solution of Potassium Arsenite, Arch. Int. Med., 51, 616, 1933.

51. FREUND, H.: Polyzythämie mit Ausgang in perniziöse Anämie, München. med. Wchnschr., 66, 84, 1919.

51a. FRIEDELL, H. L. and STORAASLI, J. P.: The Therapeutic Application of Radioactive Phosphorus with Special Reference to the Treatment of Primary Polycythemia and Chronic Myeloid Leukemia, J. Clin. Invest., 28, 1308, 1949.

51b. FROST, J. W., JONES, R., JR. and JONSSON, U.: Pyrimethamine in the Treatment of Polycythemia Vera, South. M. J., 51, 1260, 1958.

52. FUTCHER, T. B.: Clinical Aspects of Erythremia, Boston Med. & Surg. J., 191, 304, 1924.

53. GAISBÖCK, F.: Die Polyzythämie, Ergebn. inn. Med. u. Kinderh., 21, 210, 1922.

54. GANS, O.: Über spezifische Hautveränderungen bei Erythrämie, Virchows Arch., 263, 565, 1927.

55. GHIRON, M.: Considerazioni sopra un caso di eritro-leucemia, Fol. hæmat., 22, 135, 1922.

57. GIFFIN, H. Z. and ALLEN, E. V.: Experiments With Phenylhydrazine: I. Studies on the Blood, Ann. Int. Med., 1, 655, 1927–28.

58. ———— Control and Complete Remission

of Polycythemia Vera Following the Prolonged Administration of Phenylhydrazin
Hydrochloride, Am. J. M. Sc., *185*, 1, 1933.

59. GIFFIN, H. Z. and CONNER, H. M.: The Untoward Effects of Treatment by Phenylhydrazine Hydrochloride, J.A.M.A., *92*,
1505, 1929.

60. GROEN, J. and GODFRIED, E. G.: The Occurrence of Normoblasts in the Peripheral
Blood in Congestive Heart Failure, Blood,
3, 1445, 1948.

61. GÜLKE, H.: Uber Polycythämia megalosplenica hypertonica, Fol. hæmat., *38*,
396, 1929.

63. GUGGENHEIMER, H.: Röntgentherapie der
Polyzythämie, Ztschr. physik. u. diätät.
Therap., *22*, 233, 1919.

64. GUTZEIT, K.: Zur Pathologie und Genese der
Polycythaemia rubra, Deutsch Arch. klin.
Med., *141*, 30, 1923.

66. HALBERTSMA, I.: Polycythemia in Childhood:
With Report of a Case in a Boy, Six Years
Old, With Tower Head, Am. J. Dis. Child.,
46, 1356, 1933.

67. HARROP, G. A., JR.: Polycythemia, Medicine,
7, 291, 1928.

68. HARROP, G. A., JR. and HEATH, E. H.: Pulmonary Gas Diffusion in Polycythemia
Vera, J. Clin. Invest., *4*, 53, 1927.

69. HECHT, H. H. and SAMUELS, A. J.: Observations on the Oxygen Content of Sternal
Bone Marrow with Reference to Polycythemic States, Fed. Proc., *11*, 68, 1952.

70. HERRNHEISER, G.: Polycythämie rubra vera,
Deutsch. Arch. klin. Med., *130*, 315, 1919.

71. HERXHEIMER, G.: Myeloblastic Leukemia
Following Erythremia, Klin. Wchnschr.,
1, 1458, 1913.

73. HIRSCHFELD, H.: Zur Frage der Beziehungen
zwischen Erythrämie und Leukämie, Fol.
hæmat., *26*, 108, 1920.

74. HITZENBERGER, K.: Die Rolle des Magens
in der Blutbildung, Klin. Wchnschr., *13*,
1345, 1934.

75. HOWELL, W. H. and DONAHUE, D. D.: The
Production of Blood Platelets in the Lungs,
J. Exper. Med., *65*, 177, 1937.

75a. HUFF, R. L., HENNESSY, T. G., AUSTIN, R. E.,
GARCIA, J. F., ROBERTS, B. M. and LAW-
RENCE, J. H.: Plasma and Red Cell Iron
Turnover in Normal Subjects and in
Patients Having Various Hematopoietic
Disorders, J. Clin. Invest., *29*, 1041, 1950;
Cardiologia, *21*, 337, 1952.

76. ISAACS, R.: Pathologic Physiology of Polycythemia Vera, Arch. Int. Med., *31*, 289,
1923.

78. JACOBI, A.: Polycythämie und Mesenterial-
venenthrombose; ihre Beziehungen zu

Unfallverletzungen, Mitt. Grenzgeb. Med.
u. Chir., *41*, 555, 1928–30.

79. JUNG, K.: Über einen Fall von Polycythämie
mit Ausgang in Myeloblastenleukämie,
Zentralbl. Herz.- u. Gefässkr., *7*, 118, 1915.

80. KÄHLER, H.: Ein Beitrag zur Milzbehand-
lung der Erythrämien, Deutsch. Arch.
klin. Med., *167*, 105, 1930.

81. KANDEL, E. V. and LEROY, G. V.: Note on
the Lack of Hemoregulatory Effect of
Ascorbic Acid on Patients With Polycythemia Vera, Am. J. M. Sc., *196*, 392,
1938.

82. KENNEDY, A. M.: Untoward Effect of Phenylhydrazine Hydrochloride in Polycythæmia, Brit. M. J., *1*, 659, 1934.

83. v. KORANYI, A.: Die Beeinflussung der
Leukämie durch Benzol, Klin. Wchnschr.,
49, 1357, 1912.

83a. KOTNER, L. M. and TRITT, J. H.: Chorea
Complicating Polycythemia Vera, Ann.
Int. Med., *17*, 544, 1942.

84. KRATZEISEN, E.: Polycythämie und Pforta-
derthrombose, Virchows Arch., *244*, 467,
1923.

84a. LAWRENCE, J. H.: The Control of Polycythemia by Marrow Inhibition, J.A.M.A.,
141, 13, 1949.

84b. LAWRENCE, J. H., BERLIN, N. I. and HUFF,
R. L.: The Nature and Treatment of
Polycythemia, Medicine, *32*, 323, 1953;
Am. J. M. Sc., *233*, 268, 1957.

85. LOMMEL, F.: Uber Polyzythämie, Deutsch.
Arch. klin. Med., *92*, 83, 1908.

85a. LONDON, I. M., SHEMIN, D., WEST, R. and
RITTENBERG, D.: Heme Synthesis and Red
Blood Cell Dynamics in Normal Humans
and in Subjects With Polycythemia Vera,
Sickle Cell Anemia, and Pernicious Ane-
mia, J. Biol. Chem., *179*, 463, 1949.

86. LONG, P. H.: Experimental Anemia Produced by Phenylhydrazine Derivatives,
J. Clin. Invest., *2*, 239, 1926.

86a. LOUIS, J.: Treatment of Polycythemia Vera
with Busulfan (Myleran), J. A. M. A.,
168, 1880, 1958.

87. LUCAS, W. S.: Erythremia or Polycythemia
With Chronic Cyanosis and Splenomegaly,
Arch. Int. Med., *10*, 597, 1912.

88. LÜDIN, M.: Zur Kenntnis der Symptomatologie und Therapie der primären Polycythämie, Ztschr. klin. Med., *84*, 460,
1917.

90. MACKAY, W.: Observations on the Treat-
ment of Two Cases of Polycythemia Vera
With Phenylhydrazine Hydrochloride,
Lancet, *1*, 762, 1929.

91. MACKENZIE, D. W.: Perirenal Hematoma

Primary With Polycythemia, J. Urol., *23*, 535, 1930.

92. MAKAREVICZ, O. B.: A Case of Polyglobulia Turning Into Anemia, Klin. Med., *7*, 1054, 1929.

92a. MARLOW, A. A. and FAIRBANKS, V. F.: Polycythemia Vera in an Eleven-Year Old Girl, New England J. Med., *263*, 950, 1960.

93. McCANCE, R. A. and WIDDOWSON, E. M.: The Fate of the Elements Removed from the Blood-stream During the Treatment of Polycythæmia by Acetylphenylhydrazine, Quart. J. Med., *6*, 277, 1937.

93a. MENDLOWITZ, M.: The Effect of Anemia and Polycythemia on Digital Intravascular Blood Viscosity, J. Clin. Invest., *27*, 565, 1948.

93b. MERSKEY, C.: The Relationship Between Polycythemia Vera and Myeloid Leukæmia, Clin. Proc. J. Cape Town Post-Grad. M. A., *8*, 150, 1949.

95. MINOT, G. R. and BUCKMAN, T. E.: Erythremia (Polycythemia Rubra Vera), Am. J. M. Sc., *166*, 469, 1923.

97. MOSSE, M.: Polyglobulie und Lebererkrankung, Ztschr. klin. Med., *79*, 431, 1914.

97a. MYERSON, R. M. and FRUMIN, A. M.: Hyperkalemia Associated with the Myeloproliferative Disorder, Arch. Int. Med., *106*, 479, 1960.

98. NADLER, S. B. and COHN, I.: Familial Polycythemia, Am. J. M. Sc., *198*, 41, 1939.

99. NEWMAN, W., FELTMAN, J. A. and DEVLIN, B.: Pulmonary Function Studies in Polycythemia Vera, Am. J. Med., *11*, 706, 1951.

100. NORMAN, I. L. and ALLEN, E. V.: The Vascular Complications of Polycythemia, Am. Heart J., *13*, 257, 1937.

101. OERTING, H. and BRIGGS, J. F.: The Influence of Gastric Lavage on Familial and Non-familial Erythremia, Proc. Soc. Clin. Res., J.A.M.A., *104*, 250, 1935.

102. ORLOWSKI, W.: Contribution à l'étude de la "polycythemia rubra," Prog. méd., *10*, 117, 1912.

103. OSLER, W.: Chronic Cyanosis With Polycythemia and Enlarged Spleen; a New Clinical Entity, Am. J. M. Sc., *126*, 187, 1903.

104. ——— A Clinical Lecture on Erythræmia, Lancet, *1*, 143, 1908.

105. PACK, G. T. and CRAVER, L. F.: Radiation Therapy of Polycythemia Vera, Am. J. M. Sc., *180*, 609, 1930.

105a. PARKER, R. G. F.: Occlusion of the Hepatic Veins in Man, Medicine, *38*, 369, 1959.

106. PARRISIUS: Polycythaemia rubra vera mit myeloischer Leukämie, Klin. Wchnschr., *2*, 1482, 1923.

107. PASCHKIS, K. and DIAMANT, M.: Beiträge zur Pathologie der Erythrämie, zugleich I. Mitteilung über den urobilin Stoffwechsel, Deutsch. Arch. klin. Med., *169*, 180, 1930.

108. PEL, P. K.: Paroxysmale hämoglobinurie mit hyperglobulie, Abstr., Folia hæmat., *6*, 290, 1908.

109. PERLA, D. and BILLER, S. B.: Hemoblastic Sarcoma (Primitive Red Cell Type) Following Polycythemia Vera, Arch. Path., *27*, 902, 1939.

110. PICK, E. and KAZNELSON, P.: Über eine eigenartige Dermatose bei Polycythämie, Dermat. Wchnschr., p. 159, 1925; Abstr., Folia hæmat., *24*, 266, 1927.

111a. RATTO, O., BRISCOE, W. A., MORTON, J. W. and COMROE, JR., J. H.: Anoxemia Secondary to Polycythemia and Polycythemia Secondary to Anoxemia, Am. J. Med., *19*, 958, 1955.

112. REINHARD, E. H., MOORE, C. V., BIERBAUM, O. S. and MOORE, S.: Radioactive Phosphorus as a Therapeutic Agent, J. Lab. & Clin. Med., *31*, 107, 1946; J. Chron. Dis., *6*, 332, 1957.

113. RENCKI, R.: Weitere Beobachtungen über Polycythaemia rubra myelopathica (Polish), Abstr., Folia hæmat., *6*, 293, 1908.

114. REZNIKOFF, P., FOOT, N. C. and BETHEA, J. M.: Etiologic and Pathologic Factors in Polycythemia Vera, Am. J. M. Sc., *189*, 753, 1935.

115. ROSENFELD: Zur Behandlung der Polyzythämie, Klin. Wchnschr., *54*, 1050, 1917.

116. ROSENGART, J.: Milztumor und Hyperglobulie, Mitt. Grenzgeb. Med. u. Chir., *11*, 495, 1903.

117. ROSENTHAL, N. and BASSEN, F. A.: Course of Polycythemia, Arch. Int. Med., *62*, 903, 1938.

117a. ROSENTHAL, N. and ROSENTHAL, R. L.: Treatment of Polycythemia Vera with Triethylene Melamine, Arch. Int. Med., *90*, 379, 1952.

118. ROSIN, H.: Zur Lehre von der Erythrocytosis megalosplenica (Polycythämie; Polyglobulie mit Milztumor), Therap. Rundschau, *46*, 677, 1908.

119. ROTHMAN, H., STERN, J. and HOENE, P.: Influence of Excess Fat Diet on Red Blood Picture; Dietary Therapy of Polycythemia, Ztschr. klin. Med., *123*, 620, 1933.

121. SACHS, E.: Milztuberkulose bei Polycythaemia vera, Beitr. klin. Tuberk,. *69*, 699, 1928.

122. SCHMIDT, W.: Beitrag zur Pathologie und Therapie der Polyzythämie rubra, Med. Klin., *22*, 1758, 1926.

123. SCHNETZ, H.: Polycythaemia vera mit Aus-

gang in Agranulocytose und Thrombarteriitis pulmonalis, Folia hæmat., *57*, 110, 1937.

123a. SCHWARTZ, B. M. and STATS, D.: Oxygen Saturation of Sternal Marrow Blood in Polycythemia Vera, J. Clin. Invest., *28*, 736, 1949.

124. SGALITZER, M.: Röntgentotalbestrahlung bei Polycythaemia, Wien. klin. Wchnschr., *48*, 675, 1935.

125. SHELBURNE, S. A. and HANZAL, R. F.: The Endogenous Uric Acid Metabolism in Polycythemia Vera, J. Clin. Invest., *11*, 865, 1932.

126. SINGER, K.: Gibt es eine gastrogene Polyglobulie?, Klin. Wchnschr., *14*, 751, 1935.

127. SOHVAL, A. R.: Hepatic Complications in Polycythæmia Vera, Arch. Int. Med., *62*, 925, 1938.

128. SPODARO, A. and FORKNER, C. E.: Benign Familial Polycythemia, Arch. Int. Med., *52*, 593, 1933.

128a. SPURR, C. L., SMITH, T. R., BLOCK, M. and JACOBSON, L. O.: A Clinical Study of the Use of Nitrogen Mustard Therapy in Polycythemia Vera, J. Lab. & Clin. Med., *35*, 252, 1950.

129. STENSTROM, K. W., HALLOCK, P. H. and WATSON, C. J.: Negative Results of Irradiation Therapy of the Pylorus and Brunner's Gland Area in Patients With Polycythemia Vera, Am. J. M. Sc., *199*, 646 1940.

130. STEPHENS, D. J. and KALTREIDER, N. L.: The Therapeutic Use of Venesection in Polycythemia, Ann. Int. Med., *10*, 1565, 1937.

131. STONE, D. M. and WOODMAN, D.: Polycythæmia Terminating in Leucoerythroblastic Anæmia, J. Path. & Bact., *47*, 327, 1938.

132. STROEBEL, C. F., HALL, B. E. and PEASE, G. L.: Evaluation of Radiophosphorus Therapy in Primary Polycythemia, J. A. M. A., *146*, 1301, 1951; Proc. Staff Meet., Mayo Clin., *29*, 1, 1954.

132a. SZUR, L., LEWIS, S. M. and GOOLDEN, A. W. G.: Polycythaemia Vera and Its Treatment with Radioactive Phosphorus, Quart. J. Med., *28*, 397, 1959.

132b. TALBOTT, J. H.: Gout and Blood Dyscrasias, Medicine, *38*, 173, 1959.

133. TINNEY, W. S., HALL, B. E. and GIFFIN, H. Z.: Polycythemia Vera, Proc. Staff Meet. Mayo Clin., *18*, 227, 1943; *Ibid.*, *20*, 49 and 306, 1945.

134. TÜRK, W.: Beiträge zur Kenntnis des symptomenbildes Polyzythämie mit Milztumor und Zyanose, Wein klin. Wchnschr., *17*, 153, 1904.

134a. VAQUEZ, H.: Sur une forme spéciale de cyanose s'accompanant d'hyperglobulie excessive et persitente, Compt. rend. Soc. de biol., *4*, 384, 1892, and suppl. note, Bull. et mém. Soc. méd. hôp. Paris, 3 ser., *12*, 60, 1895.

135. VIDEBAEK, A.: Polycythemia Vera, Acta med. scandinav., *138*, 179, 1950.

135a. WALD, N., HOSHINO, T. and SEARS, MARY E.: Therapy of Polycythemia Vera with Myleran, Blood, *13*, 757, 1958.

135b. DE WARDENER, H. E., MCSWINEY, R. R. and MILES, B. E.: Renal Hæmodynamics in Primary Polycythæmia, Lancet, *2*, 204, 1951.

135c. WASSERMAN, L. R., DOBSON, R. L. and LAWRENCE, J. H.: Blood Oxygen Studies in Patients with Polycythemia and in Normal Subjects, J. Clin. Invest., *28*, 60, 1949.

135d. WASSERMAN, L. R., LAWRENCE, J. H., BERLIN, N. I., DOBSON, R. L. and ESTREN, S.: The Bone Marrow Picture in Polycythemia Vera before and after Treatment with Radioactive Phosphorus, Acta med. scandinav., *143*, 442, 1952.

136. WIELAND, W.: Weitere Untersuchungen über Polycythæmia vera im Kindesalter, Ztschr. Kinderh., *53*, 703, 1932.

137. WILBUR, D. L. and OCHSNER, H. C.: The Association of Polycythemia Vera and Peptic Ulcer, Ann. Int. Med., *8*, 1667, 1935.

138. WILKINSON, J. F. and KLEIN, L.: The Hæmatopoietic Activity of the Normal and the Abnormal Human Liver, Quart. J. Med., *27*, 341, 1934.

138a. WINTROBE, M. M.: Osler's Chronic Cyanotic Polycythemia with Splenomegaly, Bull. Johns Hopkins Hosp., *85*, 75, 1949.

138b. WISEMAN, B. K., ROHN, R. J., BOURONCLE, B. A. and MYERS, W. G.: The Treatment of Polycythemia Vera With Radioactive Phosphorus, Ann. Int. Med., *34*, 311, 1951.

138c. YÜ, T. F. *et al.*: On the Biosynthesis of Uric Acid from Glycine-N^{15} in Primary and Secondary Polycythemia, Am. J. Med., *21*, 901, 1956.

139. ZADEK, I.: Die Polycythämien, Ergebn. ges. Med., *10*, 355, 1927.

140. ZIMMERMAN, O.: Zur Kazuistik der Erythrämie mit Übergang in Leukämie, Klin. Wchnschr., *13*, 696, 1934.

Chapter 17

The Purpuras

In THIS and the following chapter various types of abnormal bleeding will be considered. The *causes of hemorrhage* are very numerous, as Table 17–1 indicates. By far the most common cause of hemorrhage is that resulting from injury of large vessels by trauma or by erosion from pathological processes. Bleeding due to disturbances in coagulation is, comparatively speaking, rare, even though the list of disorders characterized by alterations in platelets or in the clotting process is a long one. The physiological aspects of platelets and coagulation were discussed in detail in chapter 5 (p. 276).

In this chapter the purpuras will be considered. This includes a wide variety of conditions which have one symptom in common; namely, hemorrhage in the skin, mucous membranes, internal organs or other tissues. Their etiology and pathogenesis, vary widely and their manifestations differ considerably: from purpura with striking and characteristic changes in the blood, to conditions with no demonstrable abnormalities in the blood but associated with a variety of clinical symptoms, including erythema, joint manifestations and abdominal complaints.

It is to be expected that classification of such a variety of conditions would not be entirely satisfactory. It is convenient to classify the purpuras as thrombocytopenic and non-thrombocytopenic

(Table 17–2). Sometimes, however, etiological factors which at one time are associated with thrombocytopenia, may at other times accompany hemorrhage in the absence of platelet reduction. Again, hemorrhage is not always closely correlated with the degree of platelet reduction. The causes and fundamental nature of purpura are only gradually being elucidated.

PURPURA HEMORRHAGICA

Synonyms.—Essential, primary, or idiopathic thrombocytopenic[102] purpura, Werlhof's disease, morbus maculosus werlhofi, thrombocytolytic purpura,[53] hemogenia, hemogenic syndrome.[92]

Definition.—This is a condition of unknown etiology which is characterized clinically by petechiae or ecchymoses in the skin as well as by hemorrhage from mucous membranes and into various tissues. The onset and course of the disease are variable and may be marked by spontaneous remissions and relapses. The skin lesions are not associated with erythema, swelling or inflammation. The platelet count is reduced, the bleeding time is prolonged, the clot non-retractile and the tourniquet test positive, whereas the coagulation time is essentially normal. There is no anemia except that which can be attributed to blood loss. Leukocytic changes are insignificant.

Table 17–1—Causes of Hemorrhage

I. Vascular Abnormalities:
  A. Injury of large vessels by trauma or by erosion from pathologic processes
  B. Hereditary hemorrhagic telangiectasia
  C. Nonthrombocytopenic purpuras (Table 17–2):
    1. Allergic purpuras (Henoch-Schönlein)
    2. Symptomatic nonthrombocytopenic purpuras (infections, chemical and animal agents, avitaminosis, certain chronic diseases)
    3. Hereditary familial purpura simplex
    4. Miscellaneous: mechanical purpura, orthostatic purpura, purpura senilis, purpura cachectica

II. Extravascular and Miscellaneous Abnormalities:
  A. Atrophy of subcutaneous tissues (purpura senilis, purpura cachectica)
  B. Fragility and hyperlaxity of skin (Cushing's syndrome, Ehlers-Danlos syndrome, epidermolysis bullosa)
  C. Purpura fulminans
  D. Purpura hyperglobulinemica
  E. Purpura simplex, vicarious bleeding, "autoerythrocyte sensitization"

III. Intravascular Abnormalities
  A. Platelet abnormalities
    1. Quantitative deficiencies: symptomatic thrombocytopenic purpuras and idiopathic (Table 17–2)
    2. Qualitative abnormalities:
      a. with prolonged bleeding time: von Willebrand's disease, vascular hemophilia
      b. other thrombocytopathies, congenital and acquired
      c. with defective clot retraction: Glanzmann's thrombasthenia
      d. hemorrhagic thrombocythemia
  B. Coagulation defects
    1. Deficiency of factor VIII (AHG, AHF, hemophilia A)
    2. Deficiency of factor IX (PTC, Christmas disease, hemophilia B)
    3. Deficiency of PTA
    4. Congenital "hypoprothrombinemias"
      a. congenital hypoprothrombinemia
      b. congenital factor V deficiency (parahemophilia)
      c. congenital factor VII (SPCA) deficiency (hypoproconvertinemia)
      d. congenital factor X (Stuart-Prower) deficiency
    5. Acquired "hypoprothrombinemias"
      a. newborn (hemorrhagic disease of the newborn)
      b. vitamin K deficiency (obstructive jaundice, biliary fistula, impaired intestinal absorption, impaired bacterial growth in bowel)
      c. miscellaneous diseases (liver disease, leukemia, etc.)
      d. anticoagulant drugs (coumarin compounds, etc.)
    6. Hypofibrinogenemias
      a. congenital
      b. Acquired. Fibrinolytic purpuras (complications of pregnancy [abruptio placentae, retention of dead fetus, amniotic fluid emboli], pulmonary manipulation, neoplastic diseases, disorders of bone marrow, severe liver damage, shock)
    7. Circulating anticoagulants
      a. Drug therapy (coumarin and related compounds, heparin)
      b. In association with coagulation defects (factors VIII and IX)
      c. Idiopathic, and in association with pregnancy and various diseases

Table 17-2—Classification of Purpura

I. Thrombocytopenic purpura
 A. Idiopathic thrombocytopenic purpura (ITP) or purpura hemorrhagica
 B. Symptomatic thrombocytopenic purpura
  1. Chemical, physical, vegetable and animal agents
   a. Chemical (1) myelosuppressive agents: nitrogen mustards, TEM, busulfan, urethane, anti-metabolites, benzene
     (2) agents which in therapeutic doses produce purpura mainly because of individual sensitivity: organic arsenicals, sulfonamides, "Sedormid," quinidine, quinine, chlorothiazide (Diuril), hydrochlorothiazide, gold salts, butobarbitone; and possibly also acetazolamide (Diamox), chloramphenicol, penicillin, chlorophenothane (DDT), meprobamate (Equanil, Miltown), stibophen, oxytetracycline, para-aminosalicylic acid, streptomycin, phenylbutazone, antipyrine, sodium salicylate, tridione, meparfynol, phenobarbital, allyl-isopropylbarbituric acid, thiourea, dinitrophenol, digitoxin, mercurials, potassium iodide, bismuth, ergot, organic hair dyes, estrogens, tolbutamide (Orinase), chlorpropamide (Diabenese).
   b. Physical—ionizing radiation (X-rays, radioactive substances); heat stroke
   c. Vegetable—foods (?), orris root (?)
   d. Animal—snake venoms, insect bites, pertussis vaccine, extensive burns
  2. Disorders involving the hemopoietic system
   a. Leukemias: acute or late stages of chronic
   b. Anemias: aplastic (idiopathic or due to various agents); myelophthisic (tumors in bone marrow, myelosclerosis); acquired hemolytic anemias of immune body type; pernicious anemia
   c. Disorders involving the spleen: congestive splenomegaly, Gaucher's disease, Felty's syndrome, sarcoidosis, disseminated lupus erythematosus, etc.
   d. Thrombotic (thrombohemolytic) thrombocytopenic purpura
  3. Infections: occasionally in septicemias, subacute bacterial endocarditis, infectious mononucleosis, various exanthemata, etc.
  4. Hemangio-endothelioma
  5. Miscellaneous conditions (p. 832), including massive blood transfusions
II. Nonthrombocytopenic purpuras
 A. Allergic purpura: purpuras of Henoch and Schönlein, erythemas of Osler
 B. Symptomatic purpura:
  1. Infections: subacute bacterial endocarditis, meningococcemia, staphylococcemia, typhoid fever, rheumatic fever, scarlet fever, smallpox, measles, diphtheria, Rocky mountain spotted fever
  2. Chemical and animal agents: iodides, belladonna, atropine, quinine, procaine penicillin, bismuth, mercury, copaiba, phenacetin, salicylic acid, merbaphen, chloral hydrate and other hypnotics; snake venoms
  3. Avitaminosis: scurvy
  4. Certain skin diseases: Ehlers-Danlos syndrome, annular telangiectatic purpura, etc.
  5. Chronic diseases: renal, cardiac, hepatic; hemochromatosis, Cushing's syndrome, polycythemia vera; generalized amyloidosis, blood-borne carcinoma emboli
  6. Various forms of dysglobulinemia: multiple myeloma, cryoglobulinemia, hyperglobulinemia, macroglobulinemia; purpura hyperglobulinemica
 C. Purpuric disorders associated with qualitative abnormalities of platelets. Thrombocytopathic purpuras
  1. Prolonged bleeding time: von Willebrand's disease. Constitutional thrombopathy.
  2. Other thrombocytopathies, congenital and acquired.
  3. Defective clot retraction. Glanzmann's thrombasthenia
  4. Unclassified varieties
 D. Purpura associated with increased capillary fragility
  1. Hereditary familial purpura simplex
  2. Unclassified varieties
 E. Purpura associated with increased platelets. Hemorrhagic thrombocythemia
 F. Miscellaneous forms of purpura
  1. Purpura simplex, purpura senilis, purpura cachectica, mechanical purpura, orthostatic purpura
  2. Purpura fulminans
  3. Purpura in women. Vicarious bleeding. Autoerythrocyte sensitization

(818)

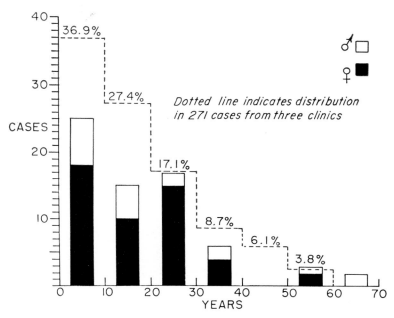

AGE AND SEX DISTRIBUTION OF 66 CASES OF I T P

FIG. 17–1.—Age and sex distribution of 66 cases of idiopathic thrombocytopenic purpura in Salt Lake City, compared with age incidence in 271 cases from New York,[15] Philadelphia[21] and Baltimore.[116]

History.[49]—Purpuric manifestations in association with pestilential fevers were described by Hippocrates and later writers, but it was not until the sixteenth century (Lusitanus) and the early part of the seventeenth century (La Riviere) that the presence of purpuric phenomena in the absence of fever was recognized. Werlhof in 1735 distinguished "morbus maculosus hemorrhagicus" as a separate entity and Willan in 1808 classified purpura under the headings (1) simplex, (2) haemorrhagica, (3) urticans and (4) contagiosa, thus separating the types later described by Schönlein (1829) and Henoch (1868) and now known by their names. The marked diminution in "hematoblasts" (platelets) in purpura hemorrhagica was recognized by Krauss (1883) and by Denys (1887), while Hayem (1895) noted the non-retractility of the blood clot. Duke (1912) demonstrated the prolonged bleeding time. The capillary fragility was observed by writers in different countries ("le signe du lacet" [Weil], Grocco-Frugoni's sign, Rumpel-Leede phenomenon, Hess capillary resistance test). Splenectomy was first performed in 1916 at the suggestion of Kaznelson who, at the time, was still a medical student.

Etiological Factors.—Purpura hemorrhagica occurs most frequently in *children and young adults.* In a series of 271 cases, which includes cases studied by others,[15,21] as well as ourselves,[116] the disease appeared before the age of twenty-one in 64.3 per cent (Fig. 17–1). In a summary of 737 cases reported in the literature[67a] 45 per cent of the patients were found to be fifteen years of age and younger. Subsequent experiences have been similar.[97c]

In childhood, purpura is most frequent between the ages of two and eight years[77c] but, in rare instances, it may occur in the

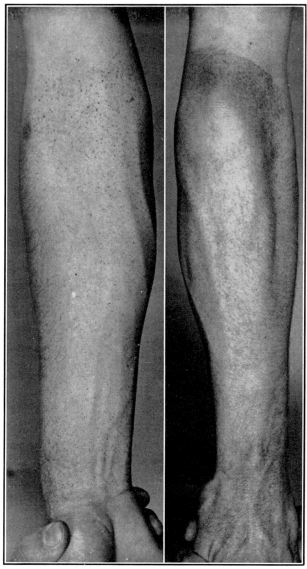

Fig. 17–2.—Strongly positive tourniquet test in a case of chronic purpura hemorrhagica. Platelet count 40,000 per c.mm., bleeding time forty-two minutes. Note that there are few petechiae in the area compressed by the blood pressure cuff

first year of life.[108] In three cases of the writer the ages of onset were seven, ten and eleven months, respectively. Purpura in the newborn will be discussed later (p. 825).

The condition is uncommon late in life. No more than 10 per cent of cases begin past the age of forty.

It is well recognized that purpura hemorrhagica occurs more frequently in *females* than males.[116] The ratio in different series has ranged from 4:3[86b] to 2:1.[107c] This sex difference is manifest chiefly after puberty. In a survey of 737 cases the ratio of females to males was 3.7:1 in those sixteen years of age and older, whereas it was only 1.3:1 below this age.[67a]

A *family history* of ready bruising, frequent epistaxes or other forms of bleeding is not unusual.[43c,86b] This was the case in 13 of our Baltimore series of 62 cases[116] and in 4 out of 41 cases in another series[104] but the significance of such a history is uncertain since familial thrombocytopenia has not been demonstrated.

Purpura hemorrhagica of the idiopathic type seems to be uncommon among Negroes.[116] The condition, thus, has suggestive constitutional manifestations: onset in early life, occasional family history and predominance in the white race. However, there is no clearly defined, sex-linked, inherited trait such as is found in hemophilia.

Symptomatology.—The onset of this disorder may be very sudden and without warning. This is especially common in children. In other cases, there is a history of ready bruising or epistaxis over a variable period of time. It is not unusual for the illness to appear following an acute upper respiratory infection.

Purpuric lesions[80] of the **skin** are the most common symptoms. These are minute, red, hemorrhages which range in size from that of a pinpoint to that of a pinhead (Fig. 17–2). Ecchymoses, larger purple areas, and even suffusions and hematomata may occur. Similar lesions may be found in the mucous membranes, especially in those of the nose and mouth. Sometimes they may occur in the absence of any noteworthy evidence of hemorrhage in the skin. Epistaxis and bleeding of the gums are frequent complaints.

Hemorrhagic bullae (blood-filled vesicles) inside the mouth and on other mucous surfaces, are particularly common in a form of acute thrombocytopenic purpura of unknown etiology observed in Africa and known as **onyalai.**[107a] With the exception of this manifestation, a possibly shorter course and tendency to affect young adult males as well as children, this form of purpura does not differ in the Bantu as compared with the purpura hemorrhagica of Europeans.[71a]

Genito-urinary Tract. — The genito-urinary tract is a frequent site of bleeding. Uterine bleeding may commence at the time expected for menstruation but differs from normal catamenia in its profuseness and duration. Menorrhagia may be the only symptom of disease. Purpura hemorrhagica may appear for the first time at puberty and may then be manifested by menorrhagia and irregularities in the cycle.[36] In other cases vaginal bleeding may appear before puberty as the initial symptom of this disorder. Again, a trivial injury or rupture of the hymen may be followed by profuse hemorrhage. Hematuria is also a common symptom. The blood may come from the renal pelvis, the bladder or the urethra. Bleeding into the kidney parenchyma is rare.

Melena or, less frequently, hematemesis indicates bleeding in the **gastrointestinal tract.** Colic and other acute abdominal symptoms, as in Henoch's purpura, or hemarthroses, as in hemophilia, are not found.

Frequently excessive bleeding following tooth extraction, tonsillectomy or other **operations or injuries** attract attention to a condition which may have been latent a long time. Subconjunctival or retinal hemorrhage is not unusual. Bleeding from the ear is rare. In severe cases there may be hemorrhage into the tongue, esophagus, larynx or vocal cords. In one of the writer's cases, bleeding occurred in the subcutaneous tissues of one side of the face and neck. In another, diaphragmatic hemorrhage developed and was the cause of death.

Nervous System. — Intracranial hemorrhage is the most serious complication. The hemorrhages are usually multiple and vary in size from petechiae to large extravasations of blood.[66] They may involve the brain, the spinal cord or the cerebrospinal meninges. Subdural hemorrhage, pachymeningitis and even hemorrhagic encephalitis have been described.

Physical Examination. — The findings on physical examination vary considerably. General glandular enlargement and bone tenderness are not found, and the spleen is palpable in only about a fifth of the cases. This organ, moreover, never extends more than one to two fingerbreadths below the costal margin. The physical signs, therefore, depend upon the extent and site of the bleeding. The condition of the patient may be very good and the color normal or, at the other extreme, there may be profound shock if bleeding has been profuse and rapid. Slight fever may be present if there is severe anemia or bleeding into the gastrointestinal tract. The pulse is usually rapid, from excitement if not because of shock. The body may be normal in appearance or it may be covered with petechiae and ecchymoses. These may be deep red, purple, brown or yellow in color, depending on their age. Swelling, erythema or urticarial lesions do not occur. When intracranial bleeding has taken place, the most frequent signs are those of hemiplegia or meningismus. Attention has been called to the occasional association of chronic leg ulcer with purpura hemorrhagica but this is rare.[118]

The Blood.—The characteristic finding is thrombocytopenia. The **platelets** may be totally absent. There is a rough correlation between the platelet count and the severity of bleeding, for the latter usually does not occur unless the platelets are fewer than 60,000 per c.mm. However, in chronic cases particularly, the platelet count may remain below this value for several months without spontaneous bleeding taking place.

Morphological changes in the platelets can often be seen: giant forms, minute platelets and deeply stained ones. Sometimes portions of megakaryocytes may be seen in the blood smear. Forms of purpura hemorrhagica (*thrombocytopathic purpura* characterized by unusual morphologic abnormalities in the platelets, will be discussed shortly (p. 847).

Prolongation of the **bleeding time** and failure of the blood clot to retract occur in conjunction with the thrombocytopenia and serve to corroborate the latter finding. The "bleeding time" may be as long as one hour or more. Rarely it is relatively short in spite of marked thrombocytopenia. The bleeding time may be markedly different in various parts of the body.[92]

Coagulation of the blood after it has been removed from the body ("coagulation time") occurs within the normal time interval but the **clot** fails to retract. Prothrombin consumption is greatly reduced[85b] but other tests of the coagulation process, including blood calcium, prothrombin time and fibrinogen are normal.[104]

The application of a tourniquet to the arm, or a suction cup to the skin (p. 299), is followed by the appearance of numerous petechiae (Fig. 17–2). The venom skin test gives a positive reaction.[80]

Anemia, if present, is proportional to the extent of blood loss and is usually normocytic. If the bleeding has been severe and long continued, it may be hypochromic and microcytic in type. Occasionally, if there has been a recent, severe hemorrhage, there may be macrocytic anemia. The characteristics of these types of anemia have been described already.

The **leukocytes** are usually normal in number and distribution; however, when there has been severe hemorrhage, slight leukocytosis with temporary "shift to the left" may occur. If the condition is of long standing, there may be relative

PLATE XIII

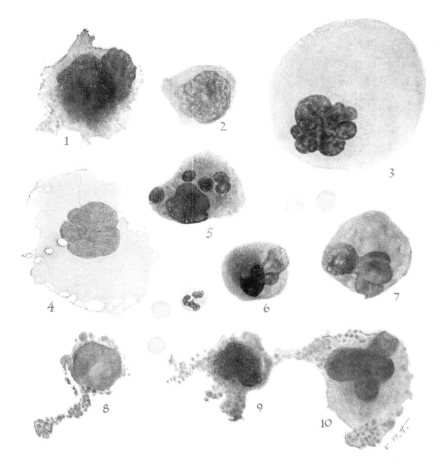

NORMAL MEGAKARYOCYTE AND MEGAKARYOCYTES FROM CASES OF IDIOPATHIC
THROMBOCYTOPENIC PURPURA (× 1200)

1. Mature megakaryocyte. Note granularity of cytoplasm, pseudopods, and the presence of platelets, which are situated chiefly at the periphery of the cell and in the pseudopods.

2. Megakaryoblast.

3. Mature megakaryocyte or intermediate form, from a case of chronic idiopathic thrombocytopenic purpura. There is well defined granularity of the cytoplasm, but no platelet formation.

4. Mature megakaryocyte from a case of chronic idiopathic thrombocytopenic purpura. There is almost complete lack of granularity and marked vacuolization and degeneration of the cytoplasm.

5. Intermediate form of megakaryocyte from an acute case of idiopathic thrombocytopenic purpura. Granule formation, without platelet development, is evident and there are some questionable nuclear bodies (asynchronism of development) in the cytoplasm.

6, 7. Lymphoid megakaryocytes from an acute case of idiopathic thrombocytopenic purpura. These are characterized by blue cytoplasm, lack of granularity, and lack of platelet formation.

8. Promegakaryocyte from an acute case of idiopathic thrombocytopenic purpura 24 hours after splenectomy. Nongranular platelet formation is present around the periphery of the cell, with a streamer containing a group of newly formed platelets.

9, 10. Intermediate form and mature megakaryocyte from an acute case of idiopathic thrombocytopenic purpura 48 hours after splenectomy. There is a striking productivity of granular (functioning) platelets, seemingly with the entire cytoplasm almost ready to break up into platelets. (*Dameshek and Miller, Blood, courtesy Grune & Stratton, Inc.*)

lymphocytosis and even slight leukopenia. A few cases of acute purpura have been described in which the leukocyte count ranged from 6000 to 16,000 and of these as many as 74 per cent were lymphocytes.[74] The latter resembled the type seen in infectious mononucleosis but adenopathy, splenomegaly and the characteristic agglutinins were lacking.[109]

Bone Marrow.—In idiopathic thrombocytopenic purpura the morphologic alterations in the bone marrow are limited to the megakaryocytes and platelets unless severe hemorrhage has taken place and anemia has developed, in which case some normoblastic hyperplasia may be observed. The leukocytic elements are essentially normal. The claim that a higher proportion of eosinophils in the bone marrow can be used as an index of good prognosis has not been confirmed.[20b,85]

Since Frank's description of the morphologic alterations in the megakaryocytes,[29] these structures have received considerable attention. It is clear that they are plentiful in number. "Young" forms of megakaryocytes, with single nuclei and relatively little or only moderately abundant cytoplasm and relatively few granules[85] as well as unusually small and exceptionally large megakaryocytes with non-lobulated nuclei, many vacuoles and few granules in the cytoplasm, have been described. In a detailed study of five cases of acute purpura hemorrhagica[18] between 366 and 734 megakaryocytes per million nucleated red cells were found as compared with not more than 300 in normal marrow. Furthermore, platelet production appeared to be greatly reduced, only 8 to 19 per cent of the megakaryocytes showing evidence of this as compared with an average of 68.6 per cent showing platelet production in normal marrow. Following splenectomy a striking increase in platelet production occurred; 69 to 85 per cent of the megakaryocytes appeared to be producing platelets. Similar findings were noted in 6 chronic cases of idiopathic thrombocytopenic purpura. They are illustrated in Plate XIII. In contrast, in cases of splenomegaly of nonleukemic origin, the megakaryocytes were somewhat increased but platelet formation appeared to be normal and, in "aplastic anemia," acute leukemia and other diseases involving the bone marrow, the megakaryocytes were conspicuously reduced although those remaining were of normal morphology.

With a few exceptions,[87] these observations have been confirmed. Phase contrast microscopy has yielded similar results.[84a] Nevertheless, examination of the bone marrow in this disorder is helpful mainly in ruling out other conditions with which idiopathic thrombocytopenic purpura may be confused rather than because of a morphologic picture which is that characteristic that it identifies the condition itself. As already indicated, bone marrow examination has not been found helpful in predicting the outcome.

In drug induced thrombocytopenias which depend on individual sensitivity, such as those caused by quinidine,[113] the bone marrow findings are similar to those described in idiopathic thrombocytopenic purpura.

Types and Clinical Course.—No student of this disorder will deny that its manifestations vary and that a rigid classification of cases is difficult to follow. There is, however, the type of case, most often seen in children, in which the onset is sudden, the manifestations mild or moderate in degree and the course limited to a few days, a few weeks or a few months.[11] There is no sex predilection. The platelets number 20,000 per c.mm. or even less but their morphology is normal.[106a] In children, particularly, eosinophilia and lymphocytosis may be present. There is no antecedent history of purpura but, in children especially, an infection may have preceded the onset; in adults, on

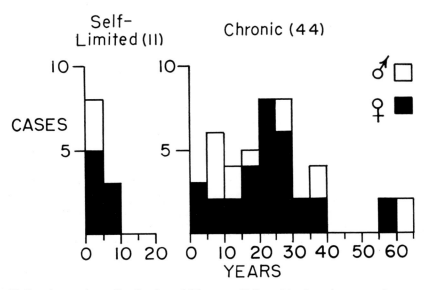

FIG. 17–3.—Age and sex distribution of 55 cases of idiopathic thrombocytopenic purpura.

the other hand, careful inquiry may reveal that some drug had been taken which previously had not been associated with any ill effects. It is rare that there is an accompanying skin rash. Mega-karyocytes in the bone marrow are usually normal in number but some have found small, non-granular or vacuolated, degenerated or immature forms to pre-dominate.[43e] The condition is **self-limited** and no other spontaneous attacks occur. Only rarely are the manifesta-tions severe or fulminating.

Other cases are more **chronic.** These may commence in the same fashion as the self-limited type and may be en-countered at all ages. In a series of 55 patients of our own, it was striking that the self-limited cases were all under ten years of age (Fig. 17–3). This does not mean that all self-limited cases are confined to this age period but only illustrates the preponderance in this age group. From the histories of these children, moreover, one could not have

predicted their course in advance. In general, however, the more chronic forms of idiopathic thrombocytopenic purpura are more likely to occur after puberty and are more often seen in females than in males. By the time the patient is first seen there is often a past history of bruising or other forms of abnormal bleeding. The history of a possible precipitating factor is obtained only rarely. Spontaneous remissions and exacerbations occur but the remissions are not likely to be complete.[43e] The severe degrees of thrombocytopenia seen in the acute form are unusual but the platelets may be large, bizarre and irregu-lar. There is no accompanying eosino-philia or lymphocytosis. The mega-karyocytes in the bone marrow tend to be mature and normal in size although they may be less granular than normal. In one study,[106a] platelet agglutinins were found in half the chronic cases, whereas they were absent in the acute ones.

Many cases will be encountered which do not readily fit either of these categories and, in any event, classification is possible only in retrospect, even though a reasonable guess can sometimes be made. In point of fact, every variation can be encountered, from the very acute cases of only a few days' duration which result in complete recovery or, rarely, sudden death, to the more protracted cases which last weeks, months or years with mild, moderate or severe manifestations. This was pointed out in our earlier study several decades ago,[116] and still holds true. Bleeding may appear suddenly and may as promptly cease. It may never return but, more often, reappears in milder or more severe form. The interval between the first bleeding episode and the second varied in our cases from one month to 26 years. In other instances there is a continuous course which may or may not be interrupted by more acute phases. Episodes of bleeding may last a few days to a few weeks. Cessation of bleeding may be associated with a rapid increase in the number of platelets, even to values above normal, or thrombocytopenia of variable degree may persist. Differences in sex incidence, degree of thrombocytopenia, platelet morphology, presence or absence of eosinophilia and lymphocytosis and morphology of the megakaryocytes unfortunately cannot be counted on as wholly dependable prognostic guides.

Purpura in Pregnancy and Congenital Purpura.—Pregnancy in a woman who has previously had thrombocytopenic purpura may run a natural course[97a] but the development of idiopathic thrombocytopenic purpura in a pregnant woman is a much more serious matter. Such purpura must be distinguished from the mild purpura without thrombocytopenia which is sometimes encountered in hyperemesis or eclampsia. Idiopathic thrombocytopenic purpura developing during pregnancy

has been reported in 81 pregnancies involving 59 mothers,[70a] to which can be added four unreported cases of our own. The overall maternal mortality rate is under 2 per cent, the fetal death rate 19 per cent. This includes more recent experience, which has been more favorable than earlier results.[97] The incidence of fetal death was approximately the same in pregnancies in which splenectomy was performed during gestation and in those in which more conservative measures were employed. When thrombocytopenia was still present at the time of delivery, postpartum hemorrhage occurred in 11.6 per cent of the cases. Thrombocytopenic purpura was observed in 40 per cent of the infants of mothers with normal platelet counts and in 73 per cent of those who were thrombocytopenic at the time of delivery.

Purpura in the newborn, both full-term and premature, now reported in more than 100 cases,[44c,76,77a] may take several forms. In most instances thrombocytopenic purpura, either idiopathic or secondary, was present in the mother. In a few, splenectomy had been performed withhout producing complete cure.[77a] An affected mother may give birth to a normal child, or may have dissimilar twins, one affected and one normal.[44c] Purpura has been observed even in the fetuses of affected mothers.[97] In many cases of congenital purpura spontaneous recovery took place in one to three weeks[76,77a] but the risk of death is nevertheless great. In one study, a mortality of 26 per cent was cited,[21a] in another it was approximately 20 per cent.[76]

In cases such as these, congenital purpura in many instances probably represents transplacental passage of the factor responsible for the thrombocytopenia in the mother.[21a] In four instances antiplatelet agglutinins were demonstrated in the serum of both the mother and her baby.[97b,100a,111]

Thrombocytopenic purpura may also be observed in the newborn of apparently normal mothers. It has been suggested in such instances that the mother developed iso-agglutinins for the baby's platelets in a manner similar to Rh iso-immunization.[42a] In one case a platelet antibody was demonstrated in the infant's blood which was active against the father's platelets but not the mother's.[31]

In a third variety of congenital thrombocytopenic purpura, in contrast to the above cases, megakaryocytes have been absent or markedly reduced in number.[44c] In most instances of such **congenital hypoplastic thrombocytopenia** recovery occurred rapidly and spontaneously. In some cases, however, other congenital abnormalities, especially absent radii, were noted,[102d] thus suggesting a relationship to Fanconi's syndrome (p. 561). Observations in one case suggested deficiency of a factor which stimulates megakaryocyte maturation.[101b]

Diagnosis.—Bleeding of more or less severity, anemia proportional to the amount of blood lost, a prolonged bleeding time, thrombocytopenia, poor clot retraction, positive tourniquet test and essentially normal coagulation time, and at the same time a lack of glandular enlargement, joint symptoms, marked fever or significant leukocytic changes, make up a clinical picture which is not readily mistaken. It is necessary to rule out, by history and examination, the recognized causes of thrombocytopenia. These will be discussed shortly. One must inquire carefully about exposure to drugs and other toxic agents. Since a thrombocytopenic reaction is not necessarily related to the quantity of drug taken but depends usually on the patient's sensitivity, complete information is needed concerning home remedies, "drugs everyone takes," hobbies, hair dyes, cleaning agents occasionally used, and other sources of exposure the patient is not likely to think are relevant.

The family history may be helpful but other members of the family may need to be examined since the history alone may be misleading. A history of bleeding in other members of the family may be encountered in 10 to 20 per cent of cases of idiopathic thrombocytopenic purpura but there is no clearly defined genetic pattern as in other disorders with which this condition may be confused. Familial bleeding is found not only in hemophilia but also in PTC deficiency (p. 875) and in a number of other well-defined disorders of coagulation discussed in the next chapter, in hereditary hemorrhagic telangiectasia (p. 888) and in certain less well delineated conditions (familial epistaxis, von Willebrand's disease, etc.) which will be considered later in the present chapter.

In hemophilia coagulation time is prolonged but the bleeding time, tourniquet test and platelet count are normal. Other conditions in which coagulation time is prolonged were listed in Table 5-2 (p. 308) where, also, the various causes of prolonged bleeding time and other bleeding functions such as prothrombin time and prothrombin consumption were tabulated. The non-thrombocytopenic purpuras (p. 844) should be distinguished and the list of causes of hemorrhage (Table 17-1, p. 817) consulted. Bone marrow examination may be needed to rule out leukemia and aplastic anemia. The L.E. test (p. 419) may be helpful in disclosing an unsuspected disseminated lupus erythematosus. Tests for platelet antibodies will be discussed in a later section (p. 840).

A condition which can be mistaken for purpura is a rare form of angiokeratoma, *angiokeratoma corporis diffusum universale (Fabry)*.[25b] Our acquaintance with this disorder came about through a patient referred because of "purpura," anemia and albuminuria. The lesions can be distinguished from those of purpura by the fact that they are more or less permanent, the larger ones are slightly raised, and they are dark-red to bluish-red rather than purple in color (Table 18–2, p. 892). They tend to be present in groups and are dense and larger on the lower trunk (scrotum, penis, buttocks, lower back, upper thighs, umbilicus [Fig. 17–4]), and more sparse on the upper parts of the trunk and upper extremities. They have no tendency to bleed and there is no thrombocytopenia or disturbance in the coagulation mechanism. This is a systemic disorder, perhaps due to a hereditary defect in lipid metabolism, in which there is widespread involvement of the media of the blood vessels, with manifestations in the renal, pulmonary and other systems of the body.[96a]

"Symptomatic" Thrombocytopenic Purpuras. Recognized Causes of Thrombocytopenia.—(See Table 17–2).

1. **Chemical, Physical, Vegetable, and Animal Agents.**—(a) *Chemical Agents.*—A number of chemical agents are capable of producing thrombocytopenia and the hemorrhagic manifestations which accompany a deficiency of platelets, without at the same time producing anemia and leukopenia. Like those which produce aplastic anemia (Table 11–3, p. 553) they can be classified, in general, in two main categories; namely, those which will regularly produce thrombocytopenia provided a large enough dose is given and those which have this effect only occasionally, depending on the sensitivity of the host. The former often produce anemia and granulocytopenia as well; the latter may never have been observed to produce other deleterious effects on the blood except thrombocytopenia (*e.g.*, "Sedormid"), while some, like the organic arsenicals, may cause this in one person or granulocytopenia or aplastic anemia in another. There are at least two apparently different mechanisms whereby drugs produce thrombocytopenia. One is by damaging the megakaryocytes,

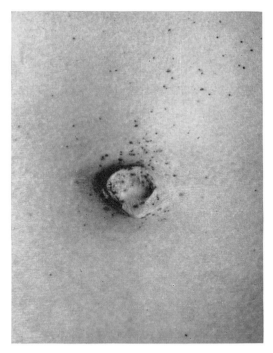

Fig. 17–4.—Lesions resembling purpura in a case of *angiokeratoma corporis diffusum universale.*

whereas the other depends mainly on the destruction of the platelets. As far as is known, the latter action depends on individual sensitivity. Megakaryocyte damage is often only a part of a reaction which, depending on unknown factors, may extend to the white and red cell forming tissues as well. This is the nature of the action of agents which regularly produce thrombocytopenia when large enough amounts are given. It can also occur, however, as a sensitivity reaction. In an earlier chapter (p. 552) a number of agents were listed which, in sensitive persons, produce aplastic anemia.

Drugs which more or less regularly are capable of producing thrombocytopenia include those used in the treatment of leukemia, Hodgkin's disease and related disorders, such as nitrogen mustard (p. 1037), triethylenemelamine (p. 974), busulfan (p. 972), urethane (p. 974) and certain antimetabolites (p. 977). Benzene falls in the same category. The most clearly demonstrated examples of drugs whose action depends upon individual sensitivity are the hypnotic Sedormid (allyl-isopropyl-acetyl-carbamide) and quinidine but the organic arsenicals and the sulfonamides come in the same category.

Of the **organic arsenicals,** sulf-arsphenamine, neoarsphenamine, silver arsphenamine and bismarsen were well known to produce thrombocytopenic purpura occasionally; and, even more infrequently, mapharsen.[102a] Tryparsamide and the inorganic arsenicals are not known to cause purpura. The deliberate administration of a small test dose of an organic arsenical to a person in whom thrombocytopenia had developed earlier, was shown to be followed within a short time by the development of purpuric and ecchymotic lesions and even varying degrees of shock.[23] Thrombocytopenic purpura as a complication of **sulfona-mide** therapy is rare[56a] but the use of sulfadiazine,[44d] sulfathiazole,[108a] sulfisoxa-zole ("Gantrisin"),[40a] sulfamezathine,[14b] sulfadimidine[67b] and sulfamethoxypyrida-zine[102b] has, nevertheless, been associated with the development of such purpura. Re-administration of sulfonamides to patients who had previously reacted with thrombocytopenia was associated with a similar reaction.[44d] In one case rapid *in vitro* agglutination and lysis of platelets followed the addition of sulfamezathine to the blood of the patient.[14b]

The observation that in a number of instances of **Sedormid** purpura the drug had been taken over many months without untoward effect and that purpura followed the ingestion of a small dose after a short abstinence, and the report[74a] that the administration of this drug to sensitive persons was followed by pronounced thrombocytopenia within thirty to sixty minutes, led to important *in vitro* experiments.[1] Ackroyd was able to

demonstrate agglutination followed by lysis of platelets when he added Sedormid, in concentrations corresponding to those to be expected with therapeutic administration of the drug, to the blood of patients who had recovered from attacks of purpura caused by it. The platelet lysis, and the reduced clot retraction caused by the platelet deficiency, were caused by some factor in the plasma acting in the presence of Sedormid and not due to any peculiarity of the platelets themselves. Normal serum had no such effect and the omission of Sedormid gave negative results. Inactivated serum produced only agglutination of platelets upon incubation with Sedormid but the addition of complement resulted in platelet lysis. It was postulated that the combination of Sedormid and platelets served as the antigen and that the presence of both is required for agglutination and lysis by the antibody. The application of Sedormid to the skin in two of three cases caused local hemorrhages without thrombocytopenia or increased capillary fragility. In their essentials, these observations have been confirmed by a number of investigators but, in some cases, sensitivity has been very brief in duration.[40]

Similar observations have been made with **quinidine.** Approximately 50 cases of quinidine-induced thrombocytopenic purpura have been reported,[12a, 99] with two deaths. No relation to the size of the dose was observed.[14b] Approximately 82 per cent of the cases were in females.[14b] Prodromal symptoms, such as chills, lethargy and pruritus have been observed and bullous lesions in the mouth, gum bleeding and epistaxis, with or without petechiae on the skin, have been described. Sensitivity has been shown *in vitro* by the demonstration of clumping of platelets when quinidine was added to the patient's platelet-rich plasma. The quinidine could be removed readily from the platelets by washing.[113] As with

Sedormid, lysis occurred only when complement was present.[99] Some investigators have been able to demonstrate agglutination of normal platelets on the addition of the patient's serum and quinidine.[14b] A very simple test of quinidine sensitivity consists in the mixture of 2 ml. of the patient's blood and 0.2 ml. of a 1:2000 quinidine sulfate solution.[99] In contrast to a similar mixture of the patient's blood with normal saline solution or with 1:2000 solution of quinine hydrochloride, no retraction of the clotted blood occurred at four, and even 24, hours in the sample containing quinidine.

The thrombocytopenia and hemorrhagic manifestations disappear in one to seven days after withdrawal of the drug but antibodies have been demonstrated in the patient's blood for as long as six months following discontinuance of quinidine therapy, even though the thrombocytopenia had subsided completely. The reaction to quinidine is so specific that negative results have been observed in quinidine sensitive cases when its levorotatory isomer, quinine, was used. In **quinine** sensitive individuals, *in vitro* agglutination and lysis of platelets following the addition of quinine has been demonstrated.[14b,55a]

Other chemical agents which have been reported to produce thrombocytopenia and purpura occasionally or rarely include *gold salts*,[109c] antibiotics such as streptomycin,[78b] oxytetracycline,[7] ristocetin[30b] and para-aminosalicylic acid,[40b] and also phenylbutazone,[25] antipyrin,[68a] sodium salicylate,[85d] tridione,[27] meparfynol ("Dormison") phenobarbital,[14] allyl-isopropyl-barbituric acid ("Alurate"), thiourea,[77b] dinitrophenol,[46] digitoxin,[10a] mercurials,[15b] chlorothiazide and hydrochlorothiazide,[6] bubaritone,[120] chlorpropamide,[37b] potassium iodide,[19c] bismuth,[12] ergot,[82] organic hair dyes,[5] estrogens,[17b] DDT[52] and possibly also meprobamate, acetazolamide and tolbuta-

mide. In some instances there is only a single case report in spite of the wide use of the agent (*e.g.*, sodium salicylate, streptomycin, digitoxin) so that one wonders about the significance of the observations but, in other reports, evidence was presented that readministration caused a return of thrombocytopenia (paraaminosalicylic acid, chlorothiazide). In the case of ristocetin, there is evidence of a direct toxic effect of the drug on circulating platelets.[30b]

Since many of these drugs are used more frequently in adults than in children, whereas purpura hemorrhagica is much more common in childhood than in adult life, the development of purpura in an adult should arouse suspicion of a chemical etiologic agent. If a drug is suspected, the effects of its readministration may be tested, provided this is done under conditions in which the patient's safety is carefully guarded or, without any risk to the subject, an *in vitro* test of sensitivity[99,113] may be carried out.

(*b*), (*c*) and (*d*) *Physical, Vegetable and Animal Agents.*—Roentgen rays and other forms of ionizing *radiation* rarely produce thrombocytopenia without leukopenia and anemia (p. 557). Their action is myelosuppressive. *Heat stroke* has been reported as causing marked thrombocytopenia and purpura.[118a] The evidence that *vegetable* substances (foods, orris root)[105] produce thrombocytopenia is not very convincing. Following **burns,** thrombocytopenia may develop within several hours after injury and purpura may be associated. *Animal* agents described as causes of thrombocytopenia include snake venoms, insect bites,[24] and pertussis vaccine.[57]

2. **Disorders Involving the Hemopoietic System.**—Thrombocytopenia, together with purpura, prolonged bleeding time, non-retractile clot and positive tourniquet test, may be only a part of an extensive involvement of the hematopoietic system. Other findings will serve

to distinguish these cases from purpura hemorrhagica and the secondary thrombocytopenic purpuras already considered.

(a) In the *acute leukemias*, even in the absence of leukocytosis, careful search of the blood smear will reveal at least a few immature leukocytes. The anemia usually will be more severe than would be expected as the result of loss of blood There may also be fever, a cachectic state, ulceration in the mouth, or glandular and sometimes hepatic enlargement and the spleen may be larger than would be expected in purpura hemorrhagica. Localized sternal tenderness is a valuable sign in leukemia. In *chronic leukemia*, marked thrombocytopenia does not usually occur until late. At this time, the leukocyte picture, splenomegaly and glandular enlargement should be sufficiently typical to make differentiation simple. When there is doubt, sternal bone marrow examination should leave no further doubt for a striking increase in immature leukocytes will be found there even when the blood picture is not convincing.

(b) In *aplastic anemia*, whether idiopathic or due to various chemical or physical agents, thrombocytopenic purpura is accompanied by pronounced leukopenia as well as relative lymphocytosis, and there is anemia which is more severe than the history of hemorrhage would lead one to expect. There are, moreover, few or no signs of attempts at red cell regeneration.

In obscure cases of purpura, roentgenograms of the bones may be helpful in making the diagnosis, for *myelophthisic anemia*, whether due to primary (multiple myeloma)[115] or metastatic tumors of the bone marrow[122] may sometimes suggest purpura hemorrhagica. The same may be said of myelosclerosis. In several instances of carcinoma of the stomach the initial complaints have been referable to purpura.[113a] In studying cases of purpura, it should be kept in mind that metastases, even extensive ones, may not always be discernible by roentgenograms.

Acquired hemolytic anemias of the immune body type (p. 615) may be accompanied by persistent thrombocytopenia and sometimes the clinical signs of purpura are prominent.[22b] In such cases the Coombs' test is likely to be positive.

In *pernicious anemia*, after a long period without treatment, moderate purpura and thrombocytopenia may develop. Such other signs and symptoms as sore tongue, achlorhydria, neurological changes, macrocytosis and bilirubinemia should make differentiation simple.

(c) Thrombocytopenic purpura may be found in a number of disorders in which *splenomegaly* is an outstanding finding (p. 1055), such as that associated with congestive splenomegaly,[70,91] Gaucher's disease,[13] chronic infections (kala-azar, tuberculosis, Felty's syndrome,[41a] histoplasmosis, etc.), sarcoidosis, lymphosarcoma and disseminated lupus. In Hodgkin's disease, when the bone marrow is extensively invaded, thrombocytopenia may develop (p. 1026). In all of these conditions additional signs will usually be present to suggest their presence, the splenomegaly will be much greater than that found in idiopathic thrombocytopenic purpura, and anemia or leukopenia, or both, may accompany the thrombocytopenia. In some of these conditions, however, the *spleen may be of normal size* or only slightly enlarged and the picture of idiopathic thrombocytopenic purpura may be closely simulated or be indistinguishable; yet microscopic examination of the spleen may reveal a histologic picture characteristic of an underlying condition. In our experience, and in that of others,[22d] this has been true particularly of *disseminated lupus*. In that disorder, splenectomy may relieve the thrombocytopenia but the L.E. test may become positive for the first time only after operation.[85c]

(d) **Thrombotic (thrombohemo-**

lytic) thrombocytopenic purpura is a disorder closely resembling thrombocytopenic purpura in certain respects, which was first described in 1925 by Moschcowitz under the title, "an acute febrile pleiochromic anemia with hyaline thrombosis of the terminal arterioles and capillaries." At first thought to be exceedingly rare, it is being recognized more and more frequently. More than 116 cases have been reported.[16a] The outstanding feature histologically is the appearance of innumerable occlusions in the terminal arterioles and capillaries of all the tissues of the body, especially the myocardium, the capsular zone of the adrenals, the renal cortex, the pancreas and the gray matter of the brain. There is increasing evidence that this is due to specific damage of the walls of the vessels rather than because of "platelet thromboses," as was originally maintained. Fibrin has been demonstrated in the vascular lesions, together with an accumulation of acidic polysaccharide similar to chondroitin sulfate or hyaluronic acid.[75] Clinically a characteristic triad is observed; namely, thrombocytopenic purpura, severe hemolytic anemia and transitory, bizarre neurologic symptoms and signs. Both sexes and all ages are affected and there is no apparent racial preference. The most common form is acute and is likely to be fatal within a few days to a few weeks from onset. A more chronic process, of a relapsing nature and lasting for several months to years, ultimately ending in most instances in death from an an acute exacerbation, has been described in 16 per cent of the cases.[16a]

The manifestations of thrombocytopenic purpura include the usual cutaneous ones as well as hemorrhage from various orifices, and prolonged bleeding time, poor clot retraction and profound thrombocytopenia. The increased blood destruction is accompanied by marked reticulocytosis and the presence of many nucleated red cells in the blood smear, but the icterus may not be striking and the existence of a hemolytic anemia may be overlooked or the signs may be confused with those of hepatic disease. The liver and spleen are usually enlarged and anorexia, nausea, diarrhea and crampy abdominal pain are frequent complaints. Fever is consistently present. The mental symptoms, which are almost always present, include restlessness, confusion, irritability, incoherent screaming, muttering delirium, stupor or coma. These symptoms are usually transitory and are followed by lucid intervals. In addition, focal lesions, such as vertigo, facial weakness, ptosis, hemiplegia, aphasia, apraxia, ataxia, dysphagia or abnormal reflexes may develop but even these signs may be transitory.

The usual pigmentary evidence of hemolytic anemia is found, but spherocytosis occurs only transiently. Since blood transfusions are not followed by sustained relief of the anemia, it is probably of the extracorpuscular variety. With only six exceptions, the Coombs' test has been found to be negative. No autohemolysin, isohemolysin, autoagglutinin or isoagglutinin has been demonstrated.[1c] The leukocyte count may be normal or, more frequently, it is elevated and there may be a leukemoid picture. No platelet autoagglutinins or isoagglutinins have been found but platelet survival appears to be shortened.[1c] In contrast to idiopathic thrombocytopenic purpura (p. 839), transfusion of the patient's plasma to normal recipients failed to produce any ill effects.[14e] Although the condition has been compared to lupus erythematosus, the L.E. test (p. 419) is negative. The bone marrow findings are nonspecific but the histologic pattern of the characteristic underlying tissue lesion has been demonstrated in paraffin sections of small fragments of material obtained by sternal marrow puncture. The characteristic lesion has also been recognized in lymph node biopsies. No satisfactory form of therapy is known. Splenectomy has been carried carried out in 18 or more cases; in eight of these the course of the disease was more protracted than usual.[16a] Whether the more prolonged course can be attributed to the operation is uncertain. Adrenocorticosteroids and ACTH have been used in many instances, without success even when associated with splenectomy, but it is claimed that massive steroid therapy may be helpful.[43d] The cause of the disorder is obscure.

3. **Infections.**—Purpura was recognized as a manifestation of the pestilential fevers two thousand years ago. Thrombocytopenia may accompany the purpura and has been observed in a few instances of septicemia, typhoid fever,[42b] typhus, tuberculosis[30a,60] (especially miliary), smallpox,[3,45] chickenpox,[16d,121] vaccinia,[86] scarlet fever,[28] measles,[44a] rubella,[25a] mumps,[56] whooping cough,[73] cat-scratch disease,[9] psittacosis, Rocky Mountain spotted fever,[82b] infectious hepatitis,[119] and subacute bacterial endocarditis.[81,91] In all of these conditions fever is an outstanding symptom and confusion with purpura hemorrhagica should rarely occur. When occurring in association with infectious mononucleosis (p. 1114), however, thrombocytopenic purpura may be confusing. Relative and absolute thrombocytopenia has been observed in association with artificially induced fever[114] and in patients given malaria (*P. vivax*) therapeutically[20a] as well as in the spontaneous disease.[103]

The degrees of thrombocytopenia and increased capillary fragility after infections of apparently equal severity vary strikingly from one patient to another and probably depend upon the susceptibility of the patient's tissues rather than upon the intensity of the primary infection.

4. **Hemangio-endothelioma.**—The naevus, in the form of the port-wine stain, and strawberry naevi in infants are commonly benign, ultimately fading or disappearing. However, the tumor has been observed to be associated with thrombocytopenia in about 20 cases, all in infants,[18a,62,98] except for one case in a girl of 13 years.[33] Because the vascular tumors have been found to contain large numbers of platelets, more than the circulating blood,[33] and because the thrombocytopenia disappears when the tumor is destroyed by radiation therapy or spontaneously regresses, it has been assumed that the hemangiomata sequester the platelets. Splenectomy has been without effect.

5. **Miscellaneous Conditions.** — Thrombocytopenic purpura has been observed in cases of hyperthyroidism[25c] in an unusual form of lipidosis associated with angiomata of the spleen,[68b] in kwashiorkor[50] and in a recurrent illness of unknown etiology, observed in children, in which hemolytic anemia and renal disease were also present.[103a] The last is to be distinguished from a constitutional disorder of childhood (*Aldrich syndrome*) which is marked by an increased susceptibility to infection and eczema,[73a] and in which thrombocytopenia is also found. This condition affects only males and is a sex-linked Mendelian recessive characteristic. Hemorrhage occurs chiefly in the skin or bowel. Still another constitutional disorder accompanied by thrombocytopenia is characterized by faulty maturation of granulocytes as well as platelets and the presence of basophilic structures (Döhle or Amato bodies) in the neutrophils and eosinophils (*Heggelin's anomaly*).[61]

Following the administration of large quantities of bank blood in a relatively short period of time, severe thrombocytopenia may develop and may persist for several days. This was observed in 14 patients who received more than 5000 ml. blood within a forty-eight hour period and in 11 of these there was clinical evidence of abnormal bleeding.[56b]

The cause of this phenomenon, which may present a serious therapeutic problem, is obscure. The severity of the thrombocytopenia is correlated with the amount of blood given. Thrombocytopenia has been observed also following severe gastro-intestinal hemorrhage but this is not likely to be severe enough to cause prolongation of bleeding.[20]

Treatment.—There is a great difference, in general, between the management of the secondary or symptomatic forms of thrombocytopenic purpura and the idiopathic variety. The proper treatment of the former depends on the cause: avoidance of the offending chemical agents, management of the leukemia, the cure of the associated infection, or some other appropriate procedure, as the case may be. The administration of BAL (2,3 dimercaptopropanol) has been associated with recovery in cases of thrombocytopenic purpura due to gold[64b] or arsphenamine.[101a] Splenectomy is obviously not indicated when the cause is a drug to which the patient is sensitive. However, in certain instances of symptomatic purpura, management is similar to that of the idiopathic form. Thus, splenectomy is helpful when thrombocytopenia complicates Gaucher's disease; again, adrenocorticosteroid therapy may be as useful in certain forms of symptomatic purpura as they are in idiopathic thrombocytopenic purpura; and blood and platelet transfusions are equally valuable in both forms.

The evaluation of therapeutic measures for the management of a disorder with a course as varied as that of idiopathic thrombocytopenic purpura is exceedingly difficult since the tendency for spontaneous improvement may be overlooked and hasty conclusions may be drawn. From time to time various remedies have been advocated which time and experience have shown to have no real value. In this group may be included foreign protein injections,[39] turpentine,

sulfuric acid, kephrine hydrochloride,[55b] ergot, iodine and coal tar,[105] ultraviolet light,[105] heliotherapy, viosterol, parathyroid extract,[67] vitamin P,[63] ascorbic acid,[77] high protein diet, liver extract, fat-soluble "T" factor,[100] toluidine blue,[44] snake venoms (tiger,[90] moccasin[80]) and antivenins (*Bothrops*). Roentgen irradiation of the spleen[71] is also no longer used.

Blood transfusions (including platelet transfusions), the use of ACTH, cortisone and related compounds such as prednisone, and splenectomy are the measures which deserve serious consideration. General measures include the administration of iron if iron deficiency has developed from chronic blood loss, a well-rounded diet suitable to the condition of the patient, and the appropriate mixture of rest and activity. It is customary to greatly restrict activity when thrombocytopenia is marked, on the assumption that rest will make the occurrence of cerebral hemorrhage less likely. For this recommendation the writer knows of no really adequate support. He has, in fact, seen fatal cerebral hemorrhage occur when the patient lay quietly in bed and observed no ill effects when a boy with severe, chronic thrombocytopenic purpura persisted in amateur boxing, contrary to advice. However, when actual bleeding is taking place, the desirability of maintaining quiet circulation is more obvious.

Blood transfusion is necessary if there has been much bleeding and shock is imminent or impending. Blood may also be administered for the purpose of supplying platelets. Studies of the fate of platelets have shown that the greatest loss occurs during collection and administration of blood by routine technics, rather than through the effects of storage. Measureable survival of platelets has been demonstrated when whole blood was transfused to thrombocytopenic patients, provided pains were taken to prevent

53

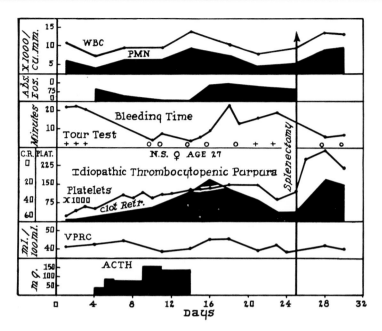

FIG. 17–5.—Increase in platelet count, reduction of bleeding time and improved clot retraction, all associated with temporary clinical improvement, in a case of purpura hemorrhagica treated with adreno-corticotrophic hormone. The effects of splenectomy are also shown.

their clumping and destruction. Thus, platelet survivals of four to six days were achieved when multiple syringes treated with silicone were used for direct transfusions from polycythemic donors.[106a] The use of plastic equipment for the preparation of platelet-rich plasma, with disodium ethylene diamine tetracetate (Na_2EDTA) as the anticoagulant, has made it possible to obtain large quantities of platelets from normal donors[30d] for administration to patients with thrombocytopenia. The technic for preparation of plasma concentrates of platelets is time-consuming, however, and the most practical procedure is the use of polycythemic or, if that is not available, normal blood, collected in plastic bags or siliconized bottles. *Transfusion of viable platelets* is indicated primarily for the treatment of severe bleeding crises. While often successful in halting hemorrhage temporarily and returning bleeding time and clot retraction to normal, these effects of platelet transfusions cannot be expected if a potent platelet destructive mechanism is at work. Furthermore, the administration of platelets may result in the formation of platelet antibodies (p. 840) with the result that their survival following transfusion becomes shorter and shorter and their value consequently less and less.[41b]

ACTH, cortisone and related compounds have been found to reduce capillary fragility in most patients with thrombocytopenic purpura and to be associated with an increase in the platelet count in about half of them.[67a,87] It has been stated that remission in this disease may be hastened by steroid therapy.[112b] The changes which may occur are illustrated in Figure 17–5.

Views concerning the place of steroid therapy in the treatment of thrombocytopenic purpura have differed.[16b,17f,41b,97c] This can be explained in part by the fact that spontaneous improvement occurs in many patients and it is difficult to know in such cases whether the observed improvement is attributable in whole, in part, or at all to the steroid therapy. Only in those cases in which relapse occurs when steroid therapy is interrupted and remission develops again on their administration can one draw conclusions with some confidence concerning the relationship of steroid therapy to the observed recovery.

Because the use of these agents is not altogether harmless, our own approach is to reserve them for special circumstances. Thus, if the hemorrhagic manifestations are mild, and especially when their short duration and the age of the patient lead one to suspect that a spontaneous remission is likely, they are not administered. In reaching this conclusion, the platelet count itself is not a criterion, for it will often be under 40,000 per c.mm. in any event. The clinical manifestations are important. The same policy is followed if the thrombocytopenia is attributable to a recognizable cause. On the other hand, if the bleeding manifestations are more pronounced, prednisone or a similar compound is employed, usually in doses of 40 mg. per day. The actual therapeutic dose, however, is that amount which appears to achieve the desired results. We have not been impressed that one compound is better than another and never use ACTH since intramuscular injections are better avoided if possible.

If the platelet count rises promptly and the bleeding manifestations disappear, steroid therapy is reduced and ultimately eliminated. This is done rapidly if improvement occurs within a few days, more slowly if steroids have been maintained for several weeks. Long term steroid therapy, in the writer's opinion, should be avoided if at all possible. It is dangerous, disfiguring and costly. The greater susceptibility to infections, the development of osteoporosis, muscle weakness and hypertension, the blossoming of latent diabetes and the many other ill effects of steroid therapy should not be, but too often are ignored by the physician. Furthermore, the psychological effects of the moon facies, hirsutism and other physical changes produced by steroids are much more serious than is sometimes appreciated. In all instances the therapeutic dose used should be reduced to the lowest possible amount consistent with the clinical condition. It does not seem reasonable to maintain high doses for several months in an attempt to achieve normality. Some increased bruisability and platelet counts of half the normal values are better than the ill effects of long term, high dosage steroid therapy. In all instances, if complete remission is not achieved with steroid therapy or if hemorrhagic manifestations are severe in the absence of steroids, splenectomy should be considered. In essence, in our view the *administration of steroids is indicated* (1) in aiding in the control of serious bleeding; (2) in the management of patients with moderately severe bleeding who, because of cardiac or other complications, cannot be submitted to splenectomy; (3) in patients who have not responded to splenectomy or have recurrences of their symptoms and these are of sufficient severity to require therapy, justifying the disadvantages of steroid therapy; and possibly (4) in the preoperative preparation of patients if bleeding is moderately severe and splenectomy is decided upon. When used in relation to operation, these agents are given for at least three days prior to surgery and for a similar period after operation, after which they are tapered off in the course of two or three days.

The value of **splenectomy** in the treatment of idiopathic thrombocytopenic purpura has long been recognized.[53] Following this operation, the platelet count may increase rapidly, even within 24 to 48 hours, and may reach very high levels in about ten days. Counts of several million platelets per c.mm. have been observed at this time. The bleeding time is reduced and the capillary resistance increases long before the platelets show any significant increase in number.[87] Usually the thrombocytosis subsides gradually. The striking increase of platelets does not follow other surgical procedures. Hysterectomy, for example, has been done in cases of purpura hemorrhagica with the object of removing a source of hemorrhage. Such treatment is not only valueless but dangerous.

Splenectomy, however, is not the infallible remedy that some have held. The earlier reports were based on only short periods of observation following operation. For example, of 213 case reports collected in one series,[21] information regarding the condition of the patients three or more years after operation was available for only 20 cases, while only five had been observed five years or longer. The course of purpura hemorrhagica, as already stated, is so varied that adequate appraisal of the effects of operation makes necessary the study of patients for many years after splenectomy, and comparison must be made with the course of the disease in unoperated cases.

In an earlier study, based on an analysis of 62 cases of our own and an additional 89 from the literature[116] we found (1) a high mortality (20.8 per cent) following splenectomy during an acute episode of thrombocytopenic purpura; and (2) more frequent long continued recovery in patients splenectomized following the first or later episodes of purpura as compared with non-splenectomized cases. The results of other studies[67a, 107c] were similar. An analysis of our cases seen and treated 20 and more years later[16b] likewise indicated an impressive superiority of splenectomy in the treatment of unremitting idiopathic thrombocytopenic purpura as compared with medical therapy, even when the latter was aided by the use of steroids. The experience of many others is similar.[20c, 41b,97c,112b] Some,[17f] however, have emphasized certain possible ill effects of splenectomy; namely (1) a "high" relapse rate, (2) the hazards of severe infections in splenectomized infants and children, and (3) the possible dissemination of lupus erythematosus.

As already stated, there is no doubt that splenectomy is unsuccessful in achieving a long term cure in a certain proportion of patients. The figure for such failures in different studies has ranged from 19 to 40 per cent of cases. Not only may relapse follow splenectomy[15,112b] but even death from intracranial hemorrhage has been observed.[69] The platelet count may not rise postoperatively, it may rise temporarily, only to return to the original low levels after a few days or a few weeks, or it may rise again to high levels but, after an interval of several months or years, it may decrease to very low levels. The thrombocytopenia, moreover may or may not be accompanied by bleeding.

Failure of splenectomy has been explained in various ways. *Accessory spleens* are mentioned frequently in this regard but there are great differences of opinion concerning their importance. Undoubtedly, at the time of the original splenectomy the surgeon should look for them carefully and remove them if found. The commonest sites are in the splenic pedicle, the pancreas and the peritoneum in the immediate neighborhood of the spleen but they have in rare instances been found in the pelvis near the ovaries in women and in the scrotum in males.[22c] In seven cases of idiopathic thrombocytopenic purpura in which relapse occurred following splenectomy, the use of thorium dioxide sol (Thorotrast) in an attempt to demonstrate accessory spleens roentgenologically failed, although this procedure had been successful in two cases of hemolytic anemia.[65] With present day knowledge of the carcinogenic effects of thorium, such examinations would no longer be attempted. In a few cases surgical exploration has revealed accessory spleens and their removal has brought about remissions.[22c] Opinions concerning the likelihood of such a successful result of exploration differ widely.[17d, 67a] Our own limited experience has not been encouraging. Certainly in many cases other explanations must be sought. Implantation splenosis as the result of rupture of the spleen at the original operation is, fortunately, not a common accident. In most cases of failure one must postulate that the spleen must not have played the major role in the production of the manifestations of the disease. This topic will be considered further shortly (p. 839).

Not everyone is agreed that splenectomy significantly increases the hazard of infection in infants or children[20c] (see p. 1051). Nor[97c] has it been a common experience that lupus erythematosus becomes exacerbated after splenectomy.[85c] It is true, as mentioned earlier (p. 830), that the manifestations of this disease may sometimes become apparent for the first time after the spleen has been removed but it is by no means certain that these events are causally related. Several of our patients improved following splenectomy when thrombocytopenic purpura was the chief manifestation of lupus.

The **indications for splenectomy** might be briefly stated as follows: (1) in those cases of idiopathic thrombocytopenic purpura in which spontaneous remission has not occurred after six or more months of observation and the clinical manifestations are moderate or severe. Thus, occasional bruising and platelet counts consistently above 100,000 per c.mm. would usually not justify splenec-

tomy or steroid therapy. More severe manifestations require consideration of splenectomy, especially in females from puberty until the menopause, since excessive menstrual bleeding carries a risk not shared by males and since recurrences seem to be more common in females than in males (see below). The estimate of "severity" is admittedly difficult to make since occasionally the course of this disorder may become unexpectedly fulminating. However, in our experience, fatal cerebral hemorrhage is unusual in a patient with disease of more than two months' duration;[16b]

(2) in patients who appear to respond to steroid therapy but require relatively large doses (more than 10 mg. prednisone daily, or its equivalent) to maintain a satisfactory clinical state devoid of serious hemorrhage and who have shown no tendency to spontaneous remission in six to 12 months of observation;

(3) in the rare patient whose growth and development or social or economic status is seriously impaired by recurrences;

(4) in the pregnant woman with this disorder, in the later stages of pregnancy, if other measures have failed.[41b] In such cases caesarian section, in addition, must also be considered. Early in pregnancy surgery endangers the fetus by the possibility of inducing abortion. It has been stated that steroids may induce congenital anomalies if employed in the first trimester.[41b] Although this has not been the universal experience and they have been used to delay splenectomy in the pregnant patient with thrombocytopenic purpura, it is probably prudent to avoid their use if at all possible;

(5) in secondary forms of thrombocytopenic purpura in which the cause cannot be treated or removed and yet the bleeding manifestations are severe. Thus, splenectomy is justified in some cases of Gaucher's disease accompanied by thrombocytopenia but is not desirable

in acute leukemia or in thrombocytopenia associated with the taking of a drug.

Some have used the presence of platelet agglutinins as a guide for splenectomy, operation having been found much more likely to be successful when they were demonstrated than in their absence.[41b] Unfortunately, techniques for demonstrating platelet agglutinins are imperfect (p. 840) and this, then, cannot be considered a dependable criterion. Possibly studies of the site of sequestration of Cr^{51}-tagged platelets will prove useful.[76a]

Splenectomy is contraindicated: (1) early in the first episode of bleeding, especially in children, since it is more probable that bleeding will subside spontaneously than that it will become more severe; (2) in most cases of symptomatic purpura, such as those due to some drug or those associated with infections; (3) in neonatal purpura, since recovery takes place naturally; (4) in cases in which the diagnosis has not been established clearly; (5) in acute, *fulminating cases.* Here the mortality following splenectomy has been high and the use of fresh, viable platelet transfusions and high dosage steroid therapy (50 to 100 mg. prednisone daily) may be more helpful. However, some consider acute fulminating thrombocytopenic purpura to be an indication for splenectomy and, in such cases, give platelet transfusions and steroids only postoperatively.[41b]

Prognosis.—As already stated, recovery, or at least improvement is the rule rather than the exception in this disease. However, relapse or recurrences do occur. It is difficult to give a satisfactory estimate of their frequency. In children ten years of age and under, the likelihood of a complete, permanent remission occurring is good. In adults the changes are less good, perhaps one out of three. In our experience, recurrences have been twice as common among female patients as compared with males.

These may appear as soon as several weeks or months following the initial symptoms of purpura, and in most instances within four years. However, in two of a total of approximately 150 of our own cases, recurrences were observed after eight and a half and 14 years, respectively, in spite of complete freedom from symptoms in the intervals.

Severe external hemorrhage and bleeding into vital tissues are the chief causes of death. Hemorrhage into various parts of the nervous system is the most common serious complication and death from this cause, as already stated, has occurred even after splenectomy. It is noteworthy, however, that recovery has been observed following intracranial hemorrhage.[16b, 32, 66, 69, 72, 112] The recovered cases include those in which large hemorrhages into the spinal meninges occurred as well as instances of multiple small hemorrhages into the substance of the brain.

Prognosis following steroid therapy and after splenectomy was discussed above in relation to the use of these therapeutic measures. Reported remission rates associated with steroid therapy range from approximately 38[16b] to 73[17f] per cent. Equally conflicting are the figures for splenectomy since the criteria for the selection of cases for operation and the duration of follow-up differ. The writer would estimate that the chance for continued recovery following splenectomy in cases selected according to the criteria outlined above are two out of three, or better.

Pathology.—The findings in the bone marrow have been described (p. 823). The spleen may be slightly enlarged. The average weight in one series was 227 Gm.,[78] while in another the range of weights was 124 to 230 Gm.[117] The increase in the size of the spleen is thought to be due to congestion of the sinusoids and an increase in the size of the follicles. The increase in the size of the germinal centers of the lymphoid follicles, although admittedly nonspecific,[43b] is the most prominent change in the spleen.[14d] In the splenic sinuses eosinophilic and neutrophilic leukocytes and megakarocytes are found.[78] The histology of the purpuric lesions has been studied.[80] In patients dying of purpura hemorrhagica, extensive hemorrhages, gross and microscopic, are found.

Pathogenesis.—In any consideration of the pathogenesis of idiopathic thrombocytopenic purpura attention must be given to the thrombocytopenia, the increased capillary permeability and the rôle of the spleen. The *thrombocytopenia* has been attributed to (1) a decreased rate of platelet formation from megakaryocytes, probably as a result of splenic inhibition.[18,29] This concept finds support in the appearance of the megakaryocytes in the bone marrow which has been interpreted as indicating arrested maturation.[29] The suggestion that the spleen is the source of an inhibitory agent was supported by the reported extraction of a substance ("thrombocytopen") from the spleens of human cases of purpura hemorrhagica which was capable of producing thrombocytopenia in rabbits.[110] In other experiments, however, the platelet reducing substance was shown to be quite nonspecific and was demonstrated in homogenates of many different organs and in the urine of normal individuals.[103c]

(2) Kaznelson's proposal of splenectomy as a form of treatment for this condition[53] was based on the assumption that the platelets are destroyed by the spleen more rapidly than is normal.[117] Comparison of platelet counts from the splenic artery and vein, which might be expected to show evidence of sequestration of platelets in the spleen, unfortunately has given equivocal results.

(3) The existence of a humoral factor in the plasma which destroys platelets and damages megakaryocytes was suggested by a number of studies. Thus, the occurrence of thrombocytopenic purpura in infants born of thrombocytopenic mothers (p. 825) was postulated as being due to the transplacental transmission of a humoral substance.[21a] Again, the rôle of antibodies in the production of thrombocytopenia was indicated by the experiments in Sedormid-induced purpura[1] which have been described already (p. 828) and was supported by studies of other drug-induced purpuras. At the same time, the presence of a platelet agglutinating factor was demonstrated in the serum of some patients with idiopathic thrombocytopenia.[22b] This was succeeded by the observation that the transfusion of plasma from some patients with idiopathic thrombocytopenic purpura into normal individuals is followed by severe thrombocytopenic purpura and even changes in the megakaryocytes suggesting immaturity.[42a,106] The presence of the thrombocytopenia-producing factor was demonstrated in the plasma of 16 out of 26 cases.[42a] This factor remained in the plasma of some of the patients even after their spleens had been removed and also after their platelet counts had returned to normal.

Studies of the survival of platelets transfused into patients with thrombocytopenia have indicated that antibodies against platelets can be formed. It was reported that platelet disappearance was extraordinarily rapid when the patient presented acute manifestations whereas, in more chronic cases and in patients with thrombocytopenia associated with leukemia or aplastic anemia, platelet survival was significantly longer.[106] These results suggested that, when platelet survival in the recipient is short, his thrombocytopenia is due to an increased rate of platelet destruction; when it is normal, decreased production may be the chief mechanism in the pathogenesis of the thrombocytopenia. The observation was also made[106] that the thrombocytopenic effect of plasma from a patient with chronic idiopathic thrombocytopenic purpura was of shorter duration in splenectomized recipients than in normal ones. This was interpreted as indicating that the spleen may be responsible for the removal of "sensitized" platelets.

It has been pointed out already (p. 834) that the survival of transfused platelets into either normal or thrombocytopenic recipients becomes progressively decreased with repeated transfusion.[30d,106] This appears to be due usually to the development of a platelet iso-agglutinin. Serologically distinguishable platelet types have been demonstrated by a number of investigators.[40c,42a,106] Actually, **platelet antibodies** of several varieties have been found, specific natural antibodies which react with the antigens A and B of the ABO blood group system, specific immune antibodies which react with antigens of the other blood groups, especially D, and specific immune antibodies independent of the erythrocyte groups.[18b] The last are of several kinds and include incomplete antibodies.[106b] Harrington found platelet agglutinins in 100 out of 132 consecutive cases of idiopathic thrombocytopenic purpura.[42] Unfortunately, of the various tests for platelet antibodies which have been devised,[18b,42a,106b] none is wholly satisfactory and the bearing of these findings on the pathogenesis of this disorder is uncertain.[42,103b]

The importance of a *capillary defect* in the etiology of purpura is indicated by clinical experience. Hemorrhage in cases of purpura hemorrhagica is not always closely correlated with the degree of thrombocytopenia. Furthermore, in aplastic anemia one may encounter severe degrees of thrombocytopenia without finding purpura. The latter, however, will develop in such cases when the capillaries are deliberately damaged, as in the tourniquet test. A number of experiments have been carried out in an attempt to understand the pathogenesis of the increased capillary fragility which

is found in purpura. Many years ago, Bedson[8] showed that thrombocytopenia may be produced experimentally by the injection of agar-serum without the development of bleeding. Only when it was administered several hours after the injection of "anti-red cell serum," a substance which produced capillary damage, did the injection of agar-serum produce purpura. Splenectomy gave his animals a measure of protection but not total immunity, for by the injection of large amounts of these antisera thrombocytopenic purpura could still be produced. These observations have been confirmed.[22,62]

Later, direct studies of the capillaries[67c] showed that they normally contract after injury. During the period of capillary contraction the blood which escapes initially has time to clot firmly in the wound. In the hemorrhagic states associated with a prolonged bleeding time, the normal capillary contraction is absent.[67c] It was also observed that splenectomy may improve capillary fragility without altering the number of platelets, and this effect in any event precedes the increase in platelets.[87] These changes were attributed at the time to a nonspecific effect of operative interference. Later it was shown that adrenocortical activity is related to capillary resistance.[87]

In the light of these observations, it seems likely that the rôle of *the spleen* in the pathogenesis of idiopathic thrombocytopenic purpura is not always the same. It is conceivable that the spleen is the site of formation of platelet agglutinins and, when it is the major source of these antibodies, its removal is followed by "cure." It may be only one of many sites of antibody production, while in other cases it may be concerned chiefly with the removal of "sensitized" platelets from the circulation. Whether or not it forms a substance which interferes with the maturation of megakaryocytes is uncertain. In any given case one or more of these mechanisms may be active and the results of splenectomy will depend on their importance.

The investigations which have been described strongly suggest that idiopathic thrombocytopenic purpura is a syndrome which may be produced in a number of different ways.[106] It is quite probable that an immunological mechanism is important in the pathogenesis of many cases. It seems likely, however, that this will not explain all the idiopathic cases. In addition to the possibilities already suggested, one must wonder about metabolic aberrations leading to deficiency of factors necessary for platelet production, or splenic dysfunction which might cause suppression of platelet formation.

The observation that some women bruise more easily before their menstrual period than after it, and that a physiological decrease in platelets may occur premenstrually (p. 284), as well as the preponderance of purpura hemorrhagica in females, led to the suggestion that some factor concerned with the menstrual cycle may stimulate thrombocytolytic activity by the spleen.[36] Minot a number of years ago described several cases in which attacks of purpura hemorrhagica recurred periodically with menstruation[74] and the injection of large doses of female sex hormone in dogs was reported to produce thrombocytopenic purpura.[4] Nevertheless, in a case such as Minot reported, no evidence of ovarian activity or cyclical variation in adrenal activity could be demonstrated, although it appeared possible that cyclical changes in pituitary function might be involved since a fall in urinary gonadotropins (FSH) was observed coincidentally with the fall in platelets.[103d]

The paradox of prolonged bleeding time in thrombocytopenic purpura and normal coagulation time was discussed in an earlier chapter (p. 309).

ALLERGIC PURPURA

Definition.—The term "allergic" refers to a group of *non-thrombocytopenic* purpuras[1b,34,79] which are characterized by purpura in association with one or more of the common *symptoms of allergy*, such as erythema, urticaria or effusions of serum into subcutaneous or submucous tissues or viscera. When accompanied by certain gastrointestinal and joint symptoms the disorder is referred to as the Henoch-Schönlein syndrome but the term allergic purpura includes purpura associated with erythema simplex, erythema multiforme, erythema bullosum, erythema vesiculosum, erythema nodosum, urticaria pigmentosa and angioneurotic edema. The true nature of these purpuras is as yet poorly understood. It must be admitted that in only a minority can an allergic cause be demonstrated.

Synonyms.—Henoch-Schönlein purpura, peliosis rheumatica, anaphylactoid purpura, hemorrhagic capillary toxicosis.

Etiology and Pathogenesis.—These conditions are not due to hematopoietic disturbances but are the result of increased permeability of the capillary endothelium, which permits the passage of plasma and blood cells. Perivascular inflammation has been demonstrated in the skin lesions and in severe cases a necrotizing arteriolitis has been observed.[30] Experimental studies have shown that a nonthrombocytopenic vascular purpura can be produced by the injection in dogs[17a] or in guinea pigs[46a] of rabbit antisera against guinea pig vascular endothelium.

The syndrome is seen most often in children, sometimes in adolescents and young adults and rarely later in life. The average age of onset in two series was 5.6 years[64] and 5.2 years,[84] respectively. While the condition is uncommon under the age of two, in a series of 139 cases the age range was from ten months to twelve and one-half years.[64] Although males predominate, more recent figures give a ratio of three males to two females[106c] rather than 2:1 or even 4:1 as earlier studies indicated. In Britain spring and autumn peaks of incidence have been observed.[16,64]

The exciting cause has most often been considered to be bacterial or an article of food. Although various infections, especially tuberculosis, and vaccines such as anti-typhoid vaccine, have been considered among the causes of the bacterial allergy, the *streptococcus*[30] has been accused most often. Comparison of the sex ratio, age of onset, seasonal trends and incidence of previous upper respiratory tract infections, particularly those associated with the hemolytic streptococcus, and similarities in the latent period before the onset of symptoms have suggested a close relationship between the Henoch-Schönlein syndrome and acute nephritis. Nephritis has been observed to develop in 22[106c] to 47[84] per cent of cases. However, antistreptolysin O titers and isolations of group A β-hemolytic streptococcus failed to provide clear evidence, as there is in rheumatic fever and nephritis, that this organism is an invariable causative factor.[16,106c,111a] A few autopsy examinations[10b] have suggested a similarity between the lesions found in cases of the Henoch-Schönlein syndrome and those seen in polyarteritis nodosa[78a] and "collagen" disorders.[19] Kidney biopsy specimens obtained at the height of the disease have revealed focal lesions of fibrinoid deposition and endothelial proliferation within scattered glomeruli. Specimens taken during clinical recovery showed focal glomerular scars.[111a] This contrasts with the diffuse and uniform changes which are observed in acute and subacute glomerulonephritis. Skin biopsies showed perivascular cellular infiltration of the dermis with numerous leukocyte-platelet thrombi in small dermal vessels. These observations give support to the view that anaphylactoid purpura is a form of diffuse vascular disease, probably caused by hypersensitivity to a variety of agents.

A few cases have been described in which hypersensitivity to certain *foods* seemed to be the cause of the disorder. Egg, milk,[59] chocolate, wheat and beans, have been implicated most often[1b,2a,51] but other foods include tomato, onion, potato, plums, blackberries, strawberries, nuts, fish, crab,[2c] pork and chicken. Hypersensitivity to cold[82a] and insect bite[15a] have also been described as etiologic agents. A close relationship in pathogenetic mechanisms between drug induced thrombocytopenic purpura (p. 828) and the Henoch-Schönlein syndrome is suggested by cases in which sensitivity to chlorothiazide[26] or to quinine was associated with a clinical picture resembling the Henoch-Schönlein syndrome. In the latter erythrophagocytosis, a serum factor that could induce erythrophagocytosis in normal blood, increased capillary fragility and transient diminution in platelet number and morphology were observed.[17c]

Symptoms depend on the site of exudation. It has been suggested that various focal lesions may account for the location of the manifestations in skin, viscera or joints.

Symptomatology.[2b] — Osler,[79] who described the symptoms in great detail, pointed out that there may be 4 types of lesions, all of an exudative character:

1. *Purpura.*—This may be simple, but more often the lesions are accompanied by swelling. Blebs may be found which have the appearance of herpes on a purpuric or hyperemic base or there may be bullae or even pemphigoid lesions. Simple edema may be present in the hands or feet or about the knees and elbows.

2. *Effusions* of serum causing urticarial wheals or angioneurotic edema.

3. *Diffuse erythema*, with or without swelling.

4. *Necrotic areas* which may be followed

by the formation of bullae or ulcers. Chronic leg ulcers have been described.[44a]

The skin lesions may "run the gamut of the skin atlas."[79] They may be of all sizes and extent, but are found most frequently in the extremities and are usually symmetrically placed. They often appear in crops and may be accompanied by itching or paresthesias. Gairdner[30] described an eruption which he regarded as very characteristic—at first small, discrete urticae appear upon the extensor surfaces of the upper and lower limbs; within a few hours these begin to change to pink maculo-papules, becoming less raised and darker in color. Dusky red macules which do not fade on pressure are found the next day and these may coalesce to form larger patches. As regression takes place, the red color becomes more purple before fading to brown. Frankly hemorrhagic lesions are less common. Small isolated red spots may be seen in the buccal mucosa but bleeding from the mouth and nose are unusual.

In contrast with most other forms of purpura, hemorrhage in this syndrome is rarely severe and even the purpura may be a relatively minor component of the clinical picture. In some attacks it may even be absent. Commonly, visceral or joint symptoms dominate the picture. The onset and course are remarkably variable. Headache, anorexia, fever, or abdominal pain may usher in an attack, or pain in and around the joints may be the first complaint. The course of the disease is characterized by a remarkable tendency to recurrences.

Henoch's name[43] is applied when abdominal symptoms predominate. Colic is the most common symptom and may be transient or very severe. Osler[79] stated that colic occurred most often at night. The pain is central, but may radiate to all parts of the abdomen, although in Osler's experience the right

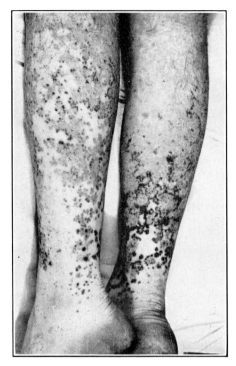

Fig. 17–6.—Hemorrhagic and erythematous lesions in a case of Henoch-Schönlein purpura.

lower quadrant was spared. Tenderness is often present but muscular rigidity is absent. Vomiting may occur and, if severe, may be accompanied by blood. Diarrhea is not very common, but with the bowel movements mucus and blood may be passed. Tenesmus may occur. Constipation may be so stubborn as to suggest obstruction. Roentgenograms may show areas of transitory edema in the small bowel.[41] Intussusception has been observed.[105b] Especially noteworthy is the fact that abdominal symptoms may develop before any purpuric eruptions appear and needless operations have been performed as a result. The lesion most commonly found at operation is an extravasation of blood or serosanguineous fluid into the wall of the small intestine.[1b] Edematous, scarlet colored, segmental lesions have been described.[5a]

Henoch pointed out that *fever* is common but that it is always moderate and usually irregular. He also stressed the association of *rheumatoid pains* with the attacks of abdominal pain or purpura, these often preceding the onset of abdominal manifestations. **Schönlein**[101] had already described the pain and tenderness about the joints or in the limbs and pointed out that the joint symptoms and the cutaneous lesions affected the lower extremities most commonly. The pain is rarely as intense as in acute rheumatic fever and is not strikingly influenced by salicylates. Periarticular effusions are common. Hemorrhages into the joints do not occur.

Nervous System and Special Sense Organs. —Involvement of the nervous system and special sense organs has been observed,[38] with the development of such symptoms as transient attacks of paresis, epileptiform convulsions, hemorrhages into the eyelids, conjunctiva or retina, optic atrophy, iritis and ophthalmitis.[10]

Renal Hemorrhages.[30] — Renal hemorrhages may occur, though very rarely. Microscopic hematuria, however, is common. Osler[79] included cases with well-marked disturbance in renal function and 5 of his cases died in uremia. Christian[17] doubted whether some of these should have been included, but he agreed that kidney lesions similar in nature to those found in the skin may develop and cause hematuria, albuminuria and profound disturbance of renal function.

Osler mentioned bronchial wheezing, asthma and dyspnea in his cases, but *respiratory symptoms* are unusual. Edema of the glottis is the chief source of danger.

Laboratory Findings. — Blood. — Hemorrhage is rarely sufficiently marked to produce anemia. There may be neutrophilic leukocytosis, sometimes eosinophilia. The blood platelets are not significantly affected, and bleeding time, coagulation time, and clot retraction are normal. The tourniquet test

and the snake venom test may be positive or negative.[80]

The *urine* may be normal, or blood or albumin may be found. Examination of the *stools* may reveal blood.

Diagnosis.—Before purpura or other skin manifestations have appeared, the symptoms may suggest a variety of conditions, depending on their location. A history of previous attacks of joint symptoms when the main complaint is referred to the abdomen, and *vice versa*, is suggestive of Henoch-Schönlein purpura. If purpura is present, the normal blood findings exclude thrombocytopenic purpura and it is only necessary to rule out **other forms of non-thrombocytopenic purpura.**

(*a*) Many **infections** may be accompanied by purpura. While, as already stated, there may be thrombocytopenia, more frequently there is no change in the blood. In subacute bacterial endocarditis the purpura is often embolic in origin. A white center may be observed in the hemorrhagic skin lesions. Purpura associated with meningococcal sepsis may also be due to emboli. In other instances hemorrhage is probably due to capillary damage produced by toxins. Substances have been obtained by autolysis of pneumococci which are capable of producing purpura experimentally.[37] The purpura may be very extensive and severe. A fulminating form of purpura associated with adrenal hemorrhage and blood stream infection, usually by the meningococcus, is known as the *Waterhouse-Friderichsen syndrome*. Infections in which purpura may occur include, in addition to those already mentioned, typhoid fever, influenza, scarlet fever[28] (Fig. 17–7), smallpox, tuberculosis,[17e] malaria, measles, diphtheria, Rocky Mountain spotted fever, and septicemias due to various organisms.[81a]

(*b*) **Chemical and Animal Agents.** —The use of iodides,[19e] copaiba, belladonna, atropine, quinine,[103] bismuth,

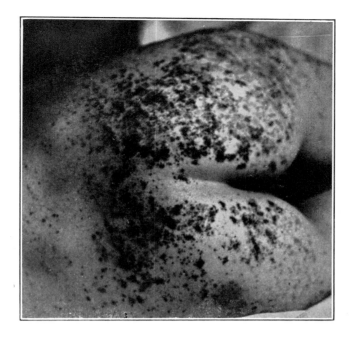

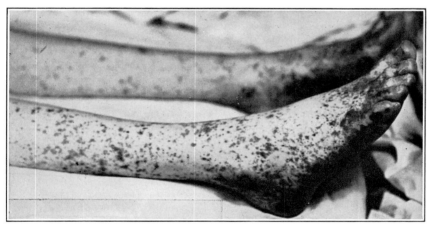

Fig. 17–7.—Purpuric lesions in a case of scarlet fever. There was no thrombocytopenia. (Fox and Enzer, courtesy of Am. J. M. Sc.)

mercury, procaine penicillin,[104a] phenacetin, acetylsalicylic acid,[29a] merbaphen, chloral hydrate and other hypnotics[14c] has been followed in some cases by the development of purpura, without thrombocytopenia. This is probably the result of idiosyncrasy. The multiple hemorrhagic lesions in the serous membranes, lungs and other viscera following poisoning by viperine and crotaline *snake venoms* is due to injury to the endothelial lining of capillaries and small veins.[55]

(*c*) **Avitaminosis.** — The hemorrhagic manifestations of scurvy are not associated with thrombocytopenia, but are attributed to increased capillary permeability. The bleeding ceases following the administration of lemon juice and similar antiscorbutic substances. This effect has been claimed to be due not to the action of ascorbic acid but to that of a second factor, "vitamin P," a flavone ("citrin"). Conclusive evidence, however, regarding the rôle of "vitamin P"[63] has yet to be furnished.

(d) In **certain skin diseases**[80] a purpuric eruption unaccompanied by thrombocytopenia may be encountered. These include annular telangiectatic purpura (Majocchi's disease), Schamberg's disease, pigmented purpuric lichenoid dermatitis, angioma serpiginosum and the Ehlers-Danlos syndrome.[88] They are distinguished by their individual characteristics.

(e) A number of **chronic diseases** may be associated occasionally with nonthrombocytopenic purpura. The purpura described in some cases of acute glomerulonephritis and rheumatic fever[47a] may, perhaps, be no different than that seen in the Henoch-Schönlein syndrome but purpura of the skin and mucous membranes as well as large subcutaneous extravasations occur also in chronic renal disease with azotemia. Purpura may also be seen in association with chronic cardiac and hepatic disease, in the Cushing syndrome and in polycythemia vera. In as many as 15 per cent of cases of hemochromatosis hemorrhagic manifestations have been noted.[107] In hepatic disease purpura is usually related to prothrombin or, more rarely, fibrinogen deficiency. In Cushing's syndrome the hemorrhagic manifestations are attributed to fragility of the skin.

Very rare causes of extensive purpura include generalized amyloidosis[85a] and blood-borne carcinoma emboli.[103e]

(f) Various forms of **dysglobulinemia,** whatever their cause, may be associated with purpura. This includes the purpura sometimes encountered in multiple myeloma (p. 1069) and in association with other instances of cryoglobulinemia, hyperglobulinemia and macroglobulinemia (p. 1078).[11a,107b] Under the title, *purpura hyperglobulinemica*, Waldenström[112a] described a unique group of cases characterized by innumerable acute episodes of purpura, especially after unusual exertion, prolonged standing or excessive pressure from garments, in which there was a considerable increase in gamma globulin and in the 7-component in the ultracentrifuge.[109b] The course was long drawn out and the skin of the lower extremities, where the purpura was more common, developed a residual mottled brown pigmentation. A great variety of cases has since been reported under this title[107b] and different hematological alterations have been described; for example, normal, decreased or increased numbers of platelets, prolonged or normal coagulation time, abnormal heparin tolerance test, hypofibrinogenemia or normal values and variable alterations in the prothrombin complex.[72a] One can hardly consider this to be a diagnositic entity. It has been suggested that the abnormalities in coagulation are the result of the complexing of unusual plasma globulins with various coagulation factors, thus interfering with the process of coagulation.[43a]

Other forms of purpura will be described in the next sections (p. 849). With the hemorrhagic disorders discussed in Chapter 18 there should rarely be any cause for confusion for many of them are characterized by prolongation of coagulation time.

Course.—A single attack of Henoch-Schönlein purpura seldom lasts more than a week. However, almost invariably, after an interval usually of days but sometimes of weeks or months, another attack begins. Any number of attacks may occur, often four or five but sometimes many more, and these may closely resemble one another or may differ considerably.

Prognosis. — The immediate prognosis is usually good unless such complications as intussusception, hemorrhage into the nervous system or kidneys, or edema of the epiglottis occur. In 50 per cent of 49 patients showing initial renal lesions, normal urine was found three months later. However, recovery was not observed in any patient in whom abnormal urinary findings were present over a period of two years or more.[106c] It has been suggested that renal sequela of anaphylactoid purpura may constitute one of the origins of chronic renal disease of "unknown etiology" seen in adults.[112c]

Treatment. — In the majority of cases only symptomatic therapy is required. If it can be discovered, the inciting agent should be removed or avoided. Elimination diets may be tried. Results of treatment with ACTH or adrenocorticosteroids have been equivocal or disappointing. In the hope of reducing the incidence and severity of nephritis, bed rest has been recommended.[1b]

PURPURIC DISORDERS ASSOCIATED WITH QUALITATIVE ABNORMALITIES OF PLATELETS

Ever since Glanzmann's rather vague description in 1918 of a purpuric disorder characterized by normal numbers of platelets and yet poor clot retraction,[134] cases of bleeding diathesis have been reported which do not fit the categories of thrombocytopenic and non-thrombocytopenic purpura just discussed. Unfortunately, in each instance the studies have been limited in scope, and often in numbers as well, and a great variety of names has been proposed. The resulting confusion is only now beginning to be cleared.

That bleeding may occur because of a qualitative rather than a quantitative platelet defect is now evident. Such bleeding disorders may be given the general designation of *thrombocytopathic purpuras*. In many instances, in addition

to the platelet abnormality, or perhaps because of it, evidence of vascular abnormality and deficiencies of certain plasma coagulation factors have been demonstrated. Several varieties can be distinguished.

Conditions Characterized by Prolonged Bleeding Time: von Willebrand's Disease, von Willebrand-Jürgens' Disease, Vascular Hemophilia. Angiohemophilia. In a number of inhabitants of the Åland Islands, von Willebrand[160] observed a hemorrhagic diathesis which was inherited as a simple Mendelian dominant and affected both sexes. This was characterized by prolonged bleeding time, normal platelet count, normal coagulation time and normal clot retraction. The tourniquet test was sometimes positive. The tendency to bleed appeared early in childhood and took the form of epistaxis, or bleeding from the gums or from the female genitalia. Hemorrhage from the gastrointestinal or urinary tract was not unusual. Six of his subjects had died of gastrointestinal or uterine bleeding. Hemarthrosis occurred only once. It was noted that there might be prolonged bleeding from injuries and operative sites, although this did not occur always. Later studies on the same patients revealed impaired agglutination of the platelets[140] and, still later, prothrombin consumption[125,138,156] and thromboplastin generation were found to be abnormal. These writers named this disorder "pseudohemophilia" and later "*constitutional thrombopathy*." In the course of time other cases were reported under a variety of confusing titles which may or may not have represented the identical condition. Thus, the fact that the platelets are numerically adequate and the clot normally retractile was confirmed[132] but in certain cases prothrombin consumption was found to be normal.[131,141] A variation in the total number of platelets has also been noted, moderate thrombocytopenia occurring at times.[132,153] In another series of similar cases, investigation of the capillaries of the skin and mucous membranes led to the conclusion that these were distorted and often bizarre in form, and failed to contract after injury.[146]

The discovery that similar cases might be associated with a deficiency of factor VIII, the antihemophilic globulin,[147,151] led to the introduction of the terms *"vascular hemophilia"* and *"angiohemophilia."*[123] Such a deficiency was subsequently demonstrated in the Åland islanders. That all of the above cases may represent a single entity is suggested by the study of a kindred of 311 individuals in Michigan which revealed that the manifestations of the bleeding diathesis among them were variable in the extreme.[150] In its fullest expression the condition was marked by a prolonged bleeding time with evidence of a morphologic defect in the platelets and a deficiency in factor VIII but any combination of these abnormalities might be encountered. Genetic analysis suggested that the hemorrhagic tendency was determined by a single dominant gene of variable penetrance and expressivity.

The relationship of the platelet abnormality and the factor VIII deficiency is obscure. It is possible that the platelet defect leads to factor VIII or other deficiencies but genetic pleiotropy has not been ruled out. The existence of still another abnormality is suggested by the observation that a plasma fraction could be prepared from fresh normal plasma which caused the bleeding time to return to normal while the factor VIII level rose.[148] However, the plasma factor correcting the bleeding time is not the same as factor VIII for it could be obtained from hemophiliac plasma. It was concluded that a specific, hitherto unrecognized, plasma factor is lacking in von Willebrand's disease.

A hemorrhagic diathesis with prolonged bleeding time and factor IX deficiency, one case associated with PTA deficiency,[133] as well as other "capillary disorders" with coagulation defects have been described.[135,159]

Jürgens and his associates found slight anisocytosis of the platelets, with many small elements of 1.3 to 1.8 μ in diameter and a few giant forms up to 5 μ in diameter. In electron microscope studies alterations in certain particles of the granulomere were observed.[140] Others, likewise noting electron microscopic abnormalities, found that the platelets contained adequate amounts of platelet factor 3 but were resistant to breakdown.[139]

The term **thrombocytopathy** can be applied to any disorder characterized by deficient platelet functional activity.[129] Several different forms have been described.[127] In addition to the above mentioned constitutional disorder in which platelet thromboplastic activity appears to be at fault, cases have been reported in which the ability of platelets to neutralize heparin was defective,[158] while in still others a decreased serotonin content was found. The last is thought to be the fundamental abnormality in Jean Bernard's *"dystrophie thrombocytaire hemorragipare congenitale."*[127] Cases have also been reported in which all known coagulation factors were normal but the platelets appeared large and lymphocyte-like and remained separated from one another in blood smears.[138]

Faulty platelet function may develop in association with various clinical conditions. Thus, *acquired thrombocytopathy* may be an important cause of the bleeding tendency which is seen in uremia.[143] This may be the consequence of poor platelet factor 3 activity.[130] There are also isolated observations of thrombocytopathy occurring in association with liver disease, sprue, scurvy[131a] and myelofibrosis.[131b]

Also characterized by prolonged bleeding time is a hemorrhagic diathesis observed in two unrelated albinos whose bone marrow contained peculiar, pigmented reticular cells.[137]

Defective Clot Retraction: Glanzmann's Thrombasthenia.[134] — This name was applied to cases of excessive hemorrhage in which the bleeding time, platelet count and coagulation time were normal but clot retraction was deficient and the platelet morphology abnormal. More recently, Braunsteiner described cases of what may be the same disorder in which, by electron microscopic examination, it was observed that the platelets were unable to form pseudopods or to spread in contact with a wettable surface.[129] Others have described similar[154] or possibly related[157] disorders. Soulier[155] subdivided cases of Glanzmann's thrombasthenia in two principal groups; namely, (a) the Glanzmann-Naegeli type which is characterized by the presence of small platelets which agglutinate imperfectly and (b) the Bernard-Soulier type in which morphological changes are found in the platelets and platelet "thromboplastin profactor" is deficient.

The studies of Gross and his associates are of special importance[134a] in that they were able to demonstrate in the platelets of one group of patients greatly reduced glyceraldehydephosphate dehydrogenase (GAPDH) and pyruvatekinase (PK) activity, decreased glucose requirement and reduced lactic acid formation, as well as low levels of adenosine triphosphate (ATP) and abnormalities in amino acid metabolism. Petechiae, ecchymoses and mucous membrane hemorrhages and bleeding following injury of a degree to produce severe anemia and low serum protein levels characterized these cases, in addition to prolonged bleeding time and normal or even increased numbers of platelets. Platelet anisocytosis, "irritation forms" of platelets and increased average platelet diameters were noted. Abnormal agglomeration and spreading

of platelets were also observed. Electron microscopy revealed an increase in vacuoles and other changes. The bone marrow megakaryocytes were approximately normal in number but possibly somewhat abnormal in morphology, and were surrounded by few platelets. In these cases, the addition of ATP and magnesium ions to the platelet-rich plasma brought about normal clot retraction.

The workers also found that there may be another form of thrombasthenia in which the clinical manifestations are the same as those described above but which may be related to defective *utilization* of ATP. In this form of the disorder, no enzyme deficiency or reduced ATP levels could be demonstrated. Nevertheless, clot retraction could be restored to normal by the addition of magnesium ions together with ATP, or even by Mg^{++} alone.

OTHER PURPURIC DISORDERS

In addition to the conditions described above, bleeding in the skin and mucous membranes and, in some cases, serious hemorrhage from internal organs may occur in a large variety of circumstances. The results of various tests of bleeding and clotting have been negative, variable or equivocal but, in one form, there is some evidence of increased capillary fragility. In another, a marked increase in the number of platelets is the chief distinguishing feature. In addition, still other types of purpura may be encountered.

Hereditary Familial Purpura Simplex.—Spontaneous ecchymoses, unassociated with abnormalities in platelets, bleeding time or coagulation factors, insofar as they were studied, but accompanied by positive tourniquet tests were observed in 88 members of 27 families.[19a] All but four were females. Rheumatoid arthritis and rheumatic fever were frequently associated. Other cases have been

54

reported[25d,155] which may or may not belong in this group.

Thrombocytosis with Repeated Hemorrhages from Mucous Membranes. Hemorrhagic Thrombocythemia.—The paradox of hemorrhagic phenomena occurring in spite of the presence of very great numbers of platelets characterizes a strange clinical syndrome which has been observed in more than 60 cases.[126,136,144,149] These are to be distinguished from cases in which very high platelet counts accompanied a recognized clinical entity, as discussed earlier (p. 285). Occurring most often over the age of 30 years and in either sex, bleeding, spontaneous in onset and of varying severity, splenomegaly and thrombocytosis mark the syndrome.[142] Gastrointestinal bleeding has been most common but hematuria, bleeding after minor trauma, dental extractions or operations, hemoptysis or menorrhagia, have been observed. Spontaneous bruising, at times with extremely large hematomas, was frequent, yet purpuric spots were not seen. The spleen has ranged greatly in size; in only a few cases was it not enlarged. Platelet counts have been in the millions and the platelets have been irregular and distorted in size, unusually large or otherwise bizarre. No functional abnormality of the platelets has been clearly established. Leukocyte counts frequently have been in the range of 10,000 to 30,000 per c.mm., occasionally above 60,000, and in only two instances were they normal in number. Polymorphonuclear cells predominate, often with eosinophilia and sometimes with basophilic leukocytosis, whereas myelocytes and myeloblasts have numbered only 1 to 3 per cent. Polycythemia of moderate degree has been seen in about a third of the cases and, at some time in the course of the illness, anemia was present in the majority. Thrombosis was encountered in a third of the cases: splenic vein thrombosis most commonly, and superficial and deep veins of the legs in others. The course, occasionally more prolonged, has usually lasted one to five years. Radioactive phosphorus or busulfan administration appeared to be helpful in some cases, splenectomy was frequently disastrous.

Both the etiology and the pathogenesis of this disorder are obscure. In some ways resembling polycythemia vera, myelocytic or megakaryocytic leukemia, neither the course nor the pathologic findings are consistent with any of these disorders, even though two cases terminated in acute leukemia. The bone marrow has been panhyperplastic with a particular abundance of megakaryocytes, except in a few instances in which some areas were found to be fibrotic. Immaturity and structural abnormalities of some of the megakaryocytes have been noted, while others appeared normal. No characteristic histologic picture has been found in the spleen. Myeloid metaplasia in the spleen, liver, lymph nodes and kidneys was reported in only a few of the cases. Tests of the coagulation mechanism have yielded no consistent pattern and the results have varied from case to case and from time to time in the same case.

Miscellaneous Forms of Purpura.[19b] **—Purpura simplex.**—This non-specific term is applied to instances of mild skin purpura unassociated with well-defined blood or capillary abnormalities and unaccompanied by mucous membrane bleeding. The condition is seen more commonly in women, often at the time of the menstrual period (See below).

Purpura Senilis and Purpura Cachectica.—In senile and extremely undernourished individuals with atrophic skin[102e] and no subcutaneous fat, the skin vessels are readily injured by minor trauma.[109a] Small petechiae and hematomas are found along the major veins and venules of the hands, feet, forearms and legs. Liver disease may be associated.[19d]

Mechanical Purpura. — Violent muscular contractions, such as occur in whooping cough or convulsions, or even constriction of a limb by a tourniquet in a normal person, may cause rupture of capillaries with extravasation of blood subcutaneously. The purpura usually involves the head, neck and upper extremities.

Orthostatic Purpura.—This term describes purpura which develops in the lower extremities in some persons after prolonged standing, presumably due to capillary weakness.

Purpura Fulminans.—This term was applied by Henoch to a very rare form of nonthrombocytopenic purpura which affects children chiefly and is characterized by sudden onset, fever, great prostration, symmetrical ecchymoses in the skin without hemorrhage from mucous membranes, and a fatal course of one to four days. The ecchymoses extend with startling rapidity and gangrene may occur. The condition has been observed in association with infections, such as scarlet fever,[16c] and with pregnancy[102c] and has been regarded as a fulminating form of allergic purpura.[35] Some include under the same category instances of extensive purpura accompanied by an extreme state of vascular collapse in meningococcemia (Waterhouse-Friderichsen syndrome, p. 844). In most instances no abnormality in coagulation has been demonstrated, but factor V deficiency, excess antithrombin[31a] and hypofibrinogenemia[64a] have been reported. Extensive intravascular thrombosis has been observed and pathological changes resembling the localized Schwartzman phenomenon have been described.[64a]

Bleeding in Women.—Severe purpura and hemorrhage from mucous membranes occurring in women was at one time ascribed to ovarian hormone deficiency,[19] without convincing supporting evidence. No adequate explanation has been presented for the "easy bruising" ("*devil's pinches*") seen in women. *Vicarious bleeding* from extragenital sites at the time of menstruation has been reported from time to time.[86a] The eyes, ears, nose, urethra, rectum and lungs have been the sites of hemorrhage. The condition is extremely rare and unexplained.

Differing from the common type of bruising in women are several cases which have been attributed to *autoerythrocyte sensitization*.[30c,37a] In these, an area of painful ecchymosis would develop at the site of trauma and this would be followed by progressive erythema and edema. In three patients episodes of abdominal pain had occurred in association with the painful bruises and, in two, there were episodes of intracranial and gastrointestinal bleeding as well. In each of these patients there was a past history of severe trauma, with bruising. This was postulated to be the circumstance which had led to autosensitization. Skin tests suggested that this might be due to some factor present in the red cell stroma. Other studies suggest that emotional factors may play an important etiologic role.[85e]

BIBLIOGRAPHY

The Purpuras

1. ACKROYD, J. F.: The Pathogenesis of Thrombocytopenic Purpura Due to Hypersensitivity to Sedormid, Clin. Sc., 7, 249, 1949; *Ibid.*, 8, 235 and 269, 1949.

1b. ACKROYD, J. F.: Allergic Purpura, Including Purpura Due to Foods, Drugs and Infections, Am. J. Med., 14, 605, 1953.

1c. ADELSON, E., HEITZMAN, E. J. and FENNESSEY, J. F.: Thrombohemolytic Thrombocytopenic Purpura, Arch. Int. Med., 94, 42, 1954.

2a. ALEXANDER, H. L. and EYERMANN, C. H.: Allergic Purpura, J.A.M.A., 92, 2092, 1929.

2b. ALLEN, D. M., DIAMOND, L. K. and HOWELL, DORIS A.: Anaphylactoid Purpura in Children (Schönlein-Henoch Syndrome), A. M. A. J. Dis. Child., 99, 833, 1960.

2c.ANCONA, G. R., ELLENHORN, M. J. and FALCONER, E. H.: Purpura Due to Food Sensitivity, J. Allergy, 22, 487, 1951.

3. ARNDT, T.: Die Pockenepidemie 1918–19 in Dresden, Ergebn. inn. Med. u. Kinderh. 20, 511, 1921.

4. ARNOLD, O., HOLTZ, F. and MARX, H.: Über Beziehungen der Sexualhormone zum Kalkstoffwechsel und zum Knochenmark, Die Naturwissenschaften, 24, 314, 1936.

5. BALDRIDGE, C. W.: Macrocytic Anemia With Aplastic Features Following the Application of Synthetic Organic Hair Dye, Am. J. M. Sc., 189, 759, 1935.

5a.BALF, C. L.: The Alimentary Lesion in Anaphylactoid Purpura, Arch. Dis. Childhood, 26, 20, 1951.

6. BALL, P.: Thrombocytopenia and Purpura in Patients Receiving Chlorothiazide and Hydrochlorothiazide, J.A.M.A., 173, 663, 1960.

7. BECKETT, A. G. and FOXELL, A. W. H.: Thrombocytopenic Purpura Associated with Oxytetracycline Therapy, Lancet, 1, 1053, 1955.

8. BEDSON, S. P.: Blood Platelet Antiserum, Its Specificity and Role in the Experimental Production of Purpura, J. Path. & Bact., 25, 94, 1922.

9. BELBER, J. P., DAVIS, A. E. and EPSTEIN, E. H.: Thrombocytopenic Purpura Associated with Cat-Scratch Disease, Arch. Int. Med., 94, 321, 1954.

10. BENEDICT, W. L.: Schönlein-Henoch's Purpura With Intra-ocular Hemorrhage and Iritis, J.A.M.A., 95, 1577, 1930.

10a.BERGER, H.: Thrombopenic Purpura Following Use of Digitoxin, J.A.M.A., 148, 282, 1952.

10b.BERGSTRAND, A., BERGSTRAND, C. G. and BUCHT, H.: Kidney Lesions Associated with Anaphylactoid Purpura in Children, Acta paediat., 49, 57, 1960.

11. BERNARD, J., AUSSANNAIRE, M., NENNA, A., et DUGAS, M.: Les purpuras thrombopéniques aigues idiopathiques, Semaine hôp. Paris, 29, 1, 1953; Sang, 27, 882, 1956.

11a.BERNARD, J., INCEMAN, S., ZARA, M., et CHRISTOL, D.: La dysglobulinémie maligne hémorragipare, Rev. hémat., 7, 264, 1952.

12. BIANCHI, A. E.: Comments on a Case of Purpura, Rev. Assoc. méd. argent., 46, 1566, 1932.

12a.BISHOP, R. C., SPENCER, H. H. and BETHELL, F. H.: Quinidine Purpura, Ann. Int. Med., 50, 1227, 1959.

13. BLOEM, T. F., GROEN, J. and POSTMA, C.: Gaucher's Disease, Quart. J. Med., 20, 517, 1936.

14. BOAS, E. P. and ERF, L. A.: Thrombocytopenic Purpura Following Medication With Sedormid and With Phenobarbital, New York State J. Med., 36, 491, 1936.

14b.BOLTON, F. G. and YOUNG, R. V.: Observations on Cases of Thrombocytopenic Purpura Due to Quinine, Sulphamezathine, and Quinidine, J. Clin. Path., 6, 320, 1953; Blood, 11, 527 and 547, 1956.

14c.BORRIE, P.: A Purpuric Drug Eruption Caused by Carbromal, Brit. M. J., 1, 645, 1955.

14d.BOWMAN, H. E., PETTIT, V. D., CALDWELL, F. T. and SMITH, E. B.: Morphology of the Spleen in Idiopathic Thrombocytopenic Purpura, Lab. Investigation, 4, 206, 1955.

14e.BRITTINGHAM, T. E., III and CHAPLIN, H., JR.: Attempted Passive Transfer of Thrombotic Thrombocytopenic Purpura, Blood, 12, 480, 1957.

15. BROWN, D. N. and ELLIOTT, R. H. E.: The results of Splenectomy in Thrombocytopenic Purpura, J.A.M.A., 107, 1781, 1936.

15a.BURKE, D. M. and JELLINEK, H. L.: Nearly Fatal Case of Schoenlein-Henoch Syndrome following Insect Bite, Am. J. Dis. Child., 88, 772, 1954.

15b.BUTT, E. M. and SIMONSEN, D. G.: Mercury and Lead Storage in Human Tissues with Special Reference to Thrombocytopenic Purpura, Am. J. Clin. Path., 20, 716, 1950.

16. BYWATERS, E. G. L., ISDALE, I. and KEMPTON, J. J.: Schönlein-Henoch Purpura, Quart. J. Med., 26, 161, 1957.

16a.CAHALANE, S. F. and HORN, R. C., JR.: Thrombotic Thrombocytopenic Purpura of Long Duration, Am. J. Med., 27, 333, 1959.

16b.CARPENTER, A. F. et al.: Treatment of Idiopathic Thrombocytopenic Purpura, J. A. M. A., 171, 1911, 1959.

16c.CHAMBERS, W. N., HOLYOKE, J. B. and WILSON, R. F.: Purpura Fulminans. Report of Two Cases following Scarlet Fever, New England J. Med., 247, 933, 1952.

16d.CHARKES, N. D.: Purpuric Chickenpox, Ann. Int. Med., 54, 745, 1961.

17. CHRISTIAN, H. A.: Visceral Disturbances in Patients With Cutaneous Lesions of the Erythema Group, J.A.M.A., 69, 325, 1917.

17a.CLARK, W. G. and JACOBS, E.: Experimental Nonthrombocytopenic Vascular Purpura: A Review of the Japanese Literature, with Preliminary Confirmatory Report Blood, 5, 320, 1950.

17b.COOPER, B. A. and BIGELOW, F. S.: Thrombocytopenia Associated with the Administration of Diethylstilbestrol in Man, Ann. Int. Med., *52*, 907, 1960.

17*c*.CREGER, W. P. and HOUSEWORTH, J.H.: Erythrophagocytosis and Thrombocytopathy Occurring during the Course of a Henoch-Schönlein Syndrome Due to Quinine, Am. J. Med., *17*, 423, 1954.

17*d*.CURTIS, G. M. and MOVITZ, D.: The Surgical Significance of the Accessory Spleen, Ann. Surg., *123*, 276, 1946.

17*e*.DALGLEISH, P. G. and ANSELL, B. M.: Anaphylactoid Purpura in Pulmonary Tuberculosis, Brit. M. J., *1*, 225, 1950.

17*f*.DAMESHEK, W. *et al.*: Treatment of Idiopathic Thrombocytopenic Purpura (ITP) with Prednisone, J. A. M. A., *166*, 1805, 1958; *ibid.*, *173*, 1025, 1960.

18. DAMESHEK, W. and MILLER, E. B.: The Megakaryocytes in Idiopathic Thrombocytopenic Purpura, a Form of Hypersplenism, Blood, *1*, 27, 1946.

18*a*.DARGEON, H. W., ADIAO, A. C. and PACK, G. T.: Hemangioma with Thrombocytopenia, J. Pediat., *54*, 285, 1959.

18*b*.DAUSSET, J. and MALINVAUD, G.: Examen critique des méthodes immunologiques employées pour l'étude des purpuras thrombopéniques, Sang, *28*, 1, 1957; Rev. franç. étud. clin. et biol., *4*, 495, 1959; Nature, *188*, 865, 1960.

19. DAVID, W.: Uber "Purpura"-Erkrankungen bei Frauen, Med. Klin., *22*, 1755, 1926.

19*a*.DAVIS, E.: Hereditary Familial Purpura Simplex, Lancet, *1*, 145, 1941.

19*b*.———— Purpura of the Skin, Lancet, *2*, 160, 1943.

19*c*.DAVIS, W. C. and SAUNDERS, T. S.: Purpura Due to Iodides, Arch. Dermat., *53*, 644, 1946.

19*d*.DERBES, V. J. and CHERNOSKY, M. E.: Senile Purpura and Liver Disease, A. M. A. Arch. Dermat., *80*, 529, 1959.

19*e*.DERHAM, R. J. and ROGERSON, M. M.: The Schönlein-Henoch Syndrome and Collagen Disease, Arch. Dis. Childhood, *27*, 139, 1952.

20. DESFORGES, J. F., BIGELOW, F. S. and CHALMERS, T. C.: The Effects of Massive Gastrointestinal Hemorrhage on Hemostasis, J. Lab. & Clin. Med., *43*, 501, 1954.

20*a*.DIGGS, L. W.: The Platelet Count, Bleeding Time, Clotting Time, Capillary Fragility, Prothrombin Concentration, and Clot Retraction in Paretics Receiving Therapeutic Malaria, Am. J. Clin. Path., *14*, 534, 1944.

20*b*.DIGGS, L. W. and HEWLETT, J. S.: A Study of the Bone Marrow from Thirty-six Patients with Idiopathic Hemorrhagic (Thrombopenic) Purpura, Blood, *3*, 1090, 1948.

20*c*.DOAN, C. A., BOURONCLE, BERTHA A. and WISEMAN, B. K.: Idiopathic and Secondary Thrombocytopenic Purpura: Clinical Study and Evaluation of 381 Cases over a Period of 28 Years, Ann. Int. Med., *53*, 861, 1960.

21. ELIASON, E. L. and FERGUSON, L. K.: Splenectomy in Purpura Hemorrhagica Ann. Surg., *96*, 801, 1932.

21*a*.EPSTEIN, R. D., LOZNER, E. L., COBBEY, T. S., JR. and DAVIDSON, C. S.: Congenital Thrombocytopenic Purpura, Am. J. Med., *9*, 44, 1950.

22. ELLIOTT, R. H. E., JR. and WHIPPLE, M. A.: Observations on the Interrelationship of Capillary, Platelet, and Splenic Factors in Thrombocytopenic Purpura, J. Lab. & Clin. Med., *26*, 489, 1940.

22*b*.EVANS, R. S. and DUANE, R. T.: Acquired Hemolytic Anemia, Blood, *4*, 1196, 1949; Arch. Int. Med., *87*, 48, 1951.

22*c*.EVANS, T. S., SPINNER, S., PICCOLO, P., SWIRSKY, M., WHITE, R. and KIESEWETTER, W.: Recurrent Hypersplenism Due to Accessory Spleen, Acta hæmat., *10*, 350, 1953.

22*d*.EVERSOLE, S. L., JR.: Cases of Disseminated Lupus Erythematosus Diagnosed as Idiopathic Thrombocytopænic Purpura, Bull. Johns Hopkins Hosp., *96*, 210, 1955.

23. FALCONER, E. H. and EPSTEIN, N. N.: Purpura Hæmorrhagica Following Neoarsphenamine and Bismarsen Therapy, Arch. Int. Med., *65*, 1158, 1940; *ibid.*, *66*, 319, 1940.

24. FATZER, H.: Schwere Thrombopenische Purpura nach Insektenstich, Folia hæmat., *63*, 145, 1939.

25. FELDMAN, L., COHNEN, F. and HIRSCH, H.: Fatal Thrombocytopenic Purpura following Phenylbutazone Therapy, Illinois Med. J., *105*, 83, 1954.

25*a*.FERGUSON, A. W.: Rubella as a Cause of Thrombocytopenic Purpura, Pediatrics, *25*, 400, 1960.

25*b*.FESSAS, P., WINTROBE, M. M. and CARTWRIGHT, G. E.: Angiokeratoma Corporis Diffusum Universale (Fabry), Arch. Int. Med., *95*, 469, 1955.

25*c*.FINOCHIETTO, R., DEL CASTILLO, E. B. and PARODI, A. S.: Exophthalmic Goiter and Hemorrhagic Thrombocytopenic Purpura, Semana méd., *43*, 1059, 1936.

25*d*.FISHER, B., ZUCKERMAN, G. H. and DOUGLASS, R. C.: Combined Inheritance of Purpura Simplex and Ptosis in Four Generations of One Family, Blood, *9*, 1199, 1954.

26. FITZGERALD, E. W., JR.: Fatal Glomerulonephritis Complicating Allergic Purpura

Due to Chlorothiazide, A. M. A. Arch. Int. Med., *105*, 305, 1960.

27. FORSTER, T. W., WATSON, J. W. and NEUMARK, E.: Agranulocytosis and Thrombocytopenia Following the Use of Tridione, Lancet, *1*, 517, 1949.

28. FOX, M. J. and ENZER, N.: A Consideration of the Phenomenon of Purpura Following Scarlet Fever, Am. J. M. Sc., *196*, 321, 1938.

29. FRANK, E.: Die essentielle Thrombopenie, Berl. klin. Wchnschr., *52*, 454, 490, 1915.

29a. FRICK, P. G.: Hemorrhagic Diathesis with Increased Capillary Fragility Caused by Salicylate Therapy, Am. J. M. Sc., *231*, 402, 1956.

30. GAIRDNER, D.: The Schönlein-Henoch Syndrome (Anaphylactoid Purpura), Quart. J. Med., *17*, 95, 1948.

30a. GALY, P., FAVRE-GILLY, J. and MOREL, P.: Purpura Thrombocytopénique au Début du Traitement d'une Tuberculose Hématogène par la Streptomycine, Sang, *20*, 357, 1949.

30b. GANGAROSA, E. J., JOHNSON, THELMA R. and RAMOS, H. S.: Ristocetin-Induced Thrombocytopenia: Site and Mechanism of Action, A. M. A. Arch. Int. Med., *105*, 83, 1960; *Antibiotics Annual*, New York, Antibiotica, Inc., 1959–1960, p. 536.

30c. GARDNER, F. H. and DIAMOND, L. K.: Auto-erythrocyte Sensitization—A Form of Purpura Producing Painful Bruising following Autosensitization to Red Blood Cells in Certain Women, Blood, *10*, 675, 1955.

30d. GARDNER, F. H., HOWELL, D. and HIRSCH, E. O.: Platelet Transfusions Utilizing Plastic Equipment, J. Lab. & Clin. Med., *43*, 196, 1954.

31. GARRETT, J. V., GILES, H. McC., COOMBS, R. R. A. and GURNER, B. W.: Neonatal Purpura with Platelet Iso-Antibody in Maternal Serum, Lancet, *1*, 521, 1960.

31a. GASSER, C. and DE MURALT, G.: Purpura fulminans mit Faktor- V-Mangel und Heilung durch Blutaustauschtransfusion, Helv. paed. acta, *5*, 364, 1950.

32. GEIGER, A. J.: Purpura Hæmorrhagica With Cerebrospinal Hemorrhage, J.A.M.A., *102*, 1000, 1934.

33. GILON, E., RAMOT, B. and SHEBA, C.: Multiple Hemangiomata Associated with Thrombocytopenia, Blood, *14*, 74, 1959.

34. GLANZMANN, E.: Die Konception der anaphylaktoiden Purpura, Jahrb. Kinderh., *91*, 391, 1920.

35. ———— Problem of Fulminating Purpura, Schweiz. med. Wchnschr., *67*, 829, 1937.

36. GOLDBURGH, H. L. and GOULEY, B. A.: Postpubertal Menorrhagia and Its Possible Relations to Thrombocytopenic Purpura Hemorrhagica, Am. J. M. Sc., *200*, 499, 1940.

37. GOODNER, K. and HORSFALL, F. L., JR.: The Purpuric Reaction Produced in Animals by Derivatives of the Pneumococcus, Proc. Soc. Exper. Biol. & Med., *37*, 178, 1937.

37a. GOTTLIEB, P. M., STUPNIKER, SONIA, SANDBERG, H. and WOLDOW, I.: Erythrocyte Auto-Sensitization, Am. J. M. Sc., *233*, 196, 1957.

37b. GRACE, W. J.: Thrombocytopenia in a Patient Taking Chlorpropamide, New England J. Med., *260*, 711, 1959.

38. GRACIE, J.: Henoch's Purpura, Practitioner, *113*, 419, 1924.

39. GRAM, H. C.: Purpura Cured by Shock Treatment, Ztschr. klin. Med., *95*, 51, 1922.

40. GRANT, D. K.: Diagnosis of "Sedormid" Purpura, Brit. M. J., *2*, 128, 1953.

40a. GREEN, T. W. and EARLY, J. Q.: Thrombocytopenic Purpura Resulting from Sulfisoxazole (Gantrisin) Therapy, J. A. M. A., *161*, 1563, 1956.

40b. GREGG, J. A. and MAYOCK, R. L.: Thrombocytopenia Induced by Administration of Sodium Para-Aminosalicylate, J. A. M. A., *172*, 1909, 1960.

40c. GUREVITCH, J. and NELKEN, D.: ABO Groups in Blood Platelets, J. Lab. & Clin. Med., *44*, 562, 1954; *ibid.*, *46*, 530, 1955.

41. HANDEL, J. and SCHWARTZ, S.: Gastrointestinal Manifestations of the Schönlein-Henoch Syndrome, Am. J. Roentgenol., *78*, 643, 1957.

41a. HANRAHAN, E. M., JR. and MILLER, S. R.: Effect of Splenectomy in Felty's Syndrome, J.A.M.A., *99*, 1247, 1932.

41b. HARRINGTON, W. J.: Therapy of the Purpuras, J. Chron. Dis., *6*, 365, 1957.

42. HARRINGTON, W. J., MINNICH, VIRGINIA and ARIMURA, GRACE: The Autoimmune Thrombocytopenias, *in Progress in Hematology*, Grune & Stratton, 1956, p. 166.

42a. HARRINGTON, W. J., MINNICH, V., HOLLINGSWORTH, J. W. and MOORE, C. V.: Demonstration of a Thrombocytopenic Factor in the Blood of Patients with Thrombocytopenic Purpura, J. Lab. & Clin. Med., *38*, 1, 1951; Ann. Int. Med., *38*, 433, 1953; Sang, *25*, 712, 1954.

42b. HARTMANN, E.: Über das Verhalten der Blutplättchen beim Typhus abdominalis, Deutsch. Arch. klin. Med., *158*, 1, 1928.

43. HENOCH, E.: Ueber eine eigenthümliche

Form von Purpura, Berl. klin. Wchnschr., *11*, 641, 1874.

43*a*.HENSTELL, H. H. and KLIGERMAN, MIRIAM: The Complexing of Euglobulin with Factor V, Factor VII and Prothrombin, Ann. Int. Med., *49*, 371, 1958; Nature, *183*, 978, 1959.

43*b*.HERTZOG, A. J.: Essential Thrombocytopenic Purpura. Autopsy Findings in 36 Cases, J. Lab. & Clin. Med., *32*, 618, 1947.

43*c*.HESS, A. F.: Blood and Blood Vessels in Hemophilia and Other Hemorrhagic Diseases, Arch. Int. Med., *18*, 203, 1916.

43*d*.HILL, J. M. and LOEB, ELLEN: Massive Hormonal Therapy and Splenectomy in Acute Thrombotic Thrombocytopenic Purpura, J. A. M. A., *173*, 778, 1960.

43*e*.HIRSCH, E. O. and DAMESHEK, W.: "Idiopathic" Thrombocytopenia, Arch. Int. Med., *88*, 701, 1951.

44. HOLOUBEK, J. E., HENDRICK, J. V. and HOLLIS, W. J.: Toluidine Blue in Bleeding Associated With Thrombopenia, J.A.M.A., *139*, 214, 1949.

44*a*.HORLER, A. R. and TRUELOVE, S. C.: Chronic Leg Ulcers in Nonthrombocytopenic Purpura, Brit. M. J., *1*, 635, 1955.

44*b*.HUDSON, J. B., WEINSTEIN, L. and CHANG, T.-W.: Thrombocytopenic Purpura in Measles, J. Pediat., *48*, 48, 1956.

44*c*.HUGH-JONES, K., MANFIELD, P. A. and BREWER, H. F.: Congenital Thrombocytopenic Purpura, Arch. Dis. Childhood, *35*, 146, 1960.

44*d*.HURD, R. W. and JACOX, R. F.: Thrombopenic Purpura Developing as a Complication of Sulfathiazole and Sulfadiazine Therapy, J.A.M.A., *122*, 296, 1943.

45. IKEDA, K.: Blood in Smallpox During Recent Epidemic, Arch. Int. Med., *37*, 660, 1926.

46. IMERMAN, S. W. and IMERMAN, C. P.: Dinitrophenol Poisoning, J.A.M.A., *106*, 1085, 1936.

46*a*.ISRAEL, L., MATHÉ, G. et BERNARD, J.: Sur le syndrome de Schönlein-Henoch, Rev. franc. études clin. et biol., *1*, 57, 1956.

47*a*.JONES, R. H., JR. and MOORE, W. W.: Purpuric Manifestations of Rheumatic Fever and Acute Glomerulonephritis, Am. Heart J., *32*, 529, 1946.

49. JONES, H. W. and TOCANTINS, L.: The History of Purpura Hemorrhagica, Ann. Med. Hist., *5*, 349, 1933 (Bibliography).

50. KAHN, E. and STEIN, H.: Purpura in Kwashiorkor, Brit. M. J., *2*, 66, 1959.

51. KAHN, I. S.: Henoch's Purpura Due to Food Allergy, J. Lab. & Clin. Med., *14*, 835, 1929.

52. KARPINSKI, F. E.: Purpura Following Exposure to DDT, J. Pediat., *37*, 373, 1950.

53. KAZNELSON, P.: Verschwinden der hämorrhagischen Diathese bei einem Falle von essentieller Thrombopenie (Frank) nach Milzextirpation, Wien. klin. Wchnschr., *29*, 145, 1916.

55. KELLAWAY, C. H.: Snake Venom, Bull. Johns Hopkins Hosp., *60*, 1, 1937.

55*a*.KISSMEYER-NIELSEN, F.: Thrombocytopenic Purpura following Quinine Medication, Acta med. scandinav., *154*, 289, 1956.

55*b*.KLIMA, R.: Treatment of Thrombopenic Purpura, Klin. Wchnschr., *15*, 921, 1936.

56. KOLARS, C. P. and SPINK, W. W.: Thrombopenic Purpura as a Complication of Mumps, J. A. M. A., *168*, 2213, 1958.

56*a*.KRACKE, R. R. and TOWNSEND, E. W.: The Effect of Sulfonamide Drugs on the Blood Platelets, J.A.M.A., *122*, 168, 1943.

56*b*.KREVANS, J. R. and JACKSON, D. P.: Hemorrhagic Disorder following Massive Whole Blood Transfusions, J. A. M. A., *159*, 171, 1955.

57. KUGELMASS, I. N.: Thrombocytopenic Purpura Induced by Pertussis Toxin in Allergic Children, J.A.M.A., *107*, 2120, 1936.

59. LANDSBERGER, M.: Allergy to Cow's Milk in Infant With Purpura, Ztschr. Kinderh., *39*, 569, 1925.

60. LAPP, R.: Purpura Thrombopénique par Tuberculose de la Rate, Rev. suisse Tubercul., *6*, 235, 1949.

61. LEITNER, S. J., NEUMARK, E. and HEERES, P. A.: Panmyelopathy with Döhle Bodies, Thrombocytopenia and Erythroblastosis (Hegglin's Syndrome), Acta hæmat., *11*, 321, 1954.

62. LEONARD, M. E. and FALCONER, E. H.: Experimental Thrombocytopenic Purpura in the Guinea Pig, J. Lab. & Clin. Med., *26*, 648, 1941.

62*a*.LEVINE, R., HOLCOMB, T. M. and LUTZNER, M. A.: Hemangioma Associated with Thrombocytopenia, A. M. A. Arch. Dermat., *82*, 94, 1960.

63. LEVITAN, B. A.: The Biochemistry and Clinical Application of Vitamin P, New England J. Med., *241*, 780, 1949.

64. LEWIS, I. C.: The Schönlein-Henoch Syndrome Compared with Certain Features of Nephritis and Rheumatism, Arch. Dis. Childhood, *30*, 212, 1955.

64*a*.LITTLE, J. R.: Purpura Fulminans Treated Successfully with Anticoagulation, J. A. M. A., *169*, 36, 1959.

64*b*.LOCKIE, L. M., NORCROSS, B. M. and GEORGE C. W.: Treatment of Two Reactions Due to Gold, J.A.M.A., *133*, 754, 1947.

65. LOEB, V., JR., SEAMAN, W. B. and MOORE, C. V.: The Use of Thorium Dioxide Sol (Thorotrast) in the Roentgenologic Demonstration of Accessory Spleens, Blood, 7, 904, 1952.

66. LONGCOPE, W. T.: Cerebral and Spinal Manifestations of Purpura Hemorrhagica, Med. Clin. North America, 3, 279, 1919.

67. LOWENBURG, H. and GINSBURG, T. M.: Induced Hypercalcemia, J.A.M.A., 106, 1779, 1936.

67a. LOZNER, E. L.: The Thrombocytopenic Purpuras, Bull. New York Acad. Med., 30, 184, 1954.

67b. MACAULAY, D.: Thrombocytopenia following Sulphadimidine, Brit. M. J., 2, 1269, 1954.

67c. MACFARLANE, R. G.: The Mechanism of Hæmostasis, Quart. J. Med., 10, 1, 1941.

68a. MALINVAUD, G., DAUSSET, J., et LAYANI, F.: Purpura thrombopénique aigue aux dérivés de l'antipyrine, Sang, 26, 130, 1955.

68b. MARSHALL, A. H. E. and ADAMS, C. W. M.: An Unusual Form of Lipidosis Associated with Thrombocytopenia and Angiomata of the Spleen, J. Path. & Bact., 76, 159, 1958.

69. MCLEAN, S., KREIDEL, K. and CAFFEY. J.: Hemorrhagic Thrombocytopenia in Childhood, J.A.M.A., 98, 387, 1932.

70. MCMICHAEL, J.: Splenic Anæmia, Edinburgh M. J., 42, 97, 1935.

70a. MENDEL, E. B. and SPARKMAN, R.: Idiopathic Thrombocytopenic Purpura in Pregnancy, J. Internat. Coll. Surgeons, 28, 156, 1957.

71. METTIER, S. R.: Classification and Treatment of the Hemorrhagic States, J.A.M.A., 108, 83, 1937.

71a. METZ, J., KRAMER, S. and CASSEL, R.: Acute Idiopathic Thrombocytopenia in the Bantu, South African J. M. Sc., 23, 93, 1958.

72. MEYER, J. and PARKER, M.: Subarachnoid Hemorrhage in a Case of Purpura Hemorrhagica, Med. Clin. North America, 13, 1205, 1930.

72a. MICHON, P., LARCAN, A., STREIFF, F. and REMIGY, E.: La diathèse hémorragique de la macroglobulinémie de Waldenstrom, Sang, 30, 477, 1959.

73. MIKULOWSKI, V.: Contributions a l'étude du purpura hémorragique de la coqueluche, Sang, 27, 461, 1956.

73a. MILLS, S. D. and WINKELMANN, R. K.: Eczema, Thrombocytopenic Purpura and Recurring Infections, A. M. A. Arch. Dermat., 79, 466, 1959.

74. MINOT, G. R.: Purpura Hemorrhagica with Lymphocytosis; an Acute Type and an Intermittent Menstrual Type, Am. J. M. Sc., 192, 455, 1936.

74a. MOESCHLIN, S.: Die Sedormid-Thrombozytopenie anhand von Sternalpunktaten, Belastungs und Transfusionsversuchen, Schweiz. med. Wchnschr., 72, 119, 1942.

75. MOORE, R. D. and SCHOENBERG, M. D.: A Polysaccharide Component in the Vascular Lesions of Thrombotic Thrombocytopenic Purpura, Blood, 15, 511, 1960.

76. MORRIS, M. B.: Thrombocytopenic Purpura in the Newborn, Arch. Dis. Childhood, 29, 75, 1954.

76a. NAJEAN, Y., LARRIEU, M. J. and BERNARD, J.: Survie des plaquettes marquées au radiochrome, Nouv. rev. fr. d'hémat., 1, 36, 1961.

77. NEUMANN, H. O.: Vitamin C Therapie bei profusen Genital-Blutungen infolge essentieller Thrombopenie, Klin. Wchnschr., 15, 368, 1936.

77a. NEVILLE, M. L. and MASTERMAN, L. M.: Neonatal Thrombocytopenic Purpura in Two Infants, Arch. Dis. Childhood, 29, 163, 1954.

77b. NEWCOMB, P. B. and DEANE, C. W.: Thiourea Causing Granulopenia and Thrombopenia, Lancet, 1, 179, 1944.

77c. NEWTON, W. A., JR. and ZUELZER, W. W.: Idiopathic Thrombopenic Purpura in Childhood, New England J. Med., 245, 879, 1951.

78. NICKERSON, D. A. and SUNDERLAND, D. A.: The Histopathology of Idiopathic Thrombocytopenic Purpura Hemorrhagica, Am. J. Path., 13, 463, 1937.

78a. NORKIN, S. and WIENER, J.: Henoch-Schönlein Syndrome, Am. J. Clin. Path., 33, 55, 1960.

78b. OPPENHEIM, M. and DE MEYER, G.: Granulo-und Thrombocytopenie infolge Streptomycin-Behandlung, Schweiz. med. Wchnschr., 79, 1187, 1949.

79. OSLER, W.: Visceral Lesions of Purpura and Allied Conditions, Brit. M. J., 1, 517, 1914.

80. PECK, S. M., ROSENTHAL, N. and ERF, L.: Purpura, Arch. Dermat., 35, 831, 1937.

81. PEPPER, O. H. P.: Hematology of Subacute Streptococcus Viridans Endocarditis, J.A.M.A., 89, 1377, 1927.

81a. PERLMAN, L. and FOX, T. A.: Hemorrhagic Diatheses, Arch. Int. Med., 68, 112, 1941.

82. PESHKIN, M. M. and MILLER, J. A.: Quinine and Ergot Allergy and Thrombocytopenic Purpura, J.A.M.A., 102, 1737, 1934.

82a. PETERS, G. A. and HORTON, B. T.: Allergic Purpura with Special Reference to Hypersensitiveness to Cold, Proc. Staff Meeting, Mayo Clinic, *16*, 631, 1941.

82*b*.PHILLIPS, C. W., JR., KIMBROUGH, G. T., WEAVER, J. A. and TUCKER, A. L.: Rocky Mountain Spotted Fever with Thrombocytopenia, South. M. J., *53*, 867, 1960.

83. PHILLIPS, R. A., ROBERTSON, D. F., CORSON, W. C. and IRWIN, G. F.: The Effect of Irradiated Ergosterol on the Thrombocytes and the Coagulation of the Blood, Ann. Int. Med., *4*, 1134, 1931.

84. PHILPOTT, M. G.: The Schönlein-Henoch Syndrome in Childhood with Particular Reference to the Occurrence of Nephritis, Arch. Dis. Childhood, *27*, 480, 1952.

84*a*.PISCIOTTA, A. V., STEFANINI, M. and DAMESHEK, W.: Morphologic Characteristics of Megakaryocytes by Phase Contrast Microscopy in Normals and in Patients with Idiopathic Thrombocytopenic Purpura, Blood, *8*, 703, 1953.

85. PRESLEY, S. J., BEST, W. R. and LIMARZI, L. R.: Bone Marrow in Idiopathic Thrombocytopenic Purpura, J. Lab. & Clin. Med., *40*, 503, 1952.

85*a*.PROPP, S., SCHARFMAN, W. B., BEEBE, R. T. and WRIGHT, A. W.: Atypical Amyloidosis Associated with Nonthrombocytopenic Purpura and Plasmocytic Hyperplasia of the Bone Marrow, Blood, *9*, 397, 1954.

85*b*.QUICK, A. J., SHANBERGE, J. C. and STEFANINI, M.: The Coagulation Defect in Thrombocytopenic Purpura, J. Lab. & Clin. Med., *34*, 761, 1949.

85*c*.RABINOWITZ, Y. and DAMESHEK, W.: Systemic Lupus Erythematosus after "Idiopathic" Thrombocytopenic Purpura, Ann. Int. Med., *52*, 1, 1960.

85*d*.RAPPOPORT, A. E., NIXON, C. W. and BARKER, W. A.: Fatal Secondary, Toxic Thrombocytopenic Purpura Due to Sodium Salicylate, J. Lab. & Clin. Med., *30*, 916, 1945.

85*e*.RATNOFF, O. D. and AGLE, D. P.: Psychiatric Patterns in Patients with a Peculiar Protracted Purpura, Tr. A. Am. Physicians, 1961.

86. REGAMEY, E.: Acute Attack of Thrombocytopenic Purpura Consecutive to a Late Vaccinial Generalization, Schweiz. med. Wchnschr., *70*, 697, 1940.

86*a*.RIVAS, F. D.: Vicarious Bleeding, Ann. Int. Med., *50*, 811, 1959.

86*b*.ROBERTS, M. H. and SMITH, M. H.: Thrombopenic Purpura, Am. J. Dis. Child., *79*, 820, 1950.

87. ROBSON, H. N.: Idiopathic Thrombocytopenic Purpura, Quart. J. Med., N. S., *18*,

279, 1949; Brit. M. J., *2*, 971, 1950; Med. J. Australia, *1*, 516, 1954.

88. RONCHESE, F.: Dermatorrhexis—With Dermatochalasis and Arthrochalasis (the Socalled Ehler-Danlos Syndrome), Am. J. Dis. Child., *51*, 1403, 1936.

90. ROSENFELD, S. and LENKE, S. E.: Tiger Snake Venom in the Treatment of Accessible Hemorrhage, Am. J. M. Sc., *190*, 779, 1935.

91. ROSENTHAL, N.: The Course and Treatment of Thrombopenic Purpura, J.A.M.A., *112*, 101, 1939.

92. ROSKAM, J.: Pathogénie de la prolongation des hémorrhagies dan les syndromes hémogéniques et dans l'hémophilie vraie, Presse méd., *31*, 972, 1923.

96. RUBIN, M. I.: Allergic Intestinal Bleeding in the Newborn, Am. J. M. Sc., *200*, 385, 1940.

96*a*.RUITER, M.: Angiokeratoma Corporis Diffusum, Excerpta Medica, *13*, 61, 1959.

97. RUSHMORE, S.: Purpura Complicating Pregnancy, Am. J. Obst. & Gynec., *10*, 553, 1925.

97*a*.SALTZMAN, G. F.: Pregnancy in Essential Thrombocytopenia, Acta med. scandinav., *133*, 221, 1949.

97*b*.SAUER, A. J. and VAN LOGHEM, J. J.: Platelet Auto-antibodies and Hæmorrhagic Disease in the Newborn, Vox sanguinis, *5*, 45, 1955.

97*c*.SCHARFMAN, W. B., HOSLEY, H. F., HAWKINS, T. and PROPP, S.: Idiopathic Thrombocytopenic Purpura, J.A.M.A., *172*, 1875, 1960.

98. SCHERZ, R. G., LOURO, J. M. and GEPPERT, L. J.: Giant Hemangioendothelioma with Associated Thrombocytopenia, J. Pediat., *52*, 212, 1958.

99. SCHEN, R. J. and RABINOVITZ, M.: Thrombocytopenic Purpura Due to Quinidine, Brit. M. J., *2*, 1502, 1958.

100. SCHIFF, E. and HIRSCHBERGER, C.: Thrombocytosis Produced by the Fat Soluble T Factor, Am. J. Dis. Child., *53*, 1, 1937.

100*a*.SCHOEN, E. J., KING, A. L. and DUANE, R. T.: Neonatal Thrombocytopenic Purpura, Pediatrics, *17*, 72, 1956.

101. SCHÖNLEIN, J. L.: Allgemeine und specielle Pathologie und Therapie, *2*, 45, 1837.

101*a*.SCHRUMPF, A.: BAL Therapy of Thrombopenic Purpura After Arsphenamine Treatment, J.A.M.A., *135*, 1152, 1947.

101*b*.SCHULMAN, I., PIERCE, MILA, LUKENS, ABBY and CURRIMBHOY, Z.: A Factor in Normal Human Plasma Required for Platelet Production; Chronic Thrombocytopenia Due to its Deficiency, Blood, *16*, 943, 1960.

102. SCHULTZ, W.: Die purpuraerkrankungen, Ergebn. inn. Med. u. Kinderh., *16*, 32, 1919 (Bibliography).

102a.SCHWARTZ, M. and VONDERHEIDE, E. C.: Thrombocytopenic Purpura Due to Mapharsen (Oxophenarsine Hydrochloride— U. S. P.), J.A.M.A., *128*, 657, 1945.

102b.SCHWARTZ, M. J. and NORTON, W. S., II: Thrombocytopenia and Leukopenia Associated with Use of Sulfamethoxypyridazine, J.A.M.A., *167*, 457, 1958.

102c.SEINFELD, R. H., HENNINGAR, G. and HELLMAN, L. M.: Purpura Fulminans Complicating Pregnancy, Am. J. Obst. & Gynec., *80*, 161, 1960.

102d.SHAW, S. and OLIVER, R. A. M.: Congenital Hypoplastic Thrombocytopenia with Skeletal Deformities in Siblings, Blood, *14*, 374, 1959.

102e.SHUSTER, and SCARBOROUGH, H.: Senile Purpura, Quart. J. Med., *30*, 33, 1961.

103. SHRAGER, J. and KEAN, B. H.: Purpura as a Complication of Malaria, Am. J. M. Sc., *212*, 54, 1946.

103a.SHUMWAY, C. N., JR. and MILLER, G.: An Unusual Syndrome of Hemolytic Anemia, Thrombocytopenic Purpura and Renal Disease, Blood, *12*, 1045, 1957.

103b SILBER, R. et al.: The Application of Fluorescent Antibody Methods to the Study of Platelets, Blood, *16*, 958, 1960.

103c.SINGER, K. and ROTTER, R.: Studies on Thrombocytopen. I. A Reliable Test for this Principle in Organ Homogenates and in Urine, J. Lab. & Clin. Med., *34*, 1336, 1949.

103d.SKOOG, W. A., LAWRENCE, J. S. and ADAMS, W. S.: A Metabolic Study of a Patient with Idiopathic Cyclical Thrombocytopenic Purpura, Blood, *12*, 844, 1957.

103e.SMITH, W. T. and WHITFIELD, A. G. W.: Intra-vascular Micro-embolic Carcinomatosis As a Cause of Purpura. Report of a Case Associated with Focal Histological Lesions in the Nervous System, Brit. J. Cancer, *8*, 97, 1954.

104. SOULIER, J. P. and LARRIEU, M. J.: Tests de l'hémostase dans l'étude des purpuras thrombopéniques, Sang, *28*, 113, 1957.

104a.SPRING, M.: Purpura and Nephritis after Administration of Procaine Penicillin, J.A.M.A., *147*, 1139, 1951.

105. SQUIER, T. L. and MADISON, F. W.: Thrombocytopenic Purpura Due to Food Allergy, J. Allergy, *8*, 143, 1937.

105a.STEINER, P. E. and GUNN, F. D.: Response of Blood Platelets to External Stimuli; Ultraviolet Light, Iodine and Coal Tar, Arch. Path., *11*, 241, 1931.

105b.STEINHARDT, I. D. and JONAS, A. F.; Coexistence of Intussusception and Henoch's Purpura, New England J. Med., *257*, 553, 1957.

106. STEFANINI, M., CHATTERJEA, J. B., DAMESHEK, W., ZANNOS, L. and SANTIAGO, E. P.: Studies on Platelets, Blood, 7, 53 and 289, 1952; Proc. Soc. Exper. Biol. & Med., *79*, 623, 1952; J. Lab. & Clin. Med., *39*, 865, 1952; Blood, 7, 700, 1952; Proc. Soc. Exper. Biol. & Med., *80*, 230, 1952; Am. J. Clin. Path., *22*, 1164, 1952; Blood, *8*, 26, 1953; J. Lab. & Clin. Med., *42*, 723, 1953; Sang, *26*, 83, 1955.

106a.STEFANINI, M. and DAMESHEK, W.: *The Hemorrhagic Disorders*, New York, Grune & Stratton, 1955.

106b.STEFFEN, C.: Isolierung von Thrombozyten-Autoantikörpern und Untersuchung über die passiv übertragbare thrombopenische Wirkung der Eluate im Tierversuch, Internat. Arch. Allergy, *13*, 348, 1958.

106c.STERKY, G. and THILÉN, A.: A Study on the Onset and Prognosis of Acute Vascular Purpura (the Schönlein-Henoch Syndrome) in Children, Acta paediat., *49*, 217, 1960.

107. STETSON, R. P. and FERRIS, H. W.: Hemochromatosis and Purpura, Arch. Int. Med., *50*, 232, 1932.

107a.STRANGWAY, W. E. and STRANGWAY, A. K.: Ascorbic Acid Deficiency in the African Disease Onyalai, Arch. Int. Med., *83*, 372, 1949.

107b.STRAUSS, W. G.: Purpura Hyperglobulinemica of Waldenström, New England J. Med., *260*, 857, 1959.

107c.STROEBEL, C. F., CAMPBELL, D. C. and HAGEDORN, A. B.: The Problem of Essential Thrombocytopenic Purpura, Med. Clin. N. Am., *33*, 1027, 1949.

108. STRÖM, J.: Thrombocytopenic Purpura (Werlhof's Disease) in the First Year of Life, Acta pædiat., *19*, 540, 1937.

108a.STRONG, P. S. and GLASSBURN, E. M.: Thrombocytopenic Purpura Following the Use of Sulfathiazole, Ann. Int. Med., *23*, 237, 1945.

109. TAGER, M. and KLINGHOFFER, K. A.: Acute Thrombocytopenic Purpura Hemorrhagica With Lymphocytosis, Ann. Int. Med., *18*, 96, 1943.

109a.TATTERSALL, R. N. and SEVILLE, R.: Senile Purpura, Quart. J. Med., *19*, 151, 1950.

109b.TAYLOR, F. E. and BATTLE, J. D., JR.: Benign Hyperglobulinemic Purpura, Ann. Int. Med., *40*, 350, 1954.

109c.THOMPSON, M., SINCLAIR, R. J. G. and DUTHIE, J. J. R.: Thrombocytopenic Purpura after Administration of Gold, Brit. M. J., *1*, 899, 1954.

110. TROLAND, C. E. and LEE, F. C.: Thrombocytopen, J.A.M.A., *111*, 221, 1938; J. Lab. & Clin. Med., *26*, 1266, 1941.

111. VANDENBROUCKE, J. and VERSTRAETE, M.: Thrombocytopenia Due to Platelet Agglutinins in the Newborn, Lancet, *1*, 593, 1955.

111a.VERNIER, R. L. *et al.:* Anaphylactoid Purpura. I. Pathology of the Skin and Kidney and Frequency of Streptococcal Infection, Pediatrics, *27*, 181, 1961.

112. WAGNER, E.: Purpura und Erythem, Deutsch. Arch. klin. Med., *39*, 431, 1886.

112a.WALDENSTRÖM, J.: Zwei interessante Syndrome mit Hyperglobulinämie, Schweiz. Med. Wchnschr., *78*, 927, 1948.

112b.WATSON-WILLIAMS, E. J., MACPHERSON, A. I. S. and DAVIDSON, S.: The Treatment of Idiopathic Thrombocytopenic Purpura, Lancet, 2, 221, 1958.

112c.WEDGEWOOD, R. J. P. and KLAUS, M. H.: Anaphylactoid Purpura (Schönlein-Henoch Syndrome)—A Long-term Follow-up Study with Special Reference to Renal Involvement, Pediatrics, *16*, 196, 1955.

113. WEISFUSE, L., SPEAR, P. W. and SASS, M.: Quinidine-induced Thrombocytopenic Purpura, Am. J. Med., *17*, 414, 1954.

113a.WILLIS, W. H.: Thrombocytopenic Purpura and Carcinoma of Stomach, Ann. Int. Med., *16*, 782, 1942.

114. WILSON, S. J. and DOAN, C. A.: The Pathogenesis of Hemorrhage in Artificially Induced Fever, Ann. Int. Med., *13*, 1214, 1940.

115. WINTROBE, M. M. and BUELL, M. V.: Hyperproteinemia Associated With Multiple Myeloma, Bull. Johns Hopkins Hosp., *52*, 156, 1933.

116. WINTROBE, M. M., HANRAHAN, E. M., JR. and THOMAS, C. B.: Purpura Hæmorrhagica With Special Reference to Course and Treatment, J.A.M.A., *109*, 1170, 1937.

117. WISEMAN, B. K., DOAN, C. A. and WILSON, S. J.: The Present Status of Thrombocytopenic Purpura, J.A.M.A., *115*, 8, 1940.

118. WITTS, L. J.: Chronic Leg Ulcer in Purpura Hæmorrhagica, Brit. M. J., *2*, 309, 1942.

118a.WRIGHT, D. O., REPPERT, L. B. and CUTTINS, J. T.: Purpuric Manifestations of Heat Stroke, Arch. Int. Med., *77*, 27, 1946.

119. WOODWARD, T. E.: Thrombocytopenic Purpura Complicating Acute Catarrhal Jaundice, Ann. Int. Med., *19*, 799, 1943.

120. YOUNG, FREIDA: Severe Post-operative Thrombocytopenic Purpura, Brit. M. J., *2*, 919, 1957.

121. WELCH, R. G.: Thrombocytopenic Purpura and Chickenpox, Arch. Dis. Childhood, *31*, 38, 1956.

122. ZUCKER, MARJORIE B. *et al.:* Thrombocytopenia with a Circulating Platelet Agglutinin, Platelet Lysin and Clot Retraction Inhibitor, Blood, *14*, 148, 1959.

Thrombocytopathic Purpuras

123. ACHENBACH, W.: Angiohämophilie, Ergebn. inn. Med. u. Kinderh., *14*, 68, 1960.

125. ALEXANDER, B. and LANDWEHR, G.: Thrombasthenia and Thrombocytopenic Purpura, New England J. Med., *241*, 965, 1949; J. Clin. Invest., *32*, 551, 1953.

126. BENNEY, W. E. and LEWIS, F. J. W.: Christmas Factor (IX) Defect in a Case of Haemorrhagic Thrombocythaemia, J. Clin. Path., *12*, 551, 1959.

127. BERNARD, J., BEAUMONT, J.-L. and CHARREYRON, M. C.: Etude de la fonction thromboplastique des plaquettes dans deux cas de dystrophie thrombocytaire hémorragipare congénitale, Rev. hémat., *8*, 20, 1953; *ibid.*, *12*, 222, 1957.

129. BRAUNSTEINER, H. and PAKESCH, F.: Thrombocytoasthenia and Thrombocytopathia— Old Names and New Diseases, Blood, *11*, 965, 1956.

130. CAHALANE, S. F., JOHNSON, S. A., MONTO, R. W. and CALDWELL, M. JUNE: Acquired Thrombocytopathy, Am. J. Clin. Path., *30*, 507, 1958.

131. CAZAL, P. and IZARN, P.: Considération sur la pseudo-hémophilie de Willebrand, Acta haemat., *4*, 357, 1950.

131a.CETINGIL, A. I., ULUTIN, O. N. and KARACA, M.: A Platelet Defect in a Case of Scurvy, Brit. J. Haemat. *4*, 350, 1958.

131b.DIDISHEIM, P.: Unpublished Observations, 1960.

132. ESTREN, S., SANCHEZ-MÉDAL, L. and DAMESHEK, W.: Pseudohemophilia, Blood, *1*, 504, 1946.

133. FRICK, P. G., BACKMANN, F. and DUCKERT, F.: Vascular Anomaly Associated with Plasma Thromboplastin Antecedent Deficiency, J. Lab. & Clin. Med., *54*, 680, 1959.

134. GLANZMANN, E.: Hereditäre hämorrhagische Thrombasthenie, Ann. Paediatrici, *88*, 113, 1918.

134a.GROSS, R. *et al.:* Über die Natur der Thrombasthenie, klin. Wchnschr., *38*, 193, 1960.

135. GUGLER, E.: Angiohämophilie, Schweiz. med. Wchnschr., *90*, 534 and 563, 1960.

136. GUNZ, F. W.: Hemorrhagic Thrombocythemia, Blood, *15*, 706, 1960.

137. HERMANSKY, F. and PUDLAK, P.: Albinism

Associated with Hemorrhagic Diathesis and Unusual Pigmented Reticular Cells in the Bone Marrow, Blood, *14*, 162, 1959.

138. HIRSCH, E. O., FAVRE-GILLY, J. and DAMESHEK, W.: Thrombopathic Thrombocytopenia, Blood, *5*, 568, 1950.

139. JOHNSON, S. A., MONTO, R. W. and CALDWELL, M. JUNE: A New Approach to the Thrombocytopathies. Thrombocytopathy A, Thromb. Diath. haemorrh., *2*, 279, 1958.

140. JÜRGENS, R.: Die erblichen Thrombopathien, Ergebn. inn. Med. u. Kinderh., *53*, 795, 1937; Schweiz. med. Wchnschr., *80*, 1098, 1950; Thromb. Diath. haemorrh.. *2*, 300, 1958.

141. LELONG, M. and SOULIER, J. P.; Sur une maladie hémorrhagique constitutionnelle caractérisée par l'allongement isolé du temps de saignement, Rev. hémat., *5*, 13, 1950.

142. LEVINSON, B., JONES, R. S., WINTROBE, M. M. and CARTWRIGHT, G. E.: Thrombocythemia and Pulmonary Intra-Alveolar Coagulum in a Young Woman, Blood, *13*, 959, 1958.

143. LEWIS, JESSICA H., ZUCKER, MARJORIE B. and FERGUSON, J. H.: Bleeding Tendency in Uremia, Blood, *11*, 1073, 1956.

144. LÜDIN, H.: Zur Klinik und Therapie der Thrombocythämie, Schweiz. med. Wchnschr., *89*, 1043, 1959.

146. MACFARLANE, J. C. W. and SIMPKISS, M. J.: The Investigation of a Large Family Affected with von Willebrand's Disease, Arch. Dis. Childhood, *29*, 483, 1954.

147. MATTER, M., NEWCOMB, T. F., MELLY, A. and FINCH, C. A.: Vascular Hemophilia: the Association of a Vascular Defect with a Deficiency of Antihemophilic Globulin, Am. J. M. Sc., *232*, 421, 1956.

148. NILSSON, INGA MARIE, BLOMBÄCK, MARGARETA and VON GRANCKEN, IRENE: On an Inherited Autosomal Hemorrhagic Diathesis with Antihemophilic Globulin(AHG)

Deficiency and Prolonged Bleeding Time, Acta med. scandinav., *159*, 35 and 179, 1957; *ibid.*, *164*, 263, 1959.

149. OZER, F. L., TRUAX, W. E., MIESCH, D. C. and LEVIN, W. C.: Primary Hemorrhagic Thrombocythemia, Am. J. Med., *28*, 807, 1960.

150. RACCUGLIA, G. and NEEL, J. V.: Congenital Vascular Defect Associated with Platelet Abnormality and Antihemophilic Factor Deficiency, Blood, *15*, 807, 1960.

151. SCHULMAN, I. *et al.:* Vascular Hemophilia, Pediatrics, *18*, 347, 1956.

153. SHARP, A. A. and ELLIS, H.: Haemoperitoneum in von Willebrand's Disease, Brit. M. J., *2*, 356, 1960.

154. SOKAL, G., VERSTRAETE, M. and VERMYLEN, C.: Diathèse hémorragique familiale par déficience qualitative des plaquettes sanguines, Acta haemat., *22*, 165, 1959.

155. SOULIER, J.-P.: Syndromes hémorrhagiques avec atteinte isolée de la résistance capillaire, Sang, *21*, 801, 1950; *ibid.*, *25*, 355, 1954.

156. SOULIER, J. P. and LARRIEU, M. J.: Syndrome de Willebrand-Jürgens et thrombopathies, Rev. d'hémat., *9*, 77, 1954.

157. ULUTIN, O. N. and KARACA, M.: A Study on the Pathogenesis of Thrombopathia Using the 'Platelet Osmotic-Resistance Test,' Brit. J. Haemat., *5*, 302, 1959.

158. VAN CREVELD, S. and PAULSSEN, M. M. P.: A Form of Haemorrhagic Diathesis Characterised by the Lack of the Third Clotting-Factor, Normally Present in Blood-Platelets (Thrombopathia haemophilica), Ann. paediat., *181*, 193, 1953.

159. VALBERG, L. S. and BROWN, G. M.: Haemorrhagic Capillary Disorder Associated with Antihaemophilic Globulin Deficiency, Medicine, *37*, 181, 1958.

160. VON WILLEBRAND, E. A.: Über hereditäre Pseudohämophilie, Acta med. scandinav., *76*, 521, 1931.

Chapter 18

Hemophilia and Other Hemorrhagic Disorders

HEMOPHILIA

Synonyms and Definition.—Since 1839 the term hemophilia has been used to refer to a constitutional anomaly of blood coagulation which depends on the hereditary transmission of a sex-linked, recessive Mendelian trait, and is characterized by a life-long tendency to prolonged hemorrhage as well as markedly delayed coagulation time in affected males. The bleeding was later found to be due to deficiency of a plasma factor (factor VIII) necessary for coagulation ("antihemophilic globulin," AHG). Later it was discovered that an essentially identical disorder develops as the result of deficiency of a different factor, factor IX ("plasma thromboplastin component," PTC) and that other conditions resembling hemophilia result from deficiency of still other components involved in coagulation or from the action of certain anticoagulants. A great variety of names have been proposed for these disorders many of which incorporate the term hemophilia, such as pseudohemophilia, deuterohemophilia, parahemophilia, and hemophilioid states A, B, C and D.[9] Confusion has arisen because different authors have used the same term in various ways; furthermore, many of the terms have not proved to be helpful since they indicate what they *resemble* rather than what they *are*. The best case for the use of the term hemophilia for more than one condition can be made for factor IX deficiency, for which the name hemophilia B was proposed, since this disorder resembles classical hemophilia (A) so completely. It seems best, however, to continue to use the term hemophilia as it has always been used and to designate the conditions resembling it by the name of the coagulation factor which is lacking.

History.—This form of hemorrhagic diathesis has been recognized for many centuries as a familial type of bleeding which tends to be severe and is sometimes fatal. This is evident from the writings of Rabbi Simon ben Gamaliel (second century A.D.) in the Talmud, of Maimonides, the Hebrew physician and philosopher and of Albucasis, the Arab (twelfth century). The disease was clearly described by Dr. John C. Otto[37] of Philadelphia in 1803, but a more complete collection of cases was furnished by Nasse[35] in 1820. Nasse formulated the law of transmission of hemophilia. The name hemophilia was given to the "bleeder's disease" by Schönlein (1839). A. E. Wright called attention to the prolonged coagulation time in 1893. Early important investigators in this field were Sahli,[50] Addis[1] and Howell.[23] Very complete monographs[7,10,51] cover the early literature. An important advance was made when the antihemophilic globulin was separated from human plasma[3b,40,41] and an unusual opportunity for study of the disorder came when an identical condition was discovered in certain dogs.[20c]

Incidence of Hemophilia and Related Disorders.—Earlier data concerning the occurrence of hemophilia include those for factor IX deficiency since these conditions are clinically indistinguishable from one another. No doubt the data exclude many of the less severe cases. Well known among the people of Europe and their descendants elsewhere, hemophilia has also been reported in Japan[18] but seems to be very rare among Chinese. It is rare in Negroes,[8a] especially in presumably full-blooded ones.[38] Hemophilia has been reported in an American Indian.[39] The existence of the trait in certain royal families of Europe is well known.[9,46a]

All studies have shown a much greater frequency of classical hemophilia than of factor IX deficiency. In an English survey there were 138 cases of hemophilia, 20 factor IX deficiency, two who had developed circulating anticoagulants, three PTA deficiency, 11 von Willebrand's disease and 13 unclassified.[5c] In other reports the ratio has ranged from two to six (average four) cases of hemophilia to one of factor IX deficiency.[21a,25,46a,48a] In several instances both hemophilia and factor IX deficiency have been demonstrated in the same subjects[52a] or in remote branches of the same family,[5c,15b] and hemophilia together with PTA deficiency has been reported.[50b] The discovery of factor VIII deficiency in association with von Willebrand's disease was mentioned earlier (p. 848) and there are also reports of factor IX deficiency accompanied by decreased capillary resistance,[52a,52c] as well as other curious combinations.[21,36a]

Inheritance.—It has long been recognized that hemophilia is a constitutional anomaly which is transmitted as a sex-linked recessive. This means that the factors or genes responsible for its development are contained in the X chromosomes of the reproductive cells (p. 76). The disease is limited to the male but is transmitted from the male through an unaffected daughter to a grandson. The sons of an affected male (Fig. 18–2) are normal themselves and cannot transmit the defect to any of their descendants. The daughters of an affected male, all outwardly normal, are capable of transmitting the trait as an evident defect to half of their sons and as a recessive or hidden characteristic to half of their daughters.

The discovery of an inherited, sex-linked bleeding disorder in dogs which in every respect appears to be identical with human hemophilia[20c] provided a means whereby the genetics of the disorder could be studied. These experiments confirmed the conclusions derived from the study of hemophiliac families and also made possible the deliberate production of **hemophilia in the female.** It had been recognized that this would be theoretically possible if the female were the daughter of a hemophiliac father and a conductor mother: she would thus acquire two X chromosomes which carry the hemophilia gene, one from her father and one from her mother. According to theory, a single chromosome carrying the hemophilia gene in the female would not produce a deficiency of factor VIII because it would be dominated by the unaffected X chromosome.

In addition to the fact that bleeder-conductor marriages could not be expected to have occurred often, it was suspected that the presence of a double quantity of the defect might be lethal and inhibit the development of the embryo.[30] That this is not true is indicated by the successful experimental production of hemophilia in a female dog.[20c] This animal was indistinguishable as far as the clotting defect was concerned from the bleeder male siblings. In retrospect, and with the knowledge that in severe hemophilia in males no factor VIII can be detected in the plasma,[9] one might have assumed that the condition in the female carrying two hemophiliac X chromosomes could not be worse.

Bona fide hemophilia in human females has now been reported in four instances.[24a,33a,45a] The father of one of these was a hemophiliac and her mother was a carrier.[24a] This patient gave birth to a healthy child and only in the puerperium did severe hemorrhage develop. In another well known hemophilia family[10] a similar union produced two female hemophiliacs who manifested symptoms and signs like those in affected male members of the family.[33a] Such cases, although exceedingly rare, are not unexpected. However, exceptions to strict sex linkage in hemophilia are suggested by cases in girls with no family histories of the disease.[8b,36,46d] In two instances sex chromatin studies were carried out. These showed that one of the patients was a male[36] but in the second instance the girl's apparent sex was confirmed.[8b] Factor VIII blood levels and hemorrhagic manifestations in female heterozygotes will be discussed shortly (p. 869).

It might be expected that, with random mating in a large general population a rare defect like hemophilia would tend to die out after several generations. The attempt to explain the lack of a progressive change in the incidence of the disease on the ground that the sex ratio of offspring in families with hemophilia is altered in such a way as to perpetuate the disorder,[6] has not been borne out by further study.[30a] It must be assumed that the defect arises *de novo* as the result of a chance mutation. Such **sporadic cases**[18a,24,46a] mark the beginning of a new hemophiliac strain.[23] It has been estimated that in at least one-third of all cases of hemophilia, no familial antecedents can be demonstrated.[52b]

Hemophilia has been observed several times in twins.[46b] Only in one somewhat equivocal instance has the disorder not appeared in both members of an identical pair.

Additional aspects of the genetics of hemophilia will be considered in connection with the discussion of female carriers of hemophilia (p. 869).

The Hemostatic Abnormality.— It is a familiar observation that normal blood, taken with adequate precautions to avoid contamination with tissue fluid, will clot in a few minutes in a test tube. When blood from a patient with hemophilia is collected in exactly the same way, it may not clot for an hour or more. The hemostatic abnormality has at one time or another been attributed to a vascular defect, a platelet defect[18,34] or a plasma clotting defect. Few investigators now believe that there is a primary vascular defect in classical hemophilia but the curious association of von Willebrand's disease with factor VIII deficiency (p. 848) deserves further study. Hemophiliac platelets were shown to be similar to normal platelets in relation to coagulation, provided a plasma factor was available.[9] The apparent resistance of hemophiliac platelets to aggregation and rupture was found to be the result rather than the cause of the delayed coagulation.[46,56a] Consequently, it is generally considered that the fundamental abnormality is a plasma defect. To explain this there are two main hypotheses; namely, a deficiency in a plasma protein, the antihemophilic factor (factor VIII), or an excess of an inhibitor.

It has been amply demonstrated that fibrinogen,[23,29] prothrombin,[23a] factors V and VII and calcium[23] are normal in hemophilia. Transfusion of normal blood or of plasma filtered free of platelets, produces marked shortening of coagulation time. Even the injection of as little as 30 or 40 ml. of blood will have this effect, which may last several hours or even one or two days.[40] This will occur even if many clotting proteins are first removed from the plasma by $BaSO_4$ adsorption.[9] Tissue extracts, even those derived from hemophiliacs, cause the coagulation of hemophiliac blood.[5b] The active substance can be precipitated from normal plasma following one-fourth saturation with ammonium sulfate or by mild acidification[41] but it is absent or greatly reduced in hemophiliac plasma. Some of the properties of the antihemophilic factor,[27b] now known as factor VIII, were discussed in an earlier chapter (p. 292). Purification factors of 20-[26] to possibly 2000-fold[7b] have been achieved. Plasma from patients with hemophilia corrects the clotting anomaly of other disorders which resemble hemophilia.[9]

According to the alternative hypothesis, an excessive amount of a plasma anticoagulant, possibly antithromboplastin, is responsible for the defect in clotting.[24b,55] Evidence for this hypothesis includes the observation that, when blood was obtained with silicone-coated syringes from hemophiliacs, and was injected without added anticoagulants into compatible normal subjects, a marked prolongation of the clotting time of the recipients occurred.[55] Since tissue thromboplastin in hemophiliacs is normal, it has been suggested that only the formation of the plasma antihemophilic factor is inhibited. However, if this should occur at different stages of its synthesis, various types of hemophilia might be produced.[41a] It has been observed that contact of hemophiliac plasma with asbestos or glass will shorten its clotting time toward normal; an inhibitor is said to be adsorbed from the hemophiliac plasma. This observation has been confirmed in hemophiliac canine plasma.[20c] However, when such plasma was reinfused into hemophiliac dogs, there was no corrective effect on the hemostatic defect. A possible explanation for this observation is that the plasma was once more subjected *in vivo* to the action of the hypothetical inhibitor. Additional experiments which are cited in support of the inhibitor theory are the seeming correction of the clotting defect in hemophiliac plasma if the plasma is diluted or if it is extracted with ether. However, ether-treated, canine hemophiliac plasma failed to correct the hemostatic defect.[20c]

The suggestion that hemophilia is attributable to both a deficiency of factor VIII and the presence of an alleged new anticoagulant ("Bridge")[36b] has not found support in the hands of others.[22c,45c]

There are vigorous proponents of both of these hypotheses. In spite of the general acceptance of the deficiency theory, it cannot as yet be regarded as fully established.

The site of synthesis of factor VIII is unknown. Neither the liver nor the lymphoid tissue seems to play an important part.[9] After intravenous administration to a patient with hemophilia it has been shown to be effective immediately. It disappears rapidly, however, half being gone from the circulation in three to six hours.[26d] With hemorrhagic crises and tissue necrosis, the loss of factor VIII may be even faster. However, *repeated* infusions, at least in canine hemophilia, showed a slower rate of fall.[20c] It has been suggested that injected factor VIII is quickly distributed between the vascular and extravascular compartments and that, once equilibrium has been established between these compartments the rate of loss from the plasma may be slower. The latter may perhaps give a truer index of its biologic half-life.

The role of factor VIII in coagulation was discussed in an earlier chapter (p. 293). The greatly reduced prothrombin consumption of hemophiliac blood is due to the lack of blood thromboplastin, which cannot be formed in the absence of one of the substances (factor VIII) on which its production depends. Observations which suggest a defect in the fibrinolytic activity of hemophiliac blood[16c, 53a] are probably best explained by assuming that antihemophilic globulin may have an action similar to that of proteolytic enzymes such as trypsin or plasmin.[5b]

The development of assay methods for factor VIII has made it possible to detect deficiencies of this substance of less severity than occurs in classical hemophilia.[5a, 9] By these means it has been possible to show that hemophilia is not always as serious a disease as is manifest in the classical condition. This topic, as well as problems related to the stability of factor VIII *in vitro* and its use in therapy, will be discussed later (pp. 869, 873).

What appears to be a mild form of hemophilia with a different mode of inheritance than human hemophilia has been observed in a breed of Poland-China *hogs*.[22a] In these animals both internal and external bleeding as well as joint hemorrhage have been described. The plasma factor VIII content was found to be slightly more than 5 per cent of the normal,[9] the coagulation time was prolonged and the clotting of recalcified plasma was delayed by rapid centrifugation. The defect appears to be inherited as a simple recessive which occurs in and is transmitted by both sexes.

Symptomatology.—Habitual *hemorrhage*, from various parts of the body, either following slight trauma or spontaneous, is the outstanding symptom of the disease.[7] The bleeding is of the nature of persistent slow oozing which is out of all proportion to the extent of the injury. Instead of minutes, hours or days or even weeks measure its duration. The tendency to prolonged bleeding appears almost invariably in early childhood, often in the first year of life but occasionally not until even 13 years of age.[13b] Hemorrhage from the umbilical cord is unusual, perhaps because of "plasma factor" derived from the mother, but prolonged bleeding after circumcision

brought the condition to the attention of the ancient Hebrews.

Subcutaneous and Intramuscular Hemorrhages.—Subcutaneous and intramuscular hemorrhages are common. Subcutaneous bleeding may spread over as much as half the body and does so in a characteristic manner. At the site of origin the tissue is hard, indurated, raised and purplish black. From this center the hemorrhage extends in all directions "like ripples on a pond,"[7] with each successive concentric extension less deeply colored. The point of origin of the hemorrhage may be entirely absorbed while the margin is still progressing.

Petechial hemorrhages are rarely seen and have been noted in only a few very severe hemophiliacs at the peak of an attack of bleeding.[7]

Hematomata may be very serious if they involve areas where the pressure of the large mass may have grave effects; *e.g.*, in the head, or neck, where airway obstruction may develop,[26f] or in a limb where pressure on an artery[32] may lead to gangrene. Volkmann's contracture has been produced by hemorrhage in the forearm. Severe pain and elevation of local and general temperature may be produced by intramuscular bleeding.

Mucous Membrane and Internal Bleeding.—Hemorrhage from the *mouth*, *gums*, *lips*, and *tongue* is common and often serious. The eruption and loss of teeth are often accompanied by bleeding which lasts for days or weeks. Epistaxis occurs in almost all cases. It is more marked before puberty. It may be moderate and frequently repeated, or fulminating.

Gastro-intestinal hemorrhage may take place and is accompanied by abdominal pain, distention, increased peristalsis, fever and leukocytosis. There may be hematemesis or melena, or both. In one of our cases such bleeding followed the ingestion of a peach stone. Even intraperitoneal hemorrhage may occur and, since it is associated with severe pain, an

55

acute abdominal condition may be simulated. Thus, there may be severe upper abdominal pain which may resemble a penetrating or perforated peptic ulcer. Pain in the midabdomen may resemble small bowel obstruction. More common than these is low abdominal pain. This has been described[13b] as being of two types: bleeding into the colon wall or mesocolon with signs of partial bowel obstruction, and bleeding into or around the ileopsoas muscle with pain of rapidly increasing severity. When on the right side the ileopsoas hemorrhage may very closely simulate acute appendicitis. The retroperitoneal hematoma, which appears within twenty-four to forty-eight hours, may be mistaken for an appendiceal abscess. Partial or complete involvement of the femoral nerve may take place with the development of pain on the anterior surface of the thigh, a positive "psoas sign" appears and the hip is held in partial flexion. Paresthesias, partial or complete anesthesia and ultimately weakness or paralysis of the thigh extensors with eventual muscular atrophy may ensue.

Pulmonary and *pleural* bleeding are uncommon, although mediastinal and pleural shadows appearing in roentgenograms, presumably from fresh or old hematomata, have been reported.[13b] Massive hemothorax[25b] and hemoptysis are rare. *Intracranial bleeding* has been reported in 2.5 to 7.8 per cent of cases in various series and tends to occur in younger hemophiliacs, especially in relation to head trauma.[52] It is frequently sub- or epidural or intracerebral. Subarachnoid bleeding occurred least commonly in the reported cases but had the best prognosis. The overall mortality from intracranial bleeding was 70 per cent. Lumbar puncture was performed with safety. Hemorrhage may develop in the spinal cord or spinal meninges. *Peripheral nerve* lesions of varying severity are common and usually complicate hemorrhage into a joint or muscle.

Hematuria is quite common. The bleeding may arise in the bladder or in one or both kidneys. The attacks of bleeding may develop gradually or very suddenly and usually persist for three to five weeks. When the hemorrhage begins to lessen and clots begin to form, severe pain resembling renal colic develops.

The most characteristic site of hemorrhage is into the joints. The typical hemophiliac possesses some deformity as the result of **hemarthrosis.** The onset as a rule, is sudden. In the acute stage the joint is swollen, warm and very painful, and is usually held in a position of flexion. Discoloration of the skin may or may not occur. It is more likely to be found about small joints. In chronic forms of hemarthrosis in hemophilia the process simulates tuberculosis and there is no skin discoloration.

Hemorrhage occurs into the joint cavity or into the diaphysis or epiphysis of the bone. One joint is generally involved at a time although eventually many joints may be attacked. Recurrences are common. The ankle is frequently the earliest joint involved but the knee is the one most often permanently crippled. Other joints which may be involved are the elbow, the hips,[56] wrists, shoulders, small joints of the hands and feet and the vertebral articulations.[54] The maxillo-mandibular joint has also been the site of bleeding.[7]

Three stages in hemophiliac hemarthrosis can be distinguished.[11] The first stage, the acute attack already described, may last a few days to a few weeks. Frequently the absorption of intra-articular blood is incomplete and the retained blood produces a chronic inflammation of the synovial membrane. This is the second stage: panarthritis. The joint remains swollen, tender and painful for months or years. Acute hemarthroses are repeated from time to time. The result is a permanently swollen joint with local deformity, contractures and muscle atrophy. Repeated hemorrhages in large joints in time tend to cause less immediate increases in the size of the joint as the articular capsule becomes thickened and restricts swelling. In the smaller articulations, however, the weaker joint structures and the thinner cortices of the smaller bones fail to hold the progressively expanding hematomas in check and complete destruction of the joints and bones may result.[17]

Folds and villi may be formed as the synovial membrane hypertrophies. The articular cartilage may be eroded at the margins of the joint. Large punched-out areas of destruction are sometimes produced by subchondral hemorrhages and, in the cancellous structure of the bone, cavitation may be caused by intra-osseous hemorrhage. Through disuse, diffuse demineralization of the involved bones may occur. Subperiosteal hemorrhages are not common.

The terminal "stage of regression" is not sharply differentiated from the pan-arthritic stage. In the larger joints fibrous or bony ankylosis may occur but in the smaller articulations complete destruction may take place, as already described. Atrophy and proliferation of bone, roughening of the articular surfaces with lipping and osteophyte formation, cyst formation, stunted growth as the result of interference with the nutrition of the bone, or accelerated development and overgrowth of the epiphyses from excessive flow of blood to the growing epiphyses,[11] are some of the permanent effects produced.

Roentgenographically, in the acute case there is distention of the joint capsule. Later, opacities are found in the soft tissues due to the deposit of iron pigment in the organizing hematomata (Fig. 18–1 *A*). In large joints, sharply defined erosions of the joint margins (Fig. 18–1 *B*), subchondrally situated rarefactions, and rarefactions in the osseous tissue unconnected with the joint surfaces result from destruction of the joint capsule,

cartilage and ends of bone by expanding hematomata.[18c] In the final stage there is subluxation and osseous ankylosis with the production of a pseudo-arthritis deformans (Fig. 18–1 *B* and *C*). In small joints the final stage may be one of complete articular and osseous destruction resembling sarcoma.[17]

Spontaneous hemorrhages are frequently cyclic. In severe cases the cycles are short and three to six weeks apart. In such cases joint hemorrhages appear early in life and crippling may be severe. In milder cases the patient may escape severe bleeding until puberty or later. In some instances the loss of blood is tremendous and shock develops, whereas in others there is time for adjustment of the circulation to the decreased blood volume.

Physical or constitutional abnormalities have not been observed in these patients, other than those produced by the hemorrhages. Mentally these patients are normal, often precocious. There is no glandular enlargement and the spleen is not palpable.

The Blood.—Other than the prolonged coagulation time and reduced prothrombin consumption, there is nothing characteristic in the blood. Anemia depends on the severity and frequency of bleeding. Usually regeneration is rapid when hemorrhage has ceased. Polymorphonuclear leukocytosis may accompany the bleeding as in other instances of acute posthemorrhagic anemia. Platelets may also be increased in number. They are never reduced below normal. Fonio, whose view that this disorder is attributable to a qualitative platelet abnormality was mentioned earlier, found them to be smaller, rounder, more sharply delineated and brighter than normal platelets.[18] Bleeding time is usually normal, the thromboplastin from tissue juice being sufficient to produce coagulation in such a small wound. During the bleeding phase of hemophilia, however, bleeding

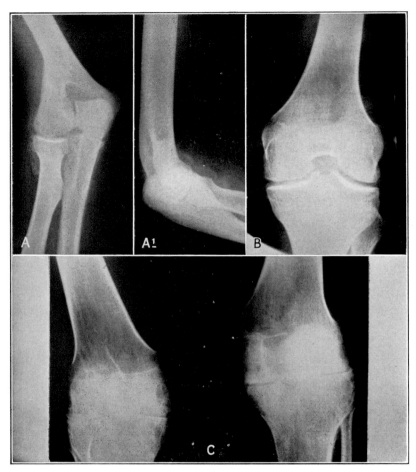

Fig. 18–1.—Roentgenograms of elbows and knee joints in 3 cases of hemophilia showing thickening of synovium with deposition of calcium in A and A^1, increased intercondylar notch in B, increased density, decreased interarticular space (A,B,C) and lipping along the borders of the joint surfaces (C).

time may sometimes be prolonged. The clot, once formed, retracts normally and the capillary resistance test is negative. Venipuncture, if skillfully executed, is without danger, the elasticity of the vessel wall being sufficient to close the wound.

The coagulation time shows spontaneous irregular variations and may range from values barely beyond the limits of normal to several hours. In some cases even normal coagulation times have been observed.[33b] Prothrombin time, as done by the Quick method (p. 302) is normal.[29] In the two-stage method (p. 302) a delay in conversion of prothrombin to thrombin is found but this is corrected when thromboplastin is added.[9] Prothrombin consumption (p. 305) is poor and, when oxalated blood is centrifuged rapidly, thus removing the platelets, the coagulation time of the plasma after recalcification is very much greater than that of plasma derived from oxalated blood centrifuged more slowly and containing more platelets. Thromboplastin generation in the thromboplastin generation test is abnormal. The significance of these findings has been discussed already (p. 307).

The *bone marrow* reflects the effects of acute blood loss, if this has occurred. The megakarycoytes are normal.

Varieties of Hemophilia.—The clinical picture which has just been described is that of classical hemophilia. For a long time little attention was paid to reports[7] of a milder form of the disease. In such cases coagulation time[33b] and even prothrombin consumption[31a] were normal and the symptoms were correspondingly mild, small wounds as a rule giving very little trouble and hemarthrosis being uncommon. However, in many instances a history of a severe bleeding episode could be obtained, particularly following tooth extraction or tonsillectomy. The blood of these patients was poor in shortening the calcium time and correcting the prothrombin consumption defect of known hemophiliac blood.[33b]

Assays of plasma factor VIII suggest that four grades of hemophilia can be distinguished:[9] (1) *classical* hemophilia, in which the plasma factor VIII is 0 per cent; (2) *moderate* hemophilia, characterized by the occurrence of subcutaneous hematomas and postoperative hemorrhages, essentially normal coagulation time, normal prothrombin consumption and less than 3 per cent plasma factor VIII; (3) *mild* hemophilia, in which coagulation time and prothrombin consumption were normal and the plasma factor VIII was approximately 16 per cent; and (4) *subhemophilia*, in which there might only be a history of prolonged postoperative oozing. Plasma factor VIII was found to be 33 per cent in this last group, as compared with the normal value of 65 to 136 per cent. The partial thromboplastin time[26c] was found prolonged only in classical and moderate hemophilia.[9]

Mild hemophilia, in particular, has been studied.[20d] Easy bruising, difficulty in stopping the bleeding from razor cuts, and prolonged bleeding after tonsillectomy or tooth extraction appear to be the major manifestations. The most reliable means for the recognition of these cases is the thromboplastin generation test[43] followed by quantitative measurement of factor VIII.

From the standpoint of prognosis as well as that of genetics, it is of interest that the study of both hemophiliac and normal families has shown that the level of plasma factor VIII is a function of the genic constitution of the individual and thus the clinical and hematologic pattern in a given individual or family is likely to be an unchanging one.[20d,44]

The unequivocal *identification of female carriers of hemophilia* cannot be made by present methods[33c] but low levels of factor VIII have been demonstrated in a number of female carriers[4,14,32a,44,47g] and it has been estimated that factor VIII assay by appropriate technics will detect with reasonable accuracy (four chances out of five) about 75 per cent of the *true* carriers in a *potential* carrier population and about 66 per cent of the normal members in a potential carrier population.[47g] It was emphasized, however, that a potential carrier with even a high level of factor VIII still retains one chance in five of being a true carrier.

Some female carriers of hemophilia have an unusual tendency to bleed.[4,15,47g,53b] It seems likely, therefore, that the gene for hemophilia may at times be only partially recessive. Prolonged bleeding time, thrombocytopenia and positive tourniquet tests, in addition to or in the absence of low levels of factor VIII, have been observed in female relatives of hemophiliacs, some of whom may not have been carriers of the trait.[5c] This would suggest that the genetic defect may cause more than a simple deficiency of factor VIII. It has also been proposed that the inheritance of factor VIII concentration may be under the control of autosomal genes and that the hemophilia gene, in its location on the X-x sex chromosome, either interferes with the normal expres-

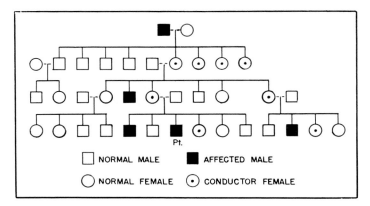

Fig. 18–2.—Hypothetical family tree of a hemophiliac (*Pt.*) with a family large enough to illustrate the mode of transmission of hemophilia.

sion of the autosomal genes controlling plasma factor VIII concentration or is itself responsible for a factor which inhibits or destroys factor VIII.[43a] The finding of low levels of factor VIII in the heterozygotes of mild hemophilia, in particular, led to the suggestion that mild hemophilia is an allelic mutant occurring at the same locus as the normal gene or the classical hemophilia gene.[20d] In another study, however, low factor VIII levels were found as frequently in female carriers of severe hemophilia as in female carriers of mild hemophilia.[14]

Diagnosis.—If a history of repeated bleeding and familial occurrence has not been obtained and the coagulation time has not been measured, a great variety of clinical conditions may be simulated, depending on the location of the hemorrhage. A deep hematoma may be mistaken for a suppurative condition and surgical drainage may be attempted. Bleeding into a small joint may produce a clinical and roentgenological picture suggesting sarcoma.[17] When larger joints are involved in a chronic process, tuberculosis, arthritis deformans, Perthe's disease or syphilis is simulated. Bleeding elsewhere will suggest local causes such as kidney tumor, pulmonary disease, peptic ulcer and so on.

Characteristic evidence in the history which suggests hemophilia is (1) habitual and immoderate hemorrhage in males, beginning early in life; (2) similar symptoms in half the brothers, maternal male cousins (if their mother was also a conductor), maternal uncles and so on, with sisters and paternal relatives usually exempt; or (3) other combinations as illustrated in Fig. 18–2.

There are a number of bleeding disorders in which a *familial* occurrence may be found. In most of these the pattern of inheritance which characterizes hemophilia, namely, transmission by females and occurrence in males, is lacking and in many there is only a very superficial resemblance to the clinical picture of hemophilia. Thus, of the conditions discussed in the preceding chapter, a familial history is sometimes encountered in idiopathic thrombocytopenic purpura but the hereditary pattern is usually vague and, in addition, thrombocytopenia, prolonged bleeding time and poor clot retraction will be found whereas coagulation time is normal. Of the other, much rarer conditions, it may be noted that in von Willebrand's disease, the bleeding time is prolonged and the inheritance of the condition is that of a simple Mendelian dominant. Either sex may be affected.

In Glanzmann's thrombasthenia and in other thrombocytopathic purpuras, it is the platelets which are abnormal. In hereditary familial purpura simplex, females rather than males are most commonly affected and there are no abnormalities in the blood. Hereditary hemorrhagic telangiectasia, which will be described later (p. 888), is identified by the characteristic skin lesions. In addition to these conditions, cases of familial epistaxis have been described in which no local or generalized abnormalities were present and in which the bleeding and coagulation times were normal.[19c]

As already indicated, the history of a patient with hemophilia does not always reveal a familial trait, for sporadic cases occur or there may be long inheritance through females with the males, by chance, being unaffected. Skipped generations or illegitimacy may be responsible for some instances while in others a mild form may have passed unnoticed from generation to generation.[18a]

In hemophilia the underlying abnormality is a defect in the process of coagulation and this, in classical cases, is manifested by a prolongation of coagulation time. In an earlier chapter the various causes of prolonged coagulation time were listed (Table 5–1, p. 308). One would hardly be confused in diagnosis by any of the conditions which, through vitamin K deficiency or impaired formation of prothrombin, result in prolonged coagulation time. Even in hemorrhagic disease of the newborn (p. 886) the very early occurrence of the bleeding, the lack of any evidence of heredity and the rapid and permanent recovery on appropriate treatment, make the differentiation from hemophilia easy enough.

There are, however, a number of disorders which more closely simulate classical hemophilia. In one of these, factor IX deficiency, even the pattern of inheritance is like that of hemophilia. These conditions will be considered in the next section (p. 875) where their differentiation from hemophilia will be discussed. Further difficulties in the recognition of hemophilia arise from the fact that sporadic cases, without any family history whatsoever, are not rare and also because of the observation that less severe cases than those presenting the classical picture may be encountered in which the coagulation time and prothrombin consumption are normal (p. 869). An example of this difficulty is found in the cases which at one time were thought to differ from true hemophilia and were tentatively classified as the "*Moëna anomaly*" but were later shown[26a] to be the same as the mild hemophilia[20d] already discussed. In cases such as these, assays of plasma factor VIII (pp. 292, 303) may be necessary before exact identification is possible.

In Table 17–1 (p. 817) the various causes of hemorrhage and in Table 17–2 (p. 818) the purpuras are classified. Causes of alterations in the various tests used in studying cases of hemorrhagic disease are listed in Table 5–2 (p. 308). Of these, coagulation time and the prothrombin consumption test, in particular, provide confirmation or exclusion of the diagnosis of hemophilia and the thromboplastin generation test (p. 306) permits differentiation of the various causes of abnormalities in the first phase of coagulation. Assay of factor VIII (p. 304) allows assessment of the severity of the disease.

Course and Prognosis.—It has been stated that hemophiliacs improve at or after adolescence.[6,10] Another analysis[7] indicated, however, that the less exciting course of older hemophiliacs can be attributed to (1) the death of the most severe cases in early life; (2) the passing of the teething period; (3) the onset of the years of discretion; and (4) increasing inactivity as the result of permanent joint deformities.

In the same study it was found that in 35 per cent of 113 cases of hemophilia, death occurred during the first year of life and in 57 per cent during the first five years. It was calculated that the life expectancy of hemophiliac babies is one-twelfth of the normal. In this investigation, factor VIII and factor IX deficiencies were not differentiated.

The greatest number of deaths (23 per cent) were due to exsanguination following surgical procedures: circumcision, tooth extraction, tonsillectomy, and lancing of hematomas. A slightly smaller proportion followed small accidental cuts. Internal hemorrhage, epistaxis, cerebral or spinal cord hemorrhage, hematuria, bleeding from the umbilical cord or lungs, gastric and intestinal hemorrhages accounted for most of the rest.

In the milder forms of hemophilia (p. 869) the prognosis is much better.

Treatment.—If the theory is accepted that hemophilia is due to the inheritance of an anomaly of coagulation, cure cannot be expected. As yet no means has been found to modify a genetically determined trait. Theoretically the number of cases might be reduced by proper restriction of marriage, or at least of propagation, even though mutations would counteract this effort to eliminate the disease. Patients and their families should be advised that only unaffected males can marry with any assurance that the hemorrhagic tendency will not be transmitted. Although it is true that only one half of the daughters of a female carrier inherit the trait and are able to transmit it, there is no reliable way of distinguishing the normal daughters from the bearers of this hereditary anomaly (p. 869).

All male children of tainted stock must be protected most carefully from wounds and abrasions. As the child grows older he should be informed of his inherited tendency and be taught to protect himself. Furthermore, even the most trivial operations should be avoided. This fact

was recognized by the ancient Jews in regard to the rite of circumcision.

While violent exertion and any trauma must be avoided, it is important that the hemophiliac live normally, participating even in moderate activity. This permits maintenance of muscle tone and joint mobility and also gives the individual a sense of equality with his associates. It is important that he be taught self reliance from early childhood and that plans be made concerning an appropriate vocation. Too often these patients are made chronic invalids. With good management they can become quite independent. In the United States, the National Hemophilia Foundation (175 Fifth Avenue, New York) provides excellent pamphlets concerning the home care of the hemophiliac child.

The use of ovarian substance was advocated[6] on the theory that the female sex hormone protects the female carrier but this, like numerous other agents which have been recommended from time to time,[23] has not withstood the test of time.[53] With a better understanding of the nature of hemophilia it has become clear that the basis of therapy in a bleeding crisis is the administration of sufficient quantities of antihemophilic factor to restore the normal coagulation of the blood and to maintain this until the crisis has passed. For local application thrombic substances which will clot the blood are required and, for special situations, as when tooth extraction or other surgery is imperative or when hemarthrosis has developed, special measures are needed. These will be discussed shortly.

Special diets have no value as far as the coagulation defect in hemophilia is concerned. It would be desirable to discover some agent which would be effective when given by mouth. None of the extracts of lung, spleen, bone marrow or placenta which have been prepared so far is of any use orally. Intramuscular injections should be avoided for not only are coagulating substances given in this way ineffective, but a hematoma may be produced, with serious consequences ensuing. Factor VIII therefore, must be given intravenously.

Factor VIII may be administered as whole blood transfusions if the patient has anemia; otherwise whole plasma, reconstituted lyophilized plasma or plasma concentrates can be used. Serum is of no value. Factor VIII is unstable in plasma kept at room temperature. It is considerably more stable in citrated (ACD) than in oxalated plasma[52e] or in EDTA.[13c] An essential factor in its preservation is the care used in the collection of the blood and the speed of its decalcification. Loss of factor VIII is due to its consumption or destruction by thrombin formed as the result of faulty collection and processing. It follows that, without measurement, no reliable statement can be made concerning the content of factor VIII in a particular preparation of blood or plasma. The blood to be used should have been decalcified and refrigerated promptly. This is perhaps more important than that it be quite fresh. Fresh whole blood may possess full potency and bank blood five to seven days old may contain 55 per cent or less[47d] but there is considerable variation. Whenever possible fresh blood or fresh, freshly frozen or freshly lyophilized plasma should be used and, failing these, the freshest available blood bank plasma. Many units of freshly frozen blood bank plasma after three months of storage were found to contain less than 50 per cent of the mean factor VIII level of the donors but lots of commerical, frozen, lyophilized plasma contained an average of 72 per cent.[45b] Slow deterioration takes place in fresh frozen plasma but in dry lyophilized plasma factor VIII remains potent for years.[26d]

Cohn fraction I of plasma, at first thought to have considerable promise as a source of concentrated factor VIII, has varied considerably in its potency and also may carry the hepatitis virus. As mentioned earlier, (p. 864) purification of factor VIII from human plasma has achieved high degrees of concentration[7b] but such preparations are as yet only available in very small amounts. Bovine plasma has about 13 times the activity of fresh human blood and 100 to 400-fold purification has been reported[31] but concentrates of bovine, or pig, plasma are antigenic and the occurrence of allergic reactions will probably prevent their continued administration for periods of time exceeding ten to 14 days.[5c] They have been employed successfully, however, in patients requiring operations.[31]

Whatever source of factor VIII is used, it is clear that its effect is not long lasting. Its biologic half-life may be of the order of nine or ten hours but, as mentioned earlier, the concentration of the initial infusion drops rapidly within three to six hours, or even more quickly if there is severe hemorrhage and tissue necrosis. The antihemophilic factor may circulate in a space two or three times the blood volume.[15a] There is disagreement as to the concentration of factor VIII which it is necessary to achieve in the treatment of a hemophiliac, the figures ranging from 10 to 30 per cent of the average normal level.[49] It is good practice to err on the side of more rather than less, if at all possible. Thus, in a 60 Kg. individual, 1500 ml. of plasma (2.5 ml./Kg./hour) or its equivalent might be needed to achieve a 30 per cent level of factor VIII. This can be done by giving 300 ml. every two hours for the first ten hours, by constant infusion, if desired. After such an initial priming dose, plasma should be given at a rate of approximately 1 ml. per Kg. per hour until there is evidence that bleeding has stopped. This can be considered the ideal or maximal dosage since, with properly collected plasma, a factor VIII concentration of about 30 per cent can be achieved in this way. In other cases 2 ml. plasma per Kg. body weight every four hours will suffice.[9] How much is to be given in a particular case will depend on the location of the hemorrhage. Thus, even the slightest bulge in the throat of a hemophiliac calls for intensive therapy, since asphyxiation may result from swelling of the soft tissues through hemorrhage. Bleeding into a joint likewise calls for intensive therapy. In all instances infusions, in decreased amounts, should be continued for several days after signs of continued bleeding have disappeared.

In the treatment of **bleeding from accessible sites,** thrombin is the hemostatic agent of choice. Bovine[45] or rabbit[29a] thrombin should be used instead of human thrombin, since the latter is frequently contaminated with the hepatitis virus. Coagulating snake venoms (Russell's viper,[5b] fer de lance[1a]) are also of some value. In an emergency a sponge soaked in normal plasma or whole blood may be applied to the bleeding site. One of a number of vehicles may be used for thrombin, such as gelatin foam or fibrin. The latter may be freshly clotted out of a fibrinogen solution, or even out of citrated plasma, thrombin being added directly to the fibrinogen just before use. Most of the fluid is expressed from the clot and it is molded, with moderate pressure, into the bleeding sites. The pressure should be maintained and the thrombin-soaked fibrin or sponge left in place since removal disturbs the clot and bleeding recurs. An ice-bag may be applied temporarily since the cold will cause contraction of the blood vessels in the injured area.

Prior to the application of thrombin it is important to remove the accumulated clots and expose the bleeding points. The clots which are found are produced through the action of the thromboplastic substance from the injured tissues but they are usually ineffective because it is only at the periphery of the wound that thromboplastic substance from the tissues

mixes with the blood.[1] The fibrin layer which is formed probably prevents the tissue element from reaching the blood flowing from the injured vessels and the latter, since it must depend only on the plasma factor VIII, continues to ooze.

Acute joint bleeding is a major bleeding episode and should be treated promptly and vigorously: full plasma therapy, bed rest and ice applied locally. Aspiration should be restricted solely to massively distended joints. Installation of hyaluronidase[30b] has been found to retard healing and may even cause intensification of pain and renewed bleeding.[49] Following arrest of hemorrhage, orthopedic rehabilitation may be required and may necessitate traction, casts and corrective braces. Details of such orthopedic management have been outlined by Jordan.[24c] Hemarthroses are apt to be recurrent and great care must be taken to avoid deformities.

Surgery should be avoided in hemophiliacs. The mortality from major surgery in 50 cases collected from the literature was 20 per cent.[42] When there appears to be an abdominal emergency, plasma therapy, antibiotics and intravenous fluids are indicated for a time, until the true nature of the intra-abdominal process is determined and an opportunity is given for it to subside. Bleeding episodes into the intestinal wall, peritoneal cavity or retroperitoneal space may simulate the rupture of an organ, or appendicitis. If surgery must be performed the factor VIII level of the blood should be raised above 30 per cent and maintained there.

The **care of the teeth** requires specia. consideration. Dental prophylaxis is of paramount importance in these patientsl Cavities can be filled without fear of hemorrhage. If dental surgery is required, plasma is given intravenously before the actual extraction in order to raise the plasma factor VIII level to 30 per cent or better. In applying local anesthesia it is better to infiltrate with a fine gauge needle the tissues at the free cuff margin of the gingivae rather than to use the more conventional type of infiltration for, by so doing, the traumatized tissue is localized in one area over which the mechanical pressure of the denture will be applied.

The extraction is done with as little trauma as possible and, after the tooth has been removed, the socket is gently sponged and cleaned. Dried thrombin, buttressed with a more solid filler such as oxidized cellulose, is firmly packed into the defect. The gum margins should not be sutured. Good hemostatic control can be maintained by individually prepared acrylic splints[33] or other suitable dentures. Some have employed, in addition, a thin, tightly fitting band of rubber (orthodontia band), placed about the neck of the tooth to be extracted about a week prior to the operation.[13b] The band progresses along the tooth root, partially separating it from the adjacent tissues. At times the band progresses rapidly so that it may be necessary to use two or three such bands in order to keep the soft tissues from reapproximating to the tooth after the band has passed. Occasionally by this means alone extraction is accomplished.

Detailed discussions concerning dental care in hemophilia have been published.[9a,33,49c]

The regular intravenous administration of plasma at weekly or semi-weekly intervals, as a prophylactic measure even in the absence of hemorrhage, is hardly justified. It is well known that even without any form of treatment, hemophiliacs may live without serious symptoms developing for greatly varying intervals of time.

A distressing complication of transfusion of blood or blood products in cases of hemophilia is the development of a **circulating anticoagulant,** rendering the patients refractory to therapy.[27] In several of these patients inhibitors against factor VIII could be demonstrated. In most instances repeated transfusions had been received by the subjects and these, in the face of complete deficiencies of factor VIII, may have led to isoimmunization against the injected globulin. However, studies of the mode of action of the inhibitor present in the blood of some patients with circulating anticoagulants indicated that the inhibitor and factor VIII react together according to a bimolecular reaction.[4b] Thus their behavior appears to be quite different from that of other antibodies.

Pathology.—The findings are those produced by the hemorrhages. The bone marrow may give signs of moderate activity as the result of the bleeding, but in hemophilia sternal puncture should be avoided. Increased numbers of megakaryoblasts and megakaryocytes in the marrow have been reported.[13]

FACTOR IX (PTC) DEFICIENCY

Synonyms and Definition.—Factor IX deficiency is a constitutional anomaly of blood coagulation which, like classical hemophilia, depends on the hereditary transmission of a sex-linked, recessive Mendelian trait which becomes manifest as a deficiency of a plasma component essential for the coagulation of blood.[1b] The disorder is also known as PTC (plasma thromboplastin component) deficiency or *Christmas disease*, after the surname of one of the first families in which it was recognized.[5a] Because it so closely resembles classical hemophilia, it has also been called *hemophilia B*.

History, Clinical Manifestations and Pathogenesis.—This disorder was first recognized in 1952,[1b,5,51a] although an observation was made five years earlier that suggested that classical hemophilia might not be a single entity; namely, it was noted that, when the plasmas of two

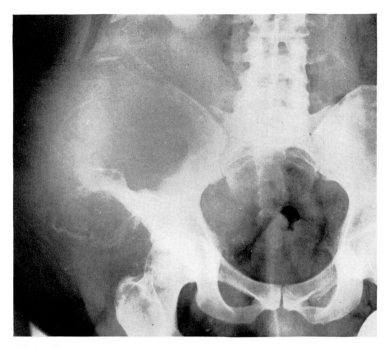

Fig. 18–3.—Roentgenogram showing pseudotumor and destruction of the ilium as the result of a hematoma in a case of factor IX deficiency.[51e]

patients with hemophilia were mixed, mutual correction of the clotting defect occurred.[41a]

Factor IX deficiency mimics classical hemophilia (factor VIII deficiency) so completely that it is now apparent that some of the original studies of hemophilia were concerned with factor IX rather than with factor VIII deficiency. This applies, for example, to the hemophiliacs of Tenna in Switzerland, the largest and oldest known family of hemophiliacs.[34a] The similarity of the two conditions includes an identical mode of inheritance and like changes in whole blood coagulation time and prothrombin consumption. Also as in hemophilia, a number of cases appear to be sporadic.[52b] The relative incidence of these two forms of hemophilia was discussed earlier (p. 862), where it was also pointed out that in several instances both types of hemophilia were demonstrated in the same subjects

and that, like factor VIII deficiency, factor IX deficiency may occur in association with a vascular defect.

The clinical manifestations of factor IX deficiency can be extremely serious, as figure 18–3 testifies. Also as in factor VIII deficiency, mild forms have been described.[4a,47b] It has been stated that the clinical manifestations tend to be of a similar degree of severity in the same family.[2e,47b] However, in the Tenna family the degree of plasma deficiency of factor IX was found to be the same and yet the clinical manifestations varied a great deal.[34a]

In mild factor IX deficiency, as in hemophilia, coagulation time may be normal or nearly so and prothrombin consumption may be normal, the defect being detectable only with the aid of the thromboplastin generation test.[4a,47b] That the trait may not always be completely recessive in the **heterozygote female**

carrier has now been demonstrated in a number of studies.[12a,14] In one of them,[2e] it was found that in 25 per cent of the heterozygotes the factor IX level was significantly reduced below the normal range. However, these females were able to withstand considerable trauma without dangerous loss of blood.

The role of factor IX in the process of coagulation and its physical and chemical properties were discussed earlier (p. 292). Methods for the assay of factor IX have also been considered (p. 304). As in the case of hemophilia, there are some grounds for considering that, contrary to the general view, the defect in factor IX deficiency may in part be due to the action of an inhibitor,[34d] rather than to the absence of this factor. A single instance of temporary, acquired factor IX deficiency has been reported.[20a]

Treatment.—Management of these patients differs little from that outlined for hemophilia (p. 872). As in that disorder, surgery, including tooth extraction, should be avoided and, when essential, must be done only after proper preparation of the patient. The relative stability of factor IX, as compared with that of factor VIII, and the fact that it is present in serum offer at least a theoretical advantage over hemophilia, in that reliance does not need to be placed on fresh blood or plasma. Stored blood is as good as fresh blood and the beneficial effect of plasma infusions may last longer than in hemophilia.[3a] On the other hand, antihemophilic globulin is of no value. It is equally important in both types of hemophilia, however, that major episodes of bleeding be treated vigorously and that the quantity of plasma used and the frequency of its administration be determined by the response of the patient.

As in hemophilia, resistance to transfusion therapy as the result of the development of an anticoagulant has been observed.[27]

PTA DEFICIENCY AND OTHER DEFICIENCIES OF THROMBO-PLASTIN FORMATION

In 1953 a hemorrhagic state resulting from the deficiency of still another substance required for thromboplastin formation was described.[49a] Although similar to hemophilia in its clinical manifestations, **PTA (plasma thromboplastin antecedent) deficiency** can occur in *either sex.* It appears to be transmitted as an autosomal dominant trait with a high degree of penetrance but variable expression. Spontaneous bleeding is rare, as are hemarthroses or purpura, and bleeding has occurred usually following trauma or a surgical procedure, including tooth extraction. Various degrees of severity have been observed, however, ranging from a severe form with prolonged coagulation time and markedly abnormal prothrombin consumption to a mild form with normal coagulation time and only slightly impaired prothrombin consumption.[11a,49] Thromboplastin generation is markedly impaired.[47a]

The properties of PTA and its role in coagulation were discussed elsewhere (pp. 293, 295). In several cases a delay in platelet viscous metamorphosis, an abnormal reaction to glass contact and some delay in the activation of factor IX was noted.[5d] This disorder is much less common than hemophilia but its occurrence apparently varies widely. In Minneapolis[19] the relative incidence of factor VIII, factor IX and PTA deficiencies was 45:6:4, in New York[49] it was 32:6:2, and in Great Britain PTA deficiency seems to be even more rare (p. 862). One family has been described as having deficiencies of factor VIII and PTA, together with vascular fragility, in various combinations.[47b]

The defect in this disorder can be corrected by plasma adsorbed with $BaSO_4$ and by serum, since PTA is present in both. In this way it can be differentiated from factor VIII deficiency, which is corrected by normal adsorbed plasma but not by serum, as well as from factor IX deficiency, which is corrected by normal serum and not by adsorbed plasma.

Treatment is similar to that for hemophilia and, as in factor IX deficiency, stored plasma or serum is an effective therapeutic agent. The beneficial effect of these agents was found to disappear gradually over the period of a week.[49a] In one instance the development of a resistant state to transfusion therapy, resulting from the appearance of an anticoagulant, was recorded.[24d]

The suggestion that there is a fourth type of thromboplastin component deficiency ("PTF-D") was later withdrawn when it was demonstrated that the patient in question had mild factor IX deficiency, probably associated with a circulating anticoagulant.[52d]

The **Hageman trait** refers to a familial trait due to deficiency of the Hageman factor (p. 293) which occurs in both sexes and is characterized by a prolonged coagulation time both in glass and in silicone-coated tubes, as well as by markedly decreased prothrombin consumption and thromboplastin generation. Yet it is unassociated with hemorrhagic symptoms.[48] Platelet viscous metamorphosis is delayed[5d] and activation of clotting by contact with glass is diminished[48] in subjects with this disorder. The condition is probably the homozygous expression of an autosomal recessive gene, the heterozygous state being undetectable by present methods.[10b]

The Thromboplastin Deficiency Syndromes.—Technical problems related to the performance of the various coagulation tests which are available, as well as the gaps in our understanding of the process of coagulation which sometimes make difficult interpretation of the results of these tests, have naturally led to the reporting of new hemorrhagic syndromes some of which prob-

ably belong in the categories already described. The hypothetical "fourth" thromboplastin component, mentioned above, is a case in point. Whether or not other new syndromes resembling hemophilia in one way or another[10a] will survive the test of time and of newer knowledge, remains to be seen. In any event, it can be considered that (1) classical hemophilia (factor VIII deficiency), (2) factor IX (PTC) deficiency and (3) PTA deficiency are well established as hemorrhagic disorders and that (4) the Hageman trait is manifested as a thromboplastin-formation defect which is unaccompanied by clinical manifestations. In addition to these abnormalities, it now appears that (5) factor VIII and factor IX deficiencies may occur simultaneously (p. 862), and that (6) a circulating anticoagulant may complicate and aggravate these conditions. Again, (7) some reduction in factor VIII or factor IX plasma levels has been observed in a proportion of the female heterozygote carriers of these disorders and (8) factor VIII deficiency of a moderate degree has been observed in women not belonging to a hemophiliac family. The last condition is usually associated with (9) a vascular defect, a form of von Willebrand's disease ("vascular hemophilia," "angiohemophilia") and may be found in either sex (p. 847). Insufficient or delayed thromboplastin formation may also be found (10) in the presence of a circulating anticoagulant in non-hemophilic men and in women, in the latter sometimes in association with a recent pregnancy. This topic will be discussed shortly (p. 884) Deficiencies of factors VIII or IX, and perhaps of PTA may also occur in the absence of an inherited trait (11) as an acquired defect, usually as the effect of an anticoagulant (p. 884). Impaired thromboplastin formation may also result from (12) thrombocytopenia and (13) in the thrombocytopathies (p. 847) as the consequence of deficiency of or faulty release of platelet factor 3; and perhaps also (14) because of a labile serum factor defect.[11d]

In addition to this rather long list one may add deficiencies of (15) factor V and (16) factor X. Here, fortunately, a distinguishing feature is found; namely the prothrombin time, which is almost never abnormal in the conditions named above, is prolonged. For this reason, these conditions have at times been classified among the hypoprothrombinemias. They will be discussed below under that heading but it should be understood that, when these factors are lacking, prothrombin consumption and thromboplastin generation, as usually measured, may also be impaired. Furthermore, these deficiencies are not always single. Thus, (17) the coexistence of factor V and factor VIII deficiencies has been observed in four patients.[51b] Still other combinations have been noted,[41b] as mentioned in the preceding pages.

From a clinical standpoint it must be emphasized that the various disorders listed may resemble one another to a greater or less degree and that a detailed personal and family history and study, together with a more or less penetrating laboratory investigation will be needed to unravel the spider's web. Fortunately, in the great majority of patients with hemorrhagic manifestations the laboratory studies do not have to be as exhaustive as is necessary in a few. Some of the main points of difference between these conditions are outlined in Table 18-1.

THE HYPOPROTHROMBINEMIAS

It was pointed out in an earlier chapter (p. 290) that what was once considered to be a single substance, "prothrombin," was shown later to represent a complex of several factors. The properties of these substances were defined and their manner of production and function were considered. Deficiencies of these factors may be acquired under certain circumstances, as will be discussed below. Congenital and idiopathic forms have also been observed and these will be discussed first. As mentioned above, the clinical manifestations of the congenital and idiopathic hypoprothrombinemias resemble those of hemophilia and, in this respect, it is of interest that the first patient to have been reported as having "congenital hypoprothrombinemia" had previously been considered to have hemophilia.[48d]

Congenital hypoprothrombinemia due to a true deficiency of prothrombin, as distinguished from deficiencies of factors V, VII or X, is exceedingly rare. At most, three cases are known.[8,46f,55a] The prothrombin level in these cases was approximately 10 per cent of normal. Whole blood clotting times were normal, slightly prolonged and markedly prolonged in the three cases, respectively, the Quick prothrombin time was prolonged in two and only slightly increased in one and prothrombin consumption, measured only in one case, was normal.

Congenital factor V deficiency[2] ("parahemophilia") has been described in about 20 families[26e] and there is a rare isolated, idiopathic case.[36d] The condition has been observed in both sexes. Its mode of inheritance appears to be that of an autosomal recessive. In some instances, the parents or children of an affected individual have had partial deficiencies of factor V. The condition varies greatly in severity, as does the degree of prolongation of prothrombin and coagulation times and the decrease in prothrombin consumption. In milder cases, spontaneous epistaxes, easy bruisability, menorrhagia and, at times, excessive bleeding after dental extractions or surgical procedures were observed; in more severe cases there were large hematomas, spontaneous gingival bleeding and bleeding into the gastrointestinal tract or central nervous system. Hemarthroses have not been described. The coexistence of factor V and VIII deficiencies in four instances,

Table 18-1.—Differentiation of Certain Congenital Deficiencies of Coagulation Factors

Factor:	Fibrinogen	V	VII	VIII	IX	X	HF	PTA
Usual Mode of Inheritance[1]	AR	AR	AR	SLR	SLR	AR	AR	AD
Sex Distribution	MF	MF	MF	M[2]	M[2]	MF	MF	MF
Clinical Severity	Moderate	Variable	Variable	Mild to severe	Mild to severe	Variable	No symptoms	Moderate
Coagulation Time Prolonged	+	±	−	±[3]	±[3]	+	+	±
Prothrombin Consumption Deficient	−	+	−	±[3]	±[3]	+	+	±
Thromboplastin Generation Deficient	−	+	+	+	+	+	+	+
Prothrombin Time Prolonged	+	+	+	−	−	+	−	−
Defect Corrected by:								
Normal Fresh Blood or Plasma	+	+	+	+	+	+	+	+
Stored Plasma	+	−	+	−	+	+	+	+
Normal Adsorbed Plasma	−	+	−	+	−	−	+	+
Normal Serum	−	−	+	−	+	+	+	+
Normal Adsorbed Serum	+	−	−	+	−	−	+	+
Dicumarol Plasma[4]	+	+	−	+	−	−	+	+

[1] AR refers to autosomal recessive; SLR, sex-linked recessive; AD, autosomal dominant
[2] Very rarely in females
[3] May be normal in mild cases
[4] Obtained from patient with markedly prolonged prothrombin time who has received Dicumarol for a week or more

mentioned above (p. 879) suggests a common step in the synthesis of these factors.[51b] Consanguinity of the parents existed in at least three of the reported cases.

Congenital Factor VII Deficiency. —This deficiency was first described under the title of SPCA (serum prothrombin conversion accelerator) deficiency.[2a] Certain cases reported earlier as instances of "idiopathic hypoprothrombinemia" can now be attributed to factor VII deficiency and restudy of some alleged SPCA or "proconvertin" deficiencies has led to their reclassification as cases of Stuart-Prower (factor X) deficiency (see below). The role of these factors in coagulation was discussed in an earlier chapter (p. 293). Factor VII deficiency probably is the most common of the congenital "hypoprothrombinemias." It is difficult to be certain about the number of acceptable cases but they probably number about 60.[10c,14c,20,26b,43a,55c] Clinical symptoms observed in these cases include spontaneous epistaxes, deep subcutaneous hematomata, genitourinary and gastrointestinal bleeding and hemarthroses. The Quick prothrombin time is prolonged whereas coagulation time, clot retraction and bleeding time have been normal in most patients. In contradistinction to factor X deficiency, prothrombin consumption and thromboplastin generation are normal. The addition of viper venom corrects the prolonged prothrombin time in factor VII deficiency but not that in factor X deficiency. Factor VII deficiency would seem to be inherited as an incompletely recessive autosomal characteristic with variable penetrance. It has been suggested that severe deficiency is due to the homozygous state.[14c]

The association of factor VII deficiency with factor VIII deficiency[12] and with factor IX deficiency[36c] has been reported.

Factor X deficiency is also known by the surnames of the patients who were first found to manifest this defect (*Stuart*[22d]

56

and *Prower*[53c]). This anomaly was distinguished from factor VII deficiency because thromboplastin generation was found to be abnormal and delayed prothrombin time was not corrected by viper venom whereas it could be corrected by plasma or serum from patients treated with a coumarin drug or phenylindanedione. Subsequently, several cases, formerly considered to be examples of factor VII deficiency, were shown to be examples of factor X deficiency[3,19b,22d] and since then a number of additional families have been reported.[48e] The clinical manifestations of this condition resemble those of factor VII deficiency. It is thought to be inherited as a highly penetrant but incompletely recessive autosomal characteristic. The heterozygotes have been found to be only mildly affected or normal, clinically, but may manifest slight abnormalities in prothrombin time and in thromboplastin generation.[22d]

Treatment of the congenital "hypoprothrombinemic" states depends on supplying the missing factor. Vitamin K does not correct the prolonged one-stage prothrombin time of factor V, factor VII, or factor X deficiency but vitamin K_1 sometimes slightly improves the prothrombin time of true hypoprothrombinemia.[46f] In factor V deficiency fresh whole blood or plasma is necessary to correct the defect. In factor VII deficiency transfusion of serum may possibly be superior to the administration of plasma. The effects of transfusions of blood or serum, however, have been only of short duration. The use of plasma concentrates of some of these factors[14a,22] has made it possible to attain hemostatic levels with the infusion of small volumes.

Acquired Deficiencies of Prothrombin, Factors V, VII and X.—The original observations on "prothrombin" did not differentiate between prothrombin and factors V, VII and X, since they were unknown. Nevertheless, certain conclusions which were drawn still hold true. Thus, it was thought that the liver is in some way concerned with the formation of "prothrombin." The fat-soluble vitamin, K, a naphthoquinone, was found to be related to this activity and it was thought that the vitamin serves as a prosthetic group for an essential enzyme. This vitamin is found abundantly in alfalfa, spinach, cabbage, cauliflower, kale and certain other vegetables. For its absorption from the gastrointestinal tract, bile salts are needed and the absorptive functions of the bowel must be adequate. It was noted that "hypoprothrombinemia" occurred (1) in the presence of vitamin K deficiency or (2) of liver disease; (3) in "sweet clover" disease; and (4) in the newborn.

Vitamin K deficiency may develop when this substance is lacking from the diet, when its absorption is impaired or when putrefactive bacteria are absent from the bowel, as occurs during treatment with certain sulfonamides and antibiotics. In mammals, vitamin K deficiency as the consequence of inadequate diet is exceedingly rare since it is synthesized by bacteria in the intestines and its absorption is good as long as bile salts are available. When bile is lacking, as in obstructive jaundice or when there is a biliary fistula, vitamin K deficiency and "hypoprothrombinemia" result. Faulty intestinal absorption secondary to hypermotility or impermeability of the bowel, as in sprue, celiac disease, intestinal fistulae and ulcerative colitis, also sometimes leads to vitamin K deficiency. In all of these conditions the parenteral administration of vitamin K restores the plasma prothrombin levels to normal.

By the more refined technics of the present day it has been shown that there is depression of prothrombin, factor VII, factor X[52f] and, in some cases, even factor IX[14d] when vitamin K is deficient. Factor V, however, is maintained at a satisfactory level. These defects can all be corrected by the intravenous administration of vitamin K.

It is now known that multiple serious plasma clotting factor defects develop *in the patient with decompensated chronic hepatocellular disease.*[47e] These include major deficiencies of prothrombin, factor VII, factor V and possibly also factor X and factor IX are deficient as well. Factor VIII remains normal. These defects are not corrected by the administration of vitamin K, as might be expected, in view of the central role attributed to the liver. The treatment of the hemorrhagic state associated with severe liver disease therefore requires the administration of blood, and this must be fresh, or at least less than a week old, since the labile factor V must be replaced. Frequently thrombocytopenia is found as well, in which case fresh blood collected in plastic bags or in silicone-treated bottles is needed.

"Sweet clover" disease is a hemorrhagic disorder of cattle which was found to be due to the ingestion of a toxic principle in spoiled sweet clover hay. This was shown to be a coumarin compound (3,3'-methylene-bis ((4-hydroxycoumarin)) which, under the trade name, "Dicumarol," became a widely used anticoagulant. "Hypoprothrombinemia" was found to occur whenever this drug or a related compound was administered. These agents produce low levels of prothrombin and of factor VII, and somewhat lesser decreases of factor V.[27a] The level of factors IX and X also fall, but more slowly than that of factor VII.[14b]

The "hypoprothrombinemia" of the *newborn* is of great significance in the pathogenesis of hemorrhagic disease of the newborn and will be discussed under that heading (p. 886).

THE HYPOFIBRINOGENEMIAS

Deficiency of plasma fibrinogen may be complete (afibrinogenemia) or partial.

The former is almost always congenital, the latter may be congenital or acquired.

Since the first report of **congenital or constitutional afibrinogenemia**[47] in 1920, approximately 29 additional cases have been described.[16d,20e,34b,55b] The hemorrhagic tendency is manifest from birth; bleeding from the umbilical cord may be profuse. Other hemorrhagic manifestations have been bleeding from cuts or after slight trauma, subcutaneous hemorrhages, epistaxis, and excessive bleeding at the eruption and casting of the deciduous teeth. Nevertheless, in spite of the complete incoagulability of the blood, these patients have been troubled with much less disability than is seen in hemophilia and hemarthroses have not been described. They have enjoyed long periods of freedom from hemorrhage. Eighteen of 28 patients have been males. Cousin marriages of parents or grandparents appeared in the kinship of 8 of the patients. Nine had siblings with bleeding disorders but only in one[2b] has this been shown to be due to afibrinogenemia. The first patient studied[47] survived to the age of thirteen. A third of the patients are known to have died in infancy or childhood as the result of hemorrhage or complications thereof but one was reported alive at 22 years of age. Various racial strains have been implicated. No significant association with other anomalies has been noted.

The blood does not coagulate. Bleeding times have ranged from five to more than forty minutes. Transitory thrombocytopenia and diminished capillary resistance have been reported. Interesting observations have been made on the events occurring in afibrinogenemic blood.[2b] Shortly after exposure of the blood to glass, morphologic changes took place in the platelets and they progressively aggregated and disappeared. Almost in parallel, plasma antihemophilic activity, originally normal, declined rapidly and practically disappeared. Factor VII evolved within a few minutes and factor V was rapidly consumed, these changes being well along before detectable amounts of prothrombin had disappeared. Prothrombin consumption proceeded at normal velocity. In other studies[21] it was shown that platelet thromboplastic principle is quantitatively consumed during the formation of blood thromboplastin. Furthermore, in contrast to the slow release of 5-hydroxytryptamine from platelets in hemophilia, liberation of this vasoconstrictor substance was normal in afibrinogenemia, presumably because thrombin was available to initiate or accelerate the process.

Delayed coagulation due to lack of fibrinogen can be distinguished from that found in factor VIII or IX deficiencies by adding to the blood a few drops of the thromboplastin solution used in the measurement of prothrombin time (p. 302). Factor VIII- or IX-deficient blood will clot promptly whereas blood containing no fibrinogen will remain fluid. Another simple procedure is to heat the plasma to 60° C. If the plasma remains clear, a diagnosis of afibrinogenemia can be made since fibrinogen coagulates at 58°. Failure of a precipitate to form when plasma is half saturated with sodium chloride or quarter saturated with ammonium sulfate also indicates the absence of this protein.

The fibrinogen level can be raised promptly by transfusion of blood or plasma but the level falls away progressively. After a transfusion of 600 ml. of plasma, measurable amounts were found after 96 hours.[21] Half to one liter of blood provides adequate coverage for most minor operative procedures in these patients.

In addition to the cases just described, five less well-defined instances of **"constitutional hypofibrinogenemia"** have been reported[2e,48f] in which the plasma fibrinogen was greatly reduced (0.018 per cent) and excessive bruising, bleeding of the gums and purpura, as well as moderate thrombocytopenia but normal bleeding and coagulation times were present. The hemorrhagic manifestations did not appear as early in these cases as in congenital afibrinogenemia, nor were their frequency or severity as great, all of the patients having reached adult life.

Acquired Hypofibrinogenemia.— The plasma concentration of fibrinogen may decrease under a variety of circumstances and as the effect of different mechanisms. Since it is formed in the liver, plasma fibrinogen may be reduced when severe destructive changes occur in this organ,[11c] as in acute yellow atrophy, and in chloroform or phosphorus poisoning. In clinical practice, however, hypofibrinogenemia much more often is the consequence of a pathological fibrinolytic state.[51a]

Natural inhibitors of coagulation, such as plasmin and its precursor, plasminogen, were discussed in an earlier chapter (p. 295). In certain pathological states, abnormal amounts of plasminogen activator may be released from the tissues into the circulation. In others, thromboplastic material may gain access to the circulation and, by bringing about intravascular clotting, consume fibrinogen and other clotting factors and set up a secondary fibrinolytic response. The clinical problem is usually complex, however, and a complete analysis of the events which take place is not yet available. The end result, in any event, is fibrinogenopenia. Other plasma coagulation factors, such as prothrombin and factors V and VIII, are often depleted as well, and thrombocytopenia may be found also, but these usually are not the primary factors involved in the development of the bleeding diathesis. In occasional instances, evidence of a circulating anticoagulant has been obtained[2d] but this appears to be an unusual cause for fibrinogenopenia.

Clinically, fibrinolysis has been observed in five main conditions: (1) under conditions of stress and in association with severe and extensive physical trauma and following extensive burns; (2) following surgery,[9b] particularly pulmonary surgery; (3) as a result of obstetric complications of abruptio placentae, intrauterine retention of a dead fetus and amniotic fluid embolism;[48b] (4) during the course of neoplastic disease,[25a] especially if the prostate[47f] or, less often, the lung,[18b] pancreas or stomach is involved; and (5) in a variety of miscellaneous disorders, such as polycythemia vera,[7a] leukemia, sarcoidosis and hepatic cirrhosis. The clinical picture may develop with great suddenness and be characterized by the appearance of extensive ecchymoses and severe bleeding from mucous membranes; or the symptoms may be of lesser severity and magnitude (*"purpura thrombolytica,"*[48c] *fibrinolytic purpura*).

The bleeding in cases of acquired fibrinogenopenia is often of extreme gravity and requires the prompt administration of whole, preferably fresh blood and fibrinogen (4 to 10 grams, occasionally even 15 to 20 grams).

CIRCULATING ANTICOAGULANTS

The natural inhibitors of coagulation were described in an earlier chapter (p. 295). Under pathologic conditions anticoagulants normally present may appear in excess or new ones may develop and produce hemorrhage. They may interfere with any phase of coagulation and can be classified in accordance with their mechanism of action.[30c]

The type of anticoagulant most frequently encountered interferes with the *first phase of coagulation.*[16a,16b] The reported cases can be divided into at least four groups; namely, (1) cases of hemophilia in which an anticoagulant opposing the action of factor VIII or factor IX developed following repeated transfusions.

These cases have been described already (p. 875); (2) cases occurring in women, usually in the childbearing period, the hemorrhagic manifestations developing some time after delivery; (3) cases of unknown etiology occurring in men, usually elderly; and (4) cases developing in association with some disease, especially disseminated lupus erythematosus.[47c]

A number of the cases of **"hemophilia-like disease in women"** which have been described from time to time fall into this category rather than being true hemophilia, which is exceedingly rare in the female (p. 862). The occurrence of symptoms such as spontaneous hemorrhage into muscles, tongue, gums, joints and rectum, and complaints such as epistaxis and hematuria suggested hemophilia but the complaints appeared for the first time in adult life and there was no familial history. Prolonged coagulation time, impaired prothrombin consumption and normal platelet counts and clot retraction were found.

Most of the women who acquired this condition before the menopause had hemorrhagic symptoms within one year of the last delivery or miscarriage and it has been suggested[18d] that the postpartum type of hemorrhagic diathesis constitutes a disease entity to be differentiated from the cases reported in postmenopausal women. In one case[18d] the anticoagulant was demonstrated in the patient's second child during his first two and one-half months of life. Such evidence of transplacental transfer of the anticoagulant and analogy with the iso-immunization against factor VIII which may occur in hemophilia (p. 875), strongly suggests that an immunological mechanism accounts for the development of this abnormality. This patient recovered eighteen months after her second delivery and sixteen months after x-ray sterilization. Others recovered spontaneously but death may occur if the bleeding is at a critical site; for example, in the base of the tongue and the mucosa of the pharynx. Blood transfusion has been found to be helpful temporarily in the management of some but not all of these cases.

Cases of abnormal bleeding as the result of the presence of an anticoagulant interfering with the formation of thromboplastin which have been observed in males[46c] form a less homogeneous group. Many of these patients were elderly and in some there was associated disease such as tuberculosis, chronic nephritis, arthritis, and syphilis, and other disorders, but others were entirely normal.[22b] The development of an anticoagulant of the antithromboplastin type has been noted particularly in association with "collagen" diseases, especially lupus erythematosus disseminatus.[50a] True hypoprothrombinemia was not infrequently present as well.[47c]

Much more rare are hemorrhagic states due to anticoagulants acting at other stages of coagulation. Bleeding associated with *heparin-like activity* has been mentioned as occurring sometimes in the course of x-ray or nitrogen mustard therapy and after exposure to ionizing radiation but there is some doubt about the validity of the original observations.[46e] It has also been described in association with disease (acute leukemia, severe liver disease,[16] chronic nephritis[11b]) and in the absence of any apparent cause,[16] when it may be congenital.[46e] Still more rare is an antithrombin unrelated to heparin[28] and different from any of the four "natural" antithrombins (p. 296).

Anticoagulants in therapeutic use can cause confusion with other hemorrhagic states if self medication is denied.[12b] In addition to coumarin derivatives and heparin, other agents which inhibit coagulation include hirudin, a substance contained in leech extract, which prevents the action of thrombin on fibrinogen; salicylates which in large doses have an effect similar to that of the coumarin compounds; cysteine, glutathione, taurine and taurocholic acid, which are thought to inhibit coagulation through an action on thrombin; and the azo dyes, such as Chicago blue and chlorazol pink, which are similar to heparin in their action.

Diagnosis.—Methods for the detection of circulating anticoagulants were discussed elsewhere (p. 305). It is possible to measure the blood level of coumarin compounds.[12b] If the anticoagulant *prevents* the formation of thromboplastin, marked impairment in the utilization of prothrombin will be found. The one-stage prothrombin time will be normal or only slightly abnormal. If the anticoagulant *antagonizes* formed thromboplastin, prothrombin consumption during clotting is impaired only slightly but the one-stage plasma prothrombin time is prolonged. When a heparin-like anticoagulant is present, all phases of the coagulation process are affected in various degrees but the hemostatic defect can be corrected by the addition of protamine sulfate or toluidin blue.

Treatment and Prognosis.—As already indicated, a hemorrhagic diathesis due to the presence of an anticoagulant not deliberately administered may be very serious and resistant to therapy, or recovery may take place spontaneously. Blood transfusions may have no striking beneficial effect other than to replace lost blood.[46c] Treatment with ACTH and adrenocorticosteroids has been stated to be beneficial.[28,46e] Toluidin blue, which can be administered by mouth in doses of 150 to 200 mg. a day, neutralizes heparin. Vitamin K preparations are effective in counteracting the effects of coumarin compounds, but they are largely ineffective when the "hypoprothrombinemia" is of the congenital or idiopathic variety. Vitamin K_1, the natural vitamin, is much more effective in counteracting Dicumarol than are the synthetic water-soluble derivatives such as menadione, although the latter are effective when used in large amounts (64 mg. intravenously). Thus, oral administration of 0.5 to 1 Gm. of the natural vitamin is effective, provided there is no serious impairment of absorption. Vitamin K_1 can be given intravenously by dissolving 200–500 or more mg. in 2 to 4 ml. of 95 per cent ethanol, suspending this solution in 250 ml. saline and administering the suspension by slow intravenous drip. Water-soluble derivatives of vitamin K have been prepared and tested[34c,51d] but clinical experience in their use is still limited.

HEMORRHAGIC DISEASE OF THE NEWBORN

Synonyms.—Melena neonatorum, hemorrhagic diathesis of the newborn, hemophilia neonatorum, morbus haemorrhagicus neonatorum.

Definition.—This is a non-hereditary, self-limited but sometimes fatal condition which occurs in the first few days of life. It is characterized by spontaneous external or internal hemorrhages and greatly prolonged prothrombin time.

History.—Danger of hemorrhage in the newborn was recognized in the Mosaic law which postponed circumcision until the eighth day after birth. In medical literature reference to a bleeding disease in newborn infants was made in 1682[61] and umbilical bleeding was reported as early as 1753.[65] The condition was given its present name in 1894 by Townsend.[69] Whipple[72] in 1912 made the important observation that "prothrombin" was completely absent, but this did not receive much attention for his study was made on postmortem blood in only 1 case. Prolonged coagulation time of the blood was described by Rodda[66] in 1920. Subsequent studies, initiated through the discovery of vitamin K, furnished understanding of the disorder.

Etiology and Pathogenesis.—This condition used to occur about once among every 118 to 333 newborn infants of both sexes.[58] It is now seldom seen because of the prophylactic use of vitamin K. By the one-stage method little hypoprothrombinemia is normally demonstrable at birth[62,65] but the prothrombin level decreases during the first two to six days of life, returning to normal spontaneously at the end of this period.[63] Likewise the thromboplastin generation test is abnormal in the majority of newborn infants. More specifically, the levels of prothrombin and of factor VII are low at birth and decrease further during the first few days of life. They then rise, and decrease again at some time in the second to sixth week of life.[59] Exogenous vitamin K was not found to alter these fluctuations. Factor IX[57] and factor X[66a] levels are also low at birth, as compared with adult values. The concentration of factor V was found to be above normal, as a rule.[59] Levels of factor VIII are similar to those found in adults. In premature infants greater reductions in "prothrombin" occur than in full term infants.[67]

In hemorrhagic disease of the newborn these normal events are accentuated. Many explanations have been offered. In some instances poor dietary intake, poor absorption or impaired utilization of vitamin K in the mother may be important.[61a] In other cases, trauma to the child at birth with hemorrhage and loss of coagulation factors may play a role. In most instances, however, functional immaturity of the liver is probably the major factor. It is plausible to assume also that there is no reserve of prothrombin in the fetus and that, since the infant's diet in the first few days of life affords little vitamin K, no prothrombin is derivable from this source. As soon as the ingestion of water or food has occurred, the entry of bacteria into the intestinal canal usually makes sufficient vitamin available to correct the deficiency.[65]

Symptomatology.—In the majority of cases of hemorrhagic disease of the newborn the onset of hemorrhage coincides with the period of transitory physiological hypoprothrombinemia, that is, two to four days after birth, rarely much later. Bleeding is spontaneous and may occur in the skin and subcutaneous tissues (about 30 per cent of cases), from the gastro-intestinal tract (70 per cent) or the umbilical cord (25 per cent), in the brain or meninges, lungs and pleura, kidneys, vagina, adrenals, or pericardial or peritoneal cavities.[58] Hemorrhages are usually multiple. The bleeding usually begins as a slow oozing and rarely is massive. Symptoms depend on the location and severity of the bleeding. They may be so slight as to attract little attention or they may be severe and may be followed by sudden death. Minor operations such as circumcision or cutting the frenulum of the tongue may be followed by slow but unremitting bleeding. If there is no external evidence of hemorrhage, only loss of appetite, listlessness or failure to gain weight may be noted; or pallor, collapse and coldness of the extremities may indicate serious internal bleeding. Drowsiness, vomiting, frequent convulsive seizures and marked respiratory embarrassment may supervene and indicate cerebral or meningeal hemorrhage.

Physical findings are variable. Extensive ecchymoses may be observed; large hematomata may appear. There may be free bleeding or simply oozing from the umbilical cord. Signs of shock or of involvement of the nervous system may develop. Petechiae are characteristically absent.

Laboratory Findings. — *Blood.* — Changes in the red cells and hemoglobin are those produced by the acute blood loss. Blood platelets are normal in number.[66] Prolonged coagulation time and bleeding time were considered characteristic by some writers but these findings are not necessary before the diagnosis is accepted.[58] As already described, the prothrombin time of the blood is greatly prolonged.[62] Severe bleeding may occur in infants whose plasma prothrombin level is below 15 per cent of normal.

Diagnosis.—Blood from an extraneous source, as from the fissured nipple of the mother, may be swallowed and subsequently vomited or may appear in the stool. Birth injuries may cause bleeding purely as a result of trauma and may produce symptoms similar to those caused by hemorrhagic disease of the newborn. In the latter condition evidence of bleeding will usually be found, in addition, in parts of the body known to have been free of injury. When hemorrhage is entirely internal, diagnosis may be very difficult.

Hemophilia and purpura hemorrhagica rarely make their appearance in the first few days of life, although "congenital purpura" is not unknown (p. 825). The marked reduction in the number of blood platelets in thrombocytopenic purpura and the hereditary features of hemophilia serve to further differentiate these conditions. Bleeding from the umbilical cord is unusual in hemophilia. In constitutional afibrinogenemia, a very rare disorder (p. 883), bleeding from the cord has been observed, the coagulation and bleeding times are prolonged, prothrombin is present but fibrinogen is lacking.

Prognosis and Treatment.—Cases with external bleeding alone are most frequently encountered and are not serious;[58] in those in which internal, or internal and external hemorrhage developed, the mortality was 70 per cent or higher. The course of the illness is rapid, death or recovery occurring in two to three days.

Blood transfusion serves the triple purpose of combatting shock, correcting the anemia and supplying prothrombin, factor VII and other coagulation factors. Vitamin K may be administered as well, even though this could not be expected to be helpful if the cause of the exceptionally low levels of coagulation factors

is hepatic functional immaturity. If the liver is adequate, however, two mg. of menadione (2-methyl-1,4-naphthoquinone) in oil, or its equivalent, given intramuscularly, will increase the prothrombin above the critical level of 20 to 25 per cent of normal within four to six hours. Vitamin K is now usually given prophylactically to all infants. It is also commonly given to the mother (2 mg. menadione) daily for one week prior to delivery, orally or parenterally, but it has not been proved that this is necessary.[60]

Pathology. — Autopsy findings are those due to hemorrhage.

HEREDITARY HEMORRHAGIC TELANGIECTASIA

Definition.—This is a vascular anomaly characterized clinically by hemorrhage and anatomically by multiple dilatations of capillaries and venules which are found in the skin and mucous membranes. Because of its clinical and familial manifestations the disorder is included among the hereditary hemorrhagic diatheses.

History. — Hereditary telangiectasia was first described by Sutton[84] in 1864 and received the attention of Rendu[82] (1896), Osler[81] (1901) and Weber[85] (1907), by whose names the condition is sometimes known.

Etiology.—The vascular abnormality appears to be transmitted as a simple dominant by both sexes. The sexes are equally affected. The telangiectases may be found in childhood but they increase in number as age advances and bleeding may not commence until adult life is reached. Some individuals rarely or never suffer from hemorrhage and this may explain the apparent skipping of individuals of a whole generation, which should not occur if the trait is transmitted as a true dominant. Painstaking examination usually reveals signs of the disease in one of the parents. Occasionally, per-

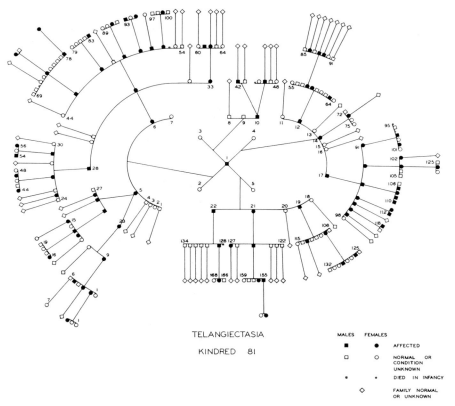

TELANGIECTASIA

KINDRED 81

	MALES	FEMALES	
	■	●	AFFECTED
	□	○	NORMAL OR CONDITION UNKNOWN
	•	•	DIED IN INFANCY
	◇		FAMILY NORMAL OR UNKNOWN

FIG. 18–4.—Family tree to show six generations of a family of "bleeders" whose progenitor had four wives.[74a] Those persons who have been examined have been found to have multiple hereditary telangiectasia. (Courtesy of Dr. F. E. Stephens.)

haps, a mutation occurs or the lesions are all internal. One instance has been reported where both parents were affected.[83c] The manifestations were severe and extensive from birth, and death occurred at eleven weeks of age.

The condition is probably not as rare as was once thought.[77] The writer has himself studied one or more members of at least 12 families afflicted with this condition including 7 at the Johns Hopkins Hospital where Osler described it in 1901. In Utah the polygamy of the pioneers led to the wide transmission of the trait, as the family tree shown in Figure 18–4 testifies. The patients studied and those described in the literature have been chiefly of Anglo-German, Latin, Scandinavian or Jewish stock, in the order named. There are three reports of the disorder in the Negro.[83b]

Symptomatology.—The symptoms are those of hemorrhage and anemia. Epistaxis is especially common, but bleeding may come from telangiectases in any location such as the tongue or mucous membranes of the mouth, or the gastro-intestinal,[80,88] respiratory or genito-urinary tracts.[76] Hemorrhage even into the brain and retina[74] has been attributed to the presence of telangiectases but telangiectactic lesions have not been demonstrated in all instances. The bleeding may arise spontaneously or following slight trauma or vasomotor disturbances.

The telangiectases may be pin-point in size or larger, they may form nodular vascular tumors the size of a split pea

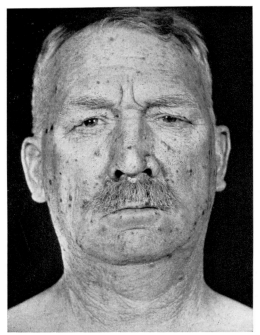

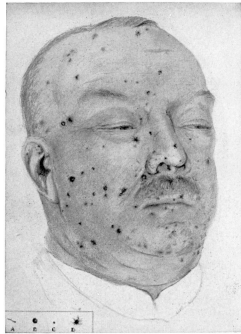

FIG. 18–5.—Photograph and drawing of a patient, aged fifty-seven years, who had suffered with hemorrhages from telangiectases since the age of twenty-four. He later developed cirrhosis of the liver. The telangiectasia was familial. Four types of vascular lesions were present. *B* is the typical telangiectasis, *D* is a "spider" angioma.

(Fig. 18–5), and sometimes they are spider-like, particularly in elderly patients. The last-named type, however, is not characteristic of the disorder. In typical cases the bright-red, violaceous or purple telangiectases may be seen on the face, lips (Fig. 18–7), tongue, conjunctivae, ears, finger-tips and even the feet (Fig. 18–6). Pallor may or may not be present. The spleen has been found enlarged in a few cases, as has also the liver.[75,83] These signs appeared late in life.

In a number of cases pulmonary arteriovenous aneurysm has been found in association with hereditary telangiectasia. In one family of 231 members, such fistulas were demonstrated in 14 individuals. This represented an incidence of 15.4 per cent among those having telangiectasia.[78] In another family, a similar syndrome of cyanosis, clubbing of the fingers and polycythemia, in the presence of a normal heart, was associated with no saccular dilatation or fistula but numerous small telangiectases were present instead.[86]

The blood findings are those which result from blood loss and the picture of acute or chronic posthemorrhagic anemia will be found if hemorrhage has occurred. Bleeding time, coagulation time, clot retraction and platelet count are practically always normal. In several cases,[83a,87,88] however, positive tourniquet tests have been found and in 2 cases the bleeding time was prolonged.

Diagnosis.—The diagnosis should be simple because the triad of habitual hemorrhage, multiple telangiectases and familial history is so characteristic. Errors may occur if the vascular anomalies are overlooked. In cases of obscure anemia they should be sought, for the cause of unexplained bleeding from the gastrointestinal tract or elsewhere may be suggested by telltale lesions of the skin.[88] When these have been overlooked, such diagnoses as pernicious or "secondary"

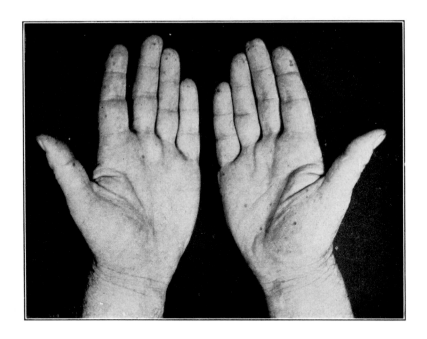

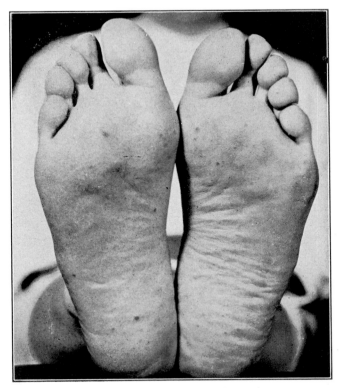

FIG. 18–6.—Hands and feet of patient shown in Figure 18–4, showing characteristic telangiectases.

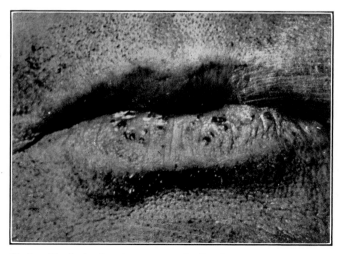

Fig. 18–7.—Typical telangiectases on the lips in another case of multiple hereditary telangiectasia.

Table 18–2.—Differentiation of Skin Lesions in Purpura, Hereditary Telangiectasia and Angiokeratoma Corporis Diffusum Universale

	Purpura	Multiple Hereditary Telangiectasia	Angiokeratoma C. D. U.
Location	Anywhere	Centrifugal	Centripetal (mainly), esp. lower trunk
Duration	Disappears	Permanent	Permanent
Color	Purple	Bright red	Dark red to blue black
Size	Variable	Pin-point to pin-head or larger	Pin-point to pin-head
Position	Flat	Flat usually	Flat or raised, in groups
Effect of pressure	Unaffected	Blanch	Some blanch
Associated skin changes	Usually none	Later, angiomas and spider telangiectases	Corn-like lesions Subcutaneous nodules

anemia, peptic ulcer or Banti's syndrome have been made. In the absence of visible lesions, however, one should hesitate to attribute bleeding of obscure cause to telangiectasia.

When the telangiectases are small they may resemble purpuric spots. They are generally brighter in color, however, and may be somewhat raised above the surface. Furthermore, they fade partially on firm pressure. To observe this, pressure may be made by means of a glass slide through which the color of the lesion may be observed. Examination with a magnifying lens usually reveals the capillary network. Unlike purpuric lesions, telangiectases are permanent.

The lack of abnormalities in the blood should further aid differentiation from purpura and from hemophilia. Unlike the latter disease, hemorrhage does not occur into joints or from areas of skin or mucous membrane in which there are no telangiectases.

Prognosis and Treatment.—The telangiectases may cause little or no inconvenience. As a rule, however, as the patient approaches middle age the telangiectases become more prominent and the bleeding increases in severity. Death from hemorrhage is not frequent, but a state of semi-invalidism as the result of frequent hemorrhagic episodes of various degrees of severity, and anemia, is common.

Oxycel, gelfoam or similar topical hemostatic agents can usually be depended on to control the hemorrhage and they have the added advantage that they do not need to be removed after the bleeding has stopped. If these alone do not suffice in the treatment of epistaxis, a useful device consists of a finger cot placed over the end of a small catheter and tied snugly with fine thread. This is lubricated, inserted well back in the nostril and inflated. Firm uniform pressure is thus applied to the entire interior of the nasal fossa. After the bleeding has stopped the cot is slowly deflated and withdrawn or allowed to drop out of the nostril.[74b]

Although it is possible to destroy the primary lesion with escharotics such as silver nitrate, chromic acid or similar agents, in general such therapy is futile for satellite lesions soon form several millimeters away. Electro-coagulation applied with persistence and gentleness has been claimed to be effective,[74b] but this is probably the exception rather than the rule. Radium, although successful immediately, eventually produces atrophy and dryness of the nasal mucosa and may be followed by perforation of the septum. Electrocoagulation has proved more satisfactory in destroying lesions about the lips, the oral cavity and on the cutaneous surface of the body than in the nasal fossae. Septal dermoplasty was reported as being effective in permanently controlling epistaxis.[82a] There has been no confirmation of the claim that hormone therapy with estrogens or combined estrogens and androgens reduces the incidence and severity of nosebleeds.[79]

Pathology.—The walls of the involved vessels have been found to be extremely thin, consisting merely of a layer of endothelium.[77] The veins are involved primarily and arterial involvement is inconspicuous. The telangiectases have been found at autopsy[81,83] in all major organ systems and in each the venous defect was diffusely distributed.[73] In 1 case,[83] multiple aneurysms of the splenic artery were also discovered. The large arteriovenous aneurysms found clinically in some cases may be only the larger counterparts of widespread telangiectases in the pulmonary tissue.[86]

BIBLIOGRAPHY

Hemophilia and Hemophilia-like Disorders

1. ADDIS, T.: Pathogenesis of Hereditary Hæmophilia, J. Path. & Bact., *15*, 427, 1910–1911.
1a. AGGELER, P. M. and LUCIA, S. P.: The Potency of Blood-coagulating Substances, Am. J. M. Sc., *199*, 181, 1940.
1b. AGGELER, P. M., WHITE, S. G., GLENDENING, M. B., PAGE, E. W., LEAKE, T. B. and BATES, G.: Plasma Thromboplastin Component (PTC) Deficiency: A New Disease Resembling Hemophilia, Proc. Soc. Exper. Biol. & Med., *79*, 692, 1952; *ibid.*, *83*, 69, 1953; Blood, *8*, 101, 1953; Science, *119*, 806, 1954; Am. J. Med., *30*, 84, 1961.
2. ALEXANDER, B. and GOLDSTEIN, R.: Parahemophilia in Three Siblings (Owren's Disease), Am. J. Med., *13*, 255, 1952.
2a. ALEXANDER, B., GOLDSTEIN, R., LANDWEHR, G. and COOK, C. D.: Congenital SPCA Deficiency, J. Clin. Invest., *30*, 596, 1951.
2b. ALEXANDER, B., GOLDSTEIN, R., RICH, L., LeBOLLOC'H, A. G., DIAMOND, L. K. and BORGES, W.: Congenital Afibrinogenemia, Blood, *9*, 843, 1954.
2c. ALLIBONE, E. C. and BAAR, H. S.: Fibrinogen Deficiency as a Factor in Haemorrhagic Disease, Arch. Dis. Childhood, *18*, 146, 1943.
2d. BAKER, S. J. and JACOB, E.: A Haemorrhagic Disorder in Pregnancy Due to an "Anticoagulant" Preventing the Conversion of Fibrinogen to Fibrin, J. Clin. Path., *13*, 214, 1960.
2e. BARROW, EMILY M., BULLOCK, W. R. and GRAHAM, J. B.: A Study of the Carrier State for Plasma Thromboplastin Component (PTC, Christmas Factor) Deficiency, Utilizing a New Assay Procedure, J. Lab. & Clin. Med., *55*, 936, 1960.

3. BEAUMONT, J. L., et BERNARD, J.: Syndrome hémorragique congénital dû au defaut du facteur de coagulation récemment isolé sous le nom de Facteur VII, Convertine, S.P.C.A., Acta med. scandinav., *145*, 200, 1953; Rev. franç. étud. clin. et biol., *3*, 161, 1958.

3a.BEAUMONT, J. L., CAEN, J., et BERNARD, J.: L'hémophilie, Semaine hôp. Paris, *31*, 1154, 1955.

3b.BENDIEN, W. M. and VAN CREVELD, S.: On Some Factors of Blood Coagulation, Especially With Regard to the Problem of Hemophilia, Acta med. scandinav., *99*, 12, 1939.

4. BENTLEY, H. P., JR. and KRIVIT, W.: An Assay of Antihemophilic Globulin Activity in the Carrier Female, J. Lab. & Clin. Med., *56*, 613, 1960.

4a.BERGSAGEL, D. E., SETNA, S. S., CARTWRIGHT, G. E. and WINTROBE, M. M.: Mild PTC (Plasma Thromboplastin Component) Deficiency Occurring in Two Brothers, Blood, *9*, 866, 1954.

4b.BIGGS, ROSEMARY and BIDWELL, ETHEL: A Method for the Study of Antihaemophilic Globulin Inhibitors with Reference to Six Cases, Brit. J. Haemat., *5*, 379, 1959.

5. BIGGS, R., DOUGLAS, A. S., MACFARLANE, R. G., DACIE, J. V., PITNEY, W. R., MERSKEY, C. and O'BRIEN, J. R.: Christmas Disease. A Condition Previously Mistaken for Hæmophilia, Brit. M. J., *2*, 1378, 1952.

5a.BIGGS, R., EVELING, J. and RICHARDS, G.: The Assay of Antihæmophilic Globulin Activity, Brit. J. Hæmat., *1*, 26, 1955.

5b.BIGGS, R. and MACFARLANE, R. G.: *Human Blood Coagulation*, Blackwell Scientific Publications, Oxford, Ed. 2, 1957.

5c.BIGGS, ROSEMARY and MACFARLANE, R. G.: Haemophilia and Related Conditions: 187 Cases, Brit. J. Haemat., *4*, 1, 1958.

5d.BIGGS, ROSEMARY *et al.:* Defects in the Early Stages of Blood Coagulation: A Report of Four Cases, Brit. J. Haemat., *4*, 177, 1958.

6. BIRCH, C. L.: Hemophilia, J.A.M.A., *99*, 1566, 1932.

7. ———— Hemophilia: Clinical and Genetic Aspects, Univ. of Illinois Bull., vol. *34*, No. 55; Illinois Med. and Dent. Monogr., vol. *1*, No. 4, University of Illinois, 1937.

7a.BJÖRKMAN, S. E.: Three Cases of Polycythemia with Fibrinopenia, Acta med. scandinav., *129*, 472, 1948.

7b.BLOMBÄCK, MARGARETA and NILSSON, INGA MARIE: Treatment of Hemophilia A with Human Antihemophilic Globulin, Acta med. scandinav., *161*, 301, 1958; Acta chem. scandinav., *12*, 1878, 1958.

8. BORCHGREVINK, C. F. *et al.:* A Study of a Case of Congenital Hypoprothrombinaemia, Brit. J. Haemat., *5*, 294, 1959.

8a.BOYLES, P. W. and CURRIE, JANE: Classic Hemophilia in a Negro Infant, Am. J. M. Sc., *235*, 452, 1958.

8b.BRAUN, E. H. and STOLLAR, D. B.: Spontaneous Haemophilia in a Female. Thromb. Diath. haemorrh., *4*, 369, 1960.

9. BRINKHOUS, K. M.: A Study of the Clotting Defect in Hemophilia; Am. J. M. Sc., *198*, 509, 1939; Proc. Soc. Exper. Biol. & Med., *66*, 117, 1947; J.A.M.A., *154*, 481, 1954; Bull. New York Acad. Med., *3*, 325, 1954; Sang, *25*, 738, 1954.

9a.BRINKHOUS, K. M., Editor: *Hemophilia and Hemophilioid Diseases*, Chapel Hill, N. C., University of North Carolina Press, 1957.

9b.BROWN, I. W., JR. and SMITH, W. W.: Hematologic Problems Associated with the Use of Extracorporeal Circulation for Cardiovascular Surgery, Ann. Int. Med., *49*, 1035, 1958.

10. BULLOCH, W. and FILDES, P.: Hemophilia, London University, Francis Galton Laboratory for National Eugenics, Treasury of Human Inheritance, *1*, 169, 1912.

10a.BÜTLER, R., RÖHRIG, S., SIEGENTHALER, P. and MOESCHLIN, S.: A Special Haemophilic Syndrome, Acta haemat., *22*, 292, 1959.

10b.CAEN, J. and BERNARD, J.: Déficit en facteur Hageman, Rev. hémat., *13*, 154, 1958.

10c.CAEN, J., YANOTTI, S., VARANGOT, J. and BERNARD, J.: Etude d'un cas d'hypoproconvertinémie vraie congénitale, Sang, *30*, 535, 1959.

11. CAFFEY, J. and SCHLESINGER, E. R.: Certain Effects of Hemophilia on the Growing Skeleton, J. Pediat., *16*, 549, 1940.

11a.CAVINS, J. A. and WALL, R. L.: Clinical and Laboratory Studies of Plasma Thromboplastin Antecedent Deficiency (PTA), Am. J. Med., *29*, 444, 1960.

11b.CETINGIL, A. I., ULUTIN, O. N. and KARACA, M.: Heparin-like Anticoagulant Occurring in Association with Chronic Nephritis, Brit. M. J., *2*, 38, 1959.

11c.CONLEY, C. L., RATNOFF, O. D. and HARTMANN, R. C.: Studies on Afibrinogenemia: I. Afibrinogenemia in a Patient with Septic Abortion, Acute Yellow Atrophy of the Liver and Bacteremia Due to E. Coli, Bull. Johns Hopkins Hosp., *88*, 402, 1951.

11d.CONNOR, W. E., WARNER, E. D. and CARTER, J. R.: A Labile Serum Factor Clotting Defect, J. Clin. Invest., *40*, 13, 1961.

12. CONSTANDOULAKIS, M.: Familial Haemophilia and Factor VII Deficiency, J. Clin. Path.. *11*, 412, 1958.

12a.Cook, I. A. and Douglas, A. S.: Demonstrable Deficiency of Christmas Factor in Two Sisters, Brit. M. J., 1, 479, 1960.

12b.Cosgriff, S. W.: Hemorrhage Due to Self-Medication with Bishydroxycoumarin, J.A. M.A., 153, 547, 1953.

13. Custer, R. P. and Krumbhaar, E. B.: The Histopathology of the Hemopoietic Tissues in Hemophilia, Am. J. M. Sc., 189, 620, 1935.

13b.Davidson, C. S., Epstein, R. D., Miller, G. F. and Taylor, F. H. L.: Hemophilia. A Clinical Study of Forty Patients, Blood, 4, 97, 1949.

13c.Didisheim, P.: An Artificial Reagent for the Diagnosis of Classical Hemophilia, Science, 129, 389, 1959.

14. Didisheim, P., Ferguson, J. H. and Lewis, J. H.: Hemostatic Data in Relatives of Hemophiliacs A and B, A. M. A. Arch. Int. Med., 101, 347, 1958.

14a.Didisheim, P., Loeb, J., Blatrix, C. and Soulier, J. P.: Preparation of a Human Plasma Fraction Rich in Prothrombin, Proconvertin, Stuart Factor and PTC and a Study of Its Activity and Toxicity in Rabbits and Man, J. Lab. & Clin. Med., 53, 322, 1959.

14b.Dische, F. E.: Blood-clotting Substances with 'Factor VII' Activity, Brit. J. Haemat., 4, 201, 1958.

14c.Dische, F. E. and Benfield, Vera: Congenital Factor VII Deficiency, Acta haemat., 21, 257, 1959.

14d.Douglas, A. S.: Some Observations on the Coagulation Defect in Vitamin K Deficiency, J. Clin. Path., 11, 261, 1958.

15. Fantl, P. and Margolis, J.: Alpha-Prothromboplastin Deficiencies (Hæmophilia) of Differing Degrees in a Mother and Son, Brit. M. J., 1, 640, 1955.

15a.Fantl, P. and Sawers, P. J.: Haemophilia, Australasian Ann. Med., 3, 245, 1954.

15b.Fantl, P. and Sawers, R. J.: Occurrence of Different Prothromboplastin Deficiencies in Related Male Bleeders, Brit. J. Haemat., 2, 102, 1956.

16. Favre-Gilly, J., Simon, Thouverez, J. P. and Diebold: Diathèse hémorragique féminine avec présence dans le sang d'une antithrombine du type de l'héparine, Sang, 29, 398, 1958.

16a.Favre-Gilly, J. and Thouverez, J. P.: Les inhibiteurs de la première phase de la coagulation en dehors de l'hémophilie, Sang, 30, 351, 1959.

16b.Ferguson, J. H., Johnston, C. L., Jr. and Howell, Doris A.: A Circulating Inhibitor (Anti-AcG) Specific for the Labile Factor-V of the Blood-Clotting Mechanism, Blood, 13, 382, 1958.

16c.Ferguson, J. H., Travis, B. L. and Gerheim, E. B.: Fibrinogenolytic Demonstration of Activation and Inhibition of Tryptase in Plasma Protein Fraction-I ("Antihemophilic Globulin"), Proc. Soc. Exper. Biol. & Med., 64, 285, 1947.

16d.Fernando, P. B. and Dharmasena, B. D.: A Case of Congenital Afibrinogenemia, Blood, 12, 474, 1957.

17. Firor, W. M. and Woodhall, B.: Hemophilic Pseudotumor: Diagnosis, Pathology and Surgical Treatment of Hemophilic Lesions in the Smaller Bones and Joints, Bull. Johns Hopkins Hosp., 59, 237, 1936.

18. Fonio, A.: Die Hämophilie, Ergebn. inn. Med. u. Kinderh., 51, 443, 1936; Schweiz. med. Wchnschr., 89, 1026, 1959.

18a.Fonio, A. und Passet, R.: Die sporadische Hämophilie in der Schweiz, Archiv. der Julius Klaus-Stiftung für Vererbungsforschung, Sozialanthropologie und Rassenhygiene, 23, 425, 1948.

18b.Fountain, J. R. and Holman, R. L.: Acquired Fibrinogen Deficiency Associated with Carcinoma of the Bronchus, Ann. Int. Med., 52, 459, 1960.

18c.Freund, E.: Die Gelenkerkrankung der Bluter, Virchows Arch., 256, 158, 1925.

18d.Frick, P. G.: Hemophilia-like Disease following Pregnancy, Blood, 8, 598, 1953. Am. J. Obst. & Gynec., 70, 328, 1955.

19. ———— The Relative Incidence of Anti-Hemophilic Globulin (AHG), Plasma Thromboplastin Component (PTC), and Plasma Thromboplastin Antecedent (PTA) Deficiency, J. Lab. & Clin. Med., 43, 860, 1954.

19b.Frick, P. G. and Hagen, P. S.: Congenital Familial Deficiency of the Stable Prothrombin Conversion Factor, J. Lab. & Clin. Med., 42, 212, 1953; J. Lab. & Clin. Med., 51, 398, 1958.

19c.Giffin, H. Z.: Familial Epistaxis without Telangiectasia, Am. J. M. Sc., 174, 690, 1927.

20. Glueck, Helen, I. and Sutherland, J. M.: Inherited Factor-VII Defect in a Negro Family, Pediatrics, 27, 204, 1961.

20a.Gollub, S., Bolton, H., Hessert, E. and Ulin, A.: Acquired Hemophilia B, J.A.M.A., 171, 1333, 1959.

20c.Graham, J. B., Buckwalter, J. A., Hartley, L. J. and Brinkhous, K. M.: Canine Hemophilia, J. Exper. Med., 90, 97, 1949; Science, 111, 723, 1950; Am. J. Physiol., 164, 710, 1951; J. Exper. Med., 106, 273,

1957; Proc. Soc. Exper. Biol. & Med., *96*, 152, 1957; Lab. Invest., *8*, 1269, 1959.

20*d*.GRAHAM, J. B., McLENDON, W. W. and BRINKHOUS, K. M.: Mild Hemophilia: An Allelic Form of the Disease, Am. J. M. Sc., *225*, 46, 1953.

20*e*.GROSSMAN, B. J. and CARTER, R. E.: Congenital Afibrinogenemia, J. Pediat., *50*, 708, 1957.

21. HARDISTY, R. M. and PINNIGER, J. L.: Congenital Afibrinogenaemia: Further Observations on the Blood Coagulation Mechanism, Brit. J. Hæmat., *2*, 139, 1956.

21*a*.HARMON, MARY C., ZIPURSKY, A. and LAHEY, M. E.: A Study of Hemophilia, A. M. A. J. Dis. Child., *93*, 375, 1957.

22. HOAG, M. SILVIJA, AGGELER, P. M. and FOWELL, A. H.: Disappearance Rate of Concentrated Proconvertin Extracts in Congenital and Acquired Hypoproconvertinemia, J. Clin. Invest., *39*, 554, 1960.

22*a*.HOGAN, A. G., MUHRER, M. E. and BOGART, R.: A Hemophilia-Like Disease in Swine, Proc. Soc. Exper. Biol. & Med., *48*, 217, 1941; Am. J. Physiol., *136*, 355 and 360, 1942; *ibid.*, *138*, 136, 1942.

22*b*.HOUGIE, C.: Pseudo-hæmophilia: An Acquired Hæmorrhagic Diathesis Due to a Circulating Anticoagulant, J. Clin. Path., *6*, 30, 1953.

22*c*.HOUGIE, C.: Pathogenesis of Haemophilia, Brit. J. Haemat., *5*, 177, 1959.

22*d*.HOUGIE, C., BARROW, EMILY M. and GRAHAM, J. B.: Stuart Clotting Defect, J. Clin. Invest., *36*, 485 and 497, 1957.

23. HOWELL, W. H.: Hemophilia, Bull. New York Acad. Med., *15*, 3, 1939.

23*a*.HOWELL, W. H. and CEKADA, E. B.: The Cause of the Delayed Clotting of Hemophilic Blood, Am. J. Physiol., *78*, 500, 1926.

24. IKKALA, E.: Haemophilia, Scandinav. J. Clin. & Lab. Invest. (Suppl. 45), *12*, 1, 1960.

24*a*.ISRAËLS, M. C. G., LEMPERT, H. and GILBERTSON, E.: Hæmophilia in the Female, Lancet, *1*, 1375, 1951.

24*b*.JOHNSON, S. A.: Activation of Purified Prothrombin with Hemophilic Plasma, Am. J. Clin. Path., *23*, 875, 1953.

24*c*.JORDAN, H. H.: *Hemophilic Arthropathies*, Springfield, Ill., C. C Thomas, 1958.

24*d*.JOSEPHSON, A. M. and LISKER, R.: Demonstration of a Circulating Anticoagulant in Plasma Thromboplastin Antecedent Deficiency, J. Clin. Invest., *37*, 148, 1958.

25. JUNG, E. G.: The Relative Frequency of Hæmophilia A and B, Thromb. Diath. hæmorrh., *4*, 331, 1960.

25*a*.JÜRGENS, R. and TRAUTWEIN, H.: Uber Fibrinopenie beim Erwachsenen nebst Bemer-

kungen über die Herkumft des Fibrinogen, Deutsch. Arch. klin. Med., *169*, 28, 1930.

25*b*.KAY, W. R. and KUPFER, H. G.: Spontaneous Hemothorax in Hemophilia, Ann. Int. Med., *47*, 152, 1957.

26. KEKWICK, R. A. and WOLF, P.: A Concentrate of Human Antihaemophilic Factor, Lancet, *1*, 647, 1957.

26*a*.KOLLER, F., KRÜSI, G. and LUCHSINGER, P.: Ueber eine besondere Form hämorrhagischer Diathese, Schweiz. med. Wchnschr., *80*, 1101, 1950; Blood, *9*, 286, 1954.

26*b*.KUPFER, H. G., HANNA, B. L. and KINNE, DIXIE R.: Congenital Factor VII Deficiency with Normal Stuart Activity, Blood, *15*, 146, 1960.

26*c*.LANGDELL, R. D., WAGNER, R. H. and BRINKHOUS, K. M.: Effect of Antihemophilic Factor on One-stage Clotting Tests, J. Lab. & Clin. Med., *41*, 637, 1953.

26*d*.————Antihemophilic Factor (AHF) Levels following Transfusions of Blood, Plasma and Plasma Fractions, Proc. Soc. Exper. Biol. & Med., *88*, 212, 1955; Arch. Path., *61*, 6, 1956.

26*e*.LARRIEU, M. J. *et al.*: Hypoaccélérinémie congénitale (parahémophilie d'Owren), Sang, *27*, 117, 1956.

26*f*.LEATHERDALE, R. A. L.: Respiratory Obstruction in Haemophilic Patients, Brit. M. J., *1*, 1316, 1960.

27. LEWIS, JESSICA H., FERGUSON, J. H. and ARENDS, T.: Hemorrhagic Disease with Circulating Inhibitors of Blood Clotting, Blood, *11*, 846, 1956.

27*a*.LEWIS, JESSICA H. *et al.*: Acquired Hypoprothrombinemia, Blood, *12*, 84, 1957.

27*b*.LEWIS, J. H., TAGNON, H. J., DAVIDSON, C. S., MINOT, G. R. and TAYLOR, F. H. L.: The Relation of Certain Fractions of the Plasma Globulins to the Coagulation Defect in Hemophilia, Blood, *1*, 166, 1946; J. Clin. Invest., *38*, 1924, 1959.

28. LOELIGER, A. and HERS, J. F. Ph.: Chronic Antithrombinaemia (Antithrombin V) with Haemorrhagic Diathesis in a Case of Rheumatoid Arthritis with Hypergammaglobulinaemia, Thromb. Diath. haemorrh., *1*, 499, 1957.

29. LOZNER, E. L., KARK, R. and TAYLOR, F. H. L.: The Coagulation Defect in Hemophilia: The Clot Promoting Activity in Hemophilia of Berkefelded Normal Human Plasma Free from Fibrogen and Prothrombin, J. Clin. Invest., *18*, 603, 1939.

29*a*.LOZNER, E. L., MacDONALD, H., FINLAND, M. and TAYLOR, F. H. L.: The Use of Rabbit Thrombin as a Local Hemostatic, Am. J. M. Sc., *202*, 593, 1941; *ibid.*, *205*, 538, 1943.

30. MACKLIN, M. T.: Heredity in Hemophilia, Am. J. M. Sc., *175*, 218, 1928.

30a.———— Sex Ratios in Families with Hemophilia, Am. J. Dis. Child., *58*, 1215, 1939.

30b. MACAUSLAND, W. R., JR. and GARTLAND, J. J.: The Treatment of Acute Hemophilic Hemarthrosis, New England J. Med., *247*, 755, 1952.

30c. MARGOLIUS, A., JR., JACKSON, D. P. and RATNOFF, O. D.: Circulating Anticoagulants: A Study of 40 Cases and A Review of the Literature, Medicine, *40*, 145, 1961.

31. MACFARLANE, R. G., BIGGS, R. and BIDWELL, E.: Bovine Antihæmophilic Globulin in the Treatment of Hæmophilia, Lancet, *1*, 1316, 1954; Brit. J. Hæmat., *1*, 35, 1955; Acta hæmat., *24*, 124, 1960.

31a. MACMILLAN, R. L., EZRIN, C. and BUTLER, A.: Prothrombin Consumption in Hæmophiliac Kindred, J. Clin. Path., *4*, 460, 1951.

32. MCCAMPBELL, S. R. and NEEDY, C. K.: Peripheral Vascular Occlusion Due to Hemorrhage in Hemophilia, Ann. Int. Med., *47*, 562, 1957.

32a. MCGOVERN, J. J. and STEINBERG, A. G.: Antihemophilic Factor Deficiency in the Female, J. Lab. & Clin. Med., *51*, 386, 1958.

33. MCINTYRE, H., NOUR-ELDIN, F., ISRAËLS, M. C. G. and WILKINSON, J. F.: Dental Extractions in Patients with Haemophilia and Christmas Disease, Lancet, *2*, 642, 1959.

33a. MERSKEY, C.: The Occurrence of Hæmophilia in the Human Female, Quart. J. Med., *20*, 299, 1951.

33b.———— The Laboratory Diagnosis of Hæmophilia, J. Clin. Path., *3*, 301, 1950; Brit. M. J., *1*, 906, 1951.

33c. MERSKEY, C. and MACFARLANE, R. G.: The Female Carrier of Haemophilia, Lancet, *1*, 487, 1951.

34. MINOT, G. R. and LEE, R. I.: Blood Platelets in Hemophilia, Arch. Int. Med., *17*, 474, 1916.

34a. MOOR-JANKOWSKI, J. K. et al.: Hemophilia B, Acta genet. statist. med., *7*, 597, 1957; ibid., *8*, 1, 1958.

34b. MORITA, H. and KAGAMI, M.: Congenital Afibrinogenemia, Acta haemat., *17*, 315, 1957.

34c. MUSHETT, C. W., KELLEY, K. L. and HIRSCHMANN, R.: Efficacy of Water-Soluble Derivatives of Vitamin K, in Counteracting Drug-Induced Hypoprothrombinemia, Blood, *14*, 37, 1959.

34d. MUSTARD, J. F.: The Serum Defect in Christmas Disease, Acta haemat., *21*, 321, 1959.

35. NASSE, C. F.: Von einer erblichen Neigung zu tödtlichen Blutungen, Arch. med. Erfahr., *1*, 385, 1820.

36. NILSSON, INGA MARIE, BERGMAN, S., REITALU, J. and WALDENSTRÖM, J.: Haemophilia A in a "Girl" with Male Sex-Chromatin Pattern, Lancet, *2*, 264, 1959.

36a. NOUR-ELDIN, F.: Different Haemostatic Defects in One Family, Brit. M. J., *2*, 502, 1960.

36b. NOUR-ELDIN, F. and WILKINSON, J. F.: Bridge Anticoagulant, Brit. J. Haemat., *4*, 38 and 292, 1958.

36c. NOUR-ELDIN, F. and WILKINSON, J. F.: Factor-VII Deficiency with Christmas Disease in One Family, Lancet, *1*, 1173, 1959.

36d. O'BRIEN, J. R.: Factor V in Blood Coagulation *in vitro* and a Report of a Case of Factor-V Deficiency, Brit. J. Haemat., *4*, 210, 1958.

37. OTTO, J. C.: An Account of an Hemorrhagic Disposition Existing in Certain Families, Med. Reposit., *6*, 1, 1803.

38. PACHMAN, D. J.: Hemophilia in Negroes, J. Pediat., *10*, 809, 1937.

39. PAINTER, S. L. and ELLETT, ROSAMOND: Hemophilia (AHG Deficiency) and Factor VII (Stable Factor) Deficiency in the American Indian, Rocky Mountain Med. J., *57*, 65, 1960.

40. PATEK, A. J., JR. and STETSON, R. P.: Hemophilia: I. The Abnormal Coagulation of the Blood and Its Relation to the Blood Platelets, J. Clin. Invest., *15*, 531, 1936.

41. PATEK, A. J., JR. and TAYLOR, F. H. L.: Hemophilia: II. Some Properties of a Substance Obtained from Normal Human Plasma Effective in Accelerating the Coagulation of Hemophilic Blood, J. Clin. Invest., *16*, 113, 1937.

41a. PAVLOVSKY, A.: Contribution to the Pathogenesis of Hemophilia, Blood, *2*, 185, 1947; Sang, *26*, 162, 1955.

41b. PERRY, S., OPFELL, R. and BAKER, MARY: Combined Deficiencies of PTA and AHG with Vascular Fragility, Blood, *16*, 1184, 1960.

42. PIEPER, G. R., PERRY, S. and BURROUGHS, J.: Surgical Intervention in Hemophilia, J.A.M.A., *170*, 33, 1959.

43. PITNEY, W. R.: Mild Haemophilia, Australasian Ann. Med., *6*, 44, 1957.

43a. PITNEY, W. R.: Congenital Deficiency of Factor VII, Australasian Ann. Med., *7*, 15, 1958.

44. PITNEY, W. R. and ARNOLD, BARBARA J.: Plasma Antihaemophilic Factor (AHF) Concentrations in Families of Patients with Haemorrhagic States, Brit. J. Haemat., *5*, 184, 1959.

45. POHLE, F. J. and TAYLOR, F. H. L.: The Use of a Globulin Substance Derived from Beef Plasma as a Local Hemostatic in Hemophilia, J. Clin. Invest., *17*, 677, 1938.

45a. POLA, V. and SVOJITKA, J.: Klassische Hämophilie bei Frauen, Folia haemat., *75*, 43, 1957.

45*b*.POOL, JUDITH G. and ROBINSON, JEAN: Observations on Plasma Banking and Transfusion Procedures for Haemophilic Patients Using a Quantitative Assay for Antihaemophilic Globulin (AHG), Brit. J. Haemat., *5*, 24, 1959.

45*c*.PUDLÁK, P., DEIMLOVÁ, E. and STARÁ, I.: The Coagulation Activity of Incomplete Thromboplastins and Bridge Anticoagulant, Brit. J. Haemat., *5*, 413, 1959.

46. QUICK, A. J.: Studies on the Enigma of the Hemostatic Dysfunction of Hemophilia, Am. J. M. Sc., *214*, 272, 1947.

46*a*.———— Sporadic Hemophilia, Arch. Int. Med., *106*, 335, 1960.

46*b*.QUICK, A. J. and CONWAY, J. P.: Hemophilia in Twins, Am. J. Med., *7*, 841, 1949.

46*c*.QUICK, A. J., DANIELS, E. R. and HUSSEY, C. V.: Acquired Antithromboplastinogenemia (Hæmophilia-like Disease): with Special Reference to Its Diagnosis, J. Lab. & Clin. Med., *44*, 94, 1954.

46*d*.QUICK, A. J. and HUSSEY, C. V.: Hemophilic Condition in a Girl, Am. J. Dis. Child., *85*, 698, 1953; Lancet, *1*, 294, 1958.

46*e*.QUICK, A. J. and HUSSEY, CLARA V.: Hyperheparinemia, Am. J. M. Sc., *234*, 251, 1957.

46*f*.QUICK, A. J., PISCIOTTA, A. V. and HUSSEY, C. V.: Congenital Hypoprothrombinemic States, Arch. Int. Med., *95*, 2, 1955.

47. RABE, F. and SALOMON, E.: Über Faserstoffmangel im Blute bei einem Falle von Hämophilie, Deutsch. Arch. klin. Med., *132*, 240, 1920.

47*a*.RAMOT, B., ANGELOPOULOS, B. and SINGER, K.: Plasma Thromboplastin Antecedent Deficiency, Arch. Int. Med., *95*, 705, 1955.

47*b*.———— Variable Manifestations of Plasma Thromboplastin Component Deficiency J. Lab. & Clin. Med., *46*, 80, 1955.

47*c*.RAPAPORT, S. I., AMES, SARA BETH and DUVALL, BARBARA J.: A Plasma Coagulation Defect in Systemic Lupus Erythematosus Arising from Hypoprothrombinemia Combined with Antiprothrombinase Activity, Blood, *15*, 212, 1960.

47*d*.RAPAPORT, S. I., AMES, SARA BETH and MIKKELSEN, SOLVEIG: The Levels of Antihemophilic Globulin and Proaccelerin in Fresh and Bank Blood, Am. J. Clin. Path., *31*, 297, 1959.

47*e*.RAPAPORT, S. I., AMES, SARA BETH, MIKKELSEN, SOLVEIG and GOODMAN, J. R.: Plasma Clotting Factors in Chronic Hepatocellular Disease, New England J. Med., *263*, 278, 1960.

47*f*.RAPAPORT, S. I. and CHAPMAN, C. G.: Co-existent Hypercoagulability and Acute Hypofibrinogenemia in a Patient with Prostatic Carcinoma, Am. J. Med., *27*, 144, 1959.

47*g*.RAPAPORT, S. I., PATCH, MARY JANE and MOORE, F. J.: Anti-Hemophilic Globulin Levels in Carriers of Hemophilia A, J. Clin. Invest., *39*, 1619, 1960.

48. RATNOFF, O. D. and COLOPY, J. E.: A Familial Hemorrhagic Trait Associated with a Deficiency of a Clot-promoting Fraction of Plasma, J. Clin. Invest., *34*, 602, 1955; Am. J. Med., *25*, 160, 1958.

48*a*.RATNOFF, O. D. and MARGOLIUS, A., JR.: On the Epidemiology of Hemophilia and Christmas Disease, New England J. Med., *256*, 845, 1957.

48*b*.REID, D. E., WEINER, A. E., ROBY, C. C. and DIAMOND, L. K.: I. Intravascular Clotting and Afibrinogenemia, the Presumptive Lethal Factors in the Syndrome of Amniotic Fluid Embolism. II. Incoagulable Blood in Severe Premature Separation of the Placenta: A Method of Management. III. Maternal Afibrinogenemia Associated with Long-standing Intrauterine Fetal Death, Am. J. Obst. & Gynec., *66*, 465, 475 and 500, 1953; J.A.M.A., *167*, 1244, 1956.

48*c*.REIMANN, F.: Purpura thrombolytica, Acta med. scandinav., *107*, 95, 1941.

48*d*.RHOADS, J. E. and FITZ-HUGH, T., JR.: Idiopathic Hypoprothrombinemia—an Apparently Unrecorded Condition, Am. J. M. Sc., *202*, 662, 1941.

48*e*.ROOS, J., VAN ARKEL, C., VERLOOP, M. C. and JORDAN, F. L. J.: A "New" Family with Stuart-Prower Deficiency, Thromb. Diath. haemorrh., *3*, 59, 1959.

48*f*.RISAK, E.: Die Fibrinopenie, Ztschr. klin. Med., *128*, 605, 1935.

49. ROSENTHAL, M. C.: The Therapy of Disorders of Coagulation, J. Chron. Dis., *6*, 383, 1957.

49*a*.ROSENTHAL, R. L., DRESKIN, O. H. and ROSENTHAL, N.: New Hemophilia-like Disease Caused by Deficiency of a Third Plasma Thromboplastin Factor, Proc. Soc. Exper. Biol. & Med., *82*, 171, 1953; Am. J. Med., *17*, 57, 1954; J. Lab. & Clin. Med., *45*, 123, 1955; Blood, *10*, 120, 1955.

49*b*.ROSENTHAL, M. C. and SANDERS, M.: Plasma Thromboplastin Component Deficiency, Am. J. Med., *16*, 153, 1954; Am. J. Clin. Path., *24*, 910, 1954.

49*c*.RUBIN, B., LEVINE, P. and ROSENTHAL, M. C.: Complete Dental Care of the Hemophiliac, Oral Surg., *12*, 665, 1959.

50. SAHLI, H.: Ueber das Wesen der Hämophilie, Ztschr. klin. Med., *56*, 264, 1905; Deutsch. Arch. klin. Med., *99*, 518, 1910.

50a. SÁNCHEZ, MEDAL, L. and LISKER, R.: Circulating Anticoagulants in Disseminated Lupus Erythematosus, Brit. J. Haemat., 5, 284, 1959.

50b. SCARDIGLI, G. and GUIDI, G.: Severe Coagulation Anomalies in a Family of Haemophiliacs, Acta haemat., 16, 338, 1956.

51. SCHLOESSMANN, H.: Die Hämophilie, Neue Deutsch. Chir., 47, 1 to 297, 1930 (Bibliography).

51a. SCHULMAN, I. and SMITH, C. H.: Hemorrhagic Disease in an Infant Due to Deficiency of a Previously Undescribed Clotting Factor, Blood, 7, 794, 1952.

51b. SEIBERT, R. H., MARGOLIUS, A., JR. and RATNOFF, O. D.: Observations on Hemophilia, Parahemophilia and Coexistent Hemophilia and Parahemophilia, J. Lab. & Clin. Med., 52, 449, 1958.

51c. SHERRY, S., FLETCHER, A. P. and ALKJAERSIG, NORMA: Fibrinolysis and Fibrinolytic Activity in Man, Physiol. Rev., 39, 343, 1959.

51d. SHOSHKES, M. and TAMI, M.: Dihydrovitamin K_1 Biphosphate in Bishydroxycoumarin Induced Hypoprothrombinemia, J. Lab. & Clin. Med., 56, 21, 1960.

51e. SILBER, R. and CHRISTENSEN, W. R.: Pseudotumor of Hemophilia in a Patient with PTC Deficiency, Blood, 14, 584, 1959.

52. SILVERSTEIN, A.: Intracranial Bleeding in Hemophilia, A. M. A. Arch. Neurol., 3, 141, 1960.

52a. SJÖLIN, K.-E.: Classical Haemophilia (AHF Deficiency) and Christmas Factor (PTC) Deficiency as Simultaneous Defects, Acta med. scandinav., 159, 7, 1957; Danish M. Bull., 3, 85, 1956.

52b. SOULIER, J.-P.: Etude génétique des syndromes hémorragiques, Sang, 25, 355, 1954; Rév. hémat., 10, 689, 1955.

52c. SOULIER, J. P. and LARRIEU, M. J.: Déficit en facteur antihémophilique B avec allongement du temps de saignment, Sang, 28, 138, 1957.

52d. SPAET, T. H., AGGELER, P. M. and KINSELL, B. G.: A Possible Fourth Plasma Thromboplastin Component, J. Clin. Invest., 33, 1095, 1954; J. Lab. & Clin. Med., 52, 634, 1958.

52e. SPAET, T. H. and GARNER, E. S.: Studies on the Storage Lability of Human Antihemophilic Factor, J. Lab. & Clin. Med., 46, 111, 1955.

52f. SPAET, T. H. and KROPATKIN, MONA: Studies on "Prothrombin Derivatives" in Vitamin K Deficiency, A. M. A. Arch. Int. Med., 102, 558, 1958.

53. STETSON, R. P., FORKNER, C. E., CHEW, W. B. and RICH, M. L.: Negative Effect of Prolonged Administration of Ovarian Substances in Hemophilia, J.A.M.A., 102, 1122, 1934; Arch. Int. Med., 55, 431, 1935.

53a. TAGNON, H. J., DAVIDSON, C. S. and TAYLOR, F. H. L.: The Coagulation Defect in Hemophilia; J. Clin. Invest., 22, 127, 1943; Blood, 1, 166, 1946.

53b. TAYLOR, K. and BIGGS, ROSEMARY: A Mildly Affected Female Haemophiliac, Brit. M. J., 1, 1494, 1957.

53c. TELFER, T. P., DENSON, K. W. and WRIGHT, D. R.: A 'New' Coagulation Defect, Brit. J. Haemat., 2, 308, 1956.

54. THOMAS, H. B.: Some Orthopedic Findings in Ninety-eight Cases of Hemophilia, J. Bone & Joint Surg., 18, 140, 1936.

55. TOCANTINS, L. M.: Demonstration of Antithromboplastic Activity in Normal and Hemophilic Plasmas, Am. J. Physiol., 139, 265, 1943; ibid., 143, 67, 1945; Blood, 1, 156, 1946; ibid., 9, 281, 1954; Fed. Proc., 15, 31, 1956.

55a. VAN CREVELD, S.: Congenital Idiopathic Hypoprothrombinemia, Acta pædiat., 43, 245, 1954 (Supp. 100).

55b. VAN CREVELD, S. and LIEM, K. H.: Congenital Afibrinogenemia, Études Néo-Natales, 7, 89, 1958.

55c. VOOS, D. and WAALER, B. A.: Congenital Hypoproconvertinemia, Thromb. Diath. haemorrh., 3, 375, 1959.

56. WINSTON, M. E.: Hæmophiliac Arthropathy of the Hip, J. Bone & Joint Surg., 34B, 412, 1952.

56a. WRIGHT, H. M. P.: Adhesiveness of Blood Platelets in Hæmophilia, Lancet, 1, 306, 1946.

Hemorrhagic Disease of the Newborn

57. BARKHAN, P.: Christmas-Factor Activity of Cord Blood, Brit. J. Haemat., 3, 215, 1957.

58. CLIFFORD, S. H.: Hemorrhagic Disease of the Newborn, J. Pediat., 14, 333, 1939.

59. FRESH, J. W. et al.: Blood Prothrombin, Proconvertin and Proaccelerin in Normal Infancy: Questionable Relationships to Vitamin K, Pediatrics, 19, 241, 1957.

60. HAY, J. D., HUDSON, F. P. and RODGERS, T. S.: Vitamin K in the Prevention of Haemorrhagic Disease of the Newborn, Lancet, 1, 423, 1951.

61. LÖVEGREN, E.: Erfahrungen und Studien über Melaena neonatorum, Jahrb. Kinderh., 78, 249, 1913 (Bibliography).

61a. MACPHERSON, A. I. S.: Observations on the Ætiology and Prophylaxis of Prothrombin Deficiency and Hæmorrhagic Disease in the New-born, J. Obst. and Gynec., Brit. Emp., 49, 368, 1942.

62. NYGAARD, K. K.: Prophylactic and Curative Effect of Vitamin K in Hemorrhagic Dis-

ease of the Newborn, Acta obst. et gynec. scandinav., *19*, 361, 1939.

63. OWEN, C. A., HOFFMAN, G. R., ZIFFREN, S. E. and SMITH, H. P.: Blood Coagulation during Infancy, Proc. Soc. Exper. Biol. & Med., *41*, 181, 1939.

65. QUICK, A. J. and GROSSMAN, A. M.: The Nature of the Hemorrhagic Disease of the Newborn, Am. J. M. Sc., *199*, 1, 1940.

66. RODDA, F. C.: Coagulation Time of Blood in the Newborn; with Especial Reference to Cerebral Hemorrhage, J.A.M.A., *75*, 452, 1920.

66a. SCHULZ, JEANETTE and VAN CREVELD, S.: Stuart-Prower Factor in Newborn Infants, Etudes Néo-Natales, *7*, 133, 1958.

67. SHETTLES, L. B., DELFS, E. and HELLMAN, L. M.: Factors Influencing Plasma Prothrombin in the Newborn Infant: II. Antepartum and Neonatal Ingestion of Vitamin K Concentrate, Bull. Johns Hopkins Hosp., *65*, 419, 1939.

68. TOCANTINS, L. M.: Probable Mechanism of the "Physiologic" Hypoprothrombinemia of the Newborn, Am. J. Dis. Child., *59*, 1054, 1940.

69. TOWNSEND, C. W.: The Hæmorrhagic Disease of the Newborn, Arch. Pediat., *11*, 558, 1894.

72. WHIPPLE, G. H.: Hemorrhagic Disease— Septicemia, Melena Neonatorum and Hepatic Cirrhosis, Arch. Int. Med., *9*, 365, 1912; *ibid.*, *12*, 637, 1913.

Hereditary Hemorrhagic Telangiectasia

73. BIRD, R. M. and JAQUES, W. E.: Vascular Lesion of Hereditary Hemorrhagic Telangiectasia, New England J. Med., *260*, 597, 1959; *ibid.*, *257*, 105, 1957.

74. CUENDET, J. F., et MAGNENAT, P.: Symptomatologie oculaire de la maladie de Rendu-Osler. Angiomatose hémorragique familiale, Schweiz. med. Wchnschr., *83*, Suppl. 38, 1531, 1955.

74a. DOLOWITZ, D. A., RAMBO, O. N., JR. and STEPHENS, F. E.: Hereditary Hemorrhagic Telangiectasia, Ann. Otol., Rhin. & Laryng., *62*, 642, 1953.

74b. FIGI, F. A. and WATKINS, C. H.: Hereditary Hemorrhagic Telangiectasia, Ann. Otol. Rhinol. & Laryngol., *52*, 330, 1943.

75. FITZ-HUGH, T., JR.: Splenomegaly and Hepatic Enlargement in Hereditary Hemorrhagic Telangiectasia, Am. J. M. Sc., *181*, 261, 1931.

76. FOGGIE, W. E.: Hereditary Hæmorrhagic Telangiectasia with Recurring Hæmaturia, Edinburgh M. J., *35*, 281, 1928.

77. HANES, F. M.: Multiple Hereditary Telangiectases Causing Hemorrhage (Heredi-

tary Hemorrhagic Telangiectasia), Bull. Johns Hopkins Hosp., *20*, 63, 1909.

78. HODGSON, C. H., BURCHELL, H. B., GOOD, C. A. and CLAGETT, O. T.: Hereditary Hemorrhagic Telangiectasia and Pulmonary Arteriovenous Fistula, New England J. Med., *261*, 625, 1959.

79. KOCH, H. J., JR., ESCHER, G. C. and LEWIS, J. S.: Hormonal Management of Hereditary Hemorrhagic Telangiectasia, J.A.M.A., *149*, 1376, 1952.

80. KUFS, H.: Über heredofamiliäre Angiomatose des Gehirns und der Retina, ihre Beziehungen zueinander und zur Angiomatose der Haut, Ztschr. ges. Neurol. u. Psychiat., *113*, 651, 1928.

81. OSLER, W.: On a Family Form of Recurring Epistaxis, Associated with Multiple Telangiectases of the Skin and Mucous Membrane, Bull. Johns Hopkins Hosp., *12*, 333, 1901.

82. RENDU, M.: Epistaxis repétées chez un sujet porteur de petits angiomes cutanés et muqueux, Bull. et mém. Soc. méd. hôp. Paris, *13*, 731, 1896.

82a. SAUNDERS, W. H.: Permanent Control of Nosebleeds in Patients with Hereditary Hemorrhagic Telangiectasia, Ann. Int. Med., *53*, 147, 1960.

83. SCHUSTER, N. H.: Familial Hæmorrhagic Telangiectasia Associated with Multiple Aneurysms of the Splenic Artery, J. Path. & Bact., *44*, 29, 1937.

83a. SINGER, K. and WOLFSON, W. Q.: Hereditary Hemorrhagic Telangiectasia, New England J. Med., *230*, 637, 1944.

83b. SMITH, J. L. and LINEBACK, M. I.: Hereditary Hemorrhagic Telangiectasia, Am. J. Med., *17*, 41, 1954.

83c. SNYDER, L. H. and DOAN, C. A.: Is the Homozygous Form of Multiple Telangiectasia Lethal?, J. Lab. & Clin. Med., *29*, 1211, 1944.

84. SUTTON, H. G.: Epistaxis as an Indication of Impaired Nutrition and of Degeneration of the Vascular System, Med. Mirror, *1*, 769, 1864.

85. WEBER, F. P.: A Case of Multiple Hereditary Developmental Angiomata (Telangiectases) of the Skin and Mucous Membranes Associated with Recurring Hemorrhages, Lancet, *2*, 160, 1907.

86. WEISS, E. and GASUL, B. M.: Pulmonary Arteriovenous Fistula and Telangiectasia, Ann. Int. Med., *41*, 989, 1954.

87. WELLS, E. B.: Hereditary Hemorrhagic Telangiectasia, Am. J. M. Sc., *211*, 577, 1946.

88. WILLIAMS, G. A. and BRICK, I. B.: Gastrointestinal Bleeding in Hereditary Hemorrhagic Telangiectasia, Arch. Int. Med., *95*, 41, 1955.

Chapter 19

Leukemia

Definition.—Leukemia is a morbid condition of unknown etiology and fatal termination which is characterized by widespread proliferation of the leukocytes and their precursors in the tissues of the body. It is usually also associated with qualitative and quantitative changes in the circulating white cells of the blood.

History.—Although descriptions of what can now be regarded as leukemia may be found recorded from the time of Hippocrates onward, the earliest microscopic observations were probably made by Donné in Barth's case (1839) at the Hôtel Dieu in Paris.[59] Leukemia was first recognized as a clinical entity by Craigie, Bennett[10] and Virchow,[213] independently, in 1845. Only Virchow appreciated that the cells involved were leukocytes and not pus cells and he proposed the name leukemia ("white blood"). Virchow later observed a type in which lymphatic enlargement predominated as well as the type in which splenomegaly was marked. A myelogenous form of leukemia was described by Neumann (1870)[163] but it was not until Ehrlich's blood staining methods came into use that the splenic and myelogenous forms were recognized as being identical.

Leukemia with an acute course was first reported by Friedreich[63] in 1857 and in 1889 Ebstein[47] gave an adequate clinical description of the outstanding symptoms of this form of the disease.

Acute leukemia, however, was considered to be only lymphocytic in type and cases of chronic leukemia in which the blood contained non-granular cells as well as granulocytes were spoken of as "mixed leukemia" until Naegeli described the myeloblast (1900).[162] Identification of this cell as a member of the myeloid series made it possible to recognize many cases of leukemia, both chronic and acute, as myelogenous in type. That there might be an additional form of leukemia was suggested by the description of an alleged case of monocytic leukemia by Reschad and Schilling-Torgau in 1913.[178] Interestingly enough this case was probably not one of monocytic leukemia as now recognized.[45]

In the succeeding years, cases of leukemia without leukocytosis ("aleukemic leukemia") have been recognized in increasing numbers, more complete clinical and morphological descriptions of various forms of leukemia have been recorded, palliative treatment has been developed and leukemia in mammals and in fowls has been studied extensively. Nevertheless, little still is known about the cause of the disease.

Varieties of Leukemia and Terminology.—As already indicated, acute and chronic forms of leukemia can be distinguished, the distinction resting on the rapidity of the course of the disease as well as the marked morphological difference between these two forms, the predominating cells in acute leukemia being much more immature than those found in chronic leukemia. Cases sometimes described as subacute usually resemble acute leukemia more than the chronic variety.

Both the acute and the chronic cases of leukemia can be further subdivided according to the predominating type of leukocyte. Here terminology is not entirely satisfactory because it is difficult to make a strict classification according to the cell type or in accordance with the site of origin of the cells. On the latter basis, myelogenous ("myeloid") and lymphogenous ("lymphatic," "lymphoid") forms are distinguished but, since the site of origin of the monocyte is disputed, this form of leukemia might be spoken of as myelogenous or histiocytic. It is perhaps best to speak of leukemia according to the predominating type of cell. Thus, reference will be made to chronic lymphocytic leukemia, acute lymphoblastic, myeloblastic or monocytic leukemia and chronic myelocytic leukemia.

The last mentioned of these terms is not altogether satisfactory because myelocytes may be neutrophilic, eosinophilic or basophilic and because a significant number of more mature forms of leukocytes are to be found in this type of leukemia in addition to myelocytes. The term chronic myelocytic leukemia is generally applied, however, to the most common variety, in which neutrophilic myelocytes are very numerous; it is synonymous with "chronic myelogenous" or chronic "myeloid" or "granulocytic" leukemia. Eosinophilic leukemia, polymorphonuclear (neutrophilic) leukemia and basophilic leukemia are names applied to those rare cases in which these cells predominate.

Aleukemic leukemia is the most common term used in referring to cases of leukemia in which there is no leukocytosis. The term "sub-leukemic" is less contradictory.

The name chloroma is applied in cases in which greenish tumor-like masses of leukemic tissue are found. This name was given because of the color of the tumors.

Many other names have been used in referring to cases of leukemia but their meaning and relation to the terms already mentioned will usually be obvious. The terms employed here are adopted because of their priority and simplicity. Mention should be made, however, of the use of the conventional nomenclature of of neoplastic diseases in referring to cases of leukemia. Thus, the terms leukosis (for leukemia), myelosis (for myelocytic leukemia), lymphadenosis (for chronic lymphocytic leukemia), myeloblastoma (for acute myeloblastic leukemia) and similar names have been adopted by some writers.

Etiology and Pathogenesis. —Mortality Statistics.—The average annual leukemia death rates[71e] among white males in the United States are shown in Figure 19–1. There has been a steady increase from 2.04 per 100,000 population in 1921–25 to 7.71 in 1951–55. For females, the corresponding figures are 1.54 and 5.32, respectively. Beginning about 1940, a decline in the rate of increase can be noted. The decline in rate of increase is very evident in the younger ages and becomes less pronounced as age advances. Among nonwhites the increase in death rates has been materially greater, with less evidence of a slackening in rate of increase. In England and Wales the leukemia death rate increased steadily from 2.6 in 1940 to 4.8 in 1953 but in Scotland the rise was more irregular.[36b] In one study no evidence could be found of an increasing incidence since 1948.[224a] A similar

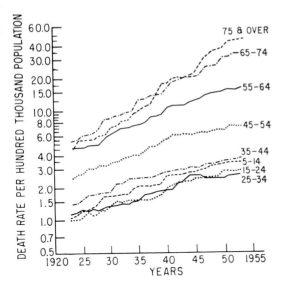

FIG. 19–1.—Trends for age-specific death rates in white males for leukemia in the death registration states, 5-year moving medians, 1921–1955 (semi-log scale). Rates for all ages were adjusted to the age distribution of the population of the United States at the 1950 census. Curves for white females are very similar. (Gilliam and Walter[71e]).

report has come from Australia.[123] It was stated that the death rates were higher in the United States and in Denmark than in various other parts of Europe, especially Germany, but a more recent report for Germany gives a figure of 6.2 per 100,000 population in 1956 for men and 4.8 for women,[163a] values which are not very different from those for the United States cited above.

It is difficult to evaluate these data. Undoubtedly, extension of medical services to larger segments of the population of a country, as well as improved accuracy of diagnosis, influence the statistics and, in part, explain the higher incidence of leukemia which has been observed among those of better economic status than among the less well to do.[86a] The former persons may, on the other hand, have been exposed to a greater extent to factors in the environment which may have favored the development of leu-

kemia. These will be discussed shortly (p. 908). The lengthening life span of the population must also be taken into consideration. More reliable, perhaps, would be the data which suggest a stabilization or actual decline in the leukemia death rates, if further observations support them, since a greater uniformity of medical services, as compared with the earlier decades of this century, is likely to be found as time goes on.

Frequency of Various Types of Leukemia.—It is difficult to determine the true incidence of the different types of leukemia. Most published series are relatively small. Other reports exclude various types of cases for one reason or another and even certain large series appear to be biased in that the cases seem to include mainly or exclusively adults[186] or children. Furthermore, the cases in a single hematology clinic or hospital do not necessarily represent the true incidence of leukemia in that community or area. Finally, criteria for differentiation of different types of leukemia differ from one clinic to another. Consequently the percentages in Table 19–1, which are derived from the four listed large series of cases, must be considered only as approximations.

It will be noted that the proportions of cases of chronic myelocytic and chronic lymphocytic leukemia are approximately equal. This is contrary to earlier published data[186,214a] and may possibly indicate a trend favoring a higher incidence of the lymphocytic form. The latter, in fact, predominated in a series published in 1953.[71a]

"Aleukemic" leukemia is relatively common. In one series of 647 cases, the total leukocyte count did not exceed 10,000 in 21.6 per cent of the cases.[71a] In another series of 123 autopsied cases, 11 per cent were "aleukemic."[125a] In acute leukemia there is a much higher incidence of "aleukemia" than in chronic leukemia, approximately one-third being

Table 19–1—Relative Frequency of Various Types of Leukemia

Author	Total No. of Cases	C L L	C M L	A L L	A M L	A Mo. L Myelo.	A Mo. L Histio.
Rosenthal[186] . .	447	104	170	32	134	. .	7
Bethell[11c] . . .	479*	158***	153	58	44	42	24
Gauld et al.[71a] .	647	207	169	144	70	57	?
Best & Limarzi[11b].	851**	278	213	170****	151	19	20
Totals	2424	747	705	404	399	118	51
Per cent . . .	100.0	30.9	29.0	16.7	16.4	4.9	2.1

C L L refers to chronic lymphocytic leukemia; C M L, chronic myelocytic; A L L, acute lymphoblastic; A M L, acute myeloblastic, and A Mo. L, acute monocytic leukemia. The last group is further subdivided into the myelo-monocytic (Naegeli) and histio-monocytic (Schilling) types. It is likely that Rosenthal included the Naegeli form among his acute myeloblastic leukemias. Gauld et al. do not specify.

* Sixteen cases of "chronic histio-monocytic" leukemia have been omitted.
** Forty-one cases of "reticulum-cell" leukemia, 21 cases of lymphocytic sarcoma, leukemic phase, and three cases of plasmocytic leukemia have been omitted.
*** Includes 80 cases of "lymphosarcoma cell" leukemia, both acute and chronic.
**** Includes 105 cases of "acute unclassified "leukemia.

more or less "aleukemic" (see p. 937). It should be added that these statistics are but rough approximations since interpretations of the meaning of the term "aleukemia" vary.

Race.—There are few data concerning the racial incidence of leukemia. It has been stated that Jews are particularly susceptible to chronic lymphocytic leukemia[169] and that this form of leukemia is relatively rare in Japanese[157b] and in Chinese.[219b] Other forms of leukemia have also been found to be relatively more common among Jews.[139a] At the Johns Hopkins Hospital, where the ratio of white to Negro admissions was about 3:1, the distribution of leukemia in the two races was 7:1. This difference was approximately the same in the chronic myelocytic, lymphocytic and acute forms of the disease. A similarly lower incidence in Negroes has been observed in some[174d] but not all[139a] studies.

Hereditary and Familial Influences.[80a,81c,211a]—There are a number of reports of leukemia occurring in several members of a family.[2,26,28,214b] These include examples of acute leukemia in two or more members of a family,[197] as well as in twins.[1e,40] In one family, acute leukemia developed in 5 of 8 siblings between the ages of five and eight.[1d] This was regarded as lymphatic in 3 and possibly "leukemic reticulo-endotheliosis (primarily myelogenous)" in 2. The writer has observed acute leukemia in two brothers which developed at the ages of three and two and a half years, respectively. Meikle[144a] reported acute leukemia in a brother and sister, myeloblastic in the latter, possibly monocytic in the former. Acute lymphoblastic leukemia has been reported in the nine month old infant of a mother who had the same type of leukemia during pregnancy.[36g] Chronic lymphocytic leukemia has been described in 6 persons comprising two generations of a family.[42a] In another family,[93b] leukemia was described in 3 sisters and developed at the ages of thirty-nine, fifty-five and fifty-five, respectively. It was chronic lymphocytic in 2, chronic myelocytic in the third. Chronic lymphocytic leukemia has been reported also in 3 brothers, in 1 of whom lymphadenopathy appeared as early as twenty-two years of age[178a] as well as in twins and in the son of one of the twins.[40]

Thus leukemia has been observed in siblings, monovular and fraternal twins, parent and child, cousins and other relatives. The total number of reported familial cases of leukemia which can be accepted as authentic is approximately 58. Thus the probability that leukemia will occur more than once in a family is very small. Nevertheless, the occurrence of a very rare disease in several members of a family cannot be due to chance alone. In a painstaking study of the pedigrees of 209 patients with leukemia, Videbaek[211a] concluded that the familial incidence of the disease is at least 8.1 per cent. It is noteworthy that lymphoid leukemia has been observed six times as frequently in the familial cases as the myeloid type.[2]

There has been some criticism of Videbaek's studies[197] but it does appear that, very rarely at least, and particularly in acute leukemia and in chronic lymphocytic leukemia, heredity may be of importance in determining susceptibility to leukemia. It seems premature to debate whether the mode of inheritance is determined by a dominant gene of low penetrance[211a] or a rare recessive gene with high penetrance.[1d,178a]

Induced leukemia in mice shows definite influences of intrinsic genetic factors.[65a,182]

Age.—Leukemia has been observed in infants at birth in at least 34 instances[39d,149a] (**"congenital" leukemia.**) An impressive feature of these cases is the predominance of the myeloblastic and myelocytic form of leukemia, the ratio of these to lymphogenous cases being 5:1.

Leukemia occurs more often in the first five years of life than at almost any other period (Fig. 19–2). Until the age of twenty the great majority of cases are acute. From this time until forty-five years of age chronic myelocytic leukemia is most common. After the age of forty-five the tide turns and chronic lymphocytic leukemia becomes the predominating form of leukemia.

It must not be assumed, however, that acute leukemia never occurs in the aged or that chronic leukemia is never to be found in children.[69a] Chronic myelocytic leukemia[7a] has been observed as early as six weeks of age and was found in about 5 per cent of a series of 294 cases of leukemia in children up to twelve years of age. In this series males predominated (3:1). Chronic lymphocytic leukemia has also been described in children[93a] but is much more unusual in childhood than the myelocytic variety. Acute leukemia has been reported even at one hundred and two years of age.[185a] Monocytic leukemia, which is more often acute than chronic, favors middle age.[110]

It is much more difficult to ascertain the relative frequencies of the various forms of acute leukemia because their differentiation is so much more a matter of opinion than that of the chronic forms. Most students of the disease would agree, however, that acute lymphoblastic leukemia predominates in childhood until about the time of puberty and approximately equals the sum of the cases of myeloblastic and monocytic leukemia until about the age of twenty-five when the latter two forms begin to appear more and more commonly.

Sex.—Chronic lymphocytic leukemia is much more common in males, who make up 67 to 75 per cent or more of all series of cases.[71a,223] Males tend to predominate also in series of cases of monocytic leukemia[167] but they exceed only slightly or moderately the number of females among cases of chronic myelocytic and acute leukemia,[11b] respectively. There appears, in fact, to have been a shift in the sex ratio among cases of chronic myelocytic leukemia from

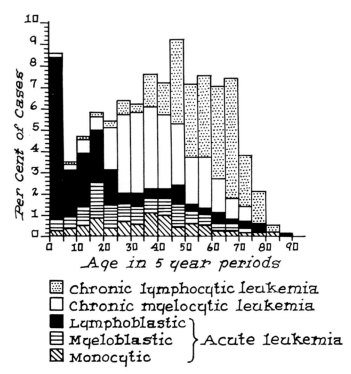

chronic lymphocytic leukemia
chronic myelocytic leukemia
Lymphoblastic ⎫
Myeloblastic ⎬ Acute leukemia
Monocytic ⎭

Fig. 19–2.—Age distribution of various common types of leukemia, based on a total of 1,539 cases.[71a, 214a, 223] The percentages have been calculated on the assumption, founded on the data presented in Table 19–1, that 40 per cent of all cases of leukemia are acute, and that chronic myelocytic and chronic lymphocytic leukemia each make up 30 per cent of all leukemias. The age distribution of the cases of acute leukemia is based on the series of 271 cases of Gauld et al.[71a]

1910 to 1948 so that the preponderance of males has almost disappeared.[194c]

Leukemia in Animals.—At this point in the discussion of the etiology and pathogenesis of leukemia it will be worthwhile to consider leukemia as seen in animals. The disease occurs spontaneously in various animals[111a] and has been studied chiefly in poultry and in mice and, to a lesser extent, in rats[194a] and in guinea pigs.[31c]

Fowl leukosis,[48] which probably is the most serious disease afflicting domestic fowl today, encompasses a number of distinct conditions; namely, visceral lymphomatosis, myeloblastosis and erythroblastosis. Visceral lymphomatosis is essentially an "aleukemic" disease. The lymphoid cells rarely reach the circula-

tion in appreciable numbers and the marrow involvement varies in degree. There is lymphocytic infiltration of organs such as the liver, lungs, intestines, periosteum, nerve trunks, and eyes. In avian myeloblastosis large numbers of young myeloid cells are predominant in the blood. In erythroblastosis normal erythroblasts enter the circulation in large numbers. Organ infiltration by the representative cell type occurs in each of these disorders. Osteopetrosis has been described as a manifestation of lymphomatosis. In the etiology of fowl leukosis, at least two agents have been identified and these do not differ in principle from other viruses.[9a] Both have been found to exist extracellularly as autonomous physical units and are susceptible to identification and examination by the same procedures employed with other filterable agents. The agents of erythroblastosis and myeloblastosis parasitize two different cell types. Age is a factor in susceptibility to inoculation. The virus can be recovered readily from leukemic cells and multiplies *in vitro* only in the presence of cells on which it apparently confers neoplastic properties.[64]

Murine leukemia varies from one strain of mouse to another in degree of involvement and ranges from single tumor growths with no changes in the blood and little or no change in the bone marrow to a full fledged picture of liver and spleen infiltration and bone marrow and blood changes. Morphologically, almost all of the mouse leukemias are lymphoid in type, only a few being myeloid, or possibly monocytic;[125] in fact, the true nature of the latter types has been questioned.[146]

Leukemia in the mouse has been the subject of extensive experimental investigation. Strains have been bred in which the incidence of spontaneous leukemia is very high, while in other strains the incidence is quite low.[65a] Genetic constitution plays an important part in mouse leukemia. Age is a significant factor in susceptibility to transmitted leukemia. In the earlier studies it was concluded that the success of transmission depends upon the transfer of viable cells.[68] The interval between inoculation and death was found to be inversely related to the number of living cells inoculated.[182]

A number of exogenous factors have been shown to play important roles both in the incidence of spontaneous leukemia and in susceptibility to inoculation. These include *x*-rays and other ionizing radiations,[68] methylcholanthrene and other hydrocarbons.[121] The importance of age as a factor is indicated by the fact that animals exposed to whole body *x*-radiation when prepubertal are much more susceptible than older animals. Nutrition is another factor.[222d] Simple caloric restriction alone inhibits leukemogenesis[189a] and feeding a diet low in cystine has a similar effect.

In addition to these factors, the thymus, the bone marrow and certain hormones influence the leukemia induction mechanism. The *thymus* is the site of origin for the lymphosarcomas and lymphatic leukemias which occur in several mouse strains.[121] Furthermore, removal of the thymus is associated with a striking reduction in the incidence of spontaneous leukemia in mice[142a] while re-implantation can restore susceptibility to thymectomized animals.[130a] The influence of the *bone marrow* is indicated by the striking inhibition of lymphoid tumor induction by whole body *x*-radiation when one hind leg is shielded or normal homologous bone marrow cell suspensions are injected intravenously into unshielded irradiated animals.[121]

The role of the *hormones* is exemplified best by the adrenal cortex. Adrenalectomy increases the percentage of "takes" of transmissible lymphogenous leukemia whereas cortisone and hydrocortisone, which are both powerfully thymolytic, very significantly depress lymphoid tumor development.[44d] It also appears that ovariectomy or progesterone mildly inhibit lymphoid tumor production whereas orchiectomy is followed by a greater incidence or shorter latent period.[121] In addition, estrogen has long been known to be leukemogenic[121] and pituitary growth hormone has a similar effect.

Evidence has been produced, however, that the transmissibility of murine leukemia is not limited to the transfer of viable cells. The possibility that a filterable agent, presumably a virus, might be concerned in the etiology of mammalian leukemia, long considered but never clearly demonstrated, was reawakened by the investigations of Gross.[80] He found that mouse leukemia could be transmitted from a high inci- dence strain (Ak) to a low incidence strain (C3H) by inoculation with cell- free filtrates. The age of the recipient mice was important to the success of these experiments; the animals in which successful takes were accomplished were less than 16 hours of age. In them, following a latent period of three to 18 months after inoculation, leukemia appeared. This work has been amplified and others have confirmed it.[84d,190c] The leukemogenic agent has been demon- strated in extracts of the normal embryos of strains of inbred mice (Ak and C58) known to have a high incidence of spontaneous leukemia, a finding which has been interpreted as an example of an egg-borne virus transmitting leukemia from one generation to the next. From fertilized ova removed from the Fallopian tubes of Ak mice and transplanted into the uteri of low leukemic strains, mice developed in which the incidence of leukemia was that of the true parent; that is, as in a high incidence strain. Again, in cell-free extracts from strains of mice in which the spontaneous occur- rence of leukemia is small and in which leukemia was induced by irradiation, a leukemogenic agent was found. The leukemogenic agent is thought by Gross to be of viral nature by virtue of its passage through appropriate filters and on grounds of physical characterization and visual- ization of the particles by electron micros- copy. Other experiments have suggested antigenic specificity.[190c] Sera from rab- bits previously injected with cell-free leukemic brain filtrate protected C3H mice from the leukemogenic action of the filtrate whereas sera obtained after the injection of nonleukemic brain filtrate into rabbits did not afford this protection. Another point of interest is the fact that exogenous factors, such as irradiation and thymectomy, which were observed to influence spontaneous leukemia in the mouse, also affect the disease which

develops following the injection of cell- free extracts.[65a,150a] A neoplastic disease, regarded by some as a form of leukemia, has also been induced in *adult* Swiss mice by the injection of cell-free tumor extracts.[63a]

Although some have assumed that these investigations give proof of the viral etiology of mouse leukemia, the concept has not gone without challenge and serious reservations have been made by competent investigators.[130a,150a]

The Nature of Leukemia in Man. —Leukemia in man has been considered to be a neoplasm.[65a,121,130a] The essential change is thought to reside in the leukemic cell and consists of an acquired inability of these leukocytes to respond to forces which normally regulate their prolifera- tion and maturation. The end result is a new type of cell with certain fixed abnormalities in appearance and be- havior. The leukemic cell is not be- lieved to be inherited as such but the change, once established, is intrinsic and is maintained. The cell fails to differ- entiate and mature in the normal manner and is capable of overcoming the forces which restrain the growth of normal immature cells. The change probably involves the enzymatic and metabolic activities of the cell. The causes of this change may be manifold and it may not be the result of an abrupt alteration from previously normal tissue but, rather, the consequence of a series of influences and alterations. The relationship of demon- strable changes in the chromosomes in leukemic cells is under active investiga- tion. It appears that in some leukemic human leukocytes small but definite chromosomal changes are demonstra- ble.[3c,164,206a]

It is noteworthy that *exogenous factors* similar to those which have been shown to affect murine leukemia, appear to play a role in the human disease. Of these, the most clearly established is **ionizing radiation.**[39,121] This was brought forcibly to attention following the detonation of the atomic bomb but was suspected long before and has been clearly confirmed since then. Among the survivors in Hiroshima and Nagasaki,[87,157c] of the 92 verified cases of leukemia, there were 52 cases of acute or subacute leukemia and 40 were chronic. Of the latter, all but one were myelocytic.

In times of peace, in the more technically advanced parts of the world, the major source of radiation exposure is derived from the medical use of x-rays. It has been noted that the frequency of leukemia in physicians is almost twice[71e] that among white males in the general population. In radiologists in the United States the incidence of leukemia was found to be eight to ten times as great as in non-radiologists.[140,209a] These differences have been attributed to exposure to radiation.[173b] In Great Britain, however, no such increased incidence of leukemia in radiologists could be demonstrated.[36c]

In patients suffering from ankylosing spondylitis who had been given x-ray therapy, the incidence of leukemia was five times higher than the number of deaths from leukemia that would be expected in the general population.[36b] The incidence was still higher among those who were given more than one course of x-ray therapy. Leukemia and other neoplasia have been reported in children who had received x-ray therapy to an enlarged thymus or for pertussis and lymphoid hyperplasia,[161] as well as in older subjects.[130] Eleven cases of acute leukemia following administration of I^{131} have been reported[25b,114] and other examples of leukemia occurring in patients exposed to various doses of x-ray have been recorded.[157d] The intravenous administration of thorium compounds has also been followed by the development of leukemia.[39,162d] It should be added, however, that when the occurrence of leukemia in 39,166 liveborn children

whose mothers were known to have been subjected to abdominal or pelvic radiation during their pregnancy was compared with the expected incidence, no evidence of a disproportionate occurrence of leukemia could be demonstrated.[36e] Neither did a study of approximately 60,000 thyrotoxic patients treated with radioiodine give any indication that this treatment induced leukemia.[174e]

There are now sufficient data to indicate that, for high level, single dose exposure of man, the incidence of leukemia is approximately linear with dose.[39] At dose levels of perhaps 100 r equivalent or greater, the incidence of leukemia is approximately 1 to $2/10^6$ persons at risk/year/rad from approximately the second to the 15th year following exposure. Below these dose levels the data are inadequate for prediction. They are also insufficient to permit reliable conclusions regarding the role of therapeutic radiation in the induction of leukemia. Still more uncertain is the question of the dangers involved in diagnostic radiation. The implication that an apparent increase in the incidence of leukemia in infancy is attributable to diagnostic radiation *in utero* has not been supported by other observers.[39,161] An important but unsolved problem is whether or not there is a threshold dose for the induction of leukemia. There are some who believe that there is a linear dose-effect relationship between radiation and leukemia which has no threshold and that doses are cumulative in their action.[25a] Others have stated that there is no good evidence to support or to deny this claim.[22,39]

From time to time various **chemical agents** have come under suspicion as an inciting cause of leukemia. Of these the evidence which suggests that chronic benzol poisoning[19] may lead to myelogenous leukemia is the most plausible. Other industrial and medicinal chemicals have been incriminated because of association with the development of sporadic cases of leukemia. In particular, various agents which have been mentioned elsewhere as causing deleterious effects on the hemopoietic system (pp. 552 and 818), such as the arsenicals and sulfonamides, have been blamed but the grounds for these charges are insecure. Other compounds which have been mentioned are hexachlorcyclohexane[113] and phenylbutazone[9] but many others could be postulated.[25a]

More than 70 cases of leukemia following *trauma* have been described.[165,225] In the majority the trauma consisted in contusion of the abdomen, while in a number the accident caused fracture of bone. The leukemia with few exceptions has been of the myelocytic variety.[165] Although judicial recognition has been granted this claim in some instances,[51] medical evidence has not been presented. Attempts to produce leukemia in animals by trauma have not been successful.[111]

Acute leukemia has been noted to occur at least three times more frequently in infants with *mongolism* than would be expected simply by fortuitous occurrence if these two rare disorders were entirely unrelated.[128] This naturally suggests the possibility that they have an etiologic agent in common. No stigmata of mongolism were found, however, in 59 children with acute leukemia.[202]

From time to time a variety of **infectious agents,** bacterial, viral and parasitic, have been suggested in relation to the etiology of leukemia, but never with convincing proof.[121] It has been pointed out frequently that a history of severe, usually nonspecific infection often antedates the discovery of acute leukemia but this may as readily mean that leukemia was already in existence at the time as that the infection was an etiologic factor. It is noteworthy that the usual channels of entry of infection, such as the gastrointestinal and respiratory tracts are generally remarkably free of evidence of disease, whereas the infiltration of the

organs and tissues, so characteristic of leukemia, is not found in diseases of recognized infectious origin. *Attempts to transmit leukemia* from man to man,[204a] or the accidental transfusion of such blood,[77] have not resulted in the development of leukemia. The reported discovery of leuko-precipitins in the blood of patients with acute leukemia[193b] may as readily be interpreted as a secondary phenomenon as that it is of primary etiologic significance. As pointed out earlier, leukemia has been reported only once in the child of a mother with leukemia,[36g] whereas delivery of a non-leukemic child by a leukemic mother has been reported many times.[11f,186c]

Attempts have been made from time to time to transmit human leukemia to animals, particularly by the inoculation of leukemic cells. The results[141] have been equivocal. It was reported that the inoculation of human leukemic cells into guinea pigs regularly elicits a severe, usually fatal anemia after a variable incubation period.[138c] The possibility that these results might be attributable to nonspecific contaminants must be considered. More recently, interest in the possibility of a viral agent being involved in the pathogenesis of human leukemia has been stimulated by the studies of the role of a replicating agent in the etiology of mouse leukemia, described above. The evidence is of several types. First, virus-like particles have been described in the lymph nodes of several patients with acute leukemia.[20b,44c] Secondly, other investigators have reported that an agent could be extracted from brain tissue of human leukemia victims which, when injected into selected strains of mice, accelerated the appearance of leukemia.[190d] The agent, contained in cell-free Berkefeld filtrates, had been passed serially through living mouse brain. The leukemogenic activity was retained, presumably by propagation through what would otherwise be dilution to an ineffectual concentration. It was also found that antiserum, obtained from human volunteers who had been inoculated with a cell-free filtrate prepared from a pool of brains from patients who had died of acute leukemia, afforded significant protection of mice challenged with cell-free filtrates of leukemic human brains. Another investigator reported that benzol extracts of organs of patients with leukemia produced leukemia and tumors in mice.[124a] Transmissible tissue culture changes, produced by fluorocarbon-extracted RNA from human leukemic and tumor cells, have also been reported.[28a] These observations are all of extreme interest and importance but they await confirmation and extension.[202a]

It is impressive that, both in murine and in human leukemia, a variety of exogenous factors appear to be associated with the development of leukemia. This has led to the suggestion that the appearance of this disease is not the consequence of a sudden, irreversible cellular change but, rather, is precipitated by certain types of injurious disturbances of growth equilibrium. These in turn initiate a train of events during the course of which an irreversible change finally takes place.[121] The leukemia induction mechanism thus is postulated as being an indirect process which reflects the complicated interrelationship of multiple factors. Physical agents such as ionizing radiation, widely different chemicals, including hormones and even self-perpetuating exogenous, virus-like agents may be responsible; or the cause may be an endogenous growth factor multiplying autocatalytically and causing abnormal differentiation of the cells. In different cases, or more likely in different types of leukemia, different factors may be responsible. In man, as in the mouse, the genetic background may play a role as well but man is, as a rule, protected

by the lack of homogeneity of his ancestral picture.

In addition to the neoplastic theory, a number of other concepts have been offered from time to time concerning the nature of leukemia. One of these postulates a *disturbance in the hemopoietic equilibrium*. Starting from the report that it was possible to produce myeloid hyperplasia and metaplasia in the organs of guinea pigs by the injection of extracts of urine from patients with leukemia,[90a] two substances were derived from the urine of patients with leukemia, Hodgkin's disease and other lymphomas. These were named myelokentric and lymphokentric acid. The former causes myeloid hyperplasia while the latter produces lymphoid hyperplasia on injection in guinea pigs. Changes which were neither lymphoid nor myeloid in character, but were nevertheless abnormal, were encountered when urine from cases of monocytic leukemia or Hodgkin's disease was in-injected or when the myeloid and lymphoid stimulating fractions were given simultaneously. The theory has been proposed that these substances are normal products which are mutually reciprocal in action, the myeloid substance stimulating myelopoiesis while the lymphoid factor inhibits the proliferation of these cells, causing them to mature, and also brings about lymphoid proliferation. The maturation of lymphoid cells, according to this hypothesis, is brought about by the action of the myeloid substance. Imbalances or deficiencies of these substances lead to the development of the various types of leukemia, and excessive production of both factors brings about Hodgkin's disease and monocytic leukemia. Convincing proof that these observations do, in fact, bear on the pathogenesis of leukemia is lacking.

Another concept of the pathogenesis of leukemia is that *failure of normal elimination* rather than excessive and disordered production is the underlying defect.[11i] This view is based on cross-transfusion experiments of blood from leukemic and non-leukemic subjects and on studies of the resistance of leukemic leukocytes to destruction. As was pointed out elsewhere (p. 243), the life span of lymphocytes in chronic lymphocytic leukemia seems to be greater than that of normal cells although the reverse has been found in regard to the cells of acute and chronic myelocytic leukemia. The hypothesis of disturbed elimination or retention of leukocytes does not explain the morphological abnormalities which are characteristic of the acute leukemias or of chronic myelocytic leukemia, nor are they compatible with many of the aspects of experimental leukemia in mice.[65a] It is quite possible, however, that all the leukemias do not have the same etiology and the hypothesis proposed may have some bearing on the manifestations of one form of leukemia, for example, the chronic lymphocytic variety.

The concept that leukemia may be, in essence, a *deficiency disease*, is based on the analogy to pernicious anemia where maturation of cells, as in some forms of leukemia, appears to be interrupted. However, attempts to demonstrate a deficiency of a maturation factor in leukemia have failed.[29] In this connection, it is of interest that serum vitamin B_{12} concentrations as well as the capacity to bind added vitamin B_{12}[149] have been found to be considerably increased in chronic myelocytic leukemia[157b] and in the acute form[145] but in chronic lymphocytic leukemia and in undifferentiated acute leukemia the values were normal. Metabolic differences between leukemic and non-leukemic cells were discussed in an earlier chapter (p. 234). It is as yet difficult to judge the significance of the interesting observations which have been made.

The cause of leukemia is, thus, unknown and the pathogenesis of the disorder is obscure. It has been generally assumed that all forms of leukemia represent variations of a single underlying abnormality due to the same etiologic factors. There are many reasons to doubt this conclusion, some of which have been touched upon already. It seems more reasonable to believe that the different forms of leukemia are the result of quite distinct pathogenetic mechanisms. In particular, chronic lymphocytic leukemia differs from the other types of leukemia but even in the acute leukemias important differences may exist.

CLINICAL MANIFESTATIONS

The clinical manifestations of leukemia are quite different in chronic and in acute leukemia. There is relatively little difference, however, between the signs and symptoms of the subvarieties of these forms of leukemia even though the chronic forms, at least, are so dissimilar in cellular morphology. The symptoms and signs of leukemia will, therefore, be discussed under the headings of chronic and acute leukemia. In this way such differences between the various types as have been observed can be emphasized.

Chronic Leukemia.— Mode of Onset and Course.—The onset of chronic leukemia is so insidious that early discovery of the disease is usually accidental. In several cases of chronic myelocytic leukemia which we had the opportunity to study from an early stage, unexplained leukocytosis was the first sign of the disease.[223] The leukocyte counts ranged from 11,000 to 77,000 and there was an increase in the granular series of leukocytes. In the case in which the lowest leukocyte count was found no immature forms were observed. The leukocytosis was discovered in these patients in the course of routine examinations, respectively, following pregnancy (M.J., Fig. 19–3), for sterility, abdominal distress and uterine myomata. In 2 of the cases

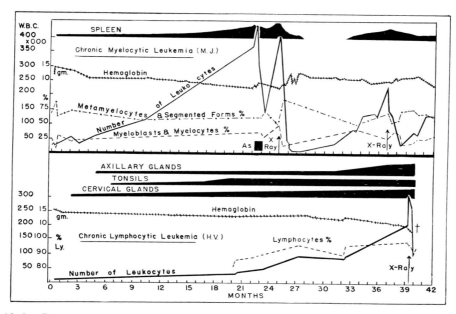

Fig. 19–3.—Progress of chief physical signs in a case of chronic myelocytic leukemia and in one of chronic lymphocytic leukemia, in which the disease was discovered very early in its course. The initial sign in the case of myelocytic leukemia, a woman, aged twenty-eight years, was unexplained leukocytosis discovered after the delivery of a normal child. This woman was carrying on her housework five years later and lived another three years. The initial sign in the case of lymphocytic leukemia, a man of fifty-nine years, was glandular enlargement. This patient died more than three years later of bronchopneumonia.

physical examination revealed no abnormality, in 1 only a few enlarged cervical lymph glands were discovered, and only in 2 cases was the spleen palpable at this stage. With one exception anemia attributable to leukemia was absent. In 1 patient it was not until three years and nine months had elapsed that the spleen was palpable whereas in another the spleen could be demonstrated one year after the discovery of leukemia. It is difficult to estimate how long a time would have elapsed before these patients would have sought medical aid because of symptoms attributable to leukemia. The patient whose initial leukocyte count was 77,000 was lost sight of and he only returned after two-and-a-half years because of weakness.

Unexplained leukocytosis was the first

evidence of leukemia only in about a third of 16 cases of the chronic lymphocytic form which we observed from an early stage, but there was lymphocytosis in a number of the cases even when the leukocyte count was relatively low.[223] In another third of the cases, glandular enlargement was the sign which first attracted attention. Only in one case was splenic enlargement the most prominent early sign.

The progress of chronic leukemia varies considerably from one case to another, but in most instances it is probably more gradual than is generally assumed. Thus, in 1 of our cases of chronic myelocytic leukemia it was twenty-two months after leukocytosis was discovered that it was deemed advisable to give treatment, and even at this time there were no complaints. In another case, as already stated, weakness caused the patient to return after two-and-a-half years. In one of the cases of lymphocytic leukemia it was more than three years after adenopathy was first discovered that the clinical picture usually associated with this disease, was present (H.V., Fig. 19–3).

When the disease is sufficiently advanced to cause the patient to seek attention, the symptoms, although varying greatly, may be classified, in general, as (1) those resulting from anemia; (2) those produced by the presence of an enlarged spleen or liver, enlarged lymph nodes, or leukemic infiltrations in various organs and tissues; or (3) symptoms attributable to the increased metabolic rate (loss of weight, nervousness, abnormal perspiration) or resulting from the generally disturbed metabolism and nutrition (cachexia). Less frequently, unusual bleeding, fever, or other symptoms are encountered. As a result, attention may be directed to the cardiovascular system, the skin, the gastro-intestinal tract or the nervous system; there may be cough and dyspnea, swelling of the abdomen, a sense of weight or actual pain in the splenic region, priapism or symptoms referring to the special sense organs.

Outward Appearance of the Patient.—The appearance of the victim of leukemia may be that of more or less perfect health; or, at the other extreme, a picture of long-continued, progressive ill health is encountered. Emaciation may be apparent and pallor may be well marked. When splenic enlargement exists, the contrast between the protuberant abdomen and the general evidences of weight loss produces a striking and characteristic picture.

Lymph. Glands—Glandular enlargement is uncommon early in myelocytic leukemia but in the latter half of the course of this disease slight or very moderate enlargement is found. Marked enlargement is very rare but has been observed.[189] In lymphocytic leukemia, on the other hand, adenopathy appears early and may be extensive and striking in degree. Rarely, however, are the huge masses seen in Hodgkin's disease or in lymphosarcoma encountered. The glands are discrete, moderately firm, freely movable and not attached to the skin. They are neither tender or painful, nor is the overlying skin reddened, unless secondary infection has supervened. It is exceedingly rare for adenopathy to be entirely absent in chronic lymphocytic leukemia, although a few such cases have been described.[227]

In most instances all accessible glands are found to be affected in some degree or become so during the course of the illness. The glands of the cervical chains are most prominent ordinarily, but on examination the axillary and inguinal glands will be found enlarged as well, and glands not usually affected in other conditions with which lymphocytic leukemia might be confused, may also be discovered. These include the post-auricular, submaxillary, epitrochlear and the pectoral group of axillary glands. Abdominal glands may be felt occasionally and enlargement of mediastinal glands may produce pressure symptoms.

In chronic lymphocytic leukemia, enlargement of the **tonsils** may be a relatively early finding and may reach extreme proportions. Very rarely the breast[83] or the **salivary and lacrimal glands** may be involved and present symmetrical painless enlargements (Mikulicz syndrome,[88,187] Fig. 19–4). In such cases dry mouth and throat, difficulty in hearing, exophthalmos and interference with vision have been prominent symptoms.

Spleen.—In chronic myelocytic leukemia the spleen is usually markedly enlarged by the time the patient presents himself to the physician. This was true in 94 per cent of a series of 82 cases.[92] The spleen is smooth and hard and preserves its characteristic shape so that

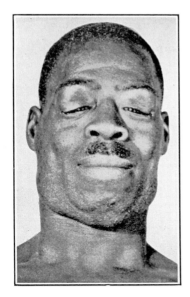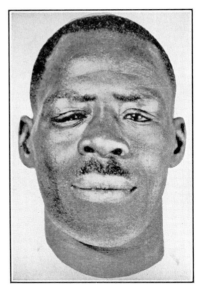

Fig. 19–4.—Milkuicz syndrome in a case of chronic lymphocytic (subleukemic) leukemia. Note the symmetrical swelling of the lacrimal and salivary glands. There was no leukocytosis (W.B.C. 7680), and only moderate lymphocytosis (lymphocytes 66 per cent). The patient died of lobar pneumonia and the diagnosis was confirmed at autopsy. (Schaffer and Jacobsen, Am. J. Dis Child.)

the notches in the border are easily felt. The size of the spleen may be extreme and the organ may extend to the ilium and even to the right anterior superior spine. The size does not appear to be related to the total number of leukocytes. In chronic lymphocytic leukemia the spleen is not as large, as a rule, as in myelocytic leukemia and may extend only 3 to 4 cm. below the costal margin. It is very rare to find in chronic leukemia that neither spleen nor lymph nodes are enlarged, but this has been observed.[90]

The entire course of development of the splenomegaly may be painless, but not infrequently there is a history of more or less distress in the left upper abdominal quadrant or in the back. Infarcts in the spleen and perisplenitis may occur and give rise to such pain and tenderness as to suggest the presence of some abdominal emergency. A friction rub may be felt and heard over the spleen at such times.

Skin and Subcutaneous Tissues.[13c] —Skin lesions in leukemia are usually

classified as (1) leukemids, or non-specific lesions which do not represent localizations of leukemic cells and may be found in other conditions; and (2) leukemic lesions which are specific for leukemia and are made up of leukemic cells. Cutaneous lesions are found in all types of leukemia but are most common in the chronic lymphocytic variety. Sometimes skin lesions are the first signs of leukemia, blood and other changes appearing later.[224]

The **leukemids** include vesicles, pustules, wheals, bullae,[192] petechiae, hematomas, papules, nodules, prurigo-like papules, pyoderma, exfoliative dermatitis and herpes zoster. Pigmentary changes may occur, as well as sensory disturbances such as itching and burning.

Bleeding into the skin is common in acute leukemia and may occur in late stages of chronic leukemia, especially in lymphocytic leukemia. Thrombocytopenia is usually present at the same time.

Herpes zoster is seen not infrequently

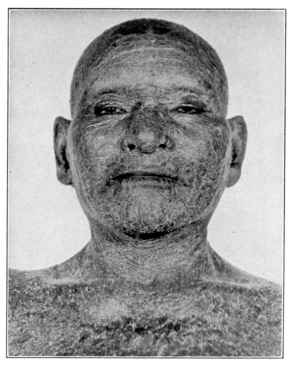

Fɪɢ. 19–5.—Leukemia cutis universalis. There was desquamation of the skin of the whole body and most of the hair was gone. The skin of the face, forehead and ears was swollen and the eyelids infiltrated. The leukocyte count was 30,000, the lymphocytes 73 per cent. All the accessible lymph nodes were greatly enlarged. On section, the cutis was found to be densely infiltrated with lymphocytes. The patient died of lobular pneumonia. None of the lymph nodes in the interior of the body were enlarged, the spleen was not increased in size and there was only slight periportal infiltration of the lymphocytes in the liver.

in the lymph node disorders, approximately in 2.8 per cent of cases.[193f] Of 42 cases of leukemia in which herpes zoster developed, 34 were lymphocytic, 3 myelocytic.[222] The herpes was followed in some cases by nerve paralysis, in others by a generalized vesicular eruption. The lesions have been attributed to involvement of the posterior nerve roots and spinal ganglia, but such changes apparently are not constant.

There is an extensive and confused literature on the specific lesions which may be found **in chronic lymphocytic leukemia** and many writers[71] regard as one group the changes found not only in leukemia but also in lymphosarcoma,

Hodgkin's disease and mycosis fungoides. *Erythrodermia*, a condition characterized by progressive reddening of the skin ("homme rouge"), together with thickening and edema or thinning and atrophy, has been described.[70,93] The involvement of the skin may be diffuse and generalized, affecting the skin of the whole body, the so-called *universal leukemia cutis* (Fig. 19–5);[91] or it may be localized, in which case the face is the seat of predilection (Fig. 19–6). The lesions may be yellowish-brown, red, bluish-red or purplish in color. Nodular lesions may be produced. Ulceration and necrosis are rare. The total leukocyte count may be very high, normal or

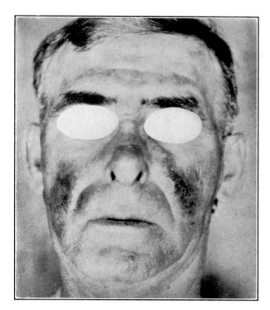

FIG. 19-6.—Reddish-purple infiltration of the skin of the face, especially the cheeks, in a case of chronic lymphocytic leukemia. The leukocyte count was only 4,850 and the lymphocytes 45 per cent, but there was moderate anemia, there were normoblasts in the blood smear, there was well-marked adenopathy even in regions where the skin was not involved, and the spleen was enlarged. Before death the leukocytes rose to 171,000, of which 84 per cent were lymphoblasts. Autopsy confirmed the diagnosis.

low but, in the latter instance, if the case is one of leukemia, the blood eventually becomes frankly leukemic. Metastatic acropachy has been reported.[27]

The lesions which have been noted in the rare cases of **chronic myelocytic leukemia**[36,124] with skin involvement are described as firm, sharply circumscribed,[169a] brownish, slaty gray or bluish cutaneous and subcutaneous nodules varying in size from that of a pinhead to that of a walnut or larger (Figs. 19-8 and 19-9). They may present a crescentic configuration.[36] It has been pointed out[172a] that the appearance of leukemic nodules in the skin in this form of leukemia is of grave prognostic import. The duration of life after the appearance of cutaneous lesions has been eleven days to four months.[74] Cutaneous lesions in chronic lymphocytic leukemia do not have such serious significance.

Gastro-intestinal System. — In addition to symptoms which might be expected to accompany any debilitating disease, such as anorexia, flatulence and the like, there may be recurring attacks of diarrhea most exhausting to the patient and occasionally accompanied by serious hemorrhages. We have been impressed by the frequency with which true peptic ulceration is associated with chronic myelocytic leukemia. However, massive gastro-intestinal hemorrhage from gastroduodenal ulcer may occur in other forms of leukemia as well.[168] Sometimes gastro-intestinal complaints[224] may so dominate the picture that an error in diagnosis may be made. There may be pain, continous or intermittent; symptoms of intestinal obstruction; or abdominal tumor. More frequently the abdominal symptoms in leukemia appear late in the course of the disease. In a small proportion of cases infiltration of parts or even the whole of the gastro-intestinal tract has been observed. This is extremely rare in myelocytic leukemia[28] but is not so unusual in the lymphocytic form. Boikan[15] described a case in which the stomach was enormously enlarged, with huge convolutions on the inner surface, giving it a brain-like appearance (Fig. 19-10), while the intestines showed polyp-like infiltrations. The leukemic infiltration is found in the mucosa and submucosa.[173a]

Outnumbering the cases in which the blood examination showed them clearly to be leukemic,[185] are reports of cases in which extensive lymphocytic infiltrations have been found in the absence of the typical clinical picture of leukemia ("*pseudoleukemia gastro-intestinalis*").[15,144]

The **liver** is usually palpable and often is decidedly enlarged. The edge is smooth and moderately firm, but it is

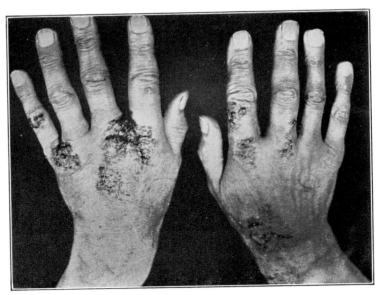

FIG. 19-7.—Skin lesions in a case of chronic lymphocytic leukemia, with inflammatory reaction superimposed on leukemia cutis. On a base of indurated skin there is a brownish encrustation due to the oozing of a pink fluid. There was marked general glandular enlargement, splenomegaly and a leukocytosis of 200,000 with 93 per cent lymphocytes.

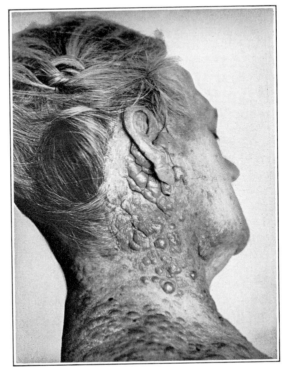

FIG. 19-8.—Myelocyticleukemia of the skin. (Ketron and Gay, courtesy of Arch. Dermat.)

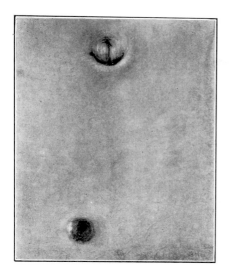

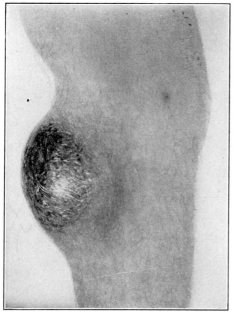

FIG. 19–9.—Purplish nodule in the skin of the abdomen and similar but larger tumor on the leg in a case of subleukemic myelogenous leukemia. (From a drawing by Mr. Jack B. Wilson.)

rarely as hard as the spleen. Jaundice due to liver damage is very unusual but it may occur as the result of nodular growths which interfere with the flow of bile. Ascites is also rare in leukemia but

has been observed in a few cases. In two of these the leukocyte changes were slight and the Banti syndrome was closely simulated.[30]

Cardiovascular System. — Anemia and anoxemia may lead to cardiac dilatation and this, together with the weight of the splenic tumor, produces symptoms such as dyspnea and palpitation. True cardiac failure may ensue. Enlargement of the heart, systolic murmurs, tachycardia and edema are found in such cases. Pericarditis may occur.[11j] Not infrequently considerable increase in pericardial fluid is found at autopsy. Infiltrations in the myocardium are not uncommon but such cases as Costa described in which rupture of the left auricle and of the descending aorta occurred as a result[35] and cases in which the conduction mechanism was disturbed,[46a] are most unusual.

Respiratory System. — When the disease is well established, cough may be present and fine crepitant rales are often heard over the bases of the lungs. These symptoms may be due to pulmonary congestion or to partial atelectasis because of compression by the enlarged organs below the diaphragm. In addition, there may be a mediastinal tumor from lymph node enlargement or due to proliferation of round cells in the thymus,[11d] or pulmonary infiltration (Fig. 19–11) or pleural effusion may occur.[77b] Such changes have been found in 30 per cent or more of cases of chronic lymphocytic leukemia,[54] but they are much less frequent in the myelocytic form.[77a] Rarely the pulmonary involvement is so pronounced that diagnostic difficulties arise.[84i]

Leukemic infiltration may occur in the upper respiratory tract in chronic as well as in acute leukemia, especially in the larynx.[193] Involvement of the tonsils has been mentioned. Their enlargement in an elderly person, if otherwise

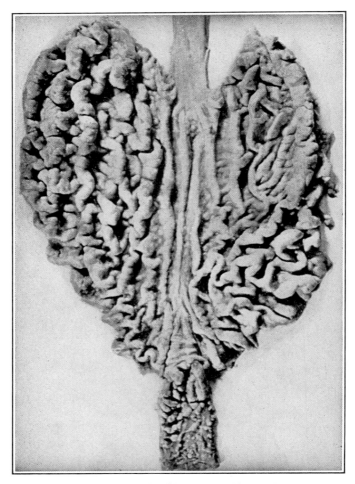

FIG. 19–10.—Enormously enlarged stomach with mucosa thickened and thrown into huge convolutions in a case of chronic lymphocytic leukemia (W.B.C. 86,000, lymphocytes 96 per cent). Some of the convolutions were as much as 2 cm. thick and 2 cm. high. (Boikan, W. S., courtesy of Arch. Int. Med.)

unaccounted for, should arouse suspicion of leukemia.

Urogenital System. — The first symptoms in a case of leukemia may direct attention to the urogenital tract: hematuria, priapism, a mass in the loin[75] or pain in the back,[7] symptoms directing attention to the prostate,[224] menorrhagia, metrorrhagia or amenorrhea.

Hemorrhage may be due to thrombocytopenia but in chronic leukemia infiltration of the kidney or congestion produced by pressure of enlarged glands

has been the cause in some cases. Hematuria has been noted in 15 to 20 per cent of cases.[136] In advanced cases, the clinical picture may resemble that of uremia.

Priapism is more common in myelocytic than in lymphocytic leukemia and may be a very troublesome, persistent and painful symptom. It is thought to be due to stasis of leukocytes or to thrombosis of the spaces of the corpora cavernosa. Priapism of the clitoris has been observed.[129]

Bones and Joints.—In chronic leu-

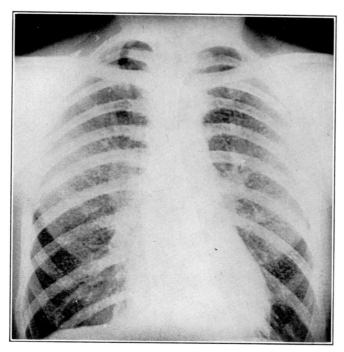

FIG. 19–11.—Diffuse, soft nodose infiltrations associated with para- and perihilar lymphadenopathy in a case of chronic lymphocytic leukemia. (Courtesy of Dr. Henry Lerner.)

kemia there may be no symptoms referable to the bones and joints. Even in such cases, however, and especially in the myelocytic form, bone tenderness can be elicited if firm pressure is made over the **sternum.** To discover such tenderness it is necessary to palpate the whole sternum systematically, for the tenderness may be limited to a small area no more than 1 cm. in diameter. This is usually found in the lower portion of the sternum, most often in the region of the fourth or fifth costal cartilages. Craver[37] noted that this sign was present in 75 per cent of cases of myelocytic leukemia and was less frequent in the lymphocytic form. This corresponds with the writer's experience. The patient is frequently unaware of any tenderness until pressure is applied at the proper point. The extensiveness of cellular hyperplasia seems to be a determining factor in the production of this sign.

One of our patients was able to detect the need for further irradiation by a return of the sternal tenderness for which he had learned to look. Tenderness over other bones is rare.

Pain, limitation of movement and other symptoms which suggest arthritis or osteomyelitis, or are due to actual fracture of bone, may occur in acute or in chronic leukemia. They are more common in acute leukemia, especially in children,[8] and may suggest rheumatic fever, brucellosis and other conditions. This subject will be discussed in the section on acute leukemia. Though less frequent in chronic leukemia,[38] these symptoms may cause much difficulty in diagnosis, particularly when they are associated with few of the classical signs of leukemia (subleukemic or "aleukemic" leukemia).[224] Sometimes symptoms arise as the result of compression by bony tumors on nerves or other structures.

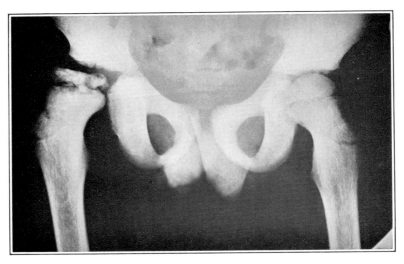

Fig. 19–12.—Extensive destructive changes in the right femur suggesting Perthe's disease in a boy, aged six years, suffering from chronic myelocytic leukemia.

The lesions may take the form of (1) tumors; (2) periosteal elevations; (3) arthritis; (4) destruction and absorption of bone leading to fracture or dislocation; (5) osteomyelitis or (6) sclerosis[222c] (Figs. 19–12, 19–13, 19–14). Chloroma is the name given to green tumors found in association with leukemia, usually the acute form, and giving rise to a clinical picture which will be described below (p. 937). The finding of a single bone tumor in cases of classical chronic myelocytic leukemia,[162c,208] is quite rare. There may be transverse bands of diminished density at the ends of the shafts of the long bones[194c] or small or extensive foci of bone destruction,[30b] moth-eaten areas, or generalized reduction of bone density. Leukemic proliferation in the juxta-articular portions of the bone may give rise to symptoms of arthritis.[9c] In one of our cases there was such extensive destruction of the head of the femur that the clinical and roentgenographic picture was that of Perthe's disease (Fig. 19–12). There may be not only absorption of bone, but also proliferation of bone tissue such as

is encountered in sarcomas of bone.[194e] The distribution of lesions of bones in leukemia is shown in Figure 19–13.

Special Senses.—Except for exophthalmos, which is so characteristic in chloroma (p. 937), symptoms referable to the *eyes* are unusual in leukemia. Examination of the fundus, however, will reveal changes in about two-thirds of cases of chronic leukemia. They are much more common in the myelocytic form (Fig. 19–14) than in the lymphocytic.[16] The changes include engorgement of veins, hemorrhages, exudates and blurring of the disk. The hemorrhages may be so small that they are difficult to find, or they may be very extensive; they may be superficial or deep; they often tend to surround the blood vessels; they may be flame-shaped or, if in the deeper retinal layers, they are roughly circular or rosette-shaped. Leukocytic infiltration may appear in the form of white lines sheathing the peripheral portions of distended veins or as white, irregular nodules surrounded by hemorrhage.

Occasionally eye symptoms give the

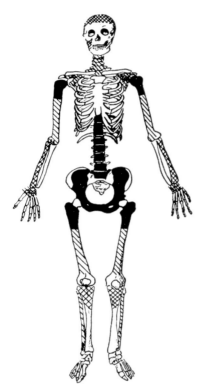

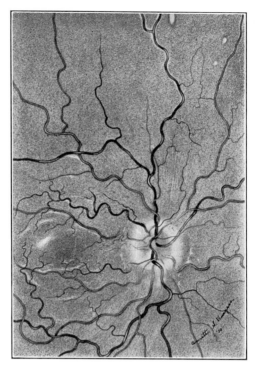

Fig. 19–13.—Distribution of lesions of bone in leukemia from the standpoint of demonstrability by roentgenography. The black areas represent the most frequent sites of changes; the checkered areas, the next most common sites; the sites occasionally involved and those rarely involved are represented by diagonal lines and white areas, respectively. (Craver and Copeland, courtesy of Arch. Surg.)

Fig. 19–14.—Fundus oculi in a case of chronic myelocytic leukemia. The disk is markedly elevated, quite red and edematous and the optic cup is practically filled. There is infiltration about the vessels, making them appear to be accompanied by white stripes. The vessels are tortuous and the veins and arteries are practically the same color. There is moderate retinal edema. In the periphery there are a few whitish plaques, many of which are surrounded by a whitish halo. (Courtesy of Dr. Alan C. Woods.)

first sign of leukemia. In one of Forkner's cases[59] of chronic myelocytic leukemia there was sudden blindness in one eye due to hemorrhage. One of our patients with chronic lymphocytic leukemia first sought attention because of pain and failing vision in one eye.[224] A leukemic nodule was present at the edge of the cornea (Fig. 19–15). Involvement of the iris, cornea, and sclera with leukemic infiltrations has been described.[220]

Infiltration of the lachrymal glands in leukemia has been mentioned (p. 914). Infiltration of the eyelids and sclerae may also occur.

Hemorrhage or infiltration in the external, middle or internal *ear*, or infiltrations along the course of the eighth nerve may produce symptoms of deafness, otitis media or Ménière's syndrome.[193d] The medullary spaces of the temporal bones and the tympanic cavities may be filled with leukemic cells.

Nervous System.—Any part of the nervous system may be involved in leukemia and the lesions[43b,176] may take the form of hemorrhage, thrombosis, infiltration with leukemic cells, or tumor-

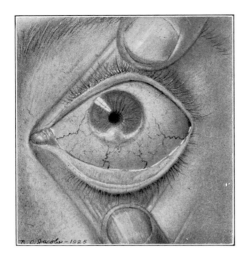

FIG. 19–15.—Lymphocytic tumor of cornea in a case of chronic lymphocytic leukemia.

like growths. In a study of 334 cases of leukemia, clinical evidence of neurological complications was found in 69 (20.5 per cent).[190] These included, in order of frequency, cranial nerve palsies or anesthesias, absent reflexes, pyramidal signs, paresthesias, meningeal signs, coma, paralysis and tremors. In a survey of the literature, Schwab and Weiss[190] found the following recorded (in order of frequency): cerebral hemorrhage, cranial meningeal involvement, invasion of cranial nerve nuclei, and cerebral involvement. Much less frequent was spinal cord invasion, spinal, meningeal, and spinal extradural or peripheral nerve involvement. The pressure of the cerebrospinal fluid may be increased, and there may be an increase in cells and protein.

Frequently it is evident from the clinical picture as a whole that one is dealing with leukemia but in some instances the symptoms and signs have directed attention chiefly or even exclusively to the nervous system. Thus, in one case of lymphocytic leukemia the first sign was pain and paralysis of both legs.[12c] Hemorrhages and infiltration of leukemic cells have been found in the brain in as many as 80 per cent of cases.[131b] In 29 per cent the hemorrhage was sufficient to cause death.

Fever.—Fever is rarely mentioned as a symptom of chronic leukemia. Sometimes it may be so high that confusion with acute leukemia may result or some complication may be suspected (Fig. 19–16).

The Blood.—In a well-advanced case one may be struck by the thickness and stickiness of the blood[198] and the difficulty in making blood smears. If the blood is mixed with an anticoagulant, allowed to stand in a hematocrit for a half hour or more and then centrifuged, a fairly clear separation of the corpuscles into three layers can be obtained. The uppermost layer is cream colored and is composed of platelets. Below this is a reddish-gray layer, composed almost entirely of leukocytes. Lowermost is the dark red layer of red corpuscles. The height of these layers roughly suggests the quantity of platelets and leukocytes and the degree of anemia. In chronic myelocytic leukemia the layer of leukocytes may be greater than the column of red corpuscles (Fig. 19–17). Above it, a layer of platelets, 1 or more mm. in depth, may be seen. The leukocyte layer in lymphocytic leukemia is rarely as great as in the myelocytic variety, not only because the total leuko cyte count may not be as high but also because lymphocytes are smaller than granulocytes. The platelet layer in chronic lymphocytic leukemia is rarely more than 0.5 mm. in thickness and may be much less.

In the early stages of chronic leukemia there may be no **anemia** (Fig. 19–3). In chronic myelocytic leukemia, in fact, there may sometimes be polycythemia (p. 802). Usually, however, by the time the diagnosis of leukemia is first made. anemia is generally present and may be quite severe. As a rule, it is normocytic. It is difficult to obtain perfect separation

PLATE XIV

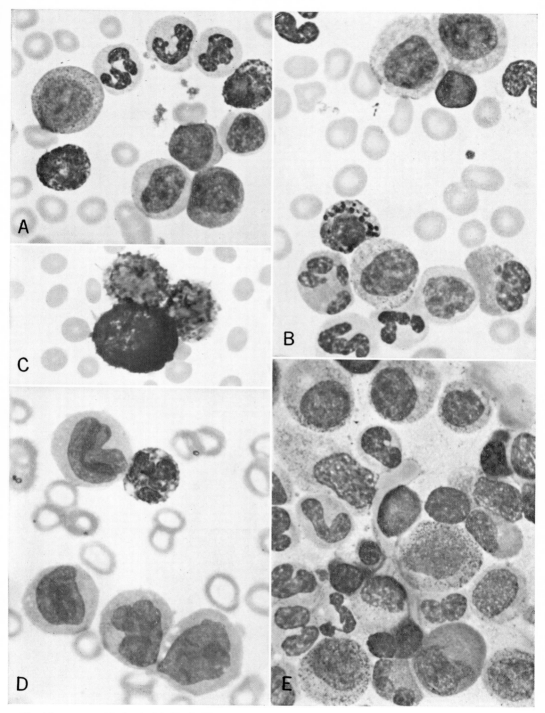

Blood from cases of leukemia (A, B, C, D) contrasted with normal bone marrow (*E*). *A* and *B* are from cases of chronic myelocytic leukemia (Wright's stain, × 1220). *C* and *D* are blood smears from cases of acute myeloid (*C*) and acute monocytic (*D*) leukemia and show a positive peroxidase reaction in all three cells from the case of myeloid leukemia and in a single cell of the monocytic leukemia. *E* shows normal bone marrow elements (Wright's stain, × 1220).

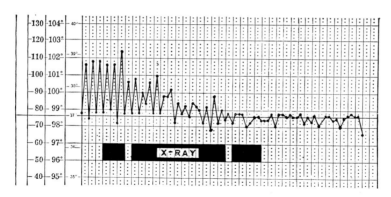

FIG. 19–16.—Fever in a case of chronic myelocytic leukemia (W.B.C. 720,000). There was diarrhea at this time but no cause for either the fever or the diarrhea could be found. Both symptoms disappeared following roentgen therapy. Maximal temperature was reached each day in the late afternoon or evening.

of red corpuscles and leukocytes in the hematocrit, so that measurements of erythrocyte size by this means carry a greater margin of error than in other forms of anemia. Anisocytosis may be well marked but poikilocytosis of any significant degree is unusual. Immature forms of the red series, such as normoblasts, polychromatophilia, basophilic stippling, and increased numbers of reticulocytes are found in myelocytic leukemia, sometimes even when there is little anemia, but they are more rare in lymphocytic leukemia unless there is an accompanying hemolytic anemia. In the later phases of chronic lymphocytic leukemia (p. 952), severe anemia develops which may or may not be associated with signs of frank hemolytic anemia. In one series of 64 cases, acquired hemolytic anemia occurred in 17.[167a] The pathogenesis of anemia in leukemia will be discussed later (p. 944).

In chronic myelocytic leukemia, blood **platelets** are usually normal in number or slightly increased in the early stages of the disease. It has been noted that a rise of platelets from a subnormal number, or a fall from an excessively high level to a normal one, is usually associated with clinical improvement.[153] A persistently

low count is often a serious omen. Fragments of megakaryocytes may be found in the blood smear. In lymphocytic leukemia, on the other hand, the platelet count is practically never increased, often is somewhat low and, if greatly reduced, suggests severe marrow insufficiency.

The blood changes already described are to be found in cases of chronic leukemia whether there be leukocytosis or not. They are valuable in recognizing the existence of a profound hematopoietic disturbance. Recognition of the type of leukemia, while it may be suspected from the clinical findings, depends in the last analysis on the study of the leukocytes.

In **chronic myelocytic leukemia,** well-marked leukocytosis is the rule, the counts ranging from 100,000 to 800,000 per c.mm. A count of 200,000 to 400,000 is frequently found at the time the disease is first discovered. Lower counts may be encountered, however, when the clinical picture and the degree of anemia indicate advanced disease, and the count actually may be normal or leukopenic (subleukemic or "aleukemic" leukemia, p. 937).

When the leukocyte count is high, the

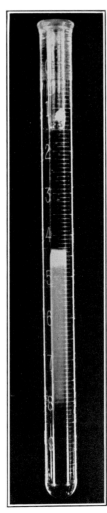

FIG. 19–17.—Blood from a case of chronic mye-locytic leukemia, centrifuged in a hematocrit and photographed against a dark background, to show the greatly increased volume of packed white cells (gray layer between 4.8 and 8.0), the increased amount of platelets (white layer between 4.3 and 4.8) and the reduced volume of packed red cells (dark layer below the "8" mark).

the leukocytes. The majority of the myelocytes are neutrophilic. Relatively few undifferentiated myelocytes and only a small number of myeloblasts (2 to 10 per cent) are found in chronic myelocytic leukemia. The appearance of the blood smear in classical cases (Plate XIV) is like that of a smear of normal sternal marrow.

Eosinophilic and basophilic myelocytes are also to be found. Eosinophils are increased, so as to maintain or even exceed their normal ratio. Basophilic granules may be found in the eosinophilic or the neutrophilic polymorphonuclear cells. Basophilic leukocytes may be greatly increased in number (3 to 20 per cent). They are more numerous in myelocytic leukemia than in any other disease. Pelger-like leukocytes (p. 224) have been described.[41]

The lymphocytes may be slightly increased in absolute numbers, but their percentage is usually relatively low. Monocytes are at first increased in number but later become less evident.

Varieties of leukemia in which eosinophils, basophils, or polymorphonuclear neutrophils predominate will be mentioned below.

In **chronic lymphocytic leukemia,** the blood smear lacks the diversity of form and type which is so characteristic of myelocytic leukemia. The total leukocyte increase is seldom as marked as in leukemia of the myelocytic type, the average being between 200,000 and 250,000 per c.mm. There is a striking uniformity in the white corpuscles, 90 to 99 per cent being small lymphocytes (Fig. 19–18). These often possess only a very narrow rim of light blue cytoplasm and some seem to be entirely devoid of cytoplasm. Azure granules are rare in the cytoplasm that may be seen, and the nuclei may stain more lightly and reveal a looser chromatin network than is found in the normal small lymphocyte. There may be some varia-

increase is found to be due to the white cells of the granular series. The segmented neutrophils comprise from 30 to 70 per cent of the leukocytes and meta-myelocytes as well as myelocytes are found in great numbers. The latter constitute 20 to 40 or even 50 per cent of

PLATE XV

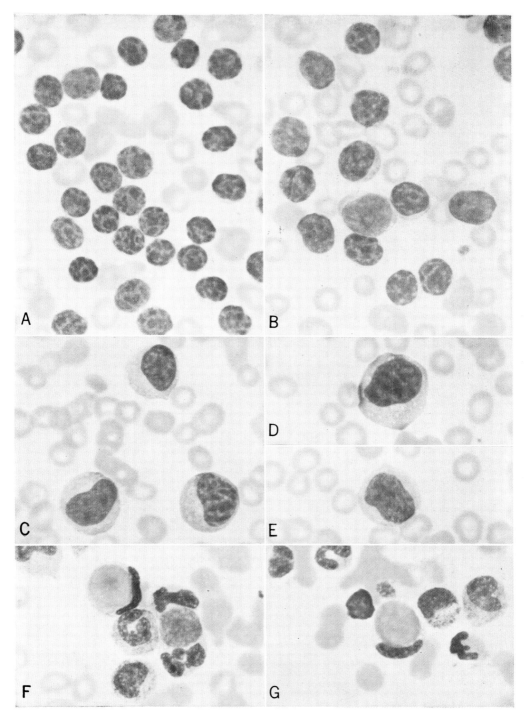

Blood of patients with *chronic lymphocytic leukemia* (*A*, *B*) contrasted with lymphocytes from cases of *infectious mononucleosis* (*C*, *D*, *E*) (Wright's stain, × 1220). In *F* and *G*, "*L. E*" (lupus erythematosus *cells*) are shown.

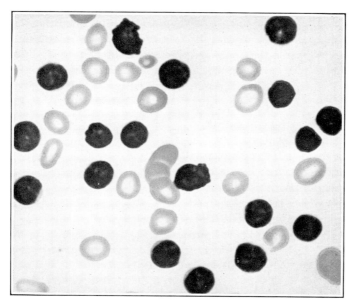

Fig. 19–18.—Photomicrograph of blood from a case of chronic lymphocytic leukemia. Wright's stain. (× 1050.) Note the "monotonous" picture of small lymphocytes, varied only by the presence of a few broken lymphocytes.

tion in size. Large lymphocytes with indented nuclei are not infrequently found. Immature lymphocytes occur less commonly. None of these cells show granules on staining by the peroxidase method.

ACUTE LEUKEMIA[184]

Mode of Onset and Course.—In comparison with chronic leukemia the onset of acute leukemia is sudden and the course is short. In some cases the first symptoms may not be alarming but signs of a grave illness nevertheless soon develop. There is fever, marked prostration and rapidly developing anemia, often there are extensive hemorrhagic manifestations, and not infrequently, if permitted to continue untreated, necrotic and gangrenous processes develop in the mucous membranes of the mouth and throat. Enlargement of lymph nodes, spleen and liver is less conspicuous than in chronic leukemia and may even be absent. The excessively high leukocyte counts of chronic leukemia are not usually reached but the leukocytes show a degree of immaturity such as is never seen in chronic leukemia. Although occasionally one sees a "spontaneous remission of varied duration, the course as a rule is rapidly progressive and eventually death ensues. The great majority of untreated patients die within six months, many in two months.

Initial Symptoms. — The initial symptoms vary, for they depend for their development on the location of hemorrhages, leukemic infiltrations and glandular enlargements, as well as on systemic manifestations such as fever, anemia, and toxemia. The first sign of acute leukemia may be the rapid develop- of weakness and pallor; or because of abnormal bleeding from the mucous membranes, or petechiae or ecchymoses in the skin, one of the hemorrhagic disorders may be suspected. In other cases attention is directed to the nasopharynx because of sore throat. Enlargement of lymph nodes may be noted or, because of infiltration or hemorrhage, cough or dyspnea resulting from enlargement of the thymus[32] or mediastinal lymph nodes, rheumatoid pains, abdominal pain or a variety of neurological manifestations may be the first noteworthy symptoms.[224] Fever, headache and general malaise may appear suddenly and produce marked prostration, thus suggesting the onset of some severe, malignantly virulent form of sepsis.[224] Some of our cases have presented features which suggested diphtheria, osteomyelitis of the jaw, acute thyroiditis, conjunctivitis, paroxysmal tachycardia, hyperthyroidism, subacute bacterial endocarditis, brucellosis, rheumatic fever, miliary tuberculosis, pelvic tumor and breast tumor.

Uncommonly, *in adults* especially,[81b] the onset may be slow and atypical. Anemia, unexplained after thorough study, thrombocytopenic purpura or leukopenia, or all three findings may be present for as long as a year, or more, before the true nature of the illness is revealed. Splenomegaly may not be detected, nor sternal tenderness and the bone marrow examination gives no certain answer. This state has been called "*pre-leukemia*" and will be discussed further shortly (p. 950).

Lymph Nodes.—Lymph node enlargement in acute leukemia is usually less conspicuous than in chronic leukemia and may be insignificant or absent in fulminating cases or in acute myeloblastic leukemia. In many cases of acute leukemia, however, and especially in the monocytic form, cervical gland enlargement, sometimes of great degree, occurs. Generalized adenopathy is more likely to be found in lymphoblastic leukemia than in the other forms.

The glands in acute leukemia may be more soft than in chronic leukemia and, as in the latter, evidence of infiltration of surrounding tissue is absent. The cervical glands may be tender, especially if there is evident oral infection. In as many as a third of cases,[32,151] glandular enlargement may be the first evidence of leukemia.

Splenomegaly. — While splenomegaly is not demonstrable clinically in all cases of acute leukemia, it is usual to find that this organ extends 1 to 4 cm. below the costal margin. The greatest enlargement has been reported in lymphoblastic leukemia where it may sometimes be as great as in chronic leukemia.

Skin.—Purpuric manifestations are the commonest lesions found in the skin. These include petechiae, ecchymoses and even necrotic changes and blisters in association with hemorrhagic areas. Specific infiltration such as is seen in chronic leukemia is less frequent in acute leukemia but in monocytic leukemia a great variety of lesions has been described.[93e] These include a diffuse exanthematous eruption consisting of slate-blue macules and papules containing monocytes, generalized pustular and even bullous lesions, generalized exfoliative dermatitis and herpes zoster.[13b]

Mucous Membranes. — Purpuric manifestations are characteristically found in the mucous membranes in acute leukemia, especially in those of the nose and the oral cavity. The first symptom may be unexpected bleeding following slight trauma, such as blowing the nose or brushing the teeth and many patients find their way to the physician *via* the dentist or the nose and throat specialist.

In addition to petechiae, large ecchymotic areas, extensive ulceration and even noma-like lesions[175] may be encountered. These may be the result of leukemic infiltration, as well as of hemorrhage and invasion of the necrotic tissue by spirochetes and other organisms found in the mouth. Such lesions may be mistaken for Ludwig's angina, diphtheria, agranulocytosis or scurvy.

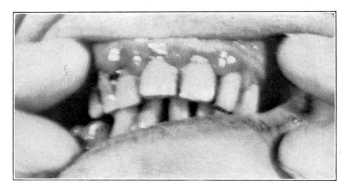

FIG. 19–19.—Swollen and spongy gums in a case of acute monocytic leukemia.

Partially clotted blood may be found at the gingival margins of the teeth and the gums themselves may be swollen and purplish in color. This swelling is sometimes so great that the gums are heaped over the teeth (Fig. 19–19). There may be ulceration and necrosis as well, the mucous membranes elsewhere in the oral cavity may be similarly involved, and there may be diffuse cellulitis which extends into the deeper tissues of the face.

It has been stated that swelling and ulceration of the mucous membranes, particularly the gingivae,[59,167] is so characteristic of monocytic leukemia that this diagnosis should be suspected on clinical grounds in such cases. Others do not agree that there exists any difference in the lesions of the mouth in the various types of acute leukemia. In the writer's experience such changes have occurred frequently, but by no means exclusively in monocytic leukemia.

Respiratory Tract. — Infiltration may occur in various parts of the respiratory tract, especially the larynx.[193] A mediastinal mass[32] may be the first sign of acute leukemia. Respiratory obstruction may occur.[134] Migratory pulmonary infiltration, small round cavities, miliary lesions resembling Boeck's sarcoid and the syndrome of "alveolar-capillary block" have been observed.[162b] Effusion into **serous cavities** especially the pleural cavities, may occur, almost always as a late manifestation.

The **cardiovascular system** is affected chiefly because of anemia and, as a result, tachycardia, dyspnea or pain may develop. These symptoms have in some instances been the first signs of leukemia.[224]

Gastro-intestinal Tract.—Specific infiltration in the gastro-intestinal tract is quite unusual in acute leukemia although leukemic nodules have been found in the appendix, cecum[28b] and rectum[59] in monocytic leukemia, and cases have been described in which the clinical picture resembled typhoid fever or dysentery.[125c] Cooke[32] referred to two children in whom severe abdominal pain with muscle spasm and vomiting was due in one instance to leukemic infiltration and perforation of the appendix and, in the other, to subserous hemorrhages. The *liver* is often enlarged. At autopsy, various degrees of portal fibrosis have been found which could not be related to age, type of leukemia, duration of disease or type of treatment.[219e]

Genito-urinary Tract. — Attention may be directed to the genito-urinary tract by hematuria[82] and pain, symptoms of nephritis,[139] or priapism. The last is more rare in acute leukemia than in the chronic disease.[59] Leukemic infiltration

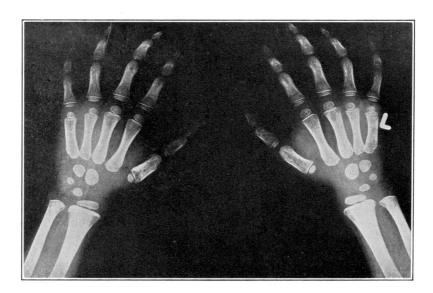

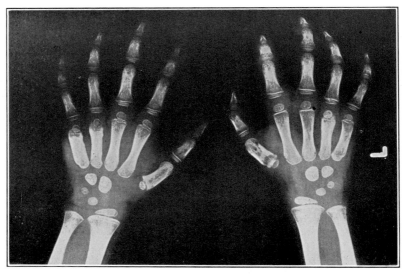

Fig. 19–20.—Roentgenograms of the hands of a child of three years with acute lymphoblastic leukemia. Note the marked prominence of the trabeculations of the metacarpal bones and phalanges, the punched out areas in the first metacarpal bone of each hand and the extensive periosteal changes and thickening of the cortex, especially in the fourth and fifth metacarpals on the left in the lower film. The latter was taken twenty-five days later than the upper film.

may produce marked elongation of the pelvis, infundibula and calices of the kidney without interfering with diodrast clearance[75] or with other renal functions.[71d] Enlargement of the kidneys sufficient to be detected by physical examination at some time in the course of the disease is not unusual.

Bones and Joints.—Manifestations referable to the bones and joints are not infrequent in acute leukemia, especially in children. The various types of lesions have been enumerated already (p. 922). The symptoms may suggest rheumatic fever, caries of the spine, brucellosis or Still's disease, and even spontaneous fractures may occur.[11e] Tenderness is usually present in the lower portion of the sternum, as in chronic leukemia, but there may also be pain and tenderness over any of the bones and there may be painful swellings of the joints. These symptoms have been shown to be due, in some instances at least, to subperiosteal leukemic proliferation in the juxta-articular portions of the bone.[87a] Bone changes can often be demonstrated by roentgenograms (Figs. 19–20, 19–21, 19–22). In children a narrow, transverse zone of diminished density just proximal to the metaphysis of the long bones is the most common finding.[8] This is not found in metastatic neuroblastoma, a disorder which may otherwise resemble leukemia radiologically.[222b]

When the leukemic tissue associated with bone assumes the form of nodules, and particularly when the bones of the skull are involved, a characteristic clinical picture (chloroma) is produced (p. 937).

Eyes and Ears.—Hemorrhages in the fundi of the eyes are usually found in acute leukemia (70 to 90 per cent of cases)[16,73] and characteristically consist of pale centers with red borders (Fig. 19–23). Hemorrhage may also occur in the conjunctivae, eyelids and other parts of the eyes. Exophthalmos is characteristic of chloroma. Deafness may occur as the result of hemorrhage into the labyrinth or infiltration of the auditory nerve, or Ménière's syndrome may be produced.

Nervous System. — Depending on their size and location, leukemic infiltrations and hemorrhages may produce a great variety of symptoms referable to the nervous system. The former are found usually in the meninges or nerve sheaths, or may produce symptoms by extension from bone.[158,219a] Cranial nerve

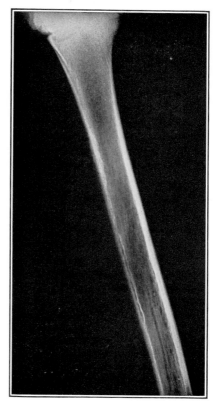

Fig. 19–21.—Roentgenograms of the humerus of a girl of eleven years with acute lymphoblastic leukemia. Note the irregular distortion of the architectural pattern and the multiple defects within the medullary portion of the bone, the decalcification of the cortex on the mesial aspect of the shaft and the periosteal proliferation.

palsies, especially those affecting the facial, oculomotor, optic, auditory and olfactory nerves, hemiplegia and other forms of paralysis, convulsions and symptoms suggesting encephalitis,[32] meningitis,[43b] and transverse myelitis may be observed. These may be the first signs of the disease but, on the other hand, numerous hemorrhages may be found in the nervous system at autopsy without physical signs of such lesions having been produced.[224] It was noted that a distinctive intracerebral lesion was present in patients with leukocyte counts greater

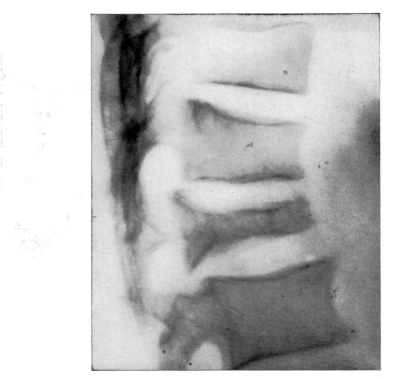

FIG. 19–22.—Compression deformity of first lumbar vertebra, partial narrowing of twelfth dorsal, in a case of monocytic leukemia.

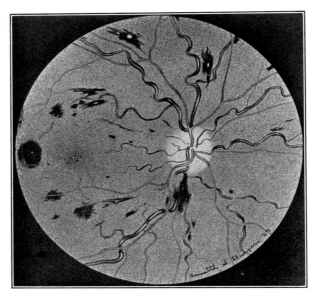

FIG. 19–23.—Fundus oculi in a case of acute leukemia. There are numerous flame-shaped hemorrhages as well as small and large irregularly round hemorrhages. Clear centers are visible in some of the hemorrhages. The caliber of the veins is greatly increased, that of the arteries decreased. (Courtesy of Dr. Alan C. Woods.)

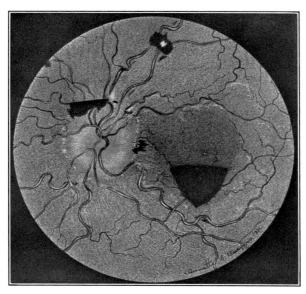

Fig. 19–24.—Fundus oculi in a case of acute lymphoblastic leukemia. The outlines of the optic disk are blurred. There are striate and subhyaloid hemorrhages. The caliber of the veins is increased, that of the arteries decreased. The vessels are tortuous and many are marked by whitish streaks. The retina has a veil-like appearance. (Courtesy of Dr. Alan C. Woods.)

than 300,000 per c.mm. who had had fatal intracranial hemorrhages.[61b] The massive hemorrhages primarily involved the white matter and within the areas of hemorrhage nodules of leukemic cells were present. The inference was drawn that proliferation of leukemic cells may result in destruction of the vessel wall with the formation of a leukemic nodule and that ultimately hemorrhage occurs about the nodule.

The Blood.—Anemia.—Anemia is characteristically found in acute leukemia and sometimes it is surprisingly severe. It has been stated that very early in the disease there may be no anemia. Although this is true, it is rare indeed that there is not some reduction below normal in the number of red corpuscles when the patient is first examined. Thus, in a review of 100 of our cases, anemia of some degree was found in every case (Table 19–2). The red corpuscles often show no marked variation from the normal in size or shape and the anemia is usually normocytic. In some cases there may be moderate macrocytosis. Polychromatophilia as well as normoblasts are frequently found.

Thrombocytopenia. — Thrombocytopenia is also characteristic of acute leukemia. It is rare that there is not some degree of reduction in the number of blood platelets and frequently their number is below 100,000 per c.mm. Exceptionally large platelets or forms which are bizarre in shape or in staining may be found. Bleeding time is prolonged, clot retraction is poor and the tourniquet test is positive, as in purpura hemorrhagica. Differentiation from the latter condition depends on the disproportion between the severity of the anemia and the amount of bleeding which has occurred, as well as on abnormalities in the leukocytes. Sometimes coagulation time is also prolonged. In some patients active fibrinolysin can be demonstrated, with fibrinogenopenia

Table 19–2—Degree of Anemia in Cases of Acute Leukemia at Time of First Blood Examination

Time between onset and first blood examination	No. of cases	R.B.C.			Average Hgb. (Gm.)
		Highest	Lowest	Average	
I. 1 week or less	5	3.20	2.03	2.81	8.3
II. Between 1 and 2 weeks .	8	2.71	1.30	2.20	6.8
III. Between 2 and 4 weeks .	13	3.10	0.89	2.04	5.8
IV. 4 to 12 weeks	39	4.08	1.21	2.58	6.3
V. More than 12 weeks . .	35	4.50	1.10	2.59	6.5
	100	4.50	0.89	2.43	6.7

as a result, plasma-thrombin clotting times may be prolonged and the levels of coagulation factors, such as factor V, may be reduced.[135] Even the presence of a heparin-like anticoagulant has been reported (p. 885).

Leukocytes.—The *leukocyte count*, particularly in the early stages, may be quite misleading. At this time it is rarely very high and may be normal or subnormal. The leukocyte count may be as low as 400 per c.mm. Persistent leukopenia, together with anemia and thrombocytopenia, should arouse suspicion of leukemia. A survey of 163 cases of acute leukemia of our own showed that the leukocyte count was less than 2500 per c.mm. in 8.4 per cent; between this value and 5,000 in 14.4 per cent; within the normal range in 13.8 per cent; between 10,000 and 25,000 in 22.7 per cent; and above 25,000 in 38.3 per cent. The last group includes 27 cases (16.1 per cent) in which the leukocyte count was greater than 100,000 per c.mm. In the absence of therapy, the leukocyte count in cases with normal or low counts often increases as the disease progresses, especially terminally. In rare cases the leukocyte count may fluctuate, from levels greatly above normal to subnormal values.

The most striking change in the blood is in the character of the leukocytes. In typical cases there is a distinct predominance of a single type of cell which is often mistaken, at first glance, for a lymphocyte. It is evident on further study, however, that these are immature leukocytes not usually found in the circulating blood. It is by the predominating leukocytes that the type of acute leukemia is recognized during life. It should be mentioned, however, that when there is no leukocytosis or there is leukopenia, the immature cells may form only a small proportion of the circulating cells. Yet it is these immature cells which are predominant in the bone marrow and it is these which increase in number as the leukocyte count rises.

In **acute myeloblastic leukemia** (Plate XVI *A*) the immature leukocytes form 30 to 60 per cent of the white cells but may be even more numerous. The remainder of the cells are those seen normally in the blood. The majority of the immature forms possess the characteristics of myeloblasts and undifferentiated myelocytes (Chapter 4): round or oval nuclei composed of fine chromatin which is not condensed about the edges so as to form a nuclear membrane; several distinct and sometimes very large nucleoli; cytoplasm which is usually deep blue and possesses few or no granules. The finding of immature cells which possess a few specific granules is very useful, for this suggests that the associated cells devoid of granules are still younger forms and that

PLATE XVI

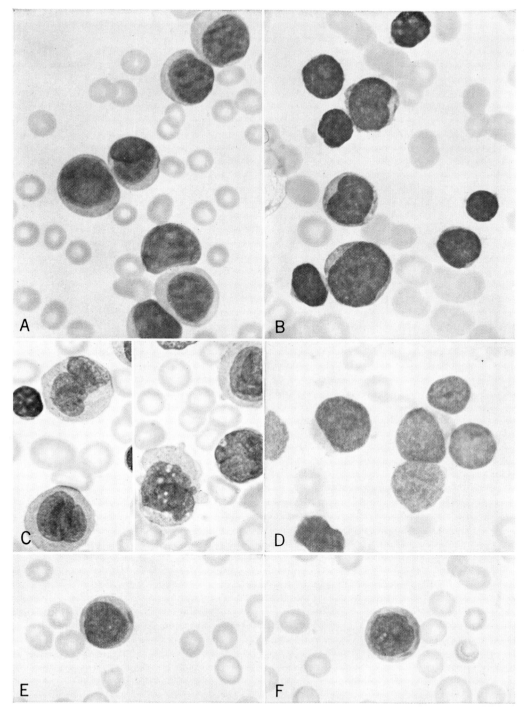

Acute leukemia and neuroblastoma. Blood smears from cases of acute leukemia: *A*, myeloblastic; *B*, lymphoblastic; *C*, monocytic. *D* is the bone marrow from a case of neuroblastoma, to show the similarity to acute leukemia, especially the lymphoblastic form. *E* and *F* show cells, each containing an Auer body, from cases of acute myeloblastic leukemia (Wright's stain, × 1220).

all of the cells are of the myeloid series. The granules can often be demonstrated in peroxidase stains or by supravital staining even when they are not easily discerned in Wright's stains.

Neutrophilic polymorphonuclear leukocytes may be scarce and eosinophilic forms are usually absent. It is only very rarely that the leukocytic picture resembles that of chronic myelocytic leukemia. The writer has seen only 2 such cases, both in children. When many myelocytes or more mature forms are found in the blood, the possibility that the case is one of acute leukemia should not be accepted too readily, even if the clinical picture suggests this diagnosis. The clinical picture during severe relapse in chronic leukemia may resemble that of acute leukemia. There may even be fever (Fig. 19–16). The presence of a greatly enlarged spleen and the lack of hemorrhagic phenomena and thrombocytopenia suggest the chronic form of the disease. Proper differentiation is important because the immediate prognosis and treatment of acute and chronic forms of leukemia are so different.

In some instances there may be numerous myeloblasts and a number of polymorphonuclear neutrophils, with few or no intermediate forms (*hiatus leukaemicus* of Naegeli).

Mitotic figures[79] may be found, as well as **Auer bodies.**[60d] The latter are rod-shaped structures in the cytoplasm, which are peroxidase-positive and may be present in myeloblasts, myelocytes or monocytes (Fig. 4–1, p. 215, Plate XVI, *E* and *F*). They have been observed in as many as 25 per cent of the cells. Auer bodies have been found by electron microscopy to be coacervates of laminated, homogeneous, crystalline plaques with the long axis of the plaques in the same plane as the long axis of the rod. They are probably formed by the coalescence of cytoplasmic granulation. It has been implied that they are present

exclusively in myelogenous and in monocytic leukemia but it remains to be proved that their formation is a phenomenon limited to leukemia. They are thought to differ from the granule-vacuole body and fibrillar formation which have also been found in leukemic cells.[1]

In **acute lymphoblastic leukemia,** the predominant cell (lymphoblast) possesses a round or oval nucleus composed of coarse, granular or "stippled" chromatin and containing usually only 1 or 2 nucleoli (Plate XVI, *B*). The chromatin tends to be arranged more compactly about the edges of the nucleus and the nucleoli, thus suggesting a distinct membrane. There may be a clear zone about the nucleus. The cytoplasm is basophilic and contains no granules. The most undifferentiated cells may be morphologically indistinguishable from myeloblasts. Lymphoblasts make up about 50 to 90 per cent of the total. Most of the remainder are readily recognizable lymphocytes, some of which contain a few azurophilic granules. Only a few neutrophilic leukocytes and perhaps an occasional myelocyte may be seen. Any appreciable number of the latter, as well as the finding of cells resembling lymphocytes but nevertheless containing a few granules in their cytoplasm and showing distinct nucleoli in their nuclei (promyelocytes), should make one suspect that one is dealing with myeloblastic rather than lymphoblastic leukemia.

Monocytic leukemia[9b] is recognized by the presence of large numbers of cells which can be definitely identified as monocytes, in addition to larger but apparently related forms (Plate XVII). The nuclei of the latter are irregular in shape, sometimes to an extreme, and are composed of very fine, reticular chromatin. The nucleus is even more lacy than in typical monocytes and it may appear to be folded or segmented. Nucleoli are inconspicuous. The cytoplasm is grayish-blue and contains innumerable, very fine, dust-like reddish-lilac granules, as well as a few larger ones. The cell boundaries may be irregular and some cells may have a serrated border due to the extrusion of short, granule-free pseudopodia. Occasional elongated or "tailed" cells[31] may be seen, some of which may contain a phagocytized red corpuscle, nucleus, or platelet. Such cells may be undifferentiated reticular cells.

In the same smear there are usually found a variable number of cells with nucleoli and few or no granules, as well as basophilic cytoplasm. These have been called "monoblasts." This term should be used only when the reticular cells are differentiated to monocytes.[45]

The cells of the monocytic series usually make up 60 or more per cent of all the leukocytes. The remaining cells are lymphocytes and polymorphonuclear leukocytes, but a few myelocytes and myeloblasts as well as plasma cells have been noted in the majority of cases. Downey[45,218] has applied *Naegeli's* name to the type of case in which a moderately large number of myelocytes has been found, because Naegeli considered the monocyte to be derived from the myeloblast. He also distinguished a *Schilling* type of monocytic leukemia, in which the large cell with lacy chromatin, bizarre nucleus and irregular cell border, already described, is found. More specifically Downey assumed that in the Schilling type the monocytes are derived from the reticulo-endothelial system whereas in the Naegeli variety they are developmental products of myeloblasts. The mature monocytes, according to this view, might have identical morphology, but the intermediate and younger cells would be different.[45] Further discussion of monocytic leukemia will be found on pages 937 and 988.

In addition to these types, cases are encountered in which the immature cells appear to be so primitive or so difficult to classify that the name **"stem cell" leukemia** is applied. These have also been referred to as hemoblastic, hemocytoblastic, lymphoidocytic, embryonal or undifferentiated cell leukemia.[115]

In spite of the differentiating criteria which have been described above, it is difficult for even an experienced hematologist to distinguish the various types of leukemia. So difficult is the differentiation that some hematologists have denied that a lymphoblastic form of leukemia exists, suggesting instead that such cells are "micromyeloblasts."[157] It should be pointed out that, in addition to careful study of blood smears stained with one of the Romanowsky stains, peroxidase staining and the supravital method should be used. The granules of myelocytes and of some monocytes can be demonstrated by the peroxidase stain, whereas the azurophil granules of lymphocytes do not give the reaction. This method may reveal granules which are not easily detected in smears stained with Wright's stain. The supravital stain affords the same advantage, and also helps to distinguish monocytes by their characteristic (although not specific) group of neutral red granules in the *hof* of the nucleus, as well as by their singular type of movement (p. 227).

Undoubtedly better methods are needed for the differentiation of the acute leukemias. Various techniques are being explored,[20c] including histochemical,[201a] enzymatic,[1g] and immunological methods, supported also by *in vivo* inoculations and *in vitro* cultures. On the basis of such biological characteristics two groups of acute leukemias were distinguished. These were independent of the morphologic appearance of the cells.[57a]

LESS COMMON TYPES OF LEUKEMIA

Subacute Leukemia. — Although one speaks generally of acute and chronic forms of leukemia, the duration of this

PLATE XVII

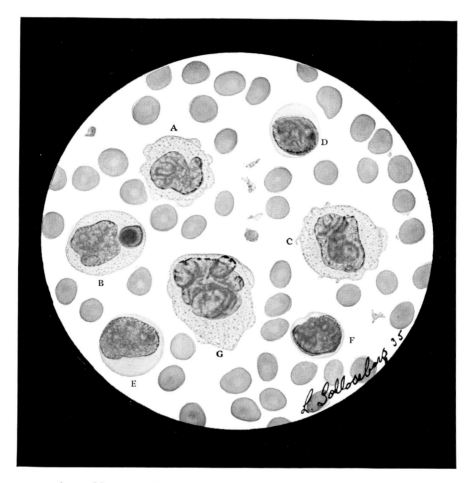

ACUTE MONOCYTIC LEUKEMIA (SCHILLING OR HISTIOMONOCYTIC TYPE).
(WRIGHT'S STAIN, × 1200.)

A, B, and C show the typical "twisted" nuclei with delicate, lacy chromatin and the bluish-gray cytoplasm containing many fine granules; A and C show the characteristic short pseudopodia; in B an inclusion, probably a nucleated red corpuscle, is present; D, lymphocyte; E, "young" monocyte—the nuclear chromatin is fine, there are two nucleoli, and only a few granules are present in the cytoplasm; F, a still less mature cell ("monoblast"?) with fine chromatin and 5 nucleoli in the nucleus and basophilic cytoplasm without granules; G, an abnormal cell of the "monocyte" series—the transparent character of the nucleus is particularly noteworthy. (*Wintrobe, Tice Practice of Medicine, courtesy of W. F. Prior Company.*)

illness varies considerably. Patients may develop the first signs of disease and die within one week, whereas in other cases the progress is much slower. It is true frequently that death occurs within six months in acute cases and not before one year in chronic cases. The term "subacute" is sometimes applied to those instances in which the duration of the disease is six to twelve months. Clinically, such cases resemble acute leukemia more than the chronic form, because such features as fever, hemorrhagic manifestations and pronounced immaturity of the leukocytes are generally present.

Aleukemic or Subleukemic Leukemia (Leukopenic Myelosis).—Few writers now restrict these terms to those cases of leukemia in which neither leukocytosis nor immature leukocytes are found in the blood ("aleukemic" in the strict sense). The terms are generally used to refer to those cases in which the leukocyte count is normal or subnormal. Almost always, persistent and repeated examinations of the blood will reveal a few immature cells ("subleukemic" leukemia).

The clinical features of leukemia without leukocytosis are similar to those of cases with leukocytosis. Acute and chronic forms are encountered and myelogenous, lymphogenous and monocytic types have been described. Leukopenia is often a manifestation of leukemia (p. 934), especially in children. In adults, lymphogenous cases are much less common than myelogenous. As mentioned earlier (p. 928), in adults especially, the clinical picture may for many months be that of refractory anemia, usually with neutropenia and thrombocytopenia and the bone marrow may appear hypoplastic, or there may be hyperplasia of erythroid elements with hypoplasia or only moderate hyperplasia of the granulocytic series.

Chloroma. — Chloroma (chloroleukemia) refers to a condition characterized by the occurrence of localized tumors in relation particularly to the periosteum and ligamentous structures of the skull, paranasal sinuses, orbits, spine, ribs and sacrum. As distinguished from myeloma, periosteal changes are found in addition to changes in the bone medulla. The growths may cause protrusion of the the eyeball, with diplopia and loss of vision, pain, deafness, and other cranial nerve palsies, as well as other phenomena caused by pressure or infiltrative growth. The general clinical manifestations are similar to those found in acute leukemia. Skin tumors have been observed[53] and even green tumors of the ovary have been described.[87b] The course of the illness is similar to that of acute leukemia and the blood changes are indistinguishable. As in leukemia, there may be no leukocytosis. The condition is seen most often in children and young adults.

The abnormal cells in the blood and tissues were considered by early observers to be lymphatic in origin.[53] Subsequent studies showed the cells in most cases to be myeloblasts.[20] In a few, myelocytes have been observed.[59] It is doubtful whether lymphocytic leukemia ever takes the form of chloroma.[119] Cases of monocytic chloroma, probably of the "Naegeli type" and thus of myelogenous origin, have been described.[81,186b]

The green coloration of the tumors, which may be evident even on superficial examination, fades on exposure to light and air, but can be restored temporarily by treatment with hydrogen peroxide. It is said that it can be preserved by placing the tumor in glycerin. The green color, at least in experimental chloroma in the rat, appears to be due principally to myeloperoxidase.[189e] Under ultraviolet light the tumor fluoresces red as the result of the presence of protoporphyrin, coproporphyrin and at least 11 other chromatographic entities.[6a,189e]

Chronic Monocytic Leukemia. — The clinical and hematological features of monocytic leukemia have been described already (p. 935). The course of monocytic leukemia is more likely to be erratic,[194f] however, than that of myeloid or lymphoid leukemia. Although the great majority of cases run an acute course, or at least take the subacute form, a few have been described which were as long as four to six years in duration.[167,218] Not everyone would agree, however, with the statement[167] that 11 per cent of cases of monocytic leukemia are chronic. Cutaneous manifestations, bone pains and relatively low or subnormal leukocyte counts have been a feature of some of the chronic cases.

The literature on monocytic leukemia reveals the difficulty in the exact classification of some cases.[45] The terms **reticulo-endotheliosis** and **reticulosis** have been used as synonymous with monocytic leukemia but other writers distinguish "leukemic" and "aleukemic reticulo-endotheliosis"[17b] from non-leukemic reticulo-endotheliosis.[160a] Downey[45] used the term *leukemic reticulo-endotheliosis* in referring to a leukemia with a primary, irreversible hyperplasia of the reticuloendothelium. In his view the great majority of "leukemic reticulo-endothelioses" show an involvement of the reticulum in which the free cells are differentiating toward some type of blood cell other than the monocyte. The majority of the monocytic leukemias which have been reported in the literature probably represent a variety of myelogenous leukemia ("Naegeli type") in which there is no disturbance in the reticulum. Only a few cases of monocytic leukemia show an involvement of the reticulum (the Schilling type). Downey pointed out that the presence of histiocytes in the blood does not necessarily indicate a monocytic leukemia. Thus, in subacute bacterial endocarditis there is an involvement of the reticulum and many undifferentiated reticular cells may

be found in the blood (p. 262), yet this does not constitute monocytic leukemia.

The term reticuloendotheliosis should probably not be employed since it is so general that, even with qualifying descriptive adjectives it does not offer a clear identification of a clinical syndrome.[125b] The same may be said of the term reticulosis.[103] As various disorders become characterized more precisely, it becomes possible to remove them from such an all-inclusive classification. Letterer-Siwe disease, which was at one time considered under this general heading, is now regarded as belonging with eosinophilic granuloma of bone and Schüller-Christian disease (p. 778).

Eosinophilic (Eosinophilocytic) Leukemia.—A number of cases have been reported in which there was marked, unexplained leukocytosis with striking eosinophilia.[10a,18] These can be classified in several categories. First of all, there are cases which in other respects fit the clinical picture of chronic myelocytic or acute myeloblastic leukemia, differing only in that large numbers of eosinophilic leukocytes are present. The eosinophilia may fluctuate in degree and may not persist. Eosinophilia is commonly seen in chronic myelocytic leukemia and some cases seem only to represent an exaggeration of the usual finding. In certain other cases which ran a more acute course, with a duration of a few days to 14 months, enlargement of the spleen, liver and lymph glands was not always present but there was anemia and thrombocytopenia and the leukocyte counts ranged from normal to 265,000 per c.mm. Death occurred in all the cases and the findings resembled those of leukemia except for infiltration by eosinophilic cells instead of other forms. In several cases the terminal morphological picture was that of acute myeloblastic leukemia[3a] but in the majority the relatively acute course was in sharp contrast to the consistent maturity of the eosinophils in the peripheral circulation. Although but 0.5 to 9.0 per cent of the cells in the blood in these cases were myeloblasts, in a number an increased proportion of myeloblasts was found in the bone marrow. It seems justified to consider these as cases of *acute* leukemia, of an *eosinophilic type*.

In a third category are cases of longer duration in which enlargement of the spleen, liver and lymph nodes have been observed more consistently.[29a] However, their clinical features and course have often been atypical for leukemia and have included a variety of visceral manifestations, edema, focal necroses, or arterial complications, or sometimes few clinical manifestations were present. The leukocyte counts have been as high as 236,000 per c.mm., of which as many as 91 per cent were eosinophils, chiefly adult forms. In many cases normoblasts have been observed in the circulating blood, as well as moderate anemia. When the terminal phase developed, cardiac insufficiency, massive pulmonary infiltration, or neurologic manifestations dominated the clinical picture. In one of our patients, myocardial fibrosis and adhesive pericarditis led to cardiac failure and death. In such cases, marked eosinophilic infiltration of the spleen, bone marrow, liver and lungs has been found at autopsy. These should probably be considered to be leukemoid rather than as examples of true leukemia. The name "*disseminated eosinophilic collagenosis*" has been applied to cases of this variety.[18]

Only examples of true leukemia should be treated by means of the chemotherapeutic or radioactive agents employed in the management of leukemia. ACTH, adrenocorticosteroids and other measures have been recommended for the remainder.

Basophilic and Mast Cell Leukemia.—*Basophilic leukemia*[175c] refers to a disorder in which the clinical picture resembles that of leukemia, chronic or acute, with the exception that basophilic leukocytes predominate. In one case as many as 96 per cent of the cells were basophilic. Among the 40 cases listed by Quattrin, values of 20 to 40 per cent were found most frequently. Ten cases were classified as acute, their course being at best four to six weeks in duration. In these cases hemorrhagic manifestations were prominent. The classification of some cases of leukemia as basophilic is rather arbitrary, however, since an increase in the number of basophilic leukocytes is characteristic of chronic myelocytic leukemia. The significance of the acute cases is more obscure. It has been pointed out that to distinguish some cases from leukemoid reactions, especially those associated with tuberculosis, is difficult.[91b]

Differing from these are cases described under the title of *mast cell leukemia*.[47a, 62a] In these the predominating cells differed from basophilic leukocytes in that they were larger, the granules were smaller and more numerous, and the nucleus was round, oval, indented, kidney-shaped or elongated and occupied from one-third to one-half of the cell's area. It is uncertain whether these cases differ fundamentally from urticaria pigmentosa, a skin disorder marked by a maculopapular skin eruption, hepatosplenomegaly and accumulations of tissue mast cells in many organs. However, the course of urticaria pigmentosa is chronic whereas that of some of the cases of mast cell leukemia was acute.

Neutrophilic Leukemia (Leukemia of Mature Cell Type, Splenomegaly with Hyperleukocytosis).— Very rare are cases resembling chronic myelocytic leukemia except for the presence in the blood of polymorphonuclear neutrophils almost to the exclusion of less mature forms.[207] As rare, and even more unusual, are cases marked by a similar blood picture but characterized by an acute course, absence of splenomegaly and the presence of severe hemorrhagic manifestations.[46b]

Megakaryocytic Leukemia. — Under this title a number of cases have been reported which have in common megakaryocyte hyperplasia, but which are not necessarily related. In chronic myelocytic leukemia, megakaryocytic elements of the bone marrow may at times be more involved than leukocytes,[153] and in the circulating blood megakaryocytes or fragments thereof may be found in relatively large numbers (5 per cent).[153] A similar hyperplasia of megakaryocytes may occur in erythremia (p. 799). The significance of thrombocythemia or piastrinemia, the flooding of the blood stream with megakaryocytes and their derivatives, was discussed earlier (p. 285).

The case of v. Boros and Korényi,[17] which was designated by them as **"acute megakaryoblastic leukemia"** had all the features of acute myeloblastic leukemia and their case is not regarded by others as representing a new entity.[46,59] Other reported cases[6,84h,142] resembled myeloid leukemia in many respects and may well have represented an exaggeration of the megakaryocyte hyperplasia which may be seen in that condition.

Cases described under such titles as "aleukemic megakaryocytic myelosis," "myeloid megakaryocytic hepato-splenomegaly"[46] and "chronic non-leukemic myelosis" are not instances of leukemia at all but fall better under the head of myelophthisic anemias (see p. 587).

Plasma Cell Leukemia. — A small number of cases have been described[21b,163b] in which plasma cells were repeatedly found in the blood and there was moderate leukocytosis as well as anemia and signs and symptoms suggestive of leukemia. Leukocyte counts have ranged from normal to about 90,000 per c.mm. and of these from 2 to 93 per cent have been plasma cells. Multiple myelomata were present in several of these cases and extraosseous plasmacytomas in a few but in most instances no discrete tumor nodules in bone were observed in roentgenograms or grossly at autopsy.[163b] In contrast to multiple myeloma, the sexes have been affected equally. The patients have ranged in age from 1.5 to 78 years but the majority have been between the ages of 45 and 60. The clinical manifestations have been similar to those of multiple myeloma and, as in that disease, hyperglobulinemia has been found in many cases. At autopsy infiltration with plasma cells has been demonstrated in the spleen, liver, bone marrow and lymph nodes. In general, duration of life after recognition of the disorder has been shorter (average, 8 months) than in multiple myeloma (two years), but that there is a true difference between these conditions may be questioned (see p. 1069).

Leukosarcoma (Sarco-leukemia). Lymphosarcoma Cell Leukemia. — The term "leukosarcoma" was applied by Sternberg[200] to those cases of lymphosarcoma in which there was a leukemic blood picture. He considered the mononuclear cells found in the blood to be leukosarcoma cells. Others have considered them to be lymphocytes, but Isaacs reaffirmed Sternberg's view and described the lymphosarcoma cell as found in the circulating blood:[100] the cell is 7.5 by 9 μ to 12 by 13.5 μ in size, the nucleus is oval or oblong, kidney-shaped or notched, and is composed of coarsely reticular, spongy chromatin. There is a large, and very prominent nucleolus which is much more prominent than is seen in lymphoblasts. The cytoplasm is sparse and deeply basophilic (Fig. 19–25).

Leukocyte counts as high as 156,000 per c.mm. have been recorded in these patients but lower values are more common. The "lymphosarcoma" cells may form 4 to 30 per cent of the cells in the earlier period of the disease when the leukocyte count is normal, but they may make up as many as 98 per cent in the

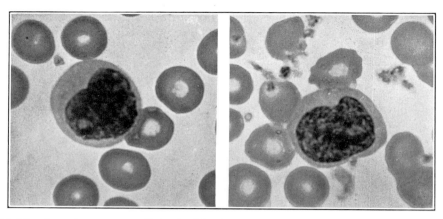

F<small>IG</small>. 19–25.—Lymphosarcoma cells in the blood. Note the very prominent nucleolus in the cell on the left. Wright's stain, × 660.

later leukocytic phase. In the latter period, anemia develops and the blood platelets, at first normal or increased in number, may be decreased.

Symptoms are produced by glandular enlargement and infiltration of surrounding tissues. In more than half the cases the primary seat has been the anterior mediastinum.[15a] Many other primary sites have been described in individual cases: the skin, eyes or eyelids, retroperitoneal and abdominal lymph nodes, pleura, breast, dura, intestines, and other tissues.[59] The clinical manifestations may be as varied as those seen in leukemia. The spleen has been found palpable in a number of cases. The duration of the disease is variable, from several months to several years. In one series of 43 cases of lymphosarcoma, leukocytosis developed at some time in the course of the disease in 15 cases.[100] The leukemic phase was of relatively short duration, two to sixty days. Passage of large numbers of tumor cells into the circulation tended to occur when there was extensive growth of these cells in moving organs, such as the lungs.

Cases of this type are not very rare. By 1948 more than 150 had been reported.[83c]

As discussed elsewhere (p. 1009), there are reasons to doubt that there is a fundamental difference between lymphocytic leukemia and lymphosarcoma.

Acute and Chronic Erythremic Myelosis and Erythroleukemia. — In 1923 di Guglielmo applied the term *acute erythremic myelosis* to a disorder characterized by a generalized proliferation of the erythropoietic cells of the bone marrow, analagous to the leukocytic proliferation in leukemia.[44] He suggested that this is a primary and specific disease, an autonomous pathologic entity. The condition is exceedingly rare and is characterized by severe, rapidly developing anemia, irregular, usually remittent fever, marked splenomegaly, enlargement of the liver, and an acute, ultimately fatal course associated with hemorrhagic manifestations. The blood contains numerous erythroblasts in all stages of maturation but the most immature forms are found in disproportionately large numbers. Atypical forms and erythroblasts with multilobed nuclei and with altered nucleo-cytoplasmic ratios are also found. Reticulocytes are not usually increased in number. There is slight leukopenia and occasional myelocytes and metamyelocytes, as well as reticulo-endothelial cells may be found in the blood smear. Platelets are decreased in number, often greatly. In contrast to the reduced proportion of erythropoietic elements which is characteristic of leukemia, these form the major part of the bone marrow cells, and basophilic forms predominate. At autopsy infiltrations of primitive erythroblasts and reticulo-endothelial cells are found not only in the hemopoietic organs but also in the kidneys, adrenals and other tissues. So fulminating is the course and so rare the cases[139b] that there has been little opportunity to study the pathogenetic mechanisms involved.

Subsequently di Guglielmo called attention to a similar but more chronic disorder, *chronic erythremic myelosis*, also marked by the presence in the blood of numerous erythroblasts but these were mainly the more mature forms. As in the acute disorder, there is irregular fever, anemia, splenomegaly and hepatomegaly but these are less striking. Hemorrhagic manifestations are less prominent. There may not be leukopenia and there is only moderate thrombocytopenia but reticulocytes are usually increased, sometimes strikingly. In the bone marrow there is erythroid hyperplasia but there is less preponderance of early forms than is seen in the acute disorder. The tissues give evidence of extramedullary hematopoiesis.

Prior to the description of these disorders, the distinguished Italian hematologist had called attention to a condition characterized by neoplastic hyperplasia of both erythroblastic and leukoblastic tissues which he named *erythroleukemia*. This too is marked by an acute course, severe anemia, moderate spleno- and hepatomegaly and numerous atypical erythroblasts in the blood but many myeloblasts containing Auer bodies, together with thrombocytopenia and prominent hemorrhagic manifestations are present as well. In the marrow there

are even larger numbers of erythroblasts than in the blood, as well as myeloblasts. The organs show infiltrations with erythropoietic cells as well as primitive myeloid cells.

In the course of time it has come to be recognized[156,190b] that, whereas cases completely fitting the descriptions of di Guglielmo are exceedingly rare, it is not so unusual to find examples of leukemia, especially of acute leukemia and of more slowly developing "aleukemic" leukemia, in which erythroid hyperplasia is pronounced and may sometimes even overshadow the myeloid proliferation. Furthermore, erythroblasts of unusual appearance may be seen, mitotic figures are numerous and even many cells suggesting megaloblasts may be found. In many instances, when there has been an opportunity to study such cases over a period of time, the erythroid hyperplasia has been seen to disappear and be replaced by the typical picture of leukemia. It is not unusual now, therefore, to speak of the *di Guglielmo syndrome* in referring to the variety of cases of leukemia in which erythroid hyperplasia is striking.

It is assumed, then, that the disorders described by di Guglielmo represent forms of leukemia. Noteworthy is the fact that a condition similar to acute erythremic myelosis has been observed in several persons chronically intoxicated with benzene.[44a] It is obviously important to distinguish erythremic myelosis from acute hemolytic anemia with marked erythroblastemia. A study of the anemia of the di Guglielmo syndrome showed somewhat shortened red cell survival time, together with some evidence of an intrinsic red cell defect, substantially increased hemolytic index, ineffective erythropoiesis as measured by erythrokinetic studies as well as low red cell iron utilization.[3d] Thus the findings differed from those of true hemolytic anemia. A high serum vitamin B$_{12}$ was found in several cases. The significance of these findings will be considered shortly (p. 946). It has been reported that the erythroblasts of patients with the di Guglielmo syndrome show strongly periodic acid-Schiff (PAS) granules in their cytoplasm[3d] and that this finding is of value in differential diagnosis.[175b] Studies with tritiated thymidine and DL-leucine indicated that there is a disturbance in both DNA and protein metabolism in the erythrocytes in erythremic myelosis.[71b]

Mixed Leukemia.—In any alleged case of mixed leukemia, one is always confronted with the possibility that there has been an error in interpretation. Thus, the presence of granular and non-granular leukocytes in large numbers in the blood at the same time, or in periods succeeding one another, might be taken as indicative of a combination of myelocytic and lymphocytic leukemia. More critical examination may reveal the non-granular cells to be myeloblasts. This is probably the explanation for most of the reported cases of "mixed" leukemia.[34,137] Nevertheless, it must be noted that a few instances of mixed leukemia were recorded many years ago by experienced hematologists.[85,89]

Pseudoleukemia.—This term was introduced by Cohnheim to refer to cases like those described by Virchow (leukemia) but in which no increase in the proportion of white to red corpuscles was observed. Later the name was applied to a variety of conditions in which no leukemic changes are found in the blood, such as lymphosarcoma, Hodgkin's disease and glandular enlargements due to infections, as well as to aleukemic leukemia. Few writers now use the term.

Leukanemia.—Leukanemia is a term which was applied by von Leube to a rapid and progressive disorder which was characterized by changes in the blood similar to those of pernicious anemia together with those of myelocytic leu-

kemia.[89] It was suggested that such a disorder could be produced by a maturation defect in the precursor of the cells of the erythroid and myeloid series.[60b] The number of cases reported is very small, perhaps 10 in all. It is noteworthy that bone marrow composed chiefly of myeloblasts and megaloblasts may be observed in the course of treatment of acute leukemia with anti-folic compounds (p. 978).

ADDITIONAL LABORATORY FINDINGS

Bone Marrow.—Hyperplasia is the characteristic feature of the bone marrow in leukemia. This is usually diffuse and may be widespread throughout the marrow spaces of the body; however, it may not involve all the marrow space, and it may be nodular in arrangement rather than evenly distributed. The duration and nature of the leukemic process probably are governing factors.

In *myelogenous leukemia* the marrow is gray, red or greenish in appearance. In *chronic* myelocytic leukemia the differential count of the material obtained by sternal puncture is remarkably similar to that of the blood. The cells may be at a slightly less mature level than in the circulating blood. The proportion of nucleated red cell elements is relatively reduced. Some observers have described an increase in the number of megakaryocytes but this is not a constant finding.[131c] In *acute* myeloblastic leukemia, the marrow is usually crowded with myeloblasts, and still more primitive types may be found. Megakaryocytes are reduced in number. In eosinophilic leukemia, a preponderance of eosinophils may not be present. In chloroma, tumor formation is the distinguishing characteristic.

In *lymphocytic leukemia* no striking abnormality in the marrow may be discovered. More often, however, there is well-marked lymphocytosis (30 to 90 per cent). A case has been described in which the marrow was crowded with lymphocytes even when there was no clinically demonstrable adenopathy or splenomegaly.[201] The finding of 50 per cent or more lymphocytes in a cellular marrow is strongly suggestive of lymphoid leukemia. In aplastic anemia there may be lymphocytosis but this is only relative and due to the absence of other cells. Lymphocytosis is not found in Hodgkin's disease and is rare in lymphosarcoma. There may be lymphocytosis in the marrow in infectious mononucleosis[102] but other features make it easy to distinguish this disease (see p. 1117).

In *monocytic leukemia* myelocytes and immature forms resembling myeloblasts may be found. In rare cases "monoblasts" and histioid monocytes (p. 936) have been reported.

There is no object in performing sternal puncture in leukemia unless the diagnosis is in question. However, for the recognition of leukemia in the absence of leukocytosis ("*aleukemic leukemia*") and the differentiation of this disease from agranulocytosis, purpura hemorrhagica and aplastic anemia, marrow examination during life achieves its greatest usefulness. Frequently the bone marrow findings in aleukemic leukemia are identical with those seen when the blood picture is clearly leukemic, and the diagnosis can be made with assurance. If the marrow picture is not frankly leukemic in such a case, however, the possibility of leukemia need not necessarily be dismissed. Sternal puncture is sometimes misleading, for few cells may be obtained.[224] This can be accounted for in some instances by a patchy distribution of cells; in such cases a second puncture may be more successful or trephining, with the removal of a large volume of marrow, may be necessary. In some cases of aleukemic leukemia, pronounced immaturity of the leukocytes has been observed even when the cellularity seemed to be reduced. In still other cases, presumably in a "preleukemic" phase (p. 950), the diagnosis cannot be made with certainty even when the bone marrow is studied. In leukopenic cases of lymphocytic leukemia, marrow lymphocytosis may be slight or absent.

The **factors which govern the release of leukocytes** into the circulating blood from the marrow are obscure and no adequate explanation has been offered for the differences in the blood picture of "aleukemic" and "leukemic" cases of leukemia. It has been stated that leukemic cells for the most part come from extramedullary foci and that the size of the latter determines the number of cells in the circulating blood.[157] Other possibilities include rapid destruction of leukocytes in the circulating blood, unusually quick passage of the cells into the tissues, or their discharge into the saliva, gastro-intestinal secretions or urine.[59]

The **mechanism of anemia** in leukemia is obscure. In acute leukemia blood loss is often a factor but this does not account for the anemia which may be encountered before there has been obvious bleeding. In chronic leukemia hemorrhage is rarely significant as a cause of anemia. Complicating infection with associated inhibition of erythropoiesis (p. 576) is rarely a factor early in the course of leukemia. That a mechanism which is intimately related to the fundamental leukemic process is involved, is suggested by cases in which severe anemia antedates the usual manifestations of leukemia by a long time (p. 950).

For many years it was assumed that crowding out of erythropoietic tissue by the leukemic cells is the cause of the anemia. This view is supported by the common observation that anemia diminishes as leukocytosis is reduced by irradiation or other means, as well as by histopathologic studies.[217a] Jaffe challenged this hypothesis because he found erythro-poiesis to be as great in many cases of myelogenous leukemia as leukopoiesis.[109] He concluded that the anemia is caused by excessive destruction of red cells and cited as evidence the hemosiderosis which may be found in leukemic tissues. From time to time various other investigators reported increased products of red cell destruction in the urine and stools and drew attention to the reticulocytosis which is sometimes observed. The latter, however, does not necessarily indicate increased blood destruction; for example, evidence has been presented that reticulocytes may be released pre-maturely from the marrow in acute leukemia.[162a] Neither does increased fecal urobilinogen output necessarily signify seriously increased destruction of circulating red cells. Heme pigment diversion or increased destruction of precursor red cells are other possible explanations, as discussed elsewhere (p. 483). These were thought to be the possible mechanisms involved in the pathogenesis of the anemia of the di Guglielmo syndrome, discussed earlier (p. 941).

Modern techniques for the study of erythrokinetics have yielded data which suggest that the development of anemia in the leukemic patient is a consequence of varying combinations of (1) decreased erythropoiesis with normal or increased red cell destruction or loss, or (2) normal or increased erythropoiesis with increased red cell destruction or loss. There is evidence that marrow reactivity in leu-kemic patients is, from an early stage of the disease, considerably impaired.[219f] This may not become apparent when red cell survival is normal but is readily brought out when even a mild hemolytic process is operating.

In acute leukemia, destruction of red cells was found to be increased in many instances,[206b] though not always.[162b] In cases of chronic myelocytic leukemia, red cell survival was normal as a rule, although not in every case. In general, no correlation has been observed between the type of leukemia or the degree of reduction in red cell life-span. In some cases evidence has been obtained of intrinsic abnormalities in the red cells, as indicated by unusual degrees of aniso-cytosis and poikilocytosis, together with increased osmotic resistance of the eryth-rocytes.[208a] More often, however, such signs are lacking. In other cases, the same workers observed increased auto-hemolysis which could be inhibited by the addition of glucose. Others have found evidence that plasma factors may be related to lysis of both autogenous and normal red cells.[39b] It appears, then, that multiple mechanisms may play a role in the pathogenesis of the anemia associated with leukemia.

With rare exceptions, only in chronic lymphocytic leukemia is a frank hemo-lytic anemia of the autoimmune type associated with a positive direct red cell antiglobulin (Coombs') test, encounter-ed.[63c] This type of anemia differs in degree and perhaps in nature from that commonly associated with chronic lym-phocytic leukemia. The latter usually occurs late in the course of the leukemia whereas the autoimmune anemia may occur at any time during the illness. The antibodies associated with the auto-immune hemolytic process are usually of the "warm" variety.[208a] It was ob-served in one case that the erythrocyte-coating protein was derived from a source endogenous to the patient.[174c] A hemolysin and agglutinin active against normal and trypsinized erythrocytes could be extracted from leukemic leukocytes but this differed from that coating the erythrocytes and the relation of these substances to the development of hemo-lytic anemia is uncertain.[174b]

There is little understanding of the reasons for the failure of leukemic mar-row to provide adequate erythropoiesis.

60

Metabolic competition between developing red cells and pathologic white cells has been suggested[10c] but the nature of the abnormality, if one exists, is obscure. It is of interest that, many years ago in biological assays in anemic dogs, the liver in leukemia was found to possess quantities of factors necessary for hemoglobin production which were at the lower limit of normal.[221] It is difficult to see what connection there may be between the anemia of leukemia and the high levels of vitamin B_{12} present in the serum of patients with chronic myelocytic leukemia (p. 933).

Hemorrhage in cases of acute leukemia is usually associated with thrombocytopenia but there is no good correlation between the deficiency of platelets, or even the levels of various plasma coagulation factors (p. 943) and clinical evidences of a bleeding tendency. Other contributing factors have therefore been sought. One of these is fever and this has been observed to be associated with elevations of protein-bound serum polysaccharide.[60c]

It is rare to observe bleeding in the absence of thrombocytopenia, however. In myelocytic leukemia such hemorrhage has been attributed to perivascular infiltration of the vessel walls by leukemic cells with consequent injury and increased permeability.

Basal Metabolic Rate.—The basal metabolic rate is increased in the great majority of cases of chronic myelocytic leukemia[183] and in acute leukemia.[132] In lymphocytic leukemia the metabolic rate was found to be increased when the disease had progressed far enough to produce more than local symptoms.[127] An increased rate has also been observed in aleukemic leukemia[92a] but, according to our own observations, it is not elevated in all cases.

The increased rate was found to be roughly proportional to the severity of the leukemic process,[183] there being a rough direct correlation between basal metabolic rate and the height of the leukocyte count, the degree of immaturity of the leukocytes and the pulse rate. This correlation is not exact,[1b] however, and there is no evidence that hyperplasia of hemopoietic tissue is the cause of the hypermetabolism; it seems more likely to be attributable to increased protein catabolism.[4] Irradiation was found to be associated with a transitory rise in metabolic rate which lasted about three days,[183] but successful therapy is accompanied by return to a normal rate. Patients in the terminal stage of leukemia continue to have an elevated oxygen consumption despite treatment.

Loss of weight may occur in leukemia and increase in pulse rate is usual,[62] but nervousness, irritability, insomnia and tremor, of a degree at all comparable to such symptoms as seen in exophthalmic goiter, are not generally found. Another point of difference between leukemia and exophthalmic goiter is the extravagance in muscular activity in the latter.[21] It is significant that patients with leukemia may be able to work and maintain their weight fairly well, in spite of an increased basal metabolic rate.

The **blood iodine** was abnormally low in 9 out of 12 cases of myelocytic leukemia and normal in the remainder. In lymphocytic leukemia, on the other hand, normal values were found in 10, high values in 7. In the same study high values were found in 14 out of 20 cases of hyperthyroidism.[209] The uptake of radioactive iodine by the thyroid gland is normal in leukemia.[1b]

Evidences of Metabolic Abnormalities.—The cellular hyperplasia of leukemia is reflected in certain chemical findings. The *uric acid* of the blood and the uric acid excretion are increased. However, the amount of uric acid excreted in the urine is not the same in all types of leukemia: it was found to be markedly increased in cases of acute lymphoblastic leukemia and moderately increased in acute myeloblastic and chronic myelocytic leukemia.[188b] In chronic lymphocytic leukemia the excretion was normal. It is noteworthy that, although there was good correlation between the magnitude of the leukocyte count and the quantity of uric acid excreted in cases of acute lymphoblastic leukemia, increased excretion was also observed in "aleukemic" cases. Uric acid elimination may be further increased temporarily when the leukocyte count is reduced by therapy, returning toward normal when the count approaches normal. Measurements of the uric acid miscible body pool have been found to be related to serum uric acid concentrations.[194] As yet, however, quantitative relationships between uric acid excretion, growth and destruction of leukemic cells remain to be defined.[92b]

Other evidences of altered purine and pyrimidine metabolism in leukemia are found in increased excretion of adenine, hypoxanthine and xanthine and the excretion of 5-ribosyl-uracil.[1a] Increased activities of certain enzymes involved in pyridine metabolism have been described.[195a]

As would be expected, the *nitrogen* balance is variable in chronic leukemia and is usually negative in acute leukemia.[132] It is an old observation that in patients with leukemia the retention of *phosphorus* and *potassium* is greater in relation to nitrogen than that seen in protein-depleted individuals with chronic non-neoplastic diseases.[56] Effective therapy is accompanied by excretion of excessive quantities of phosphorus in relation to the amount of nitrogen excreted. The blood phosphorus is high in leukemia as the result of the high phosphorus content of the leukocytes.[203] This is due to an increase in organic phosphorus. No variations in inorganic phosphorus are found.[174a]

The *serum proteins*[13e] in untreated *acute leukemia*, in the absence of fever, infection or liver disease were found to show increased levels of gamma globulins in the myeloblastic type but not in lymphoblastic leukemia.[53a] Activity of the disease process in the latter was reflected by alpha-2 globulin elevation.[78] In both types, serum albumin was significantly lowered and the beta globulin component remained essentially normal.[53a] Fever, in the absence of infection, was associated with elevation of the alpha-1 globulin component. Marked depression of the gamma globulins was unusual.

In *chronic lymphocytic leukemia* hypogammaglobulinemia has been found in 33 to 68 per cent of cases.[94,209b] This tends to occur late in the course of the disease and may be associated with an increased tendency to infectious complications, especially in the rare cases of agammaglobinemia. Very occasionally, cryoglobulinemia with marked cold sensitivity may be observed.[74b,191]

An increase in the glutamic acid, phenylalanine and "leucine" levels has been found in the blood of patients with acute leukemia and high levels of glutamic acid, phenylalanine, alanine and proline were demonstrated in chronic myelocytic and in chronic lymphocytic leukemia.[213b]

Blood *cholesterol* may be normal or reduced.[160] The total lipids and the fatty acids of the whole blood, serum and plasma have been found to be greatly elevated.[174a] The *glutathione* content of the blood is also elevated.[228] The ascorbic acid concentration is low.[213c] Abnormally elevated plasma lactic dehydrogenase (LD) and phosphohexose isomerase concentrations have been reported in acute and chronic myelocytic leukemia but they were not raised in chronic lymphocytic leukemia.[12b,138a] Plasma LD also was increased in acute lymphoblastic leukemia. Both enzymes were normal in aleukemic leukemia. The cozymase content of the blood was reported to be decreased in leukemia.[212]

Variations in the content of alkaline phosphatase in leukemic leukocytes and certain metabolic and enzymatic differences between normal and leukemic cells were discussed in an earlier chapter (p. 235). The serum alkaline phosphatase bears no discernible relationship to the leukocyte alkaline phosphatase content.

Urine.—The urine may contain traces of albumin and occasional hyaline and granular casts. In acute leukemia it is not unusual to find red cells as well, and in rare instances the diagnosis of acute nephritis may be suggested by the findings.[139] Hematuria may also occur in chronic leukemia. In a few cases Bence-Jones proteinuria has been observed.[14] Terminally the urinary findings may be those of chronic renal congestion.

Gastric Contents. — Achlorhydria has been found more frequently in lymphocytic leukemia than in the myelocytic form[42] and in the former condition its incidence is possibly greater than might be expected in persons of the age of those examined.[148]

Cerebrospinal Fluid. — Leukocytes may be found in the spinal fluid even in the absence of symptoms attributable to involvement of the central nervous system[196] and the pressure and protein content may be increased.[190]

Total Volume of Blood.—The total volume of blood was found to be increased above normal in earlier studies using Congo red dye, this being attributed to increased plasma volume.[59] These findings have been confirmed in studies with P^{32}-labelled red cells.[10b,10d] In chronic myelocytic leukemia with splenomegaly in particular, the plasma volume may be increased above normal, giving a false impression concerning the degree of anemia.

DIAGNOSIS

In the majority of cases the recognition of leukemia, particularly the chronic form, is easy. The combination of glandular enlargement, splenomegaly, striking leukocytosis and anemia is a familiar picture. In such cases, however, before the blood has been examined, diseases other than leukemia may come to mind.

Tuberculous glands differ from those in leukemia in that they tend to soften and become adherent to the skin. Hodgkin's disease usually commences in one group of glands, frequently the posterior cervical, and generalization occurs only late in the disease. The masses are larger than is common in leukemia and cause pressure symptoms more frequently. There may be recurring attacks of fever, weakness and pain. Lymphosarcoma commences in a localized area, invades the surrounding tissue spaces, forms large masses and spreads by metastasis. The glands are not distinct and the liver and spleen are not as often greatly enlarged.

Splenomegaly may suggest Hodgkin's disease, the Banti syndrome, hemolytic anemia, thalassemia, malaria, kala-azar, schistosomiasis, or trypanosomiasis. Infarction of the spleen with perisplenitis may suggest a surgical condition of the abdomen, or the finding of an abdominal mass as well as some red cells in the urine may bring renal tumor to mind. In all these cases blood examination will usually make the diagnosis evident.

The first symptoms of leukemia may direct attention[224] to the nervous system, the gastro-intestinal tract, the bones and joints, the skin or even the heart or lungs, and adenopathy or splenomegaly may be inconspicuous or absent. On the other hand, acute leukemia and even the chronic disease when there is fever, may suggest some acute inflammatory condition: endocarditis, amebiasis, tuberculosis, fulminating sepsis, quinsy, Vincent's angina, noma, diphtheria, agranulocytosis, or infectious mononucleosis. Hemorrhagic manifestations may simulate purpura hemorrhagica, aplastic anemia, or scurvy.

As regards the blood, it should be kept in mind that the immaturity of the leukocytes is of greater significance than the leukocyte count itself. With the exception of the very rare cases of leukemia in which mature cells have predominated (p. 939), and acknowledging cases of chronic lymphocytic leukemia of which the monotonous collection of small lymphoclears is so characteristic, it is the presence of immature forms of white corpuscles in numbers not seen in normal blood which suggests the disease leukemia. The "gay" collection of cells of all types, myelocytes and myeloblasts, basophils and eosinophils, as well as neutrophilic metamyelocytes and polymorphonuclears, which is so characteristic of chronic myelocytic leukemia, is rarely seen even in cases with "leukemoid" blood pictures (Chapter 4). In acute leukemia the blood has the appearance of a culture of leukocytes of a single variety and of very immature type. It should be pointed out, however, that the inexperienced observer may mistake very immature cells, devoid of granules, for lymphocytes. Careful inspection reveals nucleoli.

Anemia is characteristic of leukemia, except in early cases of chronic leukemia which may be discovered accidentally.[223] Anemia is usually found when the patient is ill enough to seek attention. At the same time nucleated red cells, as well as polychromatophilia and other evidences of profound marrow disturbance can be discovered as a rule.

Thrombocytopenia, together with such confirmatory findings as prolonged bleeding time, poor clot retraction and positive tourniquet test, is an almost invariable accompaniment of acute leukemia although sometimes it is only slight in degree in the early stages. Moderate thrombocytopenia may be found in chronic lymphocytic leukemia but occurs in chronic myelocytic leukemia only in the terminal phase. In subacute cases moderate thrombocytopenia is usually found but the bleeding time and clot retraction may not be appreciably prolonged.[224]

These facts are useful in differentiating acute leukemia from disorders with which this disease may be confused. True infectious processes, even if accompanied by a leukemoid leukocytic picture, are unlikely to be associated with severe anemia or thrombocytopenia, nor are normoblasts found in the blood smear. This is also true of agranulocytosis and infectious mononucleosis. In the latter condition the lymphocytes are of a special type (p. 1112) and the titer of heterophil antibodies is increased instead of being less than normal. In purpura hemorrhagica there is no more anemia than can be accounted for by blood loss and few or no immature leukocytes are found. Acute infectious lymphocytosis (p. 260) may cause confusion. An acute exacerbation of chronic myelocytic leukemia may suggest true acute leukemia but in the former the spleen is very large and the blood smear reveals a relatively small number of myeloblasts (roughly less than 20 per cent). The differentiation of various types of acute leukemia has been discussed (p. 934).

It is when the leukocyte count is normal or leukopenic that real difficulty in diagnosis may be encountered. Usually in "aleukemic" leukemia (see p. 937), careful examination of blood smears will reveal a number of immature leukocytes, as well as nucleated red cells, polychromatophilia, and increased reticulocytes, and anemia will be found as well. It has been noted that anemia is often more severe in such cases than in typical cases of chronic leukemia,[5] and hemorrhagic phenomena with thrombocytopenia are more likely to occur.[224] In 2 of our cases the red cell count on admission was less than 1,000,000 per c.mm.

The anemia may be macrocytic and thus pernicious anemia may be suggested.

Aleukemic leukemia should be suspected whenever there is unexplained splenomegaly, lymphadenopathy, fever, purpura or retinal hemorrhages, tumefaction of the gums, atypical symptoms of "arthritis" and deep bone pains, bone tenderness, pathological fractures, osteomyelitis of unexplained cause (or reddish-gray, non-liquefied tissue at operation) bone tumors, or acute enlargement of the breasts or ovaries.[5]

In addition to examination of the blood, other studies may have to be made in obscure cases. Sternal marrow puncture or, if necessary, trephining may reveal a typically leukemic picture. Roentgenograms of the bones may reveal subperiosteal infiltration or osteolytic or tumor-like changes. The basal metabolic rate may be increased and the blood uric acid may be high. Biopsy of an enlarged lymph node will aid differentiation of Hodgkin's disease and other conditions which may be confused with lymphocytic leukemia. Multiple myeloma, metastatic tumors involving bone marrow or acute disseminated lupus erythrematosus, in addition to the conditions already mentioned, may have to be distinguished from "aleukemic" leukemia. In children, metastatic neuroblastoma may closely simulate acute leukemia. In myelosclerosis, splenomegaly may be so great and the immaturity of the cells seen in the peripheral blood may be so striking as to strongly suggest leukemia. Examination of the bone marrow, however, will fail to reveal a leukemic picture. The confusing clinical picture and the even more confusing names applied in other cases of pseudo-leukemic disorders (aleukemic megakaryocytic myelosis, myeloid megakaryocytic hepato-spleno-megaly, chronic non-leukemic myelosis, agnogenic myeloid metaplasia) have, been discussed elsewhere (p. 582).

As mentioned earlier (p. 927), in some cases of leukemia the clinical and hematologic picture recognized as typical of that disease is preceded by a period of varied duration in which a number of different disorders are simulated. During this time, which has been as long as twenty months in a number of cases[143] and almost nine years in one,[222a] the findings have been those of unexplained leukopenia, neutropenia, thrombocytopenia or anemia, or combinations thereof. Monocytosis, nucleated red cells in the blood and reticulocytosis have also been noted.[13a] The neutropenia in some cases was accompanied by recurring infections. The anemia has been hemolytic in some instances or, much more rarely, megaloblastic. Troublesome mucous membrane lesions have been noted. In most cases there was no accompanying lymphadenopathy or splenomegaly to arouse suspicion of leukemia and, in those in which microscopic examinations were made, no histologic lesions suggesting leukemia were observed, even in a spleen removed five weeks prior to the development of recognizable signs of leukemia.[143] Immature leukocytes have not, as a rule, been found in the blood. The bone marrow has been recorded as being aplastic,[224] hyperplastic or normal, and hyperplasia, when observed, has been characterized by "maturation arrest" of the myeloid series of leukocytes, or erythroid hyperplasia and, in several instances,[84f,222a] megaloblasts were found.

Whether or not it is correct to refer to this as the **"preleukemic" stage** of leukemia cannot be decided before the nature of leukemia is better understood, since another interpretation of these findings might be that they represent a hemopoietic disorder which, for unknown reasons, has *changed* to leukemia. In any event, the ultimate occurrence in the cases described has been the appearance, often with explosive suddenness, of clear signs of leukemia and usually a rapid demise. The leukemia has been variously described as being myeloblastic, myelogenous, monocytic or of the stem cell variety. It is of interest that in certain cases the full blown picture of leukemia appeared some time following the administration of ACTH or cortisone. This calls to mind the increase in the severity of the manifestations of leukemia which has been observed to follow in certain cases after treatment with these agents (p. 983). In most cases, however, nothing was recognized which could even have been suspected as a leukemogenic agent.

These observations indicate that the existence or ultimate development of leukemia must be suspected whenever one of a variety of hematologic disorders of obscure nature is encountered. These include cases which might be classified under such titles as "splenic neutropenia," "splenic panhematopenia," hypersplenism, "agnogenic myeloid metaplasia,"[143] leukemoid reaction, aplastic anemia, primary refractory anemia with hyperplastic marrow, acquired hemolytic anemia, refractory megaloblastic anemia and thrombocytopenic purpura. The majority of the patients described were adults, many being over fifty years of age,[13a] which is a time when idiopathic thrombocytopenic purpura is unusual.

DURATION, PROGNOSIS AND COMPLICATIONS

Chronic Leukemia.—In 1939 a survey based on the study of 259 reported cases of chronic myelocytic leukemia and 152 cases of the lymphocytic type indicated an average duration of life following the onset of symptoms of 3.28 years in the former and 3.29 in the latter.[223] In another study of cases, observed and treated in a single clinic between 1936 and 1953,[131] the median survival for 152 cases of chronic myelocytic leukemia was essentially the same, namely, 3.2 years, whereas in the lymphocytic form (129

cases) the median survival was 5.4 years. However, in a statistical analysis of 1090 patients with chronic myelocytic leukemia and 685 with chronic lymphocytic leukemia reported in the literature over the period 1925 to 1951 from various clinics, it was concluded that 50 per cent of patients with either type of leukemia survive less than 2.65 years after onset of the first clinical symptoms or 1.6 years after beginning of therapy.[206]

A significant feature which was apparent even in 1924[154,155] is the great variation in individual cases. It was noted that 12 to 14 per cent of the patients treated by the methods available at that time lived five to ten years. More recent statistical analysis has indicated that 22 per cent of patients with either form of chronic leukemia will survive longer than five years after first symptoms, 6 per cent will survive longer than ten years and about 0.8 per cent twenty years or more.[206] In another study, the median duration of survival after diagnosis was 11.65 months, with 16 per cent of the patients surviving longer than 43 months and 9 per cent for five years.[55b] In one clinic four patients with chronic myelocytic leukemia were reported who lived more than ten years, another five who lived longer than fifteen years following discovery of the disease and one survived nineteen years.[157a] Of cases of chronic lymphocytic leukemia, 54 per cent survived over five years and 31 per cent over seven years.[131] The longest recorded survival is twenty-nine years.[140a] In this form of leukemia, in particular, survival may be very long. In many instances, and perhaps always, there is a phase of long duration in which there are signs of the disease and no symptoms; very occasionally, a long period may ensue in the course of this phase when even signs are minimal or absent.[214] This phase may even be preceded by a long "silent" phase in which no leukemic changes are demonstrable in lymph nodes or spleen although lymphocytic infiltration of the portal tracts of the liver and extensive lymphocytic infiltration of the bone marrow are present.[93c] The classical picture of the disease, with gross splenomegaly, adenopathy, high leukocyte count and thrombocytopenia is only the terminal phase of a disease which may run a course lasting ten to 20 years.

In general, life can be expected to be longer in cases discovered accidentally before weight loss, anemia, marked splenomegaly or adenopathy have made the disease apparent. The existence of marked anemia or thrombocytopenia are unfavorable but not necessarily discouraging signs since, with therapy, anemia may disappear and the platelet count may return to normal from excessively high or abnormally low levels. Unfavorable signs are the presence of fever, an excessively high leukocyte count or large proportions of immature leukocytes. Some degree of spontaneous remission was observed in 7.7 per cent of cases of chronic myelocytic leukemia and in 5 per cent of cases of chronic lymphocytic leukemia.[154,155] In myelocytic leukemia the disease may terminate in a picture resembling acute myeloblastic leukemia. In lymphocytic leukemia, such a termination is exceedingly rare; gradually increasing anemia is the more likely terminal event. Such anemia is usually associated with a moderately shortened red cell life span (p. 945) but in about 18 per cent of cases an overt hemolytic anemia is observed. In both types of leukemia, severe thrombocytopenia and hemorrhagic manifestations may ensue or, in chronic lymphocytic leukemia especially, recurring infections may be the most troublesome feature.

Acute Leukemia.—The duration of life varies considerably and depends on a number of factors, many of which are obscure. Clinical observation suggests that there is great variation in the intensity of the leukemic process in different cases. The occurrence of severe bleeding, especially intracranial hemorrhage, or the development of a complicating infection may lead to sudden exitus or, entirely spontaneously or following blood transfusion or some infection (see below), a **remission** may occur which is accompanied by a decrease in the size of the enlarged organs, a fall in the leukocyte count, and disappearance of anemia and thrombocytopenia. Indeed, the remission may be so complete as to defy the diagnosis of leukemia at the time. Remissions of two to twenty-one months and even four years' duration[55a] have been recorded in adults as well as in children.[12,55a] In some instances even the bone marrow was found to be normal. In one out of 14 reported cases with remissions, two remissions were observed.[12] In a series of 172 cases of acute leukemia of various types and all ages, some degree of temporary remission was observed in 8.7 per cent of the cases and in 4 per cent the remission was "complete."[195b] No patient had more than one remission.

For the evaluation of therapeutic measures, accurate information concerning **survival** in untreated leukemia is needed. In a series of 113 cases reported in 1929,[215] 21 patients survived less than two weeks, 53 between two and four weeks and 19 one to two months. Practically all the patients died within six months. However, an analysis up to May 1954 of 143 reported cases, children and adults, treated only with transfusions and antibiotics, revealed a median (50 per cent) survival of 4.5 months with as many as 10 per cent of the cases surviving eleven months.[84a] The survival of 577 patients treated with agents now regarded as not particularly useful in the management of acute leukemia, such as irradiation, nitrogen mustard, urethane or busulfan was essentially the same. In view of the frequently repeated statement that patients with acute leukemia die within six months of the onset of their disease, the long survival (nine to twenty-three months[119]) of some patients receiving only supportive therapy is noteworthy. In the largest series of cases (172) of acute leukemia of all types occurring at all ages and treated in a single clinic with only transfusions and antibiotics or only the ineffective forms of therapy mentioned above, the mean survival time from the onset of symptoms was 4.7 months.[195b] Fifty per cent of the patients were dead by four months and 90 per cent by nine months but one lived fourteen months. Survival in association with modern therapy will be discussed later (p. 985).

Death may result from intercurrent infection or from cerebral hemorrhage early in the course of leukemia, thus preventing the complete evolution of the disease. The risk of a fatal cerebral hemorrhage becomes great as thrombocytopenia persists, particularly when it is accompanied by leukocytosis of 100,000 per c.mm. or more.[63b] In relation to infection, we have found that, if it is possible to induce a remission with chemotherapy, the complication can often be overcome. On the other hand, if the disease is at a stage in which antileukemic therapy is ineffective, progress of the infection is usually not arrested by any combination of antimicrobial and surgical therapy.

In general it can be said that the prognosis is far better for leukopenic cases than in those with substantial elevations of the leukocyte count at the time the diagnosis is made; the likelihood of induction of a remission by chemotherapy and the chance of long survival is better for patients with lymphoblastic than myeloblastic leukemia; and better for children than adults.[84a] Nevertheless, there is considerable variation of acute leukemia from cases to case.

Cure of Leukemia.—There are a number of reports of cure of leukemia.

Some of these were reviewed by Forkner.[59] No more than 3 or 4 of these cases were sufficiently well studied to allow serious consideration of the accuracy of the diagnosis. Three resembled acute leukemia,[72,86,152] 1 was thought to be chloroma.[217] However, in one case[86] infectious mononucleosis and, in another,[217] xanthoma was not ruled out. In addition to these cases, a patient with acute monocytic leukemia has been reported[189c] who was still well four years after remission developed and one case each of chronic myelocytic and chronic lymphocytic leukemia have been described[189d] in which the possibility that cure was produced by therapy must be considered.

Effect of Infections.—It was once commonly stated that, as a rule, patients presenting the classic clinical and hematological signs of leukemia often exhibit in the presence of infection a marked decrease in the leukocyte count. Even the organs enlarged by the leukemic disorder have been said to decrease in size temporarily. Following a review of the observations on which this statement was based, as well as the result of our own studies,[223] we came to the conclusion that there is little evidence to support the view that such remission is the usual experience. An increase in the number of granulocytes may occur in response to infection and overshadow the blood picture produced by the leukemia. In cases of lymphocytic leukemia, an increase of lymphocytes may develop at the same time.[223] The response to infection probably depends on the persistence of sufficient normal myeloid tissue to produce mature granulocytes.[107] Jaffe found that in the absence of myeloid tissue the changes in the tissues in response to infection were similar to those seen in granulocytopenia and in aplastic anemia; that is, the normal defense reaction was lacking. Immature leukemic cells apparently do not enter exudates. In patients with acute leukemia in whom the number of circulating granulocytes was markedly reduced, acellular exudates were found.[13d]

It is nevertheless true that in cases of *acute leukemia* remarkable temporary improvement or even "complete" remission may follow such infections as streptococcal sore throat, varicella and hemolytic staphylococcus septicemia.[173c] Remission has also been described following glandular fever infection[204] and even after the deliberate injection of the feline panleukopenia virus.[11h] This is an intriguing phenomenon from the standpoint of the pathogenesis of leukemia and deserves intensive study.

More common are problems related to the *impaired resistance to infection* which is seen in patients with leukemia. In a study of the course of 55 patients with acute leukemia, we found that two-thirds of 149 febrile episodes were attributable to infection.[175d] This is similar to the experience of others.[194d] In general, as survival of our patients was achieved beyond the mean duration of life characteristic of the patient's type of leukemia, infection was more often the cause of fever than leukemia. Such patients tend to develop infections not usually encountered in otherwise healthy persons, such as pseudomonas septicemia,[60a] fungal infections (candidiasis[194e] (moniliasis), cryptococcosis, histoplasmosis, mucormycosis[196a]), cytomegalic inclusion disease,[173] and clostridial gas gangrene,[13f] in addition to those which are more common, such as pharyngitis, pyelonephritis, pneumonia, cellulitis or localized abscesses, septicemia and pyemia, due as often to gram-negative as to gram-positive bacteria. Perirectal abscess may present a serious problem which is easily overlooked.

Studies of the response to infection in patients with leukemia have included observations of the cellular composition of the inflammatory exudate, already alluded to, and the finding that the initial granulocyte response is not only diminished but also delayed.[174] There is disagreement concerning the phagocytic activity of the neutrophilic granulocytes. Most investigators have found that this is good, provided a sufficient number of leukocytes is available.[20a,194c] From time to time various observations have indicated an impaired immunological response. Thus, heterophil antibodies were found in low titer, in contrast to the findings in infectious mononucleosis.[11] An impaired antibody response was noted particularly in chronic lymphocytic leukemia[129a] and attention was called to the fact that there is a much higher incidence of infections and an unusual vulnerability to them in this type of leukemia, as compared with the chronic myelocytic variety.[223] In an earlier section (p. 947), it was pointed out that hypoglobulinemia and, very occasionally, agammaglobulinemia may be found in chronic lymphocytic leukemia. This may play a role in the impaired resistance to infection although other, undescribed factors no doubt are involved in the poor reaction of the chronically debilitated patient who, in addition to his disease, may have handicaps associated with corticosteroid and antimetabolite therapy.

Occurrence of Pregnancy. — Although the association of leukemia and pregnancy is uncommon, approximately 145 such cases have been reported[58b,61c, 83a,132b,159,163c] and the writer has observed 5 additional cases. In 35 per cent the leukemia was acute and of these the majority (approximately 60 per cent) were said to be myeloblastic in type. Of the cases of chronic leukemia almost all (95 per cent) were of the myelocytic variety. This is to be expected when one considers the most common ages of incidence of the different types of leukemia. In more than two-thirds of the chronic cases the onset of the disease was prior to pregnancy whereas this was true only in 14 per cent of the cases of acute leukemia. A few of the women with chronic leukemia, including 2 of our own patients, had become pregnant more than once in the course of the disease.

There is no conclusive evidence that pregnancy has any influence on the course of the disease although in some instances it has seemed as if there was an exceptionally rapid demise in cases of acute leukemia following delivery, or an acute terminal phase ensued in cases of chronic leukemia. Labor may begin prematurely but immediate postpartum hemorrhage is unusual, abnormal bleeding being more common somewhat later. In general, patients survive pregnancy and parturition more easily than might be expected. The prognosis for the child depends on the status of the disease in the mother; when it is such as to endanger her life or to cause premature labor, the outlook is not good. Fetal mortality has been much higher in acute than in chronic cases (64 per cent as compared with 38 per cent), even when pregnancy had progressed past seven months (39 per cent as compared with 15 per cent[163c]). As indicated earlier (p. 910), no case of transmission of leukemia to the child has been recorded.

In the management of leukemia during pregnancy, forms of therapy which may injure the child, should naturally be avoided, especially in the first trimester. Except when it is necessary to save a viable child in a terminal case, nothing is to be gained from interruption of the pregnancy.

Association with Various Diseases. —The interrelationship of chronic myelocytic leukemia and *erythremia* have been discussed (p. 809). There are many features common to both disorders and what appear to be transitions from one to the other have been described. The relationship of these disorders to "myeloid metaplasia" and to myelofibrosis (p. 581)

is obscure. They can all be considered to represent different expressions of the same underlying disturbance but it is equally possible that they have no fundamental relationship to one another.

The relationship of chronic lymphocytic leukemia to *lymphosarcoma* and *giant follicular lymphoblastoma*, and perhaps to *reticulum cell sarcoma* and even *Hodgkin's disease* may be quite close. Not only may the clinical pictures of these disorders shade from one condition to the other so that a whole spectrum can be described, but different sections of the same gland or sections of different glands may show in a given case histologic patterns ranging from that of Hodgkin's disease to that of reticulum cell sarcoma and lymphosarcoma. The histologic pattern of lymphosarcoma is indistinguishable from that of lymphocytic leukemia. Hodgkin's disease has been observed in association with acute or chronic lymphoid leukemia.[193a]

The coëxistence of *leukemia and cancer* in the same individual has been noted in a number of instances.[131a] Skin and lip cancer is the most common of the associated forms of malignancy and that of the stomach or breast comes next. We have seen carcinoma of the breast associated with acute leukemia in two instances. In the relatives of patients with leukemia the incidence of various types of cancer was found to be higher than in a control series.[211a]

It might be expected that *gout* would be a common complication of leukemia. Despite the high uric acid content of the blood in many instances of leukemia, gout is uncommon, although not as rare as was once thought.[203a]

Evidence of the coëxistence of *pernicious anemia* and leukemia in the same patient and the same family was of such a degree in one study[211a] as to suggest a relationship between the two. The occurrence of *peptic ulcer* in leukemia was mentioned earlier (p. 917).

Tuberculosis has been described in association with chronic lymphocytic[54a] and other forms of leukemia. Cases of leukemia have also been reported in which the development of tuberculosis was accompanied by disappearance or great alteration in the clinical and pathologic signs of leukemia.[84g]

TREATMENT OF LEUKEMIA

There is as yet no cure for leukemia. For many years chief reliance in the treatment of this disease was placed on irradiation by means of roentgen rays and on chemotherapy by the use of benzol or arsenical preparations. Following the introduction of the nitrogen mustards, considerable new interest in the management of the leukemias, Hodgkin's disease, lymphosarcoma and related disorders was aroused and many new forms of treatment have been introduced. These have given new hope to the patient and encouragement to the investigator. By the methods now available the symptoms of leukemia can be alleviated and remissions can be brought about which, in some cases, may be so complete as to give the appearance of unqualified well-being. The remissions in chronic leukemia may be of long duration and even in acute leukemia they may last a number of months. With the introduction of a variety of chemotherapeutic agents treatment, moreover, has become relatively inexpensive, requires a minimum of hospitalization and is associated with relatively little inconvenience so that an essentially normal existence can be achieved for a time. In the end, unfortunately, death still occurs in spite of treatment. Nevertheless, evidence is accumulating that modern therapy is significantly prolonging the life span of the majority of patients and, most certainly, wise management can make what remains of their lives much more bearable.

Some physicians have asked whether treatment is worthwile. This question can only be in the minds of those who have had little experience with diseases of this kind. It is very rare, indeed, that a patient, or the parents of children affected with acute leukemia, would not prefer to have treatment carried out to the alternative of waiting for the inevitable end without attempting therapy. Whether or not, in the end, the patient or his family is grateful for what has been accomplished by therapy depends in large measure on the physician.

The Responsibilities of the Physician.—Needless to say, it is important to make certain of the diagnosis of leukemia; some physicians are too ready to reach this conclusion and do not take sufficient steps to make sure that this is the correct diagnosis. It is by no means rare, for example, to mistake infectious mononucleosis for acute leukemia. The physician must also be aware of the desire of the patient or his family to disprove the diagnosis and hence he should never deny them the opportunity for consultation; in fact, it is his duty to assist in securing competent advice.

Next in importance is the physician's approach to the patient. The patient comes to him for help and encouragement and the doctor whose temperament is pessimistic has no place in his management. It is not very rare, furthermore, that one encounters patients who have been "frightened to death" by their physician, who seems to have considered his function to be to seal their doom rather than to give them encouragement and support. Much can be done for these patients and, for the person who has only a few years or even only a few months to live, even this limited time is precious and is grasped tenaciously. One must attempt to keep hope alive and to make the remaining time as pleasant as possible.

It is naturally necessary to give the

patient some understanding of his condition even if he is a child. This will not only insure his cooperation but may also help to dispel his fears, most of which are usually not expressed. Clearly, what one says will depend on the maturity and character of the patient. It may not be wise to present all the facts about diagnosis and prognosis, at least in the beginning. Very often the complete outlook as to prognosis is best discussed only with a responsible member of the family rather than with the patient. In some instances, however, especially when one is dealing with a mature person who carries important responsibilities, it is necessary to discuss the problem frankly with him. This naturally should be done sympathetically in a way which will minimize the trauma to the patient. In all cases it is important that some responsible person be given all the facts that are known.

The management of leukemia, like that of other ultimately fatal conditions, requires all the skill and art of the physician. Some of the psychological aspects have been touched upon already. The physician must be able to convey to the patient and his family both a feeling of understanding of the disease and appreciation of their natural reaction to such a diagnosis.

From the standpoint of the somatic problems, the physician's objectives are fivefold: (1) suppression of the leukemic cells in the blood, bone marrow and tissues; (2) prevention and control of hemorrhage; (3) control of infections and other complications; (4) relief of anemia; and (5) maintenance of appetite, weight and sense of well-being.

The principles governing treatment in the last four areas are common to all types of leukemia and will therefore be discussed first. For the suppression of the leukemic process certain chemical and physical agents are useful and these will be considered in turn. As our under-

standing of the various chemotherapeutic agents has evolved, it has become apparent that each has its special place in the treatment of a particular form of leukemia. The wise choice and the effective use of the agent often makes a very important difference in the outcome. Similarly, discrimination is necessary in the use of irradiation therapy.

Certain *general principles of therapy* deserve to be stressed. First, in so far as possible, diagnostic and therapeutic measures should be adapted to caring for the individual as an ambulatory rather than a hospitalized patient. This is helpful psychologically and, usually, financially. Secondly, the cost of the therapeutic agents employed is an important consideration. The physician must not be unmindful of the financial burdens which a long illness imposes. Thirdly, it is generally best to employ only one of the agents designed to suppress the leukemic process at one time. It has not been shown that combination therapy possesses any advantages over the use of a single agent[61] and, furthermore, the opportunity for development of resistance to therapy is limited thereby to the agent employed. As a consequence, the chance is greater that another agent may be found useful for a time. In addition, when more than one agent is being used, confusion is inevitable if toxic symptoms develop. The therapeutic armamentarium must be kept as simple as possible and the number of drugs employed should be held to the minimum.

Prevention and Control of Hemorrhage.—In leukemia, hemorrhage is usually related to the development of thrombocytopenia; fibrinolysins or deficiencies of coagulation factors are rarely the cause of bleeding (p. 933). Thrombocytopenia may be due to the disease process or may have been caused by therapy. If the latter, treatment may need to be interrupted; if the former, the choice of the therapeutic agent must be guided in part by the presence of this complication, as will be discussed further, below. When the therapeutic agent is effective in suppressing the leukemia, thrombocytopenia will usually be relieved. However, before the effect of therapy can be realized, hemorrhage must be controlled by the judicious use of local measures, such as direct pressure packs when there is epistaxis. Topical application of thrombin may be tried. When bleeding is severe, the liberal transfusion of fresh platelet-rich blood, collected no more than 3 to 4 hours before in commercially available all-plastic donor and recipient sets to minimize damage to platelets (p. 356), is usually more practical than attempts to transfuse platelet concentrates. As yet satisfactory platelet substitutes have not been found.

Control of Infections and Other Complications.—As indicated earlier (p. 953), infections pose a great problem for the patient with leukemia, especially in the later stages of acute leukemia and in chronic lymphocytic leukemia. Nevertheless, it has not been shown that prophylactic administration of antibiotics is helpful; in fact, by encouraging a change in the host's bacterial flora so that antibotic-resistant organisms, bacteria and fungi, predominate, matters are usually made worse. Even when the leukocyte count is greatly depressed it is better to withhold antibiotics and, instead, to attempt to identify the causative agent when an infection is suspected and treat with the appropriate drug. In general, it is better to use bactericidal rather than bacteriostatic agents whenever circumstances permit, and greater than customary dosage should be used. The resistance of microorganisms to antibiotics is a relative matter; thus penicillin in amounts as large as 10 to 50 Gm. (17 to 84 million units) daily may control an infection even though the organisms were judged "resistant" by the conventional antibiotic-disc sensitivity technique.

In acute leukemia in particular, **oral hygiene** requires special attention. Bleeding from the mucous membranes occurs readily. The tooth brush should be soft. The mouth should be cleansed after each meal and a mild antiseptic may be used, such as 1.5 per cent hydrogen peroxide or saturated solution of sodium perborate. Ulceration may develop in the course of the disease or, more often, as a complication of antimetabolite therapy. In patients who have received steroids for many weeks, fungus infections, such as candidiasis may occur. In such cases, interruption of therapy is by far the most effective remedy.

Anuria occurring as a consequence of crystallization of uric acid in the renal tubules and ureters may be a serious complication. Preceding the anuria, oliguria will be noted if adequate observations are made and, in many instances, pain in the abdomen or back may give warning of impending trouble. The pain, if its nature is not recognized, may lead to the consideration of other diagnoses, such as appendicitis, splenic infarction and various "surgical emergencies" of the abdomen. The serum uric acid will usually be found to be elevated and the urine will contain large quantities of uric acid. Hyperuricemia occurs in untreated leukemia and may be further augmented by any therapy that can destroy leukemic tissue rapidly. To reduce the hazard of precipitation of uric acid in the urinary tract, sodium bicarbonate administration together with large quantities of fluids orally or intravenously often suffices. Most important is the physician's awareness of the possibility of this complication ensuing and the prompt institution of therapy as soon as any signs or symptoms develop. When anuria has developed, ureteral catheterization and irrigation have been employed but these measures are not without danger in patients with a bleeding tendency. The artificial kidney has been used effectively in these circumstances.[58]

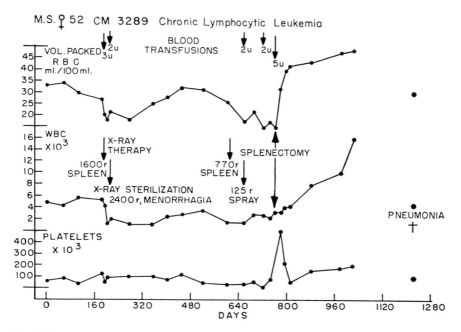

FIG. 19–26.—Dramatic relief of severe anemia and serious thrombocytopenia in a case of chronic lymphocytic leukemia (M.S.) following splenectomy. Sterilization by irradiation of the ovaries had been carried out previously in an attempt to relieve the effect of severe menorrhagia on the anemia. Following splenectomy the patient did very well but succumbed ultimately to pneumonia before she could receive appropriate therapy.

Symptoms associated with the presence of **leukemic tumor masses** are sometimes troublesome. The development of chloroma with proptosis often requires local therapy in addition to whatever systemic treatment is being given. We have found local irradiation to the area of the tumor very helpful. *Intracranial complications,* such as symptoms and signs of meningeal irritation, increased intracranial pressure, seizures or cranial nerve palsies, may be seen in patients with acute leukemia even when a successful hematological and bone marrow remission has been achieved. Examination of the eyegrounds and of the spinal fluid will give evidence of increased intracranial pressure and the protein content of the spinal fluid may be found elevated and the sugar reduced below the normal levels. In such cases the intrathecal administra-

tion of amethopterin, prepared for parenteral use (Lederle), has proved to be very useful.[36f] Amounts of 0.1 to 0.5 mg. per Kg. body weight are injected intrathecally. It may be necessary to repeat this once or twice at intervals of three or four days to achieve regression of the tumor.

The size of a *spleen* is almost never a reason for its removal. It is possible to reduce the size of this organ by local roentgen therapy or by appropriate chemotherapy. **Splenectomy,** however, has been performed successfully in cases of chronic lymphocytic leukemia when intractable pancytopenia,[1f, 58a] especially thrombocytopenia, has been present, as Figure 19–26 illustrates. In chronic lymphocytic leukemia, particularly when hemolytic anemia is the main reason for considering splenectomy, cortico-

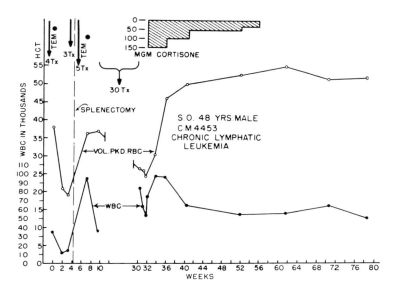

F ig. 19–27.—Failure of splenectomy to relieve hemolytic anemia complicating chronic lymphocytic leukemia (S.O.) compared with effectiveness of cortisone therapy. The anemia has not returned in the seven and a half years since interruption of cortisone therapy, but the leukocyte count has fluctuated between 58,000 and 13,000 per c.mm.

steroid therapy should be tried first, operative intervention being reserved for patients who fail to respond to medical treatment. In cases with hemolytic anemia we have observed splenectomy to fail and relief was obtained only from hormone therapy (Fig. 19–27). In other forms of leukemia there is no justification for consideration of splenectomy.

Relief of Anemia.—The relief of anemia, as a rule, is accomplished by antileukemic therapy alone, as long as this retains its effectiveness. This is the usual result in chronic myelocytic leukemia and in acute lymphoblastic leukemia and the same may happen in acute myeloblastic leukemia but there the improvement, if it occurs at all, is more likely to be delayed. In chronic lymphocytic leukemia, anemia develops only in the later stage of the disease and is not easily influenced by therapy. When the anemia is clearly hemolytic in nature, the use of adrenocorticosteroids is very valuable, as illustrated in Figure 19–27 and discussed

elsewhere (p. 628). We have found, in addition, that in a number of patients with chronic lymphocytic leukemia whose anemia is not frankly hemolytic and the Coombs' test is negative, the administration of this hormone in doses of 40 to 60 mg. of prednisone per day, will relieve the anemia in whole or in part and may be accompanied by regression of the tumor masses and decrease in the leukocyte count, following a temporary increase (Fig. 19–28). This has also been observed by others.[61c] In cases of this kind the concomitant administration of testosterone or other anabolic but less masculinizing hormones, may not only minimize osteoporosis but may possibly also further the antianemic effect. As a rule, the original doses of prednisone must be continued for at least three months, after which time a maintenance dose of 10 to 20 mg. daily may be needed. The major risk to patients receiving this form of therapy is overwhelming and undetected infection.

Other than antileukemic therapy and

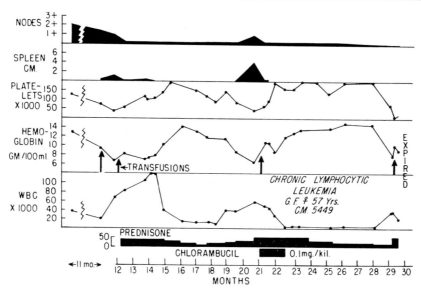

FIG. 19–28.—Course of a patient (G.F.) previously treated elsewhere with P[32], blood transfusions and 5 to 10 mg. prednisone per day who had moderately severe anemia, thrombocytopenia and moderate leukocytosis. There was no overt hemolytic anemia. The administration of prednisone in doses of 40 mg. per day was associated with relief of the anemia, a slow rise in platelets and a temporary increase in leukocytosis. These effects on the anemia and thrombocytopenia could not be maintained on smaller quantities of steroid. The addition of chlorambucil may have been beneficial. The splenomegaly and lymphadenopathy were reduced greatly. She died of cellulitis following a burn from a heating pad.

the use of hormones in the special situations described above, no antianemic measures have been shown to be helpful other than blood transfusion. Iron, liver extract, vitamin B_{12} or cobalt is of no value and folic acid may actually be detrimental.[55,84c]

Indications for *blood transfusion* were discussed in a previous chapter (p. 354). The need for transfusion should be judged largely from observation of the patient's physiological adjustment to the degree of anemia present. As a guide, it should be recalled that it is rarely necessary to give a transfusion when the hemoglobin concentration is as high as 10 Gm. per cent or more, except in the case of frank hemorrhage, when transfusion may be given to prevent or combat shock. Transfusion may be considered also in instances of thrombocytopenia with continuous bleeding and oozing, when the platelet content of fresh blood

rather than the quantity of erythrocytes is important.

The decision to give a transfusion usually does not need to be made hastily. Often the physiologic adjustment to the anemia is better than the physician would anticipate. With present day therapy of leukemia the need for transfusion early in the disease is less than it once was and, furthermore, if life span is prolonged, the need for blood in the late stages may be greater. This measure should therefore be used sparingly and held as a reserve. It must not be forgotten that the less often transfusions are given the fewer the risks of post-transfusion complications.

Of theoretical interest but of no practical value are the observations which were made of the effects of *exchange transfusions*.[11a] In a study of 60 cases, immediate improvement in the general condition was observed with relief of

61

anemia, cessation of bleeding and even healing of infections resistant to antibiotic therapy. In approximately half the cases there was, at the same time, reduction or disappearance of hepatomegaly, splenomegaly and lymphadenopathy and in about 20 per cent there was a more or less complete hematologic remission, with remarkable improvement in the bone marrow picture in a few. In those cases in which remission occurred, a precipitous drop in the leukocyte count was observed; this change affected the immature cells chiefly but the normal granulocytes disappeared as well, sometimes completely. The latter returned to normal in the course of a month but, in many cases, the pathological cells did not return at the same time. The duration of the remissions usually ranged from three weeks to three and a half months, although two patients were still alive after 11 months, one in complete remission. When relapse occurred, the beneficial effect of replacement transfusion was less marked.

We have observed, as have others, that following even simple transfusion, especially with fresh blood,[219d] the total leukocyte count is likely to fall. The explanation of this intriguing phenomenon is not apparent.

Maintenance of Appetite, Weight and Sense of Well Being.—Not to be overlooked, especially since sometimes it is all that the physician can accomplish, is the patient's approach to his illness and his sense of well being. The psychological aspects of the treatment of leukemia have been touched upon already, as has the importance of maintaining an ambulatory state out of hospital and, insofar as possible, at normal play, school or work. Naturally, when there is fever, rest is desirable but usually the patient senses his own limitations very adequately and the physician and the patient's family should avoid making an unhappy invalid of a person who would

rather make the best of things. The writer has not been impressed with any harm attending activity by patients who have leukemia. A hemorrhage is as likely to develop in a patient who lies quietly in bed as in an active one.

There is nothing in the way of specific dietary measures which needs to be prescribed other than those which the patient's appetite and the condition of his oropharynx dictate, if mucous membrane lesions are present. Effective anti-leukemic therapy will ultimately lead to an improvement in appetite and little else will help this.

"Specific" Measures. — General Remarks.—A great variety of agents have been proposed from time to time as more or less specific therapeutic measures directed toward the leukemic process. In the form of Fowler's solution (solution of potassium arsenite, U.S.P.), *arsenic* was introduced for the treatment of leukemia in 1865. The introduction of irradiation caused arsenic to be forgotten until its usefulness was demonstrated again in 1931.[60] The drug then enjoyed some popularity for a decade or more. In chronic myelocytic leukemia it can produce a remission like that caused by irradiation (Fig. 19–29). Maintenance therapy is required, since relapse soon follows if the drug was disassociated in some cases with the development of herpes zoster, widespread keratosis of the skin, tenderness of the soles of the feet, peripheral neuritis, and even ascites.[120] Organic arsenicals such as neoarsphenamine were found to be of no value in the treatment of leukemia.[59]

Benzol (C_6H_6) administered in capsules with olive oil in doses of 2 to 5 Gm. daily, was introduced for the treatment of leukemia by Korényi in 1912 following Selling's studies on the effects of benzol on the blood. Excessive dosage with corresponding deleterious effects led to its abandonment in many clinics but

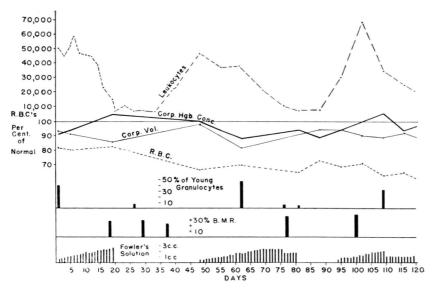

FIG. 19–29.—Drop in leukocyte count and disappearance of immature forms during three periods of administration of Fowler's solution. In this case anemia was not relieved and the basal metabolic rate eventually rose.

there is no doubt that, when correctly applied, this was a useful agent.[118]

Roentgen rays were first used successfully in the treatment of leukemia by Senn in 1903.[193c] Subsequently *radium, meso-thorium*[226] and *thorium X* were introduced. The mode of action and the physiological effects of radium are essentially the same as those of short wave roentgen rays and the indications and contraindications for treatment are also similar. Before high voltage by roentgen irradiation was available, some workers reported benefit following radium when refractoriness to roentgen rays had developed.[166] The area to be treated was outlined and marked into small squares somewhat larger than the size of the radium applicator. Radium was then applied over each area systematically. As much as 250 to 300 mg. was applied for as long as 15 hours.[170] These agents were later abandoned because they were more cumbersome and inconvenient, as well as less economical and less easily controlled than other forms of irradiation, such as

roentgen rays and radioactive phosphorus (p. 968).

The discovery of the effects of nitrogen mustard on the hemopoietic system and the lymphatic tissues[223a] initiated studies which have produced a large number of chemotherapeutic agents, some of which are very useful in the management of different forms of leukemia. Nitrogen mustard itself is now used mainly in the treatment of Hodgkin's disease (p. 1037).

Mode of Action of Antileukemic Agents.—The nature of the effects of irradiation was discussed in an earlier chapter (p. 556) and will be considered briefly later (p. 970). In a superficial way, some of the chemotherapeutic agents now in use are radiomimetic;[46c] that is, their action is similar to, although not identical[126a] with that of ionizing radiation. For example, it was observed that a combination of busulfan and chlorambucil produced effects on the blood which were similar to those caused by a single dose of whole body irradiation.[50]

In point of fact, however, much remains to be clarified concerning the mode of action of the various chemotherapeutic agents.[126b] Furthermore, the mechanisms by which these substances influence cell growth have been studied in a variety of biologic systems; for example, cellular or cell-free tissue homogenates, bacteria, mammalian cells in tissue culture, and transplanted leukemias and tumors in mice and rats. These systems have yielded valuable information but it has been found time and again that the information obtained cannot invariably be extrapolated to the treatment of the different types of leukemia or other neoplasms which occur in man.

Since nucleic acids play an important part in the regulation of cell growth, attempts to develop agents capable of modifying cell growth have focused largely on substances which might be capable of destroying or inactivating nucleic acids or inhibiting their biosynthesis. As a consequence, two types of compounds have been developed, the *polyfunctional alkylating agents* and the antimetabolites. The former are compounds possessing two or more end groups (alkyl groups) which may be either cyclic or unsaturated or can be converted to such forms. These end groups are unstable and are capable of attaching to other molecules through an oxygen, nitrogen or sulfur atom. At the concentrations used therapeutically, it is thought that this reaction occurs preferentially with deoxyribonucleic acid (DNA). The reactive groups of the alkylating agents are thought to attach to the phosphate groups of the strands of DNA, producing various types of cross linkages and thereby "denaturing" or inactivating the DNA.[126b] Three main classes of alkylating agents are in use; namely (1) the β-chloroethyl amines, such as nitrogen mustard, chlorambucil and cyclophosphamide; (2) the ethylene imines, such as triethylene melamine and

thio-phosphoramide; and (3) busulfan, which is one of a series of sulfonoxy esters.

Whereas the alkylating agents inactivate or destroy nucleic acids, the *antimetabolites* affect growing cells by inhibiting various synthetic processes on the pathways to nucleic acids. Several types of antagonists are in use; namely (1) folic acid antagonists, such as amethopterin; (2) purine analogues, such as 6-mercaptopurine; (3) glutamine antagonists, such as azaserine; and (4) pyrimidine analogues, such as 5-fluorouracil. Each of these will be discussed below in relation to its possible therapeutic usefulness.

In addition to these compounds a variety of *miscellaneous drugs* have been tried from time to time. Of these, the alkaloid demecolcin deserves mention since it has a place in modern therapy. Like colchinine, this compound produces arrest of the metaphase in cell division but this is accomplished without the severe gastrointestinal toxicity associated with colchicine. The mode of action of another compound, urethane (ethyl carbamate) is poorly understood even though this is a drug of simple molecular structure. It may possibly interfere with the utilization of pyridines for DNA synthesis. Other agents and measures which have been tested or proposed for the treatment of leukemia will be mentioned in the next section.

Choice of Therapeutic Agent.— A goal of chemotherapy is to discover substances which injure neoplastic cells selectively by virtue of chemical specificities that distinguish them from their normal analogues. Unfortunately this dream has not been realized; no qualitative biochemical differences between normal and neoplastic cells have been defined and, as a consequence, the damaging effects of chemotherapeutic agents, like that of irradiation, are widespread. Nevertheless, experience has shown that these measures, when judiciously employed, can offer dramatic benefit to the patient. Likewise, in the hands of the uninformed, they can produce untold harm and suffering.

Many factors govern the responsiveness of a given patient and of a particular form of leukemia to therapy, most of which are poorly understood. It is well known that, as a rule, children respond better to antileukemic therapy than adults and, as mentioned earlier (p. 953), the prognosis in patients with low leukocyte counts is usually better than that of those who have marked leukocytosis. Experience has also shown that certain types of leukemia respond more readily or more completely to one agent than to another, even though an effect can be achieved by the use of several modes of therapy. Again, in the chronic leukemias, in particular, irradiation is in many respects as effective and, in some situations, more useful than the chemotherapeutic agents. On the other hand, roentgen ray therapy requires special equipment, daily visits by the patient, and skin tolerance is a limiting factor. Chemotherapeutic agents may be given orally or, if administered parenterally, their effect is accomplished in one or two days.

One of the more practical accomplishments of modern antileukemic therapy is the opportunity which is provided to suit the mode of therapy to the patient and his disease in a fashion which was not possible before. It is now possible even for the physician in a community unequipped with roentgen therapy apparatus to treat his patient, provided only that he will take the trouble to become thoroughly informed concerning the proper use of the therapeutic agents he employs, including their toxic effects, and he has available adequate laboratory facilities.

In Table 19–3 are listed the various therapeutic measures which are now most generally employed and preferences are indicated. For the treatment of *chronic leukemia* the choice lies between irradiation by means of roentgen therapy or radioactive phosphorus, and chemotherapy. Busulfan or demecolcin is effective in the treatment of chronic myelocytic leukemia whereas chlorambucil or triethylene melamine is used for chronic lymphocytic leukemia. Practical considerations rather than any proved scientific differences govern the choice between irradiation and chemotherapy. Roentgen therapy is particularly useful in the local treatment of splenomegaly or enlarged lymph nodes.

It should be emphasized that the sensitivity of different patients to therapy varies and may change in the course of time. It is also noteworthy that the sensitivity of chronic lymphocytic leukemia to irradiation[61d] as well as to chemotherapeutic agents may be very great; doses much smaller than those needed in chronic myelocytic leukemia sometimes produce unexpectedly sharp decreases in the leukocyte count (Fig. 19–30). The latter effect may be associated with the development of anemia and thrombocytopenia and may produce a more serious therapeutic problem than existed before. In the management of chronic lymphocytic leukemia, in particular, restraint is sometimes more necessary than action, for in the earlier stages progression of the disease may be very slow and it is then particularly necessary to avoid doing more harm than good by the ill-advised use of therapeutic measures.

The agents which are useful for the treatment of the chronic leukemias have little or no value in the management of the *acute leukemias.* Irradiation, in fact, is in general contraindicated and the alkylating agents have no significant value. It is noteworthy, also, that the drugs used in the acute leukemias have no place in the treatment of the chronic leukemias, with only limited exceptions. In the treatment of acute leukemias, the

Table 19–3.—Choice of Therapeutic Agents for the Treatment of Leukemia

Type of Leukemia	Irradiation X-ray, P³²	Alkylating Agents			Busulfan Demecolcin	Antagonists		Adreno-cortical Hormones
		HN2	TEM	Chlor-ambucil		Amethopterin	6MP	
Chronic myelocytic	++++	+	+	+	++++	C	+¹	C
Chronic lymphocytic	++++	++	+++	+++	+	C	C	++²
Acute lymphoblastic	C	C	C	C	0	+++	+++	++++
Acute myeloblastic	C	C	C	C	0	++	++++	0
Acute monocytic	C	C	C	C	0	++	+++	0

++++ effective and the agent of choice
+++ effective
++ moderately effective but usually not the agent of choice
+ slightly effective
0 ineffective
C contarindicated

¹ temporarily useful in the "acute," terminal phase
² useful in the management of anemia

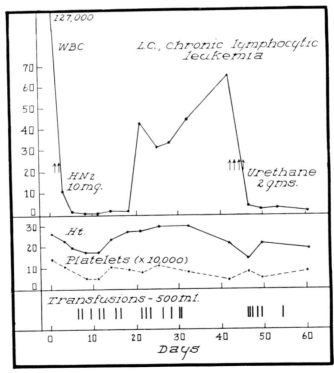

FIG. 19–30.—To illustrate the remarkable sensitivity of a patient with chronic lymphocytic leukemia to both nitrogen mustard (HN2) and urethane (Wintrobe and Huguley, Cancer, 1948).

folic acid antagonists, a purine analogue (6-mercaptopurine), and the adrenocortical hormones are the agents of choice.

As mentioned earlier (p. 957) it is better to use only one of these agents at one time. Not only is management easier but, when resistance to one drug has developed, another can be employed. Consequently, it is our practice to initiate therapy with prednisone or a similar compound if the patient has acute lymphoblastic leukemia and especially if he is acutely ill. If the condition is not so critical, treatment may be initiated with 6-MP or amethopterin. In acute myeloblastic leukemia corticosteroids are not used as a rule (see p. 983). Sometimes relatively large doses of the drug chosen are used at first to initiate a remission, after which the drug is given in smaller amounts for maintenance therapy. If signs of relapse appear the dose may be increased but, in general, we have found it better to resort to a different therapeutic agent when signs of relapse are definite rather than wait until there is marked deterioration of the clinical state. Preference is given to an agent which has not yet been used; an agent is repeated only after the others have been used once. By such a system of *continuous treatment with a succession of agents* (Fig. 19–40, p. 981) remissions can be achieved or sustained by agents used for the second or third time although they seemingly had lost their effectiveness earlier.

Details concerning the use of these various therapeutic agents will be discussed under the separate headings, below.

In addition to the therapeutic measures already discussed, a variety of others have been tried from time to time. These need only be mentioned here since they have not proved to be of any value. Thymectomy, of theoretical interest in view of the studies of leukemia in the mouse, was found to have no influence on the course of leukemia.[42b] Various organs and organ extracts (bone marrow, spleen, thyroid, lymph nodes) have been given to patients with leukemia, without benefit.[148a] The leukocyte count can be depressed by the use of antileukocytic sera,[95] Lugol's solution,[62] or antimony[138] or by the induction of malaria,[171] but nothing of benefit is gained thereby. Induced pyridoxine deficiency was not found to be of therapeutic value in the treatment of leukemia or lymphosarcoma.[71c] Myelokentric acid (p. 911) was tried in a number of cases of leukemia, with indifferent results.[150] An interesting approach is the attempt to find viruses which might have a selective affinity for some neoplastic growths, damaging them without at the same time producing appreciable injury to the host.[208b] Chemotherapeutic agents other than those mentioned above will be discussed later (p. 982).

Attempts to **transplant human bone marrow** in patients with leukemia who have been treated by irradiation with the object of destroying all the leukemic tissue deserve special mention since the concept is intriguing, even though the efforts have been unsuccessful. The problems involved in the transplantation of tissue from one person to another have been attacked experimentally with the result that much has been learned concerning the immune mechanisms which must be circumvented.[56a] Technics have been devised for securing large quantities of normal bone marrow. It has been necessary to learn what amounts of radiation are necessary in man to destroy immune responses and to permit engraftment of marrow; and how much irradiation can be given and yet permit the subject to survive. Where normal identical twins have been available as a source of bone marrow, the problem of grafting has been less great than in the more usual circumstance in which the genotype of the donor is different from that of the recipient. In leukemia, nevertheless, transplantation of allogenic hemopoietic tissue appears to be especially difficult.

As yet, cure of leukemia has not been achieved and, when survival and improvement following irradiation and marrow transplantation occurred at all, the benefit was of comparatively short duration.[83b,141a] This is a procedure which deserves further study but it must be regarded as highly experimental and should be attempted only by those who are prepared to give the patient the necessary protection against intercurrent infection, capillary bleeding and all the effects of residual radiation damage. Bone marrow transplantation must not be undertaken haphazardly and should be conducted only in an institution equipped to study the problems involved in great detail. Only under such circumstances is this sort of human experimentation justified.

Observations on Patients Undergoing Therapy.—Careful and repeated clinical and hematological examinations are necessary in patients undergoing irradiation or chemotherapy. In addition to such obvious clinical observations as those concerned with changes in the size of lymph nodes, spleen and liver and the occurrence of hemorrhagic manifestations, it is helpful to note changes in body weight, sense of well-being, and appetite and the development or disappearance of fever and bone tenderness. Examination of the blood should include volume of packed red cells or hemoglobin, leukocyte and platelet counts and careful examination of the blood smear. Bone marrow examination from time to time is helpful in cases in which there are few or no abnormal leukocytes in the blood but, since this procedure is unpleasant for the patient, it should be avoided when possible. Often it will be found that a thorough examination of the patient, supplemented by the blood studies outlined above, will make frequent bone marrow aspirations unnecessary. Depending on the condition of the patient, he may need to be observed daily, biweekly, once a week or once in several weeks. Hospitalization, as stated earlier, should be kept to a minimum; it is only necessary when there is severe anemai and thrombocytopenia or when constitutional manifestations or complications demand bed rest and constant attention.

Irradiation.—In suitable cases of *chronic leukemia*, **roentgen ray** irradiation is followed by symptomatic improvement with reduction of the leukocyte count and disappearance of immature forms (Fig. 19–3), and gain in weight, strength and color occurs. It has been aptly stated that "the patient, a pale, emaciated, anxious-looking individual with a strikingly prominent abdomen becomes plump, strong and apparently well." Large tumors in the neck, the axilla, and elsewhere, produced by enlarged lymph nodes, decrease in size or disappear. Pressure symptoms are relieved. The basal metabolic rate falls and the spleen and liver decrease in size. Other signs of a favorable effect are decreasing anemia and a return of the platelet count to normal, no matter whether this was abnormally high or greatly reduced before treatment. Relief of anemia and restitution of a normal platelet count is more often produced in chronic myelocytic leukemia than in chronic lymphocytic leukemia.[154] In *acute leukemia* irradiation may lower the leukocyte count and may relieve troublesome pressure symptoms, but anemia is not relieved, bleeding if present continues, and the general condition may be aggravated.[154] Nevertheless, small doses of roentgen rays may be helpful in the treatment of central nervous system symptoms, those related to bones and joints, cutaneous and mucosal infiltrations and any tumor masses which may be troublesome.[40a]

Indications for Irradiation.—An increased leukocyte count alone is not an indication for irradiation. A number of carefully carried out studies[92,153,154,186] showed that the duration of life is little if at all prolonged by irradiation but comfort and efficiency can be increased.[127a] Consequently the indications for treatment are loss of weight, increasing pallor and complaints attributable to anemia, pressure symptoms, invasion of tissues with the production of pain, or disfiguring and uncomfortable glandular enlargement. In other words, the history and physical findings are more important than the blood examination in determining the need for treatment. The leukocyte level, however, is often a guide to oncoming relapse, as is a falling red cell count and increasing basal metabolic rate. Roentgen therapy in the face of leukopenia is discussed below (p. 970).

As discussed elsewhere (p. 951), chronic lymphocytic leukemia frequently takes a relatively benign course. Such patients require much less irradiation than those with chronic myelocytic leukemia. Paradoxically, in spite of this sensitivity, once anemia has developed, clinical and hematological remission comparable to that observed in the myelocytic form, is quite exceptional.

Dosage.—In chronic myelocytic leukemia a total dose of 200 to 400 r, directed against the enlarged spleen[92] and given over the course of four to six days will usually suffice in early cases. The smallest possible dose which will produce a remission should be used. If the response after an interval of three to four weeks appears to have been inadequate, additional treatment may be given. As the disease progresses, larger doses may be required; even 1000 to 2000 r have been given to the spleen. Different aspects (front, back, lateral) are irradiated in order to concentrate the irradiation on the organ and to spare the neighboring tissues as much as possible. If the liver is greatly enlarged, x-ray therapy may be given over this organ but

this is likely to cause irradiation sickness. Spray x-ray therapy, in doses of 10 to 50 r may be given to the long bones.[133]

In chronic lymphocytic leukemia, enlarged nodes or the spleen may respond to doses of even 100 to 200 r. It is wise to proceed cautiously since there is wide variation in the sensitivity of patients to irradiation. Deep-seated lymph nodes must not be attacked too vigorously in the first few treatments if they are so located that edema following irradiation may lead to compression of vital areas or passages such as the trachea.

Indications for Cessation or Modification.—No arbitrary figure can be given for the leukocyte level at which treatment should be stopped, the patient's improvement being the chief guide. Unfavorable signs which are indications for cessation or modification of treatment are (1) aggravation of the patient's symptoms, rapid loss of body weight or gastro-intestinal disturbances; (2) increase of anemia; (3) increased proportion of immature leukocytes; and (4) the onset of bleeding or failure of the platelets to return to normal. The condition of the irradiated skin must be watched to prevent radionecrosis.

Irradiation Sickness.—"Irradiation sickness," manifested by anorexia, nausea, vomiting and diarrhea, may occur, particularly when the upper part of the abdomen has been treated. In the majority of patients these symptoms are not severe. Their cause is not well understood but it seems plausible that injury of the intestinal epithelium is an important factor.[82d] Injury of liver cells and disturbance in the function of that organ may be another cause. The administration of a high carbohydrate diet before commencing treatment and adequate evacuation of the bowels, as well as thorough ventilation of the rooms where treatment is administered and avoidance of excessive dosage or too rapidly repeated treatments, are measures which have been recommended for the prevention of radiation sickness. The administration of chlorpromazine may be helpful.

Signs of Imminent Relapse.—Patients should be seen at intervals after treatment has ceased. Remission following irradiation may last only a few weeks but often is many months in duration. Treatment should be resumed when anemia begins to increase, the leukocyte count rises and immature cells increase in number, the body weight begins to fall and appetite starts to fail or new symptoms appear. These are signs of imminent relapse and further aggravation of the disease can often be prevented by treatment commenced at this time.

Refractoriness to Irradiation. — There is no fixed limit to the number of times irradiation may be repeated. Eventually a time comes, however, when despite all efforts the patient's condition becomes rapidly worse. Such refractoriness to irradiation is rare early in chronic leukemia but eventually develops in all cases. Chemotherapy may be found effective in these circumstances. Eventually, however, all forms of treatment become ineffective.

Contraindications to Irradiation. —**Leukopenia** subsequent to irradiation treatment of leukemia is usually a contraindication to further therapy or at least indicates the need for caution. Leukopenia in "aleukemic" leukemia, however, need not necessarily prevent irradiation. In fact, if the case is a chronic one and particularly if pressure symptoms exist, benefit may follow roentgen-ray therapy. In some instances even anemia has been relieved. There appears to be a substantial margin of safety at leukopenic levels. Even in cases with leukocytosis it can be noted that the rapidity of fall in the count becomes less and less marked as the number of cells is reduced.

As already stated, increasing thrombocytopenia or aggravation of anemia indicate caution in therapy, but the presence of these findings before treatment does not mean that treatment by irradiation is contraindicated. With a reduction of the leukocyte level, anemia may be relieved and the platelet count may rise. Likewise the presence in the blood of some immature cells is not necessarily a contraindication to treatment if the case is one of chronic leukemia. A high proportion of such cells, however, suggests the approach of a refractory state.

Fever alone is not a contraindication to irradiation in uncomplicated chronic leukemia, as Figure 19-16 indicates. Irradiation to the abdomen should be avoided during pregnancy because of the danger of injuring the fetus.

The **mode of action of irradiation** has been discussed elsewhere (p. 556). It is well established that the cells of the peripheral blood are extremely radioresistant.[170a] The hypothesis that cells exposed to irradiation are stimulated to complete their normal life cycle more rapidly than normal does not appear to be well founded[199] but there is evidence that irradiation is capable of influencing hemopoiesis in the bone marrow even when only the spleen has been irradiated.[81a,170a] In cases of chronic myelocytic leukemia, mitotic inhibition has been observed in the marrow eighty minutes after irradiation of the spleen,[81a] as well as a reduction in cellularity as the result of a decrease in the number of cells of the granulocytic series.[170a] The ineffectiveness of roentgen therapy in acute as compared with chronic leukemias is not surprising in view of the fact that rapidly dividing and immature cells are comparatively insensitive to irradiation.[13]

Radioactive Phosphorus. — **Phosphorus** (P^{31}), made *radioactive*[177] (P^{32}) in cyclotrons, has been found useful as a weapon against leukemia. This method of treatment offers the advantage that the radioactive material is concentrated in a position where phosphorus is espe-

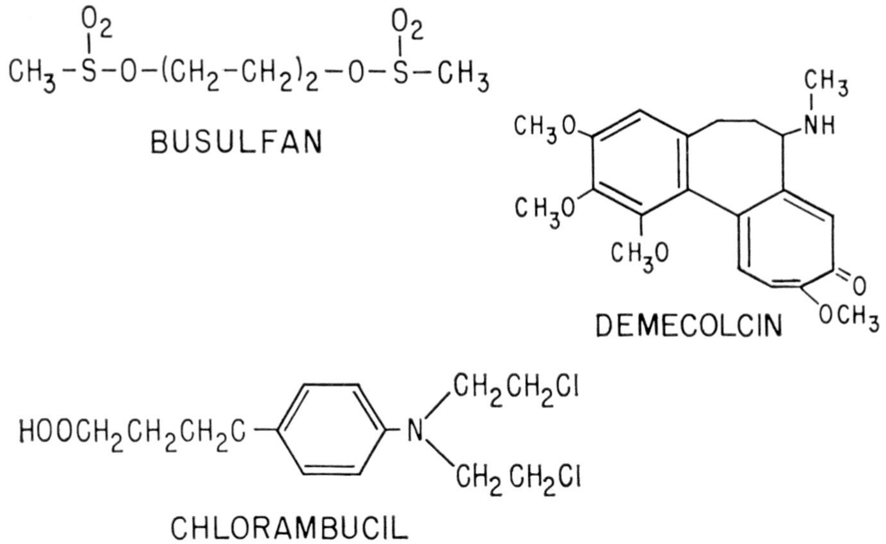

Fig. 19–31.—Chemical structures of compounds effective in the treatment of chronic leukemia.

cially required, since the activated phosphorus is found in those tissues which have a high phosphorus content and which metabolize phosphorus rapidly. The radioactive isotope is built into nucleoprotein just as is ordinary phosphorus and thus cells which are multiplying at the fastest rate use proportionately more P^{32} than do cells which are being produced more slowly. It has been found by examination of the tissues of patients dead of leukemia that the concentration of radioactive phosphorus is highest in those tissues that usually show a heavy infiltration of leukemic cells, namely the liver, spleen, kidneys and bone marrow, and is very low in slowly metabolizing tissues such as brain, fat and cartilage.[214c] Since the "half life" of radioactive phosphorus is fourteen and a half days, its action is continuous. Although it can be given orally, the intravenous route is preferred[137b] because a more accurate relationship can be maintained between the amount retained and the dose administered. The radioactive phosphorus is usually given in the form of its dibasic sodium salt, dissolved in water to make an isotonic solution.

As in the case of roentgen therapy, one cannot give enough radioactive phosphorus to destroy all leukemic cells without also destroying erythroid and megakaryocytic elements.[177] There is the advantage, however, as compared with roentgen therapy, that radiation sickness does not occur when therapeutic doses are given.

A common procedure is to inject from 1 to 2.5 millicuries of P^{32} approximately at intervals of two weeks, a total of 6 to 12 mc. being given in a single course, the actual amount depending on the extent of the leukocytosis and the degree of bone marrow hyperplasia.[177] Osgood prefers "titrated," regularly spaced therapy. By his procedure,[167a] for each patient the fewest doses and the smallest amounts which will bring the leukocyte count below 24,000 within 12 weeks are used and an attempt is made to keep the leukocyte count at 15,000 and the patient in good condition by the administration of P^{32} at intervals of four to 12 weeks. The total amount of P^{32} given during the first 12 weeks defines the threshold dose. As with other forms of therapy, approximately half as much P^{32} is usually needed to control chronic lymphocytic leukemia as compared with the myelocytic form. In the management of "aleukemic" leukemia, doses of P[32] similar to those administered to patients with elevated leukocyte counts have been used. In acute leukemia, P[32] has little value.[177]

Busulfan (1-4, dimethanesulfonyloxybutane, Myleran).—An important advance in the treatment of chronic myelo-

cytic leukemia came with the discovery[82b] of the beneficial action of busulfan (Fig. 19–31). In this disease the drug has been found superior to other chemotherapeutic agents[188] and it is now the practice of many to prescribe it in preference to radiation. In some patients who responded badly to *x*-ray therapy from the start or whose remissions had become progressively shorter, busulfan was found

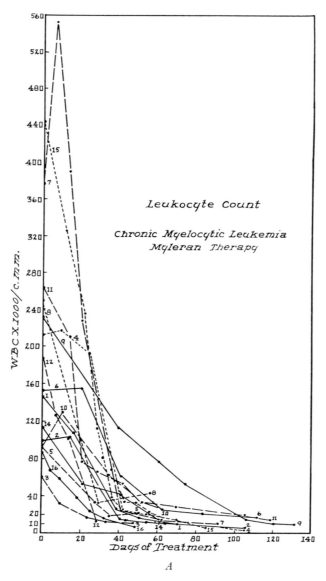

Leukocyte Count

Chronic Myelocytic Leukemia
Myleran Therapy

A

FIG. 19–32.—Legend on opposite page.

to be effective.[69] In the sense that it is recommended for the treatment of chronic myelocytic leukemia, and in view of the fact that there are better agents than busulfan for the treatment of other forms of leukemia, this drug can be thought of as being rather specific in its action. Its mode of action was discussed earlier (p. 963).

About 60 μg./Kg., generally amounting to 4 or 6 mg., is given daily in a single dose before breakfast. Treatment is continued until the number of leukocytes falls just below 10,000 per c.mm. It has been observed that the duration of therapy is roughly proportional to the logarithm of the pretreatment leukocyte count;[84] at the recommended dose it can be anticipated that the leukocyte count will be halved about every three weeks. The total duration of therapy, depending upon the height of the initial leukocyte count, usually is 70 to 90 days. Following the first course of therapy the differential leukocyte count usually returns to normal, as well as the total count, anemia is relieved without having to resort to blood transfusion (Fig. 19-32, B), the platelet count returns to normal and

the spleen is either reduced to normal size or else to less than half its initial bulk. Remissions have been maintained for as long as two years, the longer interval usually occurring in patients with a leukocyte count below 10,000 per c.mm. when therapy was stopped.

During remissions the patient is examined at one to three month intervals. When the leukocyte count has risen again to 50,000 per c.mm., treatment is repeated. With repeated treatment any residual splenomegaly is further reduced. After subsequent courses the period of remission ultimately tends to become shorter and in the end about half the patients enter a phase of the disease resembling acute myeloblastic leukemia. However, before the onset of this terminal phase we have observed as many as 12 successful remissions resulting from busulfan therapy over periods of time ranging up to six years.

When the leukocyte count returns from the post-treatment level of under 10,000 to 50,000 per c.mm. within three months, it may be well to consider maintenance therapy; for example, 2 mg. of busulfan given two or three times weekly, or more

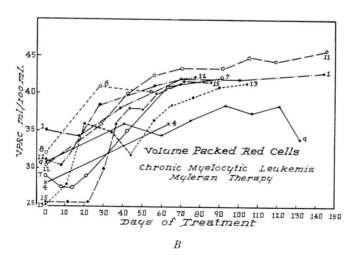

B

FIG. 19–32.—Changes in the blood in a series of cases of chronic myelocytic leukemia treated with busulfan. *A*, the rapid drop in the number of leukocytes; *B*, the simultaneous decrease of anemia as manifested by the rise in volume of packed red cells. In most instances the anemia was relieved completely.

often, as needed to prevent rapid relapse.[69] Otherwise, an important advantage of busulfan as compared with other forms of chemotherapy for this disease is the fact that maintenance therapy and, thus, constant supervision, is not required.

When the "acute" terminal phase develops, x-ray has not been found to be of any benefit but demecolcin and 6-mercaptopurine (6MP) are helpful for a time.

In the doses recommended, toxic effects from busulfan are very unusual. The chief danger is the development of pancytopenia as the consequence of prolongation of therapy beyond the recommended time, or, occasionally, with the usual course of therapy in an unexpectedly sensitive patient. The development of thrombocytopenia is a useful warning signal. In one patient who received 8 mg. daily for eight months, glossitis, anhydrosis and alopecia totalis developed. The infant born of a mother with leukemia who received 6MP and x-ray early in pregnancy and busulfan throughout most of the gestation period showed several congenital anomalies and other changes,[43a] but in two other instances no ill effects were observed.[194b]

Demecolcin (desacetylcochicine, Colcemide) (Fig. 19–31).—Isolated from the mixed alkaloid extract of *Colchicum autumnale*, this inhibitor of cell mitosis[91c] is 30 times less toxic than colchicine. It has been used in oral doses of 3 to 10 mg. daily for the treatment of chronic myelocytic leukemia.[132a] Starting with an initial dose of 3 mg., this may be gradually increased after three or four days, ultimately even to 7 or 10 mg. daily, the greater doses being used when the leukocyte count is very high. When the leukocyte count has decreased to 25,000 per c.mm., treatment is interrupted for three or four days and then a maintenance dose of 3 to 5 mg. daily is instituted. At this and lower levels of leukocyte count,

alterations in dose of 0.5 mg. or less may make the difference between satisfactory and poor control. Failure to resume therapy may result in a rising leukocyte count which may not decrease again for several weeks. It is claimed that thrombocytopenia and severe marrow hypoplasia do not develop on these doses but larger amounts will cause pancytopenia, ulcerative stomatitis, alopecia and herpetiform dermatitis.[44b]

Demecolcin has not been found effective in other forms of leukemia and, because of the need to maintain administration continuously, and to adjust the dose even to fractions of a milligram, we have preferred busulfan for the treatment of chronic myelocytic leukemia. However, as already mentioned, it has been useful for a time in doses of 3 to 5 mg. daily when busulfan has ceased to be effective, as well as in other special circumstances; for example, in some cases of leukemia cutis.[193e]

Urethane (ethyl carbamate). — Following the accidental discovery that this agent may produce leukopenia,[82a] it was shown to be capable of influencing both experimental and human leukemia.[172] As discussed elsewhere (p. 964), its mode of action is obscure. Urethane produces lymphocytopenia as well as granulocytopenia but therapeutically it was found useful only in the management of chronic myelocytic leukemia. With the availability of other agents, however, its use even in this form of leukemia has been abandoned and it now is employed only in the treatment of multiple myeloma (p. 1075).

Triethylenemelamine (TEM).—Following the discovery of the therapeutic effectiveness of nitrogen mustard, several hundred chemical congeners were prepared[139c] but only a few have earned an important place in the treatment of leukemia. TEM[121a] is similar in action to nitrogen mustard but it can be given orally as well as intravenously and pro-

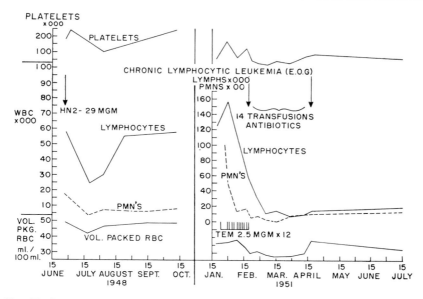

Fig. 19–33.—To illustrate the hidden danger of continouus administration of TEM. This patient with chronic lymphocytic leukemia (E.O.G.) was given 12 doses of 2.5 mg. each over a period of 26 days. A profound leukopenia developed, as well as marked marrow hypoplasia, from which he recovered only after much difficulty. Earlier in his course this patient had done relatively well on nitrogen mustard therapy.

duces relatively little nausea or vomiting. It is stable in alkaline solutions, forming the biologically active ethylenimonium ions (p. 1038) in acid solutions. For this reason, when it is administered orally it is best given two or three hours before breakfast on an empty stomach, together with 2 grams of sodium bicarbonate. The intravenous dose is approximately a third of the oral dose.

In the leukemias, TEM is now employed only in the treatment of chronic lymphocytic leukemia since better agents are available for the other forms of leukemia. The margin between therapeutic and toxic doses is narrow[3b] and the drug must be used cautiously. Preferably, it is best not used at all if thrombocytopenia is present. In contrast to nitrogen mustard (Fig. 19–33) the action of TEM is somewhat slower and there is risk of a cumulative effect from its repeated administration at short intervals. For this reason, a dose of 2.5 mg. is given at first. Thereafter, the patient and

his blood are examined once weekly, prior to succeeding doses, to determine if further treatment is necessary and to avoid bone marrow depression. Three or more weeks may elapse before the full marrow depressant action of a dose may be realized. Depending upon the response, in some cases the dose may need to be increased to 5 mg. weekly, while in other cases it may be decreased (Fig. 19–34). Nothing is gained by the intravenous administration of TEM.

Chlorambucil (p-NN-di-2-chloroethylaminophenylbutyric acid, "CB 1348," Leukeran) (Fig. 19–31).—This aromatic mustard[1c] offers a greater margin of safety than TEM and, therefore, is now preferred.[84c] Its absorption is more consistent and not related to food intake. Given in a daily dose of 0.1 to 0.2 mg./Kg., it affords a better regulated response with less chance of unexpected bone marrow depression (Fig. 19–35). Daily treatment may be continued for weeks or months but the dose should be adjusted

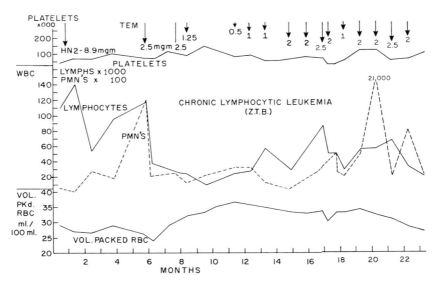

FIG. 19–34.—To illustrate the sensitivity of some patients with chronic lymphocytic leukemia to TEM. In this case (Z.T.B.) 2.5 mg. had a pronounced effect. It should be noted that absolute numbers of lymphocytes and of polymorphonuclear leukocytes are plotted rather than the total leukocyte count.

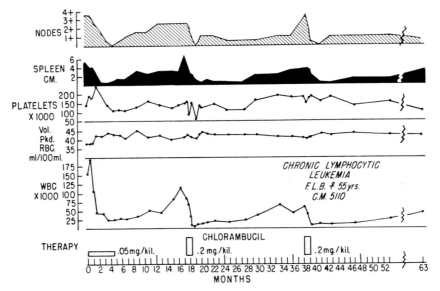

FIG. 19–35.—Course of a patient (F.L.B.) with chronic lymphocytic leukemia who had marked leukocytosis but only slight anemia and thrombocytopenia and has been treated at long intervals with chlorambucil.

according to the lymphocyte count and care must be taken to avoid the development of severe thrombocytopenia, anemia, or leukopenia as side effects of treatment. Sometimes treatment can be continued in spite of a modest thrombocytopenia and a slight drop in the hemoglobin level if the leukocyte count has not dropped sufficiently or a greater reduction in the size of the lymph nodes or spleen is desired but this, if done at all, must be carried out cautiously. Often, in such cases, when treatment has been interrupted, the anemia becomes less marked and thrombocytopenia disappears while the desired effects on the leukocyte count and physical signs are maintained. Treatment is resumed on relapse. It is our practice to restart therapy when the leukocyte count has reached 50,000 per c.mm. again, but this should be considered to be only a rough guide. The condition of the patient is the most important consideration.

Other than the potential occurrence of bone marrow hypoplasia, toxic effects after therapeutic doses have included dermatitis and one instance of jaundice and hepatomegaly attributed to the drug.[126]

Although a beneficial effect can be achieved in chronic myelocytic leukemia,[148b] busulfan is preferable in the treatment of that disease.[188] Chlorambucil has been found to be valuable, however, in the management of Hodgkin's disease and other lymph node disorders (p. 1043).[148b]

To what extent one of the newest alkylating agents, uracil-mustard (5-bis-[2'-chloroethyl]aminouracil) offers promise,[193g] remains to be demonstrated.

Folic Acid Antagonists.—The observation that folic acid deficiency (p. 132) is associated with leukopenia as well as the impression that the course of the disease in patients with acute leukemia treated with folic acid conjugates

appeared to be accelerated[55] led to the trial of metabolic antagonists of folic (pteroylglutamic) acid in leukemia. Of most interest have been those in which the substituents of the pteridine ring of folic acid (Figure 19–36) are either changed or other groups added, as well as those in which, besides these alterations, the glutamic acid is substituted by another amino acid. Aminopterin (4-aminopteroylglutamic acid), amethopterin (4-amino-N_{10}methyl-pteroylglutamic acid) and, to a lesser extent, amino-an-fol (4-amino-pteroylaspartic acid), dichloroamethopterin (3'-5' dichloroamethopterin) and other antagonists have been used in clinical trials.

There is no doubt that the use of these agents is associated in some patients with improvement, often of remarkable degree. In the hands of different investigators the results have varied to some degree and in adults, as compared with children, improvement has been observed less often. The degree of improvement has also varied, but in 18 to 56 per cent of the cases the remission was considered to be complete; that is, *no signs of the disease remained*.[84a] Anemia, thrombocytopenia and purpura disappeared, the leukocytic picture returned to normal and even the bone marrow appeared to be normal. This hematological improvement was accompanied by a sense of well-being and other signs of restoration of a normal state. Remission was achieved following two to 15 weeks of therapy. The duration of the individual remissions has varied considerably, from one month to even 30 months.[175a] Beneficial results have been observed more often in acute lymphoblastic leukemia than in the other forms. Remissions have been observed when there was initial leukopenia as well as in those cases in which leukocytosis was present. More than one remission has been produced in a number of cases although, in many, treatment on relapse was less satisfactory than initially.

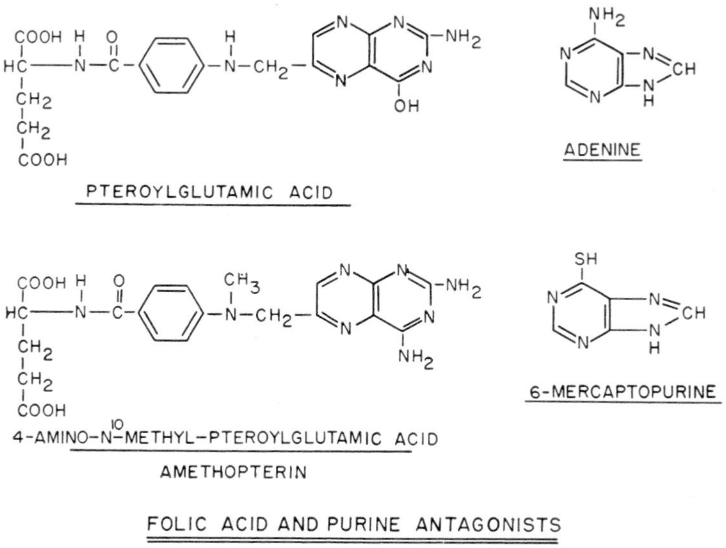

FOLIC ACID AND PURINE ANTAGONISTS

FIG. 19–36.—Chemical structures of amethopterin and 6-mercaptopurine.

Amethopterin (Methotrexate) is the folic acid antagonist which is now used, as a rule, because dose regulation is more readily achieved. However, aminopterin, in doses of 0.5 to 2. mg. daily is an equally effective agent (Fig. 19–37). The daily dose of amethopterin varies from 1.25 mg. in a small child to 10 mg. in a large adult. The average child of two to eight years receives from 2.5 to 5 mg. daily, the exact dose being individualized according to the response. Administration is continued until benefit is observed or toxic effects develop. The latter include stomatitis, diarrhea, skin and mucous membrane hemorrhage, pancytopenia and alopecia. Macrocytic anemia and even the appearance of cells resembling megaloblasts in the bone marrow may result from overdosage. It is sometimes difficult to distinguish signs of toxicity from those of acute leukemia. Repeated blood examinations and serial bone marrow studies are helpful. If the immature cells in the blood and bone marrow are reduced in number when stomatitis or diarrhea appears, the presumption is that these are indications for interruption

of therapy. If there has been no beneficial effect on the blood, administration of the drug may be continued cautiously, but only under careful supervision. Alopecia is not necessarily an indication for the cessation of therapy since the hair will return even though administration of the drug is continued. Portal cirrhosis of the liver has been reported in children following long-term therapy with amethopterin and with other forms of chemotherapy.[99]

Although second and third remissions have been achieved with this drug,[84e] these are likely to be less successful than the first course of therapy and it is better usually to resort to another agent. On the basis of observations on the effects of large, infrequent doses of amethopterin in leukemic mice, large infrequent doses (1 to 5 mg./Kg.) given parenterally and and repeated at intervals of from two to four weeks have received preliminary trial in a few patients in the hope that this may be effective when refractoriness has developed to the usual forms of therapy.[31b]

No benefit from the use of folic acid

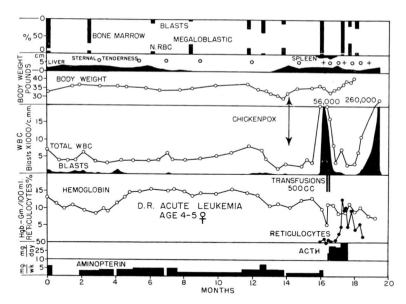

FIG. 19–37.—Course of a patient (D.R.) with acute lymphoblastic leukemia treated successfully with aminopterin for more than a year. The remission induced with ACTH, after aminopterin resistance had developed, was very brief.

antagonists has been observed in the chronic leukemias.

The intrathecal administration of amethopterin was discussed earlier (p. 959).

It has been shown in leukemic animals that the folic acid antagonists can markedly inhibit the incorporation of isotopically labelled precursors into the nucleic acid purines of normal and leukemic tissues.[195] The metabolic site of this inhibition has been shown to be in the *de novo* synthesis of purines, an effect which is accomplished by inhibiting the transfer of single-carbon (formyl) groups into certain positions of the purine ring.[126b] Different folic acid antagonists may act at different sites in the series of reactions which are involved in nucleic acid synthesis. Although amethopterin is thought to block the reduction of tetrahydrofolic acid to the N^{10}-formyl derivative, experience has not borne out the hope that its acute toxic effects could be counteracted by the administration

of citrovorum factor in a dose amounting to approximately 5 or 10 per cent of the dose of folic acid antagonist.[24]

Purine Analogues.—The first of these compounds which was given extensive clinical trial, *6-mercaptopurine*[91a] (6MP, Purinethol), (Fig. 19–36), was found effective in all forms of acute leukemia and "good" clinical and hematological remissions were observed in somewhat less than 50 per cent of children with acute leukemia[25] and in 14[25] to 54[82c] per cent of adults. The remissions lasted from one to ten months and were observed even in patients who had become resistant to folic acid antagonists or to steroid hormones (Fig. 19–38). The usual therapeutic dose is 2.5 mg./Kg. body weight per day, by mouth[25] although sometimes twice this amount has been used.[82c] A remission, once achieved, may persist for a time without therapy (Fig. 19–39) but the usual practice is to continue daily administration until either a relapse occurs or signs or symptoms of

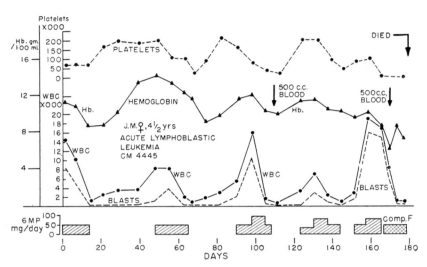

FIG. 19–38.—Effect of 6-mercaptopurine in a child (J.M.) with acute lymphoblastic leukemia who failed to respond to cortisone and amethopterin therapy after a year of successful management.

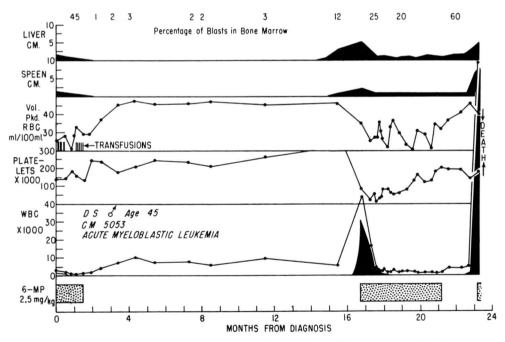

FIG. 19–39.—Long remission following administration of 6-mercaptopurine in an adult patient with acute myeloblastic leukemia.

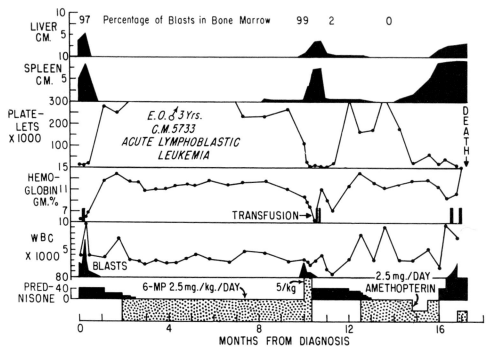

FIG. 19–40.—Course of a patient with acute lymphoblastic leukemia treated successively with predni-sone, 6-mercaptopurine, prednisone and amethopterin, illustrating the method of continuous treatment with a succession of agents.

overdosage appear (Fig. 19–40). Many patients tolerate 2.5 mg./Kg. well; in other cases smaller amounts must be given to avoid toxicity. One of our patients received the drug for 31 consecutive months, without ill effect, remaining in remission throughout. Second remissions sometimes can be obtained but they usually are less complete than the first.

The main toxic effect of overdosage is suppression of one or all of the normal cellular elements of the marrow and blood. If this occurs, administration of the drug may be stopped for a few days, then resumed at half the dose. Gradually, the dose may be raised, somewhat, to the maximum which avoids toxicity. However, a moderate leukopenia (3,000 to 4,000 leukocytes per c.mm.) is frequently encountered in patients who sustain a long remission under treatment and should not be considered sufficient ground to reduce the dose, for no harm comes from it. A lesser dose might permit the disease to escape from control earlier than would be the case if the standard dose were continued.

Another toxic effect of 6MP is the development of jaundice. In our experience this is an infrequent occurrence but others have reported this complication in as many as one-third of the patients treated with 6MP or the related compound, 6-chloropurine.[49] The pathogenesis of the jaundice is obscure. It usually clears when 6MP administration is stopped, or even when it is continued, but in some instances it has persisted. Bile-stasis and, in other cases, hepatic necrosis[30a] have been observed.

The differentiation of drug-induced cytopenia from that accompanying relapse of leukemia is based on the same

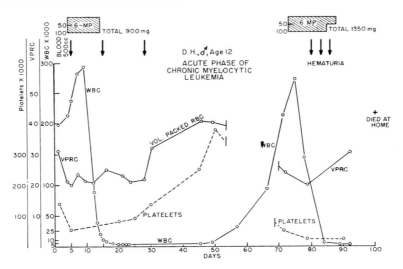

F<small>IG</small>. 19–41.—Effect of 6-mercaptopurine in a boy with chronic myelocytic leukemia of 20
months' duration in the final "myeloblastic" phase.

criteria as in the case of the folic acid antagonists, described above. The absence of immature leukocytes in the blood and lack of physical signs of developing relapse speak for toxicity. Sometimes the decision cannot be made without resorting to bone marrow examination.

Studies of toxicity in animals indicated that damage to the bone marrow and intestinal epithelium and disturbances in hepatic function may occur.[91a] In human subjects oral lesions or gastrointestinal symptoms are less common than is the case when folic acid antagonists are used, but redness and ulceration of the buccal mucosa, lips and tongue have been observed.[91a]

In chronic myelocytic leukemia improvement can be produced with 6MP but maintenance therapy is required.[25] Busulfan is therefore preferable. However, in the terminal acute stage of chronic myelocytic leukemia, the use of 6MP will bring about partial remissions, unfortunately of brief duration (Fig. 19–41).

The precise mechanism of action of 6MP is still uncertain. It is thought that its principal site of action may be in the conversion of a hypoxanthine-containing compound to an adenine-containing one.[126b]

Of the other purine analogues which have been synthesized and tested in animals and in man, some (purine and 8-azaguanine) have shown no therapeutic effect at toxic doses whereas others have been found useful in about the same degree as 6MP. The latter include 6-thioguanine and 6-chloropurine.[49] Consequently, there appears to be no reason to use them in preference to 6MP.

Glutamine Antagonists.— Neither *azaserine* nor DON (6-diazo-5-oxo-L-norleucine) has been found to be of significant value in the treatment of acute leukemia, even when given in combination with 6MP,[86b] despite the evidence of their effectiveness in leukemias in animals.[126b]

Pyrimidine Analogues. — These agents, such as 5-fluorouracil and 6-aza-uracil[61a] have been disappointing, although it was reported that, in a few children with acute leukemia resistant to other forms of therapy, complete remission occurred with 5-fluoro-2-deoxy-uridine.[39c]

Adrenocortical Hormones and Adrenocorticotrophic Hormone (ACTH).—The remarkable effects of these hormones on the blood, already referred to elsewhere (p. 49), led naturally to their trial in the treatment of the leukemias. Impressive effects have been observed in certain cases of acute leukemia and of chronic lymphocytic leukemia (p. 960). In acute leukemia, the administration of one of these agents may bring about dramatic improvement in a critically ill patient within two or three days and in the course of four to six weeks produces a complete remission which may persist for several months. This impressive effect, however, is not achieved in all cases. Of a total of 425 cases,[57] complete remissions were claimed only in approximately 30 per cent of the patients and partial remissions in another 24 per cent.

Up to that time, little attempt had been made to study the cause of differences in responsiveness to antileukemic agents. It was generally recognized that remissions are much more likely to develop in children than in adults. Little attention, however, had been paid to the possible cause of this difference or to the type of leukemia. It is noteworthy that, among the 425 above-mentioned cases, complete remissions occurred in 35 per cent of cases classified as lymphoblastic or "undifferentiated" and only in 5 per cent of those considered to be myeloblastic or monocytic.[57] In a retrospective analysis of the outcome in 50 cases of acute leukemia, classified without knowledge of the source of the blood smears and bone marrows, the writer and his associates found that complete remissions had occurred in 68 per cent of the cases of acute lymphoblastic leukemia and in none of those falling into the myeloblastic or monocytic categories.[57] In the latter, in fact, the impression was gained that these hormones sometimes even seemed

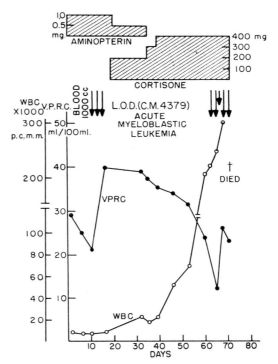

Fig. 19–42.—Course of a patient (L.O.D.), 29 years of age, with acute myeloblastic leukemia who clearly improved on aminopterin therapy. Treatment with cortisone was instituted in the hope that a prolonged remission might be produced; instead, rapid deterioration took place.

to accelerate the leukemic process (Fig. 19–42). Study of the literature tends to support this view.

In acute lymphoblastic leukemia the administration of 40 mg. of prednisone or prednisolone, corresponding amounts of methylprednisolone, triamcinolone or dexamethasone, or 150 to 250 mg. of cortisone or hydrocortisone, is associated with disappearance of fever, a return of appetite, a feeling of improvement, cessation of hemorrhagic manifestations and a decrease in the leukocyte count (Fig. 19–43). The number of leukocytes decreases in three to seven days to levels below 5000 per c.mm., the proportion of lymphoblasts decreasing at the same time. An increase in the leukocyte count after two weeks of therapy is due to the appearance

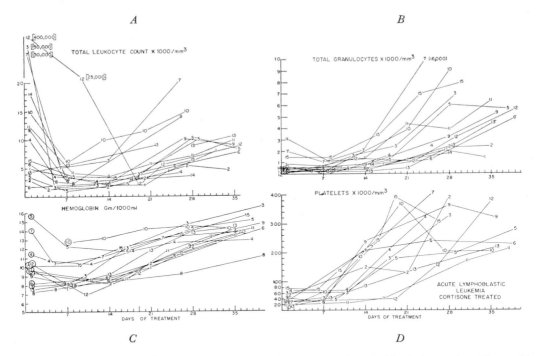

Fɪɢ. 19–43.—The effects of cortisone therapy in 15 cases of acute lymphoblastic leukemia. The rapid decrease in the number of leukocytes (*A*), often to leukopenic levels, was accompanied by the disappearance of the leukemic cells. After two weeks of therapy normal granulocytes made their appearance (*B*), erythropoiesis began to be effective (*C*) and the platelet count rose (*D*) so that an essentially normal blood picture was present in most cases at the end of five or six weeks. The numbers correspond to individual cases. Those in circles refer to patients who were given transfusions either immediately before therapy or still earlier in the course of their disease, with the exception of Case 10. This patient was transfused during therapy. The remaining cases were not transfused.

of granulocytes. For a brief period, polymorphonuclear leukocytosis of mild degree may develop. The number of platelets usually commences to increase after the first week and after two weeks the hemoglobin level will generally begin to rise. At the end of four to six weeks not only the blood but the bone marrow is likely to be normal and the patient appears well except for the signs of hypercorticism. These include, in particular, rounding of the face, some bulging of the abdomen, increased growth of hair, a "buffalo hump" on the back of the neck and sometimes, in older subjects, a "turkey wattle" in the front. In our experience, hypertension and diabetes have been rare consequences of adrenocorti-

coid therapy but edema may develop, even in children. This result is held to a minimum by the taking of a salt-poor diet and potassium chloride, 3 to 10 Gm. daily, in the form of tablets of 0.3 to 1.0 Gm. size. Osteoporosis and muscle weakness have also been observed.[57]

The adrenocortical hormones should be taken at three or four evenly spaced intervals in the course of the day. They have the advantage that they can be taken by mouth. Hydrocortisone, prednisone or ACTH (corticotropin) can be given intravenously, the latter in an eight- to twelve-hour daily infusion of glucose solution containing 25 to 50 mg. Double these amounts can be given intramuscularly but this is not desirable since it is best

Table 19–4.—Side Effects of ACTH and Steroid Therapy

Features seeen in Cushing's syndrome	Other side effects
Electrolytic	*Enjoyable*
Fluid retention—edema	Appetite increase
Hypokaliemia	Mild euphoria
Disfiguring	*Disturbing*
Round facial contour, plethoric appearance	Insomnia
Humps—cervicodorsal ("buffalo")	Polyuria
anterocervical ("turkey")	Headache
Acne, pigmentation, hirsutism, and baldness	Thin skin, striae, easy bruising, poor healing
Kyphosis	Myopathy
Disquieting	*Alarming*
Muscle wasting	Epigastric discomfort (peptic ulcer)
Hypertension	Intercurrent infections (Tbc !)
Glycosuria	Osteoporosis
Menstrual disturbances, impotence	Psychiatric symptoms
	Convulsions

to avoid parenteral injections in these patients. Neither is there any reason for intravenous administration of these compounds if the patient is able to take prednisone or a related compound orally.

Nothing is gained from interrupted or continuous administration of the adrenocorticosteroids[99a] but much is lost in the way of inviting the persistence or development of many of the untoward effects of these agents (Table 19–4), not to speak of the expense of long term therapy. For this reason, it is our practice to replace adrenocorticosteroids with 6MP or amethopterin for maintenance therapy (Fig. 19–40). This can usually be done after six weeks of hormone therapy, this being the time when maximum improvement is achieved, as a rule. The dose of the latter is reduced gradually in the course of two weeks. ACTH administration is unnecessary as a support during this weaning process.

Second remissions following administration of these hormones are usually less complete than the initial response or may not develop at all.

Others, like ourselves, have observed cases of myeloblastic and monocytic leukemia in which the administration of adrenocorticosteroids seemed to accele-

rate the process rather than being beneficial.[12a,205] However, this has not been the experience in all cases of these types of leukemia and factors other than the recognized morphological differences presumably play a role in the response to treatment. This deserves further study but it is the writer's practice to avoid the use of adrenocorticosteroids in these forms of acute leukemia, giving preference, instead, to 6MP.

Claims have been made for the beneficial effects of massive doses (250 or even 1000 mg. prednisone) of adrenocorticosteroids, especially in cases in which conventional dosage has not been helpful.[17a,175e] The subject deserves further critical study; to the writer, the evidence is as yet unconvincing. Such dosage invites serious complications, which are best avoided.

Effects of Therapy on Survival in Leukemia.—Although the beneficial effects of the antileukemic agents are clear from the standpoint of reduced morbidity, it has been less definitely established that they have increased survival. The course of leukemia, as already pointed out, varies considerably from case to case and thus makes evaluation of the long-term effects of therapy a difficult problem.

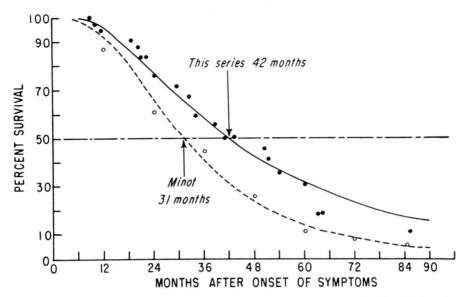

FIG. 19–44.—Comparison of survival in 30 cases treated in the writer's clinic[84] with busulfan, compared with untreated cases (Minot). Points represent original data. The lines were transcribed from log-probability plots of the data.

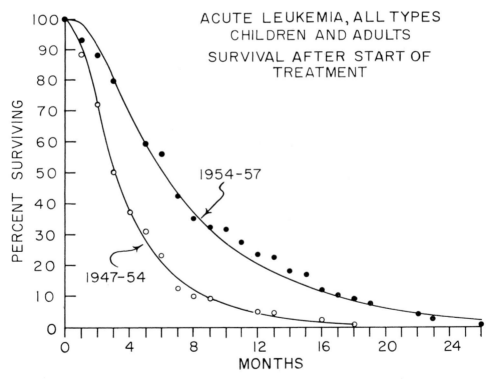

FIG. 19–45.—Survival in acute leukemia, all types and all ages, measured from the time of start of treatment. Cases treated in the author's clinic[84a] in two periods, showing the improved survival with the use of adrenocorticosteroids, 6MP and amethopterin as against a time when the effects of 6MP, in particular, could not have been included to any significant extent. Points represent original data. The lines were transcribed from log-probability plots of the data.

There are few wholly satisfactory data for the chronic leukemias. In 30 cases of *chronic myelocytic leukemia* treated with busulfan, a median survival of 42 months was observed,[84] which compares favorably with Minot's untreated cases[154] (Fig. 19–44). In comparable groups of cases treated with P[32] or X-ray therapy, the median survival was 32 to 41 and 1/2 months. For *chronic lymphocytic leukemia*, few satisfactory data are available. For a group of 100 cases of both forms of chronic leukemia a median survival of 58 months was recorded.[167b]

For *acute leukemia* there is good evidence now that survival has been prolonged by present day therapy. An analysis of our own cases showed a median survival of six as compared with three months for 89 cases of all types and ages treated between March 1954 and December 1957 as compared with 78 patients treated before that time[84a] (Fig. 19–45). In acute lymphoblastic leukemia the median survival was even better, namely ten months after the symptomatic onset of leukemia and seven and a half months after the start of treatment. Within this group there was a still greater improvement for those whose leukocyte values immediately prior to the initiation of therapy were less than 10,000 per c.mm.; half of these patients lived more than 12 months after treatment was begun. These data emphasize the relative inefficacy of chemotherapy for acute myeloblastic leukemia.

Similar but less clearly improved results have been published by others.[161a]

PATHOLOGY

The primary changes in chronic myelocytic leukemia are in the bone marrow and spleen but infiltration by leukemic cells is also found in the lymph nodes, liver, kidneys, lungs, skin and other organs, as has been indicated already. In chronic lymphocytic leukemia there is tremendous hyperplasia of lymphoid organs with disturbance of the architecture of the lymph nodes, spleen and even the bone marrow. In addition, infiltration occurs in other tissues, especially the liver, kidneys, intestine, skin and lungs. In acute leukemia the postmortem findings vary only slightly from those encountered in the chronic form save that changes such as would require greater time for their development are more prominent in the latter than in the former ailment.

Bone Marrow.—The marrow of the long bones is largely or entirely changed from fatty tissue to active marrow, usually gray in color but sometimes brown, dark red or even purulent in appearance. Although invasion or destruction of the bone is unusual, exceptions have been observed (p. 920). Nodular growths of leukemic cells are sometimes found (p. 937). In some cases of lymphocytic leukemia the bone marrow may be only slightly involved although this is unusual. Details of the microscopic picture of the bone marrow have been given (p. 943). Subperiosteal leukemic infiltration has also been discussed (p. 922).

Spleen.[128a] — The spleen is usually huge in chronic myelocytic leukemia (2 to 10 kg.). The normal splenic outline is in great measure preserved. The spleen may be adherent to the diaphragm or the abdominal wall and white areas of thickened peritoneum may be present over the sites of infarcts or perisplenitis. The consistency is firm. The normal color may be changed to a grayish tint. On section the Malpighian bodies are not to be seen, and hemorrhagic infarcts are common. On microscopic examination the splenic tissue resembles bone marrow in appearance, so great is the infiltration with myelocytes and older granulocytes. Normoblasts and megakaryocytes are also numerous.

In acute myeloblastic leukemia the enlargement is not as great as in chronic myelocytic leukemia, but infiltration with myeloblasts may be intense nevertheless.

A type of large cell, not noted hitherto, has been described.[190a] In lymphocytic leukemias the extreme enlargement of the myelocytic form is unusual. The consistence of the organ is variable, depending upon the duration of the disease. Infarcts are frequent. Few Malpighian bodies are seen on the cut surface. The microscopic architecture[108] is entirely disorganized by the lymphocytic infiltration.

Lymph Nodes.[125a]—The lymph nodes in chronic myelocytic leukemia may be of normal size or slightly enlarged. The microscopic picture is similar to that of the spleen. In chronic lymphocytic leukemia the dominant feature in the postmortem findings is the glandular enlargement, which is practically universal. The glands vary greatly in size but their outline is usually maintained. In acute lymphoblastic leukemia the glands are less firm and usually not as large as in the chronic form. Unlike leukosarcoma and lymphosarcoma, invasion of surrounding tissue is absent.

On section the glands appear soft and gray or pinkish-gray in color, smooth and homogeneous. Unlike benign hyperplasia in which the essential architecture of the glands is preserved, there is complete obliteration of normal outlines. The cells which pack the gland in the chronic disease are small lymphocytes, strikingly uniform in size and character. In acute leukemia, between the leukemic cells, vestiges of the normal architecture may still remain and hemorrhages may be observed.

Liver.—The liver is often enormous in size in chronic leukemia. The surface is pale, reddish-gray or gray. Small nodules may sometimes be seen on the cut surface. The blood vessels are tremendously distended with cells, and cells are also found about the vessels. The liver tissue itself is compressed. In lymphocytic leukemia there are, in addition, collections of cells in the portal tracts. In acute leukemia invasion of the liver is less marked.

Reference has already been made in earlier sections to the infiltration of kidneys, lungs, skin, intestines, nervous system and other tissues.

Monocytic Leukemia.—In monocytic leukemia the proliferating cells may be those of the reticulum with a liberation of free monocytic cells (Schilling type). In some of the described cases there was an unusually widespread hyperplasia of monocytic cells in the connective tissue, especially about the blood vessels, as well as hyperplasia of endothelium in the spleen, liver, lymph nodes and marrow[31] with projection of these cells into the lumens of the vessels. Many mitotic figures were found. The lymph nodes, in contrast to their state in acute myeloblastic leukemia, have been described as exhibiting destruction of the normal architecture and replacement of lymphocytes by cells of the monocyte series. In few of the cases, however, has the proportion of monocytic cells in the tissues approached the degree of specific cell infiltration seen in either lymphoblastic or myeloblastic leukemia.

In many of the cases of monocytic leukemia some degree of myeloid hyperplasia has been reported.[213a] In a large number the organ changes have been like those found in acute or subacute myeloblastic leukemia, or even like those seen in myelocytic leukemia. In some cases many eosinophilic cells have been found in the tissues. These cases with a myeloid reaction and no marked activity on the part of the reticulum have been referred to as the "Naegeli type."

Present day therapy may produce profound changes in the classical histologic pattern of leukemia, sometimes to the extent that recognition of the disease may be difficult or impossible. In cases of acute leukemia treated with a variety of antileukemic agents, epithelial atypias have been described.[219c]

BIBLIOGRAPHY

1. ACKERMAN, G. A., GRASSO, J. A. and KNOUFF, R. A.: Morphological and Histochemical Studies of the Leukemic Cells from a Patient with Atypical Myeloblastic Leukemia, Blood, *16*, 1253, 1960.

1a. ADAMS, W. S., DAVIS, FRANCES and NAKATANI, MISAE: Purine and Pyrimidine Excretion in Normal and Leukemic Subjects, Am. J. Med., *28*, 726, 1960.

1b. ALBRIGHT, E. C. and MIDDLETON, W. S.: The Uptake of Radioactive Iodine by the Thyroid Gland of Leukemic Patients, Blood, *5*, 764, 1950.

1c. ALTMAN, S. J., HAUT, A., CARTWRIGHT, G. E. and WINTROBE, M. M.: Early Experience with P-N,N-di-2-Chloroethylaminophenyl-butyric Acid ("CB 1348"), a New Chemotherapeutic Agent Effective in the Treatment of Chronic Lymphocytic Leukemia, Cancer, *9*, 512, 1956.

1d. ANDERSON, R. C.: Familial Leukemia, Am. J. Dis. Child., *81*, 313, 1951.

1e. ANDERSON, R. C. and HERMANN, H. W.: Leukemia in Twin Children, J.A.M.A., *158*, 652, 1955.

1f. ANDRE, R., DREYFUS, B. and BESSIS, M.: Lymphoid Leukemia with Leukopenia. The Presence of Anti-leukocytic Auto-antibodies. Favorable Effect of Splenectomy, Soc. med. hôp. Paris, *70*, 384, 1954.

1g. ANLYAN, A. J.: β-glucuronidase Studies in Stem-cell Leukemias, Cancer, *7*, 391, 1954.

2. ARDASHNIKOV, S. N.: Genetics of Leukemia in Man, J. Hyg., *37*, 286, 1937 (Bibliography); Brit. M. J., *2*, 957, 1947.

3a. ASTALDI, G. and CURTI, P. C.: Contributo alla conoscenza della leucemia eosinofila, Haematologica, *30*, 1, 1947.

3b. AXELROD, A. R., BERMAN, L. and MURPHY, R. V.: Clinical and Hematologic Effects of Triethylene Melamine, Am. J. Med., *15*, 684, 1953.

3c. BAIKIE, A. G., COURT BROWN, W. M., JACOBS, PATRICIA A. and MILNE, J. S.: Chromosome Studies in Human Leukaemia, Lancet, *2*, 425, 1959.

3d. BALDINI, M., FUDENBERG, H. H., FUKUTAKE, K. and DAMESHEK, W.: The Anemia of the Di Guglielmo Syndrome, Blood, *14*, 334, 1959.

4. BALDRIDGE, C. W. and BARER, A.: Relationship Between Oxygen Consumption and Nitrogen Metabolism: II. In Leukemia, Arch. Int. Med., *51*, 589, 1933.

5. BALDRIDGE, C. W. and FOWLER, W. M.: Aleukemic Myelosis, Arch. Int. Med., *52*, 852, 1933.

6. BAMFORTH, J. and KENDALL, D.: A Case of Megakaryocytic Myelosis With Paraplegia, Acta med. scandinav., *99*, 494, 1939.

6a. BARAC, G.: Rémarques sur le rôle des porphyrines dans le chlorome et le diagnostic de cette affection en clinique, Rev. med. Liège, *8*, 484, 1953.

7. BARNEY, J. D., HUNTER, F. T. and MINTZ, E. R.: Urologic Aspects of Radiosensitive Tumors of the Blood Forming Organs, J.A.M.A., *98*, 1245, 1932.

7a. BARRETT, O'N., JR., CONRAD, M. and CROSBY, W. H.: Chronic Granulocytic Leukemia in Childhood, Am. J. M. Sc., *240*, 587, 1960.

8. BATY, J. M. and VOGT, E. C.: Bone Changes of Leukemia in Children, Am. J. Roentgenol., *34*, 310, 1935.

9. BEAN, R. H. D.: Phenylbutazone and Leukaemia, Brit. M. J., *2*, 1552, 1960.

9a. BEARD, J. W.: Nature of the Viruses of Avian Myeloblastosis and Erythroblastosis, *in* Proceedings of the Third National Cancer Conference, Philadelphia, J. B. Lippincott Company, 1957, p. 336; Proc. Soc. Exper. Biol. & Med., *97*, 48, 1958; J. Nat. Cancer Inst., *24*, 395, 1960.

9b. BELDING, H. W., DALAND, G. A. and PARKER, F., JR.: Histiocytic and Monocytic Leukemia. A Clinical, Hematological, and Pathological Differentiation, Cancer, *8*, 237, 1955.

10. BENNETT, J. H.: Case of Hypertrophy of the Spleen and Liver, in Which Death Took Place From Suppuration of the Blood, Edinburgh M. & S. J., *64*, 413, 1845.

10a. BENTLEY, H. P., JR., REARDON, A. E., KNOEDLER, J. P. and KRIVIT, W.: Eosinophilic Leukemia, Am. J. Med., *30*, 310, 1961.

10b. BERLIN, N. I., LAWRENCE, J. H. and GARTLAND, J.: The Blood Volume in Chronic Leukemia as Determined by P^{32} Labelled Red Blood Cells, J. Lab. & Clin. Med., *36*, 435, 1950.

10c. BERLIN, N. I., LAWRENCE, J. H. and LEE, H. C.: The Pathogenesis of the Anemia of Chronic Leukemia: Measurement of the Life Span of the Red Blood Cell with Glycine-2-C^{14}, J. Lab. & Clin. Med., *44*, 860, 1954.

10d. BERLIN, R.: Blood Volume in Chronic Leukemia, Acta med. scandinav., *164*, 257, 1959.

11. BERNSTEIN, A.: Diagnostic Importance of the Heterophile Antibody Test in Leukemia, J. Clin. Invest., *13*, 677, 1934.

11a. BESSIS, M.: The Use of Replacement Transfusion in Diseases Other Than Hemolytic Disease of the Newborn, Blood, *4*, 324, 1949; Rev. hémat., *5*, 188, 1950.

11b.BEST, W. R. and LIMARZI, L. R.: Age, Sex, Race and Hematologic Classification of 916 Cases of Leukemia, J. Lab. & Clin. Med., 40, 778, 1952.

11c.BETHELL, F. H.: Leukemia, The Relative Incidence of Its Various Forms, and Their Response to Radiation Therapy, Ann. Int. Med., 18, 757, 1943.

11d.BICHEL, J.: Mediastinal Tumors in Leukosis, Acta radiol., 28, 81, 1947.

11e.————: Arthralgic Leukemia in Children, Acta haemat., 1, 153, 1948.

11f.BIERMAN, H. R. et al.: Leukemia and Pregnancy, J.A.M.A., 161, 220, 1956.

11g.BIERMAN, H. R., COHEN, P., McCLELLAND, J. N. and SHIMKIN, M. B.: The Effect of Transfusions and Antibiotics Upon the Duration of Life in Children With Lymphogenous Leucemia, J. Pediat., 37, 455, 1950.

11h.BIERMAN, H. R., CRILE, D. M., DOD, K. S., KELLY, K. H., PETRAKIS, N. L., WHITE, L. P. and SHIMKIN, M. B.: Remissions in Leukemia of Childhood following Acute Infectious Disease, Cancer, 6, 591, 1953.

11i.BIERMAN, H. R., KELLY, K. H. and CORDES, F.: The Behavior of Leukemic Cells during Continuous Cross-transfusions between Patients with Leukemia and Other Neoplastic Diseases, Cancer Res., 11, 236, 1951.

11j.BIERMAN, H. R., PERKINS, E. K. and ORTEGA, P.: Pericarditis in Patients with Leukemia, Am. Heart J., 43, 413, 1952.

12. BIRGE, R. F., JENKS, A. L., JR. and DAVIS, S. K.: Spontaneous Remission in Acute Leukemia, J.A.M.A., 140, 589, 1949.

12a.BJÖRKMAN, S. E.: The Effect of ACTH and Cortisone on the Leukocyte Count in Four Cases of Acute Leukemia, Acta haemat., 15, 175, 1956.

12b.BLANCHAER, M. C., GREEN, P. T., MACLEAN, J. P. and HOLLENBERG, M. J.: Plasma Lactic Dehydrogenase and Phosphohexose Isomerase in Leukemia, Blood, 8, 245, 1958.

12c.BLASCHY, R.: Polyneuritisähnliches Krankheitsbild bei Leukämie, München. med. Wchnschr., 76, 2166, 1929.

13. BLOCK, M.: Histopathologic Effects of X-Rays, Radiophosphorus, Nitrogen Mustard, Urethane and Steroids upon the Spleen in Leukemias and Lymphomas, Radiology, 71, 477, 1958.

13a.BLOCK, M., JACOBSON, L. O. and BETHARD, W. F.: Preleukemic Acute Human Leukemia, J.A.M.A., 152, 1018, 1953.

13b.BLUEFARB, S. M.: Herpes Zoster Associated with Monocytic Leukemia, Arch. Dermat. and Syphilol., 57, 319, 1948.

13c.BLUEFARB, S. M.: Leukemia Cutis, Springfield, Ill., Charles C Thomas, 1960.

13d.BOGGS, D. R.: The Cellular Composition of Inflammatory Exudates in Human Leukemias, Blood, 15, 466, 1960.

13e.BOGGS, D. R. and FAHEY, J. L.: Serum-Protein Changes in Malignant Disease. II. The Chronic Leukemias, Hodgkin's Disease, and Malignant Melanoma, J. Nat. Cancer Inst., 25, 1381, 1960.

13f.BOGGS, D. R., FREI, E., III and THOMAS, L. B.: Clostridial Gas Gangrene and Septicemia in Four Patients with Leukemia, New England J. Med., 259, 1255, 1958.

14. BOGGS, T. R. and GUTHRIE, C. G.: Bence-Jones Proteinuria in Leukemia, Bull. Johns Hopkins Hosp., 24, 368, 1913.

15. BOIKAN, W. S.: Leukemic Changes of the Gastro-intestinal Tract, Arch. Int. Med., 47, 42, 1931.

15a.BOGART, F. B.: Leukosarcoma, Am. J. Roentgenol., 55, 743, 1946.

16. BORGESON, E. J. and WAGENER, H. P.: Changes in the Eye in Leukemia, Am. J. M. Sc., 177, 663, 1929.

17. VON BOROS, J. and KORÉNYI, A.: Über einen Fall von akuter Megakaryoblastenleukämie, zugleich einige Bemerkungen zum Problem der akuten Leukamie, Ztschr. klin. Med., 118, 697, 1931.

17a.BOURONCLE, BERTHA A., DOAN, C. A. and WISEMAN, B. K.: Evaluation of the Effect of Massive Prednisolone Therapy in Acute Leukemia, Acta haemat., 22, 201, 1959.

17b.BOURONCLE, BERTHA A., WISEMAN, B. K. and DOAN, C. A.: Leukemic Reticuloendotheliosis, Blood, 13, 609, 1958.

18. BOUSSER, J.: Eosinophilie et leucémie, Sang, 28, 553, 1957.

19.BOWDITCH, M., ELKINS, H. B., HUNTER, F. T., MALLORY, T. B., GALL, E. A. and BUCKLEY, W. J.: Chronic Exposure to Benzene (Benzol), J. Indust. Hyg. & Toxicol., 21, 321, 1939.

20. BRANNAN, D.: Chloroma, Bull. Johns Hopkins Hosp., 38, 189, 1926.

20a.BRAUDE, A. I., FELTES, J. and BROOKS, M.: Differences between the Activities of Mature Granulocytes in Leukemic and Normal Blood, J. Clin. Invest., 33, 1036, 1954; Blood, 16, 1279, 1960.

20b.BRAUNSTEINER, H., FELLINGER, K. and PAKESCH, F.: On the Occurrence of Virus-Like Bodies in Human Leukemia, Blood, 15, 476, 1960.

20c.BRAUSIL, B.: Diagnostic Differences between Atypical Myeloblasts and Lymphoblasts in the Phase Contrast Microscope. A Morphologic Study of 32 Cases, Acta hæmat., 12, 276, 1954.

21. BRIARD, S. P., McCLINTOCK, J. T. and
    BALDRIDGE, C. W.: Cost of Work in Pa-
    tients With Hypermetabolism Due to
    Leukemia and to Exophthalmic Goiter,
    Arch. Int. Med., 56, 30, 1935.
21b.BRÜCHER, H. und WEICKER, H.: Beitrag zur
    lymphatischen plasmazellulären Reticu-
    lose, Acta hæmat., 13, 272, 1955.
22. BRUES, A. M.: Critique of the Linear Theory
    of Carcinogenesis, Science, 128, 693, 1958.
24. BURCHENAL, J. H.: Clinical Effects of Analogs
    of Folic Acid, Purines, Pyrimidines, and
    Amino Acids, Fed. Proc., 13, 760, 1954.
25.BURCHENAL, J. H., MURPHY, M. L., ELLISON,
    R. R., SYKES, M. P., TAN, T. C., LEONE,
    L. A., KARNOFSKY, D. A., CRAVER, L. F.,
    DARGEON, H. W. and RHOADS, C. P.:
    Clinical Evaluation of a New Antimetabo-
    lite, 6-Mercaptopurine, in the Treatment
    of Leukemia and Allied Diseases, Blood,
    8, 965, 1953; Am. J. M. Sc., 228, 371, 1954.
25a.BURNET, M.: Leukaemia As a Problem in
    Preventive Medicine, New England J.
    Med., 259, 423, 1958.
25b.BURNS, T. W., VICKERS, R. and LOWNEY, J.
    F.: Acute Leukemia after Radioactive
    Iodine (I131) Therapy for Hyperthyroidism,
    A. M. A. Arch. Int. Med., 106, 97, 1960.
26. CALDWELL, W. G. D. and AMOS, J. A. S.:
    Familial Blood Dyscrasia, Acta haemat.,
    21, 217, 1959.
27. CALVERT, R. J. and SMITH, E.: Metastatic
    Acropachy in Lymphatic Leukemia, Blood,
    10, 545, 1955.
27a.CAMPBELL, A. C. P., HENDERSON, J. L. and
    CROOM, J. H.: Monocytic Leukæmia With
    Myeloid Hyperplasia and Localized Tu-
    mour Formation, J. Path. & Bact., 42,
    617, 1936.
28. CARTER, MARY E.: Report of Two Siblings
    Diagnosed As Cases of Acute Lymphatic
    Leukaemia, Brit. M. J., 1, 265, 1957.
28a.DE CARVALHO, S., RAND, H. J. and MEYER,
    D. P.: Biologic Properties of Human
    Leukemic and Tumoral RNA, J. Lab. &
    Clin. Med., 55, 694 and 706, 1960.
28b.CAVINS, J. A., LEVIN, H. S. and DAY, H. J.:
    Chronic Myelogenous Leukemia with
    Gastric Infiltration, New England J. Med.,
    260, 1111, 1959.
29. CASTLE, W. B., MEYER, O. and CHEW, W.
    B.: Negative Results of Treatment of
    Chronic Myelogenous Leukemia as a De-
    ficiency Disease, Proc. Soc. Exper. Biol.
    & Med., 32, 660, 1935.
29a.CHEN, H. P. and SMITH, H. S.: Eosinophilic
    Leukemia, Ann. Int. Med., 52, 1343, 1960.
30. CHENEY, G.: Chronic Myelogenous Leu-
    kemia With Ascites Resembling Banti's

Syndrome, Acta med. scandinav., 81, 14,
    1934.
30a.CLARK, P. A., HSIA, Y. E. and HUNTSMAN,
    R. G.: Toxic Complications of Treatment
    with 6-Mercaptopurine, Brit. M. J., 1,
    393, 1960.
30b.CLEMENTS, D. G. and KALMON, E. H.:
    Chronic Myelogenous Leukemia; Un-
    usual Bone Changes in an Adult, Radi-
    ology, 67, 399, 1956.
31. CLOUGH, P. W.: Monocytic Leukemia, Bull.
    Johns Hopkins Hosp., 51, 148, 1932.
31a.COLSKY, J., GREENSPAN, E. M. and WARREN,
    T. N.: Hepatic Fibrosis in Children with
    Acute Leukemia after Therapy with Folic
    Acid Antagonists, Arch. Path., 59, 198,
    1955.
31b.CONDIT, P. T. and ELIEL, L. P.: Effects of
    Large Infrequent Doses of A-methopterin
    on Acute Leukemia in Children, J.A.M.A.,
    172, 451, 1960.
31c.CONGDON, C. C. and LORENZ, E.: Leukemia
    in Guinea-pigs, Am. J. Path., 30, 337, 1954.
32. COOKE, J. V.: Mediastinal Tumor in Acute
    Leukemia; Clinical and Roentgenologic
    Study, Am. J. Dis. Child., 44, 1153,
    1932; J.A.M.A., 101, 432, 1933.
33. ——— Chronic Myelogenous Leukemia in
    Children, J. Pediat., 42, 537, 1953.
34. COOKE, W. E.: A Case of Mixed Leukemia,
    Brit. M. J., 1, 895, 1934.
35. COSTA, A.: Rara forma di rottura dell'atrio
    sinistro del cuore per infiltrati leucemici
    nel miocardio, Sperimentale, Arch. di
    biol., 85, 117, 1931; ibid., 87, 7, 1933.
36. COSTELLO, M. J., CANIZARES, O., MONTAGUE,
    M., III, and BUNCKE, C. M.: Cutaneous
    Manifestations of Myelogenous Leukemia,
    Arch. Dermat., 71, 605, 1955.
36a.COURT-BROWN, W. M.: Radiation-Induced
    Leukemia in Man, J. Chron. Dis., 8, 113,
    1958.
36b.COURT-BROWN, W. M. and ABBATT, J. D.:
    The Incidence of Leukaemia in Ankyl-
    osing Spondylitis Treated with X-rays,
    Lancet, 1, 1283, 1955; Med. Res. Council,
    Spec. Rep., Series No. 295, London, His
    Majesty's Stationery Office, 1957.
36c.COURT-BROWN, W. M. and DOLL, R.: Ex-
    pectation of Life and Mortality from
    Cancer among British Radiologists, Brit.
    M. J., 2, 181, 1958.
36d.COURT-BROWN, W. M. and DOLL, R.: Adult
    Leukaemia, Brit. M. J., 1, 1063, 1959;
    ibid., 1, 1753, 1960.
36e.COURT-BROWN, W. M., DOLL, R. and HILL,
    A. B.: Incidence of Leukaemia after Ex-
    posure to Diagnostic Radiation in Utero,
    Brit. M. J., 2, 1539, 1960.

36f.CRAMBLETT, H. G.: Recognition and Treatment of Intracranial Manifestations of Leukemia, A. M. A. J. Dis. Child., 97, 805, 1959.

36g.CRAMBLETT, H. G., FRIEDMAN, J. L. and NAJJAR, S.: Leukemia in an Infant Born of a Mother with Leukemia, New England J. Med., 259, 727, 1958.

37. CRAVER, L. F.: Tenderness of Sternum in Leukemia, Am. J. M. Sc., 174, 799, 1927.

38. CRAVER, L. F. and COPELAND, M. M.: Changes of the Bones in the Leukemias, Arch. Surg., 30, 639, 1935.

39. CRONKITE, E. P., MOLONEY, W. and BOND, V. P.: Radiation Leukemogenesis, Am. J. Med., 28, 673, 1960.

39b.CROSBY, W. H. and BENJAMIN, NAOMI R.: An Abnormal Hemolytic System Associated with Leukemia and Other Disseminated Malignant Diseases, Blood, 12, 701, 1957.

39c.CURRERI, A. R. et al.: Clinical Studies with 5-Fluorouracil, Cancer Res., 18, 478, 1958.

39d.DALGAARD, J. B. and KASS, A.: Congenital Leukaemia with Cirrhosis of Liver, Acta path. et microbiol. scandinav., 37, 465, 1955.

40. DAMESHEK, W., SAVITZ, H. A. and ARBOR, B.: Chronic Lymphatic Leukemia in Twin Brothers Aged Fifty-six, J.A.M.A., 92, 1348, 1929; ibid., 164, 1323, 1957.

40a.D'ANGIO, G. J., EVANS, AUDREY E. and MITUS, ANNA: Roentgen Therapy of Certain Complications of Acute Leukemia in Childhood, Am. J. Roentgenol., 82, 541, 1959.

41. DARTE, J. M., DACIE, J. V. and McSORLEY, J. G. A.: Pelger-like Leucocytes in Chronic Myeloid Leukæmia, Acta hæmat., 12, 117, 1954.

42. DAVIS, C. L. and FITZ-HUGH, T., JR.: Achlorhydria in the Leukemias, Am. J. M. Sc., 197, 763, 1939.

42a.DECASTELLO, A.: Aspects of Familial Leukemia, Med. Klin., 35, 1255, 1939.

42b.DEAN, G. O., EARLE, A. M. and REILLY, W. A.: Failure of Thymectomy in Lymphatic Leukemia, Arch. Surg., 63, 695, 1951.

43a.DIAMOND, I., ANDERSON, MARY M. and McCREADIE, S. R.: Transplacental Transmission of Busulfan (Myleran®) in a Mother with Leukemia, Pediatrics, 25, 85, 1960.

43b.DIAMOND, I. B.: Leukemic Changes in the Brain, Arch. Neurol. & Psychiat., 32, 118, 1934.

44. DI GUGLIELMO, G.: Les Maladies Érythrémiques, Rev. hémat., 1, 355, 1946; Haematologica, 41, 605, 1956.

44a.DI GUGLIELMO, G. and IANNACCONE, A.: Inhibition of Mitosis and Regressive Changes of Erythroblasts in Acute Erythropathy Caused by Occupational Benzene Poisoning, Acta haemat., 19, 144, 1958.

44b.DITTMAN, W. A. and WARD, J. R.: Demecolcine Toxicity, Am. J. Med., 27, 519, 1959.

44c.DMOCHOWSKI, L. et al.: Studies on Human Leukemia, Proc. Soc. Exper. Biol. & Med., 101, 686, 1959.

44d.DOUGHERTY, T. F.: Effect of Hormones on Lymphatic Tissue, Physiol. Rev., 32, 379, 1952.

45. DOWNEY, H.: Monocytic Leucemia and Leucemic Reticulo-endotheliosis, in Handbook of Hematology, Hal Downey, Ed., New York, Paul B. Hoeber, Inc., 2, 1273, 1938.

46. DOWNEY, H. and NORDLAND, M.: Hematologic and Histologic Study of a Case of Myeloid Megakaryocytic Hepato-splenomegaly, Folia hæmat., 62, 1, 1939.

46a.DRESDALE, D. T., SPAIN, D. and PEREZ-PINA, F.: Heart Block and Leukemic Cell Infiltration of Interventricular Septum of Heart, Am. J. Med., 6, 530, 1949.

46b.DRUEZ, G. and DUSTIN, P.: Un cas de leucémie aigüe a polynucleaires, Sang, 29, 511, 1958.

46c.DUSTIN, P., JR.: Les poisons mitatiques "radiomimétiques" et le métabolisme des nucléoprotéines, Rev. belge path. et Med. exper., 22, 55, 1952.

47. EBSTEIN, W.: Ueber die acute Leukämie und Pseudoleukämie, Deutsch. Arch. klin. Med., 44, 343, 1889.

47a.EFRATI, P., KLAJMAN, A. and SPITZ, H.: Mast Cell Leukemia?—Malignant Mastocytosis with Leukemia-like Manifestations, Blood, 12, 869, 1957.

48. ELLERMANN, V. and BANG, O.: Experimentelle Leukämie bei Hühnern, Ztschr. Hyg. Infektionskr., 63, 231, 1909.

49a.ELLISON, ROSE RUTH, SILVER, R. T. and ENGLE, R. L., JR.: Comparative Study of 6-Chloropurine and 6-Mercaptopurine in Adult Leukemia in Adults, Ann. Int. Med., 51, 322, 1959; Blood, 13, 705, 1958.

50. ELSON, L. A.: A Comparison of the Effects of Radiation and Radiomimetic Chemicals on the Blood, Brit. J. Hæmat., 1, 104, 1955.

51. ÉMILE–WEIL, P. and BOUSSER, J.: Leucémie et traumatisme, Ann. méd., 40, 220, 1936.

53. FABIAN, E.: Über lymphatische und myeloische Chloro-Leukamie, Beitr. path. Anat. allg. Path., 43, 172, 1908.

53a.FAHEY, J. L. and BOGGS, D. R.: Serum Protein Changes in Malignant Diseases, Blood, *16*, 1479, 1960.

54. FALCONER, E. H. and LEONARD, M. E.: Pulmonary Involvement in Lymphosarcoma and Lymphatic Leukemia, Am. J. M. Sc., *195*, 294, 1938.

54a. FARBER, J. E. and BYLEBYL, H.: Lymphatic Leukemia and Tuberculosis, Am. J. Clin. Path., *12*, 253, 1942.

55. FARBER, S., DIAMOND, L. K., MERCER, R. D., SYLVESTER, R. F., JR. and WOLFF, J. A.: Temporary Remissions in Acute Leukemia in Children Produced by Folic Acid Antagonist, 4-Aminopteroyl-Glutamic Acid (Aminopterin), New England J. Med., *238*, 787, 1948.

55a. FAUVERT, R., MALLARMÉ, J. and PETIT, P. E.: "Cure" of So-called Acute Leukemia, Presse méd. *56*, 302, 1948.

55b. FEINLEIB, M. and MacMAHON, B.: Variation in the Duration of Survival of Patients with the Chronic Leukemias, Blood, *15*, 332, 1960.

56. FENNINGER, L. D., WATERHOUSE, C. and KEUTMANN, E. H.: The Interrelationship of Nitrogen and Phosphorus in Patients with Certain Neoplastic Diseases, Cancer, *6*, 930, 1953.

56a. FERREBEE, J. W. and THOMAS, E. D.: Transplantation of Marrow in Man, Arch. Int. Med., *106*, 523, 1960.

57. FESSAS, P., WINTROBE, M. M., THOMPSON, R. B. and CARTWRIGHT, G. E.: Treatment of Acute Leukemia with Cortisone and Corticotropin, Arch. Int. Med., *94*, 384, 1954.

57a. FIESCHI, A., BIANCHI, V., BIANCHINI, E., CAMBIAGGI, G., SACCHETTI, C. and SALVIDIO, E.: Ricerche sulla biologia delle cellule della leucemia acuta, XII Congresso Nazionale della Società Italiana di Ematologia, Bologna, 12–13 June, 1954; Acta haemat., *16*, 126, 1956.

58. FIRMAT, J. *et al.:* The Artificial Kidney in the Treatment of Renal Failure and Hyperuricemia in Patients with Lymphoma and Leukemia, Cancer, *13*, 276, 1960.

58a. FISHER, J. H., WELCH, C. S. and DAMESHEK, W.: Splenectomy in Leukemia and Leukosarcoma, New England J. Med., *246*, 477, 1952.

58b. FLINT, J. S.: Leukemia and Pregnancy, Rocky Mountain M. J., *56*, 59, 1959.

60. FORKNER, C. E. and SCOTT, T. F. M.: Arsenic as a Therapeutic Agent in Chronic Myelogenous Leukemia, J.A.M.A., *97*, 3, 1931.

60a. FORKNER, C. E., JR., FREI, E., III, EDG-COMB, J. H. and UTZ, J. P.; Pseudomonas Septicemia, Am. J. Med., *25*, 877, 1958.

60b. FOY, H., KONDI, A. and MURRAY, J. F.: The Syndrome of Leukanæmia, J. Path. & Bact., *58*, 157, 1946.

60c. FREEMAN, G. and BUCKLEY, E. S., JR., Serum Polysaccharide and Fever in Thrombocytopenic Bleeding of Leukemia, Blood, *9*, 586, 1954.

60d. FREEMAN, J. A.: The Ultrastructure and Genesis of Auer Bodies, Blood, *15*, 449, 1960.

61. FREI, E., III *et al.:* A Comparative Study of Two Regimens of Combination Chemotherapy in Acute Leukemia, Blood, *13*, 1126, 1958.

61a. FREIREICH, E. J., *et al.:* Evaluation of a New Chemotherapeutic Agent in Patients with "Advanced Refractory" Acute Leukemia. Studies of 6-Azauracil, Blood, *16*, 1268, 1960.

61b. FREIREICH, E. J., *et al.:* A Distinctive Type of Intracerebral Hemorrhage Associated with "Blastic Crisis" in Patients with Leukemia, Cancer, *13*, 146, 1960.

61c. FRENKEL, E. P. and MEYERS, MURIEL C.: Acute Leukemia and Pregnancy, Ann. Int. Med., *53*, 656, 1960.

61d. FREYMANN, J. G., VANDER, J. B., MARLER, ELIZABETH A. and MEYER, DOROTHY G.: Prolonged Corticosteroid Therapy of Chronic Lymphocytic Leukaemia and the Closely Allied Malignant Lymphomas, Brit. J. Haemat., *6*, 303, 1960.

61e. FRIEDELL, H. L. and STORAASLI, J. P.: The Therapeutic Application of Radioactive Phosphorus With Special Reference to the Treatment of Primary Polycythemia and Chronic Myeloid Leukemia, J. Clin. Invest., *28*, 1308, 1949.

62. FRIEDGOOD, H. B.: Relation of the Sympathetic Nervous System and Generalized Lymphoid Hyperplasia to the Pathogenesis of Exophthalmic Goiter and Chronic Lymphatic Leukemia, Am. J. M. Sc., *183*, 841, 1932.

62a. FRIEDMAN, B. I., WILL, J. J., FREIMAN, D. G. and BRAUNSTEIN, H.: Tissue Mast Cell Leukemia, Blood, *13*, 70, 1958.

63. FRIEDREICH, N.: Ein neuer Fall von Leukämie, Virchows Arch. path. Anat., *12*, 37, 1857.

63a. FRIEND, CHARLOTTE: Cell-Free Transmission in Adult Swiss Mice of a Disease Having the Character of a Leukemia, J. Exper. Med., *105*, 307, 1957; *ibid.*, *109*, 217, 1959.

63b. FRITZ, R. D. *et al.:* The Association of Fatal Intracranial Hemorrhage and "Blastic

Crisis" in Patients with Acute Leukemia, New England J. Med., *261*, 59, 1959.

63c.FRUMIN, A. M. and KOHN, A.: Autoimmune Hemolytic Disease in Acute Leukemia, Arch. Int. Med., *95*, 326, 1955.

64. FURTH, J.: Studies on Nature of Agent Transmitting Leucosis of Fowls, J. Exper. Med., *55*, 465, 479, 495, 1932; *ibid.*, *58*, 253, 1933; *ibid.*, *61*, 593, 1935; *ibid.*, *63*, 127, 1936; Arch. Path., *24*, 281, 1937; J. Exper. Med., *69*, 13, 1939; *ibid.*, *71*, 55, 1940; *ibid.*, *74*, 257, 1941.

65a.————— Recent Experimental Studies on Leukemia, Physiol. Rev., *26*, 47, 1946; Blood, *6*, 964, 1951; Cancer Res., *18*, 842, 1958; Proc. Soc. Exper. Biol. & Med., *100*, 610, 1959.

68.FURTH, J. and KAHN, M. C.: The Transmission of Leukemia of Mice With a Single Cell, Am. J. Cancer, *31*, 276, 1937.

69. GALTON, D. A. G. and TILL, M.: Myleran in Chronic Myeloid Leukemia, Lancet, *1*, 425, 1955; Brit. M. Bull., *15*, 78, 1959.

69a.GASSER, C.: 3 Fälle von chronischer myeloischer Leukämie im Kindesalter, Helv. pædiat. Acta, *1*, 299, 1946.

70. GATE, J. and CUILLERET, P.: Skin Manifestations in Leukemia, J. méd. Lyon, *18*, 283, 1937.

71. GATES, O.: Cutaneous Tumors of Leukemia and Lymphoma, Arch. Dermat., *37*, 1015, 1938.

71a.GAULD, W. R., INNES, J. and ROBSON, H. N.: A Survey of 647 Cases of Leukæmia, 1938–51, Brit. M. J., *1*, 585, 1953.

71b.GAVOSTO, F., MARAINI, G. and PILERI, A.: Radioautographic Investigations on DNA and Protein Metabolism in Two Cases of Di Guglielmo's Disease, Blood, *16*, 1122, 1960.

71c.GELLHORN, A. and JONES, L. O.: Pyridoxine Deficient Diet and Desoxypyridoxine in the Therapy of Lymphosarcoma and Acute Leukemia in Man, Blood, *4*, 60, 1949.

71d.GILBERT, ENID F., RICE, E. C. and LECHAUX, P. A.: Renal Function in Children with Leukemia, A.M.A.J. Dis. Child., *93*, 150, 1957.

71e.GILLIAM, A. G. and WALTER, W. A.: Trends of Mortality from Leukemia in the United States, 1921–55, Pub. Health Rep., *73*, 773, 1958.

72. GLOOR, W.: Ein Fall von geheilter Myeloblastenleukämie, München. med. Wchnschr., *77*, 1096, 1930.

73. GOLDBACH, L. J.: Leukemic Retinitis, Arch. Ophth., *10*, 808, 1933.

74. GOLDHAMER, S. M. and BARNEY, B. F.: Myelogenous Leukemia With Cutaneous Involvement, J.A.M.A., *107*, 1041, 1936.

74b.GOUTTAS, A. *et al.*: Uber einen Fall von Lymphatischer Leukämie mit Kryoglobulinämie, Klin. Wchnschr., *35*, 284, 1957.

75. GOWDEY, J. F. and NEUHAUSER, E. B. D.: The Roentgen Diagnosis of Diffuse Leukemic Infiltration of the Kidneys in Children, Am. J. Roentgenol., *60*, 13, 1948.

77. GRAMÉN, K.: Accident: Transfusion of Leukemic Blood, Acta chir. scandinav., *64*, 369, 1928.

77a.GREEN, R. A. and NICHOLS, N. J.: Pulmonary Involvement in Leukemia, Am. Rev. Resp. Dis., *80*, 833, 1959.

77b.GREEN, R. A., NICHOLS, N. J. and KING, E. J.: Alveolar-Capillary Block Due to Leukemic Infiltration of the Lung, Am. Rev. Resp. Dis., *80*, 895, 1959.

78. GREENDYKE, R. M. and JACOX, R. F.: A Study of Cationic Detergent Fractionation of Serum Proteins in Lymphoma and Leukemia, J. Lab. & Clin. Med., *52*, 70, 1958.

79. GROAT, W. A.: Mitosis in Myeloblasts in Peripheral Blood, Am. J. M. Sc., *180*, 607, 1930; *ibid.*, *185*, 624, 1933.

80. GROSS, L.: Mouse Leukemia: An Egg-Borne Virus Disease, Acta hæmat., *13*, 13, 1955; Cancer Res., *18*, 371, 1958; Acta haemat., *23*, 259, 1960.

80a.GUASCH, J.: Hérédité des Leucémies, Sang, *25*, 384, 1954.

81. GUMP, M. E., HESTER, E. G. and LOHR, O. W.: Monocytic Chloroma, Arch. Ophth., *16*, 931, 1936.

81a.GUNZ, F. W.: Bone Marrow Changes in Patients with Chronic Leukemia Treated by Splenic X-irradiation, Blood, *8*, 687, 1953.

81b.GUNZ, F. W. and HOUGH, R. F.: Acute Leukemia over the Age of Fifty, Blood, *11*, 882, 1956.

81c.GUNZ, F. W.: I. Leukemia: Some Present Day Problems, Ergebn. inn. Med. u. Kinderh., *14*, 1, 1960.

82. GWYN, N. B.: On Some Clinical Manifestations of Acute Leukemia, Canad. M. A. J., *23*, 35, 1930.

82a.HADDOW, A. and SEXTON, W. A.: Influence of Carbamic Esters (Urethanes) on Experimental Animal Tumours, Nature, *157*, 500, 1946; Lancet, *1*, 677, 1946.

82b.HADDOW, A. and TIMMIS, G. M.: Myleran in Chronic Myeloid Leukemia, Lancet, *1*, 207, 1953.

82c.HALL, B. H., RICHARDS, M. D., WILLET, F. M. and FEICHTMEIR, T. V.: Clinical Experience with 6-Mercaptopurine in Human

Neoplasia, Ann. New York Acad. Sc., *60*, 374, 1954.

82*d*.HALL, C. C. and WHIPPLE, G. H.: Roentgen Ray Intoxication: Disturbances in Metabolism Produced by Deep Massive Doses of the Hard Roentgen-rays, Am. J. M. Sc., *157*, 453, 1919.

83. HARAM, B. J.: Lymphatic Leukæmia With Bilateral Mammary Changes, Lancet, *1*, 1277, 1937.

83*a*.HARRIS, G.: Acute Leukæmia in Pregnancy, Brit. M. J., *2*, 101, 1955.

83*b*.HAURANI, F. I., REPPLINGER, EVALYN and TOCANTINS, L. M.: Attempts at Transplantation of Human Bone Marrow in Patients with Acute Leukemia and Other Marrow Depletion Disorders, Am. J. Med., *28*, 794, 1960.

83*c*.HAUSWIRTH, L., ROSENOW, G. and LANSMAN, W.: Lymphosarcoma Terminating in Lymphatic Leukemia (Lymphosarcoma Cell Leukemia) Acta hæmat., *1*, 45, 1948.

84. HAUT, A., ABBOTT, W. S., WINTROBE, M. M. and CARTWRIGHT, G. E.: Busulfan in the Treatment of Chronic Myelocytic Leukemia. The Effect of Long Term Intermittent Therapy, Blood, *17*, 1, 1961.

84*a*.HAUT, A., ALTMAN, S. J., CARTWRIGHT, G. E. and WINTROBE, M. M.: The Influence of Chemotherapy on Survival in Acute Leukemia, Blood, *10*, 875, 1955; *ibid.*, *14*, 828, 1959.

84*b*.———— The Use of Myleran (1-4, dimethanesulfonyloxybutane) in the Treatment of Chronic Myelocytic Leukemia, Arch. Int. Med., *96*, 451, 1955.

84*c*.HAUT, A., WINTROBE, M. M. and CARTWRIGHT, G. E.: The Clinical Management of Leukemia, Am. J. Med., *28*, 777, 1960.

84*d*.HAYS, Esther F. and BECK, W. S.: The Development of Leukemia and Other Neoplasms in Mice Receiving Cell-free Extracts from a High-Leukemia (AKR) Strain, Cancer Res., *18*, 676, 1958.

84*e*.HAYS, ESTHER F., SCANLAN, T. C. and ENGLE, R. L., JR.: Multiple Remissions in an Adult with Acute Leukemia Treated Principally with A-methopterin, Ann. Int. Med., *45*, 306, 1956.

84*f*.HEILMEYER, L. and SCHÖNER, W.: "Perniciöse Anämie" als Initialphase einer akuten Erythroleukämie, Schweiz. med. Wchnschr., *80*, 1122, 1950.

84*g*.HEINLE, R. W. and WEIR, D. R.: Morphologic Obliteration of Chronic Myeloid Leukemia by Active Tuberculosis, Am. J. M. Sc., *207*, 450, 1944.

84*h*.HEMMELER, G.: "Leucémie" mégacaryocy-

taire avec thrombocythémia, J. Suisse Med., *78*, 976, 1948.

84*i*.HEROLD, K. und MICHEL, W.: Pulmonale Veränderungen bei chronischer Leukämie, Deutsch. Arch. klin. Med., *197*, 596, 1950.

85. HERXHEIMER, G.: Ueber einen combinierten Fall von lymphatischer und Myeloblastenleukämie, Centralbl. allg. Path. path. Anat., *24*, 897, 1913.

86. HERZ, A.: Infectionen mit leukämischen Blutbild, Wien. klin. Wchnschr., *39*, 835, 1926.

86*a*.HEWITT, D.: Some Features of Leukæmia Mortality, Brit. J. Prev. & Soc. Med., *9*, 81, 1955.

86*b*.HEYN, R. M. *et al.:* The Comparison of 6-Mercaptopurine with the Combination of 6-Mercaptopurine and Azaserine in the Treatment of Acute Leukemia in Children, Blood, *15*, 350, 1960.

87. HEYSSEL, R. *et al.:* Leukemia in Hiroshima Atomic Bomb Survivors, Blood, *15*, 313, 1960.

87*a*.HINDMARSH, J. R. and EMSLIE-SMITH, D.: Monocytic Leukæmia Presenting as Polyarthritis in an Adult, Brit. M. J., *1*, 593, 1953.

87*b*.HINKAMP, J. F. and SZANTO, P. B.: Chloroma of the Ovary, Am. J. Obst. & Gynec., *78*, 812, 1959.

88. HIRD, A. J.: Mikulicz's Syndrome, Brit. M. J., *2*, 416, 1949.

89. HIRSCHFELD, H.: Ueber Leukanämie, Folia hæmat., *3*, 332, 1906.

90. ———— Uber chronische Leukämien ohne Milz und der Lymphknotenvergrosserung, Med. Klin., *28*, 1160, 1932.

90*a*.HIRSCHMANN, H., HEINLE, R. W. and WEARN, J. R.: A Characterization of a Urinary Fraction Capable of Producing Myeloid Metaplasia in Guinea Pigs, Proc. Soc. Exper. Biol. & Med., *58*, 5, 1945; Ann. Int. Med., *17*, 902, 1942.

91. HITCH, J. M. and SMITH, D. C.: Lymphatic Leukemia, Arch. Dermat., *36*, 1, 1937.

91*a*.HITCHINGS, G. H. and RHOADS, C. P.: 6-Mercaptopurine, Ann. New York Acad. Sc., *60*, 183, 1954.

91*b*.HITTMAIR, A.: Beitrag zur Basophilenleukämie, Schweiz. med. Wchnschr., *90*, 938, 1960.

91*c*.HITZIG, W. H.: Colchicum-Vergiftung bei einem Kleinkind 2. Beobachtungen über Blutbildungs- und Mitosestörungen, Acta haemat., *21*, 170, 1959.

92. HOFFMAN, W. J. and CRAVER, L. F.: Chronic Myelogenous Leukemia: Value of Irradi-

ation and Its Effect on the Duration of Life, J.A.M.A., *97*, 836, 1931.

92a. HOLBØLL, S. A.: Untersuchungen über den Grundumsatz bei Patienten mit Leukämie und Lymphogranulomatose, Acta med. scandinav., *72*, 326, 1929.

92b. HOLLAND, J. F. *et al.*: Urate Excretion in Patients with Acute Leukemia, J. Nat. Cancer Inst., *23*, 1097, 1959.

93. HOLTEN, C.: Leukemic Erythrodermia, a Survey and a Report of a Case Treated with ACTH, Acta med. scandinav., Suppl. 266, *142*, 557, 1952.

93a. HOLOWACH, J.: Chronic Lymphoid Leucemia in Children, J. Pediat., *32*, 84, 1948.

93b. HORNBAKER, J. H.: Chronic Leukemia in Three Sisters, Am. J. M. Sc., *203*, 322, 1942.

93c. HOUGIE, C.: The Early Diagnosis and Natural History of Chronic Lymphatic Leukemia, Ann. Int. Med., *45*, 39, 1956.

93e. HUBLER, W. R. and NETHERTON, E. W.: Cutaneous Manifestations of Monocytic Leukemia, Arch. Dermat., *56*, 70, 1947.

94. HUDSON, R. P. and WILSON, S. J.: Hypogammaglobulinemia and Chronic Lymphatic Leukemia, Cancer, *13*, 200, 1960.

95. HUEPER, W. C. and RUSSELL, M.: Some Immunologic Aspects of Leukemia, Arch. Int. Med., *49*, 113, 1932.

99. HUTTER, R. V. P. *et al.*: Hepatic Fibrosis in Children with Acute Leukemia, Cancer, *13*, 288, 1960.

99a. HYMAN, CAROL B. *et al.*: Prednisone in Childhood Leukemia, Pediatrics, *24*, 1005, 1959.

100. ISAACS, R.: Lymphosarcoma Cell Leukemia, Ann. Int. Med., *11*, 657, 1937.

102. ISRAËLS, M. C. G.: Lymphatic Leukæmia: The Value of Sternal Puncture in the Diagnosis of Atypical Cases, Brit. M. J., *2*, 1132, 1939.

103. ISRAËLS, M. C. G.: The Reticuloses, Lancet, *2*, 525, 1953.

107. JAFFÉ, R. H.: Morphology of the Inflammatory Defense Reactions in Leukemia, Arch. Path., *14*, 177, 1932.

108. ——— Histologic Studies on the Spleen in Cases of Leukemia, Arch. Path., *19*, 647, 1935.

109. ——— The Nature of the Anemia in Acute Leukemia, Arch. Path., *20*, 725, 1935.

110. ——— The Reticulo-endothelial System, *in Handbook of Hematology*, Hal Downey, Ed., New York, Paul B. Hoeber, Inc., *2*, 973, 1938.

111. JÁRMAI, K.: Trauma und Leukämie, zugleich ein Beitrag zur Pathologie der Milzschädigung bei den Haustieren, Beitr. path. Anat. allg. Path., *92*, 119, 1933.

111a. ——— Die Leukosen der Haustiere, Ergebn. allg. Path. path. Anat., *28*, 227, 1934.

113. JEDLIČKA, VL., HEŘMANSKÁ, Z., ŠMÍDA, I. and KOUBA, A.: Paramyeloblastic Leukaemia Appearing Simultaneously in Two Blood Cousins after Simultaneous Contact with Gammexane (Hexachlorcyclohexane), Acta med. scandinav., *161*, 447, 1958.

114. JELLIFFE, A. M. and JONES, K. M.: Leukæmia after I[131] Therapy for Thyroid Cancer, Clin. Radiol., *11*, 134, 1960.

115. JORDAN, H. E.: Hemoblastic Leukemia, Arch. Path., *23*, 653, 1937.

118. KALAPOS, I.: Die Wirkung des Benzols bei der Leukämie, Klin. Wchnschr., *14*, 864, 1935.

119. KANDEL, E. V.: Chloroma, Arch. Int. Med., *59*, 691, 1937.

120. KANDEL, E. V. and LEROY, G. V.: Chronic Arsenical Poisoning During the Treatment of Chronic Myeloid Leukemia, Arch. Int. Med., *50*, 846, 1937.

121. KAPLAN, H. S.: On the Etiology and Pathogenesis of the Leukemias: A Review, Cancer Res., *14*, 535, 1954; *ibid.*, *16*, 422, 426, 429, 434 and 890, 1956.

121a. KARNOFSKY, D. A.: Triethylene Melamine in the Treatment of Lymphomas and Leukemias, M. Clin. North America, *38*, 541, 1954.

123. KEOGH, E. V., McCALL, CYNTHIA and RANKIN, D. W.: Mortality from Leukaemia in Victoria, 1946 to 1955, Med. J. Australia, *2*, 632, 1958.

124. KETRON, L. W. and GAY, L. N.: Myeloid Leukemia of Skin, Arch. Dermat., *7*, 176, 1923.

124a. KHOKHLOVA, M. P.: Pathologic Anatomy of Experimental Leukemia Produced by Injection of Benzol Extracts from Organs of Leukemic Patients, Blood, *13*, 917, 1958.

125. KIRSCHBAUM, A.: Recent Studies on Experimental Mammalian Leukemia, Yale J. Biol. & Med., *17*, 163, 1944; J. Lab. & Clin. Med., *32*, 720, 1947; Radiology, *50*, 476, 1948; Cancer Res., *11*, 741, 1951; *in* Proceedings of the Third National Cancer Conference, Philadelphia, J. B. Lippincott Company, 1957, p. 331.

125a. KIRSHBAUM, J. D. and PREUSS, F. S.: Leukemia, a Clinical and Pathologic Study of 123 Fatal Cases in a Series of 14,400 Necropsies, Arch. Int. Med., *71*, 777, 1943.

125b. KLEMPERER, P.: Reticuloendotheliosis, Bull. New York Acad. Med., *30*, 526, 1954.

125c. KLOSTERMEYER, W.: Über eine sogenannte aleukämische Reticulose mit besonderer Beteiligung des Magen-Darmkanales, Beitr. path. Anat. allg. Path., *93*, 1, 1934.

126. KOLER, R. D. and FORSGREN, A. L.: Hepatotoxicity Due to Chlorambucil, J.A.M.A., *167*, 316, 1958.

126*a*.KOLER, P. C. and CASARINI, A.: Comparison of Cytological Effects Induced by X rays and Nitrogen Mustard, Brit. J. Cancer, *6*, 173, 1952.

126*b*.KRAKOFF, I. H.: Mechanisms of Drug Action in Leukemia, Am. J. Med., *28*, 735, 1960.

127. KRANTZ, C. Q. and RIDDLE, M. C.: The Basal Metabolism in Chronic Lymphatic Leukemia, Am. J. M. Sc., *175*, 229, 1928.

127*a*.KREBS, C. and BICHEL, J.: Results of Roentgen Treatment in Chronic Myelogenous Leucosis, Acta radiol., *28*, 697, 1947.

128. KRIVIT, W. and GOOD, R. A.: Simultaneous Occurrence of Mongolism and Leukemia, A.M.A.J. Dis. Child., *94*, 289, 1957.

128*a*.KRUMBHAAR, E. B. and STENGEL, A.: The Spleen in the Leukemias, Arch. Path., *34*, 117, 1942.

129. KULKA, H.: Leukämischer Priapismus der Klitoris unter dem Bilde eines Carcinoms, Arch. Gynäk., *149*, 450, 1932.

129*a*.LARSON, D. L. and TOMLINSON, L. J.: Quantitative Antibody Studies in Man. III. Antibody Response in Leukemia and Other Malignant Lymphomata, J. Clin. Invest., *32*, 317, 1953.

130. LATOURETTE, H. B. and HODGES, F. J.: Incidence of Neoplasia after Irradiation of Thymic Region, Am. J. Roentgenol., *82*, 667, 1959.

130*a*.LAW, L. W.: Recent Advances in Experimental Leukemia Research, Cancer Res., *14*, 695, 1954; Lancet, *1*, 154, 1959.

131. LAWRENCE, J. H.: The Treatment of Chronic Leukemia, M. Clin. North America, *38*, 525, 1954.

131*a*.LAWRENCE, J. H. and DONALD, W. G., JR.: The Incidence of Cancer in Chronic Leukemia and in Polycythemia Vera, Am. J. M. Sc., *237*, 488, 1959.

131*b*.LEIDLER, F. and RUSSELL, W. O.: The Brain in Leukemia, Arch. Path., *40*, 14, 1945.

131*c*.LEITNER, S. J.: *Bone Marrow Biopsy*, Grune and Stratton, New York, 1949.

132. LENNOX, W. G. and MEANS, J. H.: Study of Basal and Nitrogenous Metabolism in Case of Acute Leukemia During Roentgen-ray Treatment, Arch. Int. Med., *32*, 705, 1923.

132*a*.LEONARD, B. J. and WILKINSON, J. F.: Desacetylmethylcolchicine in Treatment of Myeloid Leukæmia, Brit. M. J., *1*, 874, 1955.

132*b*.LESSMANN, ELLEN M. and SOKAL, J. E.: Conception and Pregnancy in a Patient with Chronic Myelocytic Leukemia under

Continuous Colcemide Therapy, Ann. Int. Med., *50*, 1512, 1959.

133. LEUCUTIA, T.: Irradiation in Lymphosarcoma, Hodgkin's Disease and Leukemia, A Statistical Analysis, Am. J. M. Sc., *188*, 612, 1934.

134. LEVISON, V. B.: Respiratory Obstruction in Acute Leukæmia, Lancet, *1*, 1151, 1952.

135. LEWIS, JESSICA H. *et al.*: Studies of Hemostatic Mechanisms in Leukemia and Thrombocytopenia, Am. J. Clin. Path., *28*, 433, 1957.

136. LOCKE, E. A. and MINOT, G. R.: Hematuria as a Symptom of Systemic Disease, J.A.M. A., *83*, 1311, 1924.

137. LOGEFEIL, R. C.: A Study of Mixed Leukemia With the Report of a Case, Arch. Int. Med., *33*, 659, 1924.

138. LUCIA, S. P. and BROWN, J. W.: Hematopoietic Reactions to Antimonyl Antimony, Proc. Soc. Exper. Biol. & Med., *31*, 426, 1934.

138*a*.MAGILL, G. B., WROBLEWSKI, F. and LaDUE, J. S.: Serum Lactic Dehydrogenase and Serum Transaminase in Human Leukemia, Blood, *14*, 870, 1959.

138*c*.MAGRASSI, F., LEONARDI, G., NEGRONI, G. and TOLU, A.: Experimental Studies on the Aetiology of Human Leukæmias, Acta hæmat., *6*, 38, 1951; Minerva med., *2*, 1, 1953.

139. MACH, R. S.: Le syndrome urinaire dans les leucémies, Rev. méd. de la Suisse rom., *51*, 35, 1931.

139*a*.MACMAHON, B. and CLARK, D.: Incidence of the Common Forms of Human Leukemia, Blood, *11*, 871, 1956; *ibid.*, *12*, 1, 1957.

139*b*.MAGALINI, S. I. and AHSTRÖM, L.: Clinical and Hematological Aspects of Acute Erythromyelosis, J. Pediat., *52*, 501, 1958.

139*c*.MANDEL, H. G.: The Physiological Disposition of Some Anticancer Agents, Pharmacol. Rev., *11*, 743, 1959.

140. MARCH, H. C.: Leukemia in Radiologists, Radiology, *43*, 275, 1944; Am. J. M. Sc., *220*, 282, 1950.

140*a*.MARLOW, A. A. and BARTLETT, G. R.: Survival for Twenty-nine Years in Chronic Lymphocytic Leukemia, J.A.M.A., *152*, 1033, 1953.

141. MAS y MAGRO, F.: Recherches morphologiques et expérimentales sur l'étiopathogénie de la leucémie humaine, Sang. *25*, 160,516 and 633, 1954.

141*a*.MATHÉ, G.: Application of Hematopoietic Cell Grafts to the Treatment of Leukemias and Allied Diseases, Blood, *16*, 1073, 1960; Rev. hémat., *15*, 115, 1960.

142. McDONALD, J. B. and HAMRICK, J. W.:

Acute Megakaryocytic Leukemia, Arch. Int. Med., *81*, 73, 1948.

42a.McENDY, D. P., BOON, M. C. and FURTH, J.: On the Rôle of the Thymus, Spleen and Gonads in the Development of Leukemia in a High-Leukemia Stock of Mice, Cancer Res., *4*, 377, 1944.

143. MEACHAM, G. C. and WEISBERGER, A. S.: Early Atypical Manifestations of Leukemia, Ann. Int. Med., *41*, 780, 1954.

144. MEAD, C. H.: Chronic Lymphatic Leukemia Involving the Gastro-intestinal Tract, Radiology, *21*, 351, 1933.

144a.MEIKLE, R. W.: Two Varieties of Leukemia in One Family, Brit. M. J., *2*, 468, 1944.

145. MENDELSOHN, R. S. and WATKIN, D. M.: Serum Vitamin B$_{12}$ Concentrations Determined by *L. Leichmannii* Assay in Patients with Neoplastic Disease, J. Lab. & Clin. Med., *51*, 860, 1958.

146. METCALF, D., FURTH, J. and BUFFETT, RITA F.: Pathogenesis of Mouse Leukemia Caused by Friend Virus, Cancer Res., *19*, 52, 1959.

148. MEYER, O. O.: Achlorhydria in Leucemia, J. Lab. & Clin. Med., *24*, 135, 1938.

148a.MEYER, O. O., MIDDLETON, W. S. and THEWLIS, E. W.: Therapeutic Failure With Certain Organic Substances in Leukemia, Folia hæmat., *53*, 166, 1935.

148b.MILLER, D. G., DIAMOND, H. D. and CRAVER, L. F.: Clinical Use of Chlorambucil, New England J. Med., *261*, 525, 1959.

149. MILLER, A. and SULLIVAN, J. F.: Electrophoretic Studies of the Vitamin B$_{12}$-Binding Protein of Normal and Chronic Myelogenous Leukemia Serum, J. Clin. Invest., *38*, 2135, 1959.

149a.MILLER, F.: Angeborene Leukämie, Virchows Arch., *326*, 73, 1954.

150. MILLER, F. R. and TURNER, D. L.: The Action of Specific Stimulators on the Hematopoietic System, Am. J. M. Sc., *206*, 146, 1943; J. Biol. Chem., *147*, 573, 1943; Proc. Soc. Exper. Biol. & Med., *54*, 177, 1943; Am. J. Path., *21*, 233, 1945; Blood, *1*, 379, 1946; *ibid.*, *2*, 15, 1947; Acta hæmat., *2*, 80, 1949; Proc. Soc. Exper. Biol. & Med., *75*, 633, 1950; J. Nat. Cancer Inst., *14*, 439, 1953.

150a.MILLER, J. F. A. P.; Studies on Mouse Leukaemia, Brit. J. Cancer, *14*, 83 and 93, 1960.

151. MILLS, S. D.: Acute Lymphatic Leucemia in Childhood: A Study of Sixty Cases With Special Reference to the Cytologic Characteristics of the Blood, J. Pediat., *6*, 634, 1935.

152. MINOT, G. R.: A Non-fatal Case Simulating

Acute Leukemia With Anemia and Thrombopenic Purpura, Med. Clin. North America, *13*, 1, 1929.

153. MINOT, G. R. and BUCKMAN, T. E.: The Blood-platelets in the Leukemias, Am. J. M. Sc., *169*, 477, 1925.

154. MINOT, G. R., BUCKMAN, T. E. and ISAACS, R.: Chronic Myelogenous Leukemia: Age Incidence, Duration and Benefit Derived From Irradiation, J.A.M.A., *82*, 1489, 1924.

155. MINOT, G. R. and ISAACS, R.: Lymphatic Leukemia: Age Incidence, Duration and Benefit Derived From Irradiation, Boston M. & S. J., *191*, 1, 1924.

156. MOESCHLIN, S.: Erythroblastosen, Erythroleukämien und Erythroblastämien, Folia hæmat., *64*, 262, 1940.

157. MOESCHLIN, S. and ROHR, K.: Klinische und morphologische Gesichtspunkte zur Auffassung der Myelose als Neoplasma, Ergebn. inn. Med. u. Kinderh., *57*, 723, 1939.

157a.MOFFITT, H. C., JR. and LAWRENCE, J. H.: Chronic Leukemia of Long Duration: With a Report of 31 Cases With a Duration of Over Five Years, Ann. Int. Med., *30*, 778, 1949.

157b.MOLLIN, D. L. and ROSS, G. I. M.: Serum Vitamin B$_{12}$ Concentrations in Leukæmia and in Some Other Hæmatological Conditions, Brit. J. Hæmat., *1*, 155, 1955.

157c.MOLONEY, W. C.: Leukemia in Survivors of Atomic Bombing, New England J. Med., *253*, 88, 1955.

157d.MOLONEY, W. C.: Leukemia and Exposure to X-Ray, Blood, *14*, 1137, 1959.

158. MOORE, E. W., THOMAS, L. B., SHAW, R. K. and FREIREICH, E. J.: The Central Nervous System in Acute Leukemia, A.M.A. Arch. Int. Med., *105*, 451, 1960.

159. MULLA, N.: Acute Leukemia and Pregnancy, Am. J. Obst. & Gynec., *75*, 1283, 1958.

160. MULLER, G. L.: The Cholesterol Metabolism in Health and in Anemia, Medicine, *9*, 119, 1930.

160a.MUNDT, E.: Die genuine Reticulo-Endotheliose (Réticulose pure), Deutsch. Arch. klin. Med., *197*, 602, 1950.

161. MURRAY, R., HECKEL, P. and HEMPELMANN, L. H.: Leukemia in Children Exposed to Ionizing Radiation, New England J. Med., *261*, 585, 1959.

161a.MUSTACCHI, P., SHONFELD, E. M., LUCIA, S. P. and PETRAKIS, N. L.: Mortality in Acute Lymphocytic Leukemia, J. Nat. Cancer Inst., *23*, 1397, 1959; Ann. Int. Med., *52*, 1099, 1960.

162. NAEGELI, O.: Ueber rothes Knochenmark

und Myeloblasten, Deutsch. med. Wchnschr., *26*, 287, 1900.

162a. NATHAN, D. G. and BERLIN, N. I.: Studies of the Rate of Production and Life Span of Erythrocytes in Acute Leukemia, Blood, *14*, 935, 1959.

162b. NATHAN, D. J. and SANDERS, M.: Manifestations of Acute Leukemia in the Parenchyma of the Lungs, New England J. Med., *252*, 797, 1955.

162c. NESBITT, J., III, and ROTH, R. E.: Solitary Lytic Bone Lesion in an Adult with Chronic Myelogenous Leukemia, Radiology, *64*, 724, 1955.

162d. NETOUSEK, M., BOREŠ, J. and DVOŘÁK, K.: Chronic Myelosis following the Use of Thorotrast, Blood, *12*, 391, 1957.

163. NEUMANN, E.: Ein Fall von Leukämie mit Erkrankung des Knochenmarkes, Arch. d. Heilk., *11*, 1, 1870; *ibid.*, *13*, 502, 1872.

163a. NEUMANN, G.: Mortality from Leukemia in West Germany, Deutsche med. Wchnschr., *84*, 191, 1959.

163b. NEWMAN, W., DIEFENBACH, W. C. L., QUINN, M. and MEYER, L. M.: A Case of Acute Plasma-cell Leukemia Supporting the Concept of Unity of Plasmacellular Neoplasia, Cancer, *5*, 514, 1952.

163c. NEWSON, A. A., JR., BRUCE, C. H., TABLER, J. W. and STROTHER, W. K., JR.: Leukemia and Pregnancy, Am. J. Obst. & Gynec., *69*, 892, 1955.

164. NOWELL, P. C. and HUNGERFORD, D. A.: Chromosome Studies on Normal and Leukemic Human Leukocytes, J. Nat. Cancer Inst., *25*, 85, 1960.

165. OLOVSON, T.: Trauma und Leukämie, Acta chir. scandinav., *82*, 63, 1939.

166. ORDWAY, T.: Remissions in Leukemia Produced by Radium in Cases Completely Resistant to *X*-ray and Benzol Treatment, Trans. Am. Phys., *31*, 177, 1916; Boston M. & S. J., *177*, 490. 1917.

167. OSGOOD, E. E.: Monocytic Leukemia, Arch. Int. Med., *59*, 931, 1937.

167a. OSGOOD, E. E. and SEAMAN, A. J.: Treatment of Chronic Leukemias, J.A.M.A., *150*, 1372, 1952; Radiology, *64*, 373, 1955; Blood, *16*, 1104, 1960.

167b. OSGOOD, E. E., SEAMAN, A. J. and KOLER, R. D.: Results of 15 Year Program of Treatment of Chronic Leukemias with Titrated Regularly Spaced Total Body Irradiation with Phosphorus^{32} or X-ray, *in* Proceedings of the International Society of Hematology, Sixth International Congress, New York, Grune and Stratton, 1958.

168. PALMER, E. D.: Leukemia, Gastroduodenal Ulcer, and the Problem of Massive Upper Gastrointestinal Hemorrhage, Cancer, *8*, 132, 1955.

169. PANTON, P. N. and VALENTINE, F.: Chronic Lymphoid Leukæmia, Lancet, *1*, 914, 1929.

169a. PARADE, G. W. and VOEGT, H.: Zur Frage der Hautleukämie, Deutsch. Arch. klin. Med., *185*, 265, 1939.

170. PARSONS, C. G.: Radium in the Treatment of Leukæmia, Brit. J. Radiol., *10*, 573, 1937.

170a. PARSON, W. B., JR., WATKINS, C. H., PEASE, G. L. and CHILDS, D. S., JR.: Changes in Sternal Marrow following Roentgen-ray Therapy to the Spleen in Chronic Granulocytic Leukemia, Cancer, *7*, 179, 1954.

171. PASCHKIS, K.: Malariatherapie der Leukämie?, Med. Klin., *28*, 897, 1932.

172. PATERSON, E., HADDOW, A., AP THOMAS, I. and WATKINSON, J. M.: Leukemia Treated with Urethane Compared with Deep X-ray Therapy, Lancet, *1*, 677, 1946.

172a. PAUL, J. T. and LIMARZI, L. R.: Specific Cutaneous Lesions in Chronic Myeloid Leukemia, Arch. Dermat., *45*, 897, 1942.

173. PEACE, R. J.: Cytomegalic Inclusion Disease in Adults, Am. J. Med., *24*, 48, 1958.

173a. PEARSON, B., STASNEY, J. and PIZZOLATO, P.: Gastrointestinal Involvement in Lymphatic Leukemia, Arch. Path., *35*, 21, 1943.

173b. PELLER, S. and PICK, P.: Leukemia and Other Malignancies in Physicians, Am. J. M. Sc., *224*, 154, 1952.

173c. PELNER, L., FOWLER, G. A. and NAUTS, HELEN C.: *Effects of Concurrent Infections and Their Toxins on the Course of Leukemia*, Stockholm, Esselte AB, 1958.

174. PERILLIE, P. E. and FINCH, S. C.: The Local Exudative Cellular Response in Leukemia, J. Clin. Invest., *39*, 1353, 1960.

174a. PERNOKIS, E. W. and FREELAND, M. R.: Blood Chemistry Observations in Leucemias, J. Lab. & Clin. Med., *26*, 1310, 1941.

174b. PIROFSKY, B.: Studies on the Hemolysin and Agglutinin of Leukemic Leukocytes, Blood, *12*, 620, 1957.

174c. PISCIOTTA, A. V., JERMAIN, L. F. and HINZ, JEAN E.: Chronic Lymphocytic Leukemia, Hypogammaglobulinemia and Autoimmune Hemolytic Anemia, Blood, *15*, 748, 1960.

174d. PIZZOLATO, P.: Leukemia in the Negro, J. Nat. M. A., *41*, 214, 1949.

174e. POCHIN, E. E.: Leukemia following Radioiodine Treatment of Thyrotoxicosis, Brit. M. J., *2*, 1545, 1960.

175. POLLOSSON and LEBEUF, F.: Noma. Guérison par le serum antigangreneux. Apparition ulterieure d'une leucémie lymphoíde, Bull. Soc. franç. dermat. et syph., *40*, 1061, 1933.

175a.Poncher, H. G., Waisman, H. A., Richmond, J. B., Horak, O. A. and Limarzi, L. R.: Treatment of Acute Leukemia in Children with and without Folic Acid Antagonists, J. Pediat., 41, 377, 1952.

175b.Quaglino, D. and Hayhoe, F. G. J.: Periodic-Acid-Schiff Positivity in Erythroblasts with Special Reference to Di Guglielmo's Disease, Brit. J. Haemat., 6, 26, 1960.

175c.Quattrin, N., Dini, E. and Palumbo, E.: Basophile Leukämien, Blut, 5, 166, 1959.

175d.Raab, S. O., Hoeprich, P. D., Wintrobe. M. M. and Cartwright, G. E.: The Clinical Significance of Fever in Acute Leukemia, Blood, 16, 1609, 1960.

175e.Ranney, Helen M. and Gellhorn, A.: The Effect of Massive Prednisone and Prednisolone Therapy on Acute Leukemia and Malignant Lymphomas, Am. J. Med., 22, 405, 1957.

176. Reese, H. H. and Middleton, W. S.: Mechanical Compression of the Spinal Cord by Tumorous Leukemic Infiltration, J.A.M.A., 98, 212, 1932.

177. Reinhard, E. H., Moore, C. V., Bierbaum, O. S. and Moore, S.: Radioactive Phosphorus as a Therapeutic Agent, J. Lab. & Clin. Med., 31, 107, 1946; Ann. Int. Med., 50, 942, 1959.

178. Reschad, H. and Schilling-Torgau, V.: Ueber eine neue Leukämie durch echte Uebergangsformen (Splenozytenleukämie) und ihre Bedeutung für die Selbständigkeit dieser Zellen, München. med. Wchnschr., 60, 1981, 1913.

178a.Reilly, E. B., Rapaport, S. I., Karr, N. W., Mills, H. and Carpenter, G. E.: Familial Chronic Lymphatic Leukemia, Arch. Int. Med., 90, 87, 1952.

182. Richter, M. N. and MacDowell, E. C.: Experiments With Mammalian Leukemia, Physiol. Rev., 15, 509, 1935.

183. Riddle, M. C. and Sturgis, C. C.: Basal Metabolism in Chronic Myelogenous Leukemia, Arch. Int. Med., 39, 255, 1927.

184. Rietti, F.: Die akuten Leukämien, Ergebn. inn. Med. u. Kinderh., 54, 397, 1938 (Bibliography).

185. Rigler, L. G.: Leukemia of the Stomach Producing Hypertrophy of the Gastric Mucosa, J.A.M.A., 107, 2025, 1936.

185a.Rosenow, G.: Leukemia in Old Age, Acta hæmat., 7, 289, 1952.

186. Rosenthal, N. and Harris, W.: Leukemia, Its Diagnosis and Treatment, J.A.M.A., 104, 702, 1935.

186b.Ross, R. R.: Chloroma and Chloroleukemia, Am. J. Med., 18, 671, 1955.

186c.Rothberg, H., Conrad, M. E. and Cowley, R. G.: Acute Granulocytic Leukemia in Pregnancy, Am. J. M. Sc., 237, 194, 1959.

187. Rowe, S. N.: Mikulicz's Syndrome With Chronic Lymphatic Leukemia, New England J. Med., 202, 863, 1930.

188. Rundles, R. W. et al.: Comparison of Chlorambucil and Myleran® in Chronic Lymphocytic and Granulocytic Leukemia, Am. J. Med., 27, 424, 1959.

188b.Sandberg, A. A., Cartwright, G. E. and Wintrobe, M. M.: Studies on Leukemia. I. Uric Acid Excretion, Blood, 11, 154, 1956; in Proceedings of the Third National Cancer Conference, Philadelphia, J. B. Lippincott Company, 1957, p. 357.

189. Saragea, T., Walter, V. and Carstea, V.: Sur l'hypertrophie ganglionnaire dans la leucémie myélogène chronique, Bull. et mém. Soc. méd., hôp. Bucarest, 13, 1, 1931.

189a.Saxton, J. A. Boon, M. C. and Furth, J.: Observations on the Inhibition of Development of Spontaneous Leukemia in Mice by Underfeeding, Cancer Res., 4, 401, 1944.

189c.Schiro, H. S. and Weiss, H. B.: Acute Monocytic Leukemia, Am. J. Med., 1, 307, 1946.

189d.Schott, M.: Ten-year Recovery from Chronic Lymphocytic Leukæmia, Brit. M. J., 1, 877, 1955.

189e.Schultz, J. and Schwartz, S.: The Chemistry of Experimental Chloroma, Cancer Res., 16, 565 and 569, 1956; J. Biol. Chem., 234, 2486, 1959.

190. Schwab, R. S. and Weiss, S.: Neurologic Aspects of Leukemia, Am. J. M. Sc., 189, 766, 1935.

190a.Schwarz, E.: Atypical Giant Cells in the Spleen of Leukemic Conditions, Acta med. scandinav., 150, 119, 1954.

190b.Schwartz, S. O. and Critchlow, J.: Erythremic Myelosis (Di Guglielmo's Disease), Blood, 7, 765, 1952.

190c.Schwartz, S. O. and Schoolman, H. M.: The Etiology of Leukemia, Blood, 14, 279, 1959; J. Lab. & Clin. Med., 53, 233, 1959; ibid., 54, 562, 1959.

190d.Schwartz, S. O., Spurrier, Wilma, Yates, L. R. and Maduros, B. P.: Studies in Leukemia, Blood, 15, 758 and 95, 1960; Proc. Soc. Exper. Biol. & Med., 103, 420, 1960.

191. Schwartz, T. B. and Jager, B. V.: Cryoglobulinemia and Raynaud's Syndrome in a Case of Chronic Lymphocytic Leukemia, Cancer, 2, 319, 1949.

192. Scutt, R.: Bullous Lesions in Leukæmia, Brit. M. J., 1, 139, 1952.

193. Seelenfreund, B.: Veränderungen der oberen Luftwege bei Leukämie, Inaug. Diss.,

Breslau, 1925, quoted by Forkner, C. E., *Leukemia and Allied Disorders*, New York, The Macmillan Co., 1938.

193a.SEIFE, M., REICH, C. and LISA, J. R.: Chronic Lymphatic Leukemia Associated with Hodgkin's Disease, Acta hæmat., 5, 65, 1951.

193b.SELIGMANN, M., GRABAR, P. and BERNARD, J.: Presence of Precipitating Antileucocyte Antibodies in the Serum of Patients with Acute Leukæmia, Vox sanguinis, 4, 181, 1954; Sang, 26, 52, 1955.

193c.SENN, N.: Case of Splenomedullary Leukemia Successfully Treated by the Use of Roentgen Ray, Med. Rec., 64, 281, 1903.

193d.SHANBROM, E. and FINCH, S. C.: The Auditory Manifestations of Leukemia, Yale J. Biol. & Med., 31, 144, 1958.

193e.SHANBROM, E. and KAHN, D.: Treatment of Leukemia Cutis with Demecolcin, Ann. Int. Med., 47, 565, 1957.

193f.SHANBROM, E., MILLER, S. and HAAR, H.: Herpes Zoster in Hematologic Neoplasias, Ann. Int. Med., 53, 523, 1960.

193g.SHANBROM, E., MILLER, S., HAAR, H. and OPFELL, R.: Therapeutic Spectrum of Uracil-Mustard, a New Oral Antitumor Drug, J.A.M.A., 174, 1702, 1960.

194. SHAPIRO, B. and DOWBEN, R. M.: Uric Acid Body Pools and Turnover Rates in Leukemia, J. Lab. & Clin. Med., 48, 754, 1956.

194a.SHAY, H., GRUENSTEIN, M., HARRIS, C. and GLAZER, L.: Transfer of Myelogenous Leukemia Induced by Gastric Instillation of Methylcholanthrene in Wistar Rats, Blood, 7, 613, 1952; Am. J. Path., 31, 367, 1955; Blood, 8, 162, 1958.

194b.SHERMAN, J. L., JR. and LOCKE, R. B.: Use of Busulfan in Myelogenous Leukemia during Pregnancy, New England J. Med., 259, 288, 1958.

194c.SHIMKIN, M. B., METTIER, S. R. and BIERMAN, H. R.: Myelocytic Leukemia: An Analysis of Incidence, Distribution and Fatality, Ann. Int. Med., 35, 194, 1951: *ibid.*, 39, 1254, 1953.

194d.SILVER, R. T., BEAL, GRACE A., SCHNEIDERMAN, M. A. and McCULLOUGH, N. B.: The Role of the Mature Neutrophil in Bacterial Infections in Acute Leukemia, Blood, 12, 814, 1957; Am. J. Med., 24, 25, 1958.

194e.SILVERMAN, F. N.: The Skeletal Lesions in Leukemia, Am. J. Roentgenol., 59, 819, 1948.

194f.SINN, C. M. and DICK, F. W.: Monocytic Leukemia, Am. J. Med., 20, 588, 1956.

195. SKIPPER, H. E.: A Review: On the Mechanism of Action of Certain Temporary Anticancer Agents, Cancer Res., 13, 545, 1953.

195a.SMITH, L. H., JR., BAKER, FAITH A. and SULLIVAN, MARGARET: Pyrimidine Metabolism in Man, Blood, 15, 360, 1960.

195b.SOUTHAM, C. M., CRAVER, L. F., DARGEON, H. W. and BURCHENAL, J. H.: A Study of the Natural History of Acute Leukemia, Cancer, 4, 39, 1951.

196. SPRIGGS, A. I. and BODDINGTON, M. M.: Leukaemic Cells in Cerebrospinal Fluid, Brit. J. Haemat., 5, 83, 1959.

196a.STEFANINI, M. and ALLEGRA, A.: Pulmonary Mucormycosis in Acute Histiocytic Leukemia, New England J. Med., 256, 1026, 1957.

197. STEINBERG, A. G.: The Genetics of Acute Leukemia in Children, Cancer, 13, 985, 1960.

198. STEPHENS, D. J.: Relation of Viscosity of Blood to Leucocyte Count, With Particular Reference to Chronic Myelogenous Leucemia, Proc. Soc. Exper. Biol. & Med., 35, 251, 1936.

199. STEPHENS, D. J. and JONES, E.: Leucocytes in the Saliva in Normal and Abnormal Subjects, Proc. Soc. Exper. Biol. & Med., 31, 879, 1934.

200. STERNBERG, C.: Zur Kenntnis des Chloroms (Chloromyelosarkom), Beitr. path. allg. Path., 37, 437, 1905.

201. STORTI, E.: Uber einem Fall von lymphatischer Leukämie mit ausschliesslicher Lokalisation im Knochenmark und über die Bedeutung der Sternalpunktion für die Diagnose dieser Krankheitsform, Deutsch. Arch. klin. Med., 180, 612, 1937.

201a.STORTI, E. and PERUGINI, S.: Ricerche di citochimica ematologica. Le reazioni dei polisaccaridi applicate alla diagnostica citologica delle leucosi acute, Progr. med., Napoli, 2, 257, 1952.

202. SUTOW, W. W.: Incidence of Stigmata of Mongolism in Children with Acute Leukemia, Pediatrics, 21, 958, 1958.

202a.SYVERTON, J. T. and ROSS, J. D.: The Virus Theory of Leukemia, Am. J. Med., 28, 683, 1960.

203. TACHINO, T.: Observation on Blood Phosphorus Compounds in Normal Adults and Leukemiæ, Nagova J. M. Sc., 14, 122, 1951.

203a.TALBOTT, J. H.: Gout and Blood Dyscrasias, Medicine, 38, 173, 1959.

204. TAYLOR, A. W.: Effects of Glandular Fever Infection in Acute Leukæmia, Brit. M. J., 1, 589, 1953.

204a.THIERSCH, J. B.: Attempted Transmission of Human Leucemia in Man, J. Lab. & Clin. Med., 30, 866, 1945; Cancer Res., 6 695, 1946.

205. THOMPSON, R. B. and MACKAY, S. G. M.: Aleukaemic Myeloblastic Leukaemia, Brit. M. J., 1, 988, 1957.

206. TIVEY, H.: The Prognosis for Survival in Chronic Granulocytic and Lymphocytic Leukemia, Am. J. Roentgenol., 72, 68, 1954.

206a. TOUGH, I. M. et al.: Cytogenetic Studies in Chronic Myeloid Leukaemia and Acute Leukaemia Associated With Mongolism, Lancet, 1, 411, 1961.

206b. TUDHOPE, G. R.: The Survival of Red Cells and the Causation of Anaemia in Leukaemia, Scottish M. J., 4, 342, 1959.

207. TUOHY, E. L.: A Case of Splenomegaly With Polymorphonuclear Neutrophil Hyperleukocytosis, Am. J. M. Sc., 160, 18, 1920.

208. TOWNSEND, S. R.: A Single Myeloid Bone Tumour Associated With a Blood Picture of Chronic Myelocytic Leukæmia, Canad. M. A. J., 40, 352, 1939.

208a. TROUP, S. B., SWISHER, S. N. and YOUNG, L. E.: The Anemia of Leukemia, Am. J. Med., 28, 751, 1960.

208b. TURNER, J. C. and MULLIKEN, B.: Effects of Intravenous Vaccinia in Mice With Sarcoma 180 or Leukemia 9417, Cancer, 3, 354, 1950.

209. TURNER, K. B., DeLAMATER, A. and PROVINCE, W. D.: Observations on the Blood Iodine, J. Clin. Invest., 19, 515, 1940.

209a. ULRICH, H.: The Incidence of Leukemia in Radiologists, New England J. Med., 234, 45, 1946.

209b. ULTMANN, J. E., FISH, W., OSSERMAN, E. and GELLHORN, A.: The Clinical Implications of Hypogammaglobulinemia in Patients with Chronic Lymphocytic Leukemia and Lymphocytic Lymphosarcoma, Ann. Int. Med., 51, 501, 1959.

211. VERLOOP, M. C.: Anæmia in Systemic Diseases, Acta med. scandinav., 151, 367, 1955.

211a. VIDEBAEK, A.: Heredity in Human Leukemia and Its Relation to Cancer, H. K. Lewis & Co., Ltd., London, 1947. See also, Ann. Eugenics, 14, 346, 1949; Acta path. et microbiol. scandinav., 44, 372, 1958.

212. VILTER, R. W., VILTER, S. P. and SPIES, T. D.: A Note on the Blood Codehydrogenases I and II in Lymphatic or Myelogenous Leukemia, South. M. J., 32, 619, 1939.

213. VIRCHOW, R.: Weisses Blut und Milztumoren, Med. Ztg., 15, 157, 163, 1946.

213a. WAINWRIGHT, C. W. and DUFF, G. L.: Monocytic Leukemia, Bull. Johns Hopkins Hosp., 58, 267, 1936.

213b. WAISMAN, H. A., PASTEL, R. A. and PONCHER,

H. G.: Amino Acid Metabolism in Patients with Acute Leukemia, Pediatrics, 10, 653, 1952; Blood, 12, 635, 1957.

213c. WALDO, A. L. and ZIPF, R. E.: Ascorbic Acid Level in Leukemic Patients, Cancer, 8, 187, 1955.

214. WALTER, L. H., SZUR, L. and LEWIS, S. M.: Prolonged Remission in Chronic Lymphatic Leukaemia, Brit. M. J., 1, 859, 1958.

214a. WARD, G. R.: The Infective Theory of Acute Leukaemia, Brit. J. Child. Dis., 14, 10, 1917.

214b. WARD, J. E., GALINSKY, I. and NEWTON, B. L.: Familial Leukemia, Am. J. Human Genet., 4, 90, 1952.

214c. WARREN, S.: The Distribution of Doses of Radioactive Phosphorus in Leukemic Patients, Cancer Res., 3, 334, 1943.

215. WARREN, S. L.: Review of Literature and Twenty-eight New Cases of Acute Leukemia, Am. J. M. Sc., 178, 490, 1929.

217. WASHBURN, A. H.: Chloroma—Report of a Case With Recovery Following Roentgenotherapy With a Review of the Literature, Am. J. Dis. Child., 39, 330, 1930; ibid., 63, 335, 1942.

217a. WASI, P. and BLOCK, M.: The Mechanism of the Development of Anemia in Untreated Chronic Lymphatic Leukemia, Blood, 17, 597, 1961.

218. WATKINS, C. H. and HALL, B. E.: Monocytic Leukemia of the Naegeli and Schilling Types, Am. J. Clin. Path., 10, 387, 1940.

219a. WELLS, C. E. and SILVER, R. T.: The Neurologic Manifestations of the Acute Leukemias, Ann. Int. Med., 46, 439, 1957.

219b. WELLS, R. and LAU, K. S.: Incidence of Leukaemia in Singapore, and Rarity of Chronic Lymphocytic Leukaemia in Chinese, Brit. M. J., 1, 759, 1960.

219c. WESTON, J. T. and GUIN, G. H.: Epithelial Atypias with Chemotherapy in 100 Acute Childhood Leukemias, Cancer, 8, 179, 1955.

219d. WETHERLEY-MEIN, G. and COTTOM, D. G.: Fresh Blood Transfusion in Leukaemia, Brit. J. Haemat., 2, 25, 1956.

219e. WETHERLEY-MEIN, G. and COTTOM, D. G.: Portal Fibrosis in Acute Leukaemia, Brit. J. Haemat., 2, 345, 1956.

219f. WETHERLEY-MEIN, G., EPSTEIN, I. S., FOSTER, W. D. and GRIMES, A. J.: Mechanisms of Anaemia in Leukaemia, Brit. J. Haemat., 4, 281, 1958.

220. WEVE, H.: Lymphomatosis iridis bei Leukämie, Arch. Augenh., 105, 710, 1932.

221. WHIPPLE, G. H. and ROBSCHEIT-ROBBINS, F. S.: Hemoglobin Production Factors in the Human Liver: III. Anemias—Primary,

Aplastic and Secondary—Leukemias, J. Exper. Med., *57*, 671, 1933.

222. WILE, U. J. and HOLMAN, H. H.: Generalized Herpes Zoster Associated With Leukemia, Arch. Dermat., *42*, 587, 1940; *see also* BARTON, R. L. and O'LEARY, P. A.: *ibid.*, *51*, 263, 1945.

222a. WILLIAMS, M. J.: Myeloblastic Leukemia Preceded by Prolonged Hematologic Disorder, Blood, *10*, 502, 1955.

222b. WILLSON, J. K. V.: The Bone Lesions of Childhood Leukemia, Radiology, *72*, 672, 1959.

222c. WINDHOLZ, F. and FOSTER, S. E.: Bone Sclerosis in Leukemia and in Non-Leukemic Myelosis, Am. J. Roentgenol., *61*, 61, 1949.

222d. WINTROBE, M. M. *et al.:* Symposium on Nutritional Factors in Cancer Research, Texas Rep. Biol. & Med., *10*, 931, 1952.

223. WINTROBE, M. M. and HASENBUSH, L. L.: Chronic Leukemia, Arch. Int. Med., *64*, 701, 1939.

223a. WINTROBE, M. M. and HUGULEY, C. M., Jr.: Nitrogen Mustard Therapy for Hodgkin's Disease, Lymphosarcoma, the Leukemias and Other Disorders, Cancer, *1*, 357, 1948; Ann. Int. Med., *41*, 447, 1954.

224. WINTROBE, M. M. and MITCHELL, D. M.: Atypical Manifestations of Leukemia, Quart. J. Med., *9*, 67, 1940.

224a. WOOD, EILEEN, E.: A Survey of Leukaemia in Cornwall, 1948–1959, Brit. M. J., *1*, 1760, 1960.

225. YAGUDA, A. and ROSENTHAL, N.: The Relation of Trauma to Leukemia, Am. J. Clin. Path., *9*, 311, 1939.

226. ZADEK, I.: Radiothorium bei leukämischer Lymphadenose und Myelose, Folia hæmat., *47*, 418, 1932; *ibid.*, 48, 39, 210, 1932; *ibid.*, *49*, 115, 287, 1933; *ibid.*, *50*, 161, 1933.

227. ZANATY, A. F.: Zur frage der medullaren Lymphadenose, Virchows Arch. path. Anat., *292*, 356, 1934.

228. ZARA, E.: Richerche sulla quantita di glutation nel sangue dei leucemici, Gazz. internaz. med.-chir., *39*, 109, 1931.

Chapter 20

Tumors and Tumor-Like Conditions Involving the Blood-Forming Organs

REFERENCE has been made in preceding chapters to a number of conditions involving lymph nodes, the spleen or the skeleton which are either closely related to the more generally recognized "disorders of the blood" or must be differentiated from them. These will be considered more fully in this chapter. They include lymphosarcoma, Hodgkin's disease and other diseases involving lymphatic tissue, Banti's syndrome and other affections characterized by splenomegaly, and multiple myeloma. Not all of these conditions are tumors, some in fact definitely are not. The title of this chapter must therefore be interpreted in its broadest sense and as in no way implying the fundamental nature or etiology of the disorders to be discussed.

CONDITIONS CHIEFLY AFFECTING LYMPH NODES

History, Definition and Terminology.—Malpighi in 1666 described a fatal disease in which the lymphoid tissue and the spleen appeared "like a cluster of grapes" and Thomas Hodgkin[30b,50b] (1832) described the gross anatomy of seven cases, three of which would now be included under the eponym

implied by his name. It was Samuel Wilks, however, who in 1856 provided the lucid description of Hodgkin's disease as it is now recognized, a disease "characterized by a gradual progressive enlargement of the lymphatic glands beginning usually in the cervical region and spreading throughout the lymphoid tissue of the body, forming nodular growths in the internal organs, resulting in anemia and usually a fatal cachexia."[19g]

Much later Kundrat (1893)[38] outlined the picture of lymphosarcoma and Sternberg, Reed,[54] Longcope[42] and others described in detail the microscopic picture which is now accepted as characteristic of Hodgkin's disease. More recently Brill, Baehr and Rosenthal[8] as well as Symmers[64] described a malady marked by giant lymph follicle hyperplasia which is usually regarded as bearing some relation to lymphosarcoma; and Roulet[58] separated "Retothelsarkom" ("reticulum cell" sarcoma) from the general group of malignant diseases of lymphoid tissue.

The etiology of these conditions is unknown. The majority are regarded as neoplasms but Hodgkin's disease in particular has been considered by many as being of infectious origin, as the names lymphogranuloma, lymphogranulomatosis, lymphomatosis granulomatosa, by which it is also known, indicate. Nevertheless from a clinical standpoint, and in many respects histologically also, Hodgkin's disease, lymphosarcoma, "reticulum cell" sarcoma, and "giant follicular hyperplasia," as well as cases described under such names as round cell sarcoma, leukosarcoma, lymphadenosarcoma, lymphocytoma, monocytoma, pseudoleukemia, and even aleukemic lymphatic leukemia (aleukemic lymphadenosis) have much in common. Mycosis or granuloma fungoides has also been classed with this group of diseases. As pointed out in the preceding chapter (p. 955), different sections of the same gland or sections of different glands may show in a given case histologic patterns ranging from any one of these conditions to another.[64a] Some regard them all as malignant mesenchymal tumors which vary only in degree and type of differentiation.[12]

Clinically it is often impossible to distinguish these disorders from one another without the aid of lymph node biopsy. The names "malignant lymphoma," "lymphoblastoma"[50] and "lymphomatoid diseases"[37] have been suggested for the group as a whole. None of these is satisfactory because the names indicate that the conditions are all tumors ("lymphoma," "lymphoblastoma") or that all simply resemble tumors ("lymphomatoid"), neither of which statements is necessarily correct. For this reason, the non-committal designation "conditions of unknown etiology chiefly affecting lymph nodes" will be used. In the following discussion cases of frank leukemia and chloroma will not be considered because they have been discussed already in the preceding chapter.

Classification.—The classification of these disorders is a much disputed subject and a great variety of classifications has been suggested.[55] Since the clinical manifestations of each of these conditions are so varied as to make differentiation on such grounds practically impossible in most cases, resort must be made to a study of the histological picture. Though variations do occur, it has been observed[20] that there is, in general, a constancy over the period of development of the disease in individual cases as well as sufficient distinction between various types to make classification on cytological grounds practical in the majority of cases.[20]

Two general groups can be distinguished and these can be further subdivided: (I) Those cases in which the histological pattern of the lymph node is relatively simple ("reticulum cell" sarcoma, "lymphosarcoma"); (II) those in which the histological picture is more complex. The latter include (a) cases with the histological picture now recognized as typical of Hodgkin's disease; (b) those in which giant follicular hyperplasia is the outstanding characteristic; and (c) the remaining cases, including "clasmatocytic lymphoma," "monocytoma," and "Hodgkin's sarcoma," in which, even though the tumor may be composed of a single type of cell, the character of the latter is such that it generally presents a varying appearance; as a result the histological picture is more complex than in lymphosarcoma or "reticulum" cell sarcoma.

I. **Types With Simple Histological Pattern.**—In the first or **sarcoma group,** the proliferating cells tend to encroach upon, obscure and finally replace the normal architecture of the lymph node. The marginal and medullary sinuses are invaded, and the cells migrate through the nodal capsules and pass into the perinodal tissues. These have been mentioned as points of distinction from lymphocytic leukemia, although in practice they have failed in this purpose.[20] The "sarcoma group" is often referred to as "lymphosarcoma" but it has been subdivided by many writers into "large cell lymphosarcoma" and the "small cell" type and these are now often referred to as "reticulum cell" sarcoma and lymphosarcoma, respectively.

(a) **"Reticulum Cell" Sarcoma.**— The predominant cell is large, 15 to 35 μ in diameter. The nucleus is also large, two to four times that of the lymphocyte; it is round, with a thin but distinct border, the chromatin is extremely delicate, irregular in distribution and lacks points of condensation, and there is a single, prominent, dark-staining nucleolus. The cytoplasm is abundant, pale staining and amphophilic, and its outline is poorly defined. Tumors of this type have been described under the terms "stem cell lymphoma"[20] and "reticular" and "intermediary" types of lymphosarcoma[16] and include the highly undifferentiated forms of this disease.

(b) **"Lymphosarcoma."**—(1) *Lymphoblastic Lymphoma.*[20]—Although referred to as a lymphoblast, the predominant cell does not conform entirely to the characteristics of this cell as seen in the blood. It is 10 to 20 μ in diameter. The nucleus is centrally placed and round or slightly indented in shape with a sharp border and evenly distributed chromatin which is less clumped than in the lymphocyte. Nucleoli are rare. There is a uniform narrow basophilic rim of cytoplasm, spherical in outline or irregular, with psuedopod-like protuberances. Mitotic figures are usually numerous.

(2) *Lymphocytic Lymphoma.*[20]—The predominant cell resembles the lymphocyte. There are few mitotic figures, stem cells, or lymphoblasts and no multinucleated cells. The nodal architecture is obscured but the nodal capsule is usually intact.

II. **Types With Complex Histological Pattern.**—(a) **Hodgkin's Disease (Hodgkin's "Lymphoma"[20]).**— This is distinguished from the types already described by the polycellular picture of the lymph nodes: granulocytes (eosinophilic or neutrophilic), lymphocytes, plasma cells, monocytes, clasmatocytes, fibroblasts, and giant cells. The latter, the Sternberg or Dorothy Reed cells, resemble somewhat the cells of "reticulum cell" sarcoma but are prone to develop multiple and bizarre nuclei. They are 10 to 40 μ or more in diameter, with abundant cytoplasm which may be acidophilic or basophilic. The cell is often irregular in shape and cytoplasmic processes frequently extend between neighboring cells. The nucleus is multilobed or, more rarely, multiple and nucleoli are prominent. In small forms of these cells the nucleus is round or oval. The chromatin occurs in heavy clumps. Mitotic figures are not numerous. A variable amount of fibrosis may be present, in some instances, the process being highly scirrhous. Necrosis is present usually, but varies in extent from foci of microscopic size to large areas visible grossly. Often there is complete loss of the lymph node architecture. The germinal centers and the cords of lymphatic tissue as well as the sinuses are obliterated. The capsule may be invaded.

(b) **Follicular Lymphoma.** — The lymph nodes are characterized by the presence of multiple, follicle-like nodules of varied sizes (Fig. 20–1) which alter the gland structure and compress the normal tissue. The trabeculae are obscured and there is a stromal rearrangement unlike that seen in normal lymph node hyperplasia. The reticulum meshwork is distorted and condensed. Significant numbers of multinucleated cells are not seen, and there is no necrosis or inflammatory exudation. Invasive qualities are observed rarely but isolated follicle fusion occurs, and eventual complete fusion with obscured nodal architecture simulating the picture of lymphoblastic or lymphocytic lymphoma, Hodgkin's disease,[64] and very malignant forms of lymphoma has been observed.[53d, 72a]

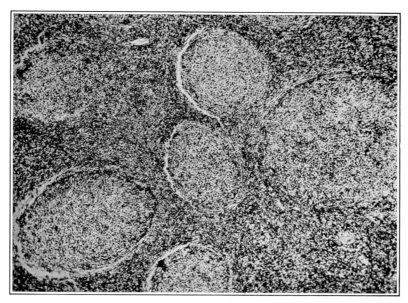

Fig. 20–1.—Follicular lymphoma. Lymph node. (× 60). (Mayer and Thomas, courtesy of Bull. Johns Hopkins Hosp.)

As distinguished from simple hyperplasia of inflammatory or toxic origin, the follicles are larger and more numerous, they are closely packed and scattered throughout the nodes instead of being arranged around the cortex in concentric rows, and they tend to fuse. The dense packing of the cells in the interfollicular tissue, the condensation of the reticulum with slight proliferation of reticular cells, and the narrowed or blocked sinuses, contrast with the scattered interfollicular cells of inflammatory hyperplasia, the loose reticulum and proliferation of reticular cells, and the open and often dilated sinuses.[3]

(c) The remaining types of lymphoma cause considerable difficulty in classification and have been described under a variety of titles. Clinically they resemble one another in their resistance to therapy. Under the name **"clasmatocytic lymphoma."** Gall and Mallory[20] described a tumor in which the predominant cells are smaller than those of "reticulum cell" sarcoma as described above, but

they are larger than lymphocytes, being 14 to 22 μ in diameter. The nucleus is often eccentric, it may be round but is more often oval, reniform, or horseshoe-shaped. The chromatin is fine and nucleoli are rare. The cytoplasm is abundant, generally eosinophilic, and the borders tend to be irregular in outline suggesting ameboid propensities. Engulfed particles and sometimes whole cells may be found in the cytoplasm. This type of tumor will be referred to as **monocytoma.**

In **"Hodgkin's sarcoma"** cells two or three times the size of a normal lymphocyte assume most of the tissue space. These cells, which may be undifferentiated forms of the Reed-Sternberg cell, are usually round but may be ovoid. They have single, spherical nuclei with prominent nucleoli. Their cytoplasm stains neutrophilic or basophilic. A variable number of Reed-Sternberg cells with multilobed nuclei are always seen. Mitotic figures are usually numerous. Generally, only scattered lymphocytes and reticulum cells are found. Neutrophils, eosinophils and plasma cells are rare. Areas of necrosis are not infrequent. The structure of the affected node is destroyed, the capsule may be invaded and there may be extension into the surrounding tissues.[32a] Those who hold that Hodgkin's disease is a granuloma, and infectious in origin, regard "Hodgkin's sarcoma" as a sarcoma developing in Hodgkin's disease, a truly neoplastic response to the exciting agent originally responsible for the chronic inflammatory reaction of the granuloma.[63]

The differentiation of "monocytoma," "Hodgkin's sarcoma" and "reticulum cell" sarcoma may be difficult. Cases have been described in the literature under such titles as "aleukemic reticulo-endotheliosis" (p. 938), "reticulo-endotheliomatosis,"[65] and "leukemic reticulo-endotheliosis" without bone marrow involvement,[72] which may be closely related to or identical with these disorders.

In some of the reports in the literature the term "lymphosarcoma" is used to include not only the "sarcoma group" ("reticulum cell" sarcoma, lymphoblastic and lymphocytic lymphoma) but also monocytoma and the other conditions which have just been mentioned. By other pathologists, the latter are included in the term "reticulum-cell sarcoma."

Hodgkin's Disease.[31b]—Jackson and Parker,[32a] who have devoted many years to the study of Hodgkin's disease, insist that this disease can and should be divided into three types and that any description that includes all three as a single form of the disease must, of necessity, be inaccurate and of little practical value. *"Hodgkin's granuloma"* refers to the familiar type and the most common. Of their 259 cases 90 per cent were classified under this heading. The manifestations of the granuloma are protean and the condition is usually fatal within a few years. *"Hodgkin's paragranuloma"* is a comparatively benign condition beginning in almost all cases in the lymph nodes of the neck and involving, in addition and at most, only the mediastinal nodes. The term "early" applied to this form is misleading because no change may take place in some cases even after two or more decades. Other cases have been observed, however, to be transformed, even after a relatively short time, to the granulomatous variety. Of Jackson and Parker's series, 10.8 per cent were classified under this heading. The experience of others has been similar.[72b] *"Hodgkin's sarcoma"* is a true neoplasm, by no means as protean in its manifestations as Hodgkin's granuloma and rarely accompanied by fever. It appears most often in the sixth and seventh decades of life. It behaves as a highly malignant, comparatively localized tumor, rapidly resulting in death. Of their cases, 19.7 per cent fell in this group. The fact that these percentages total 120.5 instead of 100 illustrates the point that paragranuloma may develop into granuloma, and the latter, as others have also recognized, may become sarcomatous.

Two features unite these three types. The first is the presence, in each, of the "Reed-Sternberg" cells. The second is the transformation, with the passage of time, of one type of the disease into another. Rarely granuloma and sarcoma have been observed coexisting in the same patient and even in the same node. In the paragranulomatous node there is found no evidence of softening or necrosis. Microscopically the predominant cell is the adult lymphocyte. The lymph follicles may be preserved or they may be partly or completely obliterated. Reed-Sternberg cells may be few in number. Reticulum cells are present in varying numbers, plasma cells are not uncommon and may be numerous but eosinophils are never present in such numbers as in Hodgkin's granuloma. Invasion of the capsule, necrosis, polymorphonuclear cell infiltration and fibrosis are minimal.

The histologic picture of Hodgkin's granuloma ("lymphoma") and of Hodgkin's sarcoma have been described in the preceding pages.

Relation to Leukemia.—From the standpoint of lymph node morphology there is no sharp distinction between leukemia and some of the conditions just mentioned. Gall and Mallory[20] attempted to predict the presence or absence of clinical leukemia on the basis of the nodal morphology but found that nodes with apparent blood vessel invasion were obtained from patients without leukemia and many with pericapsular invasion or even large invasive tumors were accompanied by leukocytosis and lymphocytosis. No attempt was made to differentiate "lymphosarcoma cell leukemia" (p. 940) from the more common lymphocytic and lymphoblastic leukemias.

Of the entire series of 618 cases which these authors studied, 50 showed frank leukemia at one time or another. Ten of these cases remained leukemic throughout the illness, 13 were non-leukemic when first observed but became leukemic later, and the remainder showed various gradations and fluctuations between the clinical picture of frank leukemia, "subleukemia," "aleukemia" and non-leukemia. Most of these changes occurred following roentgen irradiation but some developed spontaneously. The relationship between leukemia and the lymph node tumors was particularly noticeable among the cases classed by lymph node examination as lymphocytic or lymphoblastic lymphoma, for in a third of these the blood picture was subleukemic or leukemic. Again, in another series of 1269 cases of all varieties, a transition to leukemia was observed in 7.6 per cent.[56a] Among children, the leukemic transition was twice as common (13 per cent). In the whole series the incidence was highest among cases of small cell lymphosarcoma (12.6

per cent) and of these six cases developed into acute leukemia, 25 changed to chronic lymphocytic leukemia and 39 to "leukolymphosarcoma." Next in frequency were the cases of follicular lymphoma (8.6 per cent), of which two, five and seven cases, respectively, were so transformed. Showing the least tendency for leukemic modification were the cases of reticulum cell sarcoma (2.4 per cent). In another series,[73a] six out of 113 patients developed acute leukemia, of which three were of a "reticulum cell" type, two myeloblastic and one monocytoid.

When a change has taken place in cases of follicular lymphoma, the leukemic cell type, as above indicated, has usually been of the lymphocytic series. In one such case a full remission of the leukemic phase occurred.[1b] However, in two instances, acute myeloblastic leukemia was observed.[31]

It may be pointed out here that when cases are approached from the clinical angle rather than from the standpoint of lymph node histology, the distinction between leukemia and lymphoma is in most cases quite readily made. Nevertheless, the well-recognized instances in which lymphosarcoma has developed into leukemia, as well as the failure to make out any differences on the basis of nodal morphology, make one wonder whether any fundamental differences between some of the lymphomas and lymphocytic and lymphoblastic leukemias exist.

Etiology.—Incidence.— These diseases are seen in all parts of the world, sparing no race. Social conditions or occupation seem to play no part. In the United States in 1949 there were 4.2 deaths per 100,000 population which were attributable to the disorders under consideration here.[23a] Of these, 40 per cent were due to Hodgkin's disease, 38 per cent to lymphosarcoma, 6.2 per cent to reticulum cell sarcoma and 0.4 per cent to follicular lymphoma. In different

64

institutions the relative numbers of the various types of cases vary, in part as the result of differences in histologic interpretation. Thus, of 618 cases at the Massachusetts General Hospital, almost a third were Hodgkin's lymphoma, 22 per cent lymphocytic lymphoma, 14 per cent lymphoblastic lymphoma, 13 per cent clasmacytoma, 8 per cent stem cell lymphoma, 7 per cent follicular lymphoma and 6 per cent Hodgkin's sarcoma.[20] At the Memorial Hospital in New York[63] the ratio of Hodgkin's disease to "lymphosarcoma" was 4:3. Of the latter, there were equal numbers of "small cell" and "reticulum cell" sarcoma (43.6 per cent) and 12.8 per cent were classified as giant follicle lymphoma.[56a]

The recorded death rate for Hodgkin's disease in the United States rose from 0.7 per 100,000 population in 1921 to 1.7 in 1951.[61c]

Age and Sex.—It has been recognized for a long time[50] that Hodgkin's disease affects a younger age group than the other lymph node disorders. Follicular lymphoma, "reticulum cell" sarcoma and monocytoma rarely appear in youth. Hodgkin's sarcoma has been observed chiefly in the middle-aged or elderly.[32a] Lymphosarcoma[45c] like Hodgkin's disease may be seen in children but is less common.[61c] All of the diseases under discussion have been observed, however from infancy to far-advanced old age, (one hundred and seven years).[63]

In one series,[20] 22 per cent of the cases of Hodgkin's lymphoma developed before twenty years of age. Although it is uncommon in the first decade of life, nine cases have been reported even in children under two and a half years of age.[13a] The peak frequency of Hodgkin's disease, as judged by age of onset is in the third decade (twenty to twenty-nine years)[61c] but the mean age is in the next decade (thirty-one to thirty-nine years) because cases have been described even

in old age. The peak frequency of lymphosarcoma, when no distinction is made according to histologic type except for the exclusion of follicular lymphoma, was found in the same study[61c] to be during the sixth decade (fifty to fifty-nine) but the mean age was in the preceding decade (forty-eight years). In this survey, when the cases of lymphosarcoma were subdivided according to their main clinical features it was observed that the mean age at onset in cases in which peripheral lymph nodes were involved, without accompanying constitutional signs, was 49.2 years; in those whose main clinical manifestations were abdominal or thoracic masses, 43.4 years; in cases with chief involvement in the gastro-intestinal tract, skin, bone or other uncommon sites, 51.6 years; in the follicular lymphomas, 48.5 years. The results of other studies[3,20,50,63] are similar.

The age of onset and the age at death of patients with Hodgkin's disease or lymphosarcoma has shifted progressively in recent years toward an older age.[61c]

A distinction should be made between the age distribution of these diseases, as described above, and the age selection or incidence, that is *the age at risk of dying of the disease.*[23a] In Hodgkin's disease the risk progressively increases with increase in age[61c] whereas for lymphosarcoma there is only a very gradual increase in risk of death up to about forty years of age, followed by a more rapid rise to age sixty, after which risk of dying from this cause remains constant.[23a]

In all of these conditions males have been more frequently affected than females. Thus, for Hodgkin's disease the percentage of males has been recorded as 69.7 per cent,[67] 62.0 per cent[31b] and 63.4 per cent.[61c] In children the ratio increases to more than 4:1.[31b] An interesting feature is the fact that there has been a shift toward an increasing proportion of females in recent years.[61c] Figures for lymphosarcoma are similar but the preponderance of males is somewhat greater.[61c]

The age distribution of cases of Hodgkin's disease and lymphosarcoma at the Memorial Center in New York is compared with that of leukemia in Figure 20–2.

Familial Occurrence. — Sixty-three instances of familial Hodgkin's disease have been reported.[53e] Hodgkin's disease has occurred concurrently in twins,[31b] in husbands and wives and in infants and mothers.[29,31b] A very careful analysis of the familial occurrence of this condition showed it to occur more often than one might expect from chance alone. It was calculated that the probability that the immediate relatives of a proband with Hodgkin's disease will also develop the disease is three times as great as the corresponding probability for the immediate relatives of a proband without the disease. However, the chance is still small, as only a little more than 1 per cent of the probands with Hodgkin's disease had an immediate relative with this condition. A study of the familial concentration of lymphosarcoma and leukemia showed no statistically significant familial incidence.

With reference to its possible etiologic significance, it was concluded in the above study that heredity seems to play a relatively minor or indirect role in the etiology of Hodgkin's disease. Furthermore, it was considered uncertain whether the observed familial concentration was actually the consequence of heredity or the result of the greater environmental similarities for the members within a family. The evidence pointed more to environment than heredity.

Race.—It has been stated that these disorders are relatively less common in Negroes and in Orientals than in Caucasians[31b,53e] but the evidence is far from conclusive.

Pathogenesis. — Lymphosarcoma and reticulum cell sarcoma are assumed

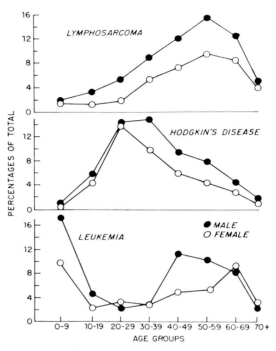

Fig. 20–2.—Comparison of the age distribution of 1269 patients with lymphosarcoma, 1102 cases of Hodgkin's disease and 220 patients with leukemia at the Memorial Center in New York. The distribution is shown according to percentages occurring in each decade. (Razis, Diamond and Craver,[53e] courtesy of Ann. Int. Med.)

generally to be true neoplasms. Experimental studies in mice and other species indicate a close relationship between lymphosarcoma and leukemia and reveal that similar factors govern the development of both types of disorder.[21] What the fundamental cause of these disorders may be, whether neoplastic, a virus-like agent[33b] or a cytoplasmic particle, is no more settled in relation to lymphosarcoma than in leukemia, nor is it known whether the conditions occurring in mice, rats[23b] or other species are identical with the human diseases. These topics have been discussed already in the preceding chapter (p. 906). Follicular lymphoma was at first considered to be a benign disease[8,64] and it was suggested that the cause, as well as that of other "lymphoid diseases," enters through mucous membranes, most often those of the gastro-intestinal tract.[64a] This hypothesis was based on the observation that in cases of lymphosarcoma the preponderant changes at autopsy are in the gastro-intestinal tract, in the thymus or in the abdominal or thoracic lymph nodes. Most students of the subject, however, now regard even follicular lymphoma as being a true neoplasm.[53d, 72a]

The histological character of Hodgkin's disease bears strong resemblance to that of an infectious granuloma.[36] The blood picture encountered in this disease is often like that associated with a non-pyogenic infection and sometimes it even resembles that of a pyogenic condition. Numerous attempts to demonstrate the etiological agent have failed, however.[65a] As Ewing aptly stated, tuberculosis has followed Hodgkin's disease like a shadow. Before the histological picture of Hodgkin's disease was clearly described, it was often confused with glandular tuberculosis. A more frequent association of tuberculosis and Hodgkin's disease was found in autopsies than of tuberculosis and pernicious anemia or cancer.[52] Yet attempts to prove that Hodgkin's disease is an atypical form of tuberculosis[18] or due to infection with avian tubercle bacilli[56] have been unconvincing.

Nor has it been shown that Hodgkin's disease is due to a diphtheroid bacillus, as was once suggested.[10a] Hodgkin's disease has never been successfully transmitted to animals. Gordon's encephalopathic agent, which can be obtained from lymph glands affected with Hodgkin's disease and was originally considered to be a virus causing the disease, was shown to be a substance derived from eosinophils which can be extracted from any tissue containing such cells.[34, 47] It is no longer considered that Brucella infection[19d] bears an etiologic relationship to Hodgkin's disease.[31a] Some workers have suggested

that Hodgkin's disease is a virus tumor analogous to avian lymphomatosis.[31a] In tissue cultures of cells from Hodgkin's disease lymph node cytoplasmic inclusions have been reported,[26] and evidence of a viral etiology for this disease has been offered on the basis of experiments in which Hodgkin's disease lymph node extracts were passed serially in embryonated chicken eggs and in suckling mice.[6b] The viral etiology of Hodgkin's disease, however, has yet to be supported by conclusive evidence.[19e, 31b] Many pathologists consider it, like lymphosarcoma and the other disorders under consideration here, to be a neoplasm.[20] It has been suggested that it is a megakaryoblastoma, a tumor arising in the bone marrow from megakaryocytes.[48] Hodgkin's sarcoma, as already stated, is classified as a neoplasm.

An intriguing concept is based on observations of homologous disease in mice, arising from interest in tissue transplantability as well as evidence of immunological inadequacy and of anergy in patients with Hodgkin's disease.[25b, 33a] It has been pointed out that homologous disease in animals and lymphoid neoplasia in man have in common wasting, anemia and lymphoid depletion.[25b, 32g] This led to the suggestion that some of the manifestations of Hodgkin's disease and of the lymphoid disorders under consideration here are the consequence of a cyto-immunological reaction of lymphoid cells against the usual hemopoietic cells of the host because of antigenic differences between the lymphoid tumor cells and the normal cells of the patient.

Symptomatology.—In the main the clinical features of the various types of disease chiefly affecting lymph nodes are similar and do not require separate description. They are also similar in many respects to those of leukemia, which have been discussed fully in the preceding chapter.

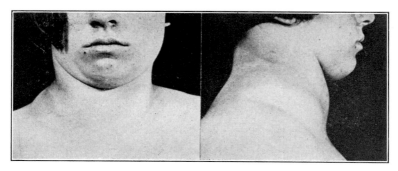

FIG. 20–3.—Enlargement of glands in the posterior triangle of the right side of the neck in a case of Hodgkin's disease.

Lymph Node Involvement. — Lymph node involvement is the most common symptom and is usually the presenting complaint (Figs. 20–3 and 20–4). Involvement of superficial nodes occurs in 60 to almost 100 per cent of cases, but it must be noted that evident adenopathy may be absent, and in rare cases of Hodgkin's disease no glandular involvement has been found even at autopsy[32,35] (Fig. 20–9). The retroperitoneal lymph nodes or the mediastinal glands (Fig. 20–6) may be enlarged and symptoms may arise from the pressure effects of such masses. Retroperitoneal enlargement is especially common in follicular lymphoma.[3,20] In this condition and occasionally in the other conditions under discussion the glands may decrease in size or even disappear spontaneously, for a time.[3,64]

The glands of the neck, at first one side and then the other, are usually the first affected in Hodgkin's disease and this is often also true of the "sarcoma" group. In Hodgkin's "paragranuloma," for many years the cervical glands may be the only ones involved. In the granulomatous type thorough examination, aided by roentgenography, will often reveal other lymph node enlargements as well. In Hodgkin's sarcoma, however, initial peripheral lymphadenopathy may be lacking in as many as half the cases.[32a] An example of the frequency of various

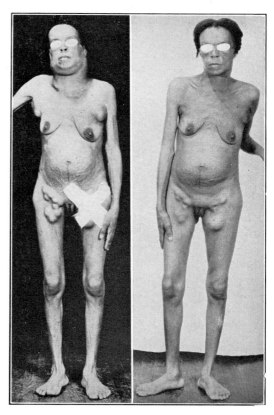

FIG. 20–4.—Extreme generalized adenopathy in a case of "reticulum cell" sarcoma. The radiosensitivity of the tumor is indicated by the change produced in thirteen days.

regions as the sites of the initial glandular enlargement in Hodgkin's disease is:[63] neck 68 per cent, axilla 20 per cent, groin 12 per cent; in the "sarcoma group,"

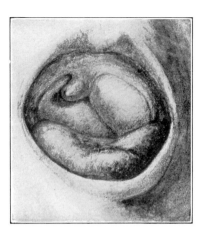

Fig. 20–5.—Nasopharyngeal tumor in a case of follicular lymphoma. The uvula is displaced to the right.

neck 59 per cent, axilla 11.4 per cent, groin 11.9 per cent, abdomen 13.1 per cent, mediastinum 1.1 per cent. Other observers[2] noted, in Hodgkin's disease, primary mediastinal and abdominal adenopathy at the expense of axillary and inguinal involvement, but in all series superficial gland enlargement, especially that of the neck, by far outnumbers primary adenopathy elsewhere. Difficulty in diagnosis arises when there is neither superficial lymphadenopathy nor definite evidence of enlargement of more deeply seated glands. As already stated, this has been seen in cases of Hodgkin's disease, and in as many as 20 per cent of cases of "reticulum cell" sarcoma and monocytoma.[20]

In most cases the enlargements are painless, except when they have developed rapidly or when nerves, such as the cervical plexus, are infiltrated as well. In Hodgkin's sarcoma, however, the superficial lymph nodes are often painful.[32a] In the "sarcoma group" the glands are characterized by a resilient firmness, somewhat like that of uncured gum rubber. Usually an entire chain is involved but the glands are discrete and movable at first, only becoming

matted together and fixed later. In Hodgkin's disease, because of the presence of connective and fibrous tissue in the nodes, they may be harder than in the "sarcoma group." They often have the consistency of cartilage. The stony hardness of carcinoma is not found, however. Redness of the skin or local heat is unusual and suppuration is rare. A characteristic appearance in advanced cases is a pyramidal swelling with its base at the clavicle and the apex at the angle of the jaw. Generally a mass of glands consists of several large ones and a number of smaller glands. Their size varies from that of a pea to that of a large orange.

Symptoms may be produced by pressure of enlarged lymph glands located in the mediastinum, abdomen or elsewhere, by development of the disease primarily in tissues other than the lymph nodes or spleen, or as the result of systemic effects.

Extranodal Primary Sites.—An extranodal primary site was observed in a third of the cases of "lymphosarcoma" (chiefly "reticulum cell" sarcoma) at the Memorial Hospital in New York.[63] Of these, 65 per cent were cranial structures, especially the tonsils and nasopharynx (Fig. 20–5), 16 per cent were in the gastro-intestinal tract (stomach, jejunum, ileum, rectum, in the order named), and 19 per cent elsewhere (bone, breast, skin, lung, thymus,[44c] ovary, testicle). Secondary sites in the same series of cases were spleen 21 per cent, lungs 12 per cent, bones 9.7 per cent, liver 8 per cent, skin 5.5 per cent, gastro-intestinal tract 5 per cent, tonsils 5 per cent.

Tonsils.—Except in Hodgkin's sarcoma, involvement of the tonsils is very uncommon in Hodgkin's disease, but is not infrequent in the other types of conditions here discussed. Of 226 cases of malignant disease of the tonsil admitted to the Huntington Hospital in Boston,[32b] 11.8 per cent were proven to be "malignant lymphoma" of one type or another. Of 36 cases, "reticulum cell" sarcoma made up 16, "lymphocytoma" and "lymphosarcoma" 15, Hodgkin's disease 4, and follicular lymphoma 1. Such tumors occupy the tonsillar fossa and often extend beyond the midline, displacing the uvula and soft palate. Ulceration has been observed in only one-third of the cases. Persistent sore throat, pain and dysphagia are common complaints.

Splenomegaly.—Splenomegaly is not as prominent a symptom in these disorders as in leukemia. It is infrequent in monocytoma, "reticulum cell" sarcoma, "Hodgkin's sarcoma"[20] and, in our experience, in "lymphosarcoma." At the Memorial Hospital in New York,[63] splenomegaly was encountered in 21 per cent of cases of "lymphosarcoma" (chiefly "reticulum cell" sarcoma) but the enlargement was never prominent "unless a leukemic picture was present." In Hodgkin's disease, splenomegaly is a more common finding and in most studies splenic enlargement has been reported in about 50 per cent of cases. It has been emphasized,[25] however, that at an early stage the incidence of splenomegaly is low even in Hodgkin's disease. In occasional cases, nevertheless, the splenic enlargement may overshadow all the other clinical features.[32] Splenomegaly is often a prominent symptom in cases of follicular lymphoma. It has been noted in 61 per cent of such cases.[3] In 1 recorded case the organ weighed as much as 6500 Gm.

Thyroid.—Although infrequent, "malignant lymphoma" involving the thyroid may be primary there and produces a characteristic clinical syndrome: rapid onset of thyroid enlargement, dysphagia, dyspnea, weakness, weight loss and hoarseness.[68a] Metastatic lesions show a predilection for the gastrointestinal tract.[67a] Secondary involvement, usually of minor extent, was found in 16.9 per cent of autopsied cases.[51a]

Respiratory Tract.—In addition to symptoms associated with involvement of the nasopharynx or tonsils, as already described, cough, stridor, dyspnea, cyanosis of the head and neck, paralysis of a vocal cord, or dysphagia may develop as the result of enlargement of mediastinal glands, infiltration of the walls of the bronchial passages, infiltration of the lungs with nodular or massive (lobular or lobar[57]) involvement, atelectasis and even secondary infection and cavitation of the lungs or pneumothorax, hydrothorax or chylous pleural effusion. Retrosternal "board-like" infiltration may develop, and this may be associated with presternal edema.[19c] Involvement of the lungs may produce a roentgenographic picture resembling that of primary neoplasm or of metastatic carcinoma or miliary tuberculosis.[49,61a] Chylous effusion is much more common in the diseases chiefly affecting lymph nodes than as the result of any other cause and of these it is most frequent in follicular lymphoma.[20a] Primary lymphosarcoma of the lung has been observed, although it is rare,[11e,62g] but preponderant or primary Hodgkin's disease of the lung is extremely rare.[64a,72c]

By roentgenographic examination intrathoracic lesions were demonstrated in 74 per cent of cases of "lymphosarcoma."[66c] In this condition involvement of the upper respiratory tract is more common than lower thoracic invasion.[63] In a series of 55 cases of Hodgkin's disease, intrathoracic involvement was found by roentgenography in 63 per cent.[70a] In half the cases there was mediastinal involvement (paratracheal, tracheobronchial and bronchopulmonary nodes); in 40 per cent the lung parenchyma was either infiltrated or, less often, isolated nodules resembling pulmonary metastases, atelectasis or cavitation were present. Pleural, osseous (ribs, sternum, vertebrae) and cardiac invasion made up the remainder.

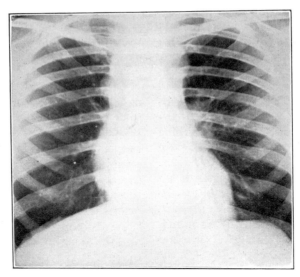

A

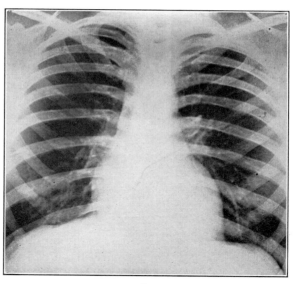

B

FIG. 20–6.—*A*, Enlargement of the glands in the upper mediastinum to the right and in the right supraclavicular region, in a case of Hodgkin's disease. *B*, Normal mediastinal shadow in the same case two and a half years following roentgen irradiation.

Digestive System.—Digestive symptoms may be due to the presence of enlarged lymph nodes or may accompany the late systemic effects of these diseases, but the digestive tract may itself be involved.

Gastric sarcoma represents approximately 3 per cent of all malignant gastric tumors.[47a] Of these approximately two-thirds have been found to be due to lymphosarcoma, the remainder being leiomyosarcomas and fibrosarcomas. The

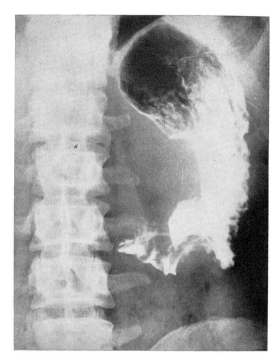

Fig. 20–7.—Extensive involvement of the stomach such as may be seen in "lymphosarcoma" or in colloid carcinoma of the stomach. The lesser curvature as well as the lower fundus and the pyloric regions of the stomach are notably affected.

age distribution of the reported cases is broad (three and one-half to ninety-one years) and the average age is somewhat lower than that of gastric carcinoma. The symptoms include pain, often like that of a peptic ulcer, weight loss, nausea, vomiting, hematemesis and melena.[19h, 53g] These have usually been less than one year in duration. An abdominal mass may be palpable. Anemia is uncommon. Roentgenographically a filling defect with smooth margins, a localized tumor or a diffuse lesion simulating linitis plastica, an annular lesion at the pylorus, pattern of giant rugae (Fig. 20–7), sluggish peristalsis, gastric retention or changes in the size of the stomach may be found. The secretory

response observed on gastric analysis has ranged from anacidity to hypersecretion.

Involvement of the bowel is about as frequent as that of the stomach if all sites in the intestines are included. The ileum is the site most often affected, with the cecum, rectum, jejunum, duodenum and other areas in the colon following next, in order of decreasing incidence.[48a, 62e] Mid-abdominal or lower abdominal pain, symptoms and signs suggestive of chronic obstruction, an abdominal mass, or a sprue syndrome when the small bowel was involved,[62f] have been the chief clinical manifestations. Hematemesis, melena or diarrhea have not been frequent in small intestinal cases but intussusception has been relatively common.[48a] Weight loss has not been as marked as in carcinoma and this has been found to contrast sharply with the large tumors visualized roentgenographically. In the small intestine single or multiple, small or large and discrete or diffuse tumors have been described; or the findings may suggest a nonspecific motor disturbance. The mucous membrane pattern may be obliterated, the intestinal walls may seem stiff, peristalsis may be absent and crescentic indentations may be observed.[12a] In the cecum the lesion has been more often polypoid, in the rectum annular, sometimes producing a stricture. As compared with carcinoma, lymphomatous involvement of the large bowel is exceedingly uncommon (0.3 per cent) but in the small intestine it forms a significant proportion of the cases (25 per cent).[62e]

In follicular lymphoma gastro-intestinal involvement is rare[3,19] but may occur. Ascites is more frequent and is often chylous.

In Hodgkin's disease the gastrointestinal tract may likewise be exclusively involved, although this is very rare,[53c] or the symptoms may be due to glandular enlargement or arise from the systemic effects of the disease. Gastro-intestinal disturbances occur in a third of the cases. Diarrhea is a common symptom even early in the course of the disease. Obstruction of the lacteals by disease of the mesenteric glands may produce the clinical picture of sprue.[2] The infiltration, as in the "sarcoma group," involves the upper gastrointestinal tract more often than the lower bowel. In the stomach,[66a] the antrum is the most common site of the disease.[53c] In the small intestine the jejunum or proximal ileum have been involved most frequently, the terminal ileum, the duodenum and the entire small intestine being next, in order of decreasing frequency. In the colon, the rectum[21b] and the esophagus[32a] Hodgkin's disease is exceedingly rare.[53c] The lesions at any of these sites are most often infiltrating and produce thickening of the wall but they may be polypoid or ulcerating. The symptoms are similar to those described for lymphosarcoma of the gastro-intestinal tract. Thus they may be those of an ulcerative lesion or of a localized or extensive tumor, or peritonitis may occur. Involvement of the digestive tract is more common in persons of middle age than in youth and diagnosis may be very difficult because of the absence of associated adenopathy or splenomegaly. The diagnosis has been made, however, by exfoliative cytology.[58a] In Hodgkin's sarcoma multiple involvement of the gastro-intestinal tract is not infrequent.[32a]

Primary "lymphosarcoma" of the *liver* has been observed.[30] Secondary invasion has been noted in 8 per cent of cases.[63] Such involvement is at least six times as common in Hodgkin's disease[64a] and has been described in 11 per cent of cases of follicular lymphoma. In the latter, dense nodules of reticulum cells in the periportal connective tissues have been described.[4a] Invasion of the *gall bladder* and the extrahepatic biliary tract[26c] and, in two cases, esophageal varices,[39a] have also been reported.

The development of *jaundice* in Hodgkin's disease is an ominous prognostic sign. Jaundice has been described in 3 to 8 per cent or more of patients. In an autopsy series of 57 cases,[39b] the cause was liver involvement with Hodgkin's disease in 70.2 per cent, unexplained in 14 per cent, hemolytic anemia in 5.2 per cent, extrahepatic bile duct obstruction due to tumor 3.5 per cent, hepatitis 3.5 per cent, choledocholithiasis 1.8 per cent and cirrhosis 1.8 per cent.

Circulatory System. — Although pathologic evidence of cardiac involvement is not uncommon, clinical manifestations are unusual. The two commonest clinical pictures are (1) intractable congestive cardiac failure as the result of invasion of the heart by a mediastinal tumor or from discrete deposits, or diffuse infiltration of the myocardium; and (2) that resulting from pericardial effusion, which is usually hemorrhagic and is the result of pericardial invasion. Various arrhythmias have been reported, as well as a syndrome resembling constrictive pericarditis.[32c] Secondary effects such as swelling and edema; venous engorgement and cyanosis of limbs as the result of compression by enlarged lymph glands; and clubbing of fingers in association with pulmonary involvement may be encountered.

Genito-urinary System. — Genito-urinary symptoms may be so prominent as to suggest primary disease of these passages.[4] As the result of invasion or by pressure from without, hematuria, pyuria, retention of urine, pain in the back, a mass in the flanks or symptoms indicative of disease of the prostate or testicles,[11a] may arise. Genito-urinary symptoms have been found in as many

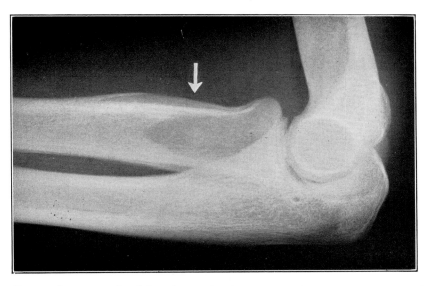

Fig. 20–8.—Destructive process involving the proximal end of the right radius with marked periosteal reaction over it, in a case of "lymphosarcoma" (lymphoblastic lymphoma).

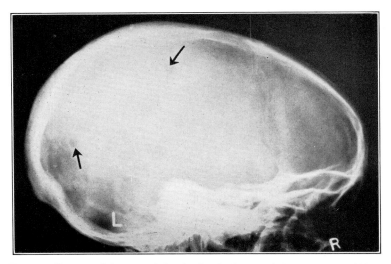

Fig. 20–9.—Two small areas of decreased density in the bones of the skull resembling metastases due to carcinoma, in a case of "bone marrow" Hodgkin's disease (p. 1024). There was severe anemia, leukopenia and thrombocytopenia without glandular enlargement or splenomegaly. The only other bone lesion was increased osteoporosis of the bones in the region of the left wrist.

as one-third of cases and involvement of the tissues of these systems has been noted in as many as 59 per cent of cases. Albuminuria, however, may be a manifestation of complicating amyloidosis.[30a,61b] Lymphosarcoma may involve the kid-neys[1a] and we have observed Hodgkin's disease with renal manifestations as the outstanding feature. Hodgkin's sarcoma has been described in the uterus[26a] and in the ovary.[27]

Osseous System. — Localized pain

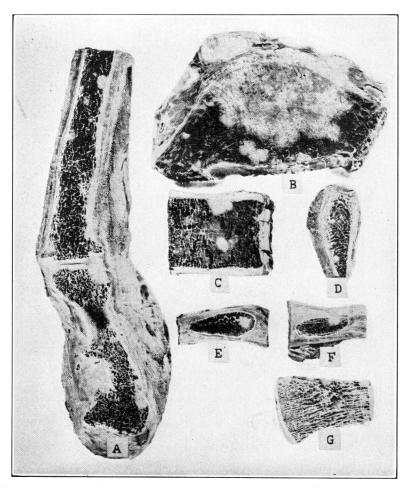

Fig. 20–10.—Lymphogranulomatous lesions in the marrow in a case of Hodgkin's disease. *A*, Manubrium and half of the sternum. *B*, Transection through the fourth lumbar vertebral body, and *C*, mid-dorsal vertebral body. *D*, Right iliac crest, and *E* and *F* the right third and second ribs. *G*, The only bone without a lesion. It is the left first metatarsal. (Steiner, courtesy of Arch. Path.)

and tenderness, less often tumors about the bone margins and neurological changes due to extension into the spinal canal from vertebral lesions, may lead to the recognition of bone involvement. Symptoms may, however, be absent; or spontaneous fractures may occur.[49] Symptoms referable to the osseous system may be the initial complaints.[14] Hodgkin's disease of the bone marrow without lymph node involvement (Fig. 20–9) and

affecting only the spleen or the liver in addition is very rare.[32,35]

Bone lesions have been demonstrated by roentgenograms in 14.8 per cent of cases of Hodgkin's disease,[66d] in 7 per cent of cases of "lymphosarcoma"[66d] and in 23 per cent of cases of "monocytoma."[20] Giant follicular lymphoma has been found to involve the skeletal system in a disproportionately low degree, reticulum cell sarcoma in a relatively high propor-

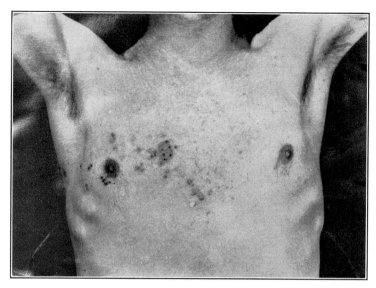

FIG. 20–11.—Herpes zoster in a case of Hodgkin's disease.

tion of cases.[11b] Determinations of serum alkaline phosphatase suggest an even higher incidence.[71] Systematic examinations at autopsy have revealed bone lesions in 50 per cent of cases of Hodgkin's disease.[18c,64a] During life the lesions are found most frequently in the pelvis, vetebrae, ribs and femora[66d] but other bones may be involved (Figs. 20–8, 20–9, 20–10). In most cases more than one bone is affected. Primary reticulum cell sarcoma of bone is uncommon.[19f,62h] In Hodgkin's disease the lesions are usually proliferative (osteoplastic) and osteolytic; in "lymphosarcoma" they are usually osteolytic.

Cutaneous Manifestations.[17]—Cutaneous manifestations constitute an important and frequently occurring part of the picture of the diseases under discussion (except follicular lymphoma) for they may be encountered in as many as 40 per cent of cases. They may be the result of infiltration of the skin by the specific cells or they may be nonspecific, the so-called "lymphomids." The latter include *pruritus*, a well-recognized sign

encountered in 10 per cent of cases of Hodgkin's disease and less frequently in the other diseases chiefly affecting lymph nodes. Pruritus may precede the onset of any other symptoms.[25] A localized or generalized brownish (*café au lait*) pigmentation of the skin may accompany or appear independently of pruritus. In Hodgkin's disease particularly, erythema, a macular morbilliform eruption, herpes zoster (Fig. 20–11), eczema, papules, wheals, vesicles, bullae, furuncles, and lichenification have been described.[17] Ulceration may occur following necrosis of glands or cutaneous tumors[61] or as the result of specific infiltration[63b] (Fig. 20–12, B).

Firm intracutaneous nodules, colorless or shiny bluish-red in appearance, are the most common specific lesions in "lymphosarcoma" and similar lesions may be seen in Hodgkin's disease (Fig. 20–12, A).[17] In the latter an exfoliative erythroderma has also been described as well as acquired ichthyosis.[55a] Lesions of the skin have been observed in 30 per

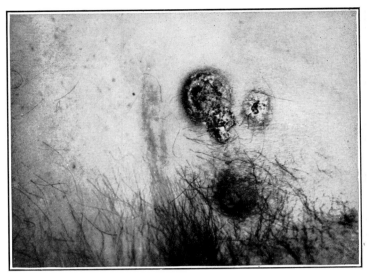

A

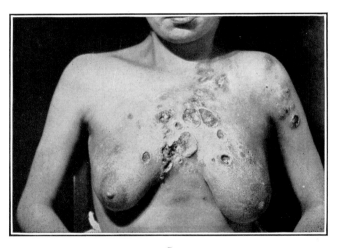

B

Fig. 20–12.—Nodular (*A*) and ulcerative (*B*) skin lesions in Hodgkin's disease. (Jackson and Parker, courtesy of New England J. Med.)

cent of cases of Hodgkin's sarcoma.[32a] Skin manifestations may be the presenting symptoms of Hodgkin's disease or of "reticulum cell" sarcoma.[6] Cutaneous touch smears may be helpful in diagnosis.[19a]

Kaposi's sarcoma has been described as occurring in association with Hodgkin's disease and lymphosarcoma.[6a]

The relation of **granuloma (mycosis) fungoides** to the diseases chiefly affecting lymph nodes has become clarified by histologic studies[64a] More and more cases formerly referred to by this name are being recognized as cases in which the cutaneous manifestations of one of the latter diseases are unusually prominent and assume a characteristic appearance. Thus, the term becomes one which applies to a conglomeration of cutaneous changes varying from variable premycotic eruptions to tumor-like growths with the histologic changes of Hodgkin's disease or of "lymphosarcoma."

Involvement of the **breast** as the principal lesion has been reported, both in Hodgkin's disease[46a] and in lymphosarcoma.[1,14a]

Nervous System.—Paresthesias and pain, which may sometimes be extreme,[49] are the most common neurological manifestations. Herpes zoster is not uncommonly the cause of such pain. Horner's syndrome from involvement of the cervical sympathetics may develop. Relatively common, also, is acute or subacute compression of the spinal cord by epidural or subdural granulomatous deposits, as the result of collapse of involved vertebrae or by obstruction of the blood and lymph supply.[68c] Paraplegia with corresponding sensory loss and sphincter paralysis develops in the course of a few days to a few months, and pain in the back or radicular pains precede or accompany these signs. There may be complete spinal block with yellow cerebrospinal fluid under low pressure, spontaneous clotting and high protein. This neurological picture, in rare instances, may exist in the absence of clinical evidence of tumor elsewhere[43a] or may precede evident involvement of other viscera.[62d]

Another neurological symptom-complex is the successive implication of cranial nerves (trigeminal, abducens, facial, auditory, glossopharyngeal) or, rarely, of the cerebral cortex. Meningeal invasion with or without cranial or spinal nerve implication or cerebral invasion, has been observed and, extremely rarely, primary cerebral involvement.[25,59a,62d]

Special Senses.—Involvement of the special sense organs is rare, more so than in leukemia. Uveitis has been described in association with Hodgkin's disease[31c] as has also involvement of the eyelids, lacrimal glands, orbit, fundus, conjunctiva and cornea.[45a]

Systemic Manifestations. — Chills, fever, lassitude, increased sweating or loss of weight are conspicuously absent until the late generalized stage of "lymphosarcoma."[63] *Fever* is sufficiently common in the more advanced stages, however, for this condition to be worth consideration in the differential diagnosis of pyrexia of unknown origin.

The absence of constitutional symptoms early in the course of "lymphosarcoma" is in contrast to Hodgkin's disease where, in the common granulomatous type, constitutional symptoms appear relatively soon. Fever is found in 30 to 50 per cent of cases.[31b] Children are especially prone to run a febrile course. The fever may be moderate in degree, irregular or continuous. It may last weeks or months with afebrile periods of variable duration. In other cases fever is more marked, ranging to 104° F. or higher. In about one-sixth of the cases irregular waves of remittent or continuous pyrexia of several days' duration interrupted by periods of remission (Murchison-Pel-Ebstein[15,51,53] fever or alternating pyrexia) can be observed.

The constitutional symptoms of Hodgkin's disease are quite varied and may resemble those of tuberculosis, undulant fever or even thyrotoxicosis. Tachycardia may be observed which is out of proportion to the degree of fever.[25] In the early stages spontaneous clinical remissions and exacerbations may occur.[32f] In follicular lymphoma, also, the enlargement of the lymph nodes may be intermittent.[68b]

A curious symptom, which has been observed in about 17 per cent of cases of Hodgkin's disease,[32d] is the occurrence of severe *pain* at the site of the active lymphogranulomatous focus *following the ingestion of alcoholic beverages,* even in small quantities, or after the intravenous injection of ethyl alcohol. The pain usually appears within five to 15 minutes and may last for ten minutes or even several hours. Except for a few cases of osteomyelitis and of fracture of bone, and several patients with carcinoma (thymus, pancreas, breast), this symptom has been observed only in Hodgkin's disease. It was noted that the patients who manifested such pain showed fewer reticulum-cell mitoses, more eosinophils and more fibrosis in their lymph nodes than those who had no alcohol-induced pain. This may be an initial sign of the disease, it may become less marked following therapy and it has not been produced by other vasodilators. This strange phenomenon has not been encountered in patients with other types of lymphoma.

Lymphosarcoma in Childhood.—While uncommon, primary malignant tumors of lymphoid origin occurring in childhood present certain special features.[56b] Superior vena-caval obstruction, involvement of bone and primary intestinal lesions appear more commonly than in adults. In particular, transitions of the disease to the typical picture of leukemia are seen about twice as often in children as compared with adults. This was observed in ten out of 69 cases in one series.[56b]

The Blood.—A good deal has been written about the blood changes in these disorders, especially those relating to the leukocytes in Hodgkin's disease, but it appears that there is nothing which can be considered as diagnostic. This is contrary to the views held several decades ago.[10] It can be said, however, that certain changes are suggestive, particularly of Hodgkin's disease.

Anemia is often conspicuously lacking in the "sarcoma group" and in follicular lymphoma, particularly at an early stage, or it is only very slight in degree.

This was true of 90 per cent of the cases of "lymphosarcoma" at the Memorial Hospital in New York.[63] In only 31 per cent of our cases was the red cell count below 4,000,000 cells per c.mm. and in these the average count was 3,210,000, the lowest count being 2,820,000. In Hodgkin's disease anemia is a more common symptom and appears earlier. A third of the cases at the Memorial Hospital in New York[63] were anemic on admission. In one-half of our cases anemia was present.[39] This is usually only mild or moderate in degree and normocytic in type. Erythrokinetic studies have shown modestly shortened Cr^{51} erythrocyte survival times, moderately increased erythropoiesis and greatly increased tissue iron stores.[22a] As in many other disorders, the bone marrow is incapable of increasing red cell production sufficiently to compensate for the increased rate of destruction.[31d]

In some cases of Hodgkin's disease, however, and, less often, in the other lymph node conditions under discussion, overt hemolytic anemia is observed. This "symptomatic" hemolytic anemia (p. 613) is similar to that found in association with chronic lymphocytic leukemia (p. 925). The anemia usually becomes macrocytic, spherocytosis and even increased osmotic red cell fragility in hypotonic saline solutions may be found, and the Coombs' test may be positive.[38a] It has been noted that, in such cases, changes characteristic of Hodgkin's disease are usually found in the spleen.

In rare cases, the anemia in untreated Hodgkin's disease is very severe. If adenopathy is absent, the correct diagnosis may not be made until autopsy, even after extensive study. A few such cases of *"bone marrow Hodgkin's"*[32,35] have been reported. One of our patients in whom this diagnosis was made antemortem complained of radiating abdominal pain, increasing weakness and loss of weight and was found to have fever of the Pel-Ebstein type. There was marked pallor and slight hepatic enlargement as well as abdominal distention, but there was no adenopathy or splenomegaly and no masses or glands could be demonstrated in the abdomen. The blood counts suggested aplastic anemia (R.B.C., 1,660,000; W.B.C., 1200; platelets, 88,000) but a moderate increase of reticulocytes (4.9 per cent), together with the presence of nucleated red cells and occasional polychromatophilic corpuscles in the blood smears, indicated the myelophthisic character of the anemia, a view supported by the demonstration of rarefied areas in the bones (Fig. 20–5). Miliary Hodgkin's disease was found at autopsy.

The total **leukocyte count** in *Hodgkin's disease* may be slightly or moderately increased or it may be normal; sometimes it may exceed 25,000 cells per c.mm., or there may be leukopenia. It has been stated that higher degrees of leukocytosis develop as the disease advances and neutrophilia has been said to be most marked in cases with deep lymph involvement[70] but these are not dependable signs. Leukocytosis, sometimes of marked degree may be present at an early stage. Leukopenia may be found even before therapy has been given.[39] Thus, every type of change in the leukocyte count, including extreme leukocytosis suggestive of leukemia,[60,73] may be encountered in Hodgkin's disease although leukocyte counts of 8000 to 16,000 are certainly the most common.

The differential count usually reveals a tendency to neutrophilia, relative and absolute lymphocytopenia, monocytosis, and eosinophilia.[39] Not infrequently all of these changes are present at the same time, but every possible combination of changes or a lack of any of them may be seen in occasional cases. Lymphocytopenia is one of the more consistent findings in the blood in Hodgkin's disease and the percentage of lymphocytes may

be reduced even to 5 per cent. Relative lymphocytosis may be observed when there is marked neutropenia but an absolute increase in lymphocytes is most unusual or never[10] occurs. Monocytosis is also a very frequent finding in Hodgkin's disease.[10,70] Values of about 10 per cent are quite common. Eosinophilia, on the other hand, though frequently mentioned, is less often found in this disease. It is rare early in the disease[10] and has been observed only in about 30 per cent of cases at any stage. Occasionally, however, extreme degrees of eosinophilia may be encountered.[60] Values as high as 90 per cent eosinophils, and even higher when the total leukocyte count was 50,000 to 100,000 per c.mm.[2,44] have been recorded. It is rare to find immature forms of leukocytes, such as myelocytes, in the blood in cases of Hodgkin's disease. Their presence suggests bone marrow involvement, as does neutropenia. In rare instances Reed-Sternberg cells have been found in the blood.[66a]

The leukocyte count in *the other forms of disease chiefly affecting lymph nodes* may be normal, or there may be leukopenia. Likewise the differential leukocyte count may be normal or there may be relative or even absolute lymphocytosis. The lymphocytes may not be remarkable, but unusual forms and "tumor" cells (p. 940) may be found.[70] The terms, "leukosarcoma" and "leukolymphosarcoma" have been used to refer to cases otherwise resembling the "sarcoma group" or follicular lymphoma in which the leukocyte count was elevated, even to 30,000 per c.mm., and in which some cells suggestive of lymphosarcoma were found in the blood or bone marrow.[53e] In follicular lymphoma, "hematogones" (cells resembling but smaller than lymphocytes, with elongated or sharply indented nuclei composed of dense chromatin masses and practically devoid of cytoplasm) have been described as being characteristically increased in the blood

65

and bone marrow; such cells are seen normally in the blood of infants and in the bone marrow of adults as well as infants.[56c] In reticulum cell sarcoma and in follicular lymphoma, in particular, monocytes may be increased in number and young forms as well as macrophages may be found. Occasionally myelocytes may be seen. Leukemoid blood pictures have been observed most frequently in association with lymphocytic and lymphoblastic lymphomas[70] but also in follicular lymphomas[8,20a] As mentioned previously (p. 1009), irradiation therapy may be followed by a change to a leukemoid picture.

The **platelet count** may be increased in Hodgkin's disease and large bizarre forms may be seen.[10] It is perhaps more common, however, to find the platelet count normal.[39] The finding of thrombocytopenia suggests bone marrow involvement. In the remaining conditions chiefly affecting lymph nodes the platelet count is usually normal but it may be reduced, especially in lymphocytic and lymphoblastic lymphoma. When thrombocytopenia is present, bleeding time is prolonged, the blood clot retracts poorly and hemorrhagic symptoms may appear. Such findings are unusual, however.

Bone Marrow.—As would be expected from the fact that lesions, if present, are likely to be focal rather than diffuse, the usual bone marrow aspiration in Hodgkin's disease and in the other diseases chiefly affecting lymph nodes reveals no characteristic changes. Thus the chief value of bone marrow study in these conditions is to rule out leukemia, especially the aleukemic form. In *Hodgkin's disease* the most constant feature is myeloid and megakaryocytic hyperplasia. There may be a shift to the left in the myeloid series of slight or moderate degree, slight monocytosis, or moderate eosinophilia, thus reflecting the findings in the blood. Lymphocytes may be reduced in number. Normal or

atypical plasma cells, eosinophils and reticulum cells may be increased in number. A pathologic type of megakaryocytopoiesis has been described with an increase in the number of immature forms and "naked" megakaryocytic nuclei.[40]

However, marrow aspiration at a site of bony tenderness may yield *Reed-Sternberg cells.*[66] These can be distinguished from megakaryocytes by their nuclear structure which, be it fine or coarse, shows a sharp distinction between basichromatin and parachromatin, in contrast to the pyknotic and pachychromatic appearance of the nucleus of megakaryocytes of a similar stage of development; their striking, large, pale to deep blue staining nucleoli, contrasting with the small and inconspicuous nucleoli of the megakaryocytes; and the absent or at most sparse granulation of the cytoplasm. Their nuclei are oval in shape but may appear to be lobulated and sometimes even segmented. The giant cells of reticulum cell sarcoma are smaller and their nuclei consist of a giant, multilobulated structure which occupies the entire cell body. It is more difficult to distinguish the large cells with striking nucleoli which may be found in cases of secondary carcinoma or amelanotic melanoma but these are likely to be found in association with other tumor cells whereas Reed-Sternberg cells are surrounded by normal marrow cells or cells of granuloma tissue, such as plasma cells, lymphocytes and even fibroblasts. The Reed-Sternberg cells have been found in films made from the aspirate[66] and in serial paraffin sections of bone marrow aspirations.[53b] Even "dry taps" have yielded noteworthy cells when they have been examined thoroughly.

In *lymphocytic lymphoma* and in *follicular lymphoma*, the bone marrow may be normal[40] or there may be an increase in lymphocytes. These may be more or less normal in appearance or they may be immature or appear otherwise abnormal: the nuclei may be irregularly shaped or indented, there may be numerous distinct nucleoli or the nuclei may be dense and hyperchromatic with but a thin rim of deeply basophilic cytoplasm surrounding them.[11f] The last correspond to the "hematogones" mentioned earlier (p. 1025). Serial paraffin sections of aspirated material may be helpful.[53b]

Aspiration of lymph nodes[43b,44b] and the study of smears of such material, as well as imprints of biopsied lymph nodes[4b] are helpful procedures in experienced hands. In Hodgkin's disease the polymorphism of the cell elements and the presence of cells not normally present are significant features.

Other Laboratory Findings.—The *basal metabolic rate* may be increased in these disorders even when there is no fever or leukocytosis. Thus in nine of our cases of Hodgkin's disease and lymphocytic, reticulum cell and follicular lymphoma the basal metabolic rate ranged from + 22 to + 36. However, it is not likely to be significantly abnormal when the disease is localized.[31b]

The electrophoretic pattern of the **serum proteins** is well established. Moderately advanced cases may reveal hypoalbuminemia and increased concentrations of alpha$_1$, alpha$_2$, and/or beta globulins, as occurs in other diseases in which there is a systemic reaction. In many cases, in addition, hypergammaglobulinemia is found in the absence of overt evidence of hepatic involvement or infection.[1c] Anomalous serum components have not been described.

The blood **uric acid** content may be considerably increased. The **alkaline serum phosphatase,** if persistently elevated, may indicate bone invasion.[71]

In Hodgkin's disease the **erythrocyte sedimentation rate** is accelerated during the active phases of the disease but may be normal in periods of remission.

Similarly C-reactive protein may appear in the blood during activity of the disease.[70c] However, it does not provide a sensitive index of the efficacy of treatment. Elevation of serum complement was thought to be a good index of activity of the disease process.[57b]

Course and Clinical Types.—From what has been said already it is apparent that the course of these diseases varies and the clinical types are innumerable. It is true of most cases, however, that there is an initial period in which the lesion is localized, and a second period in which generalization occurs. The first phase, especially in the case of the "sarcoma group," is often symptomless except for evident glandular enlargement. If the primary site is other than in superficial lymph nodes, however, symptoms are more likely to develop. These will depend on the location of the initial lesions. Hodgkin's "paragranuloma" may remain quiescent for many years and death may be due to some other cause. In other cases, within months or years transition to Hodgkin's granuloma occurs. The primary phase of follicular lymphoma is so benign that the malignant character of this disease was long denied.

Although the primary period may be of very long duration, it may be so brief as to be overlooked. Involvement of new glands takes place in an orderly manner, adjacent glands in the same region and glands in the nearest neighboring area being affected in turn, as a rule. In some cases there seems to be simultaneous involvement of many sites at the same time. Once it has broken away from the primary site, the course of all of these diseases is usually rapid and is characterized by pressure symptoms, fever, loss of weight and strength, anemia and cachexia. In Hodgkin's "granuloma," however, remissions may occur in a quite unpredictable manner—or relapse may suddenly develop in a patient who seemed to be doing well, and death may ensue in a few weeks. In Hodgkin's sarcoma a progressive course is characteristic. In all of the types of the diseases under discussion, the terminal phase finds the patient in a pitiful state, often with swelling of the face, neck and arms and imminent asphyxia from mediastinal involvement; abdominal distention or ascites, or edema of the extremities from pressure by retroperitoneal glands; or pain from pressure on nerves or bone involvement.

The clinical types which may be distinguished are about as numerous as the primary sites which may be involved. A very sharp clinical separation cannot be made for the various types tend to fuse with one another. Ziegler's classification[74] of the types of **Hodgkin's disease** illustrates the forms which this disease may take: (1) localized; (2) generalized, with very early and more or less universal lymphadenopathy, splenomegaly and cachexia; (3) mediastinal; (4) typhoidal, with retroperitoneal gland involvement, diarrhea, fever, leukopenia, and anemia; (5) splenic, with extreme splenomegaly; (6) bone and periosteal, with pain and tumor formation suggesting chloroma or multiple myeloma; and (7) an acute, rapidly advancing form (Fig. 20–15).

Likewise **lymphosarcoma** can be separated into a number of groups:[64a] (1) cases with regional collections of superficial lymph nodes, notably the cervical, less often inguinal or axillary; (2) cases in which the lymphoid structures of the thorax, especially the thymus or its remains, and the lymph nodes in the superior mediastinum and at the root of the lung are implicated; (3) those in which the lymphoid tissues of the abdomen are involved (stomach, intestines, retroperitoneal and mesenteric lymph nodes); (4) cases characterized by involvement of paired organs (breasts, ovaries, testes, adrenals, kidneys); and

(5) the "leukosarcoma" of Sternberg (p. 940).

Diagnosis.—It is necessary to differentiate the diseases under discussion from local inflammatory reactions of the lymph nodes, generalized acute and subacute lymphadenitis, tuberculosis, syphilis, infectious mononucleosis, leukemia, metastatic carcinoma, and also other causes of mediastinal tumor, abdominal growths and bone involvement. The discovery of an infected focus in the neighborhood of the affected glands, tenderness, local heat and fever, and agglutination reactions will help to separate a number of inflammatory conditions. The characteristic morphological changes in the blood and increased heterophil antibodies, as well as the benign course of the illness distinguish infectious mononucleosis. When a syphilitic chancre is extragenital and undiscovered, the neighboring glandular enlargement may be confused with that caused by one of the conditions chiefly affecting lymph nodes but the serological test for syphilis will be positive. Cervical metastases from a **nasopharyngeal tumor** usually overshadow the primary tumor, which is characteristically small and is easily overlooked unless a careful nasopharyngoscopic examination is made.

Tuberculosis. — Tuberculosis has been frequently confused with Hodgkin's disease. Differentiation may sometimes be very difficult. In the rare acute form the glands may enlarge rapidly and remain discrete and freely movable. Unlike Hodgkin's disease, however, the nodes beneath the jaw and in the anterior rather than in the posterior triangle of the neck are affected in this form of tuberculosis. In the more chronic localized glandular tuberculosis, the mass of glands tends to be fused and immobile. An open sinus or the scar of a healed one suggests tuberculous infection. Generalized caseous glandular tuberculosis does not break down as a rule and may be indistinguishable from Hodgkin's disease. The demonstration by roentgenography of calcification in the lymph nodes suggests tuberculosis. The tuberculin test is sometimes helpful.

Boeck's Sarcoid.—Boeck's sarcoid[43] (benign lymphogranulomatosis, lupus pernio) bears great clinical resemblance to Hodgkin's disease and to tuberculosis, affecting as it does not only skin, but lymph nodes, lungs, spleen (p. 1059) and bones in addition to other tissues. As in Hodgkin's disease those affected are usually young adults. There is often mediastinal glandular enlargement and there may be splenomegaly, monocytosis or eosinophilia. Leukopenia is less common than normal values but more frequent than leukocytosis.[9] Anemia is uncommon but hemolytic anemia (p. 613) and thrombocytopenic purpura[15a, 59b] have been reported in association with sarcoidosis. Distinguishing features are the frequent involvement of the preauricular and post-auricular lymph nodes, the submaxillary, submental and epitrochlear, those along the borders of the muscles of the shoulder girdles, and the paratracheal glands, all of which are less frequently involved in Hodgkin's disease or in the "sarcoma group;" the bilateral, roughly symmetrical enlargement of the hilar nodes with their sharp, lobulated outer bodies; the absence of calcification; the failure of any of the glandular enlargements to reach the size seen in the latter conditions; the occurrence in some cases of lesions in the eyes and in the lachrymal and parotid glands; the miliary pulmonary involvement; the characteristic punched-out areas in the small bones of the hands and feet; the high total serum protein content of the blood seen in some cases and the presence of renal involvement in others; and finally, the histological characteristics of affected lymph nodes. The histological picture is one of miliary epithelioid tubercles without a surrounding inflammatory zone and without areas of necrosis.

Systemic Lupus Erythematosus.[1d] —Disseminated lupus erythematosus should not be easily confused with the conditions under discussion, although such symptoms as irregular fever with remissions, glandular enlargement,[24] splenomegaly, involvement of synovial and serous membranes, skin changes and anemia as well as leukopenia are features in common. Cardiac manifestations (atypical verrucous endocarditis), signs of renal damage (acute glomerulonephritis), and articular involvement such as are found in systemic lupus are very unusual in Hodgkin's disease or in the "sarcoma group" but the leukopenia may be accompanied by a striking lymphocytopenia,[26d] as occurs in Hodgkin's disease. An additional differentiating feature is the L. E. cell of Hargraves, a phagocyte which contains within its cell membrane one or more masses of nuclear material. These masses, round or oval in outline, vary in size from a third of the size of a red blood corpuscle to three or four times that size. They stain bluish, purple or reddish-brown and may be granular, hazy or homogeneous in appearance, the chromatin network characteristic of the nuclei of cells having disappeared. The result is a large, round, bluish homogeneous body with the darker-staining lobulated nucleus of the phagocyte festooning its periphery (Plate XV, p. 926). The test for L. E. cells (p. 419) appears to be both a sensitive and a specific one.

The masses characteristic of the L. E. phenomenon are formed by the interaction of a factor present in the patient's serum which acts upon the nucleus of certain white cells and causes swelling. The swollen nucleus is then extruded into the surrounding medium and is phagocytized by another viable white cell. The latter cell, with the swollen nuclear mass within its cytoplasm as a homogeneous basophilic inclusion body, constitutes the L. E. cell. It was originally thought that the serum factor causes depolymerization of the nuclear DNA but it now appears that the serum factor acts by directly combining with the cell nucleus, most likely the nuclear nucleoprotein. The staining characteristics of the nucleus are altered as a result and the nucleus becomes subject to subsequent phagocytosis.[30c]

The **clinical differentiation of the various disorders which chiefly affect lymph nodes from one another,** as already indicated, is difficult and may times impossible. Nevertheless, certain features will suggest one more than the others. Thus, great enlargement of the spleen favors leukemia, Hodgkin's disease or follicular lymphoma rather than the "sarcoma group." The appearance of fever or anemia early in the course of the patient's illness favors Hodgkin's disease (or acute leukemia) rather than one of the other conditions under discussion. In Hodgkin's disease, neutrophilia, lymphocytopenia, monocytosis and eosinophilia may be found whereas no morphologic alterations in the blood are likely to appear in the other lymph node disorders. A uniform general glandular enlargement suggests leukemia but this may sometimes also be found in lymphocytic and lymphoblastic lymphomas and in the other conditions under discussion. When the tonsil or the alimentary canal is involved, one of the "sarcoma group" or leukemia is more probable than other forms of lymph node disease. *Follicular lymphoma* tends to attack the older age group, constitutional manifestations and visceral involvement are infrequent and abnormalities in the blood are unusual. The skeletal system in follicular lymphoma tends to be involved in a disproportionately low degree. In this disease retroperitoneal nodes become involved with possibly greater frequency than in the

other conditions named and chylous effusions, especially peritoneal, are more prone to develop. Hodgkin's sarcoma likewise attacks those of older age and advances rapidly, in contrast to the majority of cases of Hodgkin's granuloma.

Unfortunately, there are exceptions to all of these statements and, in the last analysis, determination of the cause of lymphadenopathy of obscure origin requires excision biopsy, preferably of more than one node, and study of the gland by a skilled pathologist. If a choice exists, lymph nodes of large size should be selected for biopsy from a site where the surgical risk is least, more than one node should be removed if possible, and irradiated nodes and those in the inguinal region should be avoided. A therapeutic test with roentgen irradiation or nitrogen mustard is of little diagnostic value since all of these conditions will respond in some degree to such treatment. Bone marrow examination and painstaking blood studies will usually reveal the leukemic nature of the disorder if it is "aleukemic" leukemia.

It is not as difficult, as a rule, to differentiate the **various forms of splenomegaly** discussed in the next section (p. 1055) from that caused by the conditions under discussion for in the majority of the former lymphadenopathy is absent.

The problem of diagnosis is much more difficult **when the primary lesion does not affect one of the superficial groups of lymph nodes,** for then the symptoms may attract attention to any of the systems of the body and may mimic any one of a great variety of diseases. Thus, there may be a nonstenosing tumor of the bowel; the onset may be characterized by melena, hematemesis or hemoptysis, ascites or dependent edema; or the symptoms may suggest pulmonary tuberculosis, bronchogenic carcinoma, septicemia, endocarditis, typhoid fever, rheumatic fever, pyelitis, prostatic disease or some neurological disorder. A high index of suspicion is required for the recognition of Hodgkin's disease or the "sarcoma group" when they assume one of the forms mentioned above. Various special procedures, such as biopsy of non-palpable, deeply situated nodes in the lower neck and upper mediastinum, thoracotomy and retroperitoneal pneumography, may be necessary. Even when one is dealing with a mediastinal mass the so-called therapeutic diagnostic test has no place for even bronchogenic carcinoma may in some instances regress temporarily like Hodgkin's disease or lymphosarcoma.

Prognosis.—In the series of 618 cases of "lymphomas" of all types,[20] already referred to several times, the mean duration of illness was 5.6 years for follicular lymphoma, 4.2 years for Hodgkin's "lymphoma," 3.2 years for lymphocytic lymphoma and 1.3 years each for lymphoblastic lymphoma, Hodgkin's sarcoma, "clasmatocytoma" and "stem cell" lymphoma. Fifty-three per cent of the cases of follicular lymphoma were still alive after five years, 29 per cent of the Hodgkin's "lymphomas" and 25 per cent of the lymphocytic lymphomas. In the remaining four groups death occurred during the initial two years in 80 per cent or more of the cases. This, like other available series, included treated cases.

Such other statistics as are available are in more or less agreement with these figures. Thus, in one series, the median survival of cases of follicular lymphoma was six years, lymphosarcoma 2.1 years and reticulum cell sarcoma 1.8 years.[56a] In another study, the mean duration of the illness was 4.4 years in follicular lymphoma, with 46 per cent of the patients alive after five years.[61c] In the same study, cases of "lymphoma" exclusive of follicular lymphoma and Hodgkin's disease were divided into three groups: (1) cases of lymphosarcoma with disease primarily in peripheral lymph nodes, with or without constitutional symptoms; (2) cases with abdominal or thoracic masses; and (3) cases with disease clinically limited to some specific organ or tissue, such as the gastrointestinal tract, skin or bone.[61c] The mean duration of illness in these 3 groups was 2.8, 1.4 and 3.1 years, respectively, with 23 per cent five-year survivals in the first group, 2 per cent in the second and 39 per cent in the third. That there is wide individual variation is indicated by the fact that, while a number of patients die within a year, there are others with apparently localized "lymphoma" who were alive thirteen[38b] and even twenty[28] years after treatment with no sign of recurrence. Certain writers[63] have referred to "cures" in as many as 10.6 per cent of cases of lymphosarcoma.

Some general statements can be made concerning prognosis. Thus, in children, although as many as 17.4 per cent survived five years or more, it was noted that when lymphosarcoma took a downhill course it did so at an accelerated rate.[56a] In the same study female patients did somewhat better than males. Patients with small cell lymphosarcoma survived slightly but significantly longer than did those with reticulum cell sarcoma. In another study it appeared that, if dissemination of follicular lymphoma did not occur in the first two or three years, the disease was likely to remain localized.[43c] Patients with an absolute lymphocytopenia, as a group tend to do quite poorly.[56a]

The outlook in Hodgkin's disease also varies greatly. In perhaps 2 or 3 per cent of cases the total duration of the disease is six months or less.[19b] At the other extreme are cases with long survivals and even apparent "cures."[61c] The mean duration of illness measured from clinical onset is twenty-four[25] to forty-four[61c] months according to most studies and 5-year survival figures, as measured by the "population at risk" method, range from 23 to 51 per cent.[39] However, a statement concerning mean survival in cases of Hodgkin's disease of all types is of little value. More significant, perhaps, is a consideration of cases according to "stage"[32e,37a,53a,61c] or, more appropriately, according to "class,"[11g] since one "stage" does not necessarily pass on to the other, even though it often does. Class I refers to cases with lymph node involvement in only one main group; in class II, two or more adjacent groups in either the upper or lower half of the body are involved; class III refers to cases with generalized lymph node involvement, with constitutional manifestations, with disease apparently limited to retroperitoneal lymph nodes or with involvement of structures other than lymphatic. According to three different reports there have been 88 per cent,[53a] 85[51b] and 59 per cent[32e] five-year survivals in class I, 72, 90 and 60 per cent in class II and 9, 10 and 3 per cent in class III. The difference between classes I and II is brought out by the ten-year survival figures: class I 77 per cent, class II 35 per cent, class III 2 per cent.[51b] In another study[53a] the ten-year survival for class I was only 58 per cent but the data for classes II and III were identical with those just cited.

It is rather uniformly held that the histological picture is not a satisfactory guide to prognosis.[62a] With some exceptions,[62] the paragranuloma-granuloma-sarcoma classification[32a] has been found disappointing from this point of view.[19b,32e] Some have found all proposed criteria unreliable and point out that many long term survivors did not have localized disease and that various alleged hematological criteria are valueless.[19b] Others offer statistics which indicate longer survival in females than in males,[31b,32e,61c] in patients in the third and fourth decades, and in accordance with the class of disease as described above.[32e] Exceptional survivals have

been observed in cases which exhibited primary lesions in the skin or single isolated tumors in bone or viscera, even though the histological picture indicated a less favorable outlook.[20] In our own experience, the presence of leukopenia before therapy and the early appearance of anemia or of skin involvement have been bad prognostic signs (Fig. 20–13).[39] On the other hand, the survival of patients who developed pruritus was somewhat longer than in comparable patients without this symptom.

Complications and Associated Diseases.—Secondary *infections* develop in patients with these disorders, especially as the illness progresses and repeated courses of treatment are given. Such individuals have been shown by quantitative measurements of antibody response to type-specific pneumococcus capsular polysaccharides to be poor antibody formers.[21a] A study of cutaneous reactions to various antigens suggested that there is a defect in the production or transport of the cellular antibodies concerned in these reactions.[58c] There is evidence that neoplasia,[21a,58c] and antimetabolite and steroid therapy depress *de novo* synthesis of antibody produced in response to specific antigen challenge. Tuberculosis has long been associated with Hodgkin's disease and, with the introduction of chemotherapeutic agents and steroid therapy, the danger of dissemination of latent tuberculosis has increased.[26e] The occurrence of disseminated fungus disease also appears to have increased in incidence. Cases with complicating histoplasmosis,[16a] cryptococcus meningitis,[22] aspergillosis[25a] and torulosis[50a] have been described and candidiasis is not unusual.[8a]

Secondary amyloidosis was observed in five out of a series of 1102 cases of Hodgkin's disease but in none of an even larger number of cases of lymphosarcoma or leukemia.[53f]

Malignant neoplasms of various kinds

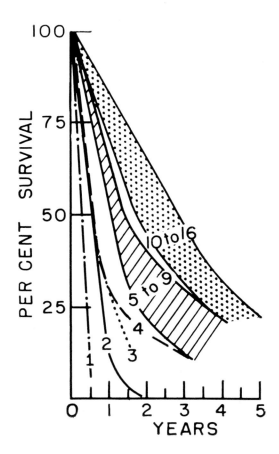

FIG. 20–13.—Survival from onset of a specific manifestation in 91 cases of Hodgkin's disease personally studied.[39] The numbers refer to: 1, skin involvement; 2, moderate anemia after therapy; 3, moderate anemia before therapy; 4, leukopenia; 5–9 (hatched area) bone involvement, liver involvement, splenomegaly, fever, lung parenchymal involvement (in that order); 10–16 (stippled area), mild anemia after therapy, mild anemia before therapy, marked leukocytosis, normal leukocyte count, mild leukocytosis, mediastinal involvement, pruritus, in that order. (Courtesy, Arch. Int. Med.)

may be encountered in association with Hodgkin's disease,[53f] including even multiple myeloma,[5] but there is no good evidence that the incidence is greater than would be found in a comparable general population. However, as discussed earlier (p. 1009), there appears to be some relationship between the other lymph node disorders under discussion and *leukemia,* just as there seems to be some connection between the different varieties of "lymphomas."

Pregnancy.—Fertility does not seem to be affected by Hodgkin's disease. Many instances of pregnancy occurring in women with Hodgkin's disease have been reported.[29,54b,62b] There is no clear evidence that pregnancy has a deleterious effect on this disease, nor does Hodgkin's disease seem to influence the pregnancy. It has been noted that Hodgkin's disease which appears for the first time during pregnancy or the puerperium carries a poor prognosis.[62c] This was explained on the ground that there would necessarily be a selection of favorable cases in the group who conceived after the development of the disease, since patients with severe or fulminating disease either would not survive or would not conceive.[62b] Spontaneous abortions have been observed in pregnancies complicated by Hodgkin's disease only when the patients had active disease before and during pregnancy, and particularly in patients with intra-abdominal or disseminated disease or both.[62c] Pathologic examination of the placentas has revealed no abnormality.[54b] As mentioned earlier (p. 1011), Hodgkin's disease in the infant born of a mother with Hodgkin's disease has been observed three times.[29]

Although a few patients have been treated with alkylating agents or by irradiation even in the first trimester without apparent ill effect, in view of the overwhelming experimental evidence that this is unwise, treatment, if required, should be postponed until the latter half of pregnancy. Conventional radiotherapy to lesions distant from the uterus seems least likely to produce any ill effects.

Advice to the patient with Hodgkin's disease, or her family, regarding pregnancy should be guided by evidence concerning the degree of apparent activity and dissemination of the disease as well as on the basis of psychologic and sociologic factors and must depend on the individual aspects of each case.

Probably the same considerations apply to cases of lymphosarcoma and the related disorders but few data are available for critical analysis.

Treatment.—As in the case of leukemia, the management of these disorders is based on the appropriate combination of (1) general supportive and symptomatic treatment, including blood transfusions when necessary; (2) irradiation; and (3) chemotherapy. In addition however, in certain cases (4) surgery may be considered.

The **general measures** are similar to those discussed in the preceding chapter (p. 957). The diet should be adequate in all respects and, if the patient is ill, should be served in a form which can be taken by an individual whose appetite is poor and who may be nauseated.

In view of the susceptibility to *infections* of various and unusual types which patients who have reached the later stages of these disorders manifest (p. 1032), the possible presence or development of one of these should constantly be kept in mind. When identified they must be treated specifically and vigorously with more than the customary doses of the appropriate therapeutic agent. As a general rule, prophylactic antibiotic therapy is undesirable. In certain instances, however, and especially when long term steroid therapy is contemplated, prophylactic anti-tuberculosis therapy deserves consideration.

The *management of the anemia* is based on the same principles as discussed in relation to leukemia (p. 960). The most effective means for the treatment of the anemia is the successful therapy of the underlying disorder. When this is accomplished, the anemia is relieved; in fact, this is an excellent index of the effectiveness of therapy. Such improvement may be preceded by a temporary and modest increase of anemia as the consequence of the action of the therapeutic measure which is being employed, whether this be irradiation or chemotherapy. It should be emphasized, however, that any substantial increase in the degree of anemia under such circumstances should serve as a warning to interrupt therapy.

Antianemic agents such as vitamin B_{12}, folic acid or iron are of no value. As a temporary measure, blood transfusions are useful but they should be employed sparingly. When there is frank hemolytic anemia, corticosteroid therapy is required. This is preferable to splenectomy, as a rule. As in chronic lymphocytic leukemia, sometimes in the lymphosarcomas the administration of these hormones is associated with reduction in the severity of the anemia even in the absence of frank signs of increased blood destruction. When they are used, however, caution is necessary as complications (p. 985) are frequent. In general, however, steroid therapy is not recommended in the treatment of Hodgkin's disease and the lymph node disorders since they have no effect on the underlying process even though they may relieve the fever and malaise and improve the appetite. As a rule, this is insufficient reward for the discomforts and complications associated with long term cortical hormone therapy.

The *pruritus* of Hodgkin's disease is a most difficult symptom to treat. Often it will respond to appropriate treatment of the disease, as outlined below, but this is not always the case. Demecolcin has been used with some success, but serious toxic symptoms may follow.[50c]

From time to time, a variety of vaccines have been proposed for the treatment of Hodgkin's disease. There has never been convincing evidence that any of them was of any value.[31b]

It should be emphasized again that here, as in the leukemias, one deals with disorders which are usually fatal. It is therefore especially important that the physician not only know what to do and when to do it but he must be an understanding human being who is prepared to help the patient to make the adjustments dictated by the development of the disease and by the many and sometimes complex events which occur during its course. It also cannot be overemphasized that one is seldom justified in delivering to the family a prognosis of certain death of the patient within a year or two. As was pointed out above, estimation of prognosis is extremely difficult in these diseases and even those who are most experienced encounter patients whose course has been much better than they would have guessed. It may be added that, although it is as yet impossible to say with certainty that survival has been prolonged by therapy, there is no doubt that morbidity has been reduced.

Surgery.—On the assumption that Hodgkin's disease and the other lymph node disorders under discussion may, in contrast to leukemia, be in some instances unicentric in their origin, surgical excision has been advocated from time to time,[2,28] especially when careful study failed to reveal evidence of spread; for example, when the lesion appeared to be localized to one side of the neck or in the stomach or intestine,[62a] radiographic examination failed to reveal disease elsewhere, anemia was absent and no other evidence of systemic disease (fever, weight loss, increased sedimentation rate) was present. It should be added that there are strong differences of opinion concerning the validity of this assumption[31b,64a] and many have held against surgical removal of affected tissue.[28]

Results have varied. In one series of 48 cases which met the criteria outlined above, 20 showed no residual evidence of disease following surgical treatment. The average total survival of these cases was nine years.[19i] In another study,[28] 24 of 30 cases of "malignant lymphoma" subjected to radical surgical attack plus irradiation were living and well five to 20 years later. Out of another 25 cases of "lymphosarcoma,"[63] six were reported as cured five or more years later whereas only 8 per cent of similar cases not treated surgically were considered cured. Similar long survivals have been reported in cases of primary lymphosarcoma of the small intestine[45] or mediastinum and even in mediastinal Hodgkin's disease.[18a] On the other hand, in a retrospective analysis of results in a total of 76 cases, selected for surgery out of a total of 1269 patients with "lymphosarcoma," five-year survivals were distinctly better among a comparable group of cases treated by non-surgical means than in those who underwent radical surgery.[56a] The conclusion that radiation therapy is the treatment of choice for this group of diseases is all the more impressive since one of the investigators earlier had favored surgery in selected cases.[11g]

Thus it appears that the place of surgery in the treatment of these disorders is very limited, indeed. The relatively rare primary disease of the stomach or bowel probably deserves surgical attack[62a] but even here the success of radiation therapy challenges that attributable to surgery alone.[10b] In any event, even when surgical excision has been carried out, radiation therapy should follow and, possibly also, the use of nitrogen mustard may be considered if the patient's condition will tolerate all these measures. By such a three-dimensional attack one might hope for cures in well-selected cases.

Splenectomy, as a rule, has no place in the treatment of these disorders. However, in carefully selected cases, particularly in those with thrombocytopenic purpura,[4c] the operation may be useful (p. 959). In cases of follicular lymphoma with manifestations primarily in the spleen, long term benefit from splenectomy was observed in two cases.[29a]

Irradiation.—For irradiation, roentgen therapy is the procedure of choice. Radioactive phosphorus has been found to be inferior to roentgen rays in the treatment of these disorders.[13,31b,54a] The value of radium is limited because of the inaccessibility of deep structures and the impracticability of application over large areas. Radium, however, has been used when the lesion was localized and superficial. Segmental or localized irradiation[23] is generally preferred as compared with total irradiation except in cases in which generalization has taken place or as a supplement to localized treatment.[63]

The greatest individualization in treatment is necessary. The response of the lesions to therapy, the general effects on the patient and the effect on the blood must be watched closely. The location of all the lesions is first determined as far as clinical examination and roentgenography allow. Where only one side of the neck is treated for what seems to be localized disease, 250 kv. roentgen rays are often used, giving 200 r in air daily or every other day to a total of not less than 2400 r and, in some cases, as high as 3000 to 3600 r in air.[11g] When disease exists in more than one site, a more moderate and "palliative" approach has usually been followed. Various areas are treated in succession and if the general condition of the patient permits, treatment is given daily, sometimes even to two ports per day. The dose given each day is that which can be tolerated by the patient without too much discomfort and which is yet powerful enough to produce substantial results. The duration of treatment depends on the extensiveness of the disease and the condition of the patient. Using 200 or 250 kv. machines with 0.5 to 1.5 mm. filter, 200 to 400 r have been given at a time over rather large rectangular portals. From 600 to 1200 r have been given in a course.[62a] In patients who are very ill, smaller doses are used at first and the amount is increased as clinical improvement takes place. The total dose may be as much as 1800 to 2000 r, measured in air, for each port, or even more[53b] in Hodgkin's disease. Giant follicular lymphoma, on the other hand, is usually very radiosensitive and as little as 400 to 600 r per field may cause complete disappearance of all palpable evidence of the disease.[62a] More will usually be required for lymphosarcoma and reticulum cell sarcoma.

Some radiotherapists restrict treatment to those parts of the body which are patently invaded. Others include regions which are suspected of invasion.[23,53b] The combination of segmental and total irradiation is one method for attempting to achieve the latter end, but total irradiation must be used very cautiously because of the danger of deleterious effects on the blood.

The *effect* on the lesions varies, but frequently the disappearance of enlarged glands is dramatic (Fig. 20–4). Large masses may melt away in the course of a week. Even adenopathy located at some distance from the site treated may decrease. The response is better in tumors of the soft type than in hard lesions, probably because the latter contain much connective tissue whereas the former consist largely of lymphocytes which are known to be very sensitive to irradiation. Pressure symptoms disappear, although it is to be kept in mind that edema may develop immediately following treatment and, where the larynx or trachea is concerned, actual asphyxia can accidentally result. Consequently, in the mediastinum only 50 to 75 r are usually given at one time.[51b] If fever or pruritis is present, relief occurs when treatment is effective. Pain caused by osseous foci is often alleviated and the lesions may become no longer discernible in roentgenograms.[23] Pulmonary lesions decrease in size and pleural effusions disappear in some instances. When treatment is fully effective the leukocyte count, if originally abnormal, becomes normal. The leukocyte count may rise to normal if leukopenia has been present. Eosinophilia may develop with irradiation. Remission of many years' duration may follow or improvement may be very brief.

Treatment is most effective in the slowly growing forms. It is sometimes stated that irradiation is contraindicated in the acute and rapidly fatal types. It may be very difficult to determine whether a given case represents such an acute form or the more or less advanced stage of a more chronic type. Treatment may be attempted in such cases but should be commenced cautiously. The same is true if there are signs of depressed bone marrow function such as severe anemia, leukopenia or thrombocytopenia. The presence of signs of renal insufficiency and nitrogen retention or of skin injury following irradiation are **contraindications** to further therapy. The presence of tuberculosis in association with these diseases is another contraindication. Pregnancy is not a contraindication if irradiation of the pelvic region and the fetus can be avoided and treatment is given in the third trimester.

Radioresistance in the early stages is seen only rarely in follicular or lymphocytic lymphoma, Hodgkin's disease or monocytoma, but has been observed in 12 to 20 per cent of cases of "reticulum cell sarcoma," lymphoblastic lymphoma and "Hodgkin's sarcoma."[20]

Treatment is *renewed* whenever there is evidence of recurrence.[23] Renewed treatment may be followed by effects which are as good as were originally obtained. In most cases a stage is reached, however, in which further treatment seems to be entirely ineffective. The cause of such radioresistance is unknown.

Nitrogen Mustard and other Al- **kylating Agents.**[23c] — During World War II it was found that the mustard gases are not only contact vesicants but, following absorption, exert powerful cytotoxic effects. The susceptibility of cells to these substances seems to be related to their proliferative activity. The nitrogen mustards manifest a type of action on cells which resembles in many ways the effect of roentgen rays. It has been found that they owe their pharmacological activity to intramolecular cyclization in a polar solvent to form a cyclic onium cation with the liberation of chloride ions. The formed elements of the blood and the mucosa of the gastrointestinal tract are the first to show the effects of this cytotoxic action. In lymphatic tisue, fragmentation has been observed within ten hours of the injection of the nitrogen mustards and this is followed by lymphoid atrophy; the bone marrow reveals swelling and alteration in the staining reaction of the hematopoietic cells. This is followed successively by disappearance of mitotic activity, progressive depletion of the marrow and ultimately aplasia. The severity of the changes produced is directly related to the amount given. At the dosage level used therapeutically the depression of hematopoiesis is reversible. The site of cellular action is the nucleus. It has been observed that nucleic acid synthesis is inhibited[61d] but a detailed understanding of the action of nitrogen mustard *in vivo* and of other "alkylating agents" is yet to be obtained.[44a]

The therapeutic value of nitrogen mustard in the treatment of *Hodgkin's disease* is clearly established.[26c,39,69a] As compared with roentgen therapy, nitrogen mustard offers the advantage that the total therapeutic dose for a course of therapy can be given in a day or two, an important economic advantage, particularly for those whose home is distant from a radiotherapy center; nitrogen mustard can, in fact, be given wherever adequate

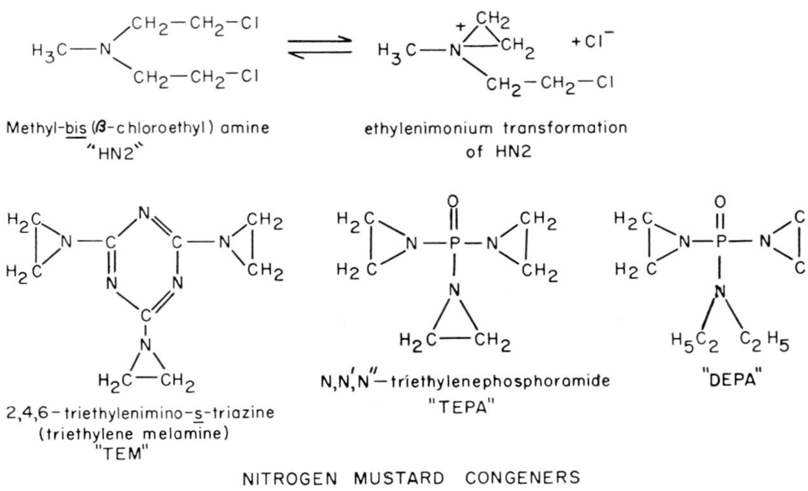

NITROGEN MUSTARD CONGENERS

FIG. 20–14.—Nitrogen mustard, TEM and other alkylating agents.

facilities for intravenous administration are available and appropriate follow-up of the patient is possible. Indications for its use will be discussed later (p. 1042). Also, when the disease is widespread, the use of a chemotherapeutic agent offers the advantage of a wide effect. On the other hand, where local therapy is the prime objective, roentgen ray therapy has obvious advantages.

Data are inadequate for a satisfactory comparison of roentgen therapy and chemotherapy alone. There is some evidence, however, that the *combined* use of the two forms of therapy may have prolonged survival in cases of generalized involvement, as compared with roentgen therapy alone.[11d] There is little doubt, furthermore, that the introduction of chemotherapy has reduced the period of morbidity. The quantity of radiation required is less, the amount of time taken up in undergoing treatment has been reduced and the economic burden of the patients has been made lighter.

Of the several agents tested, mechlorethamine hydrochloride (methyl *bis* [β-chloroethyl] amine hydrochloride [Fig. 20–14] "HN2") has received the widest use. This is a crystalline, water-soluble compound which is readily dissolved in sterile saline solution. Since it loses its activity quickly when in solution, the nitrogen mustard should be administered promptly after the powder has been dissolved. The material is best injected into the lumen of tubing through which a saline infusion is running since extravasation of the agent into the subcutaneous tissues during intravenous injection leads to severe local inflammation. Administration via a saline infusion also reduces the concentration of the mustard as it enters the vein and thus decreases the chance for the development of thrombophlebitis. The dose used ranges from 0.1 mg. per Kg. body weight to two or three times this amount and this may be repeated on the succeeding day or two to make a total of 0.2 to 0.6, rarely 0.8 mg. per Kg. body weight in a course.

Administration of the drug is followed in many cases, after one to three hours, by varying degrees of nausea and vomiting. There may be anorexia and headache. These symptoms may persist for several hours and may recur with each injection or they may occur only after the first administration. In some more robust individuals, these symptoms never appear

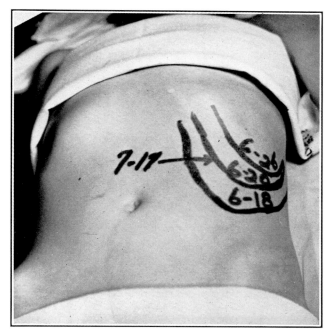

Fig. 20–15.—Reduction in the size of the spleen following nitrogen-mustard therapy in a case of Hodgkin's disease. The course of this patient is illustrated in figure 20–16.

at all. These unpleasant effects may be avoided by giving the drug at 8 P.M. Nembutal (0.1 Gm.) is given at the same time. In addition, 25 mg. chlorproma-zine is given at noon and at 4 P.M. of the same day and again at midnight if the patient is not sleeping. Adequate fluid intake and output during and following treatment should be assured in order to avoid the risk of acute renal failure as the result of uric acid precipitation.

Following the administration of nitro-gen mustard there is, as a rule, although in varying degree, relief of the systemic manifestations of Hodgkin's disease. Fever, if present, disappears; within a week a sense of well being begins to appear, the size of enlarged lymph nodes, spleen (Fig. 20–15) and other affected tissues decreases, there is gain in weight and other manifestations of improvement become manifest. Bone pain, pruritus, dyspnea, cough, dysphagia, hepatomegaly and even jaundice, as well as neurologic

symptoms of short duration may show striking regression or disappear entirely and weight is gained. In patients with mediastinal obstruction relief may be observed in twenty-four to forty-eight hours. Even in acute cases fever may disappear temporarily (Fig. 20–16).

When therapeutic doses are used, the most noteworthy change in the blood is a lowering of the leukocyte count, due to a decrease both in granulocytes and lymphocytes (Fig. 20–17). The lympho-cytopenia reaches its maximum in about six to eight days, the granulocytopenia in fifteen to twenty-one days. Recovery, often heralded by monocytosis and a "shift to the left" in the myeloid series, is usually complete within the ensuing two to three weeks.

A modest reduction in the quantity of red cells may be noted at first but, in cases in which a favorable therapeutic effect is achieved, this is restored to normal after several weeks. If anemia

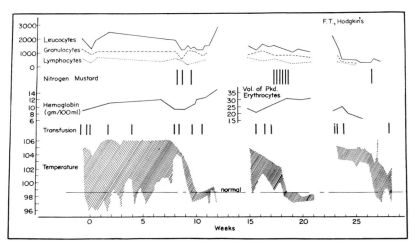

Fig. 20–16.—Course of a patient with Hodgkin's disease whose fever, ranging from 96° to 106° F. daily, ceased abruptly following three injections of nitrogen mustard. This treatment, however, became less and less effective and the patient ultimately died.

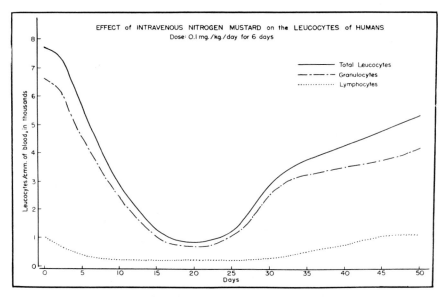

Fig. 20–17.—Effect on the leukocytes of nitrogen mustard in a dose of 0.1 mg. per kilogram per day for six days (means derived from data for 28 cases).

has been present this often decreases or may disappear entirely. A favorable effect on the anemia may be observed even in cases in which it is frankly hemolytic. Although thrombocytopenia may develop, this is rarely of such a degree as to produce serious hemorrhagic manifestations.[69] The platelet count may not reach its lowest levels until the third week after a course of therapy. The return to normal levels usually takes place within the ensuing seven to ten days.

Serial studies of bone marrow have demonstrated cytotoxic effects on both mature and immature elements but no cumulative effects have been observed

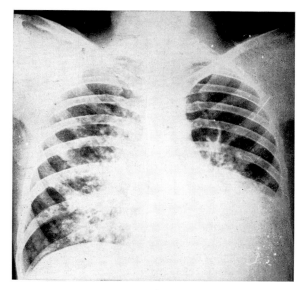

A

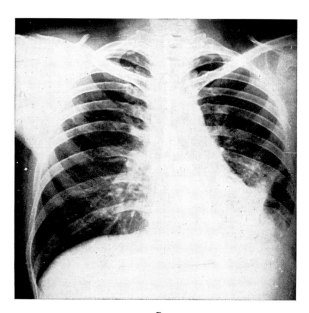

B

FIG. 20–18.—Effects of treatment with nitrogen mustard in a patient with Hodgkin's disease (A.S.) who had become resistant to roentgen therapy. There was fever (104° F.) and moderate anemia as well as a mottled diffuse infiltration of the right lung field and some infiltration in the left, together with atelectasis of the lower lobe of the left lung (*A*). Following a single course of nitrogen mustard therapy, the fever disappeared and, after a preliminary decrease in the leukocyte count from 14,000 to 1,000 per c.m.. and increase of anemia, the fever disappeared, the blood returned to normal, the patient gained 40 lb. in weight and a chest film twelve weeks later (*B*) showed evidence of marked improvement. This patient lived for fifteen months after he had become x-ray resistant and for a year of this time was in very good condition.

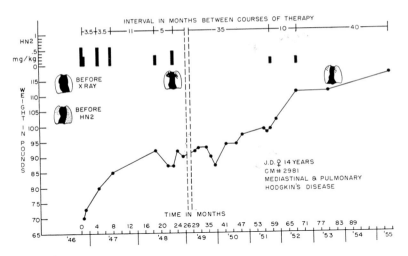

Fig. 20–19.—Course of a 14-year-old girl (J.D.) with extensive mediastinal and pulmonary Hodgkin's disease whose illness began eleven months before she was treated with nitrogen mustard as shown in the diagram. Four months before mustard therapy was instituted she received roentgen therapy (1600 r to the anterior and posterior mediastinum) with good results but, one month before, 2000 r produced no improvement. When first treated with nitrogen mustard she was dyspneic and cyanotic and had cough, dysphagia and anorexia. There was an infiltrate in the right middle lung field and in the left lung in the hilar region. The mediastinum was also shifted because of atelectasis of the right lower lobe. After three courses of mustard therapy she improved greatly and since has enjoyed long remissions.

when sufficient time was allowed for complete marrow regeneration. This may require as long as six weeks. The interesting observation has been made that the administration of l-cysteine prior to the injection of nitrogen mustard decreases and modifies the severe leukopenia and thrombocytopenia which may follow its administration.[68]

It is generally agreed that nitrogen mustard therapy is **indicated** in those cases in which the disease is widespread and signs of systemic intoxication such as fever, malaise and weight loss are present. Benefit may be achieved even when there is no obvious adenopathy and in patients with visceral involvement. Nitrogen mustard is less dangerous than radiation therapy when the superior mediastinum is compressed by tumor. A beneficial effect has been observed many times in patients "resistant" to radiation (Fig. 20–18).

The wisdom of using nitrogen mustard in cases where but one or two adjacent groups of lymph nodes appear to be involved (Classes I and II, p. 1032) is a matter of opinion. Some hold that early aggressive, local irradiation is preferable to nitrogen mustard in such cases.[62a] Our practice, even in these cases, is to use nitrogen mustard in addition to irradiation locally because one cannot be certain that undiscovered lesions do not exist elsewhere. The danger of permanent damage from the toxic effects of the drug is small when suitable amounts are given. An average dose for a course is a total of 0.4 mg. per Kg. body weight.

When there is intractable pleural effusion, the intrapleural administration of nitrogen mustard may result in effective control of the fluid accumulation. Approximately 0.3 mg. per Kg. body weight is injected intrapleurally at the completion of thoracentesis.[22]

Leukopenia is not necessarily a contraindication to nitrogen mustard therapy, provided the patient has not been treated previously. It is dangerous, on the other hand, to re-treat with nitrogen mustard if the hemopoietic system has not yet recovered from the effects of previous therapy, whether this be chemotherapy or irradiation. Impaired liver function has not been found to be a contraindication to nitrogen mustard therapy.[74a]

The duration of remission following nitrogen mustard therapy varies greatly. It may range from only several weeks to many years. It is important to bear in mind that benefit may sometimes be more apparent following a second course than after the first and that, in general, remissions following chemotherapy do not necessarily grow shorter and shorter; they vary in length from one time to another (Fig. 20–19).

In cases of **reticulum cell sarcoma, lymphocytic lymphoma** and **giant follicular lymphoma,** responses have been more variable than those in Hodgkin's disease. In some cases good results with long remissions have been observed and dramatic improvement has occurred even in well-advanced or in moribund cases. When mediastinal obstruction is present, nitrogen mustard may bring relief overnight whereas roentgen therapy would be dangerous.[62a] In cases in which roentgen therapy can be used, however, there is no evidence that results superior to those which follow such treatment can be produced by nitrogen mustard. Satisfactory remissions have been described in mycosis fungoides treated with nitrogen mustard.[5a] Therapeutic doses of nitrogen mustard for these conditions are generally somewhat lower than those for Hodgkin's disease. Lymphocytic lymphoma, in particular, should be treated at first with small doses because, when this disease is present, the hemopoietic system is sometimes found to be exceptionally sensitive to chemotherapeutic agents such as nitrogen mustard.

Of the several hundred chemical congeners of nitrogen mustard, only two, **triethylenemelamine (TEM)** and chlorambucil have earned an important place in the treatment of these disorders. The properties of TEM were discussed earlier (p. 974). Indications for its use are similar to those for nitrogen mustard. However, it is somewhat less valuable than the latter in severely ill patients who require intravenous therapy because vomiting following the injection of a single large dose of TEM may be more prolonged than after nitrogen mustard. On the other hand, there is little or no gastro-intestinal discomfort associated with its oral intake, especially if no more than 2.5 mg. is given at one time. Consequently it is particularly useful for ambulant or maintenance therapy.

There are many different dosage schedules for TEM.[33] Because of differences in sensitivity to the drug and in view of the dangers from cumulative effects (Fig. 19–33), p. 975), we prefer to give a predetermined dose in the course of two to four days and then to withhold further therapy for two or three weeks in order to observe the effect on the blood, especially the leukocyte count. Since TEM is preferably employed for the treatment of patients who are not severely ill, this delay is not harmful. After this interval, additional medication is given in accordance with the observed effects. Patients with Hodgkin's disease usually tolerate 10 to 15 mg. readily and they may be able to take 20 to 40 mg. per month. There is little evidence that TEM is effective when nitrogen mustard is not.

Chlorambucil (p. 975), has an important advantage over TEM in that absorption is more consistent and not related to food intake and the effect on the bone marrow is more easily controlled.[49a] For this reason, we give it preference. However, its action is slow, beneficial effects not appearing before three weeks as a rule. Consequently, it is our practice to use nitrogen mustard for the treatment of Hodgkin's disease when chemotherapy is indicated, reserving chlorambucil for those cases in which remission is short lived or intravenous therapy is not practicable. A dose of 0.1 mg./Kg. body weight per day can be taken for long periods of time without ill effect. Sometimes more, even twice this amount, can be used. To achieve maximum results in Hodgkin's disease an average total dose in a course was found, in one series of cases, to be 13.2 mg./Kg.[49a] In lymphosarcoma, on the other hand, as in chronic lymphocytic leukemia, smaller amounts are required, or tolerated. In all of these disorders, it should be noted, response to a second or third course of therapy may sometimes be better than in the first course (Fig. 20–19), contrary to the usual experience.

It does not appear that other alkylating agents offer any advantages, or are as useful, as those already discussed. Thus, triethylene thiophosphoramide (thio-TEPA) was thought to be less active than HN2 in the treatment of Hodgkin's disease.[74b] The advantages, if any, of cyclophosphamide[45b] (Cytoxan[11]), mannomustine (a mannitol mustard),[3a] 5-fluorouracil, vincaleukoblastine[30d] and other agents which are under trial, have yet to be demonstrated. Certain drugs, such as "R 48," an aromatic nitrogen mustard, are clearly inferior to or no better than the drugs now in use.[20b,66b] The effects of colchicine[25c] or phenylbutazone[57a] therapy are unimpressive. The antibiotic, actinomycin C, attracted interest in Germany and France but appears to be only a minor adjuvant in the treatment of Hodgkin's disease.[37a]

Attempts have been made to protect patients who have been given nitrogen mustard in single, massive doses, such as 1 mg./Kg., by the use of orthopedic tourniquets to shield their bone marrow[11c] or by withdrawing their own bone mar-row and reinfusing this after therapy.[46] The value of such procedures is obscure.

Pathology.—Many of the essential details have been given already in the preceding sections (classification, symptomatology). The findings at autopsy often reveal much more extensive disease than the clinical examination and symptoms would have led one to assume.

In the most common form of **Hodgkin's disease** one finds great collections of grayish tumors, lobulated masses composed of oval, round or irregular nodules, chiefly discrete, which are bound together by loose connective tissue. These glands may be soft, almost fluid in consistency, or quite hard. Their cut surface is pinkish-gray and semitranslucent, resembling fish-flesh. Depressed bands of yellowish tissue separate irregular bulging areas. The capsule of the glands is intact usually, but invasion of the surrounding tissue sometimes occurs. The spleen is rarely of very great size but is found involved in three-fourths of the cases. Scattered through it are yellowish-white masses which stand out against a red background and thus produce a mottled or marbled appearance. In the liver the lesions are confined to the portal tract. As already stated, the alimentary canal is usually remarkably free of lesions. Hodgkin's tissue is often found in the kidneys and in the lungs, especially about the bronchi. The characteristic microscopic picture, which has been described already (p. 1006), may be discovered even when gross examination reveals no abnormalities. As already indicated, multiple lesions are frequently found in the bones. The adrenals may be involved in 12 per cent of cases.[32a] Lesions of the nervous system proper do not occur. The histologic picture of Hodgkin's "paragranuloma" has been described already (p. 1008). In this form of the disease, involvement of the internal organs is rare. In only a few of Jackson and Parker's cases[32a] were the mediastinal nodes or the spleen, or both, affected and in no instance were other tissues involved. In Hodgkin's *sarcoma* the retroperitoneal nodes have been found to be the usual primary site. The lesion is characteristically invasive and destructive. It may not be possible to recognize the outline of the involved nodes. Instead a large, irregularly-shaped conglomerate mass may be found. The liver, the pancreas, the bones and the lungs are frequently affected and the gastro-intestinal tract has been found to be involved more often than in Hodgkin's granuloma. The spleen, on the other hand, was less frequently and less extensively affected.[32a] Invasion of the nervous system has been described.[32a] The histologic picture of Hodgkin's sarcoma has been considered already (p. 1007).

The "lymphosarcomas"[38] and "reticulum-cell" sarcomas[58] are characterized by their localized origin, the invasion and destruction of surrounding tissue, the spread to other groups of lymph nodes or collections of lymphoid tissue by way of the lymphatics, and the eventual production of distant metastases. When the primary site is in the cervical region, it may be quite small and easily overlooked.[48b] It may reside in the nasopharynx, the tonsil or the laryngeal ventricle. In the mediastinal form, there is extensive invasion of the lungs, the bronchi and other neighboring structures. Unlike Hodgkin's disease, the intestinal lymphoid tissue is not infrequently involved. The bowel may be converted into a stiff tube. At autopsy one may find extensive involvement of most of the lymphoid tissue of the body. Collections of tumor cells may be found in the liver, kidneys, spleen and bone marrow as well. The microscopic picture in the various types has been discussed already (p. 1006).

As stated previously, a conspicuous feature of follicular lymphoma frequently is enlargement of the spleen. Adhesions may be present. The cut surface is purplish-red and is studded with numerous pale, grayish, somewhat raised nodules which represent greatly hypertrophied Malpighian corpuscles.[3]

THE SPLEEN AND SPLENOMEGALY

In the preceding chapters a number of conditions were considered in which enlargement of the spleen occurs. There are several which have not as yet been discussed systematically. The following pages will be devoted to a consideration of the functions of the spleen, a classification of the splenomegalies and a discussion of "Banti's disease" as well as of other disorders of the spleen which have not been presented thus far.

Structure of the Spleen.[102]—The pulp of the spleen appears to be made up, essentially, of lymphoid cells but a more detailed examination reveals that the pulp is arranged into lobules with an artery in the middle and veins on the periphery. These lobules are further subdivided by intralobular trabeculae. The latter extend from the capsule and are made up of fibrous and elastic tissue, as well as a few flat muscle cells. Within each subdivision is a venous plexus which is made up of blood sinuses.

The *blood sinuses* are cucumber-shaped and the irregularly rod-shaped anastomosing strands of lymphoid tissue are normally stretched or squeezed between them. In addition to these structures, placed about the sinuses and intermingling with the strands of lymphoid tissue is a reticular network of *branching multipolar cells*, the representatives of the reticuloendothelial system in the spleen. In addition, some granulocytes and varying numbers of red corpuscles are found in the spleen.

The blood vessels, entering at the hilum, subdivide along the trabeculae. Each arterial branch, when it finally leaves the trabecula, is surrounded by a zone of lymphoid tissue which is often organized so as to form the Malpighian body. Beyond this corpuscle the artery ultimately subdivides into arterioles and capillaries and the majority of these terminate in a venous sinus, as described above. The histology and physiology of the vascular communications between the arteries and the veins of the spleen have been the subject of controversy for a century.[78] This is due to the extreme difficulty in getting views of the smaller vascular channels through the microscope. It has been claimed by some that the circulation of the spleen is closed whereas others insist that it is open and permits shunting of blood outside of the ordinary vascular channels. Knisely[103] interpreted his observations on the living unstimulated spleen as indicating that the vascular system is structurally closed but differs from the usual type of closed circulation in that fluid is separated from the cellular portion of the blood in the sinuses and passes into the pulp cords, leaving thick, pasty blood in the sinuses. He described ellipsoidal structures made up of club-like aggregations of cells located irregularly along the course of the arterioles. These, he thought, function as valves which can effectively close the contained arteriolar capillary. A sphincter-like structure was also described at both the efferent and afferent ends of the splenic sinuses. Others[108b] could not confirm these observations but Björkman's[78] studies favored this theory of splenic circulation and indicated that the sinus wall serves as a sort of mechanical filter. The sphincters of the sinus make possible retardation of blood flow in the sinuses while fluid is withdrawn, thus giving the appearance of an open circulation. The sinus system can be so controlled that the total volume of stored cells may be increased or decreased and blood cells may be stored in the sinuses for hours.

FUNCTIONS OF THE SPLEEN

In spite of the attention this topic has received for many decades,[104,107a] the functions of the spleen are still in many many respects obscure. It is still the *"misterii plenum organum"* of Galen, the organ of mystery.

Several clinical observations demonstrate the close relationship of the spleen to the hemopoietic system and show the need for a better understanding of the functions of this organ. First, the spleen is found to be enlarged in association with a variety of disorders of the blood; secondly, splenectomy is helpful in the treatment of some of these disorders, although this does not always occur even when the operation is performed for what appears to be the same disease; thirdly, striking changes in the blood follow the removal of this organ; and, finally, life may go on very satisfactorily in the absence of the spleen.

Changes in the Blood Following Splenectomy.[106,123a,127] — In *man*, as well as in experimental animals,[126e] alterations in all three formed elements of the blood are observed when the normal spleen is removed, and similar changes often follow splenectomy in the treatment of pathological states. The most striking effect on the *red cells* is morphologic. Nucleated red cells appear in the circulating blood, as well as corpuscles with Howell-Jolly bodies, the percentage of reticulocytes is increased and siderocytes and diffuse basophilia are found. In the splenectomized dog made anemic by bleeding or by acetylphenylhydrazine injections, the number of normoblasts in the peripheral circulation was found to be four times greater than in the non-splenectomized animal and the number of primitive erythroblasts was much higher.[80f] The cellular volume remains normal but the surface area of the red cells is larger than before splenectomy;[80e] that is, the cells are thinner and may have the form of "target cells" (p. 100). Their saline osmotic fragility is decreased.[123a] Anemia may develop but it is rarely pronounced and is usually transient. The life span of the red cells is not altered, at least to a degree which is detectable by present methods of measurement.

Leukocytosis occurs and this is sometimes quite pronounced (30,000 per c.mm.) The maximum increase in leukocytes is reached during the first week postoperatively and is due chiefly to the presence of polymorphonuclear neutrophils. Subsequently the lymphocytes and monocytes tend to increase in number and there may be some eosinophilia and an increase in basophilic leukocytes.[107g]

Thrombocytosis follows splenectomy but, contrary to the common impression, this does not necessarily occur immediately postoperatively and may begin three to ten days later to reach a peak about three weeks after splenectomy.

Abnormalities in the blood may persist for many years following the removal of a normal spleen in man.[76] There is no anemia but Howell-Jolly bodies have been observed as long as 11 years afterwards. In a few instances moderate polycythemia (6,000,000 to 7,500,000 red corpuscles per c.mm.) has developed. When examinations were made long after splenectomy, the corpuscular resistance to hypotonic saline solutions was normal and the platelet count as well as the bleeding and coagulation times were normal. In many cases there was moderate leukocytosis, and frequently there was a moderate increase in lymphocytes and monocytes. Eosinophilia was noted in half the cases. A shift to the left in the myeloid leukocytes was very unusual. In Ask-Upmark's study[76] of 100 cases of his own in which the spleen had been removed one to 27 years previously (average eight years), as well as in 94 cases from the literature, there was no evidence of increased sus-

ceptibility to infection nor to the development of malignant tumors. Nevertheless, a number of the subjects manifested a tendency to easy exhaustion, vague dyspeptic complaints and alterations in the body weight. In another study of 18 subjects[84a] similar observations were made and the additional finding was noted that the sternal marrow was entirely normal in nine out of 12 instances, there was an increase in eosinophils in one and an unusually great proportion of erythropoietic elements in two.

Congenital absence of the spleen is accompanied by all the abnormalities in the blood which appear following splenectomy; namely, target cells, decreased osmotic fragility, Howell-Jolly bodies, occasional nucleated red cells, siderocytosis, Heinz bodies, leukocytosis and a variable degree of thrombocytosis.[78b] The presence of these abnormalities, in the absence of a history of splenectomy, has therefore been used as a clue to the diagnosis of splenic agenesis, especially when congenital cardiac or other abnormalities were present as well.[92] In a few of the cases the leukocytosis was so striking that the possibility of leukemia was considered.

The *functions of the spleen* can be considered under several headings.

(1) **Role in Blood Formation.**—In embryonic life the spleen participates in blood formation (p. 33). During normal adult life lymphocytes are produced by the Malpighian corpuscles of the spleen and monocytes may also arise in the spleen, but otherwise hematopoiesis does not occur there. Nevertheless, under certain circumstances the capacity for blood formation is reawakened in the spleen. Thus, in certain chronic anemias of adult life foci of extramedullary hemopoiesis can be found in the spleen (p. 52) and erythropoiesis can also be demonstrated there by studies of radioactive iron turnover and the placement of a

scintillation counter over the spleen (p. 182).

Experimental investigations also provide evidence of hemopoiesis in the spleen in adult life. Thus, in studies of the effects of injection of radioactive strontium in normal and splenectomized mice it was found that splenectomized animals developed anemia whereas, in intact mice, no anemia occurred and ectopic erythropoiesis as well as megakaryocyte formation could be demonstrated in the spleen.[100] Again, it was shown that recovery of hemopoietic tissues following whole body irradiation of mice is significantly hastened by lead shielding of the marsupialized spleen.[99] The shielded spleen exerts its effect so promptly that it can be removed one hour following exposure of the animal to radiation. Transplantation of one or more fresh spleens immediately after radiation exposure, as well as intraperitoneal injection of spleen homogenates, also enhance survival. The protective factor was at first thought to be noncellular in nature but evidence derived from studies of the fate of injected cells carrying an immunogenetic marker strongly indicates that recovery depends on the seeding or colonization of the host by the cells of the donor tissue.[89a] Other tissues, such as bone marrow,[124c] if shielded, have a similar property although they are less active.

(2) **Destruction of Red Corpuscles.** There is good evidence that the spleen is the chief graveyard of the red cell. It is clear, also, that it sometimes becomes the slaughter-house. It was pointed out earlier (p. 167) that the spleen normally participates in the removal of effete, worn-out corpuscles by removing the products of red cell fragmentation. As the red corpuscle ages, the activity of its enzyme systems probably decreases (p. 126) with the result that the repair and restoration of the stromal lipids becomes imperfect. The corpuscle becomes brittle, mechanically fragile[124b] and hence more susceptible to fragmentation. It is thought that the unique circulation, described above, permits separation of plasma from the red corpuscles. When "sequestered" in this fashion, the red corpuscle becomes more spherical, which increases its fragility.[78] It is thought that this normal process, being tuned to the detection of cells of increased fragility, causes the rapid destruction of the abnormal cells of hereditary spherocytosis and of other hemolytic anemias. The beneficial effects produced by splenectomy in hemolytic anemias are attributed to the removal of an organ which is sensitive to and exaggerates spherocytosis and normally participates in the destruction of red corpuscles.

(3) **Reservoir Function.**—The role of the spleen as a reservoir of blood was discussed in an earlier chapter (p. 113). In some species, of which the sea lion is an outstanding example, it is extremely large and is capable of great changes in size. In such animals, the spleen, by governing the volume of blood corpuscles in the circulation, plays a part in the physiological adaptation to sudden emergencies, such as those produced by hemorrhage or asphyxia.[80d,126b] In man this reservoir function does not appear to be very important.

Nevertheless, *sequestration* of red corpuscles in the spleen probably plays a significant role in the normal process of red cell destruction, as outlined above, and is of the greatest importance in the blood destruction which occurs in certain disorders of the blood. In an adult of average size the spleen holds only about 20 to 30 ml. of red cells.[112b] It has been estimated, however, that, of the 120 days of the life span of the red corpuscle of man, about two days are spent in the spleen.

In contrast to the lungs and the kidneys, the spleen appears to be unique in the manner in which it disposes of the *iron* derived from red cell destruction. The epithelial cells of the renal tubules and the phagocytes of the lungs do not seem to be capable of returning the iron derived from corpuscular breakdown to the iron stores of the body, with the result that hemosiderin is deposited in the renal tubules and hemosiderinuria occurs, and in the lungs pulmonary siderosis can develop in the face of iron-deficiency anemia. The phagocytes that line the splenic sinusoids, on the other hand, make iron available for erythro-poiesis. The wandering phagocytes of the pulp cord, do not seem to be so efficient.[80e]

(4) **"Culling" and "Pitting."** — These apt terms, introduced by Crosby,[80e] refer to two unique roles of the spleen. "Culling" refers to the ability of this organ to scrutinize the passing red cells and to remove from circulation those which do not meet certain minimum requirements. This is most clearly exemplified by the rapid disappearance of the red cells of hereditary spherocytosis when transfused to a normal recipient, in contrast to their normal life span in a splenectomized subject (p. 653). It seems that the appearance of the circulating blood in splenectomized persons, with its nucleated red cells and other morphologic erythrocytic aberrations, can be compared to the streets of a disorganized, unregulated city. The spleen, it would appear, normally removes such cells from the circulation. However, that some of these are not destroyed but, instead, are altered by the spleen is suggested by experiments with sidero-cytes (p. 101). It was observed that, when blood containing a high proportion of siderocytes which was also tagged with Cr^{51} was transfused to two recipients, one normal and the other a splenectomized person, the siderocyte count fell rapidly in the subject with an intact spleen.[80e] In the splenectomized subject their

number was unchanged. In neither case, however, was there a great loss of transfused red cells, as judged by their radioactivity. Thus, it appeared that the number of transfused red cells in the circulation was not altered in either subject and it would follow that the spleen of the normal subject removed the iron granules from the transfused cells without destroying them; that is, they were "pitted," perhaps like the stone of a cherry is removed. It is possible that other structures may be removed from red cells by a similar process.

(5) **Control over Hemopoiesis.** — Ferrata believed that the spleen normally exerts an inhibitory effect upon bone marrow activity. This possibility has intrigued investigators for many decades but conclusive evidence is lacking. The suggestion receives support from the changes which are demonstrable in the blood following splenectomy but, as already discussed, many of these can be explained in other ways. There is no evidence that the spleen influences the enzymatic synthesis of hemoglobin or of stromal proteins but it has been suggested that the spleen determines the age at which young erythrocytes are released from the bone marrow. Thus, following splenectomy, the percentage of reticulo-cytes in the blood is increased and in dogs it was noted that this was unaccompanied by alterations in the myeloid-erythroid ratio of the bone marrow.[107j] However, this too can be explained on other grounds; for example, on the basis of splenic trapping. It was shown that immature red cells are coated with protein, at least part of which is transferrin (p. 90) or an immunologically similar substance.[100b] Such cells were found to be more agglutinable than adult corpuscles. It was suggested that this property is related to their retention in the bone marrow, as well as to their trapping in the spleen, should they be released early. Selective trapping in

the spleen of reticulocytes, rather than a splenic hormone, would then account for a hypothetical suppressive effect of the spleen on hemopoiesis.

There is comparatively little information concerning the relation of the spleen to *leukocytes and platelets* other than the changes which follow splenectomy, already described. It has not been established that the spleen normally plays a part in the destruction of platelets or leukocytes. It is possible, however, that in certain disorders, as in certain cases of "idiopathic" thrombocytopenic purpura (p. 839), platelets are destroyed by the spleen. Destruction of leukocytes and even of all three formed elements of the blood has been postulated as the underlying mechanism in the pathogenesis of "splenic neutropenia" and in "splenic panhematopenia." On the other hand, the fact that in these pathologic states a marked rise in the platelet and leukocyte counts and relief from anemia follows splenectomy has been offered as evidence that the spleen in some way exercises an inhibitory or controlling effect on the bone marrow.

The leukocytosis which develops following splenectomy in normal animals is much more pronounced than is seen after other operations.[114a] It was shown that the usual postsplenectomy leukocytosis can be prevented by leaving 25 per cent of the organ intact, within the body, or by transplanting back again as little as 10 per cent of a spleen which had been removed.[114a] Furthermore, when splenectomy was performed in one partner of parabiotic rats, no rise occurred in the leukocyte count of either animal; only when the spleen of the second partner was removed did a rise in the leukocyte count take place and this occurred in both animals. On the other hand, when rats were made leukopenic through pteroylglutamic acid deficiency, no rise in the leukocytes in the peripheral blood followed splenectomy. These observations suggest that the rate of production or liberation of leukocytes from the bone marrow may be under the control of the spleen.

The life span of rat platelets was found to be the same in normal and in splenectomized animals, as well as in animals made splenomegalic by the injection of methylcellulose.[97b] It would follow that destruction of platelets proceeds at a normal rate in the absence of the spleen and in the presence of the artificially induced splenomegaly. Comparison of thrombopoietic responses to acute platelet depletion by exchange transfusion in such animals showed the response of methylcellulose-treated animals to be approximately one-third of the normal.[108b] This would suggest, then, that the spleen exerts an effect on the level of circulating platelets through alteration in the rate of thrombopoiesis.

Thus, there are grounds for considering the possibility that the spleen in some manner influences at least leukocyte and platelet production and release from the bone marrow and for believing that its effects are not solely limited to a mechanical action within the organ itself. Clearly, however, there is room for further investigation.

(6) **Role in the Body Defense Mechanism.**—The large collection of lymphoid tissue within the spleen and the fact that the spleen is the largest single collection of reticuloendothelial cells in the body, suggest that its functions are related to the activities of these cells, some of which are thought to be concerned with defense against infections. The "acute splenic tumor" which develops in association with various infections is thought to be a manifestation of such a function.

As with other possible functions of the spleen, information on this topic is incomplete. It has long been known that rats and dogs following splenectomy may manifest serious signs of bartonellosis whereas the same animals with intact spleens, living under identical conditions, are able to control such infection without difficulty. A similar conversion of latent bacterial, protozoan and hematozoan infections into manifest disease has been observed in other species as well.[115] Evidence based on studies in parabiotic rats, however, suggests that the splenic protection is local and not mediated through a humoral substance.[83e] Thus, true parabiosis in which the interchange of blood cells amounted to about 50 per cent gave protection against Bartonellosis in carrier rats whereas false parabiosis in which there was no cross circulation afforded no protection.

The relative freedom of the spleen from tumor metastases has led to the suggestion that it plays a role in the biologic resistance of the organism to tumor formation. The phenomenon, however, can probably be explained on other grounds (see p. 1060).

Antibody production in the spleen was thought, in experimental studies, to take place mainly in the red pulp.[88b,126] In rats no difference in susceptibility to infection by a highly virulent strain of pneumococci could be demonstrated between normal and splenectomized animals.[119] The extent of production of antibodies against sheep red cells in splenectomized human subjects was found to be less than in normal persons[122a] but no difference could be detected in the antibody response to subcutaneously administered tularemia vaccine.[122b] However, the statement has been made that the *predisposition to infection* is greater in splenectomized persons, especially in young children,[123b] as compared with normal subjects. In particular, sepsis and meningitis were observed. Further investigation, however, has failed to give support to this impression.[107] It was found that when splenectomy was performed in the treatment of disorders such as hereditary spherocytosis, idiopathic

thrombocytopenic purpura or splenic rupture,[108f] the incidence of infection was not unusual. On the other hand, when the operation was carried out in the treatment of conditions which are not infrequently associated with diminished resistance to infection, such as certain cases of chronic congenital thrombocytopenia, the incidence of severe postoperative infection was high and was unrelated to the age of the patient.[117c]

Thus, although the spleen no doubt plays a role in the defense mechanism of the body, it does not appear to be essential for this purpose.

"HYPERSPLENISM"

This term, coined by Chauffard in 1907, has become popular only recently.[82,83c] Implying as it does a pathologic exuberance of splenic function, it would have been more logical to withhold the use of the term until a time when the role of this organ had become better understood. It is implied that when certain manifestations have disappeared following splenectomy, they must have been due to "hypersplenism."

As the above discussion of the functions of the spleen should have made clear, the concept is as yet on uncertain ground. Unfortunately, it has led to loose thinking and careless diagnosis. Nevertheless, the concept is useful, provided its limitations are clearly understood. Hypersplenism is conceived as being associated with neutropenia, thrombocytopenia or anemia, or with various combinations of these deficiencies in the blood. These should be accompanied by a normally cellular or hypercellular bone marrow and, usually, by splenomegaly. In cases with neutropenia the granulocytes in the bone marrow may be greatly increased; in those with thrombocytopenia the megakaryocytes are abundant and may be increased and in cases with anemia or pancytopenia the erythroblasts or the precursors of all three types of blood corpuscles are abundant. The bone marrow cellularity may be accompanied by a preponderance of the younger varieties of these precursors. This has been termed "maturation arrest" but it is equally plausible that the absence of the later forms of these cells is due to their rapid liberation into the blood stream rather than to failure of maturation.

The term hypersplenism has been applied to clinical states in which the destructive activities of the spleen and its hypothetical inhibitory actions have been presumed to have become exaggerated, with the result that a decrease of one or more formed elements of the blood has taken place. The hypersplenic syndromes have been classified as "idiopathic" or "primary," and "secondary." The latter include a number of more or less well defined entities which are associated with splenomegaly and either leukopenia, thrombocytopenia or anemia, or various combinations of these; for example, Felty's syndrome, a variety of infectious disorders involving the spleen which will be discussed in the next section, the congestive splenomegalies and even some cases of leukemia and lymphosarcoma[117a] in which leukopenia, thrombocytopenia or anemia are prominent and are relieved by splenectomy. "Hypersplenic" syndromes have even been reported in association with hyperthyroidism[92a] and with urticaria pigmentosa (p. 939).[85a]

The **"primary" hypersplenic syndromes** include "primary splenic neutropenia" and "primary splenic panhematopenia" or "pancytopenia." The clinical manifestations of the neutropenic syndrome will be discussed in the next chapter (p. 1103). "*Primary splenic panhematopenia*"[83c, 83d] was described as a disorder which develops without apparent cause; it was thought to be congenital at times. The clinical manifestations, as reported, were somewhat vague and variable and may have been present for a few weeks to many years. In a few instances they were described as recurring periodically. Complaints included lassitude, palpitation or fever and vague aches or pains in the extremities. Oral ulceration and indolent ulcers on the lower extremities were reported. There was splenomegaly but lymphadenopathy was not observed. There was little or no evidence of increased blood destruction but the reticulocyte percentage was slightly or greatly increased. Polychromatophilia as well as normal or increased osmotic fragility of the red corpuscles were sometimes seen. The bone marrow was hyperplastic. For diagnosis much stress was laid on an "*adrenalin test*"[83d] which consists in the enumeration of the corpuscular elements of the blood following the subcutaneous injection of epinephrin. An increase in their number as compared with the levels prior to injection was interpreted as incriminating the spleen in the pathogenesis of the disorder. However, changes similar to those described in cases of primary hypersplenism have been observed in normal individuals and even in those who have undergone splenectomy. The test is therefore regarded as unreliable by most investigators.[80d, 96] As discussed in an earlier chapter (p. 241), changes in the leukocyte count following the administration of adrenalin can be explained on the basis of a shift of cells from the marginal to the circulating pool of granulocytes.

It has been suggested repeatedly that neither "primary splenic panhematopenia" or "primary splenic neutropenia" is a true entity and that these conditions are manifestations of some underlying disorder the nature of which may remain obscure for a long time.[98] Nevertheless, it cannot be denied that in occasional instances splenectomy was followed by improvement[107b,126f] although this may have been gradual and prolonged rather than immediate and complete[96] and, therefore, perhaps, not really attributable to the splenectomy.

Some regard idiopathic thrombocytopenic purpura and hemolytic anemias as also representing primary forms of hypersplenism.[83c] On the basis of supravital studies of fresh splenic tissue obtained from cases of unexplained severe anemia, leukopenia or thrombocytopenia, it was concluded that excessive phagocytosis of granulocytes, platelets or red corpuscles, or of all the formed elements of the blood is the underlying mechanism whereby the spleen produces the syndrome of "hypersplenism."[127a] Others, however, denied the presence of excessive phagocytosis in the spleen and attributed the observed phenomena to excessive inhibitory action by the spleen on bone marrow function.[82]

It seems reasonable to presume that, until the functions of the spleen are better understood, the concept of "primary hypersplenism" will remain vague.

"*Secondary hypersplenism*" has been produced experimentally. Massive splenomegaly, hyperplasia of the bone marrow elements, normocytic anemia, reticulocytosis, leukopenia and mild thrombocytopenia developed in rats following the intraperitoneal administration of methyl cellulose.[114] In these animals the spleen, liver and kidneys were infiltrated with "storage-cell" macrophages. The importance of the spleen in the pathogenesis of the syndrome was indicated by the fact that the administration of methyl cellulose to rats previously splenectomized produced similar histologic lesions but failed to produce the hematologic abnormalities. Later studies suggested that the observed changes in the blood could be attributed to destruction of the blood elements by sequestration in the spleen.[112b] In another study, some evidence of a humoral factor was offered.[114b]

Indications for Splenectomy. —

Even though our understanding of splenic function is very limited, in many instances clinical experience affords a good foundation upon which a decision for or against splenectomy in a given case can be made. This can also be fitted reasonably well with what is known concerning the activities of this organ. Thus, in general, it can be stated that this operation has its greatest value when the spleen appears to be exerting a *destructive or inhibitory* effect. For example, the highest degree of success attending splenectomy in hematologic disorders is in the treatment of hereditary spherocytosis. In that condition the anemia and the icterus are relieved by splenectomy although the congenitally malformed red corpuscles are still produced by the bone marrow (p. 652). It is less valuable, as a rule, in cases of acquired hemolytic anemia for, in many of these, antibody formation and red cell destruction take place in many tissues besides the spleen. This operation is also valuable in many cases of idiopathic thrombocytopenic purpura. Failure of splenectomy in certain cases of idiopathic thrombocytopenic purpura can be explained by assuming that this condition is a syndrome which may be produced in a number of different ways and that the spleen is important only in one of these forms (p. 836). The reported beneficial effects of splenectomy in so-called "primary splenic neutropenia" and in "primary splenic pancytopenia" has been attributed either to interruption of cellular destruction within the spleen or of exaggerated inhibitory action on the part of this organ, or both. A similar explanation can be offered for those instances in which splenectomy has been helpful in cases of "secondary hypersplenism."

It follows also from these considerations that splenectomy cannot be expected to be helpful where the enlargement of this organ is associated with a *constructive*

Table 20–1.—Classification of Splenomegaly

I. *Inflammatory Splenomegaly*
   1. Acute and subacute:
      a. Acute splenic tumor of various infections (typhoid, septicemia, *etc.*)
      b. Abscess of spleen
      c. Infectious mononucleosis
      d. Subacute bacterial endocarditis, systemic lupus, *etc.*
   2. Chronic
      a. Tuberculosis
      b. Syphilis, especially congenital
      c. Felty's syndrome
      d. Malaria
      e. Leishmaniasis
      f. Trypansomiasis
      g. Amazonian and Bengal splenomegalies. Histoplasmosis
      h. Schistosomiasis
      i. Echinococcosis
      j. Cryptogenetic splenomegaly
      k. Hodgkin's disease (or neoplasm?)
      l. Boeck's sarcoid
      m. Histiocytosis X (Schüller-Christian, Letterer-Siwe diseases) (or neoplasm?)
      n. Beryllium disease

II. *Congestive Splenomegaly* ("Banti's disease," "splenic anemia")
   1. Cirrhosis of the liver
   2. Thrombosis, stenosis or cavernous transformation of the portal vein
   3. Thrombosis or other forms of obstruction of the splenic vein
   4. Less common and unrecognized causes of congestive splenomegaly
   5. Cardiac failure (occasionally)

III. *"Hyperplastic" Splenomegaly*
   1. Frankly hemolytic anemias of various types
   2. Chronic anemias with moderately increased or no increase in blood destruction
      a. Pernicious anemia and related macrocytic anemias
      b. Thalassemia, Hemoglobin C disease and combinations of C, D, E, Lepore or sickle cell hemoglobin and thalassemia
      c. Myelophthisic anemia, myelosclerosis, "aleukemic megakaryocytic myelosis," agnogenic myeloid metaplasia," *etc.*
      d. Hemolytic disease of the newborn
      e. Chronic hypochromic anemia
   2. Purpura hemorrhagica
   4. Benign lymphatic hyperplasia—Graves' disease
   5. Malignant hyperplasia: leukemias
   6. Polycythemia vera
   7. "Primary splenic neutropenia," "primary splenic panhematopenia"

IV. *"Infiltrative" Splenomegaly*
   1. Gaucher's disease
   2. Niemann-Pick's disease
   3. Amyloidosis
   4. Diabetic lipemia
   5. Gargoylism

V. *Neoplasms and Cysts*
   1. True cysts (epithelial, endothelial or parasitic: dermoids, lymphangiomas, hemangiomas, hydatid)
   2. False cysts (hemorrhagic, serous, inflammatory, degenerative)
   3. Hamartomas
   4. Sarcomas, primary or secondary (follicular lymphoma, lymphosarcoma, etc.)
   5. Metastatic

or protective function, such as that encountered in certain infectious disorders or when there is extensive myeloid metaplasia in the spleen. In the majority of cases of myelofibrosis splenectomy has been of no value, even if it has not been harmful (p. 586). In some cases, however, it has been helpful. Beneficial results have been explained by the existence of increased blood destruction in the spleen which was more harmful than the blood production was useful.

A noteworthy aspect of the physiology of the spleen is that many or perhaps all of its activities are shared by other tissues in the body. For this reason, the organ may be removed, when circumstances require it, without serious loss to the organism. Perhaps for the same reason splenectomy fails as a therapeutic procedure in certain cases in which this operation might theoretically be expected to be helpful.

CAUSES OF SPLENOMEGALY

Enlargement of the spleen is found in association with a great number of diseases of the widest variety. In a study of 2,274 patients, mostly ambulatory and seen in an office practice, the spleen was found palpable in 5.6 per cent.[107e] In 41.4 per cent of these no adequate cause was discovered. This high proportion of palpable spleens in apparently normal individuals is a surprising result and is not at all consistent with the writer's experience. Even though it can be admitted that a palpable spleen is not necessarily enlarged[83a] and occasionally an enlarged spleen may have no serious significance, it is a good principle of practice to regard the finding of a palpable spleen as a physical sign of importance and to make every effort to discover the cause since this may be the first and only symptom of disease. An enumeration of the causes of splenomegaly touches practically all the types of disease to which man is heir: infectious, metabolic, circulatory, endocrine, neoplastic, as well as purely mechanical disorders.

I. **Inflammatory Splenomegalies.** —A classification of the causes of splenomegaly is given in Table 20–1. Of the infectious splenomegalies, those of the chronic variety are of chief interest here for their clinical picture may resemble that of various hematopoietic disorders.

(a) **Tuberculous Splenomegaly** (so-called "primary tuberculosis" of the spleen) is a very rare condition and must not be confused with the common tuberculosis of the spleen seen in cases of generalized tuberculosis.[86,90a] About 100 cases have been reported.[80a] The symptoms include weakness, lassitude, loss of weight, a variable amount of fever, enlargement of the spleen, which may be very great, and, in some cases, hematemesis, ascites, jaundice and purpura. Anemia and leukopenia are the most common blood changes but there may be thrombocytopenia as well, or alone, or polycythemia may be present. Normoblasts may be found in the blood smear in the absence of anemia. Frequently tuberculosis has been discovered only following splenectomy for what was thought to be "Banti's disease," although in most of the cases which have been studied adequately tuberculous lesions have been found to exist elsewhere as well.[97] The demonstration by roentgenography of areas of calcification in the spleen is helpful in diagnosis but such calcification has not always been evident.[97] In some cases complete relief of symptoms has followed splenectomy.[80a]

(b) Splenomegaly may occur in connection with **syphilis,** especially congenital syphilis. The clinical picture is one of splenomegaly, chronic anemia, and usually leukopenia. The writer observed one such case in a young woman in whom antiluetic therapy did not influence the clinical picture. Splenectomy was followed by a very stormy course,

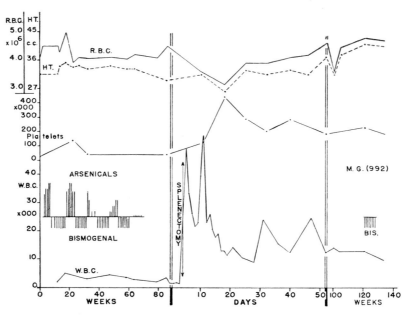

Fig. 20–20.—Congenital syphilis with splenomegaly, hypochromic microcytic anemia, leukopenia and thrombocytopenia. Antiluetic therapy was ineffectual in relieving the anemia. Splenectomy was followed by temporary and striking leukocytosis and thrombocytosis, and a gradual disappearance of anemia.

but after eight months there was complete relief of anemia (Fig. 20–20). Antiluetic therapy has been reported[90] as being beneficial, however, and we have seen this in one case. Splenomegaly may also occur in tertiary syphilis caused by huge gummata or amyloidosis. In a case of amyloid splenomegaly in congenital syphilis we found progressive hypochromic anemia but no leukopenia.

(c) Splenomegaly, chronic arthritis, anemia and leukopenia, is a combination of symptoms occurring in adults which has become known as **Felty's syndrome**.[88] The syndrome resembles Still's disease of children and has also been referred to as Chauffard-Still's disease. There is loss of weight and progressive weakness, there may be brownish pigmentation of the exposed skin and general lymphadenopathy, and the liver may be enlarged. The anemia is moderate in degree and normocytic. Leukopenia may be very pronounced

(800 to 4200, average 2500), but the differential leukocyte count is variable. Granulocytopenia and relative lymphocytosis, or lymphocytopenia and slight eosinophilia have predominated in the reported cases. The leukopenia was cyclic in one case.[107i] In the majority of the reported cases the bone marrow was found to be hyperplastic but, in a few, it was hypoplastic. Gastric achlorhydria is common. Many writers regard the condition as a variant of chronic infectious arthritis[98a] which is closely linked to systemic lupus.[78c] It is of interest that splenic enlargement was reported in 1 to 21 per cent of cases of chronic arthritis.[107h] Splenectomy has not usually produced lasting benefit although in some cases considerable improvement took place[78a, 98a] even when the bone marrow was hypoplastic.[118a]

(d) **Malaria** is a well-known cause of splenomegaly. In chronic cases[89] there may be no jaundice even when there is

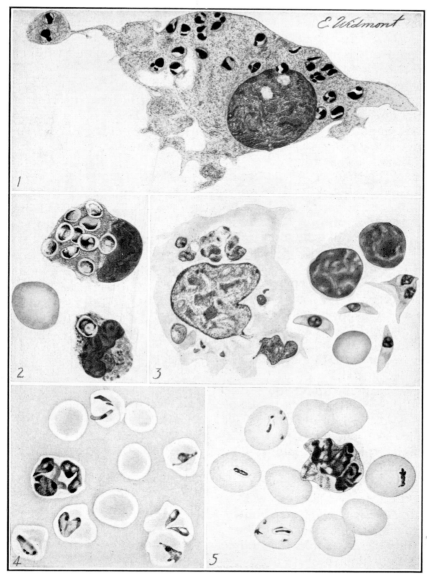

Fig. 20–21.—1. *Leishmania donovani* in a large endothelial cell. Obtained by sternal puncture in a case of kala-azar.

2. *Histoplasma capsulatum* from the spleen of a case of histoplasmosis. Note the characteristic saucer shape of the fungus, engulfed by phagocytes.

3. *Toxoplasma cuniculi* from the spleen of a rabbit. Two lymphocytes and an endothelial cell are also shown.

4. Piroplasma in red cells (cattle).

5. *Bartonella muris* in the blood of a rat. The organism is sometimes bacilliform, sometimes coccoid

substantial anemia, and parasites may be difficult to discover. The subcutaneous injection of epinephrin sometimes forces into the peripheral circulation malarial parasites harbored in the spleen. The spleen is large but is rarely huge. On cut section it is slate-blue in color and a marked increase in connective tissue can be seen.[83]

(*e*) **Leishmaniasis (kala-azar),** both the Asiatic[79] and the Mediterranean[108] or infantile form, produce splenomegaly of extraordinary degrees, irregular fever, anemia and leukopenia. Lymphadenopathy may be present, even as the primary and most important symptom.[75] The anemia is normocytic and the leukopenia is due to a reduction in all types of cells, especially neutrophils.[79] The urobilin content of the urine is increased. The diagnosis is made by the demonstration of the protozoa, *Leishmania donovani*, within the endothelial cells of the spleen, as obtained by splenic puncture. Sternal marrow puncture has also been used successfully in demonstrating these organisms[79,108] (Fig. 20–21).

(*f*) In **trypanosomiasis,** both the African and the American form (Chagas' disease), the spleen is usually enlarged but rarely is this pronounced.

(*g*) A clinical picture resembling that of kala-azar has been observed in the region of the *Amazon River* in South America,[125] in *Bengal* (India)[83] as well as in Central America and the United States. Bengal splenomegaly is attributable to a number of factors, including malaria, malnutrition, post-necrotic cirrhosis of the liver and, ultimately, the development of portal hypertension.[77a] The *American* splenomegalies[81] have been ascribed to *Histoplasma capsulatum* of Darling, a fungus morphologically resembling *Leishmania donovani*[110a] (Fig. 20–21).

Histoplasmosis has been reported in Europe[83b] and in Africa[123] as well as on the American continent.

(*h*) Infestation with the flukes *Schistosoma mansoni* or *S. japonicum* (**schistosomiasis, Egyptian splenomegaly**) results in diffuse hyperplastic periportal cirrhosis of the liver, perisplenic vein fibrosis and thrombosis within the splenic vein. Progressive splenomegaly is the consequence (p. 1062). The liver is at first enlarged, later it shrinks and ascites develops. Eosinophilia may occur in the earliest stage of the disease, anemia and leukopenia later.[118] The symptoms are produced by the deposition of the lateral-spined ova in the proximal and distal peripheral capillaries of the portal system, with resulting fibrosis.[112] Differentiation from other forms of splenomegaly presenting the "Banti syndrome" rests chiefly on the demonstration of the ova in the stools. They are rarely found in the spleen. Schistosomiasis has been observed not only in the Nile region[98] and in China and Japan but also in coastal East and West Africa, throughout the Amazon Basin and in parts of northern South America and southern Central American as well as in Puerto Rico.

(*i*) Splenomegaly may follow **echinococcus** disease of the liver. Echinococcus cysts of the spleen are rare.

(*j*) *Cryptogenetic splenomegaly* of China.[108d] A syndrome of enlargement of the spleen, commonly massive, is seen among the Chinese of Hong Kong and other parts of China and Formosa which is associated with varying degrees of liver damage. The latter is marked by features both of diffuse hepatic fibrosis and postnecrotic scarring. The splenomegaly may anticipate the liver changes. The associated anemia was found to be due both to the destructive action of the spleen and to a fault in the red corpuscles, the latter possibly the result of liver damage. An expanded plasma volume contributes to the anemia. Abnormal vascular fragility, unrelated to thrombocytopenia and chronic leg ulcers are additional features of this disorder which, like the anemia, respond favorably to splenectomy.

(*k*) The splenomegaly of **Hodgkin's disease** has been discussed (p. 1015). Some pathologists[20,48] classify Hodgkin's disease among neoplasms rather than with the infectious splenomegalies.

(*l*) In **Boeck's sarcoid** (p. 1029) the spleen may be slightly, moderately or even greatly enlarged, and sarcoidosis of the spleen with only insignificant or absent lesions elsewhere, has also been described.[43] In a small percentage of the 20 per cent of cases of sarcoidosis in which splenomegaly occurs, thrombocytopenia most frequently (p. 830), but also hemolytic anemia (p. 613), neutropenia, pancytopenia[77b] and splenic rupture have been observed.

(*m*) **Histiocytosis X.**—As discussed elsewhere (p. 778), the pathogenesis of the Letterer-Siwe and Schüller-Christian syndromes is poorly understood. The splenomegaly which is encountered in these conditions is classified here among the infectious splenomegalies because many regard them as inflammatory granulomas. Others, however, have included them among the infiltrative disorders and some emphasize the similarity between Letterer-Siwe disease and leukemia or sarcoma.

II. **Congestive Splenomegaly.** — Congestive splenomegaly will be discussed in the next section under the title of "Banti's disease."

III. **"Hyperplastic" Splenomegaly.**[102]—Enlargement of the spleen is a frequent finding in *anemia*. It is seen in acute as well as in chronic anemias of various types (Table 20–1), and in about 33 per cent of cases of purpura hemorrhagica. In none of these conditions does the splenomegaly assume great proportions as a rule. Small foci of extramedullary blood formation may be found in the spleens in many of these cases. In myelofibrosis and in a number of other instances of **myelophthisic anemia,**

however, splenomegaly may be the outstanding evidence of disease (p. 583).

The splenomegaly of leukemia (Chapter 19) and that found in polycythemia vera (Chapter 16) can also be classed under the heading, "hyperplastic splenomegaly."

"Primary splenic neutropenia" and "primary splenic panhematopenia," if they are true entities, are probably best classified among the "hyperplastic" splenomegalies. Their pathogenesis has been discussed already (p. 1052) and their clinical manifestations are considered elsewhere (pp. 1052 and 1103).

IV. **"Infiltrative" Splenomegaly.**[102] —Under this title may be grouped those instances of splenomegaly resulting apparently from excessive storage of normal and abnormal metabolic products: a cerebroside in Gaucher's disease; a phosphatid lipid, possibly sphingomyelin, in Niemann-Pick's disease. Perhaps gargoylism should be added here. These conditions were discussed in Chapter 15. The splenic enlargement found in amyloidosis and in diabetic lipemia may be added to this group of splenomegalies.

V. **Neoplasms and Cysts.**—Tumors of the spleen may be benign or malignant. The former include cysts and hamartomas. **Splenic cysts** may be lined by a specific secreting membrane (true cysts) and are then epithelial (dermoid, epidermoid), endothelial (lymphangioma, hemangioma, polycystic, serous) or parasitic (echinococcus). False cysts may be hemorrhagic, serous or inflammatory, or due to degenerating liquefaction of areas infarcted by embolism or arterial thrombosis. Some 266 non-parasitic cysts have been reported.[107b] Fulness in the epigastrium, vague digestive complaints or even epigastric pain may develop and, when the diaphragm has been elevated, dyspnea, cough and pain radiating to the shoulder have been described. The tumor may be felt in the left upper quadrant as a rounded mass which displaces the stomach downward and to the right. The splenic flexure of the colon and the left kidney may be displaced downward. Calcification is not common. Hemangioma of the spleen does not usually produce a tumor which is detectable clinically but it may rupture into the peritoneal cavity and be mistaken for perforated peptic ulcer or acute appendicitis.[124a] Non-parasitic splenic cysts have been described most frequently in women, especially in the childbearing age. Their etiology is unknown but trauma has been thought to play a dominant role.

Hamartomas are rare benign tumors composed of abnormal mixtures of normal splenic elements.[122c]

Sarcomas of the spleen most often represent only one aspect of a more widespread disorder (lymphosarcoma, follicular lymphoma, reticulum cell sarcoma, Hodgkin's sarcoma). These diseases have been discussed already. Primary sarcoma of the spleen, a tumor arising from the supporting tissues of this organ, is relatively rare. In addition to a palpable mass in the left upper quadrant of the abdomen, there may be pain there, as well as fever, anemia and general debility. More rarely, pleural effusion, gastrointestinal hemorrhage and splenic rupture have been observed.[117b,126c]

Of metastatic tumors, carcinoma is the most frequent type.[105] Although it is unusual for the spleen to be sufficiently enlarged to be palpable clinically, metastases to the spleen, from lung, breast, skin and cervix, have been observed in 2.3 per cent of autopsies in cases of carcinoma.[97a] The low incidence of splenic metastases as compared with those found in lymph nodes, liver and lungs has been attributed to inequality of exposure. Lymphatic spread has been observed.[93] No inhibiting effect of splenic tissue on carcinomatous growth has been demonstrated.

"SPLENIC ANEMIA"— "BANTI'S DISEASE"—CHRONIC CONGESTIVE SPLENOMEGALY

History and Definition.—The term "splenic anemia" was introduced in 1866[94] to refer to cases of anemia with splenomegaly which were not frank leukemia. Without doubt cases of hemolytic jaundice, "aleukemic" leukemia, Hodgkin's disease and other forms of splenic enlargement associated with anemia were not clearly differentiated at the time. At the end of the century, Banti[77] described a form of splenomegaly which was not associated with leukemia, Hodgkin's disease or hemolytic jaundice, nor was it caused by malaria, syphilis or other recognized diseases. He laid down clinical and histological criteria for the recognition of the disorder and described three stages in the disease: an anemic phase with splenomegaly, leukopenia, asthenia and occasional hemorrhagic episodes; a later intermediary phase in which hepatic enlargement occurred, urobilinuria developed and a dirty brownish discoloration of the skin sometimes appeared; and a final stage of liver atrophy and ascites. The spleen was markedly enlarged and histologically was characterized by conspicuous thickening of the fibrillar reticulum in the malpighian corpuscles and red pulp ("fibroadenie"). These changes originated either around the central artery of the follicle or about its pre-follicular division. Banti considered the spleen to be the primary seat of the disease and assumed that anemia, hepatic cirrhosis and sclerosing endophlebitis of the splenic and portal veins followed.

Osler[113] drew the attention of English-speaking clinicians to the condition and seemed to accept it at its face value but many pathologists refused to endorse the concept enunciated by Banti. Durr,[84] for example, showed that sections of spleens from Banti's own cases could not be differentiated from those found in the spleen in cases of hepatic cirrhosis. Eppinger[87] introduced the term"**hepato-lienal fibrosis**" to describe the essential pathological changes.[109] Later investigations of the pathogenesis of the disorder showed that this syndrome is associated with portal hypertension and led to the use of the term "**chronic con-gestive splenomegaly**"[106a,120] for reasons which will be given shortly.

Clinical Features.[126d] — Those affected are usually under thirty-five years of age. The disease may come on in childhood.[123c] Females were twice as numerous as males in Banti's series and this was true of Giffin's series[91] but has not been the case in all reports.[85,109] A familial incidence is very unusual but is not unknown.[109]

The onset is usually insidious but may come with explosive suddenness when vomiting of blood or the passage of large, tarry stools takes place without previous warning. Gastro-intestinal hemorrhage occurs in about half the cases.[110] In other cases abdominal pain or discomfort, the discovery of a mass in the left upper quadrant of the abdomen, or symptoms of weakness and general lassitude referable to anemia bring the patient to the physician. Flatulence, diarrhea, vague indigestion or even mild jaundice in association with abdominal pain and fever, may appear. A non-icteric type of sallow-brown pigmentation of the skin may develop. Epistaxis occurs in about a third of the cases, but other hemorrhagic manifestations such as purpura are unusual. The spleen is large and may be enormous, extending even to the pelvic brim.[91] Moderate hepatic enlargement has been observed at an early stage in perhaps a third of the cases.[80] Lymphadenopathy is absent and weight loss is not conspicuous.

Splenomegaly may precede **anemia**[91] and the latter, unless hemorrhages have occurred, is at most moderate in degree and as a rule normocytic in type.[80,106a] The average red cell count in 151 reported cases was 3,440,000 per c.mm. The red cell morphology at this stage is not remarkable. Repeated hemorrhages result in hypochromic microcytic anemia with all the morphological features of this type of anemia (p. 744). Following a hemorrhage the reticulocytes may be slightly or moderately increased in number and occasional normoblasts may be observed. The fragility of the red corpuscles to hypotonic saline solutions is normal or reduced.[110] When the condition is of long-standing and well-marked cirrhosis of the liver is present, macrocytic anemia may develop.[128] This type of anemia may also appear temporarily following an acute hemorrhage.

Leukopenia is the most constant feature of the blood picture. Leukocyte counts less than 5000 per c.mm. have been observed in about two-thirds of the cases.[91,110] A curious feature of the leukopenia is that the diminution often affects all the types of cells, the ratio of the polymorphonuclears to the lymphocytes and monocytes remaining normal as a rule. Leukocytosis has been observed following a severe hemorrhage or in association with venous thrombosis or an acute exacerbation of hepatitis.

The **platelet count** is often somewhat reduced and sometimes it is well below 100,000 per c.mm. In the latter cases prolonged bleeding time has been observed.[110] As a rule, however, bleeding and coagulation times are normal.

Findings in the **bone marrow** on sternal puncture vary. In the earlier stages, at the time when there is little or no anemia, no abnormality may be noted. However, myeloid hyperplasia has been described[107c] in the earliest stage and "maturation arrest" of the myeloid and megakaryocytic tissue later. In the last stage of the condition when cirrhosis of the liver was present, marked erythroid immaturity was found as well.

Hemorrhage causes normoblastic hyperplasia.

The relation of these changes in the blood and bone marrow to the syndrome of "hypersplenism" has been discussed already.

Course.—The disease may run a prolonged and often benign course and may appear to be spontaneously arrested, the patient living for a number of years with little or no disability. At any time, however, the uneventful course may be interrupted by one or more episodes of gastro-intestinal hemorrhage, porto-mesenteric venous thromboses or hepatitis. In other cases there is more or less steady progression with the development of symptoms of hepatic insufficiency and the signs of portal venous obstruction. Death results from one of the complications above mentioned or from intercurrent unrelated disease.

Diagnosis.—Moderate anemia and leukopenia are found in many conditions producing splenomegaly and these must be ruled out before congestive splenomegaly is considered. Hemolytic anemias, "aleukemic" leukemia, chronic hypochromic anemia, thalassemia and hookworm anemia, as well as most of the other conditions listed in Table 20–1 have been mistaken for "Banti's disease." Even when gastro-intestinal hemorrhages have occurred, the diagnosis should be made only after other possibilities have been ruled out. A "silent" duodenal ulcer, for example, may produce hypochromic microcytic anemia with slight splenic enlargement. The finding of lymphadenopathy or of immature leukocytes in the blood smear favors conditions other than "Banti's disease." Sternal marrow examination is useful in ruling out "aleukemic" leukemia.

Chronic congestive splenamegaly may result from a variety of causes. There may be obstruction of the splenic vein due to thrombosis or as the consequence of compression from pancreatic fibrosis or aneurysm of the splenic artery, or by a tumor of the pancreas, such as a cystadenoma[95] or carcinoma.[108a] The portal vein may be obliterated due to bland thrombosis or from cavernous transformation, or it may be absent ("aplasia of portal vein").[121] The obstruction, on the other hand, may be intrahepatic and result from cirrhosis. This may be of the Laennec variety or may have followed hepatitis or Schistosomiasis. In addition, in a few reported cases it was not possible to demonstrate either intra- or extrahepatic obstruction.[126a] In these cases it was postulated that the portal hypertension was caused by increased blood flow through the portal vein.

Patients in whom the portal obstruction is extra-hepatic are likely to be under eighteen years of age, they do not have gastrointestinal symptoms at times remote from bleeding and the liver is not palpable.[116] Splenomegaly associated with the *Cruveilhier-Baumgarten syndrome* should be differentiated by the presence of a prominent para-umbilical vein, as well as a venous hum and a thrill at the site of the para-umbilical circulation.[80c,100a]

A variety of relatively simple procedures is available for the study of cases of congestive splenomegaly. Liver function studies and liver biopsy are obviously necessary. It is important to note, however, that reduced bromsulfalein excretion as well as positive cephalin cholesterol flocculation and thymol turbidity tests have been found in cases of portal hypertension even when the obstruction was extra-hepatic.[116] The reduced bromsulfalein excretion has been attributed to diminished blood flow through the liver.

The extent of collateral circulation should be determined and esophageal varices looked for. The portal venous pressure may be gauged by measurement of intrasplenic pressure through percutaneous splenic puncture with a fine needle and a strain gauge.[76a] Intra-splenic pressure has been found to bear a linear relationship to the portal venous pressure. Finally, portal venography should be carried out. This is now regarded as an essential step in making a decision concerning the nature of the treatment which is to be undertaken. It may be accomplished by the percutaneous injection of the splenic pulp with radiopaque solutions[88a] or by direct injection of contrast media into the portal vein at operation.[121]

Treatment.—The chief problem is to reduce the portal hypertension and thus lessen the chance of hemorrhage. Unless this can be accomplished it is usually held that there is small chance of survival beyond a year or two at the most.[121] When signs of "secondary hypersplenism" exist (p. 1053), such as severe thrombocytopenia and leukopenia, these may require relief. If iron deficiency anemia is present from blood loss, iron therapy (p. 748) is indicated. There is no need for the administration of liver extracts or vitamin B_{12} but the diet should be nourishing and adequately supplied with vitamins. Severe hemorrhage will naturally necessitate blood transfusions and balloon tamponade may be required if early severe bleeding persists. Hepatic artery ligation together with splenectomy has been recommended in poor risk cases.[108c]

Omentopexy,[101] the production of an Eck fistula and, later, splenectomy were employed in attempts to relieve the portal hypertension. **Splenectomy** removes the evidences of "hypersplenism"[107l] and is effective in relieving obstruction close to the splenic hilum. Otherwise it has not proved to be very useful. The immediate postoperative mortality has been high and hemorrhage has recurred in as many as 50 per cent of cases.[110] In a comparative study of 51 splenectomized cases and 43 unoperated cases, no differences between the 2 groups could be demonstrated in regard to life expectancy, prevention of the progress of hepatic disease or anemia, or the occurrence of hematemesis.[97c] The implications of another study[101] are similar. It is now considered that a surgeon should not perform splenectomy in Banti's syndrome unless he is prepared to form a venovenous anastomosis, since this may be the only opportunity to construct a satisfactory shunt.[107d,120]

For relief of portal hypertension, **shunting operations** have been carried out.[107d,121] For this purpose the use of the largest caliber vessel available will usually maintain a patent shunt most efficiently and consequently portacaval shunt is preferred.[121] When there is marked splenomegaly, signs of "hypersplenism" are present and a large caliber splenic vein is available, or when the portal vein is obliterated, splenectomy and splenorenal shunt have been recommended.

Surgical intervention of this type is advocated only (1) in cases in which there is severe upper intestinal hemorrhage and in which the portal hypertension is due to extra-hepatic block; (2) in cases of portal hypertension associated with cirrhosis of the liver when there is minimal or absent ascites and icterus and a reasonable degree of hepatic reserve. When these criteria have been followed, it has been claimed that the occurrence of bleeding was markedly reduced and life was prolonged.[107d] Operative mortality was reported to be 11 per cent and the over-all mortality 29 per cent. However, it has been pointed out that little is available in the way of adequately controlled observations in which a side-by-side comparison of medical and surgical treatment in a large series of consecutive cases was made.[107k] Although the data weigh in favor of surgery, the evidence is by no means conclusive.

Pathology.—The spleen weighs 600 to 1200 Gm.[109] as a rule but may be as great as 5000 Gm.[91] The capsule is thickened and adhesions between the spleen and the stomach or diaphragm may be present. On section the spleen is grayish-red in color and firm in consistency. The trabeculae are prominent and Malpighian bodies inconspicuous. Fibrosis, dilatation of the sinuses, hyaline degenerative changes in the Malpighian bodies and the follicular arterioles, and periarterial hemorrhages are found on microscopic examination. Siderotic nodules consisting of crystalline and amorphous iron pigments deposited in the fibrous tissue around the arterioles, are found in many instances.[109]

Surgeons describe distended and tense venous radicals in the splenic pedicle and a rich venous collateral enveloping the spleen, as well as great distention of the splenic vein.[120] Endophlebitis of the splenic and portal veins is frequent, and there may be thrombosis of these veins, stenosis or cavernous transformation of the portal vein,[120] or compression of the splenic vein by tumors or scars. Cirrhosis of the liver may be evident, or this may be discovered only by microscopic examination.

Pathogenesis.—It has been shown quite conclusively that the histological picture[102,109] in the spleen described by Banti is not specific but may be seen, for example, in cases of cirrhosis of the liver and in portal or splenic vein thrombosis. The changes are of such a nature as might easily be produced by congestion of the spleen.[109] The distension in the sinuses, the hemorrhages, fibrosis, and also the siderotic nodules can be explained on this basis. In addition, definite signs of portal venous congestion are usually observed. Measurements of the pressure in the splenic vein in 14 cases presenting the clinical picture of Banti's syndrome, showed it to range from 225 to more than 500 mm. normal saline and was greater than 300 in 11 of the cases.[120] In 15 cases of splenomegaly

of other types, such as hemolytic jaundice and thrombocytopenic purpura, the pressure ranged from 70 to 275 mm., with one exception, a case of purpura in which the pressure was 360 mm. Unfortunately, it is difficult to obtain portal pressure data for normal persons. In a study carried out on 100 human adults of both sexes in whom hepatic and neoplastic disease had been excluded, the average portal pressure was found to be 215 mm. water and ranged from 100 to 300 mm.[112a]

The hematological changes observed in the Banti syndrome are attributable to the unequal distribution of the cells of the blood in the splenic vascular bed and the remaining parts of the circulation.[117] This is the consequence of stasis of the portal circulation. Although at first an obstructive factor could not be demonstrated in as many as 40 per cent of cases of the Banti syndrome, more careful study has resulted in more frequent demonstration of causes for the portal hypertension. These have been mentioned already (p. 1062). It is becoming recognized that the liver may be diseased long before significant clinical evidence is found. A very high incidence of hepatic abnormality (68 per cent or more) has been reported in cases of Banti's syndrome[80,106a,125a] It is also noteworthy that splenomegaly of some degree has been noted in as many as 79 per cent of cases of cirrhosis.[102]

No clinical or hematological differences have been found between patients with congestive splenomegaly due to intra- or extrahepatic obstruction except in cases of advanced liver disease. Furthermore, the histopathology of the spleen has been the same in all the cases, no matter what the cause of the portal hypertension happened to be. Following splenectomy the blood values usually have returned to normal. These observations strongly support the view that Banti's syndrome is the consequence of any of a variety of lesions producing chronic splenic vein hypertension.

Partial or complete occlusion of the portal vein[111] in rats and rabbits failed to produce the typical Banti syndrome, however, when hepatic cirrhosis was produced in rabbits by manganese[109] or in dogs by means of silica,[122] splenic enlargement and the picture of congestive splenomegaly did develop. The successfull production of "secondary hypersplenism" by the intraperitoneal administration of methyl cellulose[114] has been discussed already (p. 1053).

Failure to demonstrate an obstructive factor in a number of cases and the fact that portal obstruction independent of splenic disease has been observed in the absence of appreciable splenic enlargement, were reasons used to support an alternative concept[116a] which, while accepting the significance of splenic congestion, revived the theory of primary splenic disease. It was suggested that the small splenic arteries play an important role in adjusting the intake of blood into the spleen. Because of disease of these arteries, it was argued, blood enters the spleen in increased quantity, leading to congestion, and this in turn causes portal hypertension and even degenerative changes in the liver cells.

MULTIPLE MYELOMA

The bones are frequently involved in disorders of the hematopoietic system.[144] In the preceding pages attention was given to the changes to be observed in the bones in anemias characterized by bone marrow hyperplasia, especially when these diseases develop early in life, as in sickle cell anemia and in thalassemia; the osteoporosis which may occur in diseases in which fat absorption is poor and calcium is lost by the formation of soaps (sprue, idiopathic steatorrhea, celiac disease); the subperiosteal infiltration as well as the tumor-like lesions and other changes seen in the leukemias and in some of the diseases chiefly affecting lymph nodes. In other conditions which cannot be classified so readily as hematopoietic diseases, profound effects on the blood may be produced and striking changes may be demonstrable in the bones: in the infiltrative disorders (Gaucher's disease), in myelosclerosis, osteopetrosis, and in other conditions producing myelophthisic anemia. There remains to be discussed a condition which has much in common, symptomatically and perhaps also fundamentally, with a number of these disorders and particularly with leukemia.

Definition.—Multiple myeloma is a tumor characterized by multiple involvement of the skeletal trunk and the production of pain, pathological fractures and, often, by the excretion of a peculiar protein in the urine or the accumulation of an abnormal protein in the blood.

The first case was studied by McIntyre, Dalrymple, Watson and Bence-Jones in 1845 and important early contributions were made by Rustizky (1873), Kahler (1889) and Bozzolo (1897).[146]

Etiology.—The disease appears most frequently in later life, 80 per cent of all cases occurring after the age of forty. In infants and children it is very rare.[129] It is somewhat more frequent in males as compared with females Cases have been reported from all parts of the world and no race is known to be immune. The condition is probably less rare than was once thought. The mean annual death rate is about 9.0 per million.[163a] The incidence was found to be higher in non-whites than in whites. Several instances of multiple cases in the same family have been recorded.[167a] The cause of the disorder is obscure. Attempts to relate the onset of the disease to trauma or infection have been unconvincing.[146,164] A viral etiology has been suggested on the basis of the demonstration of "virus-like" particles in association with the endoplasmic reticulum of several transplantable mouse plasma-cell tumors.[169a]

Symptomatology.[168a] — Pain, tumors, deformity, pathological fractures and neuralgic or neurological symptoms are the most common complaints and one of these may be the basis of the presenting clinical picture. Less frequently complaints referable to anemia or abnormal bleeding or symptoms suggesting nephritis are the outstanding features. Fever is common but it is usually low grade and remittent.[129] Weight loss of moderate degree occurs early but in the late stages it is severe.

The *pain* is often rheumatic, wandering and intermittent at the onset and is referred to the back as a rule, less often to the chest or the extremities. Girdle sensations, or radiation down the legs may be present. Generally the onset of pain is attributed to motion or pressure. The pain may be very severe and may last for hours or days but intermittency and even remissions for several months are common.[146] In rare cases pain has not been a symptom.

The *tumors* are characteristically multiple and are confined for the most part to the sites of the red marrow: the ribs, sternum, spine, clavicles, skull, or the extremities about the shoulder or pelvic girdle. The patient may be made aware of the tumors by tenderness, a lump, pulsation or symptoms arising from pathological fractures. Generally the swellings range from the size of a pea to that of a hazelnut. They are elastic and yielding and a parchment-like crepitation may be elicited. More commonly, however, the tumors are not detected by physical examination.

Pathological fractures are frequent but, since they are confined to the trunk they may not be recognized as such but may suggest pleurisy or neurological disease. Thoracic deformity is common.

The classical changes in the bones can be demonstrated by *roentgenograms* and are revealed as rounded, punched-out areas in the sites already mentioned (Fig. 20–22). In the ribs there may be a diffuse mottling while in the spine rarefaction, globular tumor formation, shortening and twisting of the vertebral column and disappearance of intervertebral disks are found. The roentgenogram is not wholly reliable in establishing the diagnosis of myeloma.[168a] In 13 per cent of cases, or more, no significant osseous changes are found.[151] Again, instead of the typical punched-out, osteolytic lesions, diffuse osteoporosis may be seen.[173] It is also noteworthy that multiple, small, discrete osteolytic lesions may be produced by metastatic carcinoma from the breast or thyroid or by other conditions. New bone formation or periosteal reaction is most unusual in myeloma but has been observed.[152] Microradiographic studies have shown that even when standard radiographic technics reveal few or no changes, generalized thinning and destruction of trabeculae are present.[180a]

Rheumatoid manifestations are sometimes observed.[140] These have been attributed to deposition of "amyloid" in and about the joints.

Paraplegia due to compression of the spinal cord is the most common symptom referable to the *nervous system*, but intercostal neuralgia, radiculitis, diplopia, anisocoria and failing vision, or complete blindness due to thrombosis of the central artery of the retina, as well as other symptoms, have been reported.[136] Neuropathy may also result from direct infiltration of nerve roots and peripheral nerves by "amyloid" or may occur in the absence of such changes or of evidence of compression.[185b]

Gastro-intestinal symptoms may occur: diarrhea, colicky pains, nausea and vomiting. Hematemesis and melena have been described. Epistaxis may occur and ecchymoses, bleeding about the

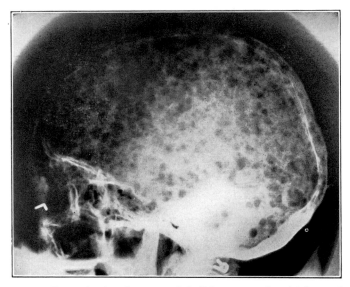

FIG. 20–22.—Extensive involvement of skull in a case of multiple myeloma.

gums and lips and petechiae have developed in some cases. Intravascular thrombosis may occur. Chronic bronchitis and pulmonary emphysema are common complications, especially if chest deformity occurs. However, in the absence of or antedating chest deformity or debilitation, *recurrent bouts of bacterial pneumonia are common.*[190] It has been shown that the antibody response of these patients is slow and feeble.[159]

Tissues other than the skeletal system may also be involved in multiple myeloma. **Extraosseous involvement** of lymph nodes,[167b] spleen,[176] tonsils, liver, thyroid, adrenal, ovary, testis, lung, pericardium and gastro-intestinal tract[149a] has been described.[136,146] Palpable hepatomegaly has been reported in 40 per cent of cases and hepatosplenomegaly in 23 per cent;[180] in another series the liver was palpable in 26 per cent of the cases and the spleen in 9 per cent.[129] The *"myeloma kidney"* will be discussed shortly (p. 1077). The extraosseous myelomatous involvement may take the form of **extramedullary plasma cell tumors.** These occur most often in the upper respiratory tract or oral cavity.[136] They have also been found in the kidney, ovary, intestine and lung. These have been regarded as benign but generalization of the disease with involvement of bone has been observed in a number of cases at variable intervals of time following discovery of the extramedullary tumor.

Occasionally, in perhaps 2 to 10 per cent of cases,[168a] a **solitary plasma cell tumor** of bone is found. This appears most often as a cystic, soap-bubble type of lesion which is much larger and more irregular than the small, discrete type characteristic of multiple myeloma. At other times it has the appearance of a solitary, destructive lesion within the medullary portion of the bone.[136] Rarely, new bone formation is seen.[160a] The solitary bone lesions have been regarded as comparatively benign and probably unrelated to multiple myeloma. However, when followed for a long period of time these patients have been found to develop diffuse plasma cell myeloma.

Cutaneous manifestations are rare but a pemphigoid eruption has been described.[154] Furthermore, hemorrhagic

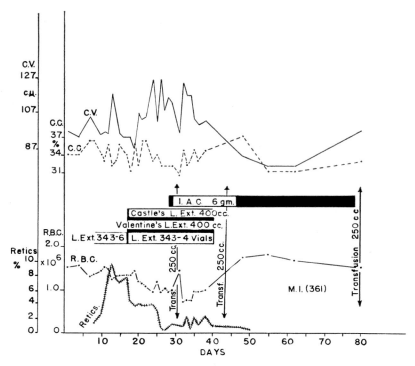

Fig. 20–23.—Macrocytic anemia in a case of multiple myeloma. Liver therapy, followed by a rise in reticulocytes, failed to relieve the anemia. Only transfusions were of value and this was but temporary. This case was mistaken for pernicious anemia at first, but differed from the latter in that the macrocytosis was not great, there was no poikilocytosis, the leukocyte count was normal, the icterus index was normal, and there was a small amount of free hydrochloric acid in the gastric juice. These findings, together with the history of stiffness followed by pain in the back, legs and chest, led to further studies which revealed Bence-Jones protein in the urine and areas of bone destruction in the ribs, spine, pelvis and skull.

manifestations such as purpura and massive subcutaneous hemorrhages may develop as the result of a disturbance in the clotting mechanism.

The Blood.—Anemia is usually moderate in degree and normocytic in type. In rare cases anemia is absent even terminally and even polycythemia may be present.[124,136,158] In other instances the anemia has been severe and, in such cases particularly, it may be moderately macrocytic (Fig. 20–23). When the classical signs of multiple myeloma are absent, the case can be mistaken for pernicious anemia. Unlike the latter, however, there is little poikilocytosis and no increased bilirubinemia. Occasional normoblasts may be found in the blood smear but no megaloblasts. There may be moderate polychromatophilia and occasional stippling. Reticulocytes may be slightly increased in number but usually they fluctuate irregularly and are not influenced by vitamin B_{12} therapy. When the anemia is less severe and normocytic, normoblasts and other immature forms of the red series are less often seen.

It has been found in a number of cases of multiple myeloma that enumeration of the red corpuscles is difficult, due to clumping. This may be caused by the presence of cold hemagglutinins, in which case it can be prevented by warming the Hayem's solution. More often it is related to the great quantity of globulin in the plasma and the marked tendency to rouleau formation. In such a case dilution with normal saline or with Gower's solution will give a more satisfactory preparation. Rouleau formation may be so pronounced that it is difficult to make satisfactory blood smears. A very rapid sedimentation rate is characteristic. Blood grouping may be difficult and the serum may need to be warmed or diluted before a satisfactory test can be made.

The **leukocyte count** may be normal, slightly increased or low. Rarely is it greatly increased (48,000).[172] The differential examination may reveal no abnormality, or there may be increased lymphocytes or eosinophils, a few myelocytes and even myeloblasts, or plasma cells and abnormal mononuclear forms. True myeloma cells such as those seen in the bone marrow (p. 1070) may be found, especially if they are looked for under low magnification.[167] In a few cases numerous plasma cells have been observed. In one of our cases 84 per cent of the 19,000 to 29,000 leukocytes per c.mm. were "myeloma cells." The separation of such cases as examples of "plasma cell leukemia" (p. 940) does not appear to serve any purpose; they would seem to be variants of multiple myeloma. Thus, in the case cited above, pain and bone tenderness were out of proportion to that seen in leukemia in adults, there were multiple lesions in the bones, including the skull, the serum contained 11 grams protein per 100 ml., chiefly globulin, and the urine was positive for Bence-Jones protein.

The **platelet count** is usually normal. In some cases it has been low.[172,187] This may be associated with prolonged bleeding time but the latter may be normal or increased without relation to the platelet count.[187] Failure of the clot to retract and difficulty in obtaining serum have been encountered in a number of cases. A disturbance in the *process of coagulation* has been observed but its true nature is obscure.[185a] The prothrombin time, thrombin time and conversion of fibrinogen to fibrin may be abnormal and in some cases an anticoagulant (antithrombin V) has been demonstrated. In the main, the abnormalities have been in the third phase of coagulation. It has been postulated that the conversion of fibrinogen to fibrin is prevented by an "abnormal" protein in the plasma[145a] which, in one instance, could be largely overcome by the addition of an excess of calcium ions.[139] Probably another factor in the development of hemorrhagic manifestations is capillary damage from impaired blood flow due to the greatly increased *blood viscosity*.[182]

Bone Marrow.—The characteristic finding is the "myeloma cell." These cells may make up 3 to 96 per cent of all the cells in the marrow. The remainder of the marrow constituents are not remarkable.

In the older literature reference was made to myelomas of various types: myeloblastic, lymphoblastic, lymphocytic, myelocytic, erythroblastic,[183] and even hemocytoblastic,[178] lipoblastic[142] and megakaryoblastic,[142,148] There is good reason to doubt these designations because they depended for the most part on examinations of tissue sections,[135] an uncertain basis for finer identification. It is significant that, since sternal aspiration has become popular, the older designations have been dropped and disagreement remains only in regard to the relationship of the "myeloma cell" and the plasma cell which is found in normal individuals and in pathological states other than multiple myeloma.

Myeloma Cell.—The typical myeloma cell[172,188] as seen in smears is moderately large (15 to 30 μ), round or ovoid, and contains a nucleus about 5 to 7 μ in diameter. The latter is round, eccentrically placed and contains one, sometimes two, nucleoli. The chromatin is not as fine as in the myeloblast nor as coarse

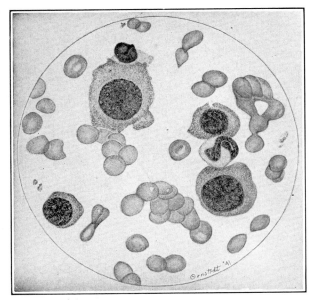

FIG. 20–24.—Drawing of "myeloma cells" in the material obtained by sternal puncture in a case of multiple myeloma. From a preparation stained with Wright's and magnified × 960. One metamyelocyte with a distorted nucleus is also shown. Note the clumping of the red corpuscles.

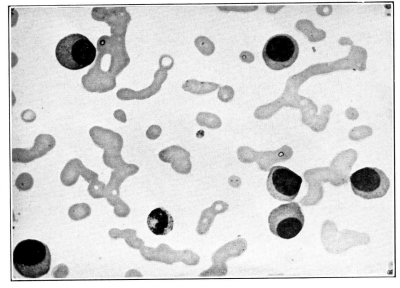

FIG. 20–25.—Photomicrograph showing "myeloma cells" in material obtained by sternal puncture in a case of multiple myeloma. The eccentricity of the nuclei is well shown and the dark, "ground-glass," vacuolated cytoplasm is evident.

PLATE XVIII

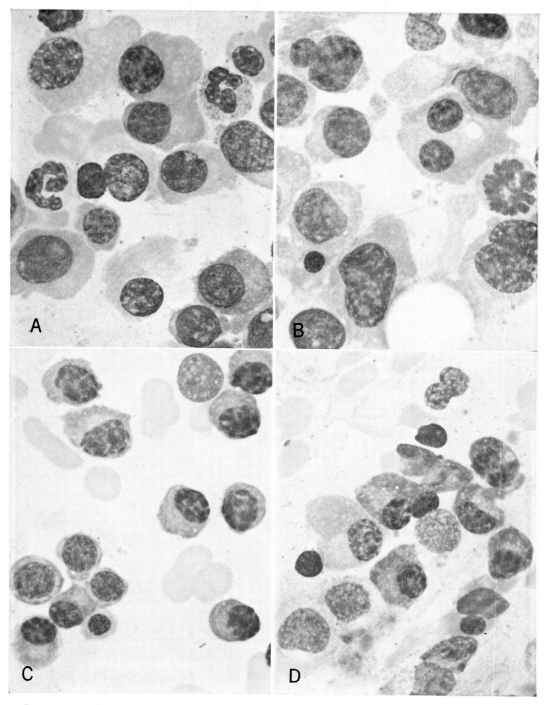

Bone marrow from cases of *multiple myeloma* (*A, B*) contrasted with normal *plasma cells* (*C, D*) (Wright's stain, × 1220). In *C*, lower left, the two plasma cells should be contrasted with the normoblasts lying beside them. *C* is from a patient with agranulocytosis, *D* is from a patient with chronic infection.

as in the plasma cell, nor is the wheel-spoke arrangement of the latter present. The cytoplasm is basophilic and bright blue, not blue-green as in the plasma cell. It may contain a few azure granules and, occasionally, acidophilic inclusions (Russell bodies) or clear globules (Mott bodies) may be observed. A perinuclear clear zone is unusual. The myeloma cell does not take the "specific" plasma cell stains. It is oxidase negative.

The cells seen in different cases range, however, from a very anaplastic, immature form to one closely resembling if not identical with the plasma cell seen normally. Some writers differentiate a mature variety, 7 to 12 μ in diameter, which resembles the typical plasma cell, and a "malignant" variety, a large cell 20 to 30 μ in diameter with a dark blue, somewhat scroll-like cytoplasm and a round or oval nucleus occupying much of the cell and possessing several nucleoli[129] (Plate XVIII).

Still other myeloma cells may be extraordinarily large and may contain two or three nuclei. Azurophilic, crystalloid, rod-like and thromboid inclusions, somewhat resembling Auer bodies, have been observed within myeloma cells in the marrow and in the circulating blood.[181] These inclusions have been found to be protein crystals.

It has not been possible to correlate the morphological characteristics of myeloma cells and the type of abnormal protein (α-, β- or γ-globulin) in the serum.[186]

Protein Abnormalities.—A striking feature of multiple myeloma is the evidence of a disturbance in protein synthesis. This takes three forms: the excretion in the urine of a protein with characteristic physical properties, recognized more than a century ago (Bence-Jones); hyperproteinemia, first noticed by Ellinger in 1899 and studied intensively only many decades later; and a peculiar protein deposition in the tissues, particularly amyloidosis, which Magnus-Levy recognized as a unique feature in 1938.[164]

The **hyperproteinemia** may be of extreme degree, values as high as 18.7 and even 23.3 Gm. per cent having been recorded.[187] In many cases the plasma protein has been greater than 10.0 Gm. per 100 ml. The average value in a series of 91 cases was 8.97 Gm. as compared with 7.23 Gm. in normal individuals.[171] The increase in practically all cases has been due to the globulin fraction and the albumin : globulin ratio has been reversed.

A positive *formol-gel reaction*[133] serves to indicate that hyperglobinemia exists. This test is carried out by adding 2 drops of 40 per cent formalin to 1 ml. of serum If the tube is allowed to stand at room temperature for three hours, a milky gel will be seen when the result is positive. A positive reaction is also found in kala-azar and in certain chronic infections.

Fractionation of serum from patients with multiple myeloma by the Howe method[149] demonstrated that the solubility characteristics of globulin fractions varies considerably from one patient to another. These observations were extended and clarified by the development of the Tiselius electrophoretic technic which permitted separation of the myeloma proteins of the serum into those having the mobilities of α-, β-, and γ-globulins, respectively. In one series of 91 cases, 55 per cent were found to have abnormal components of the general range of γ-globulin mobility, 15.4 per cent showed major peaks of β-globulin mobility and 6.6 per cent manifested abnormal components in the range of α-globulin mobility. An additional 22 per cent showed only minor anomalies which were not distinctive for myeloma.[171] The results of other studies are in essential agreement with these figures except that others have found even fewer examples of the α-globulin anomaly.[150,155a] Still another abnormal component ("M fraction"), which has a mobility intermediate between that of beta and gamma has also been described.[149]

Although hyperproteinemia is encountered in only approximately 50 to 65 per cent of cases,[149] the study of electrophoretic patterns reveals characteristic abnormalities in approximately 75 per cent of cases.[169] The diagnostic patterns in multiple myeloma are characterized by a tall, narrow, sharply defined peak due to the presence of large amounts of a relatively homogeneous abnormal protein. Filter paper electrophoresis also affords a sensitive and specific means for recognition of the plasma protein anomalies and, as compared with the Tiselius method, offers the advantage of simplicity, low cost and speed.[138,169]

Much more rare is the presence of a protein in the plasma which precipitates at temperatures less than 37° C. Such an anomaly was discovered accidentally by the writer in 1933 in a patient with extensive purpura, Raynaud's phenomena and retinal vein thrombosis.[187] The protein was first observed in the hematocrit above the layer of packed red cells where it occupied 10 mm. of the column. The peculiar, yellowish-gray, gelatinous material always precipitated out from the blood, even when it was collected in a warm needle and syringe. Furthermore, when the hematocrit was placed in a refrigerator, an additional cloudy, white material appeared in the supernatant plasma above the gelatinous protein, but this cloudy substance disappeared at room temperature in ten to fifteen minutes. It was this phenomenon which first brought multiple myeloma to mind, a diagnosis which was then promptly confirmed by appropriate examinations.

A similar observation was not made until fourteen years later, when the term **"cryoglobulin"** was proposed for the cold-precipitable protein of the serum.[160] Cryoglobulins in large quantities are encountered almost exclusively in multiple myeloma but in smaller amounts they have been found in cases of chronic lymphocytic leukemia, lymphosarcoma, kala-azar, lupus erythematosus, rheumatoid arthritis, polyarteritis nodosa, Sjögren's syndrome, subacute bacterial endocarditis, coronary artery disease, polycythemia vera, portal cirrhosis and malignant tumors.[143a,163]

Rarely the abnormal myeloma globulin is found to exhibit the opposite type of thermolability to that of the cryoglobulins; namely, precipitation when serum is heated to 56° C. ("*pyroglobulinemia*").[135a,164a] The protein responsible is not identical with Bence-Jones protein and, unlike cryoglobulinemia, the reaction is not reversible.

In approximately 40[159] to 47[129] per cent of cases of multiple myeloma *Bence-Jones protein* can be demonstrated in the urine by the simple heat test, and in 61 per cent by paper electrophoresis.[168a]

When the urine is heated, a white cloudy precipitate appears at temperatures of 50° to 60° C., sometimes even at 45°. On further heating, this precipitate goes into solution at about boiling and reappears on cooling. If the precipitate does not clear on boiling, the addition of a few drops of 5 per cent acetic acid usually will dissolve the turbidity. If the common form of proteinuria is present, the protein should be coagulated and filtered off at boiling. Following this the test for Bence-Jones protein can be made. It is helpful to heat the urine in a water bath slowly, raising the temperature from 40° C. to 100° in the course of fifteen to twenty minutes. If Bence-Jones protein is present, cloudiness will appear at a temperature of 45° to 65° C. and will disappear on boiling and reappear on cooling to between 85° and 65° C.[129] It has been pointed out that care in the examination of the urine, especially care to avoid confusion with other forms of proteinuria and to insure appropriate dilution of the specimen, will yield a high percentage of positive results.[175,179a] A sensitive salting-out test has been described[141a] and a simple serological method was devised for the detection of Bence-Jones protein in urine,[137] but especially helpful is simultaneous filter paper electrophoresis of serum and urine. In the urine, Bence-Jones proteins appear as sharply defined homogeneous bands between the ranges of the α- and γ-globulins.[189] In starch gel they were found to consist of several fractions.[145b]

Very rarely Bence-Jones protein has been found in disorders other than multiple myeloma: leukemia, both myelocytic and lymphocytic, polycythemia vera, metastatic carcinoma in bone, senile osteomalacia, multiple fractures in bones, and inactive tuberculosis.[134] In multiple myeloma, Bence-Jones protein may be found in the urine when the serum is normal.[182] This has been observed in 18 per cent of cases.[169]

Atypical amyloidosis or **paramyloidosis** has been observed upon histologic examination in 6 to 10 per cent of cases of multiple myeloma.[162] Its distribution is that of primary amyloidosis; namely, in the mesenchymal tissues of the gastrointestinal tract, subcutis, subendocardium and subendothelial areas of blood vessels. It has also been found within myeloma cells.[184] Unlike the substance found in amyloidosis secondary to chronic infectious and wasting diseases, the protein stains poorly with metachromatic dyes.

Other Chemical Changes in the Blood.—**Hypercalcemia** has been observed in 20[134] to 53[129] per cent of cases. Values of 12 to 16 mg. per 100 ml. are not unusual and higher levels have been recorded.[136] With progression of the disease, the hypercalcemia may increase. The high serum calcium levels have been attributed to the resorption of bone which takes place in multiple myeloma but they are further increased by secondary hyperplasia of the parathyroids caused by renal impairment.[162] As a rule the hypercal-

cemia is not accompanied by a decrease in the inorganic serum phosphorus and the serum alkaline phosphatase is normal,[166] thus differing from the changes found in primary hyperparathyroidism.[149] However, exceptions have been reported[129,136,180] and confusion with primary hyperparathyroidism is not uncommon.[166a]

The serum **uric acid** is not infrequently increased (4.5 to even 31.1 mg. per 100 ml.).[136,182] **Nitrogen retention** also has been noted in a number of cases and can be ascribed to the renal damage associated with the deposits of Bence-Jones protein. This occurs not only in the distal tubules but in the entire nephron up to the proximal convoluted tubules.[136] In no other renal disease are such large extensive casts formed. They are characteristically lamellated and large multinucleated foreign body giant cells surround them. Eosinophilic globular material may be found in the epithelial cells of the convoluted tubules. The resulting distension and obstruction to renal flow lead to glomerular atrophy and ultimate renal failure.[145] In association with the *"myeloma kidney"* an "atypical nephritis" thus develops which is not usually associated with hypertension or edema. The **urine** may contain albumin, casts and renal epithelial cells but it is unusual to find red cells.[164] There is impairment in the concentrating function of the kidneys and dye excretion is lowered. It has been stated[131] that glomerular dysfunction may sometimes be more severe than the failure in tubular excretory capacity, but this has been disputed.[129] In two instances signs of the adult form of the Fanconi syndrome, with amino-aciduria and other typical changes, were observed in association with multiple myeloma.[141b]

Lower than normal values for β_1- and α_1-serum lipoproteins and for serum cholesterol concentrations have been reported.[162]

Diagnosis.—The clinical manifestations of multiple myeloma are so varied and the disorder is so uncommon that the initial diagnosis is often incorrect. Lumbago, Pott's or Paget's disease, nephritis, pleurisy, pernicious anemia, tabes dorsalis, and visceral carcinoma are only a few of the erroneous diagnoses which have been made. When extra-osseous tumors exist (p. 1067) still other conditions are simulated. The following signs are of cardinal diagnostic importance, for taken in pairs, triads, or collectively as a group, these symptoms are strongly suggestive of multiple myeloma: (1) multiple involvement of the skeletal trunk of an adult, (2) pathological fracture of a rib, (3) the excretion of Bence-Jones protein, (4) characteristic backache with signs of early paraplegia (beginning loss of sexual potentia, difficulty in starting urination, or loss of power in the legs), (5) an otherwise inexplicable anemia and (6) chronic nephritis with nitrogen retention and low blood pressure and usually unaccompanied by marked edema, hypertension or retinitis.[146] Unlike many other bone diseases, the extremities alone are never affected in multiple myeloma and bowing of the extremities does not occur. Unlike metastatic carcinoma, more than one vertebra is usually involved. To these criteria may be added (7) hyperproteinemia. The last is a very helpful sign since **hyperglobulinemia,** to which it is usually due, is found in a limited number of conditions many of which are readily differentiated from multiple myeloma: lymphogranuloma venereum, sarcoid, systemic lupus, kala-azar, leprosy, subacute bacterial endocarditis, cirrhosis, leukemia, chronic nephritis, tuberculous lymphadenitis and a few miscellaneous infections. Only in the first four or five of these, furthermore, are marked increases like those seen in multiple myeloma usually encountered.

Sternal puncture is usually of great assistance in diagnosis. In a number of instances[172] this procedure has clarified an otherwise obscure clinical picture. In some instances, however, several punctures, sometimes at different sites, have had to be made before the characteristic myeloma cells were found. It should also be added that *the finding of plasma cells in the bone marrow in excessive numbers* is not of itself evidence of the presence of multiple myeloma; increased numbers have been observed in rheumatoid arthritis,[155] acute rheumatic fever,[147] in various "collagen disorders" and hypersensitivity reactions,[136b] in hepatic cirrhosis and in Hodgkin's disease.[135,143] Morphologic differences (p. 1069) between the myeloma cell and the plasma cell observed in the latter conditions are sometimes helpful in recognizing multiple myeloma. In particular, it has been pointed out that the ratio of nucleolus to nucleus is greater in the myeloma cell than in the plasma cell.[130a]

Paper electrophoresis of serum and urine now provides a means for the ready detection of the characteristic protein abnormalities of multiple myeloma. When both serum and urine were examined, a significant abnormality could be demonstrated in 97 per cent of cases of multiple myeloma.[169] Now it is rarely, if ever, necessary to resort to biopsy in making a diagnosis of multiple myeloma, although this is still needed to identify the solitary tumor. However, new syndromes have been uncovered by the use of modern methods for the study of the serum proteins. Idiopathic macroglobulinemia in many ways resembles multiple myeloma and must be differentiated (p. 1078).

Prognosis and Treatment.—The prognosis is uniformly unfavorable when there are multiple lesions, the duration being one and a half to two years after the date of recognition or less.[129,134,146] The median duration of survival from the time of diagnosis in a series of 238 residents of Brooklyn, New York, was only 3.5 months, although 16 per cent of the patients survived longer than 18 months and 8 per cent for three years.[144a] The median duration of symptoms in these cases prior to diagnosis was five months. Nevertheless, sometimes the course may be very prolonged,[136,164] even 11 years and longer,[153] and may be characterized by remissions and exacerbations. Weakness, pain and incapacity eventually progress, and in the end failure sets in with cachexia, anemia, flaccid paralysis, or renal impairment with nitrogen retention. Decubitus ulcers, secondary infections, ascending urinary infection, hemorrhages, or agonizing pains, mark the terminal course until one of these or some other complication leads to death. Prognosis is better in cases with an apparently solitary bone lesion but, after several years, sometimes after eight or ten years and often sooner, dissemination occurs.[136] It should be noted that prognosis is not necessarily bad in cases in which very large quantities of myeloma protein are found in the plasma or in those in which the lesions are widespread. Of more significance are the vigor of the malignant process, the extent to which the kidneys are being damaged, the altered viscosity of the blood, and the development of complications such as infection and hemorrhage.

Nursing care to avoid unnecessary pain and pathological fractures, and the usual treatment of the latter when they occur, as well as supportive measures, are obvious therapeutic procedures. If there is a single bone lesion, local **irradiation** is often helpful and may be strikingly so. Excision is sometimes feasible. When there has been compression of the spinal cord, laminectomy and decompression may sometimes be helpful,[134] though rarely.[130] The effects of irradiation on multiple myeloma are rather unpredictable but even in cases of widespread disease relief of pain and healing of pathologic fractures have been reported.[136] Some relief of pain may also be associated with the use of radioactive phosphorus but, as a whole, this agent has not been found very useful.[54a] Radioactive iodine and radioactive iodinated serum albumin have also been employed in the treatment of multiple myeloma with palliative benefit in some cases.[157]

Urethane (p. 974) is perhaps the best therapeutic agent for multiple myeloma which is currently available but even its value is limited. Subjective improvement is associated with its administration in less than half the cases and objective improvement has been observed in about a fifth.[162a] Increase in hemoglobin concentration and decrease in erythrocyte sedimentation rate are the most commonly encountered objective signs of improvement. In some instances reduction in the number of myeloma cells in the bone marrow and decrease in the concentration of serum proteins as well as in Bence-Jones proteinuria have been reported.[173] This, however, is unusual.[162a] No changes take place in the destructive lesions. The drug may be given orally as a 10 per cent aqueous solution flavored with syrup, or in suppository form. Enteric-coated tablets are unsatisfactory because of irregular absorption. The usual daily dose is 2 to 4 grams, given in 3 or 4 divided amounts. It has also been given intravenously in the same amounts over the course of eight to ten hours by adding the medication, prepared in sterile saline, to 1000 ml. physiological saline or 5 per cent dextrose. Relief of pain may occur within a week of institution of therapy but objective signs of remission are usually not evident until the fourth or fifth week. Leukopenia develops but moderate degrees of leukopenia, such as 2500 cells per c.mm., do not necessarily demand interruption of therapy. However, because of the frequency of unpleasant gastrointestinal side effects, such as nausea and vomiting, and the hazard of hepatic toxicity,[186a] some consider it desirable to discontinue urethane therapy after four to six weeks.[168a] Others continue treatment for seven to ten weeks, if possible.[173] Remissions may last a few months or even several years. Treatment is reinstituted when signs of relapse appear.

ACTH and, particularly, prednisone or similar **corticosteroids** have been found by some investigators to relieve bone pain and cause a rise in hemoglobin and volume of packed red cells[130] as well as a decrease in the hypercalcemia.[166b] Consequently they favor such therapy in preference to urethane. In a given case it is likely to be found that each of these agents will be given a trial as neither will be very effective, as a rule.

Other chemotherapeutic agents, such as those used in the treatment of various forms of leukemia and the various lymph node disorders have not been found effective in multiple myeloma. *Stilbamidine* enjoyed a brief period of popularity[179,180] but has been abandoned because of its serious toxic effects, such as trigeminal neuralgia and a detrimental effect on the already damaged kidneys.

The development of hypercalcemia, with its attendant symptoms, such as anorexia, nausea, vomiting, apathy, polydipsia, polyuria and other signs, is best treated by assuring a high fluid intake, but sometimes additional measures, such as the administration of sodium citrate and chelating agents may be required.[130]

Pathology.—The tumor cuts readily with the knife, for the bone shell is extremely thin. The cortex of the bone may be entirely resorbed and the spongiosa rarefied. Rarely the tumor is extraskeletal, the cells infiltrating about the periosteum.[146] A dark red or gray-red mass of gelatinous substance makes up the tumor, which often bleeds freely. Microscopically, it is composed of round or oval cells, about 9 to 11 μ in diameter, with an eccentrically placed nucleus often containing 1 to 3 nucleoli. In stained sections a spoke-like arrangement of the

nuclear chromatin may be seen. The appearance of these cells in smears of bone marrow has been described already (p. 1069). In addition to these "plasma" or myeloma cells, fat cells, giant cells and eosinophils are found, especially at the outskirts of the tumor. The myeloma tissue is rich in blood vessels and there is often profuse hemorrhage into the tumor. This may account for the pulsation sometimes seen in the tumors and absorption of blood may account for spontaneous regression in the size of the tumor mass.

The distribution of the lesions in the bones has been described (p. 1066) and extraosseous involvement as well as extramedullary plasma cell tumors have also been discussed (p. 1067). The "myeloma kidney" and the occurrence of paramyloidosis have been considered (p. 1073).

Pathogenesis.—As stated earlier, the cause of multiple myeloma is unknown. The manifestations of the disease appear to be related to the growth of the myeloma cell, a structure which greatly resembles or perhaps is a variant of the normal plasma cell. It seems likely that multiple myeloma and "plasma cell leukemia" are closely allied disorders and that both are fundamentally akin to leukemia.

As judged by ultraviolet microscopy and spectrophotometric analyses, the myeloma cell, like the plasma cell, is an intensely protein-producing cell. As the plasma cell differentiates from its reticulum-cell precursor, ribonucleic acid accumulates in the cytoplasm.[168] Electron microscope studies of plasma cells show the cytoplasmic ribonucleoprotein to be distributed in the form of granules in association with the cytoplasmic reticulum;[183a] this is thought to be the specific locus of protein synthesis. By means of the fluorescent antibody technic it has been shown that myeloma cells contain cytoplasmic concentrations of gamma globulin.[185] Protein with ultracentrifugal and electrophoretic properties similar to those of the abnormal components present in the plasma has been extracted from myeloma tumor tissue.[165] It is uncertain whether the protein is released from intact cells or whether cellular degeneration is invariably required.

Proteins isolated from the serum of different cases of multiple myeloma usually have had molecular weights of 160,000 or greater. The possibility has been considered that the abnormality of myeloma proteins consists only in the fact that there is produced an abundance of a highly homogeneous representative which is otherwise present only in small proportion in the family of normal globulins.[170,177] However, in immunological studies, myeloma proteins of various electrophoretic mobilities appear to be related to one another but are not identical. Immunologically even myeloma proteins of γ-globulin mobility often differ significantly from the γ-globulin of normal serum. The nature of the cross reactions has suggested that the multiple myeloma globulins lack antigenic determinants that are present in the γ-globulins of human fraction II.[156] The carbohydrate content of myeloma proteins is considerably higher than that of the γ-globulin of normal serum.[169,174]

Likewise investigation of amino acid composition, of N-terminal groups and of the peptides derived by tryptic hydrolysis has provided evidence for the hypothesis that the tumor produces a new type of globulin that differs structurally from normal gamma globulin.[169b] Although large segments of the polypeptide structure of normal gamma globulin and the myeloma proteins are identical, interchanges of amino acids may occur in the N-terminal position and in various other loci characteristic of the protein of the individual patient.

Bence-Jones protein is, like the myeloma serum proteins, not a single substance.[187] The term actually designates a group of substances.[135b,170] Molecula weights of about 37,000 have been calculated from ultracentrifuge and diffusion experiments.[149] The electrophoretic mobility of the Bence-Jones proteins has been observed to range from 0.8 to 3.8; that is, between the speeds of α_2-globulin and γ-golublin.[180] Contrary to an earlier view, Bence-Jones proteins are not derived by renal cleavage of the myeloma globulins but, in fact, may be their precursors.[169b] The interesting suggestion has been made that Bence-Jones proteins are constituent proteins of a virus causing multiple myeloma.[141]

A number of the manifestations of multiple myeloma, other than the bone tumors themselves, may be ascribed to the hyperproteinemia and the extreme viscosity of the blood; for example, the autohemagglutination, excessive rouleau formation, extremely rapid sedimentation rate of the blood, and the intravascular thrombosis.[187]

It is thought that the "myeloma kidney" is the consequence of damage to the renal tubules by the Bence-Jones proteins. These proteins have been demonstrated within the tubular epithelium and their presence is thought to impair grossly the function of the tubules and ultimately lead to cellular atrophy and degeneration. At the same time, large obstructing casts are found along the entire length of the renal tubule and the whole nephron ultimately becomes nonfunctional.[168a]

The paramyloidosis has been attributed to the production of proteins of such low molecular weight that they are capable of diffusing through the capillary beds of many, if not all, tissues. In those tissues in which these proteins find complementary polysaccharides which they can bind, insoluble complexes are formed and the proteins remain.[168a] Some of the hemorrhagic manifestations of multiple myeloma have been attributed to protein-protein complexing between the abnormal globulins and one or more of the proteins concerned in the coagulation process.

MACROGLOBULINEMIA

The general use of paper electrophoretic analysis of serum and the utilization of the ultracentrifuge in the study of certain clinical problems, like the earlier introduction of the Tiselius electrophoretic technic, has revealed the existence of syndromes which had not been clearly distinguished before and has led to a series of investigations which will undoubtedly greatly clarify our understanding of disease processes. The syndrome of macroglobulinemia first described by Waldenström in 1944[216] in many ways resembles multiple myeloma and to some extent has features suggestive of chronic lymphocytic leukemia and lymphosarcoma. It is to be distinguished from purpura hyperglobulinemica (p. 846), a syndrome to which Waldenström's name is also attached but is unassociated with discrete components demonstrable by electrophoresis or in the ultracentrifuge.

Definition and Classification.[163,213] —Macroglobulins are carbohydrate and lipid-containing proteins (glycolipoproteins) of exceptionally high molecular weight (1,000,000 or higher) which, in the ultracentrifugal field, have a sedimentation constant above 15 Svedberg (S) units, usually 19 or 20. Trace amounts (2 to 5 per cent) of a protein of high molecular weight are present in normal sera. The Wassermann antibody, the red cell iso-agglutinins, properdin and the rheumatoid factor are macroglobulins.[208] Electrophoretically the normal macroglobulins are found in the α fraction. Pathological macroglobulins move with any one of the several globulin fractions. Their concentration varies and may change in the same patient from time to time.

As already stated, macroglobulins may be found normally ("physiological macroglobulinemia"), they may be observed in association with certain disorders ("secondary macroglobulinemia") and they characterize the syndrome described by Waldenström ("primary", "essential" or "idiopathic" macroglobulinemia).

Symptomatology of Waldenström's Macroglobulinemia.[204,208,213] —This is a relatively rare, chronic disorder observed more particularly in men over the age of 50, which is characterized by vague complaints such as lassitude, weakness and weight loss; disturbances of vision and bizarre neurologic manifestations (radiculitis, myelitis, encephalitis);[207a] Raynaud's phenomena and cold sensitivity; modest lymphadenopathy, hepato- and splenomegaly; anemia and a hemorrhagic diathesis; a tendency to frequent infections; excessively high sedimentation rate, hyperproteinemia and, sometimes, Bence-Jones proteinuria and/or cryoglobulinemia; and the presence of lymphocytes in excessive numbers in the bone marrow.

In contrast to multiple myeloma, which this disorder closely resembles, bone pain is not a prominent symptom and, instead of punched-out bone lesions, diffuse osteoporosis is seen. Renal manifestations are unusual. The anemia is generally normocytic and unremarkable but hemolytic anemia, with or without a positive direct Coombs' test, has been described. As a rule, the leukocyte count is normal but in some cases neutropenia or pancytopenia has been reported and, in other cases, thrombocytopenia has been observed. Bleeding may be massive, from the nose, mouth, stomach or lower gastro-intestinal tract but purpura is unusual. The *bone marrow* contains many lymphoid cells more closely resembling lymphocytes than plasma or myeloma cells. They are characteristically small and often possess little cytoplasm. When the latter is more abundant, it may be very basophilic or it may contain abundant polysaccharide, as manifested by a positive periodic acid-Schiff staining reaction. The PAS-staining material sometimes takes the form of globules ("grape cells"). Occasionally one or two nucleoli are seen in the nucleus of the cells. Basophils or mast cells may be somewhat increased in number, and in this connection it is of interest that the macroglobulin may be specifically precipitable by heparin.[210] In some cases eosinophilia has been reported.

As in other hyperglobulinemic states, the Sia or water-test,[213] or the formol-gel test (p. 1071) will be found positive and the viscosity of the serum is increased. On paper electrophoresis, a symmetrical gradient with a narrow, sharp and high peak in the globulin fraction will be found, most often in the γ-position. However, in macroglobulinemia serums of β mobility, the Sia test was found to be negative.[207] The ultracentrifuge is the ultimate criterion for the identification of macroglobulinemia. In multiple myeloma, S-values like those of normal globulins are found, usually 7 or less, whereas in macroglobulinemia S values of 15 or higher are characteristic.

Secondary Macroglobulinemia. — A diagnosis of primary macroglobulinemia requires exclusion of the various disorders in which macroglobulinemia has sometimes been observed;[213] namely: (1) neoplastic diseases: multiple myeloma, extramedullary plasmacytoma, reticuloses, cancer of the uterus, bronchi, skin, larynx, biliary tract, prostate; (2) collagen disorders: polyarteritis nodosa, lupus erythematosus, rheumatoid arthritis, Felty's syndrome, Sjögren's syndrome; (3) chronic infections: chronic hepatitis, kala-azar, toxoplasmosis, congenital syphilis; (4) miscellaneous conditions: liver cirrhosis, amyloidosis.

Prognosis and Course.—The average life expectancy of the idiopathic disorder is 38 to 40 months from the time of the first complaints.[204] However, this figure is somewhat misleading since the process in some patients appears to be quite malignant, resulting in a shorter survival time, whereas in others it is comparatively benign (ten years). In the secondary form, the prognosis is that of the underlying disease. It should be added, also, that many "atypical" cases have been described[203] in which, for example, the manifestations simulated more closely those of multiple myeloma or of lymphocytic leukemia than those described above. Thus cases with a leukemic blood picture have been described.[208] Again, in about 8 per cent of the reported cases,[204] carcinomatous lesions were observed; it is difficult in some instances to be certain whether the neoplastic diseases were the cause of the macroglobulinemia or merely present coincidentally. Finally, three cases were described in which all the features of the primary syndrome were present except the macroglobulinemia.[205]

Death is usually due to anemia, hemorrhagic manifestations, failure to combat infections, and complications due to cold sensitivity and increased plasma viscosity, including precipitation of protein in the lymph spaces of the nervous system and ensuing "coma paraproteinemicum."

Treatment.—There is no clear evidence that adrenocorticosteroids, alkylating agents, stilbamidine, irradiation or splenectomy are of value. However, benefit from chlorambucil therapy has been reported.[199] Treatment with penicillamine was tried because the sulfhydryl concentration in the serum of two patients was observed to be low and the macroglobulin did not contain any free sulfhydryl radicals. This led to attempts to depolymerize the macroglobulins by the oral administration of the low molecular weight mercaptan. A decrease in the total protein and gamma globulin concentrations was observed which was associated with clinical improvement.[200] Intensive plasmapheresis has also been reported as beneficial.[215]

Pathology.[202,208]—Proliferation of cell

components of the lymphoid system results in enlargement of the spleen and lymph nodes, and dense infiltrations in the periportal zones of the liver, in the kidney and throughout other viscera. In the bone marrow the infiltrations are rarely in clumps or aggregates. The appearance of the cells has been described already (p. 1078).

Etiology and Pathogenesis.—The underlying pathological process appears to be a proliferation of those elements of the mesenchymal tissue responsible for the synthesis of immune globulins. The picture is that of reticuloendothelial hyperplasia or neoplasia. It has been suggested that the macroglobulins are the products of clones of genetically identical cells within the antibody-producing system, such clones arising through a mutation process which ultimately assumes frankly neoplastic properties, although occasionally macroglobulinemia is the sole evidence of the existence of the aberrant clone.[208] The secondary forms may be caused by benign, reversible alterations in the activities of the reticuloendothelial system. It is noteworthy that a condition similar in many respects to Waldenström's syndrome has been observed in a transplantable mouse leukemia.[201]

As in the case of multiple myeloma, there is some uncertainty concerning the identity of the macroglobulins encountered in the clinical disorder and in normal serum components. The weight of evidence, however, suggests that they are truly abnormal proteins, antigenically different from normal gamma globulins.[169b,206]

The manifestations of macroglobulinemia are readily attributable to the presence in the plasma of large quantities of the high molecular weight proteins with consequent alterations in blood viscosity, the formation of protein-protein complexes which interfere with normal physiological processes, the deposition of protein in a manner which interferes with circulation, and perhaps also competition with normal mechanisms, such as those concerned with antibody production. Thus, coating of platelets by macroglobulins may interfere with release of platelet factor 3, resulting in poor prothrombin consumption time accompanied by very little residual prothrombin in the serum.[211] It has been postulated that even leukocyte and red cell function may be impaired as the result of coating with macroglobulin.

Hypogammaglobulinemia Associated with Hematological Abnormalities.[225]

Unusual susceptibility to infections has been noted in patients with certain hematological disorders; namely, chronic lymphocytic leukemia (954), lymphosarcoma (p. 1032), the terminal stages of Hodgkin's disease (p. 1032), multiple myeloma (p. 1075) and idiopathic macroglobulinemia (p. 1079). It has been postulated that in these conditions the growth of the neoplastic process interferes in some manner with the normal mechanisms for antibody production. In a few instances of chronic lymphocytic leukemia, agammaglobulinemia has been reported.[221]

In addition to these more or less well defined conditions, cases of hypogammaglobulinemia have been described in which no underlying disease was recognized and in which splenomegaly, lymphadenopathy, hemolytic anemia and neutropenia were also present, in various combinations.[219,224] Histologically there was evidence of diffuse reticuloendothelial hyperplasia and, in some cases, a virtual absence of plasma cells. Splenectomy was associated with marked hematological improvement.

In all of these cases the disorder seems to have been acquired. In congenital agammaglobulinemia splenomegaly, if it occurs at all, is unusual but leukopenia and also hemolytic anemia and lympho-penia have been observed.[220] The con-genital condition is thought to be due to hereditary transmission of a sex-linked recessive gene.

Splenomegaly and leukopenia, asso-ciated with hypogammaglobulinemia, characterize a unique family in which the father and half his children were af-fected.[222] Here a hereditary disorder seemed to be present which was trans-mitted as an autosomal dominant gene.

In these various cases of hypo- and agammaglobulinemia the splenomegaly and the various hematological manifesta-tions have been thought to be the conse-quence of reticulum cell hyperplasia caused by the lack of gamma globulin and the resulting repeated infections. Clearly further study is needed.

BIBLIOGRAPHY

Conditions Chiefly Affecting Lymph Nodes

1. Adair, F. E. and Herrmann, J. B.: Primary Lymphosarcoma of the Breast, Surgery, *16*, 836, 1944.
1a. Allen, D. H., Berg, O. C. and Rosenblatt, W.: Lymphosarcoma of the Kidney, Radi-ology, *55*, 731, 1950.
1b. Anday, G. J. and Schmitz, H. L.: Follicular Lymphoma with Transient Leukemic Phase, Arch. Int. Med., *89*, 621, 1952; *ibid.*, *97*, 631, 1956.
1c. Arends, T., Coonrad, C. V. and Rundles, R. W.: Serum Proteins in Hodgkin's Dis-ease and Malignant Lymphoma, Am. J. Med., *16*, 833, 1954.
1d. Armas-Cruz, R. *et al.*: Clinical Diagnosis of Systemic Lupus Erythematosus, Am. J. Med., *25*, 409, 1958.
2. Baker, C. and Mann, W. N.: Hodgkin's Disease, Guy's Hosp. Rep., *89*, 83, 1939.
3. Baggenstoss, A. H. and Heck, F. J.: Folli-cular Lymphoblastoma (Giant Lymph Follicle Hyperplasia of Lymph Nodes and Spleen), Am. J. M. Sc., *200*, 17, 1940.
3a. Barlow, A. M., Leeming, J. T. and Wilkin-son, J. F.: Mannomustine in Treatment of Leukaemias, Polycythaemia, and Malig-nant Disorders, Brit. M. J., *2*, 208, 1959.
4. Barney, J. D., Hunter, F. T. and Mintz, E. R.: The Urological Aspects of Radio-

sensitive Tumors of the Blood-forming Organs, Trans. Am. Assn. Genito-Urin. Surg., *24*, 413, 1931.
4a. Bässler, R.: Leberveränderungen bei Mor-bus Brill-Symmers, Arch. path. Anat., *332*, 335, 1959.
4b. Berman, L.: Malignant Lymphomas, Blood, *8*, 195, 1953.
4c. Berman, L., Klein, A. A., Linn, H. J. and Bates, G. S.: Hypersplenism Associated With Follicular Lymphoblastoma, Blood, *5*, 286, 1950.
5. Bichel, J.: Coincidence of Hodgkin's Disease and Myelomatosis, Acta med. scandinav., *157*, 399, 1957.
5a. Bierman, H. R., Shimkin, M. B., Mettier, S. R., Weaver, J., Berry, W. C. and Wise, S. P., III.: Methyl-bis (Beta-Chloroethyl) amine in Large Doses in the Treatment of Neoplastic Diseases, Cali-fornia Med., *71*, 1, 1949.
6. Bingham, C. T. and Quarrier, S. S.: Re-ticulum Cell Sarcoma, Arch. Dermat., *41*, 722, 1940.
6a. Bluefarb, S. M. and Webster, J. R.: Kaposi's Sarcoma Associated with Lym-phosarcoma, Arch. Int. Med., *91*, 97, 1953.
6b. Bostick, W. L. and Hanna, L.: Experi-mental Studies on the Etiology of Hodg-kin's Disease, Cancer Research, *11*, 505, 1051; Fed. Proc., *13*, 424, 1954; Cancer Res., *15*, 650, 1955.
8. Brill, N. E., Baehr, G. and Rosenthal, N.: Generalized Giant Lymph Follicle Hyper-plasia of Lymph Nodes and Spleen, J.A.M.A., *84*, 668, 1925; Trans. A. Am. Physicians, *47*, 330, 1932.
8a. Brody, J. I. and Finch, S. C.: Candida-Reacting Antibody in the Serum of Pa-tients with Lymphomas and Related Dis-orders, Blood, *15*, 830, 1960.
9. Bruschi, M. and Howe, J. S.: Classification of the Hematologic Variations and Ab-normalities Associated with Boeck's Sar-coid, Blood, *5*, 478, 1950.
10. Bunting, C. H.: The Blood Picture in Hodg-kin's Disease, Bull. Johns Hopkins Hosp., *25*, 173, 1914.
10a. Bunting, C. H. and Yates, J. L.: Cultural Results in Hodgkin's Disease, Arch. Int. Med., *12*, 236, 1913.
10b. Burnett, H. W. and Herbert, E. A.: The Role of Irradiation in the Treatment of Primary Malignant Lymphoma of the Stomach, Radiology, *67*, 723, 1956.
11. Coggins, P. R., Ravdin, R. G. and Eisman, S. H.: Clinical Evaluation of a New Alkyl-

ating Agent: Cytoxan (Cyclophosphamide), Cancer, *13*, 1254, 1960.

11a. COHEN, B. B., KAPLAN, G., LIBER, A. F. and ROSWIT, B.: Reticulum-cell Sarcoma with Primary Manifestation in the Testis, Cancer, *8*, 136, 1955.

11b. COLES, W. C. and SCHULZ, M. D.: Bone Involvement in Malignant Lymphoma, Radiology, *50*, 458, 1948.

11c. CONRAD, M. E., JR. and CROSBY, W. H.: Massive Nitrogen Mustard Therapy in Hodgkin's Disease with Protection of Bone Marrow by Tourniquets, Blood, *16*, 1089, 1960.

11d. COOK, J. C., KRABBENHOFT, K. L. and LEUCUTIA, T.: Combined Radiation and Nitrogen Mustard Therapy in Hodgkin's Disease As Compared with Radiation Therapy Alone, Am. J. Roentgenol., *82*, 651, 1959.

11e. COOLEY, J. C., McDONALD, J. R. and CLAGETT, O. T.: Primary Lymphoma of the Lung, Ann. Surg., *143*, 18, 1956.

11f. COOPER, T. and WATKINS, C. H.: An Evaluation of Sternal Aspiration as an Aid in Diagnosis of the Malignant Lymphomata, Blood, *4*, 534, 1949.

11g. CRAVER, L. F.: Some Aspects of the Treatment of Hodgkin's Disease, Cancer, *7*, 927, 1954.

12. CUSTER, R. P. and BERNHARD, W. G.: The Interrelationship of Hodgkin's Disease and Other Lymphatic Tumors, Am. J. M. Sc., *216*, 625, 1948.

12a. DEEB, P. H. and STILSON, W. L.: Roentgenologic Manifestations of Lymphosarcoma of the Small Bowel, Radiology, *63*, 235, 1954.

13. DIAMOND, H. D., CRAVER, L. F. and WOODARD, HELEN Q.: Radioactive Phosphorus, Cancer, *10*, 143, 1957.

13a. DOUGLAS, D. M. and CLAIREAUX, A. E.: Hodgkin's Disease in Childhood, Arch. Dis. Childhood, *28*, 222, 1953.

14. DRESSER, R. and SPENCER, J.: Hodgkin's Disease and Allied Conditions of Bone, Am. J. Roentgenol., *36*, 809, 1936.

14a. DuROY, R. M. and SAWYER, K. C.: Lymphosarcoma of the Breast, Am. Surgeon, *25*, 489, 1959.

15. EBSTEIN, W.: Das chronische Rückfallsfieber, eine neue Infektionskrankheit, Berl. klin. Wchnschr., *24*, 565, 837, 1887.

15a. EDWARDS, M. H., WAGNER, J. A. and KRAUSE, L. A. M.: Sarcoidosis with Thrombocytopenia, Ann. Int. Med., *37*, 803, 1952.

16a. ENDE, N., PIZZOLATO, P. and ZISKIND, J.:

Hodgkin's Disease Associated with Histoplasmosis, Cancer, *5*, 763, 1952.

17. EPSTEIN, E. and MacEACHERN, K.: Dermatologic Manifestations of the Lymphoblastoma-leukemia Group, Arch. Int. Med., *60*, 867, 1937.

18. L'ESPERANCE, E. S.: Experimental Inoculation of Chicken With Hodgkin's Nodes, J. Immunol., *16*, 37, 1929; *ibid.*, *18*, 127, 1930.

18a. EVANS, B. H. and HAIGHT, C.: Surgical Removal of Unsuspected Mediastinal Lymphoblastomas, Arch. Surg., *57*, 307, 1948.

18c. FALCONER, E. H. and LEONARD, M. E.: Skeletal Lesions in Hodgkin's Disease, Ann. Int. Med., *29*, 1115, 1948.

19. FAULKNER, J. W. and DOCKERTY, M. B., Lymphosarcoma of the Small Intestine: Surg., Gynec. & Obst., *95*, 76, 1952.

19a. FELDAKER, M., KIERLAND, R. R. and MONTGOMERY, H.: Cutaneous Lymphoblastoma, Arch. Dermat., *70*, 583, 1954.

19b. FINKBEINER, J. A., CRAVER, L. F. and DIAMOND, H. D.: Prognostic Signs in Hodgkin's Disease, J.A.M.A., *156*, 472, 1954.

19c. FLEISCHNER, F. G., BERNSTEIN, C. and LEVINE, B. E.: Retrosternal Infiltration in Malignant Lymphoma, Radiology, *51*, 350, 1948.

19d. FORBUS, W. D. and GUNTER, J. U.: The Pathogenicity of Strains of Brucella, Obtained From Cases of Hodgkin's Disease, South. M. J., *34*, 376, 1941; Am. J. Path., *18*, 745, 1942; *ibid.*, *22*, 35, 1946.

19e. FRAJOLA, W. J., GREIDER, M. H. and BOURONCLE, B. A.: Nature of Virus-like Structures in Red Cells of Patients with Hodgkin's Disease, Proc. Soc. Exper. Biol. & Med., *88*, 507, 1955.

19f. FRANCIS, K. C., HIGINBOTHAM, N. L. and COLEY, B. L.: Primary Reticulum Cell Sarcoma of Bone, Surg., Gynec. & Obst., *99*, 142, 1954.

19g. FRENKEL, RHODA S.: The History of Hodgkin's Disease, U. Michigan Med. Bull., *25*, 390, 1959.

19h. FRIEDMAN, A. I.: Primary Lymphosarcoma of the Stomach, Am. J. Med., *26*, 783, 1959.

19i. GALL, E. A.: The Surgical Treatment of Malignant Lymphoma, Ann. Surg. *118*, 1064, 1943.

20. GALL, E. A. and MALLORY, T. B.: Malignant Lymphoma, Am. J. Path., *18*, 381, 1942.

20a. GALL, E. A., MORRISON, H. R. and SCOTT, A. T.: The Follicular Type of Malignant Lymphoma, Ann. Int. Med., *14*, 2073, 1941.

20b. GARDIKAS, C. and WILKINSON, J. F.: Trial of

β-Naphthyl-di-2-chloroethylamine in Leukæmia, Hodgkin's Disease, and Allied
Disorders, Lancet, *1*, 137, 1951.

21. GARDNER, W. U. and RYGAARD, J.: Further
Studies on the Incidence of Lymphomas
in Mice Exposed to X-rays and Given Sex
Hormones, Cancer Res., *14*, 205, 1954.

21a.GELLER, W.: A Study of Antibody Formation
in Patients with Malignant Lymphomas,
J. Lab. & Clin. Med., *42*, 232, 1953.

21b.GECHMAN, E., BLUTH, I. and GROSS, J. M.:
Hodgkin's Disease of the Rectum, Arch.
Int. Med., *97*, 483, 1956.

22. GELLHORN, A.: Management of the Patient
with Hodgkin's Disease, J. Chron. Dis.
1, 698, 1955.

22a.GIANNOPOULOS, P. P. and BERGSAGEL, D. E.:
The Mechanism of the Anemia Associated
with Hodgkin's Disease, Blood, *14*, 856,
1959.

23. GILBERT, R.: Radiotherapy in Hodgkin's
Disease (Malignant Granulomatosis) Am.
J. Roentgenol., *41*, 198, 1939.

23a.GILLIAM, A. G.: Age, Sex, and Race Selection
at Death from Leukemia and the Lymphomas, Blood, *8*, 693, 1953.

23b.GILLMAN, J., GILLMAN, T. and GILBERT, C.:
The Pathogenesis of Experimentally Produced Lymphomata in Rats (Including
Hodgkin's-Like Sarcoma), Cancer, *5*, 792,
1952.

23c.GILMAN, A. and PHILIPS, F. S.: The Biological
Actions and Therapeutic Applications of
the B-Chloroethyl Amines and Sulfides,
Science, *103*, 409, 1946.

24. GOLD, S. C. and GOWING, N. F. C.: Systemic
Lupus Erythematosus, Quart. J. Med., *22*,
457, 1953.

25. GOLDMAN, L. B.: Hodgkin's Disease: An
Analysis of 212 Cases, J.A.M.A., *114*, 1611,
1940.

25a.GOWING, N. F. C. and HAMLIN, IRIS M. E.:
Tissue Reactions to Aspergillus in Cases of
Hodgkin's Disease and Leukaemia, J.
Clin. Path., *13*, 396, 1960.

25b.GREEN, I. and CORSO, P. F.: A Study of Skin
Homografting in Patients with Lymphomas, Blood, *14*, 235, 1959; Lancet, *1*, 30,
1960.

25c.GROLLMAN, A., JOHNSON, R. L. and REGAN,
W. W.: A Clinical Evaluation of Colchicine in the Treatment of Hodgkin's Disease, Ann. Int. Med., *42*, 154, 1955.

26. GRAND, C. G.: Cytoplasmic Inclusions and
the Characteristics of Hodgkin's Diseased
Lymph Nodes in Tissue Culture, Cancer
Res., *9*, 183, 1949.

26a.HAHN, G. A.: Gynecologic Considerations in
Malignant Lymphomas, Am. J. Obst. &
Gynec., *75*, 673, 1958.

26b.HALL, C. A. and OLSON, K. B.: Therapy of
the Malignant Lymphomas, Am. J. Med.,
20, 392, 1956.

26c.HARRELL, G. T.: Hodgkin's Disease with Invasion of Pericardium and Gall Bladder,
Arch. Path., *28*, 58, 1939.

26d.HASERICK, J. R.: Modern Concepts of Systemic Lupus Erythematosus, J. Chron.
Dis., *1*, 317, 1955.

26e.HAYNES, W. F., JR. and BEGG, C. F.: Miliary
Tuberculosis Occurring in Patients with
Malignant Lymphoma, Cancer, *10*, 1221,
1957.

27. HELLER, E. L. and PALIN, W.: Ovarian Involvement in Hodgkin's Disease, Arch.
Path., *41*, 282, 1946.

28. HELLWIG, C. A.: Malignant Lymphoma. The
Value of Radical Surgery in Selected
Cases, Surg. Gynec. & Obst., *84*, 950, 1947.

29. HENNESSY, J. P. and ROTTINO, A.: Hodgkin's
Disease in Pregnancy with a Report of
Twelve Cases, Am. J. Obst. & Gynec.,
63, 756, 1952.

29a.HICKLING, R. A.: Giant Follicle Lymphoma
of the Spleen, Brit. M. J., *1*, 1464, 1960.

30. HIRSCH, E. F.: Primary Lymphosarcoma of
the Liver With Metastases to the Marrow
and Secondary Anemia, Arch. Path., *23*,
674, 1937.

30a.HOCHMAN, A. and CZERNIAK, P.: Hodgkin's
Disease and Amyeloidopathia, Radiology,
63, 716, 1954.

30b.HODGKIN, T.: On Some Morbid Appearances
of the Absorbent Glands and Spleen,
Trans. Roy. Med.-Chir. Soc., Glasgow,
17, 68, 1832.

30c.HOLMAN, H. R., DEICHER, H. R. G. and
KUNKEL, H. G.: The L. E. Cell and the
L. E. Serum Factors, Bull. New York
Acad. Med., *35*, 409, 1959.

30d.HODES M. E., ROHN, R. J. and BOND, W. H.:
Vincaleukoblastine. I. Preliminary Clinical
Studies, Cancer Res., *20*, 1041, 1960; Proc.
4th Canad. Cancer Conf. (in press).

31. HORNBAKER, J. H.: Giant Follicular Lymphoblastoma Terminating in Acute Myelogenous Leukemia, Ann. Int. Med., *53*,
221, 1960.

31a.HOSTER, H. A., DOAN, C. A. and SCHU-
MACHER, M.: Studies in Hodgkin's Syndrome. II. A Search for Brucella in Hodgkin's Syndrome, Proc. Soc. Exper. Biol.
& Med., *57*, 86, 1944; J. Lab. & Clin.
Med., *30*, 675, 1945; Ohio State M. J., *43*,
721, 1947; Cancer Res., *9*, 473, 1949; *ibid.*,
10, 467 and 530, 1950.

31b.HOSTER, H. A. and DRATMAN, M. B.: Hodgkin's Disease 1832–1947, Cancer Res., *8*, 1, 1948 (Bibliography).

31c.HUGGERT, A.: Uveitis in Hodgkin's Disease, Acta med. scandinav., *151*, 155, 1955.

31d.HYMAN, G. A.: Studies on Anemia of Disseminated Malignant Neoplastic Disease. I. The Hemolytic Factor, Blood, *9*, 911, 1954.

32. ISAACSON, N. H., SPATT, S. D. and GRAYZEL, D. M.: Primary Splenic Hodgkin's Disease Without Lymph Node Involvement, Ann. Int. Med., *27*, 294, 1947.

32a.JACKSON, H., JR. and PARKER, F., JR.: Hodgkin's Disease, New England J. Med., *230*, 1, 1944; *ibid.*, *231*, 35 and 639, 1944; *ibid.*, *232*, 547, 1945; *ibid.*, *233*, 369, 1945.

32b.JACKSON, H., JR., PARKER, F., JR. and BRUES, A. M.: Malignant Lymphoma of the Tonsil, Am. J. M. Sc., *191*, 1, 1936.

32c.JAKOB, H. G. and ZIRKIN, R. M.: Hodgkin's Disease with Involvement of the Heart and Pericardium, J.A.M.A., *173*, 338, 1960.

32d.JAMES, A. H.: Hodgkin's Disease with and without Alcohol-Induced Pain, Quart. J. Med., *29*, 47, 1960.

32e.JELLIFFE, A. M. and THOMSON, A. D.: The Prognosis in Hodgkin's Disease, Brit. J. Cancer, *9*, 21, 1955.

32f.JOHNSTON, A. W.: Spontaneous Regression of the Glands in Hodgkin's Disease, Brit. M. J., *1*, 916, 1954.

32g.KAPLAN, H. S. and SMITHERS, D. W.: Auto-Immunity in Man and Homologous Disease in Mice in Relation to the Malignant Lymphomas, Lancet, *2*, 1, 1959.

33. KARNOFSKY, D. A., BURCHENAL, J. A., ARMISTEAD, C. C., JR., SOUTHAM, C. M., BERNSTEIN, J. L., CRAVER, L. F. and RHOADS, C. P.: The Use of Oral and Intravenous Triethylene Melamine, a Compound with Nitrogen Mustard-Like Activity, in the Treatment of Neoplastic Disease, Arch. Int. Med., *87*, 477, 1951; M. Clin. North America, *38*, 541, 1954.

33a.KELLY, W. D., GOOD, R. A. and VARCO, R. L.: Anergy and Skin Homograft Survival in Hodgkin's Disease, Surg. Gynec. & Obst., *107*, 565, 1958.

33b.KIDD, J. G.: Regression of Transplanted Lymphomas Induced *in Vivo* by Means of Normal Guinea Pig Serum, J. Exper. Med., *98*, 565, 1953; Proc. Soc. Exper. Biol. & Med., *86*, 781 and 865, 1954.

34. KING, L. S.: Some Properties of the Encephalopathic Agent in Primate Bone Marrow (the Gordon Agent), J. Exper. Med., *71*, 603, 1940.

35. KRUMBHAAR, E. B.: Hodgkin's Disease of Bone Marrow and Spleen Without Ap-

parent Involvement of Lymph Nodes, Am. J. M. Sc., *182*, 764, 1931.

36. ————— Is Typical Hodgkin's Disease an Infection or Neoplasm?, Am. J. M. Sc., *188*, 597, 1934.

37. —————: The Lymphomatoid Diseases (the So-called Lymphoblastomas), J.A.M.A., *106*, 286, 1936.

37a.KUENTZ, M.: Etude Statistique, Clinique et Thérapeutique de la Granulomatose maligne, 1955, Imprimerie des Beaux-Arts, Lyon (France).

38. KUNDRAT, H.: Ueber Lymphosarkomatosis, Wien, klin. Wchnschr., *6*, 211, 1893.

38a.KYLE, R. A., KIELY, J. M. and STICKNEY, J. M.: Acquired Hemolytic Anemia in Chronic Lymphocytic Leukemia and the Lymphomas, A. M. A. Arch. Int. Med., *104*, 61, 1959.

38b.LAWRENCE, K. B. and LENSON, N.: Reticulum Cell Sarcoma, J.A.M.A., *149*, 361, 1952.

39. LEVINSON, B., WALTER, B. A., WINTROBE, M. M. and CARTWRIGHT, G. E.: A Clinical Study in Hodgkin's Disease, A. M. A. Arch. Int. Med., *99*, 519, 1957.

39a.LEVITAN, R., DIAMOND, H. D. and CRAVER, L. F.: Esophageal Varices in Hodgkin's Disease Involving the Liver, Am. J. Med., *27*, 137, 1959.

39b.LEVITAN, R., DIAMOND, H. D. and CRAVER, L. F.: Jaundice in Hodgkin's Disease, Am. J. Med., *30*, 99, 1961.

40. LIMARZI, L. R. and PAUL, J. T.: Sternal Marrow Studies in Hodgkin's Disease, Am. J. Clin. Path., *19*, 929, 1949.

42. LONGCOPE, W. T.: On the Pathological Histology of Hodgkin's Disease, Bull. Ayer Clin. Lab., Pennsylvania Hosp., No. 1, p. 3, 1903; *ibid.*, No. 4, p. 18, 1907.

43. LONGCOPE, W. T. and FREIMAN, D. G.: A Study of Sarcoidosis, Medicine, *31*, 1, 1952.

43a.LOVE, J. G., MILLER, R. H. and KERNOHAN, J. W.: Lymphomas of Spinal Epidural Space, Arch. Surg., *69*, 66, 1954.

43b.LUCAS, P. F.: Lymph Node Smears in the Diagnosis of Lymphadenopathy, Blood, *10*, 1030, 1955.

43c.LUMB, G. and NEWTON, K. A.: Prognosis in Tumors of Lymphoid Tissue, Cancer, *10*, 976, 1957.

44. MAJOR, R. H. and LEGER, L. H.: Marked Eosinophilia in Hodgkin's Disease, J.A.M. A., *112*, 2601, 1939.

44a.MANDEL, H. G.: The Physiological Disposition of Some Anticancer Agents, Pharmacol. Rev., *11*, 743, 1959.

44b.MARCHAL, G. et DUHAMEL, G.: L'adénogramme de la maladie de Hodgkin, Sang, *26*, 542, 1955.

44c. MARSHALL, A. H. E. and WOOD, C.: The Involvement of the Thymus in Hodgkin's Disease, J. Path. & Bact., 73, 163, 1957.

45. MARCUSE, P. M. and STOUT, A. P.: Primary Lymphosarcoma of the Small Intestine, Cancer, 3, 459, 1950.

45a. MATTEUCCI, P.: Corneal Lesions in Hodgkin's Disease, Am. J. Ophth., 30, 136, 1947.

45b. MATTHIAS, J. Q., MISIEWICZ, J. J. and SCOTT, R. B.: Cyclophosphamide in Hodgkin's Disease and Related Disorders, Brit. M. J., 2, 1837, 1960.

45c. MAXWELL, G. M.: Twelve Cases of Lymphoblastomata in Children, Arch. Dis. Childhood, 29, 155, 1954.

46. McFARLAND, W., GRANVILLE, NORMA B. and DAMESHEK, W.: Autologous Bone Marrow Infusion as an Adjunct in Therapy of Malignant Disease, Blood, 14, 503, 1959.

46a. McGREGOR, J. K.: Hodgkin's Disease of the Breast, Am. J. Surg., 99, 348, 1960.

47. McNAUGHT, J. B.: The Gordon Test for Hodgkin's Disease, J.A.M.A., 111, 1280, 1938.

47a. McNEER, G. and BERG, J. W.: The Clinical Behavior and Management of Primary Malignant Lymphoma of the Stomach, Surgery, 46, 829, 1959.

48. MEDLAR, E. M., HORNBAKER, J. H. and ORDWAY, W. H.: An Interpretation of the Nature of Hodgkin's Disease, Folia haemat., 57, 52, 1937.

48a. MESTEL, A. L.: Lymphosarcoma of the Small Intestine in Infancy and Childhood, Ann. Surg., 149, 87, 1959.

48b. VAN METRE, T. E., JR.: Malignant Tumors of the Nasopharynx, Bull. Johns Hopkins Hosp., 82, 42, 1948.

49. MIDDLETON, W. S.: Some Clinical Caprices of Hodgkin's Disease, Ann. Int. Med., 11, 448, 1937.

49a. MILLER, D. G., DIAMOND, H. D. and CRAVER, L. F.: Clinical Use of Chlorambucil, New England J. Med., 261, 525, 1959.

50. MINOT, G. R. and ISAACS, R.: Lymphoblastoma and Malignant Lymphoma, J.A.M.A., 86, 1185, 1265, 1926.

50a. MISCH, K. A.: Torulosis Associated with Hodgkin's Disease, J. Clin. Path., 8, 207, 1955.

50b. MORRISON, H.: Thomas Hodgkin, New England J. Med., 251, 946, 1954.

50c. MOSCHELLA, S. L. and KRETZSCHMAR, H. O.: The Treatment of Pruritus in Hodgkin's Disease with Demecolcine (Colcemid), A. M. A. Arch. Dermat., 79, 536, 1959.

51. MURCHISON, C.: Case of "Lymphadenoma" of the Lymphatic System, etc., Trans. Path. Soc. London, 21, 372, 1870.

51a. NAYLOR, B.: Secondary Lymphoblastomatous Involvement of the Thyroid Gland, A. M. A. Arch. Path., 67, 432, 1959.

51b. NICE, C. M. and STENSTROM, K. W.: Irradiation Therapy in Hodgkin's Disease, Radiology, 62, 641, 1954.

52. PARKER, F., JR., JACKSON, H., JR., BETHEA, J. M. and OTIS, F.: The Co-existence of Tuberculosis With Hodgkin's Disease and Other Forms of Malignant Lymphoma, Am. J. M. Sc., 184, 694, 1932.

53. PEL, P. K.: Zur Symptomatologie der sogenchnten Pseudo-leukämie, Berl. klin. Wchnsanr., 22, 3, 1885.

53a. PETERS, M. V.: A Study of Survivals in Hodgkin's Disease Treated Radiologically, Am. J. Roentgenol., 63, 299, 1950; ibid., 79, 114, 1958.

53b. PETTET, J. D., PEASE, G. L. and COOPER, T.: An Evaluation of Paraffin Sections of Aspirated Bone Marrow in Malignant Lymphomas, Blood, 10, 820, 1955.

53c. PORTMANN, U. V., DUNNE, E. F. and HAZARD, J. B.: Manifestations of Hodgkin's Disease of the Gastrointestinal Tract, Am. J. Roentgenol., 72, 772, 1954.

53d. RAPPAPORT, H., WINTER, W. J. and HICKS, ETHEL B.: Follicular Lymphoma, Cancer, 9, 792, 1956.

53e. RAZIS, D. V., DIAMOND, H. D. and CRAVER, L. F.: Familial Hodgkin's Disease: Its Significance and Implications, Ann. Int. Med., 51, 933, 1959.

53f. RAZIS, D. V., DIAMOND, H. D. and CRAVER, L. F.: Hodgkin's Disease Associated with Other Malignant Tumors and Certain Non-Neoplastic Diseases, Am. J. M. Sc., 238, 327, 1959.

53g. REDD, B. L., JR.: Lymphosarcoma of the Stomach, Am. J. Roentgenol., 82, 634, 1959.

54. REED, D.: On the Pathological Changes in Hodgkin's Disease, Johns Hopkins Hosp. Rep., 10, 133, 1902.

54a. REINHARD, E. H., MOORE, C. V., BIERBAUM, O. S. and MOORE, S.: Radioactive Phosphorus as a Therapeutic Agent. J. Lab. & Clin. Med., 31, 107, 1946.

54b. RIVA, H. L., ANDRESON, P. S. and O'GRADY, J. W.: Pregnancy and Hodgkin's Disease, Am. J. Obst. & Gynec., 66, 866, 1953.

55. ROBB-SMITH, A. H. T.: Reticulosis and Reticulosarcoma: A Histological Classification, J. Path. & Bact., 47, 457, 1938.

55a. RONCHESE, F. and GATES, D. C.: Ichthyosiform Atrophy of the Skin in Hodgkin's Disease, New England J. Med., 255, 287, 1956.

56. VAN ROOYEN, C. E.: Ætiology of Hodgkin'

Disease With Special Reference to B. Tuberculosis Avis, Brit. M. J., *1*, 50, 1933.

56a.Rosenberg, S. A., Diamond, H. D. and Craver, L. F.: Lymphosarcoma: The Effects of Therapy and Survival in 1269 Patients in a Review of 30 Years' Experience, Ann. Int. Med., *53*, 877, 1960; Medicine, *40*, 31, 1961.

56b.Rosenberg, S. A., Diamond, H. D., Dargeon, H. W. and Craver, L. F.: Lymphosarcoma in Childhood, New England J. Med., *259*, 505, 1958.

56c.Rosenthal, N., Dreskin, O. H., Vural, I. L. and Zak, F. G.: The Significance of Hematogones in Blood, Bone Marrow and Lymph Node Aspiration in Giant Follicular Lymphoblastoma, Acta hæmat., *8*, 368, 1952.

57. Rottino, A. and Hoffman, G.: The Pathology of the Lung in Hodgkin's Disease, Am. J. Surg., *89*, 550, 1955.

57a.Rottino, A., Joffe, A. and Hoffmann, G.: Phenylbutazone (Butazolidin), a Useful Chemotherapeutic Agent for Hodgkin's Disease, Arch. Int. Med., *93*, 561, 1954.

57b.Rottino, A. and Levy, A. L.: Behavior of Total Serum Complement in Hodgkin's Disease and Other Malignant Lymphomas, Blood, *14*, 246, 1959.

58. Roulet, F.: Weitere Beiträge zur Kenntnis des Retothelsarkoms der Lymphknoten und anderer Lymphoiden-Organe, Virchows Arch. path. Anat., *286*, 702, 1932.

58a.Rubin, C. E. and Massey, B. W.: The Preoperative Diagnosis of Gastric and Duodenal Malignant Lymphoma by Exfoliative Cytology, Cancer, *7*, 271, 1954.

58c.Schier, W. W.: Cutaneous Anergy and Hodgkin's Disease, New England J. Med., *250*, 353, 1954; Am. J. Med., *20*, 94, 1956.

59a.Schricker, J. L., Jr. and Smith, D. E.: Primary Intracerebral Hodgkin's Disease, Cancer, *8*, 629, 1955.

59b.Schrijver, H. and Schillings, P. H. M.: Thombocytopenic Purpura with Sarcoidosis, Cured after Splenectomy, Acta med. scandinav., *144*, 213, 1952.

60. Sears, W. G.: The Blood in Hodgkin's Disease, With Special Reference to Eosinophilia, Guy's Hosp. Rep., *82*, 40, 1932.

61. Senear, F. E. and Caro, M. R.: Ulcerative Hodgkin's Disease of the Skin, Arch. Dermat., *35*, 114, 1937.

61a.Sheinmel, A., Roswit, B. and Lawrence, L. R.: Hodgkin's Disease of the Lung, Radiology, *54*, 165, 1950.

61b.Sherman, M. J., Morales, J. B., Bayrd, E. D. and Schierman, W. D.: Amyloid

Nephrosis Secondary to Hodgkin's Disease, Arch. Int. Med., *95*, 618, 1955.

61c.Shimkin, M. B., Oppermann, K. C., Lowbeer, B. V. A. and Mettier, S. R.: Hodgkin's Disease and Lymphosarcoma: An Analysis of Frequency, Distribution and Mortality at the University of California Hospital, Ann. Int. Med., *40*, 1095, 1954; ibid., *42*, 136, 1955; Blood, *10*, 1214, 1955.

61d.Skipper, H. E., Mitchell, J. H., Jr., Bennett, L. L., Jr., Newton, M. A., Simpson, L. and Edison, M.: Observations on Inhibition of Nucleic Acid Synthesis Resulting from Administration of Nitrogen Mustard, Urethan, Colchicine, 2,6-Diaminopurine, 8-Azaguanine, Potassium Arsenite, and Cortisone, Cancer Res., *11*, 145, 1951.

62. Smetana, H. F. and Cohen, B. M.: Mortality in Relation to Histologic Type in Hodgkin's Disease, Blood, *11*, 211, 1956.

62a.Slaughter, D. P. and Craver, L. F.: Hodgkin's Disease, Am. J. Roentgenol., *47*, 596, 1942; Radiology, *50*, 486, 1948; M. Clin. North America, *33*, 527, 1949; Ann. Surg., *148*, 705, 1958.

62b.Smith, R. B. W., Sheehy, T. W. and Rothberg, H.: Hodgkin's Disease and Pregnancy, A. M. A. Arch. Int. Med., *102*, 777, 1958.

62c.Southam, C. M., Diamond, H. D. and Craver, L. F.: Pregnancy During Hodgkin's Disease, Cancer, *9*, 1141, 1956.

62d.Sparling, H. J., Jr., Adams, R. D. and Parker, F., Jr.: Involvement of the Nervous System by Malignant Lymphoma, Medicine, *26*, 285, 1947 (Bibliography).

62e.Spellberg, M. A. and Zivin, S.: Lymphosarcoma of the Gastrointestinal Tract, Arch. Int. Med., *83*, 135, 1949.

62f.Sleisenger, M. H., Almy, T. P. and Barr, D. P.: The Sprue Syndrome Secondary to Lymphoma of the Small Bowel, Am. J. Med., *15*, 666, 1953.

62g.Sternberg, W. H., Sidransky, H. and Ochsner, S.: Primary Malignant Lymphomas of the Lung, Cancer, *12*, 806, 1959.

63. Sugarbaker, E. D. and Craver, L. F.: Lymphosarcoma, J.A.M.A., *115*, 17, 112, 1940.

63b.Sweitzer, S. E. and Winer, L. H.: Ulcerative Hodgkin's Disease and Lymph Node Imprints, Arch. Dermat., *51*, 229, 1945.

64. Symmers, D.: Giant Follicular Lymphadenopathy With or Without Splenomegaly, Arch. Path., *26*, 603, 1938; ibid., *31*, 385, 1942.

64a.————Clinical Significance of the Deeper

Anatomic Changes in Lymphoid Diseases, Arch. Int. Med., *74*, 163, 1944; Arch. Path., *45*, 73, 1948.

65. SYMMERS, D. and HUTCHESON, W.: Reticuloendotheliomatosis, Arch. Path., *27*, 562, 1939.

65a.UHLENHUTH, R. and WURM, K.: Untersuchungen zum Problem der Hodgkinschen Krankheit, Ztschr. ges. exper. Med., *105*, 205, 1939.

66. VARADI, S.: Hodgkin's Disease: Specific Findings in Sternal Puncture Material, Brit. J. Hæmat., *1*, 184, 1955.

66a.VARADI, S.: Reed-Sternberg Cells in the Peripheral Blood and Bone-Marrow in Hodgkin's Disease, Brit. M. J., *1*, 1239, 1960.

66b.VIDEBAEK, A. A. and KAAE, S.: β-Naphthyl-di-chloroethylamine in the Treatment of Malignant Diseases, Particularly Hodgkin's Disease, Acta med. scandinav., *149*, 361, 1954.

66c.VIETA, J. O. and CRAVER, L. F.: Intrathoracic Manifestations of the Lymphomatoid Diseases, Radiology, *37*, 138, 1941.

66d.VIETA, J. O., FRIEDELL, H. L. and CRAVER, L. F.: A Survey of Hodgkin's Disease and Lymphosarcoma in Bone, Radiology, *39*, 1, 1942.

66e.WAHL, H. R. and HILL, J. H.: Gastric Lesions in Hodgkin's Disease and Leukemia, Am. J. Path., *32*, 235, 1956.

67. WALLHAUSER, A.: Hodgkin's Disease, Arch. Path., *16*, 522, 672, 1933.

67a.WALT, A. J., WOOLNER, L. B. and BLACK, B. M.: Primary Malignant Lymphoma of the Thyroid, Cancer, *10*, 663, 1957.

68. WEISBERGER, A. S., HEINLE, R. W. and LEVINE, B.: The Effect of L-Cysteine on Nitrogen Mustard Therapy, Am. J. M. Sc., *224*, 201, 1952; J. Lab. & Clin. Med., *43*, 246, 1954.

68a.WELCH, J. W., CHESKY, V. E. and HELLWIG, C. A.: Malignant Lymphoma of the Thyroid, Surg. Gynec. & Obst., *106*, 70, 1958.

68b.WETHERLEY-MEIN, G., SMITH, P., GEAKE, M. R. and ANDERSON, H. J.: Follicular Lymphoma, Quart. J. Med., *21*, 327, 1952.

68c.WILLIAMS, H. M., DIAMOND, H. D. and CRAVER, L. F.: The Pathogenesis and Management of Neurological Complications in Patients with Malignant Lymphomas and Leukemia, Cancer, *11*, 76, 1958.

69. WINTROBE, M. M. and HUGULEY, C. M., JR.: Nitrogen Mustard Therapy for Hodgkin's Disease, Lymphosarcoma, the Leukemias, and Other Disorders, Cancer, *1*, 357, 1948.

69a.WINTROBE, M. M., CARTWRIGHT, G. E.,

FESSAS, P., HAUT, A. and ALTMAN, S. J.: Chemotherapy of Leukemia, Hodgkin's Disease and Related Disorders, Ann. Int. Med., *41*, 447, 1954.

70. WISEMAN, B. K.: The Blood Pictures in the Primary Diseases of the Lymphatic System, J.A.M.A., *107*, 2016, 1936.

70a.WOLPAW, S. E., HIGLEY, C. S. and HAUSER, H.: Intrathoracic Hodgkin's Disease, Am. J. Roentgenol., *52*, 374, 1944.

70c.WOOD, H. F. *et al.*: Determination of C-Reactive Protein in the Blood of Patients with Hodgkin's Disease, Ann. Int. Med., *48*, 823, 1958.

71. WOODWARD, H. Q. and CRAVER, L. F.: Serum Phosphatase in the Lymphomatoid Diseases, J. Clin. Invest., *19*, 1, 1940.

72. WRIGHT, C. B. and NORRIS, E. H.: Leukemic Reticulo-endotheliosis, Arch., Path., *24*, 626, 1937.

72a.WRIGHT, C. J. E.: Macrofollicular Lymphoma, Am. J. Path., *32*, 201, 1956.

72b.————: The "Benign" Form of Hodgkin's Disease (Hodgkin's Paragranuloma), J. Path. & Bact., *80*, 157, 1960.

72c.YARDUMIAN, K. and MYERS, L.: Primary Hodgkin's Disease of the Lung, Arch. Int. Med., *86*, 233, 1950.

73. YATES, J. L. and BUNTING, C. H.: Results of Treatment in Hodgkin's Disease, J.A.M.A., *68*, 747, 1917.

73a.ZEFFREN, J. L. and ULTMANN, J. E.: Reticulum Cell Sarcoma Terminating in Acute Leukemia, Blood, *15*, 277, 1960.

74. ZIEGLER, K.: *Die Hodgkinsche Krankheit*, Jena, Gustav Fischer, 1911.

74a.ZIMMERMAN, H. J., ALPERT, L. K. and HOWE, J. S.: The Effect of Nitrogen Mustard (Bis-B-Chloroethylamine) on Liver Function and Structure in Patients with Neoplastic Disease, J. Lab. & Clin. Med., *40*, 387, 1952.

74b.ZUBROD, C. G. *et al.*: Appraisal of Methods for the Study of Chemotherapy of Cancer in Man, J. Chron. Dis., *11*, 7, 1960.

Splenomegaly

75. ANGEVINE, D. M., HAMILTON, T. R., WALLACE, F. G. and HAZARD, J. B.: Lymph Nodes in Leishmaniasis, Am. J. M. Sc., *210*, 33, 1945.

76. ASK-UPMARK, E.: The Remote Effects of Removal of the Normal Spleen in Man, Acta Soc. med. Suecanæ, Stockholm, Isaac Marcus Boktryckeri-Aktiebolag, *61*, 197, 1935.

76a.ATKINSON, M. and SHERLOCK, S.: Intrasplenic Pressure as Index of Portal Venous Pressure, Lancet, *1*, 1325, 1954.

77. BANTI, G.: Splenomegalie mit Lebercirrhose, Beitr. path. Anat. allg. Path., 24, 21, 1898.

77a.BASU, A. K.: Chronic Splenomegaly and Its Relation to Hepatic Pathology, Brit. M. J., 2, 947, 1958.

77b.BERTINO, J. and MYERSON, R. M.: The Role of Splenectomy in Sarcoidosis, A. M. A. Arch. Int. Med., 106, 213, 1960.

78. BJÖRKMAN, S. E.: The Splenic Circulation, With Special Reference to the Function of the Spleen Sinus Wall, Almqvist and Wiksells Boktryckeri Ab, Uppsala, 1947; (also Suppl. 191, Acta med. scandinav.).

78a.BLAU, J. N. and WILLCOX, A.: Splenic Neutropenia in Felty's Syndrome, Brit. M. J., 2, 1094, 1957.

78b.BUSH, J. A. and AINGER, L. E.: Congenital Absence of the Spleen with Congenital Heart Disease, Pediatrics, 15, 93, 1955.

78c.CALABRESI, P., EDWARDS, E. A. and SCHILLING R. F.: Fluorescent Antiglobulin Studies in Leukopenic and Related Disorders, J. Clin. Invest., 38, 2091, 1959.

79. CARTWRIGHT, G. E., CHUNG, H. L. and CHANG, A.: Studies on the Pancytopenia of Kala-Azar, Blood, 3, 249, 1948.

80. CHANEY, W. C.: Splenic Anemia: A Clinical and Pathological Study of 69 Cases, Am. J. M. Sc., 165, 856, 1923.

80a.CHAPMAN, A. Z., REEDER, P. S. and BAKER, L. A.: Neutropenia Secondary to Tuberculous Splenomegaly, Ann. Int. Med., 41, 1225, 1954.

80b.CHATTERJEA, J. B., DAMESHEK, W. and STEFANINI, M.: The Adrenalin (Epinephrin) Test as Applied to Hematologic Disorders, Blood, 8, 211, 1953.

80c.CHENG, T. O., SUTTON, G. C. and SUTTON, D. C.: Cruveilhier-Baumgarten Syndrome, Am. J. Med., 17, 143, 1954.

80d.COOK, S. F. and ALAFI, M. H.: Role of the Spleen in Acclimatization to Hypoxia, Am. J. Physiol., 186, 369, 1956.

80e.CROSBY, W. H.: Normal Functions of the Spleen Relative to Red Blood Cells, Blood, 14, 399, 1959.

80f.CRUZ, W. O. and ROBSCHEIT-ROBBINS, F. S.: Relationship between the Spleen and the Morphologic Picture of Blood Regeneration, Am. J. M· Sc., 203, 28, 1942.

81. CURTIS, A. C. and GREKIN, J. N.: Histoplasmosis, J.A.M.A., 134, 1217, 1947.

82. DAMESHEK, W.: Hypersplenism, Bull. New York Acad. Med., 31, 133, 1955.

83. DE, M. N. and TRIBEDI, B. P.: The Pathogenesis of the Commoner Types of Splenomegaly Met With in India, Indian Med. Gaz.. 74, 9, 1939.

83a.DELL, J. M., JR. and KLINEFELTER, H. F., JR.: Roentgen Studies of the Spleen, Am. J. M. Sc., 211, 437, 1946.

83b.DERRY, D. C. L., CARD, W. I., WILSON, R. and DUNCAN, J. T.: Histoplasmosis of Darling, Lancet, 1, 224, 1942.

83c.DOAN, C. A.: Hypersplenism, Bull. New York Acad. Med., 25, 625, 1949.

83d.DOAN, C. A. and WRIGHT, C. S.: Primary Congenital and Secondary Acquired Splenic Panhematopenia, Blood, 1, 10, 1946.

83e.DOMÉNICO, A. D. and ANDREOTTI, HEBE T.: Mechanism of Splenic Protection against Bartonella muris in the Parabiotic Rat, Am. J. Physiol., 197, 795, 1959.

84. DÜRR, R.: Bantimilz und hepatolienale Fibrose, Beitr. path. Anat., 72, 418, 1924.

84a.EK, J. I. and RAYNER, S.: An Analytical Study of Splenectomized Cases after Traumatic Rupture of Healthy Spleens, Acta med. scandinav., 137, 417, 1950.

85. ELIASON, E. L. and JOHNSON, J.: Splenectomy, Surgery, 2, 823, 1937; ibid., 13, 177, 1943.

85a.ENDE, N. and CHERNISS, E. I.: Splenic Mastocytosis, Blood, 13, 631, 1958.

86. ENGELBRETH-HOLM, J.: A Study of Tuberculous Splenomegaly and Splenogenic Controlling of the Cell Emission From the Bone Marrow, Am. J. M. Sc., 195, 32, 1938.

87. EPPINGER, H.: Die Hepato-Lienalen Erkrankungen, Berlin, Julius Springer, 1920.

88. FELTY, A. R.: Chronic Arthritis in the Adult, Associated With Splenomegaly and Leucopenia, Bull. Johns Hopkins Hosp., 35, 16, 1924.

88a.FIGLEY, M. M.: Splenoportography: Some Advantages and Disadvantages, Am. J. Roentgenol., 80, 313, 1958.

88b.FITCH, F. W., BARKER, P., SOULES, K. H. and WISSLER, R. W.: A Study of Antigen Localization and Degradation and the Histologic Reaction in the Spleen of Normal, X-irradiated, and Spleen-shielded Rats, J. Lab. & Clin. Med., 42, 598, 1953.

89. FONDÉ, G. H. and FONDÉ, E. C.: Chronic Malaria, Arch. Int. Med., 64, 1156, 1939.

89a.FORD, C. E., HAMERTON, J. L., BARNES, D. W. H. and LOUTIT, J. F.: Cytological Identification of Radiation-Chimaeras, Nature, 177, 452, 1956.

90. GATE, J. and RIOU, J.: Banti Syndrome of Syphilitic Origin Ameliorated by Specific Treatment, Lyon méd., 157, 438, 1936.

90a.GELIN, G.: Les splénomégalies tuberculeuses, Sang, 25, 172, 1954.

91. GIFFIN, H. Z.: Clinical Observations Concerning Twenty-seven Cases of Splenectomy, Am. J. M. Sc., 145, 781, 1913.

92. GILBERT, ENID F., NISHIMURA, KINSUKE and WEDUM, BERNICE G.: Congenital Malformations of the Heart Associated with Splenic Agenesis, Circulation, *17*, 72, 1958.

92a. GIRSH, L. S. and MYERSON, R. M.: Thyrotoxicosis Associated with Thrombocytopenia and Hypersplenism, Am. J. Clin. Path., *27*, 328, 1957.

93. GOLDBERG, G. M.: Metastatic Carcinoma of the Spleen Resulting from Lymphogenic Spread, Lab. Invest., *6*, 383, 1957.

94. GRETSEL: Ein Fall von Anæmia splenica bei einem Kinde, Berl. klin. Wchnschr., *3*, 212, 1866.

95. GRUNBERG, A., BLAIR, J. L. and ST. HILL, C. A.: Congestive Splenomegaly Due to Pancreatic Cystadenoma, Brit. M. J., *2*, 265, 1952.

96. HEINLE, R. W. and HOLDEN, W. D.: Primary Splenic Panhematopenia, Surg. Gynec. & Obst., *89*, 79, 1949.

97. HICKLING, R. A.: Tuberculous Splenomegaly, With Miliary Tuberculosis of the Lungs, Quart. J. Med., *7*, 263, 1938.

97a. HIRST, A. E., JR. and BULLOCK, W. K.: Metastatic Carcinoma of the Spleen, Am. J. M. Sc., *223*, 414, 1952.

97b. HJORT, P. F. and PAPUTCHIS, Helen: Platelet Life Span in Normal, Splenectomized and Hypersplenic Rats, Blood, *15*, 45, 1960.

97c. HOWELLS, L.: Treatment of Splenic Anæmia and Banti's Syndrome, Lancet, *1*, 1320, 1938.

98. HUTCHISON, H. S., HAMILTON, P. K., JR., JAMESON, P. W. and JONES, H. L.: Evaluation of Splenectomy in the Treatment of Egyptian Splenomegaly, Surg. Gynec. & Obst., *102*, 588, 1956.

98a. HUTT, M. S. R., RICHARDSON, J. S. and STAFFURTH, J. S.: Felty's Syndrome. A Report of Four Cases Treated by Splenectomy, Quart. J. Med., *20*, 57, 1951.

99. JACOBSON, L. O.: Modification of Radiation Injury, Bull. New York Acad. Med., *30*, 675, 1954; Proc. Soc. Exper. Biol. & Med., *91*, 135, 1956.

100. JACOBSON, L. O., SIMMONS, E. L. and BLOCK, M. H.: The Effect of Splenectomy on the Toxicity of SR[89] to the Hematopoietic System of Mice, J. Lab. & Clin. Med., *34*, 1640, 1949.

100a. JAHNKE, E. J., JR., PALMER, E. D. and BRICK, I. B.: The Cruveilhier-Baumgarten Syndrome, Ann. Surg., *140*, 44, 1954.

100b. JANDL, J. H.: The Agglutination and Sequestration of Immature Red Cells, J. Lab. & Clin. Med., *55*, 663, 1960.

101. JORDAN, G. L., JR. and HECK, F. J.: Fate of Patients with Splenomegaly and Hypersplenism Not Treated by Splenectomy, Ann. Surg., *143*, 29, 1956.

101a. KIMBRELL, O. C., JR.: Sarcoidosis of the Spleen, New England J. Med., *257*, 128, 1957.

102. KLEMPERER, P.: The Spleen, in *Handbook of Hematology*, Hal Downey, Ed. New York, Paul B. Hoeber, Inc., *3*, 1587, 1938.

103. KNISELY, M. H.: Microscopic Observations of the Circulatory System of Living Unstimulated Mammalian Spleens, Anat. Rec., *65*, 23, 131, 1936.

104. KRUMBHAAR, E. B.: Functions of the Spleen, Physiol. Rev., *6*, 160, 1926.

105. ———The Incidence and Nature of Splenic Neoplasms, Ann. Clin. Med., *5*, 833, 1927.

106. ———The Changes Produced in the Blood Picture by Removal of the Normal Mammalian Spleen, Am. J. M. Sc., *184*, 215, 1932.

106a. LARRABEE, R. C.: Chronic Congestive Splenomegaly and Its Relationship to Banti's Disease, Am. J. M. Sc., *188*, 745, 1934.

107. LASKI, B. and MACMILLAN, A.: Incidence of Infection in Children after Splenectomy, Pediatrics, *24*, 523, 1959.

107a. LAUDA, E.: *Die normale und pathologische Physiologie der Milz*, Berlin, Urban u. Schwartzenberg, 1933.

107b. LEE, R. E. and ARNSPIGER, L. A.: Epidermoid Cyst of the Spleen, A.M.A. Arch. Surg., *77*, 10, 1958.

107c. LIMARZI, L. R., JONES, R. M., PAUL, J. T. and PONCHER, H. G.: Sternal Marrow in Banti's Syndrome and Other Splenomegalic States, Am. J. Clin. Path., *13*, 231, 1943.

107d. LINTON, R. R.: The Surgical Treatment of Bleeding Esophageal Varices by Portal Systemic Venous Shunts With a Report of 34 Cases, Ann. Int. Med., *31*, 794, 1949; New England J. Med., *254*, 931, 1956.

107e. LIPP, W. F., ECKSTEIN, E. H. and AARON, A. H.: The Clinical Significance of the Palpable Spleen, Gastroenterology, *3*, 287, 1944.

107g. LIPSON, R. L., BAYRD, E. D. and WATKINS, C. H.: The Postsplenectomy Blood Picture, Am. J. Clin. Path., *32*, 526, 1959.

107h. LOCKIE, L. M., SANES, S. and VAUGHAN, S. L.: Chronic Arthritis; Associated With Neutrophilic Leukopenia, Splenomegaly and Hepatomegaly, Am. J. Clin. Path., *12*, 372, 1942.

107i. LÖFFLER, W. and MAIER, C.: Über einen Fall von Feltyschem Syndrom mit cyclischer Agranulocytose, Cardiologia, *12*, 17, 1947,

69

107j. LORBER, M.: The Effects of Splenectomy on the Red Blood Cells of the Dog with Particular Emphasis on the Reticulocyte Response, Blood, 13, 972, 1958.

107k. MACPHERSON, A. I. S.: Assessment of the Results of Surgical Treatment in Portal Hypertension, Gastroenterology, 38, 142, 1960.

107l. MACPHERSON, A. I. S. and INNES, J.: Peripheral Blood Picture after Operation for Portal Hypertension, Lancet, 1, 1120, 1953.

108. MALAMOS, B.: Beitrag zur Klinik, Therapie und Epidemiologie der Mittelmeer-Kala-Azar, Ergebn. inn. Med. u. Kinderh., 52, 1, 1937.

108a. MARKS, L. J., WEINGARTEN, B. and GERST, G. R.: Carcinoma of the Tail of the Pancreas Associated with Bleeding Gastric Varices and Hypersplenism, Ann. Int. Med., 37, 1077, 1952.

108b. MATTER, M. et al.: A Study of Thrombopoiesis in Induced Acute Thrombocytopenia, Blood, 15, 174, 1960.

108c. McFADZEAN, A. J. S. and COOK, J.: Ligation of the Splenic and Hepatic Arteries in Portal Hypertension, Lancet, 1, 615, 1953.

108d. McFADZEAN, A. J. S., TODD, D. and TSANG, K. C.: Observations on the Anemia of Cryptogenetic Splenomegaly, Blood, 13, 513 and 524, 1958; Brit. J. Hæmat., 2, 355, 1956; Tr. Roy. Soc. Trop. Med. & Hyg., 52, 354, 1958.

108e. McKENZIE, D., WHIPPLE, A. O. and WINTERSTEINER, M. P.: Studies on Microscopic Anatomy and Physiology of Living Transilluminated Spleens, Am. J. Anat., 68, 397, 1941; Angiology, 6, 350, 1955.

108f. McKINNON, W. M. P., BOLEY, S. J. and MANPEL, J.: Infection in Children following Splenectomy for Traumatic Rupture, A. M. A. J. Dis. Child., 98, 710, 1959.

109. McMICHAEL, J.: The Pathology of Hepatolienal Fibrosis, J. Path. & Bact., 39, 481, 1934.

110. ———Splenic Anaemia, Edinburgh M. J., 42, 97, 1935.

110a. MELENEY, H. E.: Histoplasmosis, Am. J. Trop. Med., 20, 603, 1940.

111. MENON, T. B.: Venous Splenomegaly: A Study in Experimental Portal Congestion, J. Path. & Bact., 46, 357, 1938.

112. MOHAMED, A. S.: Critical Study of the Different Theories on the Ætiology of Egyptian Splenomegaly, J. Egyptian M. A., 19, 652, 1936.

112a. MORENO, A. H., CHIESA, D. and AFFANI, J.: Studies on the Portal Tension of Human Adults, Surg. Gynec. & Obst., 104, 25, 1957.

112b. MOTULSKY, A. G. et al.: Anemia and the Spleen, New England J. Med., 259, 1164 and 1215, 1958.

113. OSLER, W.: On Splenic Anæmia, Am. J. M. Sc., 119, 54, 1900.

114. PALMER, J. G., EICHWALD, E. J., CARTWRIGHT, G. E. and WINTROBE, M. M.: The Experimental Production of Splenomegaly, Anemia and Leukopenia in Albino Rats, Blood, 8, 72, 1953.

114a. PALMER, J. G., KEMP, I., CARTWRIGHT, G. E. and WINTROBE, M. M.: Studies on the Effect of Splenectomy on the Total Leukocyte Count in the Albino Rat, Blood, 6, 3, 1951.

114b. PÉREZ-TAMAYO, R., MORA, J. and MONTFORT, IRMGARD: Humoral Factor(s) in Experimental Hypersplenism, Blood, 16, 1145, 1960.

115. PERLA, D. and MARMORSTON, J.: The Spleen and Resistance, Baltimore, The Williams & Wilkins Co., 1935.

116. RATNOFF, O. D., CONLEY, C. L. and BERTHRONG, M.: The Differentiation between Extrahepatic and Intrahepatic Obstruction of the Portal Circulation, Bull. Johns Hopkins Hosp., 87, 305, 1950.

116a. RAVENNA, P.: Banti Syndrome (Fibrocongestive Splenomegaly), Arch. Int. Med., 66, 879, 1940; ibid., 72, 786, 1943.

117. REIMANN, F., ERDOGAN, G. and ULAGAY, I.: Untersuchungen über die Genese des Syndroms der "Hypersplenie" bei portalem Hochdruck, Acta hepato-splen., 7, 230, 1960.

117a. REINHARD, E. H. and LOEB, V., JR.: Dyssplenism Secondary to Chronic Leukemia or Malignant Lymphoma, J.A.M.A., 158, 629, 1955.

117b. RIPSTEIN, C. B. and VIRSHUP, M.: Sarcoma Involving the Spleen, Am. J. Surg., 86, 422, 1953.

117c. ROBINSON, T. W. and STURGEON, P.: Post-Splenectomy Infection in Infants and Children, Pediatrics, 25, 941, 1960.

118. RODRIGUEZ MOLINA, F. and PONS, J. A.: Hematological Studies on Schistosomiasis Mansoni in Puerto Rico, Puerto Rico J. Pub. Health & Trop. Med., 11, 369, 1936.

118a. ROGERS, H. M. and LANGLEY, F. H.: Neutropenia Associated With Splenomegaly and Atrophic Arthritis (Felty's Syndrome), Ann. Int. Med., 32, 745, 1950.

119. ROTHBERG, H. and CORALLO, L. A.: Influence of Splenectomy on Resistance to Pneumococcal Infection in Rats, Proc. Soc. Exper. Biol. & Med., 100, 220, 1959.

120. ROUSSELOT, L. M.: Congestive Splenomegaly

(Banti's Syndrome), Bull. New York Acad. Med., *15*, 188, 1939; J.A.M.A., *140*, 282, 1949; Surgery, *8*, 34, 1940; Ann. Surg., *150*, 384, 1959.

121. ROUSSELOT, L. M.: The Present Status of Surgery for Portal Hypertension, Am. J. Med., *16*, 874, 1954.

122. ROUSSELOT, L. M. and THOMPSON, W. P.: Experimental Production of Congestive Splenomegaly, Proc. Soc. Exper. Biol. & Med., *40*, 705, 1939.

122a. ROWLEY, D. A.: The Formation of Circulating Antibody in the Splenectomized Human Being Following Intravenous Injection of Heterologous Erythrocytes, J. Immunol., *65*, 515, 1950.

122b. SASLAW, S., BOURONCLE, BERTHA A., WALL, R. L. and DOAN, C. A.: Studies on the Antibody Response in Splenectomized Persons, New England J. Med., *261*, 120, 1959.

122c. SCHRIJVER, H. and VERDONK, G. J.: Hamartoma of the Spleen with Inhibition of the Bone Marrow, Acta med. scandinav., *158*, 235, 1957.

123. SIMSON, F. W. and BARNETSON, J.: Histoplasmosis, J. Path. & Bact., *54*, 299, 1942.

123a. SINGER, K., MILLER, E. B. and DAMESHEK, W.: Hematologic Changes Following Splenectomy in Man, Am. J. M. Sc., *202*, 171, 1941.

123b. SMITH, C. H., ERLANDSON, MARION, SCHULMAN, I. and STERN, GERTRUDE: Hazard of Severe Infections in Splenectomized Infants and Children, Am. J. Med., *22*, 390, 1957.

123c. SMITH, R. M. and HOWARD, P. J.: The Early Occurrence of Gastric Hemorrhage in Children With Splenomegaly, Am. J. Dis. Child., *34*, 585, 1927.

124. SPICKARD, A.: Multiple Myeloma with Myelofibrosis and with Polycythemia Vera, Bull. Johns Hopkins Hosp., *107*, 234, 1960.

124a. STEWART, E. H., JR.: Cavernous Hemangioma of the Spleen, Am. J. Surg., *71*, 536, 1946.

124b. STEWART, W. B., STEWART, J. M., IZZO, M. J. and YOUNG, L. E.: Age as Affecting the Osmotic and Mechanical Fragility of Dog Erythrocytes Tagged with Radioactive Iron, J. Exper. Med., *91*, 147, 1950.

124c. STORER, J. B., LUSHBAUGH, C. C. and FURCHNER, J. E.: The Protective Effect of Shielded Ectopic Bone Marrow against Total Body X-radiation, J. Lab. & Clin. Med., *40*, 355, 1952.

125. STRONG, R. P., SHATTUCK, G. C., BEQUAERT, J. C. and WHEELER, R. E.: Hamilton Rice Seventh Expedition to the Amazon, etc., Contrib. from the Harvard Inst. for Trop.

Biol. and Med., Cambridge, Harvard Univ. Press, No. IV, 1926.

125a. THOMPSON, W. P.: The Pathogenesis of Banti's Disease, Ann. Int. Med., *14*, 255, 1940.

126. THORBECKE, G. J. and KEUNING, F. J.: Antibody Formation *in Vitro* by Hæmopoietic Organs after Subcutaneous and Intravenous Immunization, J. Immunol., *70*, 129, 1953.

126a. TISDALE, W. A., KLATSKIN, G. and GLENN, W. W. L.: Portal Hypertension and Bleeding Esophageal Varices, New England J. Med., *261*, 209, 1959.

126b. TURNER, A. W. and HODGETTS, V. ELIZABETH: The Dynamic Red Cell Storage Function of the Spleen in Sheep, Australasian J. Exper. Biol. & M. Sc., *37*, 399, 1959; *ibid.*, *38*, 79, 1960.

126c. WACHSTEIN, M.: Primary Hemangiosarcoma of the Spleen Diagnosed by Needle Biopsy, J.A.M.A., *152*, 237, 1953.

126d. WAGLEY, P. F.: A Consideration of the Banti Syndrome, Bull. Johns Hopkins Hosp., *85*, 87, 1949.

126e. WALDMANN, T. A., WEISSMAN, S. M. and BERLIN, N.: The Effect of Splenectomy on Erythropoiesis in the Dog, Blood, *15*, 873, 1960.

126f. WELCH, C. S. and DAMESHEK, W.: Splenectomy in Blood Dyscrasias, New England J. Med., *242*, 601, 1950.

127. WOLLSTEIN, M. and KREIDEL, K.: Blood Picture After Splenectomy in Children, Am. J. Dis. Child., *51*, 765, 1936.

127a. WRIGHT, C. S., DOAN, C. A., BOURONCLE, B. A. and ZOLLINGER, R. M.: Direct Splenic Arterial and Venous Blood Studies in the Hypersplenic Syndromes Before and After Epinephrine, Blood, *6*, 195, 1951.

128. WRIGHT, D. O.: Macrocytic Anemia in Banti's Disease, Ann. Int. Med., *8*, 814, 1935.

Multiple Myeloma

129. ADAMS, W. S., ALLING, E. L. and LAWRENCE, J. S.: Multiple Myeloma, Am. J. Med., *6*, 141, 1949; J. Lab. & Clin. Med., *40*, 519, 1952.

130. ADAMS, W. S. and SKOOG, W. A.: The Management of Multiple Myeloma, J. Chron. Dis., *6*, 446, 1957.

130a. AHERNE, W. A.: The Differentiation of Myelomatosis from Other Causes of Bone Marrow Plasmacytosis, J. Clin. Path., *11*, 326, 1958.

131. ARMSTRONG, J. B.: A Study of Renal Function in Patients With Multiple Myeloma, Am. J. M. Sc., *219*, 488, 1950.

133. BING, J.: The Formolgel Reaction and Other

Globulin Reactions, Acta med. scandinav., 91, 336, 1937.

134. BAYRD, E. D. and HECK, F. J.: Multiple Myeloma, J.A.M.A., 133, 147, 1947; ibid., 153, 784, 1953.

135. BAYRD, E. D.: The Bone Marrow on Sternal Aspiration in Multiple Myeloma, Blood, 3, 987, 1948.

135a.BRACHFELD, J. and MYERSON, R. M.: Pyroglobulinemia, J.A.M.A., 161, 865, 1956.

135b.BURTIN, P., HARTMANN, L., FAUVERT, R., et GRABAR, P.: Recherches sur les protéines du myélome: I. Étude critique des techniques d'identification de la protéine de Bence-Jones et de leur valeur diagnostique, Rev. franç. études clin. et biol., 1, 17, 1956.

136. CARSTON, C. P., ACKERMAN, L. V. and MALTBY, J. D.: Plasma Cell Myeloma, Am. J. Clin. Path., 25, 849, 1955.

136b.CLARK, H. and MUIRHEAD, E. E.: Plasmacytosis of Bone Marrow, Arch. Int. Med., 94, 425, 1954.

137. COLLIER, F. C., REICH, A. and KING, J. W.: The Value of Precipitin Tests for Bence-Jones Protein in Early Diagnosis, New England J. Med., 247, 60, 1952.

138. CONN, H. O. and KLATSKIN, G.: Filter Paper Electrophoretic Patterns of Serum in Multiple Myeloma, Am. J. Med., 16, 822, 1954.

139. CRADDOCK, C. G., JR., ADAMS, W. S. and FIGUEROA, W. G.: Interference with Fibrin Formation in Multiple Myeloma by an Unusual Protein Found in Blood and Urine, J. Lab. & Clin. Med., 42, 847, 1953.

140. DAVIS, J. S., JR., WEBER, F. C. and BARTFELD, H.: Conditions Involving the Hemopoietic System Resulting in a Pseudorheumatoid Arthritis, Ann. Int. Med., 47, 10, 1957.

141. DENT, C. E. and ROSE, G. A.: The Bence-Jones Protein of Multiple Myelomatosis: Its Methionine Content and Its Possible Significance in Relation to the Aetiology of the Disease, Biochem. J., 44, 610, 1949.

141a.EFFERSØE, P. and TIDSTRØM, B.: Detection of Myeloma Protein in Urine by a New Quick Method, J. Lab. & Clin. Med., 50, 134, 1957.

141b.ENGLE, R. L., JR. and WALLIS, LILA A.: Multiple Myeloma and the Adult Fanconi Syndrome, Am. J. Med., 22, 5, 1957.

142. ERF, L. A. and HERBUT, P. A.: Comparative Cytology of Wright's Stained Smears and Histologic Sections in Multiple Myeloma, Am. J. Clin. Path., 16, 1 and 13, 1946.

143. FADEM, R. S. and McBIRNIE, J. E.: Plasmacytosis in Diseases Other Than the Primary Plasmacytic Diseases. A Report of Six Cases, Blood, 5, 191, 1950.

143a.FARMER, R. G., COOPER, T. and PASCUZZI, C. A.: Cryoglobulinemia, Arch. Int. Med., 106, 483, 1960.

144. FARRERAS VALENTI, P., and VILASECA SABATER, J. M.: Etudes générales sur la pathologie, la clinique et la radiologie des localisations osseuses et articulaires dans les maladies du sang, Acta haemat., 2, 43, 1949.

144a.FEINLEIB, M. and MACMAHON, B.: Duration of Survival in Multiple Myeloma, J. Nat. Cancer Inst., 24, 1259, 1960.

145. FORBUS, W. D., PERLZWEIG, W. A., PARFENTJEV, I. A. and BURWELL, J. C., JR.: Bence-Jones Protein Excretion and Its Effect Upon the Kidney, Bull. Johns Hopkins Hosp., 57, 47, 1935.

145a.FRICK, P. G.: Inhibition of Conversion of Fibrinogen to Fibrin by Abnormal Proteins in Multiple Myeloma, Am. J. Clin. Path., 25, 1263, 1955.

145b.FLYNN, F. V. and STOW, ELIZABETH A.: Fractionation of Bence-Jones Protein by Starch Gel Electrophoresis, J. Clin. Path., 11, 334, 1958.

146. GESCHICKTER, C. F. and COPELAND, M. M.: Multiple Myeloma, Arch. Surg., 16, 807, 1928 (Bibliography).

147. GOOD, R. A. and CAMPBELL, B.: Relationship of Bone Marrow Plasmacytosis to the Changes in Serum Gamma Globulin in Rheumatic Fever, Am. J. Med., 9, 330, 1950.

148. GUNN, F. D. and MAHLE, A. E.: Megakaryoblastic Myeloma With Crystalline Protein in the Renal Tubes, Arch. Path., 26, 377, 1938.

149. GUTMAN, A. B., MOORE, D. H., GUTMAN, E. B., McCLELLAN, V. and KABAT, E. A.: Fractionation of Serum Proteins in Hyperproteinemia, With Special Reference to Multiple Myeloma, J. Clin. Invest., 20, 765, 1941; ibid., 22, 67, 1943.

149a.HAMPTON, J. M. and GANDY, J. R.: Plasmacytoma of the Gastro-intestinal Tract, Ann. Surg., 145, 415, 1957.

150. HEINIVAARA, O. and EISALO, A.: Multiple Myeloma, Acta med. scandinav., 168, 211, 1960.

151. HEISLER, S. and SCHWARTZMAN, J. J.: Variations in the Roentgen Appearance of the Skeletal System in Myeloma, Radiology, 58, 178, 1952.

152. HODLER, J.: Uber das Vorkommen osteoplastischer Knochenveränderungen bei der Kahlerschen Krankheit, Schweiz. med. Wchnschr., 88, 1065, 1958.

153. KENNY, J. J. and MOLONEY, W. C.: Long-

Term Survival in Multiple Myeloma, Ann. Int. Med., *45*, 950, 1956.

154. KINGERY, F. A. J. and MONTES, L. F.: A Nonacantholytic Bullous Dermatosis Associated with Multiple Myeloma, A. M. A. Arch. Dermat., *78*, 293, 1958.

155. KLEIN, H. and BLOCK, M.: Bone Marrow Plasmocytosis, Blood, *8*, 1034, 1953.

155a. KÖNIG, E. and KNEZEVIĆ, M.: Über ein Alpha-Myelom mit retothelialer Tumorbildung, Acta haemat., *23*, 172, 1960.

156. KORNGOLD, L. and LIPARI, R.: Multiple-Myeloma Proteins. I. Immunological Studies, Cancer, *9*, 183, 1956.

157. KRISS, J. P., BIERMAN, H. R., THOMAS, S. F. and NEWELL, R. R.: Treatment of Multiple Myeloma with Radioactive Iodine and Radioactive Iodinated Serum Albumin, Radiology, *65*, 241, 1955.

158. LAWRENCE, J. H. and ROSENTHAL, R. L.: Multiple Myeloma Associated With Polycythemia, Am. J. M. Sc., *218*, 149, 1949.

159. LAWSON, H. A., STUART, C. A., PAULL, A. M., PHILLIPS, A. M. and PHILLIPS, R. W.: Observations on the Antibody Content of the Blood in Patients with Multiple Myeloma, New England J. Med., *252*, 13, 1955.

160. LERNER, A. B. and WATSON, C. J.: Studies on Cryoglobulins, Am. J. M. Sc., *214*, 410 and 416, 1947.

160a. LEWIN, H. and STEIN, J. M.: Solitary Plasma Cell Myeloma with New Bone Formation, Am. J. Roentgenol., *79*, 630, 1958.

162. LICHTENSTEIN, L. and JAFFE, H. L.: Multiple Myeloma, Arch. Path., *44*, 207, 1947.

162a. LUTTGENS, W. F. and BAYRD, E. D.: Treatment of Multiple Myeloma with Urethane, J.A.M.A., *147*, 824, 1951.

163. MACKAY, I. R., ERIKSEN, N., MOTULSKY, A. G. and Volwiler, W.: Cryo- and Macroglobulinemia, Am. J. Med., *20*, 564, 1956.

163a. MACMAHON, B. and CLARK, D. W.: The Incidence of Multiple Myeloma, J. Chron. Dis., *4*, 508, 1956.

164. MAGNUS-LEVY, A.: Multiple Myeloma (XII), Acta med. scandinav., *95*, 218, 1938; J. Mt. Sinai Hosp., *19*, 8, 1952.

164a. MARTIN, W. J., MATHIESON, D. R and EIGLER, J. O. C.: Pyroglobulinemia: Further Observations and Review of 20 Cases, Proc. Staff Meet., Mayo Clin., *34*, 95, 1959.

165. MARTIN, N. H.: A Study of the Plasma and Tissue Globulins in Myelomatosis, J. Clin. Invest., *26*, 1189, 1947.

166. MARTIN, N. H. and SCULTHORPE, H.: The Non-Protein Constituents of the Plasma in Myelomatosis, J. Clin. Path., *11*, 330, 1958.

166a. McGEOWN, MARY G. and MONTGOMERY, D. A. D.: Multiple Myelomatosis Simulating Hyperparathyroidism, Brit. M. J., *1*, 86, 1956.

166b. MERIGAN, T. C., JR. and HAYES, R. E., III: Treatment of Hypercalcemia in Multiple Myeloma, A.M.A. Arch. Int. Med., *107*, 389, 1961.

167. MORISSETTE, L. and WATKINS, C. H.: Multiple Myeloma, Proc. Staff. Meet. Mayo Clinic, *17*, 433, 1942.

167a. NADEAU, L. A., MAGALINI, S. I. and STEFANINI, M.: Familial Multiple Myeloma, A. M. A. Arch. Path., *61*, 101, 1956.

167b. NELSON, M. G. and LYONS, A. R.: Plasmacytoma of Lymph Glands, Cancer, *10*, 1275, 1957.

167c. NIKKILÄ, E. A. and PESOLA, R.: Serum Protein-Bound Carbohydrate Pattern in Normal Subjects and in Patients with Multiple Myeloma, Scandinav. J. Clin. & Lab. Invest.. *12.* 209, 1960.

168. OLHAGEN. B.. THORELL, B. and WISING, P.: The Endocellular Nucleic Acid Distribution and Plasma Protein Formation in Myelomatosis, Scandinav. J. Clin. & Lab. Invest., *1*, 49, 1949.

168a. OSSERMAN, E. F.: Plasma-Cell Myeloma, New England J. Med., *261*, 952 and 1006, 1959.

169. OSSERMAN, E. F. and LAWLOR, D. P.: Abnormal Serum and Urine Proteins in Thirty-five Cases of Multiple Myeloma, as Studied by Filter Paper Electrophoresis, Am. J. Med., *18*, 462, 1955; J. Clin. Invest., *36*, 352, 1957.

169a. POTTER, M., FAHEY, J. L. and PILGRIM, H. I.: Abnormal Serum Protein and Bone Destruction in Transmissible Mouse Plasma Cell Neoplasm (Multiple Myeloma), Proc. Soc. Exper. Biol. & Med., *94*, 327, 1957; Proc. Am. Assn. Cancer Res., *3*, 14, 1959; Blood, *15*, 103, 1960.

169b. PUTNAM, F. W.: Plasma-Cell Myeloma and Macroglobulinemia, New England J. Med., *261*, 902, 1959.

170. PUTNAM, F. W. and UDIN, B.: Proteins in Multiple Myeloma, J. Biol. Chem., *202*, 727, 1953; *ibid.*, *203*, 347, 1953; *ibid.*, *212*, 361 and 371, 1955; Science, *120*, 848, 1954.

171. REINER, M. and STERN, K. G.: Electrophoretic Studies on the Protein Distribution in the Serum of Multiple Myeloma Patients, Acta hæmat., *9*, 19, 1953.

172. ROSENTHAL, N. and VOGEL, P.: Value of the Sternal Puncture in the Diagnosis of Multiple Myeloma, J. Mt. Sinai Hosp., *4*, 1001, 1938.

173. RUNDLES, R. W., DILLON, M. L. and DILLON, E. D.: Multiple Myeloma. III. Effect of Urethane Therapy on Plasma Cell Growth,

Abnormal Serum Protein Components and Bence-Jones Proteinuria, J. Clin. Invest. *29*, 1243, 1950; Blood, *4*, 201, 1949; Am. J. Roentgenol., *64*, 799, 1950; J. Clin. Invest. *30*, 1125, 1951; Proc. Third National Cancer Conference, Philadelphia, J. B. Lippincott Company, 1957, p. 389.

174. SACHS, B. A., CADY, P. and Ross, G.: An Abnormal Lipid-like Material and Carbohydrate in the Sera of Patients with Multiple Myeloma, Am. J. Med., *17*, 662, 1954.

175. SANDKÜHLER, S.: A Simple and Sensitive Test for Bence-Jones Protein, Am. J. Clin. Path., *22*, 282, 1952.

176. SHAPIRO, H. D. and WATSON, R. J.: Splenic Aspirations in Multiple Myeloma, Blood, *8*, 755, 1953.

177. SMITH, E. L., BROWN, D. M., McFADDEN, M. L., BUETTNER-JANUSCH, V. and JAGER, B. V.: Physical, Chemical, and Immunological Studies on Globulins from Multiple Myeloma, J. Biol. Chem., *216*, 601, 1955.

178. SMITH, R. P. and SILBERBERG, M.: Multiple Myeloma of Hemocytoblastic Type, Arch. Path., *21*, 578, 1936.

179. SNAPPER, I.: Treatment of Multiple Myeloma With "Stilbamidine," J.A.M.A., *137*, 513, 1948; Acta hæmat., *3*, 9, 1950.

179a. SNAPPER, I. and ORES, R. O.: Determination of Bence Jones Protein in the Urine, J.A.M.A., *173*, 1137, 1960.

180. SNAPPER, I., TURNER, L. B. and MOSCOVITZ, H. L.: *Multiple Myeloma*, New York, Grune & Stratton, 1953.

180a. STARCICH, R.: Histopathological and Microradiographical Observations on Myelomatous Osteopathy, Acta haemat., *18*, 113, 1957.

181. STEINMANN, B.: Über azurophile, stäbchenförmige Einschlüsse in den Zellen eines multiplen Myeloms, Deutsch. Arch. klin. Med., *185*, 49, 1939.

182. STEWART, A. and WEBER, F. P.: Myelomatosis, Quart. J. Med., *7*, 211, 1938.

183. TAYLOR, C. E.: Erythroid Multiple Myeloma, Am. J. Clin. Path., *17*, 222, 1947.

183a. THIÉRY, J. P.: Etude sur le plasmacyte en contraste de phase et en microscope électronique, Rev. hémat., *13*, 61, 1958.

184. TRUBOWITZ, S.: The Sternal Marrow Aspiration of Amyloid in Multiple Myeloma, Blood, *5*, 581, 1950.

185. VAZQUEZ, J. J.: Immunocytochemical Study of Plasma Cells in Multiple Myeloma, J. Lab. & Clin. Med., *51*, 271, 1958.

185a. VERSTRAETE, M. and VERMYLEN, C.: Recherches sur l'antithrombine V dans la maladie de Kahler, Acta haemat., *22*, 240, 1959.

185b. VICTOR, M., BANKER, BETTY Q. and ADAMS,

R. D.: The Neuropathy of Multiple Myeloma, J. Neurol., Neurosurg. & Psychiat., *21*, 73, 1958.

186. WEISE, H. and LOHSE, H.: Über Plasmazellen bei Plasmocytomen, Folia haemat., *2*, 11, 1958.

186a. WEISS, D. L. and DE LOS SANTOS, R.: Urethane-Induced Hepatic Failure in Man, Am. J. Med., *28*, 476, 1960.

187. WINTROBE, M. M. and BUELL, M. V.: Hyperproteinemia Associated With Multiple Myeloma, Bull. Johns Hopkins Hosp., *52*, 156, 1933.

188. ZADEK, I.: Herkunft und hämatologischer Nachweis der "Myelomzellen," Folia hæmat., *58*, 196, 1937.

189. ZINNEMAN, H. H., GLENCHUR, H. and GLEASON, D. F.: The Significance of Urine Electrophoresis in Patients with Multiple Myeloma, A. M. A. Arch. Int. Med., *106*, 172, 1960.

190. ZINNEMAN, H. H. and HALL, W. H.: Recurrent Pneumonia in Multiple Myeloma and Some Observations on Immunologic Response, Ann. Int. Med., *41*, 1152, 1954; A. M. A. Arch. Int. Med., *103*, 173, 1959.

Macroglobulinemia

199. BAYRD, E. D.: Continuous Chlorambucil Therapy in Primary Macroglobulinemia of Waldenström, Proc. Staff Meet., Mayo Clin., *36*, 135, 1961.

200. BLOCH, H. S., PRASAD, ANANDA, ANASTASI, ADA and BRIGGS, D. R.: Serum Protein Changes in Waldenström's Macroglobulinemia during Administration of a Low Molecular Weight Thiol (Penicillamine), J. Lab. & Clin. Med., *56*, 212, 1960.

201. CLAUSEN, J.: Macroglobulinemia in a Transplantable Mouse Leukemia, Proc. Soc. Exper. Biol. & Med., *103*, 802, 1960.

202. DUTCHER, T. F. and FAHEY, J. L.: The Histopathology of the Macroglobulinemia of Waldenström, J. Nat. Cancer Inst., *22*, 88, 1959.

203. GOLDBERG, A. F.: An Unusual Lymphomatous Disease Associated with Intracytoplasmic Crystals in Lymphoplasmocytoid Cells, Blood, *16*, 1693, 1960.

204. KAPPELER, R., KREBS, A. and RIVA, G.: Klinik der Makroglobulinämie Waldenström: Beschreibung von 21 Fällen und Übersicht der Literatur, Helvet. med. acta, *25*, 54, 1958.

205. KAPPELER, R., GUGLER, E. and RIVA, G.: Zur Frage des atypischen Morbus Waldenström, Schweiz. med. Wchnschr., *89*, 1331, 1959.

206. KORNGOLD, L. and VAN LEEUWEN, GERDA:

Macroglobulinemia, J. Exper. Med., *106*, 467 and 477, 1957; *ibid.*, *110*, 1, 1959.

207. LAURELL, C.-B., LAURELL, H. and WALDEN-ström, J.: Glycoproteins in Serum from Patients with Myeloma, Macroglobulinemia and Related Conditions, Am. J. Med. *22*, 24, 1957.

207a. LOGOTHETIS, J., SILVERSTEIN, P. and COE, J.: Neurologic Aspects of Waldenström's Macroglobulinemia, Arch. Neurol., *3*, 564, 1960.

208. MACKAY, K. R., TAFT, L. I. and WOODS, E. F.: Clinical Features and Pathogenesis of Macroglobulinaemia, Brit. M. J., 1, 561, 1957; Australasian Ann. Med., *8*, 158, 1959.

210. MILLER, D.: Heparin Precipitability of the Macroglobulin in a Patient with Waldenström's Macroglobulinemia, Blood, *16*, 1313, 1960.

211. PACHTER, M. R., JOHNSON, S. A., NEBLETT, T. R. and TRUANT, J. P.: Bleeding, Platelets, and Macroglobulinemia, Am. J. Clin. Path., *31*, 467, 1959.

213. RITZMANN, S. E., THURM, R. H., TRUAX, W. E. and LEVIN, W. C.: The Syndrome of Macroglobulinemia, A. M. A. Arch. Int. Med., *105*, 939, 1960.

214. RITZMANN, S. E., COLEMAN, S. L. and LEVIN, W. C.: The Effect of Some Mercaptanes upon a Macrocryogelglobulin; Modifications Induced by Cysteamine, Penicillamine and Penicillin, J. Clin. Invest., *39*, 1320, 1960.

215. SCHWAB, P. J. and FAHEY, J. L.: Treatment of Waldenström's Macroglobulinemia by Plasmapheresis, New England J. Med., *263*, 574, 1960.

216. Waldenström, J.: Incipient Myelomatosis or "Essential" Hyperglobulinemia with Fibrinogenopenia—A New Syndrome? Acta med. scandinav., *117*, 216, 1944.

Hypogammaglobulinemia Associated with Hematological Abnormalities

219. CITRON, K. M.: Agammaglobulinaemia with Splenomegaly, Brit. M. J., *1*, 1148, 1957.

220. GOOD, R. A. and ZAK, S. J.: Disturbances in Gamma Globulin Synthesis as "Experiments of Nature", Pediatrics, *18*, 109, 1956.

221. JIM, R. T. S. and REINHARD, E. H.: Agammaglobulinemia and Chronic Lymphocytic Leukemia, Ann. Int. Med., *44*, 790, 1956.

222. KUSHNER, D. S., DUBIN, A., DONLON, W. P. and BRONSKY, D.: Familial Hypogammaglobulinemia, Splenomegaly and Leukopenia, Am. J. Med., *29*, 33, 1960.

224. PRASAD, ANANDA S., REINER, E. and WATSON, C. J.: Syndrome of Hypogammaglobulinemia, Splenomegaly and Hypersplenism, Blood, *12*, 926, 1957.

225. ULTMANN, J. E., FISH, W., OSSERMAN, E. and GELLHORN, A.: The Clinical Implications of Hypogammaglobulinemia in Patients with Chronic Lymphocytic Leukemia and Lymphocytic Lymphosarcoma, Ann. Int. Med., *51*, 501, 1959.

Chapter 21

Agranulocytosis and Infectious Mononucleosis

AGRANULOCYTOSIS

History.—In 1922 Werner Schultz[43] drew attention to a syndrome of unknown etiology which he had observed in women of middle age especially, and which was characterized by severe sore throat, marked prostration, extreme reduction or even complete disappearance of the granulocytes from the blood, and, in rapid succession, sepsis and death. He considered this to be a clinical entity. A detailed report of a similar condition had been published by Brown[6] in 1902 and by Türk[53] in 1907. It was not until the description of 6 cases by Schultz, however, that general interest in this disorder was aroused. After 1922 a large number of cases was described and a more comprehensive picture of the disease was formed. In recent years the relationship of the condition to the taking of certain drugs has been demonstrated.

Terminology and Definition.—A great variety of names has been used in referring to this condition: agranulocytosis, agranulocytic angina, granulocytosis, idiopathic, malignant or pernicious leukopenia, and granulocytic hypoplasia.

The chief characteristic of the blood in this disorder is a reduction in the number of granulocytes, but in many instances there is also a diminution in the absolute number of other types of leukocytes. There is justification, therefore, for the names malignant or pernicious leukopenia but many writers dislike the designation leukopenia or even granulocytopenia because these terms are used in referring to a reaction of the blood which occurs in a great variety of diseases. To refer to the disorder which is characterized by an acute course, fever, and usually necrotic lesions in the throat and elsewhere, as well as leukopenia with pronounced granulocytopenia but without significant changes in the red corpuscles or platelets, usage in Europe[35,39] as well as in this country continues to favor the name suggested by Schultz, namely, agranulocytosis.

Etiology.—Although the majority of cases have been reported in the United States and Europe, agranulocytosis has been observed in all parts of the world.[35] The disease makes its appearance everywhere in the form of isolated cases.

Relatively few cases were described between 1922 and 1929, but in the next five years many cases were reported.[39] In 1931 Kracke[26] pointed out that the sudden appearance of many cases of agranulocytosis corresponded with the introduction of certain coal-tar derivatives. The disorder was especially common in the countries in which such drugs were in great use, those affected were chiefly women of good economic status, as well as nurses and other medical workers to whom these drugs were easily accessible. He noted that a history of the use of one of the coal-tar derivatives was often obtainable in cases of agranulocytosis. Shortly afterwards, several reports[30,35,54] appeared which incriminated **amidopyrine** ("Pyramidon") as the offending drug. It was noted that the majority of patients who developed agranulocytosis were adults, usually past middle age.[35] In proportion to other causes, agranulocytosis was a relatively frequent cause of sore throat among people over forty years of age, whereas it was very rare under twenty-five years of age. Satisfactory accounts of typical agranulocytosis were found in only 9 children.[35] It was observed again that the condition was much more frequent among females than males, the ratio being about two or three to one.[35] In relation to amidopyrine, it was reported[30] that the mortality in 6 patients who continued the use of drugs containing amidopyrine, was 100 per cent, whereas in a group of 8 patients who took no more amidopyrine, only 2 died. The increased incidence of agranulocytosis in Denmark until 1934 corresponded exactly with the increased sale of amidopyrine.[35]

After 1934 the number of cases of agranulocytosis decreased. This coincided with the reduced sales of amidopyrine following reports of its injurious effects.[35] Later, however, as new drugs were introduced new cases appeared. A pattern was repeated which has now become a familiar one. A new agent is described and in a few years it is widely used. At first it is hailed as being nontoxic; ultimately a report appears describing the development of agranulocytosis in association with its use. This is followed by another case, and another, and the circumstantial evidence becomes impressive. The drug loses popularity and is employed with more discrimination than before. The number of cases of agranulocytosis due to this agent decreases sharply, only to be replaced by others as new drugs are added to the therapeutic armamentarium.

It seems clear that the explanation for this train of events depends mainly on the fact that the syndrome first recognized in association with the taking of amidopyrine develops only in a very small proportion of those taking the offending drug. As was pointed out in an earlier chapter (p. 255), among the many different causes of leukopenia, certain chemical and physical agents can be included. The chemical agents can, in general, be classified in two groups (Table 21–1); namely, those which, like certain physical agents, can be expected to produce leukopenia regularly provided a sufficiently large dose is given. Some of these have been discussed already since they are used in the treatment of the leukemias and "lymphomas."

There is another group of compounds which is associated with the development of untoward reactions in only a small proportion of persons taking them. Many of these were listed in earlier chapters dealing with pancytopenia (p. 553) and thrombocytopenia (p. 818). Some have been associated with the development of one or both of these hematological changes rather than leukopenia. Others have more often been associated with the occurrence of leukopenia (Group B, Table 21–1). The low incidence of the untoward effects on the hemopoietic system is indicated by various studies. Thus, in a series of 400 cases of arthritis in which amidopyrine was given, agranulocytosis developed in four.[36] In another series of 103 cases, agranulocytosis was not encountered at all.[46] Similar statistics have been reported by others.[12] In association with the administration of thiouracil, a reduction in the leukocyte count to less than 3000 per c.mm., with slight to marked granulocytopenia, was observed in 3.4 per cent of 781 patients taking this agent and a depression or absence of granulocytes together with

Table 21–1—Agents Associated with the Occurrence of Leukopenia

A. *Agents which regularly produce* leukopenia if a sufficient dose is given:
   (1) Ionizing radiation (roengten rays, radioactive P, Au, etc.)
   (2) Mustards (sulfur and nitrogen mustards, triethylenemelamine (TEM), etc.)
   (3) Urethane, busulfan, Demecolcin
   (4) Benzene
   (5) Antimetabolites (antifolic compounds, 6-mercaptopurine, etc.)

B. *Agents occasionally associated* with leukopenia (granulocytopenia):

analgesics	*Amidopyrine* and drugs containing it (amidophen, amytal compound, causaline,[2,32] cibalgin,[12] neonal compound, neurodyne, peralga, pyraminal, yeast-vite,[27] etc.) Antipyrine,[24d] novaldin (novalgin)[20b,25,27] Phenylbutazone (butazolidin)[24d,48,48a]
antithyroid drugs	Thiouracil,[33b,52a] propylthiouracil,[8a] methylthiouracil,[35a] methimazole,[38a] carbimazole[51a]
anticonvulsants	Trimethadione (tridione),[32a] phethenylate,[21b] phenacemide,[21b] diethazine[20c], diphenylhydantoin sodium[50a]
sulfonamides	Sulfanilamide,[1c,5,51] prontosil,[4] sulfapyridine,[41] salicylazosulfapyridine,[38c] sulfathiazole,[24c] sulfadiazine,[20d] succinylsulfathiazole,[24a] sulfisoxazole (Gantrisin),[31a] sulfamethoxypyridazine (Kinex)
antihistaminics	Pyribenzamine,[7a] methaphenilene (diatrin),[12a] phenothiazine,[54a] thenalidine[1]
antimicrobial agents . . .	Organic arsenicals,[14,29b] chloramphenicol,[53b] thiosemicarbazone (tibione),[11a] ristocetin[34a]
miscellaneous	Dinitrophenol,[18] tolbutamide,[50a] chlorpropamide,[24b] carbutamide (antidiabetic drugs), phenindione[51b] (anticoagulant), gold salts,[35] industrial chemicals[21a]
tranquilizers	Chlorpromazine and other phenothiazine derivatives[13a,25a,34e] (mepazine, promazine, prochlorperazine, etc.)
Compounds mentioned only in one or two reports . .	Procaine amide,[32b] barbiturates,[54] "new allonal,"[19] acetophenetidin (phenacetin), acetanilid,[27] pyrithyldione (presidon),[53a] quinine,[35] cincophen,[49a] plasmochin,[35] salol,[56] antimony (neostibasan),[57] bismuth,[35] fumagillin,[31] diamox,[34d] thioglycolic acid ("cold wave"),[8b] D.D.T.,[56a] mercurial diuretics,[25c] novobiocin[45]

infection in the throat and neck developed in 1.7 per cent of 1,091 cases.[33b] Leukopenia was observed in 1.5 per cent of 672 patients treated with propylthiouracil[1e] and was stated to have occurred in 4.1 per cent of 1,886 patients given methylthiouracil.[35a] Neutropenia was noted in only three of 460 patients given sulfadiazine[13] and acute agranulocytosis has been stated as occurring in 1 per cent of patients treated with tibione.[11a] In the case of the phenothiazine derivatives, published data differ widely but a ratio of 1:700 for the occurrence of agranulocytosis and perhaps twice as often for uncomplicated leukopenia is probably a reasonable approximation.[13a] The incidence of leukopenia in association with certain other drugs is so low that one wonders whether in these cases the occurrence of the leukopenia is not purely coincidental. Thus, the reports incriminating the barbiturates are very few[19,54] in comparison to their wide use. Nevertheless, in two subjects a new attack of agranulocytosis was reported to have developed following readministration of amytal.[54]

In the case of most of the agents which are only occasionally associated with the development of leukopenia, the quantity of drug employed appears to be of no importance. Thus, in a number of instances fatal agranulocytosis was observed to occur following the taking of even a single dose of amidopyrine. A number of investigators showed that, following recovery from an attack of agranulocytosis, the administration of small amounts of the suspected agent (amidopyrine, thiouracil) was followed within six to ten hours by disappearance of all the neutrophils from the blood.[1d,3,30,35,39] Preceding the granulocytopenia a sensation of general malaise as well as a chill and fever were sometimes observed.

That the mechanism of action may differ with different drugs and in different individuals is suggested by the observation that with some drugs changes in the blood have not developed before several weeks of administration, in contrast to the prompt effect in the case of amidopyrine and some other agents. Thus, when granulocytopenia followed thiouracil administration, it usually developed after four to eight weeks of treatment.[33b] This slow effect had also been noted with sulfonamide compounds,[5,13,27,41] although exceptions were observed.[38b] Again, in the case of phenothiazine derivatives, granulocytopenia was found to be of gradual onset.[34e] Leukopenia was noted only after 13 to 171 days (average 50 days) of continuous administration.[25a] We noted in cases treated with thiouracil that transient, moderate leukopenia sometimes occurred in three weeks to five months after initiation of therapy but the leukocyte count returned to normal in seven out of nine instances even though thiouracil was continued. Others had similar experiences.[1d,31b] Transient leukopenia of slight degree was described as developing after one to three weeks of therapy with sulfanilamide in as many as 46 per cent of patients.[5] This has also been noted in patients treated with mepazine.[13a] Re-

administration of the phenothiazine derivatives has often failed to induce granulocytopenia or has done so only after several months of administration.[13a]

It has not been possible to incriminate drugs in all cases of agranulocytosis. The proportion of cases in which no etiologic agent could be suspected has been estimated to be 44 per cent,[32] 38 per cent,[39] or much smaller.[26,35] In a certain number of cases a more adequate history perhaps would have revealed the cause but undoubtedly there are some in which another type of etiologic factor must be postulated.

Pathogenesis.—Although there is obvious evidence of *infection* when the full-blown picture of agranulocytosis has developed, and blood cultures have been positive in a number of cases, there is reason to assume that the infection is secondary to the granulocytopenia rather than its cause. There is no seasonal incidence of agranulocytosis nor has there been evidence of spread by contact. Attempts to produce agranulocytosis in animals by the injection of organisms isolated from patients have failed.

Kracke pointed out that the drugs producing agranulocytosis were those of the "benzamine" group (benzene ring with an attached amine) and suggested that their action might be a *leukotoxic effect* due to an oxidation product. No evidence has been produced, however, that the action of drugs such as amidopyrine is a simple toxic effect. It is noteworthy that numerous attempts to produce agranulocytosis in animals have failed. The feeding or injection of amidopyrine to rabbits, guinea pigs, dogs, rats and monkeys[8,20,21,27,55] has been unsuccessful. Neutropenia was reported only in two animals.[7,30] The syndrome produced in dogs fed amidopyrine and a black-tongue-producing diet[33] differed from agranulocytosis in man. There appears to be no relationship between feline agranulocytosis, which is caused by a virus,[29] and human agranulocytosis. Extensive unpublished studies in our own laboratory have met with similar failure.

It has been noted that the drugs which may produce agranulocytosis occasionally in man are frequently the cause of other manifestations of idiosyncrasy, such as rash, urticaria, edema and asthma. Furthermore, as already stated, the amount consumed when agranulocytosis has occurred has often been very small, although frequently the affected person has taken the same agent before. These observations, together with the fever, chills, headache and dizziness which have been associated with the development of agranulocytosis, suggest that the reaction is that of an *allergic process*. Nevertheless, with the exception of one report of a strongly positive skin reaction following the intradermal injection of a mixture of amidopyrine and blood serum in 3 patients,[9] scratch tests, patch tests, passive transfers and intradermal tests with the offending drugs in patients who had recovered from agranulocytosis, have been negative.[21]

A noteworthy advance in the study of the pathogenesis of agranulocytosis was made when it was demonstrated that the transfusion of blood withdrawn three hours after administration of a test dose of amidopyrine to a sensitive patient, produced outspoken granulocytopenia in two subjects which lasted three to five hours.[33a] Furthermore, in the plasma and serum of the patient a substance was found which produced agglutination of homologous and heterologous leukocytes *in vitro*. The leukocyte-agglutinating substance was found to be a globulin. Subsequent studies indicated that destruction of the agglutinated leukocytes occurs *in vivo*, probably in the lung capillaries. The changes in the bone marrow were attributed to a precipitate depletion and exhaustion of the bone marrow due to the greatly increased peripheral destruction of the granulocytes. The same investi-

gator was able to produce an antileukocytic serum which was capable of producing agranulocytosis in guinea pigs. It was postulated that the offending drug combines with a protein in the serum to form an antigen. This causes sensitization and the antibodies so formed become attached to the leukocytes which are then agglutinated and destroyed when the leukocyte-bound antibody and antigen come in contact.

These investigators were able to demonstrate **leukocyte agglutinins** not only in drug-sensitive cases, but also in cases of leukopenia associated with a large variety of disorders.[33a] Further investigation has demonstrated that the interpretation of leukocyte agglutinins is complex.[11] They are found in persons who have had blood transfusions and occur with greater frequency as the number of transfusions increases.[1a] Such agglutinins appear to be isoantibodies[40] and are not related to the presence of leukopenia.[1a, 34c] Transfusion reactions have been observed which may have been due to sensitization against leukocytes given in earlier transfusions (p. 360). Incomplete white cell isoantibodies are found more frequently than complete ones.[18a] They are rare, however, in persons who have not been transfused although they have been reported in patients with collagen disorders[24e] and in pregnant women.[34c] In the latter, feto-maternal leukocyte incompatibility has been postulated to be the cause. In the absence of these various circumstances the demonstration of leukocyte agglutinins is quite uncommon and to what extent such agglutinins are "auto-aggressive"[24e] and cause leukopenia is uncertain.[1a] Thus their role in the pathogenesis of agranulocytosis remains to be demonstrated. The role of leuko-agglutinins in the pathogenesis of neonatal neutropenia will be considered shortly (p. 1103).

As suggested earlier, the mode of action of the various types of drugs occasionally associated with the development of agranulocytosis may not be the same. In contrast with the findings described in cases attributable to amidopyrine administration, in patients who developed granulocytopenia while receiving chlorpromazine the marrow picture suggested temporary aplasia.[34e] No leukoagglutinins or leukolysins could be demonstrated. In these and in other cases[13a] a higher frequency in women than in men was noted and it has been claimed that the Negro is relatively immune to agranulocytosis associated with the taking of drugs. Whether or not this claim can be supported, it must be conceded that constitutional factors may play a role in the pathogenesis of some instances of agranulocytosis. No convincing evidence has ever been produced that such individual factors as the onset of the menstrual cycle[52] or the operation of other endocrine factors,[23,78] fatigue,[38] traumatic shock[13] or infection[38] are of any etiologic importance. There is nothing, furthermore, to indicate that patients who develop agranulocytosis have suffered previous bone marrow damage. In fact, in many instances they have responded normally to infections before or after the attack of agranulocytosis and, as a rule, have been able to take drugs which, in other individuals, have produced agranulocytosis. For example, those sensitive to one sulfonamide are not necessarily sensitive to other sulfonamides.

The changes which have been observed in the blood and bone marrow have been interpreted in various ways. The observation that there is a scarcity of juvenile and segmented neutrophilic leukocytes in the bone marrow in cases of agranulocytosis, less mature forms being plentiful (p. 1104), led to the suggestion that the primary disturbance is a failure of maturation of granulocytes ("maturation arrest"[15]). That this might not be a correct interpretation was suggested by various bone marrow studies. Thus, in a patient who had had agranulocytosis following the use of amidopyrine, the administration of a test dose was associated with a change in two days from normal bone marrow findings to practically complete loss of promyelocytes, myelocytes and metamyelocytes, while the number of more mature granulocytes was normal. At this stage the blood was still normal and complete granulocytopenia did not develop until five days later.[35] Whereas in some patients leukopenia may develop in an interval as short as six hours following ingestion of amidopyrine,[35] this sort of reaction is not always found. Thus, in a patient who was sensitive to salicylazolsulfapyridine, a slow fall in granulocytes in the blood occurred which was associated with a decrease in marrow granulocyte precursors at all stages.[12c]

Some of the observations which have been recorded are consistent with the action of a toxic agent which inhibits cell metabolism and division or the effect of an antibody on dividing cells in the bone marrow. However, failure of leukocyte production alone could not account for the very rapid depletion of cells from the blood which has been noted in many instances, since the bone marrow stores are so abundant. To explain the rapid disappearance of granulocytes from the blood, abnormal peripheral destruction of polymorphonuclear leukocytes[39] or segregation of the cells, as would occur if they should stick to the capillary endothelium,[13] has been postulated. As already indicated, it is likely that different pathogenetic mechanisms are involved in the various circumstances in which granulocytopenia is encountered.

Symptomatology.—The type of case described by Schultz presents a dramatic picture. The onset of the illness is sudden and is marked by a chill, high fever and necrotizing angina. Prostration is extreme. The patients often look pale, yet the mucous membranes are of normal color or cyanotic. Jaundice is often present. Gangrenous ulceration may be found on the gums, tonsils, soft palate, lips, pharynx or buccal mucous membranes, and somewhat less frequently in the skin, nose, vagina, uterus, rectum or anus. A dirty yellow, gray or greenish-black membrane covers an underlying ulcer but the surrounding tissue may show little reaction. Regional adenopathy is present in such cases but generalized lymphadenopathy does not occur. Splenomegaly and bone tenderness are very unusual and the liver is rarely enlarged. The fever is high, the pulse rapid and weak and death ensues in a few days. Plum[35] noted that the duration of the illness in fatal cases was three to nine days with few exceptions. Three-fourths of his cases died within three days following admission.

When it is possible to obtain an adequate history, it is often found that a sensation of fatigue and overpowering weakness has preceded by two or three days the onset of the illness. Sore throat may not appear until twelve to twenty-four hours after the onset[35] of other symptoms. Painful deglutition, headache, rigors and chilly sensations are common and vomiting, dyspnea, mental confusion and pain in different parts of the body may occur. Dermatitis or a rash has been observed in about 10 per cent of cases.[35]

The train of events in these cases may be divided into three periods: (1) malaise, fever and perhaps a chill, prodromal symptoms which are often forgotten; (2) a period of freedom from symptoms except for fatigue and prostration, during which time the leukocyte count falls and the granulocytes disappear; (3) the final and frequently fatal stage when, the resistence being lowered by the absence of granulocytes, infection occurs in those regions normally harboring bacteria and progresses with the extreme rapidity to be expected in defenseless tissues.

Cases have been described in which the course was less rapid and the symptoms not as fulminating. These cases should perhaps not be classed with those presenting the typical Schultz syndrome. In certain cases permanent injury of the bone marrow may have been the cause, rather than the temporary effects of what appears to be an allergic reaction. In other instances anemia was present. The latter cases were discussed in an earlier chapter (p. 549). In general the "atypical" cases have been more chronic than those which Schultz described.

More Chronic Forms of Granulocytopenia.—These cases are, in the main, ill-defined and their differentiation from one another is difficult. Nevertheless, for descriptive purposes at least, they may be separated into several groups:

(1) **Periodic or Cyclic Neutropenia.**[37]—The disorder may begin in infancy or becomes evident at any age, even after sixty. It persists for decades. The striking feature is the regularity with which the episodes of neutropenia, together with symptoms of malaise, fever, chills, stomatitis and various infections, especially of the oral, pharyngeal and anal mucosa, recur. The average cycle is twenty-one days but extremes of fourteen and forty-five days have been described. Splenomegaly, adenopathy, arthralgia and abdominalgia may occur. The episodes may last ten days. The leukopenia is moderately severe (2000 to 4000 leukocytes per c.mm.) and the granulocytopenia has often been extreme (0 to 16 per cent neutrophils). Monocytosis often compensates for the neutropenia and eosinophilia frequently appears in the recovery phase. The bone marrow according to different observers has been normally cellular, hypoplastic or hyperplastic with, however, a reduced number of mature forms of granulocytes. Serial bone marrow examinations in one case revealed a cyclic arrest of production of the entire neutrophil series.[34b] Some 34

cases have been reported.[1f] Nothing has been found which will interrupt the cylic changes and their cause is a mystery.

(2) **"Primary Splenic Neutropenia."**[56]—This syndrome is characterized by fever, pain over the splenic region and splenic enlargement as well as essentially normal, or somewhat hyperplastic, bone marrow. In the few cases which have been reported[12b,28,38d,42a] the manifestations were acute, subacute or chronic and in one instance were recurrent. The splenomegaly ranged from slight to quite marked. Thrombocytopenia and hepatic dysfunction were observed in one case.[38d] Relief of all symptoms followed splenectomy. The removed organ showed extreme clasmatocytosis with excessive phagocytosis of granulocytes in the majority of the cases. Consequently the disorder was attributed to excessive lysis of neutrophils by the spleen.[34] This is considered by Doan to be a form of "hypersplenism" (p. 1051) in which the leukocytes rather than the erythrocytes are the object of splenic hyperactivity. The related syndrome, "primary splenic panhematopenia," has been discussed already (p. 1052).

(3) **Chronic Hypoplastic Neutropenia.**[42,47]—This syndrome in many ways resembles "primary splenic neutropenia" except that marked *hypoplasia* of the granulocytic elements is found on marrow aspiration and splenectomy is of no therapeutic value. The course is extremely chronic and is characterized by repeated infections. There may be slight or moderate splenomegaly. The neutropenia may be severe, absolute lymphocytosis and monocytosis are common and slight anemia and thrombocytopenia have been noted at times in addition to the neutropenia.

(4) **Chronic Granulocytopenia in Childhood.**[17,53b,53c]—These cases have been characterized by recurrent febrile episodes of upper respiratory tract infection, moderate lymphadenopathy and occasionally slight enlargement of the liver and spleen. There is marked neutropenia with usually a shift to the left and toxic granulation, relative and sometimes absolute lymphocytosis and, in a few instances, anemia and thrombocytopenia. The condition has extended over months or years but most commonly spontaneous remission has occurred.

(5) **Familial Neutropenia.**[4a,7c] — Cases somewhat similar to those described above have been reported in which there appeared to be a familial disposition. In one type, described among inbred families in a geographically isolated area of northern Sweden, the condition is thought to be transmitted genetically by a single autosomal recessive gene and is usually fatal.[25b] Similar cases, but associated with eosinophilia, have been reported.[1b]

(6) **Transitory Neonatal Neutropenia.**—Several instances of neutropenia in the newborn have been described which appear to be isoimmune in character.[4b,41a] In one family in which multiple cases were observed, a potent leukoagglutinin was found in the maternal serum which agglutinated leukocytes obtained from the father and all three available children but failed to agglutinate the mother's own cells.[27a] The symptoms in the infants ranged from mild manifestations with minor infections to a fulminating process with death due to overwhelming bacteremia. Severe neutropenia accompanied by monocytosis was present and the bone marrow showed numerous neutrophil precursors. A leukoagglutinin identical with that found in the mother was present in the youngest baby's serum and disappeared when the baby recovered. In two other cases, the mothers as well as the newborn infants were leukopenic and their bone marrows showed hyperplasia with "maturation arrest."[48b] One mother's serum contained a leukoagglutinin which could be transferred by transfusion to a normal person.

(7) **Miscellaneous Cases.**—Still other cases have been described which do not fit into the above categories.[6a,27,49] Common features are the vague complaints, the recurring infections, the neutropenia and the obscure etiology.

Among the various syndromes described above, "primary splenic neutropenia" differs from the rest in that the bone marrow is said to be hyperplastic and splenectomy has been reported to be curative. Splenectomy has been of little value in the other groups of cases. However, the appearance of the bone marrow is not alone an adequate criterion for splenectomy since bone marrow hyperplasia has been observed in patients who were not benefited by splenectomy. In some cases splenectomy has been followed by a rise in the leukocyte count and less tendency to recurring infection but the neutropenia has not been affected to any great degree. Cases such as these are probably more common than published reports indicate. The writer has seen several. It is likely that some cases of this type, if followed long enough, will be found to have leukemia, lymphosarcoma or disseminated lupus but there remain a significant number which have been studied for long periods of time and even at autopsy without the underlying cause having been discovered.

The Blood.—In typical agranulocytosis, granulocytopenia is the outstanding finding but usually other types of leukocytes are also reduced in number. In fulminating cases the leukocyte count when first made is usually less than 2000 per c.mm. and frequently it is below 1000. Counts as low as 50 have been recorded. The granulocytes may be completely absent or 1 to 2 per cent may be found. These cells may possess a pyknotic nucleus and vacuolated cytoplasm with poorly staining granules. Myelocytes are seen only when recovery begins.

The majority of the cells which are to be found are lymphocytes. In some cases monocytes may be increased relatively and even in absolute numbers. It was suggested that this represents a special type ("*leukopenic infectious monocytosis*").[40] In other instances a number of cells of the Türk "irritation" type have been described.[35]

In chronic or recurrent types, the leukocyte count is rarely below 2000 cells per c.mm. and the granulocytopenia is less pronounced.

In typical cases there is no anemia or thrombocytopenia and bleeding and coagulation times are normal. In a number of cases a slight or moderate degree of anemia has been observed but there is no evidence that this did not exist before the attack. The appearance of the red cells is normal and the number of reticulocytes is normal. The sedimentation rate, however, is greatly accelerated. The icterus index may be moderately raised.

Bone Marrow.—The bone marrow, examined by biopsy or postmortem, shows normal erythropoietic tissues and normal numbers of megakaryocytes. The picture as a whole may be one of moderate hypoplasia or of hyperplasia.[33a,39] The striking feature often has been a lack of granulocytes, including polymorphonuclear cells, metamyelocytes and myelocytes. The observation that promyelocytes and myeloblasts were found in the bone marrow at the time of examination led to the designation "maturation arrest"[15] which has been discussed already (p. 1101). Plasma cells, lymphocytes and reticulum cells may be increased in number.[10]

Other Laboratory Findings.—The urine may contain traces of albumin but it is otherwise normal. Blood cultures have been positive in a number of instances and a great variety of organisms has been found in these as well as in throat cultures. As already stated, there is no evidence that such organisms are to be regarded other than as secondary invaders.

Diagnosis.—Although it is most important that diagnosis in cases of acute agranulocytosis be made in the early stage before septicemia has developed, the early symptoms are so much like those of many other illnesses that early recognition is unlikely unless the physician has a high index of suspicion and obtains a leukocyte count whenever he is confronted with symptoms of unexplained weakness and profound exhaustion, or those of a severe acute infection. It is to be remembered that local symptoms in the buccal cavity may not always be present in agranulocytosis.[35] Where drugs are being employed which are known to be associated with granulocytopenia, it is important that the physician be alert for the possible development of this syndrome.

Once the blood has been examined, it should not be difficult to rule out the various types of pharyngitis and other infections occurring in the mouth or throat because these are generally accompanied by leukocytosis. Infections such as typhoid fever, measles, rubella and undulant fever, which are associated with leukopenia, can be readily distinguished from agranulocytosis by their more gradual onset and characteristic symptoms and signs; but influenza is not so easily differentiated. In cases of sepsis with leukopenia the course is less fulminating than in agranulocytosis. It is most unusual in any of these conditions for the leukocyte count to reach the low levels seen in agranulocytosis.

Of disorders of the blood which might be confused with agranulocytosis, acute "aleukemic" leukemia and aplastic anemia can be recognized by the presence of anemia and thrombocytopenia. The former is also characterized by the presence of immature leukocytes in the blood as well as by adenopathy and splenomegaly. If doubt still remains, bone marrow examination should make the diagnosis clear. Like agranulocytosis,

infectious mononucleosis is marked by changes which are confined to the leukocytes but extreme leukopenia is unusual, the typical lymphocytes are found and the heterophil antibody test is positive.

Prognosis and Course.—Before the sulfonamides and antibiotics became available, the prognosis was very poor. In Plum's series[35] of 88 cases, the mortality was 84 per cent. In 7 per cent death occurred after temporary improvement. Statistics by other authors[39] gave the mortality as 70 to 90 per cent. Unfavorable signs are confusion and drowsiness, great prostration, jaundice, necrosis of the skin, a leukocyte count less than 1000 with absence of all granulocytes, or the onset of complications such as pneumonia. Mortality is greatest in patients of advanced age.

Death may occur as the result of sepsis, pneumonia, hemorrhage following necrosis, or other causes even after hematological improvement has set in. Before the importance of drugs as etiological agents was recognized, relapses were common.

Improvement is heralded by the reappearance of leukocytes of the granular series in the blood. These at first are myelocytes and metamyelocytes. Myeloblasts may be seen. Segmented neutrophils are the last of this series to make their appearance. The presence of monocytes,[39] especially if they persist,[38] is said to be a good sign. The leukocytic reaction may be very rapid and marked degrees of leukocytosis, even of "leukemoid" character, may be reached although counts of about 15,000 per c.mm. have been recorded most often.[39]

With the availability of potent antibiotics to control the complicating infection, the outlook even in severe cases now is far better than when agranulocytosis was first discovered, provided the potential offending agent is sought out and, if found, its further use interdicted.

Treatment. — The most important

measure is to discover, if possible, the **offending agent** and to **prohibit its further use.** It is of almost equal importance to prevent overwhelming sepsis from developing before the leukocytes reappear. Through their action as bacteriostatic agents, therefore, **antibiotics** such as penicillin are the most important agents for the treatment of agranulocytosis. It may be added that, although the sulfonamides are known to produce granulocytopenia in some cases, this fact need not prevent their use in cases in which they are not the offending agents.

When the granulocytopenia is due to the action of arsenic or gold[29a] BAL (British Anti-Lewisite, 2,3-dimercaptopropanol) should be given in doses of approximately 150 mg. (1.5 ml.) of a 10 per cent solution in oil, intramuscularly, every four hours for the first two days and then in this dosage twice daily for another eight to ten days. This agent will facilitate excretion of the toxic metal.

The general care of the patient is of great importance since the mouth, particularly, and local lesions wherever they may be situated, must be given scrupulous attention to prevent the development of painful and serious ulcerations.

No means has been found which effectively stimulates granulocyte formation and, furthermore, it may be questioned whether the hemopoietic mechanism is capable of producing these cells more rapidly than occurs once there is no further exposure to the causative agent.[39] The evidence that pentnucleotide[24] is valuable in the treatment of agranulocytosis was never convincing[13,35,39] and there certainly is no indication for its use now that the antibiotics are available. Transfusions, even of blood from patients with leukemia[3] or leukocytosis resulting from some infection, were not found to be of value.[24,35] Injections of leukocytes, "leukocytic cream,"[50] liver extracts[15] and various vitamins, the feeding of bone marrow, especially yellow marrow[7b] and

marrow extracts, and the irradiation of the long bones with "stimulating doses" of x-rays,[16] all had their brief popularity but never earned a place in the management of this disorder.

Reports to the effect that the administration of adrenocorticotropic hormone (ACTH) is a valuable therapeutic adjunct[20b,31a] are difficult to evaluate since it cannot be said how well or poorly the patients would have done without the hormone.

The use of splenectomy in the treatment of the more or less chronic neutropenias of obscure etiology has been discussed already (p. 1103).

Pathology. — The most significant feature revealed by autopsy is a lack of granulocytes. Polymorphonuclear leukocytes are conspicuously absent about the necrotic lesions which may be found in the oral cavity, skin, vagina, uterus or the gastro-intestinal tract, and only plasma cells and lymphocytes are seen. Enormous collections of bacteria are to be found. In the lungs there may be pneumonic lesions with a similar lack of granulocytes, or gangrene. The liver is often enlarged and cloudy swelling, fatty degeneration or small areas of necrosis may be present. The spleen is frequently somewhat heavier than normal. There is marked engorgement with blood, the lymph follicles are small, granulocytes are absent and there may be small areas of necrosis. Of the lymph nodes, only those draining infected areas are enlarged. Microscopically they show hyperemia, hemorrhage and necrosis with some obliteration of the normal structure.

The bone marrow has been described already (p. 1104).

INFECTIOUS MONONUCLEOSIS

Definition.—This is an acute infection, benign in nature and of unknown etiology, which is characterized clinically by irregular fever, sore throat, lymphadenopathy, especially in the neck, and enlargement of the spleen, as well as by an absolute lymphocytosis due largely to the appearance of abnormal, though chiefly mature lymphocytes. The blood serum contains heterophil antibodies against sheep erythrocytes in high concentrations.

History and Terminology.—An illness characterized by cervical glandular swelling, failure of the glands to suppurate and enlargement of the liver and spleen, which appeared in epidemic form in children and ran a favorable course, was described by Emil Pfeiffer[95] in 1889 under the title, *"glandular fever."* Similar cases were described in various parts of the world,[59] including the United States where the disease was first reported in 1896 by West.[110] Attention was called to an increase in the small mononuclear elements ot the blood by Burns[63] who described an epidemic in a Baltimore hospital in 1909.

Somewhat later, notice was gradually taken of a sporadically occurring infection which has from time to time been thought to be related to the glandular fever of Pfeiffer. Türk[105] in 1907 recorded his surprise at finding a young man well, to whose family he had expressed the opinion the that illness was acute leukemia and that death would soon follow. Reports of similar cases characterized by glandular enlargement, mononuclear cell increase and sore throat were made by Cabot,[64] Marchand[86] and others.[80] Some of these cases were described as examples of acute leukemia with apparent cure. It remained for Sprunt and Evans,[99] in 1920, to classify these cases as well as 6 they had observed under the title *"infectious mononucleosis"* and to point out that abnormal cells of a peculiar type were present in the blood.

Tidy and Morley[104] suggested that glandular fever and infectious mononucleosis were one and the same, a view accepted with reservation by Longcope[85]

in 1922 who presented additional cases of the sporadic type and described the morphological abnormalities in the blood as well as the histology of excised lymph nodes. The hematological aspects of the disease were studied in minute detail by Downey and McKinlay[72] in 1923.

Cases of a similar character have been described under the title of *"acute benign lymphoblastosis,"*[61] *"acute lymphadenosis,"*[71] *"monocytic angina"*[98] and *"lymphocytic angina."* An important advance was made when Paul and Bunnell[94] discovered, in 1932, that the blood serum of patients with the sporadic form of this disease may contain antibodies against sheep erythrocytes in concentrations far above a normal titer. The demonstration of positive serological reactions in the blood of a number of cases of epidemic glandular fever by Nolan[90] in 1935 has been interpreted as demonstrating the relationship of the sporadic and the epidemically occurring cases. This conclusion is not necessarily correct, as will be discussed below.

Etiology and Pathogenesis.—Infectious mononucleosis has been recognized throughout Europe and America as well as in Australia, China, Japan and elsewhere.[59] In Japan a number of epidemic fevers (tosa-netsu, tokushima-netsu and kagami-netsu) have been compared to infectious mononucleosis and glandular fever.[59]

Until an opportunity arose in army camps during World War II to examine many Negroes with symptoms for which they would not ordinarily have been examined thoroughly, it had appeared that infectious mononucleosis was rare in this race.[79a,85] It has been stated repeatedly that the sporadic form is more frequent in individuals working about a hospital, but the apparently high incidence in this group is due no doubt to the fact that blood examinations are more likely to be done on medical students and nurses even when they have a mild illness than in the population at large. Only one-third of

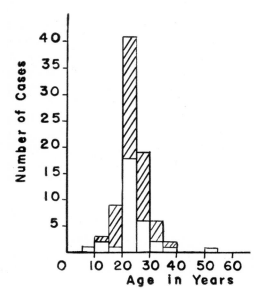

Fig. 21–1.—Age and sex of 82 cases of infectious mononucleosis (sporadic type) at the Johns Hopkins Hospital. Males are indicated by hatched columns, females by open columns. All the patients were white.

Bernstein's[59] 65 cases were limited to the "hospital class." Many cases were seen in the United States Army during World War II.[96d]

Age.—The epidemic disorder, until World War II, had been confined, with few exceptions, to children. Tidy and Morley[104] calculated that at least 80 per cent of all cases of the epidemic type reported up to 1921 occurred in children under thirteen years of age. In Nolan's[90] series of 220 cases in California only 5 were adults. Nevertheless, in an isolated community (Falkland Islands) 10 per cent of the sufferers were between forty-five and sixty-five years of age.[89] In a nursery epidemic, infants as young as seven months of age were affected.[70] With many young persons collected together in the armed forces during World War II, a number of instances of the epidemic condition were observed in young adults.[88,96d,109]

The sporadic cases may occur in older children and in young adults.[59] In Bernstein's series the youngest patient was six years old, the oldest thirty-six; 81 per cent of the patients were between the ages of fifteen and thirty years. The age incidence in 82 cases at the Johns Hopkins Hospital is shown in Figure 21-1. Infectious mononucleosis is quite uncommon over the age of 40 but has been encountered occasionally.[98a]

Sex.—The condition has been reported more often in males than in females (3 to 2).[59]

Epidemiology.—Epidemics have usually appeared in the spring.[59] There seems to be little evidence for a seasonal incidence of sporadic cases.[65] The contagiousness of the sporadic disease is low, it being quite exceptional for members of a patient's family or his intimate associates to contract the infection.[65,79b] It has been stated that it is acquired by the intimate oral exchange of saliva.[79b] In a survey of a dormitory of 63 residents in which 5 cases had occurred within a period of a month, no evidence of "inapparent" or subclinical infections in others of this group could be found.[73a]

These differences in the apparent epidemiology of epidemic glandular fever and sporadic infectious mononucleosis cause one to wonder whether they are identical disorders. The clinical manifestations of many of the patients described in the epidemics, whether in children[90] or in adults,[109] were not typical of the sporadic disease. The validity of the reported positive heterophil antibody tests in many epidemics is in doubt because the guinea pig absorption technique was not used. When this was done in an epidemic in Japan, the results were indefinite and irregular.[92]

Suspected Etiological Agents. — There can be no doubt that infectious mononucleosis is a specific entity rather than a peculiar reaction to a variety of infectious agents. Affected individuals have been observed to respond to other infections with the usual polymorpho-nuclear reaction.[98]

Attempts to discover the cause of infectious mononucleosis, however, by culture or by animal inoculation, have on the whole been fruitless. Wising[111] stated that the injection in monkeys of emulsified material from lymph nodes of patients with infectious mononucleosis caused a mild febrile illness similar to this disease. The infection could be transmitted from one monkey to another and a laboratory worker after accidentally piercing his finger with infected material developed the complete disease picture. It was also reported that the intravenous administration of 250 ml. of the blood of a patient produced in the recipient a suggestive clinical and hematological picture with a rise in heterophil antibodies. The subcutaneous inoculation of the blood of an affected child was found to produce in monkeys[106] a suggestive morphologic and serologic picture. Furthermore, a Seitz filtrate of blood from patients was found to produce a similar disorder in successive passages from monkey to monkey, and cultures in tissue were successful in preserving the virulence of the infective agent. Others,[80b] however, failed to produce significant changes in monkeys or other animals when blood, gargle washings and material from excised lymph nodes were used. Likewise, in human volunteers, gargling with the throat washings of a patient, spraying the throat with a saline extract of lymph nodes removed from a patient during the febrile period of the disease, and the intramuscular injection of such an extract, failed to reproduce the disease. Inoculation of serum, throat washings or stool preparations from patients with the disease in still another study[73] yielded only suggestive clinical or hematological signs of infectious mononucleosis.

Suspected etiological agents range from various forms of cocci and bacilli to spirochetes, protozoa and viruses. *Bacterium* or *Listerella monocytogenes*, a small slowly-growing Gram-positive bacillus has been isolated from the blood of several cases of infectious mononucleosis.[91,96] This organism injected into dogs,[91] rabbits, guinea pigs and white mice, [96] produces an increase in mononuclear leukocytes as well as an acute generalized infection. It does not, however, appear to produce agglutinins for sheep erythrocytes nor the complement-fixing or flocculating reagins which give false-positive Wassermann reactions in cases of infectious mononucleosis.[83] The titer of *Listerella* agglutination tests has been found slightly elevated in the sera of patients with infectious mononucleosis as compared with control sera but no significant trend in the titer in relation to the course of the disease could be demonstrated.[80a] Moreover, other attempts to isolate the organism from the blood of patients have failed.[80a] The intracutaneous inoculation of mouse-lethal suspensions of this organism in two human subjects failed to produce a disorder simulating infectious mononucleosis.[80b]

Invasion of the oral cavity by Vincent's organisms is very frequent in infectious mononucleosis. Nevertheless, there is little to indicate that this is more than a fortuitous occurrence.[77a]

Bland[60] produced a febrile disease in rabbits by the injection of the blood of patients affected with infectious mononucleosis. In monkeys injected with the blood of such infected rabbits a febrile disease with anemia, lymphocytosis, lymphadenopathy and splenomegaly developed. In the laked blood of the rabbits Bland found a protozoön, *Toxoplasma*, to which he attributed the disease. Protozoa were not demonstrated in the organs of the monkeys. The significance of their presence in rabbits is doubtful since such organisms (*T. cuniculi*) may infect rabbits presumably not in contact with infectious mononucleosis. Furthermore, these results could not be confirmed.[87]

Isolation of the etiologic agent of epidemic glandular fever in Japan, *Rickettsia sennetsu*, has been reported[80c] and it has been suggested that the Sendai virus is related antigenically to the etiologic agent of infectious mononucleosis.[70a]

Symptomatology.—In the absence of a demonstrable etiologic agent, various students of this disease have allowed themselves more or less liberty in its definition. Thus, many have held that the manifestations of infectious mononucleosis are protean[59] and that a great variety of disorders may be simulated by this condition. Some would make the diagnosis in the absence of a positive heterophil antibody test or even in the presence of only equivocal morphologic changes in the blood, basing their diagnosis on the presence of more or less typical clinical findings or even on little more than the lack of any better explanation for a self-limited febrile disorder in a young person. Others,[79b] on the other hand, would restrict the diagnosis to cases in which lymphocytes constitute more than 50 per cent of the leukocytes, "atypical" lymphocytes are present, and both of these features have been present over a period of at least ten days. When circumscribed in this manner and when a titer of at least 1:28 for heterophil antibodies was obtained, after guinea pig absorption, Hoagland found that the clinical picture is a very consistent one and not protean.

The clinical manifestations can be described in three stages, (1) the prodromal period, characterized by nonspecific features similar to those of other infections, during which diagnosis may be difficult because enlarged lymph nodes, a suggestive blood picture or a significant rise in sheep cell agglutinin titers may not develop until the end of the first week of illness; (2) a mid-stage lasting four to 20 days during which the full-blown disease presents itself; and (3) the stage of convalescence.[77]

The **incubation period** is uncertain and may be as long as 33 to 49 days.[79b] The *onset* is gradual: malaise during the first two days, then fever, chilliness and finally slight posterior cervical and axillary lymph node enlargement and pharyngeal inflammation. Symptoms are usually mild or moderate in the first week. A *pharyngeal syndrome* is most common (80 per cent of cases). In 12 per cent of cases the picture is "*typhoidal*" with fever, malaise and headache predominating. Still less common (8 per cent of cases) is the *icteric* form.[79b]

Lymph node enlargement is invariably present at some time and is bilateral.[79b] The cervical glands were always enlarged in two large series of cases.[65,79b] The enlarged posterior chains are often palpable down to the clavicle. Enlargement of axillary and inguinal nodes is usually but not invariably present. A "bull neck" is quite exceptional.[79b] Local heat, redness or marked tenderness, fluctuation and suppuration are conspicuously absent.

The **spleen** probably is enlarged in at least 50 per cent of cases[103] but the exact figure is difficult to determine since splenic enlargement has no doubt been looked for with varying degrees of diligence. Generally the spleen extends 2 to 3 cm. below the costal margin but it may protrude a whole hand's breadth and enlargement to the iliac crest has been described.[59] Splenomegaly may be found even when lymphadenopathy is not impressive.

Pharyngeal inflammation varies in intensity but hyperplasia of pharyngeal lymphoid tissue is almost always present. The palatal arch and uvula often have a gelatinous appearance, but significant edema of the uvula is unusual. Laryngeal edema with obstruction is very rare.[96c] Vincent's infection is a common complication. The gums may become tender, swollen and ulcerated, and may bleed.

The **fever** is of no characteristic type.

It may be very transient and slight in degree but in 14 to 33 per cent of cases it reached a peak of 103° to 104° F.[59,79b] This may come at the end of four to eight days, rising in a remittent manner. A secondary rise after an initial drop to normal may accompany the onset of glandular swelling or sore throat. In one series of 196 cases, 11 per cent of all the patients had no fever.[65] In another group of 200 cases, fever was present in all but five patients.[79b] In the most seriously ill patient the writer has seen, a temperature of 106.6° F. was reached following a chill and levels of 104° F. were attained on three other days. In this case the throat was comparatively innocent in appearance. The temperature curve may, very occasionally, suggest malaria. In other cases it may suggest typhoid fever, especially since the pulse may be relatively slow.

The **typhoidal syndrome** is characterized by feverishness, malaise and headache. The headache may be so severe as to suggest meningitis. Cervical lymphaadenopathy is usually found but the enlargement of the glands may be delayed for a week or two and, if a rash appears, the similarity to typhoid fever may be quite great. Gastrointestinal symptoms, however, are unusual.

Jaundice may be present, even in the absence of hepatic enlargement. The liver is palpable in about 12 per cent of cases.[59] Jaundice may develop five to 14 days after the onset of the illness. The urine becomes dark and gives a positive reaction for bile but the stools rarely become acholic. In the majority of cases, however, **hepatitis** occurs in the absence of jaundice. Positive flocculation tests (cephalin-cholesterol flocculation, thymol turbidity) and increased serum alkaline phosphatase activity are found in the majority of cases of infectious mononucleosis.[57a,89c,108,112] More sensitive reflectors of the hepatic involvement are measurements of serum glutamic pyruvic

and oxalacetic transaminase.[97a] Hepatic involvement, however, although very common, is usually mild.[79b] With some exceptions,[107] histologic examinations of liver biopsies have revealed lymphocytic infiltration and relatively slight changes in hepatic cells, with no change in hepatic architecture,[79b] in contrast to the evidence of necrosis and inflammatory exudate which is found in infectious hepatitis.

Skin and Mucous Membranes.—
Edema of the eyelids[93] has been described in 36 per cent of cases.[79b] This consists of drooping of the swollen orbital portion of the upper eyelid upon the palpebral portion and sagging of the latter. As a result, the ocular aperture is narrowed.

A *palatal enanthem*, consisting of approximately five to 20 pinhead sized red spots which darken in about 48 hours and disappear after about three or four days may be seen in about 25 per cent of cases, usually at the junction of the soft and hard palate.[79b] This appears in crops, usually between the fifth and 12th day of the illness.

Contrary to earlier reports,[101] when diagnosis was probably less exact, faint erythema or, rarely, a maculopapular eruption represents the extent of the cutaneous eruptions in this disease.[79b]

Hemorrhagic manifestations include epistaxis and, much less frequently, petechial hemorrhages and purpura.[71,93] Thrombocytopenic purpura[79] has been described in a total of 33 cases In one of our patients a circulating fibrinolysin caused extensive ecchymoses to appear.

Gastrointestinal symptoms such as nausea, vomiting and diarrhea are uncommon. Abdominal pain of a type to suggest acute appendicitis has been reported. This may be due to swelling of mesenteric lymph nodes. Pancreatitis may possibly occur in some cases since elevated values for serum amylase and lipase have been observed.[89b]

Cardiac, Pulmonary and Renal

Symptoms. — Cardiac or pulmonary symptoms are uncommon. In one of our cases, however, tachycardia and cyanosis became so pronounced as to suggest acute cardiac dilatation. Pericarditis[97b,98b] and other cardiac manifestations have been described but, in some of the reported cases,[73b] the diagnosis must be regarded as in doubt. In a few instances transient T wave changes in the electrocardiogram have been reported.[79b]

Enlargement of mediastinal lymph nodes[79b] or pulmonary parenchymal changes demonstrable by X-ray are infrequent but have been described.[86a] Nephritis has been reported but this has not usually been accompanied by all the customary signs. Red cells, leukocytes and albumin may be found in the urine but hyaline or granular casts are quite rarely seen. Hematuria was reported in 6 per cent in Tidy's series[104] but has been rare in other series. Vaginitis and endocervicitis have been seen in one case.[84b]

Nervous System. — It has been estimated that central nervous system involvement occurs in 0.7 to 1.0 per cent of cases[109] but this figure may be high since some cases were probably included which would now be excluded by the differential absorption heterophil antibody test. Headache and blurring of vision are the most common symptoms but convulsions, stupor, coma and bradycardia, stiff neck and positive Romberg and Babinski signs have been described. Toxic psychosis resembling schizophrenia has been reported. Grand mal seizures,[84a,98c] partial ocular motor paralysis or paresis, nystagmus, optic neuritis, bilateral papilledema, anosmia, facial paralysis, left upper extremity paresis, ataxia, skin hyperesthesia and signs of diffuse lower motor neurone involvement have also been reported. The Guillain-Barré syndrome with multiple involvement of peripheral nerves, ascending paralysis, high spinal fluid

protein and no cells has been described in a number of instances.[96a] Encephalitis has been reported[96e] as well as syndromes resembling acute meningitis and meningoencephalitis.[75] Death from respiratory paralysis has occurred in several cases with neurologic complications.

"Glandular fever," especially as seen in children, may present a somewhat different picture.[103] Following a prodromal period of one to four days, lymph node enlargement becomes pronounced. All or any group of glands may be involved but those posterior to the sternomastoid muscles are preeminently affected. The glands are single or in clumps but they are usually discrete. They have a firm elastic consistency and are only slightly tender unless they drain an area which is secondarily infected, such as the throat. Enlargement is rarely symmetrical. The glands vary in size from 1 to 3 or 4 cm. in diameter. The enlargement may develop suddenly and a large lymph node may be found where none was felt the day before. Axillary and inguinal glands are less frequently involved than those in the cervical region but in some cases these have been the primary and only sites of lymphadenopathy.

The Blood. — The characteristic feature is an increase in mononuclear cells. These are of three types: (1) small lymphocytes; (2) monocytes, both of these appearing normally in blood; and (3) large mononuclear leukocytes which are not normally observed in the blood. The "mononucleosis" is due mainly to the presence of these abnormal cells (Plates XV and XIX).

The abnormal cells vary greatly in size and shape. They possess a nucleus which may be oval, kidney-shaped or slightly lobulated and cytoplasm which most frequently is non-granular and vacuolated or foamy in appearance. The nuclear chromatin forms a coarse network of strands and masses and is not clearly differentiated from the parachromatin. The identity of these cells has been disputed but most hematologists regard them as highly differentiated, mature lymphocytes.[71] They do not show granules when stained by the peroxidase method and can thus be distinguished from cells of the granulocytic series and, to some extent, from monocytes.

These "leukocytoid lymphocytes,"[71] the form most frequently seen, were classed as Type I by Downey.[71] He described two other types of abnormal lymphocytes in infectious mononucleosis. Type II cells are less varied but larger than Type I cells, their nuclear chromatin is not as condensed, and their cytoplasm is more homogeneous and not vacuolated. Type III cells resemble somewhat those of lymphoblastic leukemia. Their nuclei show a diffuse sieve-like arrangement of the chromatin and possess 1 or 2 nucleoli. The cytoplasm of the Type III cells is vacuolated and may be quite basophilic. Excellent illustrations of these cells were published by Downey and McKinlay.[71]

The **total leukocyte count** is usually increased but it may be normal or even lower than normal.[74] In Bernstein's series[59] of 65 cases, the leukocyte count was between 10,000 and 15,000 cells per c.mm. in 39.5 per cent and between 15,000 and 20,000 in 22 per cent. In almost a third of the cases it did not exceed 10,000 and in 7 cases the leukocyte count at one time was below 4000. Similar observations have been made by others.[74,93]

During the first week there may be a well-marked leukopenia. This was true in 40 per cent of the cases in one series.[77] When the leukocyte count is low at the onset of the disease it generally rises before the temperature falls to normal, but it rarely exceeds the normal range. The leukocyte count generally parallels the course of the infection, a recrudescence of symptoms being associated with a secondary leukocyte increase. In exceptional cases the most marked leukocyte changes may be coincidental with the fall of the temperature or follow it.

In 10 reported cases the leukocyte count was greater than 40,000 (up to 63,000)[103] but 7 of these patients were children less than ten years of age.[59] At the other extreme, exceptional cases have been reported in which the leukocyte count was as low as 2000[103] and even 1500.[67]

The polymorphonuclear cells may be increased early in the disease, but in the fully developed stage a relative reduction in the number of granulocytes and a marked increase in the number of nongranular cells is a characteristic feature of the differential count. The latter cells often (87 per cent of cases) make up 60 per cent or more of all the leukocytes[59] and frequently they are still more numerous. Values as high as 97 per cent mononuclear cells have been observed.[59] The rise in non-granular cells usually begins on the fourth or fifth day and attains a peak by the seventh or tenth day. The characteristic blood changes have been noted as early as the second day of the illness and as late as the twelfth to fourteenth day.[79b] Consequently, since patients frequently do not consult a physician until the fourth or fifth day of the illness or later, the blood is usually characteristic when they are first seen.

In exceptional cases the polymorphonuclear cell increase persists until the fever has disappeared. In other unusual cases granulocytopenia may be extreme, suggesting the picture of agranulocytosis.[103] The myeloid leukocytes present may be chiefly young and stab forms. Eosinophils do not disappear entirely during the acute phase[74] and may even be increased in number.[82] Eosinophilia is common during convalescence. Mitoses have been observed in the peripheral blood.[62] In supravitally stained preparations it has been noted that the number of lymphocytes containing refractive granules is reduced.[76]

The hematologic changes usually persist for one to two months. However, they have been observed to disappear in two weeks or to remain even longer than three months.[79b]

The changes in the blood described above have not been found as consistently in epidemic glandular fever as in sporadic infectious mononucleosis. This may be due to the fact that only the most typical instances of the sporadic type are recognized, deviations from the customary findings being more readily accepted when many cases are encountered.[59] It is also possible, as already stated, that the sporadic and the epidemic disorders are not identical.

Anemia is so extremely rare that the report[96d] of anemia in 6 cases out of a series of 300 still permits the statement to be made that the finding of anemia makes the diagnosis of infectious mononucleosis highly improbable. Several instances of hemolytic anemia complicating infectious mononucleosis have been reported, however.[78] The Coombs' test was positive in some of these cases.

The **platelet count** is usually normal but thrombocytopenia has been reported in a total of 35 cases, of which 20 can be accepted as genuine cases of infectious mononucleosis.[70b] In addition to purpura, epistaxis, gastrointestinal bleeding, hematuria and hemoptysis occurred in some of these patients. As a rule the purpura developed about a week following the appearance of the first symptoms of infectious mononucleosis and the bleeding manifestations lasted about ten days, the thrombocytopenia a month. The *bleeding time* may be prolonged without relation to the platelet count.[59,103] *Coagulation time* is normal. In one of our patients, marked thrombocytopenia was accompanied by fibrinogenopenia and a circulating fibrinolysin, with startling hemorrhagic manifestations resulting

even though the coagulation time remained within normal limits.[70b]

When there is jaundice, the icterus index may be as high as 50 units and the **serum bilirubin** 8 mg. per 100 ml.,[59] with a significant proportion giving the direct reaction.

The **serological test for syphilis** may become transiently positive in approximately 7 per cent[114] of cases and occasionally this may persist for several months.[81] This effect is independent of the presence of sheep cell antibodies, for the positive reaction can be demonstrated in equally high titer even when the sheep cell antibodies have been absorbed out. Falsely positive trichina skin tests,[57b] and significant increases of agglutinins for a variety of organisms have also been observed.[59] Increased titers of cold hemagglutinins may be present and may produce false-positive heterophil agglutination tests.[115]

The principal abnormalities demonstrated by electrophoretic analyses of the serum were diminution of the albumin fraction and elevation of the gamma-globulin.[100] The heterophil antibodies were contained predominantly in the gamma-globulin fraction.

Significant reductions in high density lipoprotein fractions and the standard $S_f O$—12 lipoproteins have been described.[97c] These changes were found to contrast sharply with those occurring in infectious hepatitis.

Urine.—It has been mentioned already that albumin may be found in the urine as well as red cells, the latter even in sufficient numbers to produce gross hematuria. Renal function is unimpaired. When there is jaundice, urobilinogen and bile will be found.

Cerebrospinal Fluid.—The cerebrospinal fluid pressure may be moderately elevated. Pleocytosis may be present, even several hundred cells, mostly lymphocytes.[116] There may be changes in the spinal fluid even in the absence of

Table 21–2—Heterophil Antibody Test

Tube No.	Saline solution (ml.)	Patient's serum (ml.)	2 per cent sheep cells (ml.)	Final dilutions of serum
1	0.4	0.1	0.1	1:7
2	0.25	0.25 from tube 1	0.1	1:14
3	0.25	0.25 from tube 2	0.1	1:28
4	0.25	0.25 from tube 3	0.1	1:56
5	0.25	0.25 from tube 4	0.1	1:112
6	0.25	0.25 from tube 5	0.1	1:224
7	0.25	0.25 from tube 6	0.1	1:448
8	0.25	0.25 from tube 7	0.1	1:896
9	0.25	0.25 from tube 8	0.1	1:1792
10	0.25	0.25 from tube 9	0.1	1:3584
11	0.25	0.25 from tube 10*	0.1	1:7168
12 (Control)	0.25		0.1	

* Discard 0.25 ml. from this tube.

signs of nervous system involvement.[59b] The sugar content is normal, the protein may be increased and the Pandy test may be strongly positive. In a few instances heterophil antibodies have been demonstrated in the spinal fluid.[75]

Heterophil Antibodies.—*Paul-Bunnell Test.*—The discovery by Paul and Bunnell[94] that the serum in cases of infectious mononucleosis contains agglutinins against sheep red cells in high titer has proved to be of the greatest value in the study of this disease and has been demonstrated to be very useful in diagnosis. The proportion of cases in which the test has been reported to be positive depends upon the extent to which the test was relied upon for diagnosis. Thus, while in some series[59] positive values in as many as 92 and even 100[79b] per cent of cases have been reported, Paul himself reported negative results in more than half of the cases during the first week of the disease, 40 per cent negative during the second week and a return to more than half negative in the third week.[77]

Method.[67] — The patient's blood serum is inactivated for thirty minutes at 56° C. to destroy the complement. Only 0.1 ml. is required for the test. A 2 per cent suspension of sheep red corpuscles is needed. These cells should not be less than twenty-four hours old, nor more than a week old. They must be washed the day of the test. This is done three times by mixing them well with two to three times as much physiologic solution of sodium chloride. The third centrifugalization should take twice as long as the others, that is about fifteen minutes, and should concentrate the cells to about half the original volume. The supernatant fluid must be clear after the third centrifugalization.

The test is set up in 11 test tubes (75 mm. by 10 mm.), and a twelfth tube is used for the control. The dilutions are made up as shown in Table 21–2. The test tubes are well shaken and allowed to stand at room temperature for two hours. They are then shaken again until the sediment is suspended. Agglutination of the corpuscles indicates the presence of heterophil antibody in that tube. The highest dilution in which this can be detected with the naked eye, or with the low power microscope objective, is taken as the end point.

It has been reported that goat red cells can be used in the place of sheep cells.[107a]

Interpretation.[68]—The heterophil antibody test, as above described, is non-

Table 21–3.—Differential Test for Infectious Mononucleosis

	Absorption of Antisheep Agglutinins by	
Serum Derived From	Guinea Pig Kidney	Beef Red Cells
Persons without serum disease or infectious mononucleosis	+	±
Serum disease	+	+
Infectious mononucleosis	—	+

+ indicates complete absorption
— indicates incomplete absorption
± indicates complete or partial absorption

specific. The term "heterophil" refers to the condition in which antibodies react with an antigen that seemingly has had nothing to do with their development. Antisheep agglutinins are present in titers up to 1:28 in most normal persons, and occasionally even in a titer of 1 : 56. In various infections a titer of 1 :112 and occasionally of 1 : 224 may be seen. Persons receiving injections of horse serum and horse immune serum may develop titers as high as any seen in infectious mononucleosis. After various kinds of known or unknown antigenic stimulation a titer of 1 : 448 and higher is occasionally found.

For these reasons the test for heterophil antibodies has been called "*presumptive.*" In the presence of clinical and hematologic findings suggestive of infectious mononucleosis, a titer of 1 : 224 or higher can be interpreted as confirming the diagnosis. In this disease, positive heterophil reactions almost always appear during the first two weeks of the illness.[79b] Highest titers are found usually during the second and third weeks of illness. As a rule positive reactions last four to eight weeks. They have been observed to persist as short a time as seven to nine days or as long as eighteen weeks.[68] The titer bears no relation to the severity of the disease or to the leukocyte changes. Wide variations in the agglutinability of erythrocytes from different sheep have been demonstrated.[115]

If the titer of the presumptive test is less than 1 : 224 in the presence of clinical and hematologic findings suggestive of infectious mononucleosis, or if the titer is 1 : 224 or higher in the absence of such findings, or if the patient gives a history of a recent horse serum injection, the results should be checked by a differential test.

The **differential test** is based on the observation that heterophil antibodies in normal serum, in horse serum sensitization and in a variety of infections can be absorbed completely by guinea pig kidney. On the other hand, antisheep agglutinins in infectious mononucleosis are never completely removed by treating the serum with guinea pig kidney although they are, as a rule, completely removed by beef red cells. Beef red cells also completely remove the antisheep agglutinins in horse serum sensitization but do so less regularly and less completely in normal, apparently healthy individuals and in persons with diseases other than infectious mononucleosis or horse serum sensitization (Table 21–3). The differential test is carried out by absorbing a portion of the patient's serum with guinea pig kidney and another portion with beef red cells. After this the absorbed specimens are tested for sheep red cell agglutination.

An alternative procedure to the differential absorption test which has been found to be both simple and accurate involves the inactivation of the receptor for the antibody of infectious mononucleosis in the sheep erythrocyte by *papain.*[89a] Another procedure which was found to compare favorably with the Paul-Bunnell test is the *ox cell hemolysin test.*[86b]

Bone Marrow.—Sternal puncture is chiefly of value from a negative standpoint, in the sense that the findings characteristic of leukemia are absent. However, the bone marrow cannot be said to be entirely normal. Thus, there may be a moderate "shift to the left" of the myeloid leukocytes. An increase in eosinophils and in reticular and leukocytoid lymphocytes has been described and, in sectioned particles of aspirated bone marrow, granulomatous lesions have been demonstrated as well as epithelioid cells morphologically identical with those seen in imprints of lymph nodes from this disease.[79d]

Clinical Course.—The irregular fever persists in most cases for one to three weeks and subjective symptoms disappear as a rule in two to four weeks. Sometimes the duration of the disease is still shorter, in other cases it may be longer. Recrudescences are infrequent.[79b] *Relapse* is rare. *Recurrence* has been observed but is very rare. Adenopathy, splenomegaly and the characteristic blood findings may persist for months.[59] There may be a long period of slight but definite debility following an attack of infectious mononucleosis. A true chronic form of the disease, however, has not been recognized.

Diagnosis.—Since infectious mononucleosis is relatively uncommon whereas many of its manifestations are similar to those seen in more common illnesses, the diagnosis may be overlooked unless the physician's suspicions are aroused by the lymphadenopathy or splenomegaly, by fever of unexplained etiology or by unusual findings in the blood. Cases with severe sore throat may be mistaken for follicular tonsillitis, diphtheria, herpetic pharyngitis or aphthous stomatitis. The fever and systemic symptoms may suggest typhoid fever, undulant fever, influenza, bacterial endocarditis, or even acute rheumatic fever, while symptoms and signs of meningeal irritation and abnormalities in the cerebrospinal fluid may make it necessary to rule out pyogenic or benign lymphocytic meningitis, encephalitis or poliomyelitis. Fever or glandular enlargement in a child or young adult which are out of proportion to any local inflammatory manifestations, should indicate the need for a blood examination and the test for heterophil antibodies.

Lymphocytosis, relative or absolute, may, of course, be encountered regularly or occasionally in a number of diseases, all of which may be and have been confused with infectious mononucleosis: leukemia, agranulocytosis, Vincent's angina, tuberculosis, tularemia, pertussis, dengue, mumps, chickenpox, German measles, typhoid fever, benign lymphocytic meningitis, infectious hepatitis, acute appendicitis, serum disease and various allergic states.[96b] In some of these conditions, abnormal lymphocytes suggesting those of infectious mononucleosis have been observed.[72] Marked leukocytosis, due chiefly to the presence of small lymphocytes of normal appearance, and associated neither with splenomegaly, lymphadenopathy nor a positive heterophil agglutination reaction, suggests acute infectious lymphocytosis (p. 260). Differentiation from infectious hepatitis is sometimes difficult but the test for heterophil antibodies is negative in the latter. A false positive serological test for syphilis, or a false positive Widal test or agglutination for *B. melitensis,* may occur in infectious mononucleosis[59] thus making the differentiation from secondary syphilis, typhoid or undulant fever a problem.

The clinical picture may suggest acute leukemia but this diagnosis should not be made in the absence of red cell changes, platelet reduction, hemorrhagic phenomena and immature leukocytes. Although many of the leukocytes seen in infectious mononucleosis appear abnormal, very few of them contain nucleoli. Hemorrhagic phenomena and thrombocytopenia occur very occasionally in infectious mononucleosis but are not seen in association with lymphoblasts and severe anemia. Moderate or severe anemia is almost always present when acute leukemia is first discovered (p. 933).

As already stated, cases of infectious mononucleosis have been observed which closely simulated purpura hemorrhagica.[59] When there is leukopenia and severe sore throat, agranulocytosis must be considered. It is noteworthy that abnormal cells like those of infectious mononucleosis have been seen in agranulocytosis in a few instances.[72] The older age of the patients, as a rule, the history of drug ingestion which may be obtained, and the absence of lymphadenopathy or splenomegaly, are valuable differentiating features in agranulocytosis. Finally, in all of the blood disorders which have been mentioned, the Paul-Bunnell test is negative. In leukemia the titer of heterophil antibodies may be even lower than normal.

The reverse may also occur. *Other disorders may be mistaken for infectious mononucleosis.* It has been pointed out that some clinicians are not sufficiently discriminating and are willing to include under this heading a miscellaneous variety of illnesses.[79b] As discussed earlier (p. 1110) the diagnosis should be restricted to cases in which there are both a positive heterophil antibody reaction and a characteristic blood picture. There should be a minimum of 20 per cent "atypical" lymphocytes near the time of the fever peak.[58] The paradox of a positive heterophil test unaccompanied by characteristic clinical and hematological features of infectious mononucleosis can be explained by persistence of the antibodies from an earlier unrecognized attack and, in rare instances, by a resurgence of

heterophil antibodies with another illness.[58] From the clinical standpoint, certain symptoms are so unusual in infectious mononucleosis that their presence militates against the diagnosis; namely, nasal discharge or congestion, paroxysmal harassing cough, sputum, chest pain, joint pains, painful or extremely tender lymph nodes, watery diarrhea, hematuria or dysuria, or signs suggesting acute appendicitis.[79b]

Treatment.—There is no specific therapy. Sodium perborate mouth washes are recommended since Vincent's infection is so frequently associated with infectious mononucleosis. Agents such as arsenicals and emetine,[59] penicillin and Aureomycin[97d] were tried, without benefit. Convalescent serum, obtained from patients one or two weeks after they had become free from fever, and given intravenously in total doses of 50 to 300 ml., was found useful in bringing about symptomatic relief and fall of temperature, and in preventing complications.[84] It is difficult to evaluate such claims, or other reports, such as the beneficial effects of chloroquine[77b] or adrenocorticosteroid therapy,[65a] since no controlled observations were carried out. Nevertheless, in the rare instances of more than average severity, the corticosterids can at least be expected to provide symptomatic relief without harm resulting if treatment is continued only for five to ten days.[59a]

Strict isolation of cases of the sporadic type does not seem necessary. Cross infection has never been seen in such cases.[59,79b] In epidemic glandular fever contagiousness is high and therefore strict isolation should be practiced.

Prognosis.—In the experience of most physicians the prognosis has been excellent.[59,79b] In a report from a Danish hospital,[84] however, a mortality rate of 1 to 2 per cent in over 500 cases was reported. Undoubtedly the disease may sometimes assume so fulminating a course that a fatal outcome may be feared. Death has been known to occur from pneumonia, edema of the glottis, hemorrhage from a deep tonsillar ulceration, septic complications and, as pointed out earlier, from respiratory paralysis in cases with neurologic complications. One of the commonest of all of these rare complications is splenic rupture, which has led to death in several cases.[79c] The development of pain in the upper left quadrant of the abdomen which is referred to the left shoulder blade, together with shifting dulness and signs of hemorrhage, call for prompt surgical intervention.

It has been observed that, despite the intensity of the changes which may be present, the hepatic lesion in infectious mononucleosis is more benign than its counterpart in infectious hepatitis. Likewise the prognosis in cases with nervous system involvement is good.[59b]

Pathology.—Infectious mononucleosis is a generalized disease with perivascular infiltration of normal and abnormal lymphocytes in almost every organ of the body. At autopsy gross changes have been reported as being confined almost exclusively to enlargement of lymphoid tissues, especially the spleen.[66] Nasopharyngeal lymphoid hyperplasia was constant in the cases examined and hepatic enlargement was consistently present. The abnormal lymphocyte characteristic of the disease can be identified in thin, lightly-stained sections. In the lymph nodes,[66,72,85,97] the pattern ranges from a predominantly follicular hyperplasia to a blurred picture simulating that of a malignant lymphoma, the latter being due to lymphocytic and reticulo-endothelial proliferation in the medullary cords. In the spleen, lymphocytic infiltration in the thinned capsule and trabeculae, frequently dissolving the latter, explains the unusual liability to splenic rupture in this disease. The pattern is partially effaced in most instances and the follicles widely spaced.

In the liver, periportal lymphoid collars sometimes attaining the proportions seen in leukemia have been observed[66] and only rarely has there been evidence of hepatocellular involvement.[107] The finding of meningoencephalitis,[66] and of focal infiltrations in the myocardium,[66] kidneys and lungs[116] explains some of the clinical manifestations of this disorder.

BIBLIOGRAPHY

Agranulocytosis

1. ADAMS, D. A. and PERRY, S.: Agranulocytosis Associated with Thenalidine (Sandostene) Tartrate Therapy, J.A.M.A., *167*, 1207, 1958.
1a. ANDRÉ, R., DREYFUS, B. and SALMON, CH.: Iso-immunisation antileucocytes après transfusions anticorps antileucocytes et leucopénies, Rev. franç. étud. clin. et biol., *3*, 33, 1958.
1b. ANDREWS, J. P., McCLELLAN, J. T. and SCOTT C. H.: Lethal Congenital Neutropenia with Eosinophilia Occurring in Two Siblings, Am. J. Med., *29*, 358, 1960.
1c. ARROWSMITH, W. F., BINKLEY, B. and MOORE, C. V.: Fatal Agranulocytosis Following the Intraperitoneal Implantation of Sulfanilamide Crystals, Ann. Int. Med., *21*, 323, 1944.
1d. ASTWOOD, E. B.: Thiouracil Treatment in Hyperthyroidism, J. Clin. Endocrinol., *4*, 229, 1944.
1e. BARTELS, E. C.: Agranulocytosis During Propylthiouracil Therapy, Am. J. Med. *5*, 48, 1948.
1f. BECKER, F. D., COVENTRY, W. D. and TUURA, J. L.: Recurrent Oral and Cutaneous Infections Associated with Cyclic Neutropenia, A. M. A. Arch. Dermat., *80*, 731, 1959.
2. BERGHAUSEN, O.: Fatal Leukopenia Following Internal Administration of Causalin, J.A.M.A., *114*, 1547, 1940.
3. BOCK, H. E.: Treatment of Agranulocytosis, Fortschr. d. Therap., *13*, 537, 1937.
4. BORST, J. G. G.: Death From Agranulocytosis After Treatment With Prontosil Flavum, Lancet, *1*, 1519, 1937.
4a. BOUSSER, J. and NEYDÉ, R.: La neutropénie familiale, Sang, *18*, 521, 1947.
4b. BRAUN, E. H., BUCKWOLD, A. E., EMSON, H. E. and RUSSELL, A. V.: Familial Neonatal Neutropenia with Maternal Leukocyte Antibodies, Blood, *16*, 1745, 1960.
4c. BRITTINGHAM, T. E. and CHAPLIN, H., JR. The Antigenicity of Normal and Leukemic Human Leukocytes, Blood, *17*, 139, 1961.
5. BRITTON, C. J. C. and HOWKINS, J.: Action

of Sulphanilamide on Leucocytes, Lancet, 2, 718, 1938.

6. BROWN, P. K. and OPHULS, W.: A Fatal Case of Acute Primary Infectious Pharyngitis With Extreme Leukopenia, Am. Med., 3, 649, 1902.

6a. BUTLER, J. J.: Chronic Idiopathic Immuno-neutropenia, Am. J. Med., 24, 145, 1958.

7. BUTT, E. M., HOFFMAN, A. M. and SOLL, S. N.: Experimental Production of Neutro-penia With Aminopyrine, Arch. Int. Med., 64, 26, 1939.

7a. CAHAN, A. M., MEILMAN, E. and JACOBSON, B. M.: Agranulocytosis Following Pyri-benzamine, New England J. Med., 241, 865, 1949; see also J.A.M.A., 143, 741, 742, 1950.

7b. CALDWELL, J. E., SIFFERD, R. H., PORSCHE, J. D. and FENGER, F.: Recent Studies on Yellow Bone Marrow Extracts, Am. J. M. Sc., 209, 717, 1945.

7c. CESAR, A. B.: Familial Chronic Malignant Neutropenia, Bol. Soc. Cubana Pediatria, 15, 900, 1943.

8. CLIMENKO, D. R.: The Modification of the Hematopoietic Function in the Rabbit by Certain Cyclic Compounds, J. Lab. & Clin. Med., 21, 913, 1936.

8a. COLWELL, A. R., JR., SANDO, D. E. and LANG, S. J.: Propylthiouracil-induced Agranulocytosis, Toxic Hepatitis, and Death, J.A.M.A., 148, 639, 1952.

8b. COTTER, L. H.: Thioglycolic Acid Poisoning in Connection With the "Cold Wave" Process, J.A.M.A., 131, 593, 1946.

9. DAMESHEK, W. and COLMES, A.: The Effect of Drugs in the Production of Agranulo-cytosis With Particular Reference to Amidopyrine Sensitivity, J. Clin. Invest., 15, 85, 1936.

10. DARLING, R. C., PARKER, F., JR. and JACK-SON, H., JR.: The Pathological Changes in the Bone Marrow, Am. J. Path., 12, 1, 1936.

11. DAUSSET, J. and NENNA, A.: Présence d'une leuco-agglutinine dans le sérum d'un cas d'agranulocytose chronique, Compt. rend. Soc. de biol., 146, 1539, 1952; Rev. hémat., 8, 316, 1953; Sang, 24, 410, 1953; Vox sanguinis, 4, 190, 1954; Sang, 30, 634, 1959; Brit. J. Haemat., 5, 225, 1959.

11a. DAVIS, J. A., VIEHMAN, A. J., FROMMEYER, W. B., JR.: Acute Agranulocytosis during the Use of Tibione, South. M. J., 45, 861, 1952.

12. DISCOMBE, G.: Agranulocytosis Caused by Amidopyrine, Brit. M. J., 1, 1270, 1952.

12a. DRAKE, T. G.: Agranulocytosis During Therapy with the Anti-Histaminic Agent Methaphenilene (Diatrin), J.A.M.A., 142, 477, 1950.

12b. ERF, L. A. and FRY, K. E.: Primary Splenic Neutropenia, Am. J. Clin. Path., 19, 48, 1949.

12c. EVANS, R. S. and FORD, W. P., JR.: Studies of the Bone Marrow in Immunological Granulocytopenia, A. M. A. Arch. Int. Med., 101, 244, 1958.

13. FINLAND, M., PETERSON, O. L. and GOOD-WIN, R. A., JR.: Sulfadiazine; Further Studies of Its Efficacy and Toxic Effects in 460 Patients, Ann. Int. Med., 17, 920, 1942.

13a. FIORE, J. M. and NOONAN, F. M.: Agranulo-cytosis Due to Mepazine (Phenothiazine), New England J. Med., 260, 375, 1959.

14. FISHER, S., HOLLEY, H. L. and FEIN, G.: Agranulocytosis, Arch. Dermat., 55, 57, 1947.

15. FITZ-HUGH, T. and KRUMBHAAR, E. B.: Myeloid Cell Hyperplasia of Bone Marrow in Agranulocytic Angina, Am. J. M. Sc., 183, 104, 1932.

16. FRIEDEMANN, U. and ELKELES, A.: Roentgen Treatment of Agranulocytosis, Deutsch. med. Wchnschr., 56, 947, 1930.

17. GASSER, C.: Die Pathogenese der essentiellen chronischen Granulocytopenie im Kindes-alter auf Grund der Knochenmarksbe-funde, Helvet. pædiat. acta, 7, 426, 1952.

18. GOLDMAN, A. and HABER, M.: Acute Com-plete Granulopenia With Death Due to Dinitrophenol Poisoning, J.A.M.A., 107, 2115, 1936.

18a. GOUDSMIT, R. and VAN LOGHEM, J. J., JR.: Studies on the Occurrence of Leucocyte-antibodies, Vox sanguinis, 3, 3, 1953; ibid., 3, 203, 1958.

19. HADLER, A. J.: Granulocytopenia Following Barbiturate Therapy, New England J. Med., 222, 755, 1940.

20. HANSEN, A. B.: Some Investigations on Experimental Agranulocytosis in Rabbits, Acta med. scandinav., 98, 307, 1939.

20b. HART, F. D., WRAITH, D. G. and MANSELL, E. J. B.: Agranulocytosis Successfully Treated with A.C.T.H., Brit. M. J., 1, 1273, 1952.

20c. HELLER, G. C. and SIME, D. A.: Agranulo-cytosis during Treatment with Diethazine Hydrochloride, Lancet, 1, 192, 1952.

20d. HETTIG, R. A. and STURGIS, C. C.: Sulfa-diazine Agranulocytosis, J. Mich. State Med. Soc., 42, 959, 1943.

21. HOLTEN, C.: Considerations and Experiments on the Hypersensitive Nature of Amido-

pyrine Agranulocytosis, Am. J. M. Sc., *194*, 229, 1937.

21*a*.HUNTER, D.: Industrial Toxicology, Quart. J. Med., *12*, 185, 1943.

21*b*.HUSSAR, A. E. and ROGERS, H. B.: Agranulocytosis Occurring during Phethenylate ("Thiantoin") Sodium Therapy, J.A.M.A., *149*, 1312, 1952.

22. ISRAËLS, M. C. G. and WILKINSON, J. F.: Observations on Agranulocytosis, Quart. J. Med., *6*, 35, 1937.

23. JACKSON, H., JR.: Relation of Amidopyrin and Allied Drugs to Etiology of Agranulocytic Angina, Am. J. M. Sc., *188*, 482, 1934.

24. JACKSON, H., JR. and TIGHE, T. J. G.: An Analysis of the Treatment and Mortality of 390 Cases of Acute Agranulocytic Angina, New England J. Med., *220*, 729, 1939.

24*a*.JOHNSON, S. A. M.: Acute Agranulocytosis Due to Administration of Succinylsulfathiazole, J.A.M.A., *122*, 668, 1943.

24*b*.KARLIN, H.: Fatal Agranulocytosis Following Chlorpropamide Treatment of Diabetes, New England J. Med., *262*, 1076, 1960.

24*c*.KENNEDY, P. C. and FINLAND, M.: Fatal Agranulocytosis From Sulfathiazole, J.A. M.A., *116*, 295, 1941; J. Pediat., *22*, 432, 1943.

24*d*.KIELY, J. M. and STICKNEY, J. M.: Agranulocytosis Caused by Phenylbutazone and 4-amino-antipyrine, Proc. Staff Meet., Mayo Clin., *28*, 341, 1953.

24*e*.KILLMANN, S. A.: Auto-Aggressive Leukocyte Agglutinins in Leukaemia and Chronic Leukopenia, Acta med. scandinav., *163*, 207, 445, and 449, 1959.

25. KLUMPP, T. G.: Agranulocytosis Associated With the Administration of "Novaldin," a derivative of Aminopyrine, J.A.M.A., *108*, 637, 1937.

25*a*.KORST, D. R.: Agranulocytosis Caused by Phenothiazine Derivatives, J.A.M.A., *170*, 2076, 1959.

25*b*.KOSTMANN, R.: Infantile Genetic Agranulocytosis, Acta paediat. (Suppl. 105), *45*, 6, 1956.

25*c*.KOSZEWSKI, B. J. and HUBBARD, T. F.: Immunologic Agranulocytosis Due to Mercurial Diuretics, Am. J. Med., *20*, 958, 1956.

26. KRACKE, R. R.: Recurrent Agranulocytosis, Am. J. Clin. Path., *1*, 385, 1931.

27. ———Relation of Drug Therapy to Neutropenic States, J.A.M.A., *111*, 1255, 1938.

27*a*.LALEZARI, P., NUSSBAUM, M., GELMAN, S. and SPAET, T. H.: Neonatal Neutropenia Due to Maternal Isoimmunization, Blood, *15*, 236, 1960.

28. LANGSTON, W., WHITE, O. A. and ASHLEY, J. D., JR.: Splenic Neutropenia, Ann. Int. Med., *23*, 667, 1945.

29. LAWRENCE, J. S., SYVERTON, J. T., SHAW, J. S., JR. and SMITH, F. P.: Infectious Feline Agranulocytosis, Am. J. Path., *16*, 333, 1940; J. Exper. Med., *77*, 41 and 57, 1943.

29*a*.LOCKIE, L. M., NORCROSS, B. M. and GEORGE, C. W.: Treatment of Two Reactions Due to Gold, J.A.M.A., *133*, 754, 1947.

29*b*.LOVEMAN, A. B.: Toxic Granulocytopenia, Purpura Hemorrhagica and Aplastic Anemia Following the Arsphenamines, Ann. Int. Med., *5*, 1238, 1932; KASICH M.: Agranulocytosis Following Mapharsen Therapy, Arch. Dermat., *50*, 302, 1944.

30. MADISON, F. W. and SQUIER, T. L.: Etiology of Primary Granulocytopenia (Agranulocytic Angina), J.A.M.A., *102*, 755, 1934; J. Allergy, *6*, 9, 1934.

31. MALEWITZ, E. C.: Leukopenia following Fumagillin Treatment for Amebiasis, J.A.M.A., *153*, 1446, 1953.

31*a*.McCLUSKEY, H. B.: Corticotropin (ACTH) in Treatment of Agranulocytosis following Sulfisoxazole Therapy, J.A.M.A., *152*, 232, 1953.

31*b*.McGAVACK, T. H., GERL, A. J., VOGEL, M. and SCHWIMMER, D.: Treatment of 26 Thyrotoxic Patients With Thiouracil and a Review of Toxic Reactions in All (135) Reported Cases, J. Clin. Endocrinol., *4*, 249, 1944.

32. McGOVERN, F. H.: Granulocytopenia Following Ingestion of Causalin, J.A.M.A., *115*, 1359, 1940.

32*a*.MICHELSTEIN, I. and WEISER, N. J.: Fatal Agranulocytosis Due to Trimethadione (Tridione), Arch. Neurol. & Psych., *62*, 358, 1949.

32*b*.MILLER, H., POLLOCK, R. C. and GRIFFITH, G. C.: Fatal Agranulocytosis Resulting from a Procaine Derivative, J. Lab. & Clin. Med., *38*, 850, 1951.

33. MILLER, D. K. and RHOADS, C. P.: The Effect of Diet on the Susceptibility of the Canine Hematopoietic Function to Damage by Amidopyrine, J. Exper. Med., *66*, 367, 1937.

33*a*.MOESCHLIN, S. and WAGNER, K.: Agranulocytosis Due to the Occurrence of Leukocyte-Agglutinins, Acta hæmat., *8*, 29, 1952; *ibid.*, *11*, 73, 1954; Klin. Wchnschr., *32*, 799, 1954; Arztl. Forsch., *8*, 229, 1954; Sang, *26*, 32, 1955.

33b. MOORE, F. D.: Toxic Manifestations of Thiouracil Therapy. J.A.M.A., *130*, 315, 1946.

34. MUETHER, R. O., MOORE, L. T., STEWART, J. W. and BROUN, G. O.: Chronic Granulocytopenia Caused by Excessive Splenic Lysis of Granulocytes, J.A.M.A., *116*, 2255, 1941.

34a. NEWTON, R. M. and WARD, V. G.: Leukopenia Associated with Ristocetin (Spontin) Administration, J.A.M.A., *166*, 1956, 1958.

34b. PAGE, A. R. and GOOD, R. A.: Studies on Cyclic Neutropenia, A.M.A.J. Dis. Child., *94*, 623, 1957.

34c. PAYNE, ROSE: Leukocyte Agglutinins in Human Sera, A.M.A. Arch. Int. Med., *99*, 587, 1957; J. Clin. Invest., *37*, 1756, 1958.

34d. PEARSON, J. R., BINDER, C. I. and NEBER, J.: Agranulocytosis following Diamox Therapy, J.A.M.A., *157*, 339, 1955.

34e. PISCIOTTA, A. V. *et al.*: Agranulocytosis Following Administration of Phenothiazine Derivatives, Am. J. Med., *25*, 210, 1958.

35. PLUM, P.: *Clinical and Experimental Investigations in Agranulocytosis*, London, H. K. Lewis & Co., Ltd., 1937.

35a. PULVER, W. und SPILLMANN, W.: Agranulocytose und Methylthiouracil, Schweiz. med. Wchnschr., *83*, 538, 1953.

36. RAWLS, W. B.: The Effect of Amidopyrin Upon the Red, White and Polymorphonuclear Blood Cells of a Series of 100 Patients, Am. J. M. Sc., *192*, 175, 1936.

37. REIMANN, H. A. and DEBARARDINIS, C. T.: Periodic (Cyclic) Neutropenia, Blood, *4*, 1109, 1949; Medicine, *30*, 219, 1951; Arch. Int. Med., *92*, 494, 1953.

38. REZNIKOFF, P.: The Etiologic Importance of Fatigue and the Prognostic Significance of Monocytosis in Neutropenia (Agranulocytosis), Am. J. M. Sc., *195*, 627, 1938.

38a. RICH, M. and BELLE, M. S.: Agranulocytosis Resulting from Methimazole (Tapazole), J.A.M.A., *167*, 573, 1958.

38b. RINKOFF, S. S. and SPRING, M.: Toxic Depression of the Myeloid Elements Following Therapy With the Sulfonamides, Ann. Int. Med., *15*, 89, 1941.

38c. RITZ, N. D. and FISHER, M. J.: Agranulocytosis Due to Administration of Salicylazosulfapyridine (Azulfidine), J.A.M.A., *172*, 237, 1960.

38d. ROGERS, H. M. and HALL, B. E.: Primary Splenic Neutropenia, Arch. Int. Med., *75*, 192, 1945.

39. ROHR, K.: Der heutige Stand der Agranulozytoseforschung, Helvet. med. acta, *6*, 611, 1939.

40. ROSENTHAL, N. and ABEL, H. A.: The Significance of the Monocytes in Agranulocytosis (Leukopenic Infectious Monocytosis), Am. J. Clin. Path., *6*, 205, 1936.

41. ROSENTHAL, N. and VOGEL, P.: Granulocytopenia Caused by Sulfapyridine in Children, J.A.M.A., *113*, 584, 1939.

41a. ROSSI, J. P. and BRANDT, I. K.: Transient Granulocytopenia of the Newborn Associated with Sepsis Due to Shigella Alkalescens and Maternal Leukocyte Agglutinins, J. Pediat., *56*, 639, 1960.

42. ROSSMAN, P. L. and HUMMER, G. J.: Chronic Neutropenia in Siblings: the Effect of Steroids, Ann. Int. Med., *52*, 242, 1960.

42a. SALZER, M., RANSOHOFF, L. and BLATT, H.: Primary Splenic Neutropenia, Ann. Int. Med., *22*, 271, 1945.

43. SCHULTZ, W.: Über eigenartige Halserkrankungen, Deutsch. med. Wchnschr., *48*, 1495, 1922.

45. SIMON, H. J. and ROGERS, D. E.: Agranulocytosis Associated with Novobiocin Administration, Ann. Int. Med., *46*, 778, 1957.

46. SIMON, S. D. and METZ, M. H.: Amidopyrine and the Circulating Leucocytes, J. Lab. & Clin. Med., *21*, 1154, 1936.

47. SPAET, T. H. and DAMESHEK, W.: Chronic Hypoplastic Neutropenia, Am. J. Med., *13*, 35, 1952.

48. STEEL, S. J. and MOFFATT, J. L.: Stevens-Johnson Syndrome and Granulocytopenia after Phenylbutazone, Brit. M. J., *1*, 795, 1954.

48a. STEINBERG, C. L., BOHROD, M. G. and ROODENBURG, A. I.: Agranulocytosis following Phenylbutazone (Butazolidin) Therapy, J.A.M.A., *152*, 33, 1953.

48b. STEFANINI, M., MELE, ROSE H. and SKINNER, D.: Transitory Congenital Neutropenia, a New Syndrome, Am. J. Med., *25*, 749, 1958.

49. STEPHENS, D. J. and LAWRENCE, J. S.: Cyclical Agranulocytic Angina, Ann. Int. Med., *9*, 31, 1935.

49a. STERNLIEB, P. and EISMAN, S. H.: Toxic Hepatitis and Agranulocytosis Due to Cinchophen, Ann. Int. Med., *47*, 826, 1957.

50. STRUMIA, M. M.: Effect of Leukocytic Cream Injections in Treatment of Neutropenias, Am. J. M. Sc., *187*, 527, 1934.

50a. Subcommittee on Blood Dyscrasias, Committee on Research, Council on Drugs, Tabulation of Therapeutic and Other Agents Involved in Blood Dyscrasias, American Medical Association, Vol. 4, No. 2, 1960, Chicago.

51. SWEENEY, J. S. and ALLDAY, L. E.: Granulo-

cytopenia From Sulfanilamide With Unusual Blood Crisis and Recovery, Ann. Int. Med., *13*, 1241, 1940.

51*a*.TAIT, G. B.: Fatal Agranulocytosis During Carbimazole Therapy, Lancet, *1*, 303, 1957.

51*b*.TASHJIAN, A. H., JR. and LEDDY, J. P.: Agranulocytosis Associated with Phenindione, A.M.A. Arch. Int. Med., *105*, 121, 1960.

52. THOMPSON, W. P.: Observations on Possible Relation Between Agranulocytosis and Menstruation With Further Studies on a Case of Cyclic Neutropenia, New England J. Med., *210*, 176, 1934.

52*a*.TRASOFF, A., WOHL, M. G. and MINTZ, S. S.: Fatal Agranulocytosis With Autopsy Following the Use of Thiouracil, Am. J. M. Sc., *211*, 62, 1946.

53. TÜRK, W.: Septische Erkrankungen bei Verkümmerung des Granulocytensystems, Wien. klin. Wchnschr., *20*, 157, 1907.

53*a*.TYSON, T. L.: Agranulocytosis Following Pyrithyldione (Presidon) Therapy, J.A.M.A., *141*, 128, 1949.

53*b*.VAHLQUIST, B., et ANJOU, N.: Granulocytopénie chronique bénigne, Acta hæmat., *8*, 199, 1952.

53*c*.VRTILEK, M. R.: Das Bild der chronischen Granulocytopenie im Kindesalter, Helvet. pædiat. acta, *7*, 207, 1952.

54. WATKINS, C. H.: The Possible Rôle of Barbiturates and Amidopyrine in the Causation of Leucopenic States, Proc. Staff Meet., Mayo Clin., *8*, 713, 1933.

54*a*.WENDEROTH, H. und LENNARTZ, H.: Agranulocytose nach Phenothiazin, Med. Klin., *50*, 818, 1955.

55. WILSON, S. J.: Effects of Aminopyrine and Phenobarbital on Blood Cell Count of White Rats, Kansas Med. Soc. J., *36*, 500, 1935.

56. WISEMAN, B. K. and DOAN, C. A.: A Newly Recognized Granulopenic Syndrome Caused by Excessive Splenic Leukolysis and Successfully Treated by Splenectomy, J. Clin. Invest., *18*, 473, 1939; Ann. Int. Med., *16*, 1097, 1942.

56*a*.WRIGHT, C. S., DOAN, C. A. and HAYNIE, H. C.: Agranulocytosis Occurring After Exposure to a D.D.T. Pyrethrum Aerosol Bomb, Am. J. Med., *1*, 562, 1946.

57. ZIA, L. S. and FORKNER, C. E.: Syndrome of Acute Agranulocytosis and Its Occurrence as Complication of Kala-azar, Am. J. M. Sc., *188*, 624, 1934.

Infectious Mononucleosis

57*a*.BARONDESS, J. A. and ERLE, H.: Serum Alkaline Phosphatase Activity in Hepatitis of Infectious Mononucleosis, Am. J. Med., *29*, 43, 1960.

57*b*.BASSEN, F. A., THOMSON, A. E. and SILVER, A.: The Occurrence of False Positive Trichina Precipitin Tests in Infectious Mononucleosis, J. Lab. & Clin. Med., *34*, 543, 1949.

58. BENDER, C. E.: Interpretation of Hematologic and Serologic Findings in the Diagnosis of Infectious Mononucleosis, Ann. Int. Med., *49*, 852, 1958.

59. BERNSTEIN, A.: Infectious Mononucleosis, Medicine, *19*, 85, 1940 (Bibliography).

59*a*.BERNARD, J., MATHE, G. and SIGAL, SUZANNE: Traitement par la cortisone de 22 cas de mononucléose infectieuse avec réaction de Paul et Bunnell positive, Sang, *27*, 545, 1956.

59*b*.BERNSTEIN, T. C. and WOLFF, H. G.: Involvement of the Nervous System in Infectious Mononucleosis, Ann. Int. Med., *33*, 1120, 1950.

60. BLAND, J. O. W.: Glandular Fever, II: The Protozoal Nature of the Experimental Disease, Brit. J. Exper. Path., *12*, 311, 1931.

61. BLOEDORN, W. A. and HOUGHTON, J. E.: The Occurrence of Abnormal Leukocytes in the Blood in Acute Infections, Arch. Int. Med., *27*, 315, 1921.

62. BOWCOCK, H.: Mitotic Leucoblasts in the Peripheral Blood in Infectious Mononucleosis, Am. J. M. Sc., *198*, 384, 1939.

63. BURNS, J. E.: Glandular Fever: Report of an Epidemic in the Children's Ward of the Union Protestant Infirmary, Arch. Int. Med., *4*, 118, 1909.

64. CABOT, R. C.: The Lymphocytosis of Infection, Am. J. M. Sc., *145*, 335, 1913.

65. CONTRATTO, A. W.: Infectious Mononucleosis, Arch. Int. Med., *73*, 449, 1944.

65*a*.CREDITOR, M. C. and McCURDY, H. W.: Severe Infectious Mononucleosis Treated with Prednisolone, Ann. Int. Med., *50*, 218, 1959.

66. CUSTER, R. P. and SMITH, E. B.: The Pathology of Infectious Mononucleosis, Blood, *3*, 830, 1948.

67. DAVIDSOHN, I.: Serologic Diagnosis of Infectious Mononucleosis, J.A.M.A., *108*, 289, 1937.

68. DAVIDSOHN, I., STERN, K. and KASHIWAGI, C.: The Differential Test for Infectious Mononucleosis, Am. J. Clin. Path., *21*, 1101, 1951; J. Lab. & Clin. Med., *45*, 561, 1955.

70. DAVIS, C. M.: Acute Glandular Fever of Pfeiffer, J.A.M.A., *92*, 1417, 1929.

70*a*.DeMEIO, J. L. and WALKER, D. L.: Sendai Virus Antibody in Acute Respiratory Infections and Infectious Mononucleosis, Proc. Soc. Exper. Biol. & Med., *98*, 453, 1958.

70*b*.DIDISHEIM, P. and LEE, G. R.: Thrombocytopenia, Fibrinogenopenia and Fibrinolysin in Infectious Mononucleosis, (to be published).

71. DOWNEY, H. and McKINLAY, C. A.: Acute Lymphadenosis Compared With Acute Lymphatic Leukemia, Arch. Int. Med., *32*, 82, 1923.

72. DOWNEY, H. and STASNEY, J.: The Pathology of the Lymph Nodes in Infectious Mononucleosis, Folia hæmat., *54*, 417, 1936.

73. EVANS, A. S.: Further Experimental Attempts to Transmit Infectious Mononucleosis to Man, J. Clin. Invest., *29*, 508, 1950; Proc. Soc. Exper. Biol. & Med., *82*, 437 1953.

73*a*.EVANS, A. S. and ROBINSON, E. D.: An Epidemiologic Study of Infectious Mononucleosis in a New England College, New England J. Med., *242*, 492, 1950.

73*b*.FISH, M. and BARTON, H. R.: Heart Involvement in Infectious Mononucleosis, A.M.A. Arch. Int. Med., *101*, 636, 1958.

74. FOORD, A. G. and BUTT, E. M.: The Laboratory Diagnosis of Infectious Mononucleosis, Am. J. Clin. Path., *9*, 448, 1939.

75. FREEDMAN, M. J., ODLAND, L. T. and CLEVE, E. A.: Infectious Mononucleosis with Diffuse Involvement of Nervous System, Arch. Neurol. & Psychiat., *69*, 49, 1953.

76. GALL, E. A.: Diagnostic Value of Supravital Staining in Infectious Mononucleosis, Am. J. M. Sc., *194*, 546, 1937.

77. GARDNER, H. T. and PAUL, J. R.: Infectious Mononucleosis at the New Haven Hospital, 1921 to 1946, Yale J. Biol. & Med., *19*, 839, 1947.

77*a*.GORHAM, L. W., SMITH, D. T. and HUNT, H. D.: The Experimental Reproduction of the Blood Picture of Infectious Mononucleosis in the Guinea Pig. J. Clin. Invest., *7*, 504, 1929.

77*b*.GOTHBERG, L. A.: Severe Infectious Mononucleosis Treated with Chloroquine Phosphate, J.A.M.A., *173*, 53, 1960.

78. GREEN, N. and GOLDENBERG, G.: Acute Hemolytic Anemia and Hemoglobinuria Complicating Infectious Mononucleosis, A. M. A. Arch. Int. Med., *105*, 108, 1960.

79. GROSSMAN, L. A. and WOLFF, S. M.: Acute Thrombocytopenic Purpura in Infectious Mononucleosis, J.A.M.A., *171*, 2208, 1959.

79*a*.HARLEY, J. F.: Infectious Mononucleosis in the Negro, J. Pediat., *39*, 303, 1951.

79*b*.HOAGLAND, R. J.: Infectious Mononucleosis, Am. J. Med., *13*, 158, 1952; Ann. Int.

Med., *43*, 1019, 1955; Am. J. M. Sc., *232*, 252, 1956; *ibid.*, *240*, 21, 1960; Blood, *16*, 1045, 1960.

79*c*.HOAGLAND, R. J. and HENSON, H. M.: Splenic Rupture in Infectious Mononucleosis, Ann. Int. Med., *46*, 1184, 1957.

79*d*.HOVDE, R. F. and SUNDBERG, R. D.: Granulomatous Lesions in the Bone Marrow in Infectious Mononucleosis, Blood, *5*, 209, 1950.

80. IRELAND, R. A., BAETJER, W. A. and RUHRÄH, J.: A Case of Lymphatic Leukemia With Apparent Cure, J.A.M.A., *65*, 948, 1915.

80*a*.JANEWAY, C. A. and DAMMIN, G. J.: Infectious Mononucleosis: II. The Relationship of the Organisms of the genus *Listerella* to the Disease, J. Clin. Invest., *20*, 233, 1941.

80*b*.JULIANELLE, L. A., BIERBAUM, O. S. and MOORE, C. V.: Studies on Infectious Mononucleosis, Ann. Int. Med., *20*, 281, 1944.

80*c*.KAGEYAMA, T.: Morphological Studies on the Pathogenic Agent of Glandular Fever, Fukuoka acta med., *49*, 1056 and 1072, 1958.

81. KAHN, R. L.: Are There Paradoxic Serologic Reactions in Syphilis? Arch. Dermat., *39*, 92, 1939.

82. KAUFFMAN, R. E.: Eosinophilia in Infectious Mononucleosis, Am. J. M. Sc., *219*, 206, 1950.

83. KOLMER, J. A.: *Listerella Monocytogenes* in Relation to the Wassermann and Flocculation Reactions in Normal Rabbits, Proc. Soc. Exper. Biol. & Med., *42*, 183, 1939.

84. LASSEN, H. C. A. and THOMSEN, S.: Treatment of Infectious Mononucleosis With Specific Convalescent Serum, Acta med. scandinav., *104*, 427, 1940.

84*a*.LAZAR, H. P., MANFREDI, R. and HAMMOND, J. H.: Seizures in Infectious Mononucleosis, Am. J. Med., *21*, 990, 1956.

84*b*.LI, J. G. and MORTON, D. G.: Infectious Mononucleosis, Am. J. Obst. & Gynec., *67*, 184, 1954.

85. LONGCOPE, W. T.: Infectious Mononucleosis (Glandular Fever), With a Report of Ten Cases, Am. J. M. Sc., *164*, 781, 1922.

86. MARCHAND, F.: Über ungewöhnlich starke Lymphocytose im Anschluss an Infektionen, Deutsch. Arch. klin. Med., *110*, 359, 1913.

86*a*.McCORT, J. J.: Infectious Mononucleosis, Am. J. Roentgenol., *62*, 645, 1949.

86*b*.MIKKELSEN, W., TUPPER, C. J. and MURRAY, JEAN: The Ox Cell Hemolysin Test As a Diagnostic Procedure in Infectious Mononucleosis, J. Lab. & Clin. Med., *52*, 648, 1958.

87. MINKENHOF, J. E.: La réaction de Paul et Bunnell, Sang, *9*, 87, 1935.

88. MITCHELL, R. H. and ZETZEL, L.: Infectious Mononucleosis in the Army, War Med., *5*, 356, 1944.

89. MOIR, J. I.: Glandular Fever in the Falkland Islands, Brit. M. J., *2*, 822, 1930.

89a.MUSCHEL, L. H. and PIPER, D. R.: Enzyme-Treated Red Blood Cells of Sheep in the Test for Infectious Mononucleosis, Am. J. Clin. Path., *32*, 240, 1959.

89b.MYHRE, J. and NESBITT, S.: Pancreatitis in Infectious Mononucleosis, J. Lab. & Clin. Med., *34*, 1671, 1949.

89c.NELSON, R. S., and DARRAGH, J. H.: Infectious Mononucleosis Hepatitis, Am. J. Med., *21*, 26, 1956.

90. NOLAN, R. A.: Report of So-called Epidemic of Glandular Fever (Infectious Mononucleosis), U. S. Nav. Med. Bull., *33*, 479, 1935.

91. NYFELDT, A.: Klinische und experimentelle Untersuchungen über die Mononucleosis infectiosa, Folia hæmat., *47*, 1, 1932; Ugesk. f. læger, *13*, 1, 1938; *ibid.*, *100*, 336, 1938.

92. OGINO, T.: Infectious Mononucleosis in Japan, Kobe J. M. Sc., *4*, 59, 1958.

93. PAUL, J. R.: Infectious Mononucleosis, Bull. New York Acad. Med., *15*, 43, 1939.

94. PAUL, J. R. and BUNNELL, W. W.: The Presence of Heterophile Antibodies in Infectious Mononucleosis, Am. J. M. Sc., *183*, 90, 1932.

95. PFEIFFER, E.: Drüsenfieber, Jahrb.f. Kinderh., *29*, 257, 1889.

96. PONS, C. A. and JULIANELLE, L. A.: Isolation of *Listerella Monocytogenes* From Infectious Mononucleosis. Proc. Soc. Exper. Biol. & Med., *40*, 360, 1939.

96a.RAFTERY, M., SCHUMACHER, E. E., JR., GRAIN, G. O. and QUINN, E. L.: Infectious Mononucleosis and Guillain-Barré Syndrome, Arch. Int. Med., *93*, 246, 1954.

96b.RANDOLPH, T. G. and GIBSON, E. B.: Blood Studies in Allergy, Am. J. M. Sc., *207*, 638, 1944; *ibid.*, *209*, 306, 1945.

96c.RAVENNA, P. and SNYDER, J.: The Occurrence of Edema of the Pharynx and Larynx in Infectious Mononucleosis, Ann. Int. Med., *28*, 861, 1948.

96d.READ, J. T. and HELWIG, F. C.: Infectious Mononucleosis, Arch. Int. Med., *75*, 377, 1945.

96e.REAM, C. R. and HESSING, J. W.: Infectious Mononucleosis Encephalitis, Ann. Int. Med., *41*, 1231, 1954.

97. REINAUER, H.: Morphologische Befunde an Lymphknoten bei infektiöser Mononukleose, Arch. path. Anat., *332*, 56, 1959.

97a.RENNIE, L. E. and WROBLEWSKI, F.: The Clinical Significance of Serum Transaminase in Infectious Mononucleosis Complicated by Hepatitis, New England J. Med., *257*, 547, 1957.

97b.ROSEMAN, D. M. and BARRY, R. M.: Acute Pericarditis As the First Manifestation of Infectious Mononucleosis, Ann. Int. Med., *47*, 351, 1957.

97c.RUBIN, L.: The Serum Lipoproteins in Infectious Mononucleosis, Am. J. Med., *17*, 521, 1954.

97d.SCHULTZ, A. L. and HALL, W. H.: Clinical Observations in 100 Cases of Infectious Mononucleosis and the Results of Treatment with Penicillin and Aureomycin, Ann. Int. Med., *36*, 1498, 1952.

98. SCHULTZ, W.: Ueber eigenartige Halserkrankungen: (*a*) Monozytenangina, Deutsch. med. Wchnschr., *48*, 1495, 1922.

98a.SHAPIRO, C. M. and HORWITZ, H.: Infectious Mononucleosis in the Aged, Ann. Int. Med., *51*, 1092, 1959.

98b.SHUGOLL, G. I.: Pericarditis Associated with Infectious Mononucleosis, A.M.A. Arch. Int. Med., *100*, 630, 1957.

98c.SILVER, H. K., ROBERTSON, W. O., WRAY J. D. and GRUSKAY, F. L.: Involvement o the Central Nervous System in Infectious Mononucleosis in Childhood, A.M.A. Am. J. Dis., Child., *91*, 490, 1956.

99. SPRUNT, T. P. and EVANS, F. A.: Mononuclear Leucocytosis in Reaction to Acute Infections ("Infectious Mononucleosis"), Bull. Johns Hopkins Hosp., *31*, 410, 1920.

100. STERLING, K.: The Serum Proteins in Infectious Mononucleosis. Electrophoretic Studies, J. Clin. Invest., *28*, 1057, 1949.

101. TEMPLETON, H. J. and SUTHERLAND, R. T.: The Exanthem of Acute Mononucleosis, J.A.M.A., *113*, 1215, 1939.

103. TIDY, H. L.: Glandular Fever and Infectious Mononucleosis, Lancet, 2, 180 and 236, 1934.

104. TIDY, H. L. and MORLEY, E. B.: Glandular Fever, Brit. M. J., *1*, 452, 1921.

105. TÜRK, W.: Septische Erkrankungen bei Verkümmerung des Granulozytensystems, Wien. klin. Wchnschr., *20*, 157, 1907.

106. VAN DEN BERGHE, L. and LIESSEN, P.: Transmission de la mononucleose infectieuse au Macacus rhesus, Compt. rend. Soc. de biol., *131*, 156, 1939.

107. WADSWORTH, R. C. and KEIL, P. G.: Biopsy of the Liver in Infectious Mononucleosis, Am. J. Path., *28*, 1003, 1952.

107a. WANG, S.-P. and GRAYSTON, J. T.: Goat Red Blood Cells in Agglutination Test for Infectious Mononucleosis, Proc. Soc. Exper. Biol. & Med., *101*, 111, 1959.

108. WATSON, J., JOHNSON, P., KAHN, J. and STONE, F. M.: Subclinical Infectious Mononucleosis with Hepatitis, Arch. Int. Med., *88*, 618, 1951.

109. WECHSLER, H. F., ROSENBLUM, A. H. and SILLS, C. T.: Infectious Mononucleosis— Report of an Epidemic in an Army Camp, Ann. Int. Med., *25*, 113 and 236, 1946.

110. WEST, J. P.: An Epidemic of Glandular Fever, Arch. Pediat., *13*, 889, 1896.

111. WISING, P. J.: Some Experiments With Lymph Gland Material From Cases of Infectious Mononucleosis, Acta med. scandinav., *98*, 328, 1939; *ibid.*, *109*, 507, 1942.

112. YI-YUNG, HSIA, D. and GELLIS, S. S.: Hepatic Dysfunction in Infectious Mononucleosis in Children, Am. J. Dis. Child., *84*, 175, 1952.

114. ZARAFONETIS, C. J. and KENT, J. F.: Serologic Tests for Syphilis in Infectious Mononucleosis, J. Lab. & Clin. Med., *43*, 253, 1954.

115. ZARAFONETIS, C. J. D., OSTER, H. L. and COLVILLE, V. F.: Cold Agglutination of Sheep Erythrocytes as a Factor in False-Positive Heterophile Agglutination Tests, J. Lab. & Clin. Med., *41*, 906, 1953.

116. ZIEGLER, E. E.: Infectious Mononucleosis, Fatal Case With Autopsy, Arch. Path., *37*, 196, 1944.

Appendix A

COMPARATIVE HEMATOLOGY— TABULATED DATA AND BIBLIOGRAPHY

In Tables A–1 and A–2 are listed blood counts as recorded by a number of different observers in a large variety of animals. The tabulated data are representative but not exhaustive. Some blood counts are not given in the tables but will be found in the references cited, especially in the monographs on comparative hematology which are listed. Descriptions of cells and excellent illustrations will be found in the articles cited.

Leukocyte counts, both total and differential, fluctuate much more in animals than in man in the absence of disease. The data recorded give only average values and a considerable range about these means should be expected.

Table A-1—Blood Counts in Twenty-Four Species of Mammals

Species	Author	R.B.C.	Hgb.	Ht.	M.C.V.	M.C.H.	M.C.H.C.	Diam.	W.B.C.	N.	E.	B.	L.	Mo.	Pl.	No. of animals
Camel	Ponder et al.[22]	10.62	..	..	..	..	..	7.3 x 3.8	11.4	61.0	21.0	2.5	9.5	6.0	..	..
Cat	Landsberg[31]	7.24±1.01	10.5±2.1	40.2±6.1	57±6	15±2.2	27±4.1	..	17.2±6.6	59.3	6.9	0	33.0	0.8	232±62	52
	Scarborough[18]	8.43±1.40	..	..	..	..	..	..	13.8	57.1	5.3	0.1	32.5	5.9	..	130±
	Vaulont[17]	7.85	12.8	..	..	..	..	5.9	9.2–24.0	42–84	1–18	1.0	8–45	1–3	..	20
Chimpanzee	Wintrobe[9][41]	5.11	12.3	41.6	82	25	30	..	12.0–22.0	53.0	7.0	0	40.0	0	290	10
	Ponder et al.[41]	6.30	..	..	..	..	..	7.4	10.4	58.0	5.0	20.0	16.0	1.0	..	1
Cow	Kushner[23] (Cows, bulls and calves of different ages).	5.6–8.9	..	..	..	..	..	5.0–5.9	..	..	..	..	..	..	..	219
	Delaune[24] (to six months of age)	8.70	..	..	..	..	..	..	..	3.5	0.5	0	96.0	0	..	6
	(three to six and a half years of age)	6.39	..	..	..	..	..	..	..	..	..	..	..	..	..	5
	Drastisch[10]	6.41	10.6	33.0	52	19	32	..	10.7	19.6	3.3	0	64.4	12.2	..	1
	Wintrobe[9]	6.96	13.5	40.0	58	20	34	..	10.2	25.9	7.0	0	58.1	8.0	160	2
Deer	Wintrobe[9]	8.37	13.9	40.5	48	17	34	..	7.5	27.0	7.0	2.0	63.0	1.0	..	1
Dog	Ashley and Guest[25]	6.87	16.0	45.6	67	24	35	..	14.2±5.2	..	..	..	..	..	..	50
	Bruner and Wakerlin[27]	6.45±0.76	13.6±1.6	44.3±1.4	69±5	21±1.6	31±1.4	7.0	8.8	..	..	..	..	..	..	34
	Leichsenring et al.[26]	7.17	14.1	..	..	..	..	..	11.2	74.0	2.0	..	20.0	4.0	..	32
	Mayerson[20] (Adults)	6.49	13.0	47.7	67	20	30	..	11.5	71.8	5.4	..	21.8	1.0	621	60
	Morris et al.[26a] (2 to 8 mos. of age)	6.20	15.1	38.6	59	24	34	..	12.2	62.5	4.0	..	33.3	0.2	..	35
		5.30	12.6	..	..	24	..	..	..	..	..	..	..	..	..	31
	Scarborough[18]	7.20±0.80	..	..	..	..	..	..	..	..	..	..	..	..	..	700±
	Wintrobe et al.[30]	7.02±0.66	14.6±1.4	47.3±4.7	68±4	21±1.4	31±1.6	7.0	11.8±5.0	69.0	5.0	0.7	20.0	6.1	400	54
Ferret	Wintrobe[21]	9.98	15.2	51.0	48	16	30	..	..	..	..	..	..	..	..	3
Fox	Wintrobe[9]	7.99	12.8	42.4	53	16	30	..	..	60.0	7.0	2.0	25.0	6.0	..	1
Goat	Drastisch[10]	18.70	9.8	30.0	16	8	32	..	..	..	..	..	..	..	..	4
	Wintrobe[9]	17.33	11.4	33.2	19	7	35	..	7.4	36.5	3.5	0	58.0	2.0	2500	2
Guinea-pig	Drastisch[10]	6.41	14.2	45.4	71	22	31	..	..	..	..	..	..	..	..	5
	King and Lucas[24]	5.06	..	..	..	..	..	..	17.4	31.1*	3.5	0.2	63.4	1.8	..	9
	Scarborough[18]	5.75±1.20	14.5	47.7	83	25	30	7.1	10.8	41.8*	4.8	0.8	45.3	8.4	..	500±
	Wintrobe[9]	5.75	..	..	..	..	..	..	5.5	..	..	..	..	..	..	4
Hamster	Stewart et al.[31c]	7.5±0.5	17.6±1.0	47.4±2.4	63	23	37	6.6	8.56±1.54	29.0	0.7	0.5	67.9	2.4	500	318
Horse	Scarborough[18]	6.0–8.5	..	..	..	..	..	..	..	..	..	..	..	..	250	53
	Kushner[34]	5.4–7.4	..	..	..	..	..	..	..	..	..	..	..	..	..	20
	Vaulont[17]	6.5–8.3	11–15	..	..	..	..	5.7	6.0–12.0	56.8	3.7	..	30.4	8.5	..	3
	Drastisch[10]	6.05	10.7	31.6	52	18	34	..	..	..	..	..	..	..	..	5
	Macleod and Ponder[34a]	10.35	13.9	43.5	42	13	33	5.9–6.3	6.4–8.9	..	..	..	..	..	..	..

Animal	Authority	R.B.C.	Hgb.	V.P.C.	M.C.V.	M.C.H.	M.C.H.C.	Diam.	W.B.C.	N.	E.	B.	L.	Mo.	Pl.	Ref.
Jackal	Wintrobe	5.06	12.2	35.5	70	24	34	··	··	54.0	5.0	0	41.0	0	··	1
Kinkajou	Wintrobe[9]	6.52	10.9	36.0	55	17	30	··	··	32.0	15.0	0	53.0	··	··	··
Llama	Wintrobe[9]	15.00	14.9	36.9	25	10	40	··	··	47.5	1.5	0	50.0	1.0	··	2
	Knoll[14,14]	··	··	··	··	··	··	··	··	66.0	4.8	4.0	21.9	3.3	··	··
	Ponder et al.[25]	15.35	··	··	··	··	··	7.4 x 4.0	11.2	57.0	7.4	24.0	7.4	4.3	··	4
Monkey	Hall[0]	4.94	··	··	··	··	··	··	14.2	42.6	2.8	0.3	52.1	1.2	··	8
	Ponder et al.[41]	5.50	··	··	··	··	··	··	8.4	71.5	2.5	2.5	22.0	1.5	··	3
	Shukers et al.[41]	5.20	12.2	40.0 (36–44)	··	··	59.0	7.2	15.1	36.0	··	··	59.0	2.0	475	19
	Wintrobe[9]	5.44 (4.6–5.8)	13.2 (10.9–13.5)	43.5	··	··	70.5	··	(9.7–20.5)	23.0	··	··	70.5 (44–74)	··	··	4
Mouse	Petri[30]	7.81	14.3	38.7	48	··	··	··	6.6	28.0	··	··	65.0	7.0	698	44
	Drastisch[10]	9.24	··	47.1	51	··	··	··	··	··	··	··	··	··	··	7
	Scarborough[18]	9.70±1.70	15.1	43.0	49	··	··	··	8.5	26.2	2.0	0.5	67.8	7.5	270	60±1
	Wintrobe[9]	8.88	··	··	··	··	··	··	··	··	··	··	··	··	··	1
	Kamenoff[28]	9.55	··	··	··	··	··	··	11.0	··	··	··	··	··	··	118
Opossum	Wintrobe[21]	4.00	10.1	31.9	79	··	··	··	12.0	39.0	4.7	1.0	46.0	9.3	250	4
	Jordan[4]	5.90	10.0	35.0	··	··	··	··	15.3	26.0	3.3	1.0	62.8	7.0	··	··
Pig	Wintrobe[21,48]	7.93	15.0	46.3	58	19	33	5.5	7.0–20.0	28.0	··	··	52.1	3.3	300	··
	Götze[43]	7.09♂ / 6.90♀	13.0	43.2	60	18	30	··	··	··	··	··	··	··	··	··
	Scarborough[18]	6.74	11.8	38.9	57	17	30	6.1	8.0–20.0	39.0	··	··	··	··	215	··
Rabbit	Wintrobe et al.[20]	6.29±0.60	13.0±1.5	39.8±4.3 (males only)	64±4	21±1.6	33±1.7	··	7.7	49.4*	1.5	6.7	32.9	9.5	500	61
	Casey et al.[47]	5.37	11.9 (?)	49.4*	··	··	··	6.7	7.9	··	··	··	··	··	500	180
	Scarborough[18]	5.62±1.20	··	43.4*	··	··	··	··	··	43.4*	2.0	4.3	41.8	9.0	900±	··
Rat	Wintrobe et al.[20]	6.60±0.76	13.0±1.2	39.4±3.6	61±4	20±2.1	33±2.3	6.3	8.5	4.0	0	0.8	90.0	5.3	330	73
	Scarborough[18]	8.50±1.50	··	··	··	··	··	5.9	8.0–15.0	27.0	··	··	67.9	0–4	800	200±
	Wills and Mehta[44]	9.55	14.0	43.5	··	··	··	5.98	21.4	52	17	··	··	··	673	··
	Cameron and Watson[49]h	♂8.58 / ♀8.70	14.6 / 13.8	41.8	··	··	··	6.14	20.4	49	16	··	70–89	··	532	··
Sheep	Wintrobe[9]	10.50	12.9	35.7	34	12	36	··	8.0	28.0	8.0	0	62.0	2.0	350	4
	Drastisch[10]	10.90	11.8	38.5	35	11	31	··	··	··	··	··	··	··	··	1
Skunk	Wintrobe[9]	10.00	15.1	51.4	51	15	29	··	16.0	48.0	7.0	0	42.0	3.0	540	2
Woodchuck	Jordan[4]	7.33	13.9	48.0	66	19	30	7.4	15.7	70.2	1.7	0.4	26.2	0.7	··	3

R.B.C., red cell count in millions per c.mm.; Hgb., hemoglobin in grams per 100 cc. blood; Ht., volume of packed red cells in cc. per 100 cc.; M.C.V., mean corpuscular volume in cubic microns; M.C.H., mean corpuscular hemoglobin in micromicrograms; M.C.H.C., mean corpuscular hemoglobin concentration in per cent; Diam., mean erythrocyte diameter (in dry smears) in microns; W.B.C., leukocyte count in thousands per c.mm.; N., neutrophils; E., eosinophils; B., basophils; L., lymphocytes; Mo., monocytes, all in per cent; Pl., platelets in thousands per c.mm. Values following ± in most instances represent 1 standard deviation.

*In rabbits and in guinea pigs the cells listed under "N" are "pseudo-eosinophils," "amphophils," or "heterophils." The granules are eosinophilic for the most part, rounded and of fairly uniform size but are not as densely packed as in true eosinophils. In these animals the granules in the true eosinophils are very abundant, large and ovoid or bluntly fusiform.

Table A-2—Blood Counts in Various Vertebrates Other than Mammals

Class and species	Author	R.B.C.	Hgb.	Ht.	M.C.V	M.C.H.	M.C.H.C.	Diam.	W.B.C.	N or P.E.G.	E or P.E.R.	B.	L.	Mo.	Thr.
Birds															
Duck	Magath and Higgins[62]	3.06	15.6	...	127	37	...	11.2 x 6.7	23.4	24.3	2.1	1.5	61.7	10.8	30.7
Fowl	Wintrobe[9]	2.81	10.3	35.8	...	...	29	11.2 x 6.9	4.0	19.0	30.0	3.0	48.0		
(Domestic)	Palmer and Biely[63]	2.61	...	...	...	...	...	...	45.0						35.0
	Blain[34]		...	...	...	...	...	...	18.6						
	Forkner[49]	3.27	...	...	...	...	...	...	24.6						
Guinea	Wintrobe[9]	3.69	14.0	50.0	136	38	28	12.5 x 6.5	8.0	8.7	49.4	3.6	32.8	5.7	
Goose	Wintrobe[9]	2.82	12.7	44.6	160	45	29	12.2 x 7.2	8.0	1.8	34.7	4.2	41.8	17.1	
Pigeon	Wintrobe[9]	3.22	12.8	42.3	131	40	30	13.2 x 6.9	4.0	20.0	64.0	2.0	14.0		
	Riddle and Braucher[65]	3.13	14.8										92.0		
	Magath and Higgins[62]	3.53*	14.4												
Turkey	Wintrobe[21]	1.93	11.2	39.2	203	58	29	14.2 x 9.7	16.7	3.8	35.2	4.0	54.0	3.0	37.0
Reptiles.															
Alligator	Wintrobe[9]	0.67	8.2	30.0	450	123	27	23.2 x 12.1	3.0						
Lizard	Wintrobe[9]	0.81	4.4	13.8	171	54	32								
Snake, hog nose	Wintrobe[9]	0.56	5.6	18.7	324	97	30	16.4 x 9.6							
Snake, garter	Wintrobe[9]	1.05	8.5	28.0	267	82	31	18.1 x 10.4							
Snake, water	Wintrobe[9]	0.77	10.0	35.5	465	131	28	19.6 x 11.0							
Turtle	Wintrobe[9]	0.74	6.2	22.1	300	85	28	18.1 x 8.7							
Amphibia.															
Frog	Wintrobe[9]	0.44	7.8	29.3	670	179	27	24.8 x 15.3	3.0	5.0	7.0		88.0	0	
	Freidsohn[80]									12.6	5.2	4.4	77.8		
Amphiuma	Wintrobe[9]	0.03	9.4	40.0	13,860	3,290	24	62.5 x 36.5	8.0	50.0	5.0	5.0	40.0		7.0
Cryptobranchus	Wintrobe[9]	0.07	13.3	49.0	7,425	2,010	27	40.5 x 21.0	1.9						
Necturus	Wintrobe[9]	0.02	4.6	21.4	10,070	2,160	22	52.8 x 28.2	2.5	25.7	10.0		64.3		
Salamander	Freidsohn[20]	...	...	...											
Fishes.															
Carp	Field et al.[55a]	0.84	10.5	31.3	311	72	34	12.3 x 8.6							
Mackerel	Wintrobe[9]†	4.20	15.2	59.0	140	36	26	11.3 x 8.6							
Rock cod	Wintrobe[9]	1.49	5.2	23.8	159	35	22	10.7 x 7.3	6.0	2.0	6.0	10.0	84.0	4.0	
Rusty flounder	Wintrobe[9]	0.78	2.1	8.4	108	28	25								
Trout	Field et al.[55a]	1.01	8.5	27.2	314	75	31								
Dogfish	Wintrobe[9]	0.07	1.4	7.3	1,010	195	19	22.5 x 17.1	45.0		6.0		94.0		
Skate	Reznikoff and Reznikoff[64]	0.39	4.4	9.9	952	153	16	25.2 x 17.3	83.5	5.0	17.5	0	66.5	1.0	13.5
Cyclostomes.															
Hagfish	Wintrobe[9]	0.13	4.2	19.8	1,560	330	21	26.8 x 16.2	33.0						

* Average of 14 authors quoted by Magath and Higgins.

† The values given are only a few representative determinations. In the article cited, erythrocyte values or a great variety of animals, especially fishes, are reported.

Legends: Same as in Table 64. In addition, N refers to polymorphonuclear leukocytes without granules; P.E.G. refers to leukocytes with polymorphonuclear nuclei and eosinophilic granules; P.E.R. refers to similar cells with eosinophilic rods; Thr. refers to thrombocytes in thousands per c.mm. In birds and in certain selachians and reptiles there is no finely granular "special" cell corresponding to the polymorphonuclear neutrophil o. man; and amphibia. Its place is taken by a leukocyte with ellipsoidal or bacillary granules. The differential leukocyte counts recorded above give only an approximate indication of the findings. Full descriptions of cells together with drawings will be found in the excellent monograph by Jordan and in the other references cited 1. 3. 55 60 62. 67)

BIBLIOGRAPHY

Comparative Hematology

General and Miscellaneous Papers

1. Didisheim, P., Hattori, K. and Lewis, Jessica H.: Hematologic and Coagulation Studies in Various Animal Species, J. Lab. & Clin. Med., *53*, 866, 1959.
1a. George, W. C.: Comparative Hematology and the Functions of the Leucocytes, Quart. Rev. Biol., *16*, 426, 1941.
1b. Grünberg, C.: Beiträge zur vergleichenden Morphologie der Leukocyten, Virchows Arch. path. Anat., *163*, 303, 1901.
2. Gulliver, G.: Observations on the Sizes and Shapes of the Red Corpuscles of the Blood of Vertebrates, With Drawings of Them to a Uniform Scale, and Extended and Revised Tables of Measurements, Proc. Zoölogical Soc., London, p. 474, 1875.
3. Herzog, D.: *In* Hirschfeld, H. and Hittmair, A., *Handbuch der allgemeine Hämatologie*, Berlin, Urban und Schwarzenburg, *1*, Pt. 2, 1229, 1932–33.
4. Jordan, H. E.: Comparative Hematology, *in* Downey, H., *Handbook of Hematology*, New York, Paul B. Hoeber, Inc., *2*, 703, 1938 (Bibliography).
5. Kalabukhov, N. and Rodionov, V.: Changes in the Blood of Animals According to Age (Rodents and Birds), Folia hæmat., *52*, 145, 1934.
6. Romieu, M.: Blood of Annelids, Arch. morphol. gén. et expér., *17*, 1, 1923–24.
7. Warner, E. D., Brinkhous, K. M. and Smith, H. P.: Plasma Prothrombin Levels in Various Vertebrates, Am. J. Physiol., *125*, 296, 1939.
8. Wells, J. J. and Sutton, J. E.: Blood Counts in the Frog, the Turtle and Twelve Different Species of Mammals, Am. J. Physiol., *39*, 31, 1916.
9. Wintrobe, M. M.: Variations in the Size and Hemoglobin Content of Erythrocytes in the Blood of Various Vertebrates, Folia hæmat., *51*, 32, 1933.

Mammals
Miscellaneous and Rarer Mammals as well as Articles Describing More Than One Species

9a. Depelchin, A.: Hématologie Animale, Ann. méd. vétérin., *100*, 325, 1956.
10. Drastich, L.: Ist die Konzentration des Blutfarbstoffes im Blutkörperchen bei allen Tieren Konstant? Arch. ges. Physiol., *219*, 227, 1928.
10a. Gordon, A. S. and Charipper, H. A.: The Endocrine System and Hemopoiesis, Ann.

N. Y. Acad. Sc., *48*, 615, 1947 (Bibliography).
11. Hirschfeld, H.: Beiträge zur vergleichenden Morphologie der Leukocyten, Virchows Archiv., *149*, 22, 1897 (well illustrated).
11a. Hoitink, A. W. J. H.: Hæmatologische Onderzœkingen bij Zebus, Tijdschr. v. diergeneesk., *79*, 812, 1954.
11b. Holman, H. H.: A Negative Correlation between Size and Number of the Erythrocytes of Cows, Sheep, Goats and Horses, J. Path. & Bact., *64*, 379, 1952.
12. Kalabuchow, N.: Über das Verhältnis zwischen Grösse und Zahl der Erythrocyten, Hämoglobingehalt und Körpergrösse bei Citellus pygmaeus Pall(Rodentia), Ztschr. Zellforsch. u. mikr. Anat., *17*, 1, 1933.
13. Kennedy, W. P. and Climenko, D. R.: Studies on the Arneth Count: XVIII. The Normal Count in Various Mammals, Quart. J. Exper. Physiol., *21*, 253, 1931.
14. Knoll, W.: Das morphologische Blutbild der Säugetiere, Ztschr. mikr.-anat. Forsch., *30*, 116, 1932. (A variety of the less common mammals. Bibliography and drawings in color.)
15. ——— Untersuchungen über die Morphologie des Säugetierblutes, Folia hæmat., *47*, 201, 1932. (Includes red cell diameters of many mammals.)
15a. Ottis, K. and Tauber, O. E.: Blood Platelet Counts of the Golden Hamster, *Cricetus auratus*, Blood, 7, 948, 1952.
16. Scarborough, R. A.: The Blood Picture of Normal Laboratory Animals, Yale J. Biol. & Med., *3*, 63, 168, 282, 359, 431, 547, 1931.
17. Vaulont, H.: Untersuchungen des Katzen- und Pferdeblutes, Ztschr. Biol., *96*, 241, 1935 (Bibliography).
18. Welsch, W.: Das Blut der Haustiere mit neueren Methoden untersucht: V. Untersuchung des Schweine-, Schaf-, und Ziegenblutes, Arch. ges. Physiol., *198*, 37, 1923.
19. Wintrobe, M. M. and Shumacker, H. B., Jr.: Erythrocyte Studies in the Mammalian Fetus and Newborn: Erythrocyte Counts, Hemoglobin and Volume of Packed Red Corpuscles, Mean Corpuscular Volume, Diameter and Hemoglobin Content, and Proportion of Immature Red Cells in the Blood of Fetuses and Newborn of the Pig, Rabbit, Rat, Cat, Dog and Man, Am. J. Anat., *58*, 313, 1936.
20. Wintrobe, M. M., Shumacker, H. B., Jr., and Schmidt, W. J.: Values for Number, Size and Hemoglobin Content of Erythrocytes in Normal Dogs, Rabbits and Rats, Am. J. Physiol., *114*, 502, 1936.

21. Wintrobe, M. M. and Wintrobe, Becky Z.: Unpublished Observations. *See also* References 2, 9.

Camel

22. Ponder, E., Yeager, J. F. and Ch{ARIPPER, H. A.: Studies in Comparative Hæmatology: I. Camelidæ, Quart. J. Exper. Physiol., *19*, 115, 1928.

Cat

23. Landsberg, J. W.: The Blood Picture of Normal Cats, Folia hæmat., *64*, 169, 1940 (Bibliography).
23a.Sawitsky, A. and Meyer, L. M.: The Bone Marrow of Normal Cats, J. Lab. & Clin. Med., *32*, 70, 1947.

See also References 8, 9, 16, 17, 19.

Cattle

24. Delaune, E.: Observations on the Bovine Blood Picture in Health and Under Parasitism, Proc. Soc. Exper. Biol. & Med., *41*, 482, 1939.
24a.Ferguson, L. C., Irwin, M. R. and Beach, B. A.: On Variation in the Blood Cells of Healthy Cattle, J. Infect. Dis., *76*, 24, 1945.
24b.Kupferschmied, H.: Untersuchungen über den Hämoglobin- und Erythrozytengehalt des Rinderblutes, Zentralbl. Veterinärmed., *4*, 983, 1957.
25. Kushner, H. F.: Investigation of the Blood Value of the Yaroslav Breed of Cattle With Reference to Productivity, Compt. rend. Acad. d. sc., *20*, 393, 1938.
25a.Afonsky, D.: Blood Picture in Normal Dogs, Am. J. Physiol., *180*, 456, 1955.

See also References 8, 9, 33e.

Dog

26. Ashley, A. and Guest, G. M.: Distribution of Blood Phosphorus After Suppression of Renal Function, J. Clin. Invest., *13*, 219, 1934.
27. Bruner, H. D. and Wakerlin, G. E.: The Blood Picture of the Normal Dog, Proc. Soc. Exper. Biol. & Med., *36*, 667, 1937.
27a.Ederstrom, H. E. and DeBoer, B.: Changes in the Blood of the Dog with Age, Anat. Rec., *94*, 663, 1946.
28. Gibson, J. G., 2d, Keeley, J. L. and Pijoan, M.: The Blood Volume of Normal Dogs, Am. J. Physiol., *121*, 800, 1938.
28a.Hamilton, A. S.: Study of *in vitro* Methods for the Demonstration of Iso-agglutination With the Bloods of Normal and of Ill Dogs, Am. J. Physiol., *154*, 525, 1948.
29. Leichsenring, J. M., Biester, A., Hönig, H. H., Furnas, S. M., Foss, E. S. and

Routt, M. V.: Observations on the Blood of Normal Dogs With Special Reference to the Measurement of Volume, Erythrocytes, Leucocytes and Nitrogenous Constituents, Am. J. Physiol., *99*, 391, 1932.
30. Mayerson, H. S.: The Blood Cytology of Dogs, Anat. Rec., *47*, 239, 1930.
31. Meyer, L. M. and Bloom, F.: The Bone Marrow of Normal Dogs, Am. J. M. Sc., *206*, 637, 1943.
31a.Morris, M. L., Stelton, N. J., Allison, J. B. and Green, D. F.: Blood Cytology of the Normal Dog, J. Lab. & Clin. Med., *25*, 353, 1940.
31b.Mulligan, R. M.: Quantitative Studies on the Blood and Bone Marrow of Newborn Mongrel Puppies, Anat. Rec., *91*, 161, 1945.
31c.Rekers, P. E. and Coulter, M.: A Hematological and Histological Study of the Bone Marrow and Peripheral Blood of the Adult Dog, Am. J. M. Sc., *216*, 643, 1948.
31d.Smith, S. G.: Evidence That the Physiologic Normal Hemoglobin Value for Adult Dog Blood Is 18 Grams per 100 ml., Am. J. Physiol., *142*, 476, 1944; *ibid.*, *182*, 433, 1955.
31e.Van Loon, E. J., Clark, B. B. and Blair, D.: Hematology of the Peripheral Blood and Bone Marrow of the Dog, J. Lab. & Clin. Med., *28*, 1575, 1943.
31f.Weissman, S. M., Waldmann, T. A. and Berlin, N. I.: Quantitative Measurement of Erythropoiesis in the Dog, Am. J. Physiol., *198*, 183, 1960.

See also References 8, 9, 16, 19, 20.

Guinea pig

32. Babudieri, B.: Presenza di forme degenerative di linfociti nel sangue circolante di cavia, Folia hæmat., *52*, 159, 1934.
32a.Cruz, W. O. and Ubatuba, F.: Blood Picture of Adult Gold Hamster (*Cricetus auratus*) After Castration, Proc. Soc. Exper. Biol. & Med., *65*, 321, 1947.
32b.Epstein, R. D. and Tompkins, E. H.: A Comparison of Techniques for the Differential Counting of Bone Marrow Cells (Guinea Pig), Am. J. M. Sc., *206*, 249, 1943.
32c.Hudson, G.: Eosinophil Populations in Blood and Bone Marrow of Normal Guinea Pigs, Am. J. Physiol., *198*, 1171, 1960.
33. King, E. S. and Lucas, M.: A Study of the Blood Cells of Normal Guinea Pigs, J. Lab. & Clin. Med., *26*, 1364, 1941.
33a.Sawitsky, A. and Meyer, L. M.: Bone Marrow of Normal Guinea Pigs, Blood, *3*, 1050, 1948.
33b.Smith, E.: Certain Characteristics of the Leukocytes of Guinea Pig Blood With

Particular Reference to the Kurloff Body, Blood, Supp. No. 1, 1947, p. 125.

33c. STEWART, M. O., FLORIO, L. and MUGRAGE, E. R.: Hematological Findings in the Golden Hamster (Cricetus Auratus), J. Exper. Med., *80*, 189, 1944.

See also References 9, 16.

Horse

33d. FEGLER, G.: Hæmoglobin Concentration, Haematocrit Value, and Sedimentation Rate of Horse Blood, Quart. J. Exper. Physiol. & Cognate M. Sc., *34*, 129, 1948.

33e. CALHOUN, M. L.: A Cytological Study of Costal Marrow, Am. J. Vet. Research, *15*, 181 and 395, 1954; *ibid.*, *16*, 297, 1955.

34. KUSHNER, H. F.: The Connection Between Heterosis in Mules and Their Blood Composition, Compt. rend. Acad. d. sc., *19*, 747, 1938.

34a. MACLEOD, J. and PONDER, E.: An Observation on the Red Cell Content of the Blood of the Thoroughbred Horse, Science, *103*, 73, 1946.

See also References 8, 16, 17.

Marsupials

35. PONDER, E., YEAGER, J. F. and CHARIPPER, H. A.: Studies in Comparative Hæmatology: III. Marsupialia, Quart. J. Exper. Physiol., *19*, 273, 1929.

See also Reference 4.

Mouse

35a. EHRENSTEIN, G. v.: The Life Span of the Erythrocytes of Normal and of Tumour-Bearing Mice as Determined by Glycine-2-^{14}, Acta physiol. scandinav., *44*, 80, 1958.

36. FRANCIS, L. D. and STRONG, L. C.: Hemoglobin Studies on the Blood of Female Mice of the CBA Strain: Effects of Age, Diet, Strain, and Reproduction, Am. J. Physiol., *124*, 511, 1938.

37. GRÜNEBERG, H.: The Growth of the Blood of the Sucking Mouse, J. Path. & Bact., *52*, 323, 1941.

38. KAMENOFF, R. J.: Erythrocyte Count in Four Inbred Strains of Mice, Proc. Soc. Exper. Biol. & Med., *36*, 411, 1937.

39. PETRI, S.: Morphologie und Zahl der Blutkörperchen bei 7—ca. 30 g. schweren normalen weissen Laboratoriumsmäusen, Acta path. et microbiol. scandinav., *10*, 159, 1933. (Bibliography and drawings in color.)

39a. RUSSELL, E. S., NEUFELD, E. F. and HIGGINS, C. T.: Comparison of Normal Blood Picture of Young Adults from 18 Inbred Strains of Mice, Proc. Soc. Exper. Biol. & Med., *78*, 761, 1951.

See also Reference 5, 16.

Monkey and Other Primates

40. HALL, B. E.: The Morphology of the Cellular Elements of the Blood of the Monkey, Macacus rhesus, Folia hæmat., *38*, 30, 1929. (Bibliography and drawings in color.)

40a. JONES, E. S., McCALL, K. B., ELVEHJEM, C. A. and CLARK, P. F.: The Effect of Diet on the Hemoglobin, Erythrocyte, and Leukocyte Content of the Blood of the Rhesus Monkey (Macaca Mulatta), Blood, *2*, 154, 1947.

41. PONDER, E., YEAGER, J. F. and CHARIPPER, H. A.: Studies in Comparative Hæmatology: II. Primates, Quart. J. Exper. Physiol., *19*, 181, 1928.

42. SHUKERS, C. F., LANGSTON, W. C. and DAY, P. L.: The Normal Blood Picture of the Young Rhesus Monkey, Folia hæmat., *60*, 416, 1938 (Bibliography).

42a. SUÁREZ, R. M., DIAZ RIVERA, R. S., HERNANDEZ MORALES, F.: Hematological Studies in Normal Rhesus Monkeys (Macaca mulatta), Puerto Rico J. Pub. Health & Trop. Med., *18*, 212, 1942.

See also Reference 9.

Pig

43. GÖTZE, R.: Zuchterisch-biologische Studien über die Blutausrüstung der landwirtschaftlichen Haustiere, Ztschr. Konstitutionslehre, *9*, 217, 1924.

44. KERNKAMP, H. C. H.: The Blood Picture of Pigs Kept Under Conditions Favorable to the Production and to the Prevention of So-called "Anemia of Suckling Pigs," Univ. Minnesota Agric. Exper. Station Bull., *86*, 3, 1932.

45. WINTROBE, M. M., SAMTER, M. and LISCO, H.: Morphologic Changes in the Blood of Pigs Associated With Deficiency of Water-soluble Vitamins and Other Substances Contained in Yeast, Bull. Johns Hopkins Hosp., *64*, 399, 1939.

See also References 8, 9, 16, 18, 19.

Rabbit

46. BOTZARIS, A.: Contribution à l'étude de l'hématocytologie des cobayes normaux, Folia hæmat., *60*, 222, 1938.

47. CASEY, A. E., ROSAHN, P. D., HU, C. and PEARCE, L.: The Hemocytological Constitution of Adult Male Rabbits From Fifteen Standard Breeds, J. Exper. Med., *64*, 453, 1936. (Data for different breeds.)

48. CHENG, S. C.: Leucocyte Counts in Rabbits: Observations on the Influence of Various Physiological Factors and Pathological Conditions, Am. J. Hyg., *11*, 449, 1930.

48a.DIETZ, A. A.: Composition of Normal Bone Marrow in Rabbits, J. Biol. Chem., *165*, 505, 1946.

48b.FARR, R. S., SCHORK, P. K. and GAYHART, C. H.: The Spontaneous Leukocyte and Temperature Variation in Untreated Rabbits Studied Under Controlled Conditions, Naval Medical Research Institute, 28 July 1948, Project NM 007 039, Report No. 12.

48c.PINTOR, P. P. and GRASSINI, V.: Individual and Seasonal Spontaneous Variations of Haematological Values in Normal Male Rabbits, Acta haemat., *17*, 122, 1957.

49. ROSAHN, P. D., PEARCE, L. and HU, C.: Comparison of the Hemocytological Constitution of Male and Female Rabbits, J. Exper. Med., *60*, 687, 1934.

See also References 8, 9, 16, 19, 20.

49a.SAUERBIER, W.: Die normale Lebenszeit und die Kinetik des Auf- und Abbaus der Erythrocyten beim Kaninchen, Folia haemat., *76*, 258, 1959.

49b.SUTHERLAND, D. A., MINTON, P. and LANZ, H.: The Life Span of the Rabbit Erythrocyte, Acta haemat., *27*, 36, 1959.

Rat

49c.ASCHKENASY, A.: Le Myélogramme du Rat Blanc Adulte, Sang, *17*, 399, 1946.

49d.BELCHER, E. H. and HARRISS, EILEEN B.: Studies of Red Cell Life Span in the Rat, J. Physiol., *146*, 217, 1959.

49e.BERLIN, N. I.: A Simple Method for Repeated Bone Marrow Aspirations in Rats, Proc. Soc. Exper. Biol. & Med., *69*, 53, 1948.

49f.BURKE, W. T. and HARRIS, C.: Total Cell Counts of the Bone Marrow of Normal Albino Rats from 1 to 50 Weeks of Age, Blood, *14*, 409, 1959.

49g.CAMERON, D. G. and WATSON, G. M.: Femoral Bone Marrow Biopsy in the Albino Rat, Blood, *3*, 292, 1948.

49h.———— The Blood Counts of the Adult Albino Rat, Blood, *4*, 816, 1949.

50. DRABKIN, D. L. and FITZ-HUGH, T., JR.: A Comparison of the Normal Blood Picture of Rats (at Various Ages) of Two Different Colonies Reared Upon Different Stock Rations, Am. J. Physiol., *108*, 61, 1934.

50a.DUVOLON, S.: Contribution à l'Étude Hématologique du Rat Blanc Normal. Données Morphologiques et Numériques, Sang, *18*, 205, 1947.

51. ENZMANN, E. V.: The Changes in Hemoglobin Concentration of Blood of Growing Rats, Am. J. Physiol., *108*, 373, 1934.

51a.GOLDECK, H. and HEINRICH, W. D.: Die tagesperiodischen Spontanschwankungen der Blutmauserung bei der Laboratoriumsratte, Acta hæmat., *2*, 167, 1949.

51b.LATTA, J. S. and NELSON, W. W.: The Effects of Experimental Hyperpyrexia and Restraint on the Blood and Hemopoietic Organs of the Albino Rat, Am. J. Anat., *82*, 321, 1948.

52. ORTEN, J. M. and SMITH, A. H.: The Proportion of Reticulocytes in the Blood of Albino Rats, Am. J. Physiol., *108*, 66, 1934.

52a.VAN PUTTEN, L. M.: The Life Span of Red Cells in the Rat and the Mouse as Determined by Labeling with DFP[32] *in Vivo*, Blood, *13*, 789, 1958.

52b.QUIMBY, F. H., SAXON, P. A. and GOFF, L. G.: Total White Cell Counts of Peripheral and Heart Blood of the Rat, Science, *107*, 447, 1948.

53. SCHMIDT-REUTER: Cytologische Studien über die Zusammensetzung des normalen Rattenblutes in verschiedenen Lebensaltern, Folia hæmat., *55*, 368, 1936.

53a.THEWLIS, E. W. and MEYER, O. O.: The Blood Count of Normal White Rats, Anat. Rec., *82*, 115, 1942.

54. WILLS, L. and MEHTA, M. M.: Determination of Normal Blood Standards for the Nutritional Laboratory's Stock Albino Rat, Indian J. Med. Res., *18*, 307, 1930–31.

See also References 9, 16, 19, 20.

Various Vertebrates Other Than Mammals

55. ALDER, A. and HUBER, E.: Untersuchungen über Blutzellen und Zellbildung bei Amphibien und Reptilien, Folia hæmat., *29*, 1, 1923. (Good illustrations in color.)

55a.BERGMAN, R. A. M.: The Erythrocyte of Snakes, Folia haemat., *75*, 92, 1957.

56. BLAIN, D.: A Direct Method for Making Total White Blood Counts on Avian Blood, Proc. Soc. Exper. Biol. & Med., *25*, 594, 1928.

56a.CATTON, W. T.: Blood Cell Formation in Certain Teleost Fishes, Blood, *6*, 39, 1951.

57. CHARIPPER, H. A. and DAVIS, D.: Studies on the Arneth Count: XX. A Study of the Blood Cells of *Pseudemys Elegans* With Special Reference to the Polymorphonuclear Leucocytes, Quart. J. Exper. Physiol., *21*, 371, 1932.

58. CULLEN, E. K.: A Morphological Study of the Blood of Certain Fishes and Birds, With Special Reference to the Leucocytes o Birds, Bull. Johns Hopkins Hosp., *153*, 352, 1903.

58a.FIELD, J. B., ELVEHJEM, C. A. and JUDAY, C.: A Study of the Blood Constituents of Carp and Trout, J. Biol. Chem., *148*, 261, 1942.

59. FORKNER, C. E.: Blood and Bone Marrow

Cells of the Domestic Fowl, J. Exper. Med. 50, 121, 1929.

60. FREIDSOHN, A.: Zur Morphologie des Amphibienblutes, Zugleich ein Beitrag zur Lehre der Differenzierung der Lymphocyten, Arch. mikr. Anat., 75, 435, 1910.

60a.GEORGE, W. C. and NICHOLS, J.: A Study of the Blood of Some Crustacea, J. Morph., 83, 425, 1948.

60b.HARBOE, A. and SCHRUMPF, A.: The Red Blood Cell Diameter in Blue Whale and Humpback Whale, Acta hæmat., 9, 54, 1953.

60c.JAKOWSKA, SOPHIE: Morphologie et nomenclature des cellules du sang des téléostéens, Rev. hémat., 11, 519, 1956.

60d.JOHNSTON, P. M.: Hematocrit Values for the Chick Embryo at Various Ages, Am. J. Physiol., 180, 361, 1955.

60e.KAPLAN, H. M.: Sex Differences in the Packed Cell Volume of Vertebrate Blood, Science, 120, 1044, 1954.

60f.KATZ, M.: The Number of Erythrocytes in the Blood of the Silver Salmon, Tr. Am. Fish. Soc., 80, 184, 1951.

60g.KEILIN, D. and RYLEY, J. F.: Hæmoglobin in Protozoa, Nature, 172, 451, 1953.

60h.KISCH, B.: Hemoglobin Content, Size and Amount of Erythrocytes in Fishes, Exper. Med. & Surg., 7, 118, 318, 1949.

61. LATORRE, A.: Untersuchungen über Blut und Lymphe einiger chilenischer Anuren, Folia hæmat., 61, 36, 1938.

61a.LIEBMAN, E.: On Trephocytes and Trephocytosis: A Study on the Rôle of Leucocytes in Nutrition and Growth, Growth, 10, 291, 1946.

62. MAGATH, T. B. and HIGGINS, G. M.: The Blood of the Normal Duck, Folia hæmat., 51, 230, 1934. (Also fowl and pigeon.)

62a.MARVIN, H. N. and LUCY, D. D.: The Survival of Radiochromium-Tagged Erythrocytes in Pigeons, Ducks and Rabbits, Acta haemat., 18, 239, 1957.

62b.OTTESEN, J.: Life-Span of Red and White Blood Corpuscles of the Hen, Nature, 162, 730, 1948.

63. PALMER, E. I. and BIELY, J.: Studies of Total Erythrocyte and Leucocyte Counts of Fowls: I. Repeated Erythrocyte and Leucocyte Counts, Folia hæmat., 53, 143, 1935.

64. REZNIKOFF, P. and REZNIKOFF, D. G.: Hematological Studies in Dogfish (Mustelus Canis), Biol. Bull., 66, 115, 1934.

65. RIDDLE, O. and BRAUCHER, P. F.: Hemoglobin and Erythrocyte Differences According to Sex and Season in Doves and Pigeons, Am. J. Physiol., 108, 554, 1934.

66. RIDDLE, O. and CAUTHEN, G. E.: Erythrocyte Number in Young Pigeons and Its Relation to Heredity, Growth and Metabolism, Am. J. Physiol., 122, 480, 1938.

66a.RODNAN, G. P., EBAUGH, F. G., JR. and FOX, M. R. S.: The Life Span of the Red Blood Cell and the Red Blood Cell Volume in the Chicken, Pigeon and Duck as Estimated by the Use of $Na_2Cr^{51}O_4$, Blood, 12, 355, 1957.

66b.RYERSON, D. L.: Separation of the Two Acidophilic Granulocytes of Turtle Blood, With Suggested Phylogenetic Relationships, Anat. Rec., 85, 25, 1943.

66c.VAN DAM, L. and SCHOLANDER, P. F.: Concentration of Hemoglobin in the Blood of Deep Sea Fishes, J. Cell. & Comp. Physiol., 41, 1, 1953.

67. WERZBERG, A.: Studien zur vergleichenden Hämozytologie einiger Poikilothermer Vertebraten, Folia hæmat., 11, 17, 1911. (Amphibia, Reptiles, Fishes.)

See also References 1, 2, 5, 8, 9.

Appendix B

From Wintrobe—Clinical
Hematology, 5th Edition

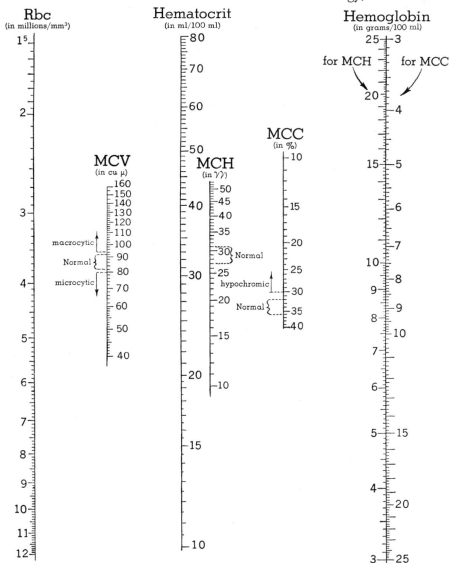

FIG. B-1.—Nomographic alignment chart for reading of corpuscular constants. (Prepared by Dr. Robert E. Mason.) For mean corpuscular volume (M.C.V.) join the value for red cell count and volume of packed cells ("hematocrit") by means of a ruler, preferably a transparent one. (A very satisfactory one is prepared by scratching a straight line on a strip of clear x-ray film and filling it in with ink.) The reading is made where the line intersects M.C.V. Similarly where a line joining R.B.C. and Hemoglobin intersects M.C.H. the reading for mean corpuscular hemoglobin is made; where a line joining Hemoglobin and Hematocrit intersects M.C.C. the reading for mean corpuscular hemoglobin concentration is made. Note that the left side of the Hemoglobin scale is used for M.C.H., the right side for M.C.C.

FIG. 8–12 is reprinted here so that it can be torn out and fixed permanently on a desk.

© Lea & Febiger

(1137)

Index